the calorie carb and fat bible 2016

Juliette Kellow BSc RD, Lyndel Costain BSc RD & Rebecca Walton

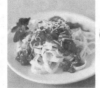

The UK's Most Comprehensive Calorie Counter

The Calorie, Carb & Fat Bible 2016

© Weight Loss Resources 2016
Lyndel Costain's contributions © Lyndel Costain

Published by:
Weight Loss Resources Ltd
2C Flag Business Exchange
Vicarage Farm Road
Peterborough
PE1 5TX.

Tel: 01733 345592
www.weightlossresources.co.uk

Companies and other organisations wishing to make bulk purchases of the Calorie, Carb and Fat Bible should contact their local bookstore or Weight Loss Resources direct.

ISBN 978-1-904512-15-8

Authors: Lyndel Costain BSc RD
          Juliette Kellow BSc RD
          Rebecca Walton, Weight Loss Resources

Database Editor: Tim Sharp

Design and Layout: Joanne Putney

Printed and bound in the UK

Contents

Losing weight – the easy way

Juliette Kellow BSc RD

PIZZA, curries, chocolate, chips and the odd glass of wine! Imagine being told the best diet to help you lose weight can include all these foods and more. It sounds too good to be true, doesn't it? But the truth is, these are exactly the types of foods you can still enjoy if you opt to lose weight by counting calories.

But you'd be forgiven for not knowing you can still eat all your favourite foods *and* lose weight. In recent years, endless trendy diets that cut carbs, or skip entire groups of foods, have helped to make dieting a complicated business. Added to this, an increasing number of celebrities and so-called nutrition experts have helped mislead us into thinking that dieting is all about restriction and denial. Is it any wonder then that most of us have been left feeling downright confused and miserable about what we should and shouldn't be eating to shift those pounds?

Dieting doesn't have to be complicated or an unhappy experience. In fact, there's really only one word you need to remember if you want to shift those pounds healthily and still eat all your favourite foods. And that's CALORIE!

It's calories that count

When it comes to losing weight, there's no getting away from the fact that it's calories that count. Ask any qualified nutrition expert or dietitian for advice on how to fight the flab and you'll receive the same reply: quite simply you need to create a calorie deficit or shortfall. In other words, you need to take in fewer calories than you use up so that your body has to draw on its fat stores to provide it with the energy it needs to function properly. The result: you start losing fat and the pounds start to drop off!

Fortunately, it couldn't be easier to create this calorie deficit. Regardless of your age, weight, sex, genetic make up, lifestyle or eating habits, losing weight is as simple as reducing your daily calorie intake slightly by modifying your diet and using up a few more calories by being slightly more active each day.

Better still, it's a complete myth that you need to change your eating and exercise habits dramatically. You'll notice I've said you need to reduce your calorie intake 'slightly' and be 'slightly' more active. It really is just LITTLE differences between the amount of calories we take in and the amount we use up that make BIG differences to our waistline over time. For example, you only need to consume one can of cola more than you need each day to gain a stone in a year. It's no wonder then that people say excess weight tends to 'creep up on them'.

10 simple food swaps you can make every day (and won't even notice!)

Make these simple swaps every day and in just 4 weeks you'll lose 7lb!

SWAP THIS...	FOR THIS...	SAVE...
300ml full-fat milk (195 calories)	300ml skimmed milk (100 calories)	95 calories
1tsp butter (35 calories)	1tsp low-fat spread (20 calories)	15 calories
1tbsp vegetable oil (100 calories)	10 sprays of a spray oil (10 calories)	90 calories
1tsp sugar (16 calories)	Artificial sweetener (2 calories)	14 calories
1tbsp mayonnaise (105 calories)	1tbsp fat-free dressing (10 calories)	95 calories
Regular sandwich (600 calories)	Low-fat sandwich (350 calories)	250 calories
Can of cola (135 calories)	Can of diet cola (1 calorie)	134 calories
Large (50g) packet of crisps (250 calories)	Small (25g) packet of crisps (125 calories)	125 calories
1 chocolate digestive (85 calories)	1 small chocolate chip cookie (55 calories)	30 calories
1 slice thick-cut wholemeal bread (95 calories)	1 slice medium-cut wholemeal bread (75 calories)	20 calories
	TOTAL CALORIE SAVING:	868 calories

The good news is the reverse is also true. You only need to swap that daily can of cola for the diet version or a glass of sparking water and you'll lose a stone in a year – it really is as easy as that!

Of course, most people don't want to wait a year to shift a stone. But there's more good news. To lose 1lb of fat each week you need to create a calorie deficit of just 500 calories a day. That might sound like a lot, but you can achieve this by simply swapping a croissant for a wholemeal fruit scone, a regular sandwich for a low-fat variety, a glass of dry white wine for a gin and slimline tonic and using low-fat spread on two slices of toast instead of butter. It is also important to become more active and increase your level of exercise. Losing 1lb a week, amounts to a stone in 14 weeks, or just under 4 stone in a year!

Taking control of calories

By now you've seen it really is calories that count when it comes to shifting those pounds. So it should be no surprise that a calorie-controlled diet is the only guaranteed way to help you shift those pounds – and that's a scientific fact! But better still, a calorie-controlled diet is one of the few that allows you to include anything, whether it's pizza, wine or chocolate. A healthy diet means including a wide range of foods (see 'Healthy Eating Made Easy' page 32).

And that's where this book can really help. Gone are the days when it was virtually impossible to obtain information about the calorie contents of foods. This book provides calorie information for more than 22,000 different branded and unbranded foods so that counting calories has never been easier.

The benefits of counting calories

- *It's guaranteed to help you lose weight providing you stick to your daily calorie allowance*

- *You can include favourite foods*

- *No foods are banned*

- *It's a great way to lose weight slowly and steadily*

- *Nutrition experts agree that it's a proven way to lose weight*

Calorie counting made easy

Forget weird and wacky science, complicated diet rules and endless lists of foods to fill up on or avoid every day! Counting calories to lose weight couldn't be easier. Quite simply, you set yourself a daily calorie allowance to help you lose between ½-2lb (¼-1kg) a week and then add up the calories of everything you eat and drink each day, making sure you don't go over your limit.

To prevent hunger from kicking in, it's best to spread your daily calorie allowance evenly throughout the day, allowing a certain amount of calories for breakfast, lunch, dinner and one or two snacks. For example, if you are allowed 1,500 calories a day, you could have 300 calories for breakfast, 400 calories for lunch, 500 calories for dinner and two snacks or treats of 150 calories each. You'll find more detailed information on p26-31 (Your step-by-step guide to using this book and shifting those pounds).

QUESTION
What affects the calorie content of a food?

ANSWER:
Fat, protein, carbohydrate and alcohol all provide the body with calories, but in varying amounts:

- *1g fat provides 9 calories*

- *1g alcohol provides 7 calories*

- *1g protein provides 4 calories*

- *1g carbohydrate provides 3.75 calories*

The calorie content of a food depends on the amount of fat, protein and carbohydrate it contains. Because fat provides more than twice as many calories as an equal quantity of protein or carbohydrate, in general, foods that are high in fat tend to contain more calories. This explains why 100g of chips (189 calories) contains more than twice as many calories as 100g of boiled potato (72 calories).

DIET MYTH:
Food eaten late at night stops you losing weight

DIET FACT:

It's not eating in the evening that stops you losing weight. It's consuming too many calories throughout the day that will be your dieting downfall! Providing you stick to your daily calorie allowance you'll lose weight, regardless of when you consume those calories. Nevertheless, it's a good idea to spread your calorie allowance throughout the day to prevent hunger from kicking in, which leaves you reaching for high-calorie snack foods.

Eat for good health

While calories might be the buzz word when it comes to shifting those pounds, it's nevertheless important to make sure your diet is healthy, balanced and contains all the nutrients you need for good health. Yes, you can still lose weight by eating nothing but, for example, chocolate, crisps and biscuits providing you stick to your calorie allowance. But you'll never find a nutrition expert or dietitian recommending this. And there are plenty of good reasons why.

To start with, an unbalanced diet is likely to be lacking in essential nutrients such as protein, vitamins, minerals and fibre, in the long term putting you at risk of nutritional deficiencies. Secondly, research proves that filling up on foods that are high in fat and/or salt and sugar can lead to many different health problems. But most importantly, when it comes to losing weight, it's almost impossible to stick to a daily calorie allowance if you're only eating high-calorie foods.

Filling up on lower-calorie foods also means you'll be able to eat far more with the result that you're not constantly left feeling unsatisfied. For example, six chocolates from a selection box contain around 300 calories, a lot of fat and sugar, few nutrients – and are eaten in just six mouthfuls! For 300 calories, you could have a grilled skinless chicken breast (packed with protein and zinc), a large salad with fat-free dressing (a great source of fibre, vitamins and minerals), a slice of wholemeal bread with low-fat spread (rich in fibre and B vitamins) and a satsuma (an excellent source of vitamin C). That's a lot more food that will take you a lot more time to eat! Not convinced? Then put six chocolates on one plate, and the chicken, salad, bread and fruit on another!

Bottom line: while slightly reducing your calorie intake is the key to losing weight, you'll be healthier and far more likely to keep those pounds off if you do it by eating a healthy diet *(see 'Healthy Eating Made Easy' page 32).*

Eight steps to a healthy diet

1 *Base your meals on starchy foods.*

2 *Eat lots of fruit and vegetables.*

3 *Eat more fish.*

4 *Cut down on saturated fat and sugar.*

5 *Try to eat less salt - no more than 6g a day.*

6 *Get active and try to be a healthy weight.*

7 *Drink plenty of water.*

8 *Don't skip breakfast.*

SOURCE: www.nhs.uk/Livewell/Goodfood/Pages/eatwell-plate.aspx

Fat facts

Generally speaking, opting for foods that are low in fat can help slash your calorie intake considerably, for example, swapping full-fat milk for skimmed, switching from butter to a low-fat spread, not frying food in oil and chopping the fat off meat and poultry. But don't be fooled into believing that all foods described as 'low-fat' or 'fat-free' are automatically low in calories or calorie-free. In fact, some low-fat products may actually be higher in calories than standard products, thanks to them containing extra sugars and thickeners to boost the flavour and texture. The solution: always check the calorie content of low-fat foods, especially for things like cakes, biscuits, crisps, ice creams and ready meals. You might be surprised to find there's little difference in the calorie content when compared to the standard product.

Uncovering fat claims on food labels

Many products may lure you into believing they're a great choice if you're trying to cut fat, but you need to read between the lines on the labels if you want to be sure you're making the best choice. Here's the lowdown on what to look for:

LOW FAT	by law the food must contain less than 3g of fat per 100g for solids. These foods are generally a good choice if you're trying to lose weight.
REDUCED FAT	by law the food must contain 25 percent less fat than a similar standard product. This doesn't mean the product is low-fat (or low-calorie) though! For example, reduced-fat cheese may still contain 14g fat per 100g.
FAT FREE	the food must contain no more than 0.5g of fat per 100g or 100ml. Foods labelled as Virtually Fat Free must contain less than 0.3g fat per 100g. These foods are generally a good choice if you're trying to lose weight.
LESS THAN 8% FAT	this means the product contains less than 8g fat per 100g. It's only foods labelled 'less than 3% fat' that are a true low-fat choice.
X% FAT FREE	claims expressed as X% Fat Free shall be prohibited.
LIGHT OR LITE	claims stating a product is 'light' or 'lite' follows the same conditions as those set for the term 'reduced'.

10 easy ways to slash fat (and calories)

1 Eat fewer fried foods – grill, boil, bake, poach, steam, roast without added fat or microwave instead.

2 Don't add butter, lard, margarine or oil to food during preparation or cooking.

3 Use spreads sparingly. Butter and margarine contain the same amount of calories and fat – only low fat spreads contain less.

4 Choose boiled or jacket potatoes instead of chips or roast potatoes.

5 Cut off all visible fat from meat and remove the skin from chicken before cooking.

6 Don't eat too many fatty meat products such as sausages, burgers, pies and pastry products.

7 Use semi-skimmed or skimmed milk instead of full-fat milk.

8 Try low-fat or reduced-fat varieties of cheese such as reduced-fat Cheddar, low-fat soft cheese or cottage cheese.

9 Eat fewer high-fat foods such as crisps, chocolates, cakes, pastries and biscuits.

10 Don't add cream to puddings, sauces or coffee.

Getting Ready for Weight Loss Success

Lyndel Costain BSc RD

THIS BOOK not only provides tools to help you understand more about what you eat and how active you are, but guidance on how to use this information to develop a weight loss plan to suit your needs. Getting in the right frame of mind will also be a key part of your weight control journey, especially if you've lost weight before, only to watch the pounds pile back on.

The fact is that most people who want to lose weight know what to do. But often there is something that keeps stopping them from keeping up healthier habits. The same may be true for you. So what's going on? For many it's a lack of readiness. When the next diet comes along with its tempting promises it's so easy to just jump on board. But if you have struggled with your weight for a while, will that diet actually help you to recognise and change the thoughts and actions that have stopped you shifting the pounds for good?

Check out your attitude to weight loss programmes

Before starting any new weight loss programme, including the Weight Loss Resources approach, ask yourself:

Am I starting out thinking that I like myself as a person right now?	(YES or NO)
OR I feel I can only like myself once I lose weight?	(YES or NO)
Do I want to stop overeating, but at the same time find myself justifying it – in other words I want to be able to eat what I want, but with no consequences?	(YES or NO)
Do I believe that I need to take long-term responsibility for my weight?	(YES or NO)
OR Am I relying on 'it' (the diet) to do it for me?	(YES or NO)

Keep these questions, and your replies, in mind as you read through this chapter.

Next Steps

You may have already assessed the healthiness of your weight using the BMI guide on page 37. If not, why not do it now, remembering that the tools are a guide only. The important thing is to consider a weight at which you are healthy and comfortable – and which is realistic for the life you lead *(see opposite - What is a healthy weight?)*.

The next step is to have a long hard think about why you want to lose weight. Consider all the possible benefits, not just those related to how you look. Psychologists have found that if we focus only on appearance we are less likely to succeed in the long-term. This is because it so often reflects low self-esteem or self-worth – which can sabotage success – as it saps confidence and keeps us stuck in destructive thought patterns. Identifying key motivations other than simply how you look - such as health and other aspects of physical and emotional well being - is like saying that you're an OK person right now, and worth making changes for. Making healthy lifestyle choices also has the knock on effect of boosting self-esteem further.

Write down your reasons for wanting to lose weight in your Personal Plan *(see page 42)* – so you can refer back to them. This can be especially helpful when the going gets tough. It may help to think of it in terms of what your weight is stopping you from doing now. Here's some examples: to feel more confident; so I can play more comfortably with my kids; my healthier diet will give me more energy; to improve my fertility.

What is a Healthy Weight?

With all the 'thin is beautiful' messages in the media it can be easy to get a distorted view about whether your weight is healthy or not. However, as the BMI charts suggest, there is no single 'ideal' weight for anybody. Research also shows that modest amounts of weight loss can be very beneficial to health and are easier to keep off. Therefore, health professionals now encourage us to aim for a weight loss of 5-10%. The ideal rate of weight loss is no more than 1-2 pounds (0.5-1kg) per week – so averaging a pound a week is great, and realistic progress.

The health benefits of modest weight loss include:

- *Reduced risk of developing heart disease, stroke and certain cancers*
- *Reduced risk of developing diabetes and helping to manage diabetes*
- *Improvements in blood pressure*
- *Improvements in mobility, back pain and joint pain*
- *Improvements with fertility problems and polycystic ovarian syndrome*
- *Less breathlessness and sleep/snoring problems*
- *Increased self esteem and control over eating*
- *Feeling fitter and have more energy*

Are You Really Ready to Lose Weight?

When you think of losing weight, it's easy just to think of what weight you'd like to get to. But weight loss only happens as a result of making changes to your usual eating and activity patterns – which allow you to consume fewer calories than you burn *(see 'It's calories that count' page 5).*

So here comes the next big question. Are you really ready to do it? Have you thought about the implications of your decision? If you have lost weight in the past, and put it all back on - have you thought about why that was? And how confident do you feel about being successful this time?

To help you answer these questions, try these short exercises.

Where would you place yourself on the following scales?

Importance

How important is it to you, to make the changes that will allow you to lose weight?

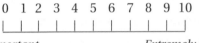

Not at all important   *Extremely important*

If you ranked yourself over half way along the scale then move on to the next question. If you were half way or less along the scale, you may not be mentally ready to make the required changes to lose weight. To further explore this, go to *'The Pros and Cons of Weight Loss' (page 17)*.

Confidence

How confident are you in your ability to make the changes that will allow you to lose weight?

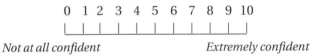

Not at all confident   *Extremely confident*

Now ask yourself (regarding your confidence ratings):

1. Why did I place myself here?
2. What is stopping me moving further up the scale (if anything)?
3. What things, information, support would help me move further up the scale? (if not near 10)

If you aren't sure about answers to question 3, then keep reading for some pointers.

The Pros and Cons of Weight Loss

Making lifestyle changes to lose weight is simpler if there are lots of clear benefits or pros, for example, clothes fit again, more energy, helps back pain - but there will also be associated downsides or cons. For example, some may feel it interferes with their social life, or don't have the time to plan meals or check food labels. Or overeating can help, if only temporarily, as a way of coping with unwanted feelings. Being overweight allows some people to feel strong and assertive, or to control their partner's jealousy. So in these cases there are downsides to losing weight, even if the person says they are desperate to do it.

If you are aware of the possible downsides, as well as the pros, you will be better prepared to deal with potential conflicts. Understanding what could be (or were with past weight loss efforts) barriers to success gives you the chance to address them. This boosts confidence in your ability to succeed this time, which in turn maintains your motivation.

Have a go at weighing up the pros and cons using the charts below and on page 18. Some examples are included. If you decide that the pros outweigh the cons, then great. You can also use the cons as potential barriers to plan strategies for *(see page 42)*. If you find it's the other way around, this may not be the best time to actively lose weight. Try the exercise again in a month or so.

Making Lifestyle Changes to Lose Weight Now

CONS *e.g. Must limit eating out, take aways*	PROS *e.g. Feel more energetic, slimmer*

Not Making Changes Now – how would I feel in 6 months time?

PROS *e.g. Haven't had to worry about failing;* *Still able to eat take aways a lot*	CONS *e.g. Probably gained more weight;* *Back pain may be worse*

To change your weight, first change your mind

To lose weight you may already have a list of things to change, such as eating more fruit and veg, calculating your daily calorie intake, going for a walk each morning or buying low fat options. Others could also give you tips to try. But knowing what to do isn't the same as feeling motivated or able to do it. To be effective, you have to believe the changes are relevant, do-able and worth it.

What you think, affects how you feel, and in turn the actions you take.

Self-efficacy

In fact, research is telling us that one of the most important factors that influences weight loss success are your feelings of 'self-efficacy'. Self-efficacy is a term used in psychology to describe a person's belief that any action they take will have an effect on the outcome. It reflects our inner expectation that what we do will lead to the results we want. Not surprisingly, high levels of self-efficacy can enhance motivation, and allow us to deal better with uncertainty and conflict, and recovery from setbacks. But low levels, can reduce our motivation. We fear that whatever we do will not bring about our desired goal. This can lead self-defeating thoughts or 'self-talk', which make it hard to deal with set-backs, meaning we are more likely to give up. Here's some examples.

Examples: Low self-efficacy

'*No matter how carefully I diet, I don't lose weight ...*'

'*I have eaten that chocolate and as usual blown my diet, so I may as well give up now.*'

'*I had a rich dessert – I have no willpower to say no. I can't stand not being able to eat what I want.*'

If you have a strong sense of self-efficacy, your mindset and 'self-talk' will be more like:

Examples: High self-efficacy

'*I know from previous weight loss programmes, that if I stay focussed on what I am doing I do lose weight. I have always expected to lose too much too quickly which frustrates me. I know that I will lose weight if I keep making the right changes, and this time it is important to me.*'

'*The chocolate bar won't ruin my diet, but if I think it has and keep on eating, then my negative self-talk will. So I will get back on track.*'

'*I don't like having to eat differently from others, but losing weight is very important to me, so I **can** stand it. After all, the world won't stop if I say no to dessert, and I will feel great afterwards. If I think about it, I am not hungry so would just feel bloated and guilty if I ate it.*'

Willpower is a Skill

Many people feel that they just need plenty of willpower or a good telling off to lose weight. But willpower isn't something you have or you don't have. Willpower is a skill. Like the dessert example on page 19, it's a sign that you've made a conscious choice to do something, because you believe the benefits outweigh any downsides. In reality everything we do is preceded by a thought. This includes everything we eat. It just may not seem like it because our actions often feel automatic *(see 'Look out for trigger eating' page 21)*.

When it comes to weight loss, developing a range of skills – including choosing a lower calorie diet, coping with negative self-talk and managing things that don't go to plan - will boost your sense of self-efficacy to make the changes you want. This is especially important because we live in such a weight-promoting environment.

Our weight-promoting environment

We are constantly surrounded by tempting food, stresses that can trigger comfort eating and labour-saving devices that make it easy not to be physically active. In other words, the environment we live in makes it easy to gain weight, unless we stop and think about the food choices we make and how much exercise we do. In fact, to stay a healthy weight/maintain our weight, just about all of us need to make conscious lifestyle choices everyday. This isn't 'dieting' but just part of taking care of ourselves in the environment we live in.

It is also true that some people find it more of a challenge than others to manage their weight, thanks to genetic differences in factors such as appetite control, spontaneous activity level and emotional responses to food – rather than metabolic rate, as is often believed. The good news is that with a healthy diet and active lifestyle a healthier weight can still be achieved. But do talk to your doctor if you feel you need additional support.

Coping with Common Slimming Saboteurs

Lyndel Costain BSc RD

Look out for 'trigger' eating

Much of the overeating we do or cravings we have are actually down to unconscious, habitual, responses to a variety of triggers. These triggers can be external, such as the sight or smell of food, or internal and emotion-led, such as a response to stress, anger, boredom or emptiness. Your food diary (see page 43) helps you to recognise 'trigger' or 'non-hungry' eating which gives you the chance to think twice before you eat (see below).

Get some support

A big part of your success will be having someone to support you. It could be a friend, partner, health professional, health club or website. Let them know how they can help you most.

Make lapses your ally

Don't let a lapse throw you off course. You can't be, nor need to be perfect all the time. Doing well 80-90% of the time is great progress. Lapses are a normal part of change. Rather than feel you have failed and give up, look at what you can learn from a difficult day or week and use it to find helpful solutions for the future.

Understand why you eat

When I ask people what prompts them to eat, hunger usually comes down near the bottom of their list of reasons. Some people struggle to remember or appreciate what true hunger feels like. We are lucky that we have plenty of food to eat in our society. But its constant presence makes it harder to control what we eat, especially if it brings us comfort or joy.

If you ever find yourself in the fridge even though you've recently eaten, then you know hunger isn't the reason but some other trigger. The urge to eat can be so automatic that you feel you lack willpower or are out of control. But it is in fact a learned or conditioned response. A bit like Pavlov's dogs. He rang a bell every time he fed them, and from then on, whenever they heard the bell ring they were 'conditioned' to salivate in anticipation of food.

Because this 'non-hungry' eating is learned, you can reprogramme your response to the situations or feelings that trigger it. The first step is to identify when these urges strike. When you find yourself eating when you aren't hungry ask yourself 'why do I want to eat, what am I feeling?' If you aren't sure think back to what was happening before you ate. Then ask yourself if there is another way you can feel better without food. Or you could chat to your urge to eat in a friendly way, telling it that you don't want to give into it, you have a planned meal coming soon, and it's merely a learned response. Whatever strategy you choose, the more often you break into your urges to eat, the weaker their hold becomes.

Practise positive self-talk

Self-talk may be positive and constructive (like your guardian angel) or negative and irrational (like having a destructive devil on your shoulder).

If you've had on-off battles with your weight over the years, it's highly likely that the 'devil' is there more often. 'All or nothing' self-talk for example, 'I ate a "bad food" so have broken my diet', can make you feel like a failure which, can then trigger you into the action of overeating and/or totally giving up *(see 'Diet-binge cycle' page 23)*. One of the most powerful things about it is that the last thoughts we have are what stays in our mind. So if we think 'I still look fat' or 'I will never be slim', these feelings stay with us.

To change your self-talk for the better, the trick is to first recognise it's happening (keeping a diary really helps, *see Keep a Food Diary, page 29*). Then turn it around into a positive version of the same events *(see Self-efficacy, page 18)* where the resulting action was to feel good and stay on track. Reshaping negative self-talk helps you to boost your self-esteem and feelings of self-efficacy, and with it change your self-definition - from someone who can't 'lose weight' or 'do this or that', to someone 'who can'. And when you believe you can…

The Diet – Binge Cycle

If this cycle looks familiar, use positive self-talk, and a more flexible dietary approach, to help you break free.

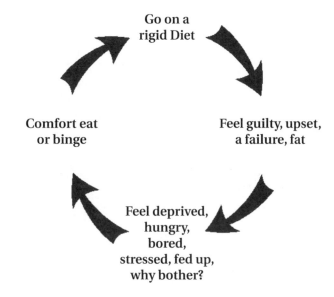

Go on a
rigid Diet

Feel guilty, upset,
a failure, fat

Feel deprived,
hungry,
bored,
stressed, fed up,
why bother?

Comfort eat
or binge

Really choose what you want to eat

This skill is like your personal brake. It also helps you to manage 'trigger/non-hungry' eating and weaken its hold. It legalises food and stops you feeling deprived. It helps you to regularly remind yourself why you are making changes to your eating habits, which keeps motivation high. But it doesn't just happen. Like all skills it requires practise. Sometimes it will work well for you, other times it won't – but overall it will help. Basically, ask yourself if you really want to eat that food in front of you. This becomes the prompt for you to make a conscious choice, weighing up the pros and cons or consequences of making that choice, and feeling free to have it, reject it or just eat some. Remembering all the while that you can eat this food another time if you want to.

Action Planning

Successful people don't just wait for things to happen. They believe in themselves, plan ahead, take action and then refine their plan until it gets, and keeps on getting the results they want. Successful slimmers use a very similar approach. They don't rely on quick-fixes or magic formulas, but glean information from reliable sources to develop a plan or approach that suits their needs, tastes and lifestyle. Thinking of weight management as a lifelong project, which has a weight loss phase and a weight maintenance phase, is also a route to success.

When the Going Gets Tough - Staying on Track

If things start to go off track, don't panic. Learning new habits takes time. And life is never straightforward so there will be times when it all seems too much, or negative 'self- talk' creeps in to try and drag you back into old ways. So if the going gets tough:

- Value what you've achieved so far, rather than only focus on what you plan to do.
- Look back at your reasons to lose weight and refer to the list often.
- Don't expect to change too much, too quickly. Take things a step at a time.
- Accept difficulties as part of the learning and skill building process.
- Enjoy a non-food reward for achieving your goals (including maintaining your weight).
- Use recipes and meal ideas to keep things interesting.
- Talk to your supporters and get plenty of encouragement. This is really vital!

Strategies of Successful Slimmers

Thanks to research conducted by large studies such as the US National Weight Control Registry and the German Lean Habits Study, we now know more about what works best for people who have lost weight and successfully kept it off. So be inspired!

The key elements of success are to:

- Believe that you can control your weight and the changes involved are really worth it.

- Stay realistic and value what you have achieved rather than dwell on a weight you 'dream' of being.

- Be more active – plan ways to fit activity into your daily life – aim for 1 hour of walking daily.

- Plan ahead for regular meals and snacks, starting with breakfast.

- Choose a balanced, low-fat diet with plenty of fruit and vegetables *(see Healthy Eating Made Easy, page 32)*.

- Watch portion size and limit fast food.

- Sit down to eat and take time over meals, paying attention to what you are eating.

- Have a flexible approach – plan in and enjoy some favourite foods without guilt.

- Recognise and address 'all or nothing' thinking and other negative 'self-talk'.

- Keep making conscious choices.

- Learn to confront problems rather than eat, drink, sleep or wish they would go away.

- Enlist ongoing help and support from family, friends, professionals or websites.

- Regularly (at least once a week but not more than once daily) check your weight.

- Take action before your weight increases by more than 4-5lb (2kg).

- Accept that your weight management skills need to be kept up long-term.

- Take heart from successful slimmers, who say that it gets easier over time.

Your step-by-step guide to using this book and shifting those pounds

Juliette Kellow BSc RD and Rebecca Walton

1. Find your healthy weight

Use the weight charts, body mass index table and information on pages 36-43 to determine the right weight for you. Then set yourself a weight to aim for. Research shows it really helps if you make losing 10% of your weight your first overall target. It also brings important health benefits too *(see 'What is a Healthy Weight?' page 15)*. You can break this down into smaller manageable steps, for example, 3kg/6.5lbs at a time. If 10% is too much, then go for a 5% loss – this has important health benefits too. In fact, just keeping your weight stable is a great achievement these days, because of our weight-promoting environment *(see page 20)*.

Waist Management

In addition to BMI, another important way to assess your weight is by measuring your waist just above belly button level. It is especially useful for men as they tend to carry more excess weight around their bellies, but women should test it out too. Having excess weight around your middle (known as being 'apple-shaped') increases your risk of heart disease and type 2 diabetes. A simple way to stay aware of your waist is according to how well, or otherwise, skirts and trousers fit. Talk to your doctor about any weight and health concerns.

WAIST MEASUREMENT

	Increased Health Risk	High Risk to Health
Women	32-35in (81-88cm)	more than 35in (88cm)
Men	37-40in (94-102cm)	more than 40in (102cm)

2. Set a realistic time scale

With today's hectic lifestyles, everything tends to happen at breakneck speed, so it's no wonder that when it comes to losing weight, most of us want to shift those pounds in an instant. But it's probably taken years to accumulate that extra weight, with the result that it's unrealistic to expect to lose the excess in just a few weeks! Instead, prepare yourself to lose weight slowly and steadily. It's far healthier to lose weight like this. But better still, research shows you'll be far more likely to maintain your new, lower weight.

If you only have a small amount of weight to lose, aim for a weight loss of around 1lb (½kg) a week. But if you have more than 2 stone (28kg) to lose, you may prefer to aim for 2lb (1kg) each week. Remember though, it's better to keep going at 1lb (½kg) a week than to give up because trying to lose 2lb (1kg) a week is making you miserable! The following words may help you to keep your goal in perspective:

'Never give up on a goal because of the time it will take to achieve it – the time will pass anyway.'

Weight Fluctuations

Weight typically fluctuates on a day to day basis. You know that shock/horror feeling when you weigh yourself in the morning then later in the day, or after a meal out, and it looks like youve gained pounds in hours! But this is due to fluid not fat changes. Real changes in body fat can only happen more gradually (remember, to gain 1lb you need to eat 3500 calories more than you usually do). Don't be confused either by seemingly very rapid weight loss in the first week or so.

When calorie intake is initially cut back, the body's carbohydrate stores in the liver and muscles (known as glycogen) are used up. Glycogen is stored with three times its weight in water, meaning that rapid losses of 4.5- 6.6lb (2 -3 kg) are possible. These stores can be just as rapidly refilled if normal eating is resumed. True weight loss happens more gradually and this book helps you to lose weight at the steady and healthy rate of no more than 1-2 lbs per week.

---

3. Calculate your calorie allowance

Use the calorie tables on pages 39-40 to find out how many calories you need each day to maintain your current weight. Then use the table below to discover the amount of calories you need to subtract from this amount every day to lose weight at your chosen rate. For example, a 35 year-old woman who is moderately active and weighs 12 stone (76kg) needs 2,188 calories a day to keep her weight steady. If she wants to lose ½lb (¼kg) a week, she needs 250 calories less each day, giving her a daily calorie allowance of 1,938 calories. If she wants to lose 1lb (½kg) a week, she needs 500 calories less each day, giving her a daily calorie allowance of 1,688 calories, and so on.

TO LOSE...	Cut your daily calorie intake by	In three months you could lose...	In six months you could lose...	In one year you could lose...
½lb a week	250	6.5lb	13lb	1st 12lb
1lb a week	500	13lb	1st 12lb	3st 10lb
1½lb a week	750	1st 5.5lb	2st 11lb	5st 8lb
2lb a week	1,000	1st 12lb	3st 10lb	7st 6lb

TO LOSE...	Cut your daily calorie intake by	In three months you could lose...	In six months you could lose...	In one year you could lose...
¼kg a week	250	3.25kg	6.5kg	13kg
½kg a week	500	6.5kg	13kg	26kg
¾kg a week	750	9.75kg	19.5kg	39kg
1kg a week	1,000	13kg	26kg	52kg

4. Keep a food diary

Writing down what you eat and drink and any thoughts linked to that eating helps you become more aware of your eating habits. Recognising what is going on helps you feel in control and is a powerful way to start planning change. Keeping a food diary before you start to change your eating habits will also help you identify opportunities for cutting calories by substituting one food for another, cutting portion sizes of high-calorie foods or eating certain foods less often. Simply write down every single item you eat or drink during the day and use this book to calculate the calories of each item. Then after a few days of eating normally, introduce some changes to your diet to achieve your daily calorie allowance. Remember to spread your daily calorie allowance fairly evenly throughout the day to prevent hunger. You'll find a template for a daily food and exercise diary on page 43. Try to use it as carefully as you can as research shows that people who do, do best.

 Top Tip

If you only fill in your main food diary once a day, keep a pen and notepad with you to write down all those little extras you eat or drink during the day – that chocolate you ate in the office, the sliver of cheese you had while cooking dinner and the few chips you pinched from your husband's plate, for example! It's easy to forget the little things if they're not written down, but they can make the difference between success and failure.

QUESTION: Why are heavier people allowed more calories than those who have smaller amounts of weight to lose?

ANSWER: This confuses a lot of people but is easily explained. Someone who is 3 stone overweight, for example, is carrying the equivalent of 42 small packets of butter with them everywhere they go – up and down the stairs, to the local shops, into the kitchen. Obviously, it takes a lot more energy simply to move around when you're carrying that extra weight. As a consequence, the heavier you are, the more calories you need just to keep your weight steady. In turn, this means you'll lose weight on a higher calorie allowance. However, as you lose weight, you'll need to lower your calorie allowance slightly as you have less weight to carry around.

5. Control your portions

As well as making some smart food swaps to cut calories, it's likely you'll also need to reduce your serving sizes for some foods to help shift those pounds. Even 'healthy' foods such as brown rice, wholemeal bread, chicken, fish and low-fat dairy products contain calories so you may need to limit the amount you eat. When you first start out, weigh portions of foods like rice, pasta, cereal, cheese, butter, oil, meat, fish, and chicken rather than completing your food diary with a 'guesstimated' weight! That way you can calculate the calorie content accurately. Don't forget that drinks contain calories too, alcohol, milk, juices and sugary drinks all count.

6. Measure your success

Research has found that regular weight checks do help. Weighing yourself helps you assess how your eating and exercise habits affect your body weight. The important thing is to use the information in a positive way – to assess your progress - rather than as a stick to beat yourself up with. Remember that weight can fluctuate by a kilogram in a day, for example, due to fluid changes, premenstrually, after a big meal out, so weigh yourself at the same time of day and look at the trend over a week or two.

People who successfully lose weight and keep it off, also tend to continue weighing themselves at least once a week, and often daily (but not in an obsessive way), because they say it helps them stay 'on track'. Probably because they use it as an early warning system. People who weigh themselves regularly (or regularly try on a tight fitting item of clothing) will notice quickly if they have gained a couple of kilograms and can take action to stop gaining more. Checking your weight less often can mean that you might discover one day that you gained 6kg. That can be pretty discouraging, and it might trigger you to just give up.

Top Tip

Don't just focus on what the bathroom scales say either – keep a record of your vital statistics, too. Many people find it doubly encouraging to see the inches dropping off, as well as the pounds!

7. Stay motivated

Each time you lose half a stone, or reach your own small goal – celebrate! Treat yourself to a little luxury – something new to wear, a little pampering or some other (non-food) treat. It also helps replace the comfort you once got from food and allows you to take care of yourself in other ways. Trying on an item of clothing that used to be tight can also help to keep you feeling motivated. Make sure you keep in touch with your supporters, and if the going gets tough take another look at the *'Coping with Common Slimming Saboteurs' section on page 21*. Once you've reviewed how well you've done, use this book to set yourself a new daily calorie allowance based on your new weight to help you lose the next half stone *(see point 3 - page 28 - Calculate your calorie allowance)*.

8. Keep it off

What you do to stay slim is just as important as what you did to get slim. Quite simply, if you return to your old ways, you are likely to return to your old weight. The great thing about calorie counting is that you will learn so much about what you eat, and make so many important changes to your eating and drinking habits, that you'll probably find it difficult to go back to your old ways – and won't want to anyway. It's still a good idea to weigh yourself at least once a week to keep a check on your weight. The key is to deal with any extra pounds immediately, rather than waiting until you have a stone to lose *(see page 30)*. Simply go back to counting calories for as long as it takes to shift those pounds and enjoy the new slim you. Page 25 has more information about how successful slimmers keep it off.

QUESTION: Do I need to stick to exactly the same number of calories each day or is it OK to have a lower calorie intake during the week and slightly more at the weekend?

ANSWER: The key to losing weight is to take in fewer calories than you need for as long as it takes to reach your target, aiming for a loss of no more than 2lb (1kg) a week. In general, most nutrition experts recommend a daily calorie allowance. However, it's just as valid to use other periods of time such as weeks. If you prefer, simply multiply your daily allowance by seven to work out a weekly calorie allowance and then allocate more calories to some days than others. For example, a daily allowance of 1,500 calories is equivalent to 10,500 calories a week. This means you could have 1,300 calories a day during the week and 2,000 calories a day on Saturday and Sunday.

Healthy Eating Made Easy

Juliette Kellow BSc RD

GONE ARE THE DAYS when a healthy diet meant surviving on bird seed, rabbit food and carrot juice! The new approach to eating healthily means we're positively encouraged to eat a wide range of foods, including some of our favourites – it's just a question of making sure we don't eat high fat, high sugar or highly processed foods too often.

Eating a healthy diet, together with taking regular exercise and not smoking, has huge benefits to our health, both in the short and long term. As well as helping us to lose or maintain our weight, a healthy diet can boost energy levels, keep our immune system strong and give us healthy skin, nails and hair. Meanwhile, eating well throughout life also means we're far less likely to suffer from health problems such as constipation, anaemia and tooth decay or set ourselves up for serious conditions in later life such as obesity, heart disease, stroke, diabetes, cancer or osteoporosis.

Fortunately, it couldn't be easier to eat a balanced diet. To start with, no single food provides all the calories and nutrients we need to stay healthy, so it's important to eat a variety of foods. Meanwhile, most nutrition experts also agree that mealtimes should be a pleasure rather than a penance. This means it's fine to eat small amounts of our favourite treats from time to time.

To help people eat healthily, the Food Standards Agency recommends eating plenty of different foods from four main groups of foods and limiting the amount we eat from a smaller fifth group. Ultimately, we should eat more fruit, vegetables, starchy, fibre-rich foods and fresh products, and fewer fatty, sugary, salty and processed foods.

The following guidelines are all based on the healthy eating guidelines recommended by the Food Standards Agency.

Bread, other cereals and potatoes

Eat these foods at each meal. They also make good snacks.

Foods in this group include bread, breakfast cereals, potatoes, rice, pasta, noodles, yams, oats and grains. Go for high-fibre varieties where available, such as wholegrain cereals, wholemeal bread and brown rice. These foods should fill roughly a third of your plate at mealtimes.

TYPICAL SERVING SIZES

• *2 slices bread in a sandwich or with a meal*

• *a tennis ball sized serving of pasta, potato, rice, noodles or couscous*

• *a bowl of porridge*

• *around 40g of breakfast cereal*

Fruit and vegetables

Eat at least five portions every day.

Foods in this group include all fruits and vegetables, including fresh, frozen, canned and dried products, and unsweetened fruit juice. Choose canned fruit in juice rather than syrup and go for veg canned in water without added salt or sugar.

TYPICAL PORTION SIZES

• *a piece of fruit eg: apple, banana, pear*

• *2 small fruits eg: satsumas, plums, apricots*

• *a bowl of fruit salad, canned or stewed fruit*

• *a small glass of unsweetened fruit juice*

• *a cereal bowl of salad*

• *3tbsp vegetables*

Milk and dairy foods

Eat two or three servings a day.

Foods in this group include milk, cheese, yoghurt and fromage frais. Choose low-fat varieties where available such as skimmed milk, reduced-fat cheese and fat-free yoghurt.

TYPICAL SERVING SIZES

* *200ml milk*

* *a small pot of yoghurt or fromage frais*

* *a small matchbox-sized piece of cheese*

Meat, fish and alternatives

Eat two servings a day

Foods in this group include meat, poultry, fish, eggs, beans, nuts and seeds. Choose low-fat varieties where available such as extra-lean minced beef and skinless chicken and don't add extra fat or salt.

TYPICAL SERVING SIZES

* *a piece of meat, chicken or fish the size of a deck of cards*

* *1-2 eggs*

* *3 heaped tablespoons of beans*

* *a small handful of nuts or seeds*

Healthy Eating on a plate

A simple way to serve up both balance and healthy proportions is to fill one half of your plate with salad or vegetables and divide the other half between protein-rich meat, chicken, fish, eggs or beans, and healthy carbs (potatoes, rice, pasta, pulses, bread or noodles).

Fatty and sugary foods

Eat only small amounts of these foods

Foods in this group include oils, spreading fats, cream, mayonnaise, oily salad dressings, cakes, biscuits, puddings, crisps, savoury snacks, sugar, preserves, confectionery and sugary soft drinks.

TYPICAL SERVING SIZES:

- *a small packet of sweets or a small bar of chocolate*

- *a small slice of cake*

- *a couple of small biscuits*

- *1 level tbsp mayo, salad dressing or olive oil*

- *a small packet of crisps*

Useful Tools

Body Mass Index

The Body Mass Index (BMI) is the internationally accepted way of assessing how healthy our weight is. It is calculated using an individual's height and weight. Use the Body Mass Index Chart to look up your BMI, and use the table below to see what range you fall into.

BMI Under 18.5	Underweight
BMI 18.5-25	Healthy
BMI 25-30	Overweight
BMI 30-40	Obese
BMI Over 40	Severely Obese

This is what different BMI ranges mean.

- **Underweight:** you probably need to gain weight for your health's sake. Talk to your doctor if you have any concerns, or if you feel frightened about gaining weight.

- **Healthy weight:** you are a healthy weight, so aim to stay in this range (note that most people in this range tend to have a BMI between 20-25).

- **Overweight:** aim to lose some weight for your health's sake, or at least prevent further weight gain.

- **Obese:** your health is at risk and losing weight will benefit your health.

- **Severely obese:** your health is definitely at risk. You should visit your doctor for a health check. Losing weight will improve your health.

Please note that BMI is not as accurate for athletes or very muscular people (muscle weighs more than fat), as it can push them into a higher BMI category despite having a healthy level of body fat. It is also not accurate for women who are pregnant or breastfeeding, or people who are frail.

Body Mass Index Table

HEIGHT IN FEET / INCHES

	4'6	4'8	4'10	5'0	5'2	5'4	5'6	5'8	5'10	6'0	6'2	6'4	6'6	6'8	6'10
6st 7	22.0	20.5	19.1	17.8	16.7	15.7	14.7	13.9	13.1	12.4	11.7	11.1	10.6	10.0	9.5
7st 0	23.7	22.1	20.6	19.2	18.0	16.9	15.9	15.0	14.1	13.3	12.6	12.0	11.4	10.8	10.3
7st 7	25.4	23.6	22.0	20.6	19.3	18.1	17.0	16.0	15.1	14.3	13.5	12.8	12.2	11.6	11.0
8st 0	27.1	25.2	23.5	22.0	20.6	19.3	18.1	17.1	16.1	15.2	14.4	13.7	13.0	12.3	11.8
8st 7	28.8	26.8	25.0	23.3	21.8	20.5	19.3	18.2	17.1	16.2	15.3	14.5	13.8	13.1	12.5
9st 0	30.5	28.4	26.4	24.7	23.1	21.7	20.4	19.2	18.1	17.2	16.2	15.4	14.6	13.9	13.2
9st 7	32.2	29.9	27.9	26.1	24.4	22.9	21.5	20.3	19.2	18.1	17.1	16.2	15.4	14.7	14.0
10st 0	33.9	31.5	29.4	27.4	25.7	24.1	22.7	21.4	20.2	19.1	18.0	17.1	16.2	15.4	14.7
10st 7	35.6	33.1	30.8	28.8	27.0	25.3	23.8	22.4	21.2	20.0	18.9	18.0	17.0	16.2	15.4
11st 0	37.3	34.7	32.3	30.2	28.3	26.5	24.9	23.5	22.2	21.0	19.8	18.8	17.9	17.0	16.2
11st 7	39.0	36.2	33.8	31.6	29.6	27.7	26.1	24.6	23.2	21.9	20.7	19.7	18.7	17.8	16.9
12st 0	40.7	37.8	35.2	32.9	30.8	28.9	27.2	25.6	24.2	22.9	21.6	20.5	19.5	18.5	17.6
12st 7	42.3	39.4	36.7	34.3	32.1	30.1	28.3	26.7	25.2	23.8	22.5	21.4	20.3	19.3	18.4
13st 0	44.0	41.0	38.2	35.7	33.4	31.4	29.5	27.8	26.2	24.8	23.5	22.2	21.1	20.1	19.1
13st 7	45.7	42.5	39.6	37.0	34.7	32.6	30.6	28.8	27.2	25.7	24.4	23.1	21.9	20.8	19.8
14st 0	47.4	44.1	41.1	38.4	36.0	33.8	31.7	29.9	28.2	26.7	25.3	23.9	22.7	21.6	20.6
14st 7	49.1	45.7	42.6	39.8	37.3	35.0	32.9	31.0	29.2	27.6	26.2	24.8	23.5	22.4	21.3
15st 0	50.8	47.3	44.0	41.2	38.5	36.2	34.0	32.0	30.2	28.6	27.1	25.7	24.4	23.2	22.0
15st 7	52.5	48.8	45.5	42.5	39.8	37.4	35.2	33.1	31.2	29.5	28.0	26.5	25.2	23.9	22.8
16st 0	54.2	50.4	47.0	43.9	41.1	38.6	36.3	34.2	32.3	30.5	28.9	27.4	26.0	24.7	23.5
16st 7	55.9	52.0	48.5	45.3	42.4	39.8	37.4	35.2	33.3	31.4	29.8	28.2	26.8	25.5	24.2
17st 0	57.6	53.6	49.9	46.6	43.7	41.0	38.6	36.3	34.3	32.4	30.7	29.1	27.6	26.2	25.0
17st 7	59.3	55.1	51.4	48.0	45.0	42.2	39.7	37.4	35.3	33.3	31.6	29.9	28.4	27.0	25.7
18st 0	61.0	56.7	52.9	49.4	46.3	43.4	40.8	38.5	36.3	34.3	32.5	30.8	29.2	27.8	26.4
18st 7	62.7	58.3	54.3	50.8	47.5	44.6	42.0	39.5	37.3	35.3	33.4	31.6	30.0	28.6	27.2
19st 0	64.4	59.9	55.8	52.1	48.8	45.8	43.1	40.6	38.3	36.2	34.3	32.5	30.8	29.3	27.9
19st 7	66.1	61.4	57.3	53.5	50.1	47.0	44.2	41.7	39.3	37.2	35.2	33.3	31.7	30.1	28.6
20st 0	67.8	63.0	58.7	54.9	51.4	48.2	45.4	42.7	40.3	38.1	36.1	34.2	32.5	30.9	29.4
20st 7	69.4	64.6	60.2	56.3	52.7	49.4	46.5	43.8	41.3	39.1	37.0	35.1	33.3	31.6	30.1
21st 0	71.1	66.2	61.7	57.6	54.0	50.6	47.6	44.9	42.3	40.0	37.9	35.9	34.1	32.4	30.9
21st 7	72.8	67.7	63.1	59.0	55.3	51.9	48.8	45.9	43.3	41.0	38.8	36.8	34.9	33.2	31.6
22st 0	74.5	69.3	64.6	60.4	56.5	53.1	49.9	47.0	44.4	41.9	39.7	37.6	35.7	34.0	32.3
22st 7	76.2	70.9	66.1	61.7	57.8	54.3	51.0	48.1	45.4	42.9	40.6	38.5	36.5	34.7	33.1
23st 0	77.9	72.5	67.5	63.1	59.1	55.5	52.2	49.1	46.4	43.8	41.5	39.3	37.3	35.5	33.8
23st 7	79.6	74.0	69.0	64.5	60.4	56.7	53.3	50.2	47.4	44.8	42.4	40.2	38.2	36.3	34.5
24st 0	81.3	75.6	70.5	65.9	61.7	57.9	54.4	51.3	48.4	45.7	43.3	41.0	39.0	37.0	35.3
24st 7	83.0	77.2	71.9	67.2	63.0	59.1	55.6	52.3	49.4	46.7	44.2	41.9	39.8	37.8	36.0
25st 0	84.7	78.8	73.4	68.6	64.2	60.3	56.7	53.4	50.4	47.6	45.1	42.8	40.6	38.6	36.7
25st 7	86.4	80.3	74.9	70.0	65.5	61.5	57.8	54.5	51.4	48.6	46.0	43.6	41.4	39.4	37.5
26st 0	88.1	81.9	76.3	71.3	66.8	62.7	59.0	55.5	52.4	49.5	46.9	44.5	42.2	40.1	38.2
26st 7	89.8	83.5	77.8	72.7	68.1	63.9	60.1	56.6	53.4	50.5	47.8	45.3	43.0	40.9	38.9
27st 0	91.5	85.1	79.3	74.1	69.4	65.1	61.2	57.7	54.4	51.5	48.7	46.2	43.8	41.7	39.7
27st 7	93.2	86.6	80.8	75.5	70.7	66.3	62.4	58.7	55.4	52.4	49.6	47.0	44.7	42.4	40.4
28st 0	94.9	88.2	82.2	76.8	72.0	67.5	63.5	59.8	56.4	53.4	50.5	47.9	45.5	43.2	41.1
28st 7	96.5	89.8	83.7	78.2	73.2	68.7	64.6	60.9	57.5	54.3	51.4	48.7	46.3	44.0	41.9
29st 0	98.2	91.4	85.2	79.6	74.5	69.9	65.8	62.0	58.5	55.3	52.3	49.6	47.1	44.8	42.6
29st 7	99.9	92.9	86.6	80.9	75.8	71.1	66.9	63.0	59.5	56.2	53.2	50.5	47.9	45.5	43.3

WEIGHT IN STONES / LBS

Weight Chart

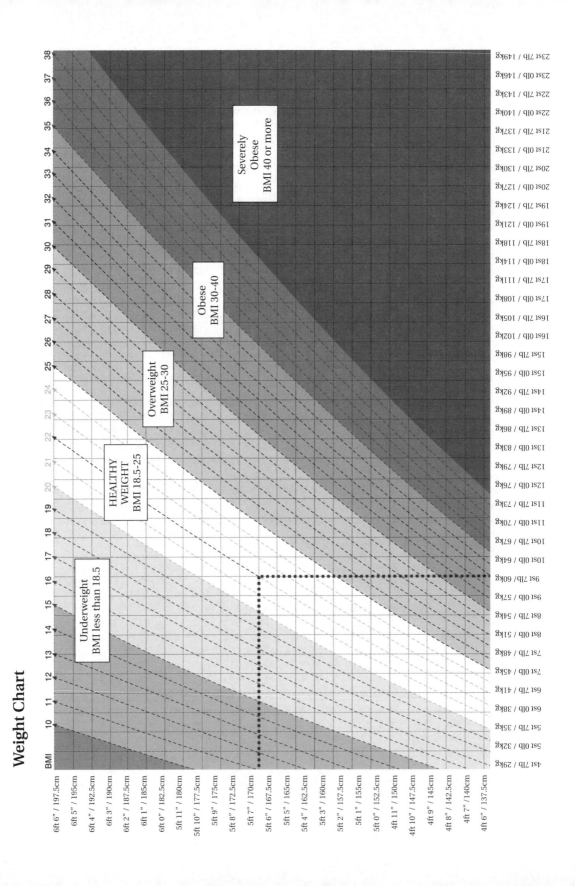

Calories Required to Maintain Weight
Adult Females

ACTIVITY LEVEL / AGE

WEIGHT IN STONES / LBS	VERY SEDENTARY			MODERATELY SEDENTARY			MODERATELY ACTIVE			VERY ACTIVE		
	<30	30-60	60+	<30	30-60	60+	<30	30-60	60+	<30	30-60	60+
7st 7	1425	1473	1304	1544	1596	1412	1781	1841	1630	2138	2210	1956
8st 0	1481	1504	1338	1605	1629	1450	1852	1880	1673	2222	2256	2008
8st 7	1537	1535	1373	1666	1663	1487	1922	1919	1716	2306	2302	2059
9st 0	1594	1566	1407	1726	1696	1524	1992	1957	1759	2391	2349	2111
9st 7	1650	1596	1442	1787	1729	1562	2062	1996	1802	2475	2395	2163
10st 0	1706	1627	1476	1848	1763	1599	2133	2034	1845	2559	2441	2214
10st 7	1762	1658	1511	1909	1796	1637	2203	2073	1888	2644	2487	2266
11st 0	1819	1689	1545	1970	1830	1674	2273	2111	1931	2728	2534	2318
11st 7	1875	1720	1580	2031	1863	1711	2344	2150	1975	2813	2580	2370
12st 0	1931	1751	1614	2092	1897	1749	2414	2188	2018	2897	2626	2421
12st 7	1987	1781	1648	2153	1930	1786	2484	2227	2061	2981	2672	2473
13st 0	2044	1812	1683	2214	1963	1823	2555	2266	2104	3066	2719	2525
13st 7	2100	1843	1717	2275	1997	1861	2625	2304	2147	3150	2765	2576
14st 0	2156	1874	1752	2336	2030	1898	2695	2343	2190	3234	2811	2628
14st 7	2212	1905	1786	2397	2064	1935	2766	2381	2233	3319	2858	2680
15st 0	2269	1936	1821	2458	2097	1973	2836	2420	2276	3403	2904	2732
15st 7	2325	1967	1855	2519	2130	2010	2906	2458	2319	3488	2950	2783
16st 0	2381	1997	1890	2580	2164	2047	2976	2497	2362	3572	2996	2835
16st 7	2437	2028	1924	2640	2197	2085	3047	2535	2405	3656	3043	2887
17st 0	2494	2059	1959	2701	2231	2122	3117	2574	2449	3741	3089	2938
17st 7	2550	2090	1993	2762	2264	2159	3187	2613	2492	3825	3135	2990
18st 0	2606	2121	2028	2823	2298	2197	3258	2651	2535	3909	3181	3042
18st 7	2662	2152	2062	2884	2331	2234	3328	2690	2578	3994	3228	3093
19st 0	2719	2182	2097	2945	2364	2271	3398	2728	2621	4078	3274	3145
19st 7	2775	2213	2131	3006	2398	2309	3469	2767	2664	4162	3320	3197
20st 0	2831	2244	2166	3067	2431	2346	3539	2805	2707	4247	3366	3249
20st 7	2887	2275	2200	3128	2465	2383	3609	2844	2750	4331	3413	3300
21st 0	2944	2306	2235	3189	2498	2421	3680	2882	2793	4416	3459	3352
21st 7	3000	2337	2269	3250	2531	2458	3750	2921	2836	4500	3505	3404
22st 0	3056	2368	2303	3311	2565	2495	3820	2960	2879	4584	3552	3455
22st 7	3112	2398	2338	3372	2598	2533	3890	2998	2923	4669	3598	3507
23st 0	3169	2429	2372	3433	2632	2570	3961	3037	2966	4753	3644	3559
23st 7	3225	2460	2407	3494	2665	2608	4031	3075	3009	4837	3690	3611
24st 0	3281	2491	2441	3554	2699	2645	4101	3114	3052	4922	3737	3662
24st 7	3337	2522	2476	3615	2732	2682	4172	3152	3095	5006	3783	3714
25st 0	3394	2553	2510	3676	2765	2720	4242	3191	3138	5091	3829	3766
25st 7	3450	2583	2545	3737	2799	2757	4312	3229	3181	5175	3875	3817
26st 0	3506	2614	2579	3798	2832	2794	4383	3268	3224	5259	3922	3869
26st 7	3562	2645	2614	3859	2866	2832	4453	3307	3267	5344	3968	3921
27st 0	3618	2676	2648	3920	2899	2869	4523	3345	3310	5428	4014	3973
27st 7	3675	2707	2683	3981	2932	2906	4594	3384	3353	5512	4060	4024
28st 0	3731	2738	2717	4042	2966	2944	4664	3422	3397	5597	4107	4076
28st 7	3787	2768	2752	4103	2999	2981	4734	3461	3440	5681	4153	4128

Calories Required to Maintain Weight
Adult Males

ACTIVITY LEVEL / AGE

WEIGHT IN STONES / LBS	VERY SEDENTARY			MODERATELY SEDENTARY			MODERATELY ACTIVE			VERY ACTIVE		
	<30	30-60	60+	<30	30-60	60+	<30	30-60	60+	<30	30-60	60+
9st 0	1856	1827	1502	2010	1979	1627	2320	2284	1878	2784	2741	2254
9st 7	1913	1871	1547	2072	2026	1676	2391	2338	1933	2870	2806	2320
10st 0	1970	1914	1591	2134	2074	1724	2463	2393	1989	2955	2871	2387
10st 7	2027	1958	1636	2196	2121	1772	2534	2447	2045	3041	2937	2454
11st 0	2084	2001	1680	2258	2168	1820	2605	2502	2100	3127	3002	2520
11st 7	2141	2045	1724	2320	2215	1868	2677	2556	2156	3212	3067	2587
12st 0	2199	2088	1769	2382	2262	1916	2748	2611	2211	3298	3133	2654
12st 7	2256	2132	1813	2444	2310	1965	2820	2665	2267	3384	3198	2720
13st 0	2313	2175	1858	2506	2357	2013	2891	2719	2322	3470	3263	2787
13st 7	2370	2219	1902	2568	2404	2061	2963	2774	2378	3555	3329	2854
14st 0	2427	2262	1947	2630	2451	2109	3034	2828	2434	3641	3394	2920
14st 7	2484	2306	1991	2691	2498	2157	3106	2883	2489	3727	3459	2987
15st 0	2542	2350	2036	2753	2545	2205	3177	2937	2545	3813	3525	3054
15st 7	2599	2393	2080	2815	2593	2253	3248	2992	2600	3898	3590	3120
16st 0	2656	2437	2125	2877	2640	2302	3320	3046	2656	3984	3655	3187
16st 7	2713	2480	2169	2939	2687	2350	3391	3100	2711	4070	3721	3254
17st 0	2770	2524	2213	3001	2734	2398	3463	3155	2767	4155	3786	3320
17st 7	2827	2567	2258	3063	2781	2446	3534	3209	2823	4241	3851	3387
18st 0	2884	2611	2302	3125	2828	2494	3606	3264	2878	4327	3917	3454
18st 7	2942	2654	2347	3187	2876	2542	3677	3318	2934	4413	3982	3520
19st 0	2999	2698	2391	3249	2923	2591	3749	3373	2989	4498	4047	3587
19st 7	3056	2741	2436	3311	2970	2639	3820	3427	3045	4584	4112	3654
20st 0	3113	2785	2480	3373	3017	2687	3891	3481	3100	4670	4178	3721
20st 7	3170	2829	2525	3434	3064	2735	3963	3536	3156	4756	4243	3787
21st 0	3227	2872	2569	3496	3112	2783	4034	3590	3211	4841	4308	3854
21st 7	3285	2916	2614	3558	3159	2831	4106	3645	3267	4927	4374	3921
22st 0	3342	2959	2658	3620	3206	2880	4177	3699	3323	5013	4439	3987
22st 7	3399	3003	2702	3682	3253	2928	4249	3754	3378	5098	4504	4054
23st 0	3456	3046	2747	3744	3300	2976	4320	3808	3434	5184	4570	4121
23st 7	3513	3090	2791	3806	3347	3024	4392	3862	3489	5270	4635	4187
24st 0	3570	3133	2836	3868	3395	3072	4463	3917	3545	5356	4700	4254
24st 7	3627	3177	2880	3930	3442	3120	4534	3971	3600	5441	4766	4321
25st 0	3685	3220	2925	3992	3489	3168	4606	4026	3656	5527	4831	4387
25st 7	3742	3264	2969	4054	3536	3217	4677	4080	3712	5613	4896	4454
26st 0	3799	3308	3014	4116	3583	3265	4749	4135	3767	5699	4962	4521
26st 7	3856	3351	3058	4177	3630	3313	4820	4189	3823	5784	5027	4587
27st 0	3913	3395	3103	4239	3678	3361	4892	4243	3878	5870	5092	4654
27st 7	3970	3438	3147	4301	3725	3409	4963	4298	3934	5956	5158	4721
28st 0	4028	3482	3191	4363	3772	3457	5035	4352	3989	6042	5223	4787
28st 7	4085	3525	3236	4425	3819	3506	5106	4407	4045	6127	5288	4854
29st 0	4142	3569	3280	4487	3866	3554	5177	4461	4101	6213	5354	4921
29st 7	4199	3612	3325	4549	3913	3602	5249	4516	4156	6299	5419	4987
30st 0	4256	3656	3369	4611	3961	3650	5320	4570	4212	6384	5484	5054

Calories Burned in Exercise

This table shows the approximate number of extra* calories that would be burned in a five minute period of exercise activity.

ACTIVITY	CALORIES BURNED IN 5 MINUTES	ACTIVITY	CALORIES BURNED IN 5 MINUTES
Aerobics, Low Impact	25	Situps, Continuous	17
Badminton, Recreational	17	Skiing, Moderate	30
Cross Trainer	30	Skipping, Moderate	30
Cycling, Recreational, 5mph	17	Squash Playing	39
Dancing, Modern, Moderate	13	Tennis Playing, Recreational	26
Fencing	24	Toning Exercises	17
Gardening, Weeding	19	Trampolining	17
Hill Walking, Up and Down, Recreational	22	Volleyball, Recreational	10
Jogging	30	Walking, Uphill, 15% Gradient, Moderate	43
Kick Boxing	30	Walking Up and Down Stairs, Moderate	34
Netball Playing	23	Walking, 4mph	24
Rebounding	18	Weight Training, Moderate	12
Roller Skating	30	Yoga	13
Rowing Machine, Moderate	30		
Running, 7.5mph	48		

*Extra calories are those in addition to your normal daily calorie needs.

My Personal Plan

Date: _____

Body Mass Index: _____

Weight: _____

Waist Measurement: _____

Height: _____

Body Fat % (if known) _____

10% Weight Loss Goal: _____

Current weight	16stone (224lb)	100kg
- 10% weight	1stone 8½lb (22½lb)	10kg
= 10% loss goal	14stone 5½lb (201½lb)	90kg

My smaller weight targets on the way to achieving my 10% goal will be:

_____ _____ _____ _____

Reasons why I want to lose weight:

_____

Changes I will make to help me lose weight:

Diet: _____

Activity: _____

_____   _____

_____   _____

Potential saboteurs or barriers will be:

Ways I will overcome these:

_____   _____

_____   _____

My supporters will be:

_____

I will monitor my progress by:

_____   _____

_____   _____

I will reward my progress with:

In the short term: _____

In the long term: _____

_____   _____

_____   _____

Food and Exercise Diary

Date: ___/___/___

Daily Calorie Allowance: [_____] **A**

Food/Drink Consumed	Serving Size	Calories

You are aiming for your Calorie Balance (Box D) to be as close to zero as possible - ie. you consume the number of calories you need.

Your Daily Calorie Allowance (Box A) should be set to lose ½-2lb (¼-1kg) a week, or maintain weight, depending on your goals.

Total calories consumed [_____] **B**

Daily Calorie Allowance (A) *plus* Extra Calories used in Exercise (C) *minus* Total Calories Consumed (B) *equals* Calorie Balance (D)

Exercise/Activity	No. mins	Calories

Calories used in exercise [_____] **C**

$A + C - B = D$

Calorie balance [_____] **D**

You can also write down any comments or thoughts related to your eating if you want to.

Food Information

Nutritional Information

CALORIE AND FAT values are given per serving, plus calorie and nutrition values per 100g of product. This makes it easy to compare the proportions of fat, protein, carbohydrate and fibre in each food.

The values given are for uncooked, unprepared foods unless otherwise stated. Values are also for only the edible portion of the food unless otherwise stated. ie - weighed with bone.

Finding Foods

The Calorie, Carb & Fat Bible has an Eating Out section which is arranged alphabetically by brand. In the General Foods and Drinks A-Z most foods are grouped together by type, and then put in to alphabetical order. This makes it easy to compare different brands, and will help you to find lower calorie and/or fat alternatives where they are available.

This format also makes it easier to locate foods. Foods are categorised by their main characteristics so, for example, if it is bread, ciabatta or white sliced, you'll find it under "Bread".

Basic ingredients are highlighted to make them easier to find at a glance. You'll find all unbranded foods in bold - making the index easier to use, whether it's just an apple or all the components of a home cooked stew.

There are, however, some foods which are not so easy to categorise, especially combination foods like ready meals. The following pointers will help you to find your way around the book until you get to know it a little better.

FILLED ROLLS AND SANDWICHES - Bagels, baguettes, etc which are filled are listed as "Bagels (filled)" etc. Sandwiches are under "Sandwiches".

CURRIES - Popular types of curry, like Balti or Jalfrezi, are listed under their individual types. Unspecified or lesser known types are listed under their main ingredient.

BURGERS - All burgers, including chicken-type sandwiches from fast-food outlets, are listed under "Burgers". CHIPS & FRIES - Are listed separately, depending on the name of the particular brand. All other types of potato are listed under "Potatoes".

SWEETS & CHOCOLATES - Well-known brands, eg. Aero, Mars Bar, are listed under their brand names. Others are listed under "Chocolate" (for bars) and "Chocolates" (for individual sweets).

READY MEALS - Popular types of dishes are listed under their type, eg. "Chow Mein", "Casserole", "Hot Pot", etc. Others are listed by their main ingredient, eg. "Chicken With", "Chicken In", etc.

EATING OUT & FAST FOODS - By popular demand this edition has the major eating out and fast food brands listed separately, at the back of the book. They are alphabetised first by brand, then follow using the same format as the rest of the book.

Serving Sizes

Many ready-meal type foods are given with calories for the full pack size, so that an individual serving can be worked out by estimating the proportion of the pack that has been consumed. For example, if you have eaten a quarter of a packaged pasta dish, divide the calorie value given for the whole pack by 4 to determine the number of calories you have consumed. Where serving sizes are not appropriate, or unknown, values are given per 1oz/28g. Serving sizes vary greatly from person to person and, if you are trying to lose weight, it's very important to be accurate – especially with foods that are very high in calories such as those that contain a fair amount of fat, sugar, cream, cheese, alcohol etc.

Food Data

Nutrition information for basic average foods has been compiled by the Weight Loss Resources food data team using many sources of information to calculate the most accurate values possible. Some nutrition information for non-branded food records is from The Composition of Foods 6th Edition (2002). Reproduced under licence from The Controller of Her Majesty's Stationary Office. Where basic data is present for ordinary foodstuffs such as 'raw carrots'; branded records are not included.

Nutrition information for branded goods is from details supplied by retailers and manufacturers, and researched by Weight Loss Resources staff. The Calorie Carb & Fat Bible contains data for over 1400 UK brands, including major supermarkets and fast food outlets.

The publishers gratefully acknowledge all the manufacturers and retailers who have provided information on their products. All product names, trademarks or registered trademarks belong to their respective owners and are used only for the purpose of identifying products.

Calorie & nutrition data for all food and drink items are typical values.

Caution
The information in The Calorie, Carb and Fat Bible is intended as an aid to weight loss and weight maintenance, and is not medical advice. If you suffer from, or think you may suffer from a medical condition you should consult your doctor before starting a weight loss and/or exercise regime. If you start exercising after a period of relative inactivity, you should start slowly and consult your doctor if you experience pain, distress or other symptoms.

Weights, Measures & Abbreviations

ABBREVIATIONS

kcal	*kilocalories / calories*
prot	*protein*
carb	*carbohydrate*
sm	*small*
med	*medium*
av	*average*
reg	*regular*
lge	*large*
tsp	*teaspoon*
tbsp	*tablespoon*
dtsp	*dessertspoon*
gf	*gluten free*

BRAND ABBREVIATIONS USED

ASDA

Good for You	*GFY*
Chosen by You	*CBY*

MARKS & SPENCER — *M & S*

Count on Us	*COU*

MORRISONS

Better For You	*BFY*

SAINSBURY'S

Be Good to Yourself	*BGTY*
Way to Five	*WTF*
Taste the Difference	*TTD*

TESCO

Healthy Eating	*HE*
Healthy Living	*HL*
Light Choices	*LC*

WAITROSE

Perfectly Balanced	*PB*

	Measure INFO/WEIGHT	per Measure KCAL	FAT	Nutrition Values per 100g / 100ml KCAL	PROT	CARB	FAT	FIBRE
ABSINTHE								
Average	**1 Pub Shot/35ml**	**127**	**0.0**	**363**	**0.0**	**38.8**	**0.0**	**0.0**
ACKEE								
Canned, Drained, Average	**1oz/28g**	**43**	**4.3**	**151**	**2.9**	**0.8**	**15.2**	**0.0**
ADVOCAAT								
Average	**1 Pub Shot/35ml**	**91**	**2.2**	**260**	**4.7**	**28.4**	**6.3**	**0.0**
AERO								
Creamy White Centre, Nestle*	1 Bar/46g	244	13.8	530	7.6	57.4	30.0	0.0
Milk Chocolate, Bubbles, Sharing Bag, Aero, Nestle*	1 Bag/113g	610	34.7	540	6.5	57.8	30.7	0.0
Milk, Giant, Bar, Nestle*	1 Bar/125g	674	38.6	539	6.6	57.7	30.9	2.2
Milk, Medium, Bar, Nestle*	1 Bar/43g	232	13.3	539	6.6	57.7	30.9	2.2
Milk, Snacksize, Bar, Nestle*	1 Bar/21g	110	6.5	537	6.6	55.9	31.9	2.2
Milk, Standard, Bar, Nestle*	1 Bar/31g	165	9.6	531	6.3	56.9	30.9	0.8
Minis, Nestle*	1 Bar/11g	57	3.2	518	6.8	58.1	28.7	0.8
Mint, Bubbles, Aero, Nestle*	1 Bubble/3g	16	0.9	538	5.4	60.5	30.1	1.4
Mint, Nestle*	1 Bar/41g	221	12.3	538	5.1	61.5	29.9	0.9
Mint, Snack Size, Nestle*	1 Bar/21g	112	6.7	548	7.7	55.3	32.8	0.9
Mint, Standard, Aero, Nestle*	1 Bar/43g	233	13.2	542	5.2	60.5	30.8	0.9
Orange, Nestle*	6 Squares/22g	119	6.8	542	5.1	60.7	30.7	0.9
ALFALFA SPROUTS								
Raw, Average	**1 Serving/33g**	**8**	**0.3**	**24**	**3.0**	**3.0**	**0.9**	**3.0**
ALLSPICE								
Ground, Schwartz*	1 Tsp/3g	11	0.1	358	6.1	74.3	4.0	0.0
ALMONDS								
Blanched, Average	**1 Serving/100g**	**617**	**54.3**	**617**	**25.1**	**6.9**	**54.3**	**8.1**
Candied, Sugared	1 Serving/100g	458	16.3	458	8.4	69.2	16.3	2.2
Flaked, Average	**1oz/28g**	**172**	**15.2**	**613**	**24.9**	**6.5**	**54.3**	**7.6**
Flaked, Toasted, Average	**1oz/28g**	**176**	**15.8**	**629**	**24.6**	**5.8**	**56.4**	**7.5**
Ground, Average	**1 Serving/10g**	**62**	**5.6**	**625**	**24.0**	**6.6**	**55.8**	**7.4**
Marcona, Average	**1 Serving/100g**	**608**	**53.7**	**608**	**22.1**	**13.0**	**53.7**	**9.7**
Toasted, Average	**1oz/28g**	**178**	**15.8**	**634**	**25.0**	**6.6**	**56.4**	**6.6**
Wasabi, Roasted, Deluxe, Lidl*	1 Serving/25g	160	13.6	639	19.2	14.3	54.6	6.6
Whole, Average	**1 Serving/20g**	**122**	**11.0**	**612**	**23.4**	**6.9**	**54.8**	**8.4**
Yoghurt Coated, Holland & Barrett*	1 Pack/100g	536	37.0	536	10.9	45.3	37.0	2.8
ALOO								
Bombay, M&S*	½ Pack/114g	108	5.2	95	1.8	10.3	4.6	2.3
Gobi Sag, Retail	1oz/28g	27	1.9	95	2.2	7.1	6.9	1.4
Saag, Canned, Tesco*	½ Can/200g	124	3.8	62	1.8	9.3	1.9	2.0
Saag, Fresh, Sainsbury's*	1 Pack/400g	388	13.2	97	2.0	14.7	3.3	4.8
Saag, Gobi, Indian Takeaway, Sainsbury's*	1 Pack/334g	164	3.7	49	1.7	8.0	1.1	1.5
Saag, Gobi, Indian, Tesco*	1 Pack/225g	225	16.4	100	2.1	6.5	7.3	1.8
Saag, Gobi, M Kitchen, Morrisons*	1 Pack/225g	130	6.1	58	2.0	4.6	2.7	3.8
Saag, Gobi, Tesco*	1 Serving/175g	166	8.9	95	2.1	9.5	5.1	1.9
Saag, Gobi, Waitrose*	½ Pack/150g	147	7.5	98	2.1	9.0	5.0	3.9
Saag, Sainsbury's*	1 Pack/300g	441	31.8	147	2.1	10.7	10.6	3.5
Saag, Tesco*	1 Serving/200g	144	7.0	72	2.1	8.0	3.5	2.0
Tikki, Average	**1 Serving/25g**	**48**	**2.0**	**191**	**4.5**	**25.2**	**8.0**	**3.5**
ANCHOVIES								
Drained, Finest, Tesco*	1 Fillets/3g	7	0.4	220	21.3	0.8	14.6	0.5
Fillets, Flat, John West*	1 Can/50g	113	7.0	226	25.0	0.1	14.0	0.0
Fillets, in Olive Oil, Salted, Deluxe, Lidl*	1 Serving/100g	197	9.0	197	28.0	1.0	9.0	0.0
Fillets, Tesco*	1 Serving/15g	34	2.1	226	25.0	0.0	14.0	0.0
in Oil, Canned, Drained	1 Anchovy/4g	8	0.5	195	23.4	0.0	11.3	0.0
Marinated, Sainsbury's*	¼ Pot/44g	78	4.0	177	22.0	2.0	9.0	0.1

A

	Measure INFO/WEIGHT	per Measure KCAL	per Measure FAT	Nutrition Values per 100g / 100ml KCAL	PROT	CARB	FAT	FIBRE
ANCHOVIES								
Salted, Finest, Tesco*	1 Serving/10g	9	0.2	93	18.2	0.0	2.2	0.0
White, Flat, Tesco*	1 Serving/100g	130	3.2	130	22.9	1.5	3.2	0.0
ANGEL DELIGHT								
Butterscotch Flavour, No Added Sugar, Kraft*	1 Sachet/47g	226	11.3	480	4.5	61.0	24.0	0.0
Chocolate Flavour, Kraft*	1 Sachet/67g	305	12.1	455	3.7	69.5	18.0	0.4
Strawberry Flavour, Kraft*	1 Sachet/59g	286	12.4	485	2.5	71.0	21.0	0.0
ANGEL HAIR								
Pasta, Dry	1 Serving/50g	181	1.1	362	12.4	73.6	2.2	4.4
ANTIPASTO								
Coppa, from Selection Platter, TTD, Sainsbury's*	1 Serving/100g	255	17.1	255	25.2	0.1	17.1	0.0
Italian, Specially Selected, Aldi*	¼ Pack/30g	97	6.9	323	28.0	0.0	23.0	0.0
Mixed Mushroom, Sainsbury's*	¼ Jar/72g	70	6.5	97	2.7	1.4	9.0	3.7
Parma Ham, from Selection Platter, TTD, Sainsbury's*	1 Serving/100g	236	12.9	236	29.9	0.1	12.9	0.0
Parma, Salami Milano, Bresaola, Finest, Tesco*	¼ Pack/30g	104	7.9	345	26.4	0.5	26.3	0.0
Roasted Pepper, Drained, Tesco*	1 Jar/170g	128	9.4	75	0.9	5.5	5.5	4.1
Sun Dried Tomato, Sainsbury's*	¼ Jar/70g	275	25.0	393	4.5	13.4	35.7	6.2
APPLES								
Bites, Average	*1 Pack/118g*	*58*	*0.1*	*49*	*0.3*	*11.6*	*0.1*	*2.2*
Braeburn, Average	*1 Apple/123g*	*52*	*0.1*	*42*	*0.3*	*10.2*	*0.1*	*1.8*
Cape, Tesco*	1 Apple/100g	50	0.1	50	0.4	11.8	0.1	1.8
Cooking, Baked with Sugar, Flesh Only, Average	*1 Serving/140g*	*104*	*0.1*	*74*	*0.5*	*19.2*	*0.1*	*1.7*
Cooking, Raw, Peeled, Average	*1oz/28g*	*10*	*0.0*	*35*	*0.3*	*8.9*	*0.1*	*1.6*
Cooking, Slices, Frozen, Asda*	1 Serving/80g	33	0.1	41	0.3	8.9	0.1	1.6
Cooking, Stewed with Sugar, Average	*1 Serving/140g*	*104*	*0.1*	*74*	*0.3*	*19.1*	*0.1*	*1.2*
Cooking, Stewed without Sugar, Average	*1 Serving/140g*	*46*	*0.1*	*33*	*0.3*	*8.1*	*0.1*	*1.5*
Cox, English, Average	*1 Apple/108g*	*47*	*0.1*	*43*	*0.4*	*10.2*	*0.1*	*1.8*
Discovery, Average	*1 Apple/182g*	*82*	*0.9*	*45*	*0.4*	*10.6*	*0.5*	*1.0*
Dried, Average	*1 Pack/250g*	*537*	*0.7*	*215*	*0.8*	*52.8*	*0.3*	*5.9*
Empire, Average	*1 Apple/120g*	*52*	*0.1*	*44*	*0.4*	*10.7*	*0.1*	*1.8*
Fuji	1 Apple/132g	64	0.1	48	0.4	11.8	0.1	1.8
Gala, Average	*1 Apple/152g*	*66*	*0.2*	*43*	*0.3*	*10.4*	*0.1*	*1.4*
Golden Delicious, Average	*1 Med/102g*	*44*	*0.1*	*43*	*0.3*	*10.1*	*0.1*	*1.6*
Granny Smith, Average	*1 Sm/125g*	*56*	*0.1*	*45*	*0.3*	*10.7*	*0.1*	*1.8*
Green, Raw, Average	*1 Med/182g*	*86*	*0.2*	*48*	*0.4*	*11.3*	*0.1*	*1.8*
Kanzi, Tesco*	1 Apple/134g	71	0.1	53	0.4	11.8	0.1	1.8
Mackintosh, Red, Average	*1 Apple/165g*	*81*	*0.5*	*49*	*0.2*	*12.8*	*0.3*	*1.8*
Pink Lady, Average	*1 Apple/125g*	*56*	*0.1*	*45*	*0.4*	*10.6*	*0.1*	*1.9*
Red, Average	*1 Med/149g*	*71*	*0.2*	*48*	*0.3*	*11.8*	*0.1*	*2.0*
Sliced, Average	*1oz/28g*	*14*	*0.0*	*49*	*0.4*	*11.6*	*0.1*	*1.8*
APPLETISER*								
Juice Drink, Sparkling, Appletiser, Coca-Cola*	1 Glass/200ml	94	0.0	47	0.0	11.0	0.0	0.4
APRICOTS								
Canned, in Syrup, Average	*1oz/28g*	*18*	*0.0*	*63*	*0.4*	*16.1*	*0.1*	*0.9*
Dried, Average	*1 Apricot/10g*	*17*	*0.1*	*171*	*3.6*	*37.4*	*0.5*	*6.3*
Dried, Soft, Average	*1 Serving/50g*	*104*	*0.2*	*208*	*2.4*	*48.5*	*0.4*	*5.2*
Halves, in Fruit Juice, Average	*1 Can/221g*	*87*	*0.1*	*40*	*0.5*	*9.2*	*0.1*	*1.0*
Milk Chocolate Coated, Graze*	1 Pack/35g	158	8.6	450	6.1	55.9	24.7	5.0
Raw, Flesh Only, Average	*1 Apricot/37g*	*19*	*0.2*	*52*	*1.5*	*12.0*	*0.4*	*2.2*
Raw, Weighed with Stone, Average	*1 Apricot/40g*	*19*	*0.2*	*47*	*1.4*	*10.8*	*0.4*	*1.9*
ARANCINI								
Mozzarella & Pecorino, World Cafe, Waitrose*	½ Pack/75g	223	10.9	314	8.0	34.8	15.3	2.5
ARCHERS*								
& Lemonade, Premixed, Canned, Archers*	100ml	86	0.0	86	0.0	13.2	0.0	0.0

	Measure INFO/WEIGHT	per Measure		Nutrition Values per 100g / 100ml				
		KCAL	FAT	KCAL	PROT	CARB	FAT	FIBRE
ARCHERS*								
Aqua, Peach, Archers*	1 Bottle/275ml	206	0.0	75	0.3	7.7	0.0	0.0
Peach (Calculated Estimate), Archers*	1 Shot/35ml	91	0.0	260	0.0	0.0	0.0	0.0
ARTICHOKE								
Chargrilled, in Olive Oil, Cooks Ingredients, Waitrose*	1 Serving/40g	52	4.9	129	1.7	2.7	12.3	2.7
Chargrilled, Italian, Drained, Sainsbury's*	1/3 Tub/43g	40	2.7	92	3.1	2.8	6.1	6.5
Fresh, Raw, Average	*1oz/28g*	*13*	*0.0*	*47*	*3.3*	*10.5*	*0.2*	*5.4*
Hearts, Canned, Drained, Average	*½ Can/117g*	*35*	*0.1*	*30*	*1.9*	*5.4*	*0.0*	*2.2*
Hearts, Marinated & Grilled, Waitrose*	1 Serving/50g	57	5.0	114	3.0	3.0	10.0	3.0
Hearts, Sliced with Extra Virgin Olive Oil, Waitrose*	1 Serving/40g	24	1.6	59	1.3	4.4	4.0	7.0
in Oil, Grilled, Cucina, Aldi*	¼ Jar/43g	41	3.7	96	1.1	2.3	8.6	2.2
in Oil, Tesco*	1 Piece/15g	18	1.6	120	2.0	2.2	11.0	7.5
Marinated in Oil with Parsley & Garlic, Drained, M&S*	1 Serving/100g	115	11.9	115	1.5	0.5	11.9	4.7
Marinated, Roasted, M&S*	1 Pack/200g	300	26.6	150	1.9	5.0	13.3	2.3
ASPARAGUS								
Boiled, in Salted Water, Average	*5 Spears/125g*	*16*	*0.5*	*12*	*1.6*	*0.7*	*0.4*	*0.7*
Canned, Average	*1 Can/250g*	*41*	*0.4*	*16*	*2.0*	*1.8*	*0.2*	*1.4*
Trimmed, Raw, Average	*1 Serving/80g*	*20*	*0.4*	*24*	*2.9*	*1.9*	*0.6*	*1.7*
AUBERGINE								
Baby, Tesco*	1 Aubergine/50g	8	0.2	15	0.9	2.2	0.4	2.3
Baked Topped, M&S*	1 Serving/150g	165	11.6	110	2.4	7.4	7.7	0.9
Fried, Average	*1oz/28g*	*85*	*8.9*	*302*	*1.2*	*2.8*	*31.9*	*2.3*
in Hot Sauce, Yarden*	1 Serving/35g	96	9.0	273	1.5	8.8	25.8	0.0
Marinated & Grilled, Waitrose*	½ Pack/100g	106	10.0	106	1.0	3.0	10.0	2.0
Parmigiana, M&S*	1 Pack/350g	332	18.6	95	4.6	7.6	5.3	1.1
Raw, Fresh, Average	*1 Small/250g*	*36*	*1.0*	*14*	*0.9*	*2.1*	*0.4*	*1.9*
AVOCADO								
Flesh Only, Average	*1 Med/145g*	*276*	*28.3*	*190*	*1.9*	*1.9*	*19.5*	*3.4*
Weighed with Stone, Raw	*½ Avocado/101g*	*120*	*11.4*	*119*	*1.5*	*5.5*	*11.3*	*3.7*

A

INFO/WEIGHT	Measure	per Measure KCAL	per Measure FAT	Nutrition KCAL	PROT	CARB	FAT	FIBRE

BACARDI*

	Measure INFO/WEIGHT	per Measure KCAL	FAT	KCAL	PROT	CARB	FAT	FIBRE
& Diet Cola, Bacardi*	1 Bottle/275ml	85	0.0	31	0.0	1.0	0.0	0.0
*37.5% Volume, Bacardi**	*1 Pub Shot/35ml*	*72*	*0.0*	*207*	*0.0*	*0.0*	*0.0*	*0.0*
*40% Volume, Bacardi**	*1 Pub Shot/35ml*	*78*	*0.0*	*222*	*0.0*	*0.0*	*0.0*	*0.0*
Breezer, Lime, Bacardi*	1 Bottle/275ml	182	0.0	66	0.0	9.1	0.0	0.0

BACON

Back, Dry Cured, Average	*1 Rasher/31g*	*77*	*4.7*	*250*	*28.1*	*0.3*	*15.1*	*0.3*
Back, Dry Fried or Grilled, Average	*1 Rasher/25g*	*72*	*5.4*	*287*	*23.2*	*0.0*	*21.6*	*0.0*
Back, Lean, Average	*1 Rasher/33g*	*57*	*4.0*	*174*	*16.3*	*0.1*	*12.0*	*0.5*
Back, Smoked, Average	*1 Rasher/25g*	*66*	*5.0*	*265*	*20.9*	*0.0*	*19.9*	*0.0*
Back, Smoked, Lean, Average	*1 Rasher/25g*	*41*	*1.2*	*163*	*28.2*	*1.1*	*5.0*	*0.2*
Back, Smoked, Rindless, Average	*1 Rasher/25g*	*60*	*4.3*	*241*	*21.0*	*0.1*	*17.4*	*0.0*
Back, Tendersweet, Average	*1 Rasher/25g*	*63*	*3.6*	*250*	*29.8*	*0.4*	*14.4*	*0.0*
Back, Unsmoked, Average	*1 Rasher/32g*	*78*	*5.5*	*242*	*21.3*	*0.4*	*17.3*	*0.0*
Back, Unsmoked, Rindless, Average	*1 Rasher/23g*	*56*	*3.9*	*241*	*22.5*	*0.0*	*16.9*	*0.0*
Bits, Average	*1oz/28g*	*75*	*5.9*	*268*	*18.6*	*0.7*	*21.2*	*0.1*
Chops, Average	*1oz/28g*	*62*	*4.2*	*222*	*22.3*	*0.0*	*14.8*	*0.0*
Collar Joint, Lean & Fat, Boiled	*1oz/28g*	*91*	*7.6*	*325*	*20.4*	*0.0*	*27.0*	*0.0*
Collar Joint, Lean & Fat, Raw	*1oz/28g*	*81*	*7.4*	*290*	*13.3*	*0.0*	*26.3*	*0.0*
Collar Joint, Lean Only, Boiled	*1oz/28g*	*53*	*2.7*	*191*	*26.0*	*0.0*	*9.7*	*0.0*
Fat Only, Cooked, Average	*1oz/28g*	*194*	*20.4*	*692*	*9.3*	*0.0*	*72.8*	*0.0*
Fat Only, Raw, Average	*1oz/28g*	*209*	*22.7*	*747*	*4.8*	*0.0*	*80.9*	*0.0*
Gammon Rasher, Lean Only, Grilled	*1oz/28g*	*48*	*1.5*	*172*	*31.4*	*0.0*	*5.2*	*0.0*
Lardons, Smoked, Sainsbury's*	1 Serving/200g	476	30.8	238	21.4	0.1	15.4	0.1
Lean Only, Fried, Average	*1 Rasher/25g*	*83*	*5.6*	*332*	*32.8*	*0.0*	*22.3*	*0.0*
Lean Only, Grilled, Average	*1 Rasher/25g*	*73*	*4.7*	*292*	*30.5*	*0.0*	*18.9*	*0.0*
Lean, Average	*1 Rasher/33g*	*47*	*2.2*	*142*	*19.6*	*0.9*	*6.7*	*0.2*
Loin Steaks, Grilled, Average	*1 Serving/120g*	*229*	*11.6*	*191*	*25.9*	*0.0*	*9.7*	*0.0*
Medallions, Average	*1 Rasher/18g*	*27*	*0.6*	*151*	*29.4*	*0.9*	*3.3*	*0.1*
Middle, Fried	*1 Rasher/40g*	*140*	*11.4*	*350*	*23.4*	*0.0*	*28.5*	*0.0*
Middle, Grilled	*1 Rasher/40g*	*123*	*9.2*	*307*	*24.8*	*0.0*	*23.1*	*0.0*
Middle, Raw	*1 Rasher/43g*	*95*	*7.9*	*222*	*14.0*	*0.0*	*18.4*	*0.0*
Rashers, Lean Only, Trimmed, Average	*1 Rasher/20g*	*24*	*0.8*	*119*	*20.6*	*0.0*	*4.0*	*0.0*
Rindless, Average	*1 Rasher/20g*	*30*	*1.7*	*150*	*18.5*	*0.0*	*8.5*	*0.0*
Smoked, Average	*1 Rasher/28g*	*46*	*2.1*	*166*	*24.8*	*0.2*	*7.4*	*0.0*
Smoked, Crispy, Cooked, Average	*1 Rasher/10g*	*46*	*2.7*	*460*	*53.0*	*2.1*	*26.9*	*0.0*
Smoked, Rindless, Average	*1 Rasher/20g*	*21*	*0.6*	*106*	*19.8*	*0.0*	*3.0*	*0.0*
Streaky, Average	*1 Rasher/12g*	*32*	*2.5*	*266*	*19.7*	*0.0*	*20.7*	*0.0*
Streaky, Cooked, Average	*1 Rasher/20g*	*68*	*5.6*	*342*	*22.4*	*0.3*	*27.8*	*0.0*

BACON VEGETARIAN

Rashers	*1 Rasher/16g*	*33*	*1.7*	*206*	*19.5*	*8.6*	*10.4*	*2.8*
Rashers, Cheatin', The Redwood Co*	1 Rasher/16g	32	1.2	196	25.9	7.3	7.3	0.5
Rashers, Tesco*	1 Rasher/20g	41	2.2	203	22.5	3.3	11.1	3.9
Streaky Style Rashers, Tesco*	1 Rasher/8g	17	0.8	215	23.7	5.0	10.6	2.2
Strips, Morningstar Farms*	1 Strip/8g	30	2.3	375	12.5	12.5	28.1	6.2

BAGUETTE

Brie, Tomato & Rocket, Freshly Prepared, M&S*	1 Baguette/219g	570	21.7	260	10.3	33.2	9.9	1.9
Cheese & Ham, Average	*1 Baguette/203g*	*593*	*20.8*	*292*	*14.0*	*35.9*	*10.3*	*1.4*
Cheese, & Ham, Snack 'n' Go, Sainsbury's*	1 Baguette/178g	383	9.1	215	12.6	29.6	5.1	1.9
Cheese, & Tomato, Tesco*	1 Baguette/108g	243	8.3	225	9.7	29.3	7.7	1.8
Cheese, Mixed, & Spring Onion, Asda*	1 Pack/190g	629	34.8	331	9.5	32.1	18.3	1.3
Chicken, & Mayonnaise, Asda*	1 Pack/190g	407	16.5	214	9.7	30.5	8.7	1.3
Chicken, & Salad, Asda*	1 Serving/158g	326	9.5	206	9.0	29.0	6.0	2.1
Chicken, & Salad, Boots*	1 Baguette/132g	202	2.4	153	11.0	23.0	1.8	2.0

INFO/WEIGHT	Measure	per Measure		Nutrition Values per 100g / 100ml				
		KCAL	FAT	KCAL	PROT	CARB	FAT	FIBRE
BAGUETTE								
Chicken, Tikka, Asda*	1 Pack/190g	439	17.9	231	10.4	32.8	9.4	1.3
Egg Mayonnaise, & Cress, Cafe, Sainsbury's*	1 Pack/100g	480	20.4	480	13.8	60.2	20.4	0.0
Egg, & Tomato, Oldfields*	1 Pack/198g	416	15.0	210	8.7	27.0	7.6	0.0
Egg, Bacon & Tomato, Freshly Prepared, M&S*	1 Baguette/182g	455	17.3	250	12.9	28.0	9.5	1.7
Ham & Cheese, Freshly Prepared, M&S*	1 Baguette/231g	555	11.3	240	13.4	35.9	4.9	2.4
Ham &Salad with Mustard Mayonnaise, Sainsbury's*	1 Baguette/100g	412	15.9	412	17.6	49.6	15.9	0.1
Ham, & Turkey, Asda*	1 Baguette/360g	774	18.4	215	11.6	30.7	5.1	1.3
Mozzarella, Tomato, & Pesto, Darwins Deli*	1 Serving/210g	531	20.4	253	11.7	29.7	9.7	0.0
Prawn Mayonnaise, Asda*	1 Pack/190g	399	9.3	210	9.1	32.5	4.9	1.3
Smoked Salmon & Egg, Freshly Prepared	**1 Baguette/178g**	**455**	**17.3**	**255**	**13.7**	**28.4**	**9.7**	**1.6**
Steak, & Onion, Snack 'n' Go, Sainsbury's*	1 Baguette/177g	398	8.8	225	14.3	30.6	5.0	2.2
Tuna, Crunch, Shapers, Boots*	1 Pack/138g	315	4.8	228	14.0	35.0	3.5	3.1
Tuna, Melt, Sainsbury's*	1 Serving/204g	373	8.0	183	11.3	25.8	3.9	0.0
BAILEYS*								
Irish Cream, Original, Baileys*	**1 Serving/50ml**	**164**	**6.5**	**327**	**3.0**	**25.0**	**13.0**	**0.0**
BAKE								
Aubergine & Mozzarella Cheese, BGTY, Sainsbury's*	1 Pack/360g	194	7.2	54	3.0	6.0	2.0	1.3
Aubergine & Mozzarella, Finest, Tesco*	1 Pack/400g	288	13.6	72	3.6	6.7	3.4	2.6
Bolognese Pasta, Annabel Karmel*	1 Pack/200g	180	7.6	90	6.8	7.2	3.8	1.8
Broccoli & Cheese, Asda*	1 Bake/132g	269	15.4	204	5.3	19.3	11.7	2.5
Broccoli & Cheese, M&S*	1 Pack/400g	480	31.2	120	6.5	5.4	7.8	1.6
Butternut Squash & Parsnip, Tesco*	½ Pack/124g	144	7.8	116	3.3	10.5	6.3	2.1
Chicken Pasta, Chilled, Light Choices, Tesco*	1 Pack/400g	425	7.2	106	8.2	13.5	1.8	1.4
Chicken, Bacon & Potato, British Classics, Tesco*	½ Pack/375g	435	16.5	116	7.0	12.2	4.4	1.4
Cod & Prawn, 327, Oakhouse Foods Ltd*	1 Meal/340g	466	23.5	137	8.6	10.3	6.9	0.3
Cod & Prawn, COU, M&S*	1 Pack/400g	320	8.0	80	6.5	8.8	2.0	1.0
Corned Beef, 379, Wiltshire Farm Foods*	1 Bake/290g	322	11.2	111	3.8	15.2	3.9	2.1
Courgette & Butternut Squash, Meat Free, Tesco*	1 Pack/375g	367	13.7	98	2.5	12.8	3.6	1.8
Fish, Haddock, Average	**1 Serving/400g**	**312**	**9.2**	**78**	**6.4**	**8.0**	**2.3**	**0.9**
Fish, Haddock, Smoked, Light & Easy, Youngs*	1 Pack/310g	242	7.1	78	6.4	8.0	2.3	0.9
Haddock, Smoked, Luxury, Light & Easy, Youngs*	1 Pack/355g	390	17.0	110	7.5	9.2	4.8	0.6
Lentil, Spiced, Vegetarian, TTD, Sainsbury's*	1 Bake/132g	245	8.4	186	4.8	27.3	6.4	4.2
Mediterranean Vegetable Bistro, Cauldron Foods*	1 Bake/100g	190	10.0	190	4.0	21.0	10.0	3.0
Mediterranean Vegetable, CBY, Asda*	1 Bake/120g	279	13.2	232	8.4	22.8	11.0	4.2
Mushroom, Leek & Cheddar, CBY, Asda*	½ Pack/199g	181	8.8	91	3.7	8.1	4.4	1.9
Penne Bolognese, BGTY, Sainsbury's*	1 Pack/400g	492	10.8	123	7.0	17.7	2.7	1.3
Penne Bolognese, Sainsbury's*	1 Pack/397g	603	27.8	152	7.6	14.8	7.0	2.0
Potato with Cheese & Leek, Aunt Bessie's*	½ Pack/275g	300	13.8	109	3.4	12.7	5.0	2.7
Potato, Cheese, & Bacon, Homepride*	1 Serving/210g	277	26.2	132	1.6	3.2	12.5	0.0
Potato, Cheese, & Onion, Tesco*	1 Pack/400g	376	19.6	94	2.4	10.0	4.9	1.0
Potato, Leek & Gruyere, M&S*	½ Pack/200g	240	15.4	120	2.2	10.3	7.7	1.4
Potato, Mushroom & Leek, M&S*	1 Serving/225g	225	13.3	100	3.5	10.0	5.9	2.0
Roast Onion & Potato, COU, M&S*	1 Pack/450g	338	5.8	75	1.9	13.6	1.3	1.5
Roast Potato, Cheese & Onion, Asda*	½ Pack/200g	288	16.0	144	4.2	14.0	8.0	1.1
Roasted Butternut Squash & Mushroom, BFY, M&S*	1 Pack/390g	339	10.5	87	6.1	8.4	2.7	2.1
Three Fish Roast, Deluxe, Lidl*	1 Portion/300g	498	29.7	166	12.6	6.2	9.9	0.6
Vegetable, M&S*	½ Lge Pack/255g	181	6.9	71	1.9	8.9	2.7	1.6
BAKING POWDER								
Average	**1 Tsp/2g**	**3**	**0.0**	**163**	**5.2**	**37.8**	**0.0**	**0.0**
BAKLAVA								
Average	**2 Pieces/50g**	**239**	**14.2**	**478**	**8.0**	**47.4**	**28.4**	**2.8**
BALTI								
Chick Pea & Spinach, Cauldron Foods*	1 Pack/400g	356	8.0	89	2.3	15.5	2.0	1.0

B

INFO/WEIGHT	Measure	per Measure		Nutrition Values per 100g / 100ml				
		KCAL	FAT	KCAL	PROT	CARB	FAT	FIBRE
BALTI								
Chicken & Mushroom, Tesco*	1 Serving/350g	326	10.5	93	12.3	4.2	3.0	0.7
Chicken Ceylon, Finest, Tesco*	1 Pack/400g	588	38.0	147	14.4	0.9	9.5	5.0
Chicken Tikka, Finest, Tesco*	½ Pack/200g	280	17.2	140	15.8	1.1	8.6	3.2
Chicken with Pilau Rice & Naan Bread, Tesco*	1 Meal/550g	660	19.8	120	6.1	15.5	3.6	1.4
Chicken with Pilau Rice, Asda*	1 Pack/504g	625	24.7	124	5.0	15.0	4.9	1.2
Chicken with Pilau Rice, Light Choices, Tesco*	1 Pack/400g	440	5.2	110	6.3	17.4	1.3	1.8
Chicken with Pilau Rice, Weight Watchers*	1 Pack/329g	306	4.3	93	6.9	13.4	1.3	1.2
Chicken, Asda*	1 Pack/450g	324	9.9	72	8.0	5.0	2.2	0.0
Chicken, M&S*	½ Pack/175g	245	15.2	140	13.0	2.0	8.7	1.7
Chicken, Morrisons*	1 Pack/350g	441	26.6	126	12.1	2.3	7.6	1.5
Chicken, Take Away, Tesco*	½ Pack/200g	170	7.6	85	8.1	4.6	3.8	1.9
Chicken, Takeaway, Sainsbury's*	1 Pack/400g	404	18.0	101	10.4	4.8	4.5	1.4
Chicken, Tesco*	1 Pack/460g	662	25.8	144	6.1	17.4	5.6	1.6
Lamb, Bhuna, Tesco*	1 Pack/400g	360	14.8	90	9.2	4.8	3.7	1.1
Prawn, Budgens*	1 Pack/350g	374	24.8	107	5.6	5.2	7.1	1.3
Vegetable & Rice, Tesco*	1 Pack/450g	378	7.2	84	2.0	15.6	1.6	1.3
Vegetable, Asda*	½ Can/200g	206	12.0	103	2.2	10.0	6.0	2.5
Vegetable, Average	**1 Serving/200g**	**182**	**8.3**	**91**	**1.9**	**11.3**	**4.1**	**1.7**
Vegetable, GFY, Asda*	1 Pack/450g	324	4.0	72	1.9	14.0	0.9	1.5
BAMBOO SHOOTS								
Canned, Average	**1 Sm Can/120g**	**10**	**0.1**	**8**	**1.0**	**0.8**	**0.1**	**0.8**
BANANA								
Chips, Average	**1oz/28g**	**143**	**8.8**	**511**	**1.0**	**59.9**	**31.4**	**1.7**
Raw, Flesh Only, Average	**1 Med/100g**	**95**	**0.3**	**95**	**1.2**	**20.9**	**0.3**	**4.2**
Raw, Weighed with Skin, Average	**1 Med/152g**	**98**	**0.3**	**65**	**0.8**	**14.2**	**0.2**	**2.9**
Slices, Dried, LL, Waitrose*	1 Serving/25g	74	0.2	295	4.8	66.5	0.6	5.2
BARLEY								
Quick Cook, Wholefoods, Tesco*	1 Portion/83g	291	1.2	351	8.0	70.7	1.4	11.6
BARS								
All Bran, Honey & Oat, Kellogg's*	1 Bar/27g	99	2.2	366	6.0	67.0	8.0	12.0
All Fruit, Frusli, Passion Fruit, Jordans*	1 Bar/30g	92	0.2	307	1.3	74.0	0.7	5.0
All Fruit, Frusli, Strawberry, Jordans*	1 Bar/30g	94	0.1	313	2.3	81.3	0.3	5.0
Almond, Apricot, & Mango, M&S*	1 Bar/50g	205	7.4	410	9.0	60.2	14.8	5.0
Am, Breakfast Muffin, Apple & Sultana, McVitie's*	1 Bar/45g	168	7.5	373	4.4	54.9	16.7	1.6
Am, Cereal, Apricot, McVitie's*	1 Bar/30g	146	6.2	486	6.5	68.8	20.5	0.5
Am, Cereal, Raisin & Nut, McVitie's*	1 Bar/35g	148	5.8	422	6.4	62.1	16.4	2.4
Am, Granola, Almond, Raisin & Cranberry, McVitie's*	1 Bar/35g	133	4.0	380	7.1	62.9	11.4	4.0
Am, Muesli Fingers, McVitie's*	1 Bar/35g	154	6.9	440	6.0	59.8	19.6	3.1
Apple, Fruit Bake, Go Ahead, McVitie's*	1 Bar/35g	124	2.5	354	2.7	73.8	7.2	1.2
Apricot & Almond, Eat Natural*	1 Bar/50g	202	8.1	403	11.2	53.3	16.1	0.0
Apricot & Almond, Yoghurt Coated, Eat Natural*	1 Bar/35g	162	9.3	471	7.5	39.7	27.0	5.0
Apricot & Peach, Multigrain, BGTY, Sainsbury's*	1 Bar/25g	70	0.6	282	6.6	58.2	2.5	23.1
Apricot, Dried Fruit, Sunsweet*	1 Bar/33g	96	0.0	292	3.6	72.5	0.1	0.0
Berry Delight, Gluten Free, Nak'd*	1 Bar/35g	135	5.2	385	9.0	52.0	15.0	6.0
Berry, Nut Free, Get Buzzing*	1 Bar/62g	173	8.7	279	3.2	50.0	14.0	2.9
Biscuit, Choc 'n' Oat, Fox's*	1 Bar/21g	22	4.9	104	1.4	13.6	22.8	4.0
Biscuit, Chocolate, Mint, Penguin, McVitie's*	1 Bar/25g	133	6.9	531	5.4	65.0	27.7	1.5
Biscuit, Chocolate, Orange, Penguin, McVitie's*	1 Bar/25g	133	6.9	531	5.4	65.0	27.7	1.5
Biscuit, Chocolate, Original, Penguin, McVitie's*	1 Bar/20g	106	5.6	515	5.1	61.4	27.1	2.4
Biscuit, Groovy, Aldi*	1 Bar/27g	123	5.3	457	4.9	64.2	19.7	1.8
Blue Riband, Double Choc, Nestle*	1 Bar/22g	113	5.6	513	4.8	66.4	25.3	1.1
Blueberry & Yoghurt Nougat, Shapers, Boots*	1 Bar/23g	85	3.0	369	1.8	76.0	13.0	1.7
Blueberry, Fruit & Grain, Asda*	1 Bar/37g	124	2.6	335	4.1	64.0	7.0	3.9

BARS

INFO/WEIGHT	Measure per Measure		Nutrition Values per 100g / 100ml				
	KCAL	FAT	KCAL	PROT	CARB	FAT	FIBRE
Brazil, Sultanas, Almonds & Hazelnuts, Eat Natural* — 1 Bar/50g	227	11.3	454	11.2	40.0	22.6	5.0
Breakfast, Chocolate Chip, Crisp, Morning Start, Atkins* — 1 Bar/37g	137	7.0	370	31.8	22.5	18.8	15.0
Breakfast, Vitality, Fruit & Fibre, Asda* — 1 Bar/29g	113	2.9	390	6.0	69.0	10.0	4.1
Caramel Crisp Bite, Tesco* — 1 Bar/15g	72	3.5	483	4.3	64.4	23.1	1.3
Caramel Nougat, Soft, Shapers, Boots* — 1 Bar/25g	86	2.5	343	2.9	60.4	10.0	0.6
Caramel, Nut Chew, Endulge, Atkins* — 1 Bar/34g	130	2.7	382	5.0	5.9	8.0	6.0
Cashew Cookie, Raw Fruit & Nut, Gluten Free, Nak'd* — 1 Bar/35g	143	8.0	410	10.0	46.0	23.0	5.0
Cereal & Milk, Nesquik, Nestle* — 1 Bar/25g	108	3.7	433	6.2	68.5	14.9	1.0
Cereal, 3 Berries & Cherries, Dorset Cereals* — 1 Bar/35g	127	1.7	363	5.7	73.9	4.9	5.2
Cereal, 3 Fruit, Nuts & Seeds, Dorset Cereals* — 1 Bar/35g	136	3.6	389	7.4	66.6	10.3	6.2
Cereal, Apple & Blackberry with Yoghurt, Alpen* — 1 Bar/29g	117	3.1	404	5.4	71.8	10.6	5.0
Cereal, Apple & Cinnamon, Fruit 'n' Grain, Asda* — 1 Bar/37g	131	2.6	353	4.5	68.0	7.0	2.9
Cereal, Apple & Sultana, Light, Alpen* — 1 Bar/20g	63	0.7	330	4.1	59.4	3.6	21.7
Cereal, Banana, Apricot, & Milk Chocolate, Eat Natural* — 1 Bar/30g	108	2.0	362	3.7	71.8	6.7	4.0
Cereal, Banoffee, Light, Alpen, Weetabix* — 1 Bar/19g	66	1.3	346	4.7	54.0	7.0	24.0
Cereal, Banoffee, Vitality, Asda* — 1 Bar/22g	73	0.6	331	6.5	69.6	2.9	13.5
Cereal, Chewy & Crisp with Choc Chips, Tesco* — 1 Bar/27g	125	6.3	463	9.2	54.0	23.4	3.8
Cereal, Chewy, BGTY, Sainsbury's* — 1 Bar/25g	85	0.5	342	4.9	75.8	2.1	1.9
Cereal, Choc Chip, Brunch, Cadbury* — 1 Bar/35g	156	6.2	445	6.0	64.0	17.6	4.1
Cereal, Chocolate & Banana, Lidl* — 1 Bar/25g	110	4.0	440	6.4	67.2	16.0	0.0
Cereal, Chocolate & Fudge, Light, Alpen* — 1 Bar/18g	62	1.2	344	4.9	55.4	6.5	22.0
Cereal, Chocolate & Orange, Light, Alpen* — 1 Bar/21g	71	1.2	339	4.8	56.0	5.5	23.1
Cereal, Chocolate Chip, Special K, Kellogg's* — 1 Bar/21g	84	1.5	401	9.0	76.0	7.0	1.5
Cereal, Chocolate, Geobar, Traidcraft* — 1 Bar/32g	130	2.7	407	4.3	78.5	8.4	0.0
Cereal, Chocolate, Milk, Double, Special K, Kellogg's* — 1 Bar/20g	79	1.8	396	9.0	66.0	9.0	10.0
Cereal, Chocolate, Milk, Double, Special K, Kellogg's* — 1 Bar/20g	80	2.0	400	10.0	65.0	10.0	10.0
Cereal, Chocolate, Milk, Oaty, Weetabix* — 1 Bar/23g	80	1.5	342	6.9	51.7	6.5	24.3
Cereal, Chocolate, Mint, Kellogg's* — 1 Bar/22g	88	2.2	401	4.5	74.0	10.0	3.5
Cereal, Citrus Fruits, Light, Alpen* — 1 Bar/21g	59	0.9	283	5.6	55.9	4.1	22.4
Cereal, Cranberry & Yoghurt, Harvest Morn, Aldi* — 1 Bar/29g	117	2.6	403	6.5	71.9	9.0	4.1
Cereal, Crunchy Granola, Apple Crunch, Nature Valley* — 1 Bar/21g	92	3.2	440	7.3	69.0	15.0	5.7
Cereal, Crunchy Granola, Ginger Nut, Nature Valley* — 1 Bar/42g	189	7.1	451	7.9	64.2	16.9	2.3
Cereal, Double Chocolate, Light, Alpen, Weetabix* — 1 Bar/19g	65	1.2	344	5.0	56.0	6.2	22.0
Cereal, Fruit & Fibre, Asda* — 1 Bar/29g	111	2.8	390	6.0	69.0	10.0	4.1
Cereal, Fruit & Nut Break, Jordans* — 1 Bar/37g	138	3.8	374	7.0	63.2	10.4	8.1
Cereal, Fruit & Nut, Alpen* — 1 Bar/28g	109	2.3	390	5.8	73.0	8.3	2.9
Cereal, Fruit & Nut, Chewy Trail Mix, Nature Valley* — 1 Bar/30g	114	3.2	379	7.7	63.2	10.6	7.3
Cereal, Fruit & Nut, with Milk Chocolate, Alpen* — 1 Bar/29g	123	3.8	425	6.4	70.5	13.0	2.2
Cereal, Fruit, Average — ***1 Bar/34g***	***130***	***3.9***	***382***	***5.9***	***64.7***	***11.5***	***6.5***
Cereal, Fruity Granola, EAT* — 1 Bar/67g	282	14.7	421	5.5	51.7	22.0	4.8
Cereal, Frusli, Blueberry, Jordans* — 1 Bar/30g	113	2.1	375	5.2	70.2	7.1	4.9
Cereal, Frusli, Cranberry & Apple, Jordans* — 1 Bar/30g	113	2.1	376	5.1	75.6	7.1	5.0
Cereal, Frusli, Raisin & Hazelnut, Jordans* — 1 Bar/30g	117	3.7	390	5.8	64.3	12.2	4.5
Cereal, Frusli, Red Berries, Jordans* — 1 Bar/30g	112	2.2	374	4.8	75.1	7.2	5.4
Cereal, Granola, Alpen* — 1 Bar/29g	119	3.1	410	5.9	72.4	10.7	0.0
Cereal, Hazelnut, Brunch, Cadbury* — 1 Bar/35g	160	7.4	460	7.0	60.5	21.4	2.2
Cereal, Muesli Break, Breakfast in a Bar, Jordans* — 1 Bar/46g	178	5.0	387	5.9	66.6	10.8	4.3
Cereal, Muesli, Apple, No Added Sugar, Crownfield, Lidl* — 1 Bar/25g	96	2.8	386	6.3	67.9	11.2	6.7
Cereal, Multigrain, Peach & Apricot, BGTY, Sainsbury's* — 1 Bar/28g	77	0.6	274	6.4	57.0	2.3	24.2
Cereal, Nut & Seed, Organic, Green & Black's* — 1 Bar/50g	258	16.3	516	8.4	47.2	32.6	10.0
Cereal, Oat & Raisin, Basics, Sainsbury's* — 1 Bar/25g	98	2.2	391	5.1	72.8	8.8	3.8
Cereal, Oaty, Toffee Dazzler, Weetabix* — 1 Bar/23g	80	1.5	348	6.2	54.9	6.7	21.5
Cereal, Peanut Butter & Oat, Organic, Meridian Foods* — 1 Bar/50g	204	9.2	407	12.6	50.9	18.4	5.0

BARS

INFO/WEIGHT	Measure	per Measure KCAL	FAT	Nutrition Values per 100g / 100ml KCAL	PROT	CARB	FAT	FIBRE
Cereal, Raisin & Coconut, Value, Tesco*	1 Bar/21g	84	2.4	400	5.5	67.2	11.6	5.0
Cereal, Raisin, Raisin, Cadbury*	1 Bar/35g	150	5.4	430	5.6	66.4	15.5	1.8
Cereal, Strawberry with Yoghurt, Alpen*	1 Bar/29g	119	3.1	409	5.7	72.6	10.6	0.0
Cereal, Strawberry, Fruit 'n' Grain, Asda*	1 Bar/37g	126	2.6	340	4.2	65.0	7.0	4.5
Cereal, Summer Fruits, Light, Alpen*	1 Bar/21g	70	0.9	334	4.4	58.7	4.1	22.4
Cereal, White Chocolate & Strawberry, Value, Tesco*	1 Bar/21g	85	1.7	405	6.2	76.2	8.1	2.4
Cereal, White Chocolate Chip, Chewy, Harvest Morn, Aldi*	1 Bar/22g	88	2.0	400	5.9	71.8	9.1	2.7
Cereal, White Chocolate, Oaty, Weetabix*	1 Bar/23g	78	1.4	341	6.4	52.4	6.3	24.3
Choco & Biscuit, Orange, Choceur, Aldi*	1 Bar/33g	176	9.9	533	7.6	59.0	30.0	1.1
Chocolate & Caramel, Rice Krispies Squares, Kellogg's*	1 Bar/36g	155	5.0	430	4.5	71.0	14.0	2.0
Chocolate Brownie, Average	***1 Bar/68g***	***240***	***4.0***	***353***	***14.7***	***60.3***	***5.9***	***8.8***
Chocolate Caramel, Weight Watchers*	1 Bar/20g	80	2.5	400	5.0	70.0	12.5	0.0
Chocolate Chip Granola, Advantage, Atkins*	1 Bar/48g	200	8.0	417	35.4	37.5	16.7	12.5
Chocolate Crisp, Weight Watchers*	1 Bar/25g	94	2.6	378	4.8	66.8	10.2	1.6
Chocolate Flavour, Protein, Diet Chef Ltd*	1 Bar/60g	225	7.1	375	29.3	37.5	11.9	4.2
Chocolate Orange, Montana*	1 Bar/25g	131	6.8	523	7.0	62.2	27.4	0.0
Chocolate Twist Shortcake, Breakaway, Nestle*	1 Bar/19g	97	4.6	510	5.6	66.7	24.2	1.5
Chocolate, Caramel, & Biscuit, Asda*	1 Bar/30g	150	8.3	508	8.0	56.0	28.0	2.5
Chocolate, Caramel, Wacko, Belmont, Aldi*	1 Bar/21g	102	4.6	485	5.3	65.0	22.0	1.7
Chocolate, Dark, Chewy Delight, Special K, Kellogg's*	1 Bar/24g	97	3.4	404	4.5	57.0	14.0	17.0
Chocolate, Decadence, Atkins*	1 Bar/60g	233	12.0	388	30.0	27.3	20.0	9.8
Chocolate, Fruit & Nut, M&S*	1 Bar/50g	235	12.0	470	6.5	57.1	24.1	2.5
Chocolate, Milk, Chewy Delight, Special K, Kellogg's*	1 Bar/24g	95	3.1	397	5.0	57.0	13.0	17.0
Chocolate, Milk, Crispy, Endulge, Atkins*	1 Bar/30g	141	9.6	469	13.0	48.0	32.0	2.0
Chocolate, Polar, Sainsbury's*	1 Bar/25g	133	7.2	533	5.5	63.0	28.6	1.2
Chocolate, Racer, Dairyfine, Aldi*	1 Bar/38g	185	9.5	486	8.6	54.0	25.0	4.2
Chocolate, Soya, Dairy Free, Free From, Sainsbury's*	1 Bar/50g	274	17.5	548	10.8	47.5	35.0	4.3
Chocolate, Wafer, Blue Riband, 99 Calories, Nestle*	1 Bar/19g	99	4.7	514	5.5	66.5	24.6	2.0
Chocolate, Wafer, Caramel, Penguin, McVitie's*	1 Bar/21g	106	5.4	492	5.1	60.7	25.2	1.4
Chocolate, Wild & Whippy, Tesco*	1 Bar/18g	78	2.8	447	3.7	72.0	16.0	0.8
Club, Fruit, Jacob's*	1 Biscuit/25g	124	6.2	496	5.6	62.2	25.0	2.3
Club, Milk Chocolate, Jacob's*	1 Biscuit/24g	123	6.3	511	5.8	62.6	26.4	2.0
Club, Mint, Jacob's*	1 Biscuit/24g	124	6.5	517	5.6	62.5	27.2	1.7
Club, Orange, Jacob's*	1 Biscuit/23g	117	6.1	509	5.7	61.8	26.5	2.3
Coco Pops, & Milk, Kellogg's*	1 Bar/20g	85	2.6	423	7.0	70.0	13.0	1.0
Cocoa Brownie, Trek, The Natural Health Company*	1 Bar/68g	223	4.1	328	17.0	53.0	6.0	8.0
Cocoa Crunch, Nak'd*	1 Bar/30g	105	2.6	351	18.4	47.2	8.8	6.3
Cocoa Delight, Wholefood, Gluten Free, Nak'd*	1 Bar/35g	135	5.3	386	9.4	49.4	15.1	6.8
Cocoa Loco, Wildly Different, Nak'd*	1 Bar/30g	106	2.9	354	7.9	55.4	9.8	7.5
Cocoa Mint, Gluten Free, Raw, Wholefood, Nak'd*	1 Bar/35g	135	5.3	386	9.4	49.4	15.1	6.8
Cocoa Orange, Gluten Free, Nak'd*	1 Bar/35g	145	7.0	415	11.0	45.1	20.0	6.4
Coconut Chocolate Crisp, Weight Watchers*	1 Bar/25g	89	2.6	356	3.6	71.2	10.4	3.2
Cookie, Apple Crumble, COU, M&S*	1 Bar/27g	90	0.7	335	5.8	72.6	2.6	2.3
Corn Flakes, & Chocolate Milk, Kellogg's*	1 Bar/40g	176	6.4	440	9.0	66.0	16.0	2.0
Cranberry & Macadamia Porridge Oat, Stoats*	1 Bar/85g	385	22.9	453	6.9	71.8	26.9	5.9
Crazy Caramel, Tesco*	1 Bar/40g	192	9.2	480	3.9	64.0	23.0	1.0
Crunchy Nut, Chocolate Peanut Crisp, Kellogg's*	1 Bar/35g	169	8.8	483	12.0	53.0	25.0	3.5
Dark Chocolate & Mint Crunch, Weight Watchers*	1 Bar/23g	85	3.0	371	2.7	48.7	13.1	23.7
Dark Chocolate, Cranberries, & Macadamias, Eat Natural*	1 Bar/45g	215	11.1	478	4.7	41.0	24.6	5.9
Dark Chocolate, Cranberry, Organic, Biona*	1 Bar/40g	162	5.9	405	6.2	53.5	14.7	0.0
Date & Walnut, with Pumpkin Seeds, Eat Natural*	1 Bar/50g	206	7.8	411	7.5	48.8	15.5	4.2
Digestive, Milk Chocolate, McVitie's*	1 Bar/23g	118	5.8	511	6.6	64.6	25.1	1.9
Digestive, Milk Chocolate, Tesco*	1 Bar/19g	96	4.9	506	6.8	61.6	25.8	2.4

BARS

	Measure INFO/WEIGHT	per Measure KCAL	FAT	Nutrition Values per 100g / 100ml KCAL	PROT	CARB	FAT	FIBRE
Digestive, Milk Chocolate, Value, Tesco*	1 Bar/19g	96	4.9	505	6.6	61.8	25.8	3.0
Energy, Cool Mint, Chocolate, Clif*	1 Bar/68g	256	5.0	377	14.7	63.2	7.3	7.4
Energy, Ride, Power Bar*	1 Bar/55g	213	9.1	387	18.6	40.9	16.6	7.4
Flapjack, Apple & Sultana, Organic, Dove's Farm*	1 Bar/40g	178	7.8	446	4.7	61.1	19.6	3.5
Food Bar, Apple & Walnut, The Food Doctor*	1 Bar/35g	117	4.0	333	10.8	46.8	11.4	15.3
Forest Fruit, Yoghurt, Breaks, Go Ahead, McVitie's*	1 Pack/36g	144	3.6	402	5.4	72.6	10.0	2.2
Frosties, & Milk, Kellogg's*	1 Bar/25g	102	2.8	408	7.0	71.0	11.0	1.0
Frosties, Snack Bar, Kellogg's*	1 Bar/25g	104	2.8	414	7.0	72.0	11.0	1.0
Fruit & Fibre, Coconut, Apricots, Oats & Spelt, Eat Natural*	1 Bar/40g	165	7.0	413	6.4	51.6	17.5	6.1
Fruit & Fibre, Plums, Peanuts, Oats & Spelt, Eat Natural*	1 Bar/40g	176	7.8	441	9.4	53.3	19.6	6.8
Fruit & Grain, Apple, Harvest Morn, Aldi*	1 Bar/37g	129	3.0	349	4.2	65.0	8.0	4.5
Fruit & Grain, Strawberry, Harvest Morn, Aldi*	1 Bar/37g	130	2.6	349	4.2	65.0	7.0	4.5
Fruit & Nut, Eat Natural*	1 Bar/50g	223	11.2	446	11.6	49.8	22.3	5.3
Fruit & Nut, Organic, Eat Natural*	1 Bar/50g	244	15.3	488	10.2	42.9	30.6	0.0
Fruit Muesli, Morning, Oat So Simple, Quaker Oats*	1 Bar/35g	139	3.2	398	7.7	68.1	9.1	6.6
Fruit 'n' Fibre, Kellogg's*	1 Bar/25g	95	2.2	380	5.0	71.0	9.0	5.0
Fruit, Apple, Trimlyne*	1 Bar/27g	92	0.7	342	4.5	69.6	2.7	3.8
Fruit, Nut & Seeds Cereal, Eat Well, M&S*	1 Bar/24g	88	2.6	365	6.1	60.8	10.9	6.9
Ginger Bread, Nak'd*	1 Bar/35g	157	10.7	450	10.0	35.4	30.8	9.4
Golden Syrup, Morning, Oat So Simple, Quaker Oats*	1 Bar/35g	142	3.5	407	8.2	67.6	10.0	6.8
Goodies, Cereal & Fruit, Apricot, Organic, Organix*	1 Bar/30g	122	6.1	408	7.2	55.3	20.4	6.2
Granola, Crunchy, Oats & Chocolate, Nature Valley*	2 Bars/42g	195	8.3	464	8.3	59.8	19.8	7.1
Granola, Crunchy, Roasted Almond, Nature Valley*	1 Bar/42g	193	7.6	459	8.1	65.6	18.2	3.7
Granola, Maple Syrup, Twin Pack, Tesco*	2 Bars/42g	204	9.4	485	6.0	64.7	22.3	4.1
Granola, Oats & Hazelnuts, Nature Valley*	2 Bars/42g	195	8.4	465	8.4	58.9	20.1	7.5
Granola, Peanut Butter, Quaker Oats*	1 Bar/28g	110	3.5	393	7.1	64.3	12.5	3.6
Harvest Cheweee, Choc Chip, Quaker Oats*	1 Bar/22g	95	3.5	430	5.5	68.0	16.0	3.5
Harvest Cheweee, Toffee, Quaker Oats*	1 Bar/22g	94	3.3	427	5.0	68.0	15.0	3.0
Harvest Cheweee, White Chocolate Chip, Quaker Oats*	1 Bar/22g	94	3.4	425	6.0	67.0	15.5	3.5
Hobnobs, Raisin & Chocolate, Medley, McVitie's*	1 Bar/31g	131	4.1	422	5.5	69.4	13.3	3.6
Honeycomb, Club, Jacob's*	1 Bar/23g	116	6.0	512	5.7	61.9	26.3	2.3
Luxury, Absolute Nut, Jordans*	1 Bar/45g	251	18.6	557	12.7	33.3	41.4	7.0
Marshmallow, Chewy, Rice Krispies Squares, Kellogg's*	1 Bar/28g	119	3.4	424	3.0	76.0	12.0	0.9
Muesli, Peanut, No Added Sugar, Crownfield, Lidl*	1 Bar/25g	98	3.3	391	7.9	65.7	13.2	4.7
Nine Bar, Mixed Seed with Hemp, Original, Wholebake*	1 Bar/40g	222	16.2	555	18.3	29.2	40.5	5.2
Nine Bar, Nutty, Wholebake*	1 Bar/50g	279	20.4	558	15.3	32.3	40.8	4.9
Noisettes & Amandes, Special K, Kellogg's*	1 Bar/21g	83	2.1	397	8.0	66.0	10.0	7.0
Nougat, Cool Mint, & Dark Chocolate, Shapers, Boots*	1 Bar/23g	83	3.2	362	2.6	70.0	14.0	1.1
Nougat, Summer Strawberry, Shapers, Boots*	1 Bar/23g	83	3.0	361	2.7	73.0	13.0	0.6
Nut, Dark Chocolate & Apricot, Natural, Nice & Natural*	1 Bar/35g	163	10.2	465	15.2	35.2	29.1	5.4
Nutri-Grain, Apple, Kellogg's*	1 Bar/37g	131	3.3	355	4.0	67.0	9.0	4.0
Nutri-Grain, Apple, Soft & Fruity, Kellogg's*	1 Bar/37g	133	3.0	359	4.0	70.3	8.1	4.0
Nutri-Grain, Blackberry & Apple, Soft & Fruity, Kellogg's*	1 Bar/37g	133	3.0	359	4.0	70.3	8.1	4.0
Nutri-Grain, Blueberry, Kellogg's*	1 Bar/37g	133	3.0	359	3.5	69.0	8.0	3.5
Nutri-Grain, Blueberry, Soft & Fruity, Kellogg's*	1 Bar/37g	133	3.0	359	4.0	70.3	8.1	4.0
Nutri-Grain, Elevenses, Choc Chip Bakes, Kellogg's*	1 Bar/45g	179	5.8	397	4.0	66.0	13.0	2.0
Nutri-Grain, Elevenses, Ginger Bakes, Kellogg's*	1 Bar/45g	168	4.0	373	5.0	68.0	9.0	3.0
Nutri-Grain, Elevenses, Raisin Bakes, Kellogg's*	1 Bar/45g	168	4.0	374	4.5	68.0	9.0	2.5
Nutri-Grain, Oat Bakes, Totally Oaty, Kellogg's*	1 Bar/50g	206	7.5	411	5.0	64.0	15.0	3.0
Nutri-Grain, Strawberry, Kellogg's*	1 Bar/37g	133	3.0	359	3.5	69.0	8.0	3.5
Nutri-Grain, Strawberry, Soft & Fruity, Kellogg's*	1 Bar/37g	133	3.0	359	4.0	70.3	8.1	4.0
Nutty Nougat Caramel, Tesco*	1 Bar/40g	200	11.1	490	8.7	52.7	27.2	3.8
Oaty, Strawberry Crusher, Weetabix*	1 Bar/23g	79	1.4	345	6.1	55.2	6.1	22.2

	Measure INFO/WEIGHT	per Measure KCAL	FAT	Nutrition Values per 100g / 100ml KCAL	PROT	CARB	FAT	FIBRE

BARS

	Measure INFO/WEIGHT	KCAL	FAT	KCAL	PROT	CARB	FAT	FIBRE
Original Muesli, Diet Chef Ltd*	1 Bar/50g	199	6.9	398	6.1	59.0	13.8	6.4
Original, Crunchy, Honey & Almond, Jordans*	1 Bar/30g	139	6.8	463	8.3	56.7	22.7	6.7
Original, Nut Free, Get Buzzing*	1 Bar/62g	248	12.0	400	6.8	51.6	19.4	3.7
Peach & Apricot, Special K, Kellogg's*	1 Bar/21g	80	1.3	383	8.0	75.0	6.0	2.5
Peanut & Caramel Whip, Weight Watchers*	1 Bar/20g	76	2.7	381	4.4	73.7	13.7	1.2
Peanut & Popcorn, Dark Chocolate Chunks, Eat Natural*	1 Bar/45g	204	9.9	453	10.7	50.6	21.9	5.2
Peanut, Mr Toms*	1 Bar/40g	210	13.0	525	20.0	42.5	32.5	2.5
Pecan Pie, Gluten Free, Nak'd*	1 Bar/35g	156	10.3	477	7.6	36.4	31.4	8.9
Protein, Chocolate Peanut, Musclefood*	1 Bar/42g	173	4.0	411	35.7	33.0	9.5	0.0
Protein, Flapjack, Oat Crunch, Natural Balance Foods*	1 Bar/56g	249	12.9	444	18.0	43.0	23.0	3.0
Protein, Peanut Blast, Natural Energy, Ball, Bounce*	1 Ball/49g	210	8.0	429	28.6	38.8	16.3	4.1
Protein, Premium, Ball, Bounce*	1 Ball/49g	209	9.0	426	30.6	40.8	18.4	2.0
Protein, Whey, Sculptress, Maxitone*	1 Bar/60g	203	5.6	339	33.9	30.6	9.3	8.5
Raisin & Oatmeal, Breakfast Snack, Tesco*	1 Bar/38g	133	4.4	355	5.6	56.8	11.7	2.8
Raisin, Munch, Tesco*	1 Bar/30g	126	4.4	420	5.4	66.3	14.8	3.8
Raspberry, Yoghurt Breaks, Go Ahead, McVitie's*	1 Pack/35g	143	3.6	408	5.4	73.6	10.2	2.3
Rice Krispies & Milk, Kellogg's*	1 Bar/20g	83	2.4	416	7.0	71.0	12.0	0.3
Rice Krispies, Snack, Kellogg's*	1 Bar/20g	83	2.0	415	7.0	70.0	10.0	0.5
Rich Toffee, Weight Watchers*	1 Bar/26g	83	2.8	319	3.6	52.3	10.6	0.8
Rocky Road, Rice Krispies Squares, Kellogg's*	1 Square/34g	143	3.7	420	4.0	76.0	11.0	1.5
Sandwich, Chocolate Viennese, Fox's*	1 Biscuit/14g	76	4.4	542	6.9	57.4	31.6	1.6
Sandwich, Milk Chocolate Orange, Tesco*	1 Biscuit/25g	136	7.4	536	6.2	62.2	29.1	1.8
Sesame Snaps in Chocolate, Anglo-Dal*	1 Pack/40g	211	11.9	527	9.3	55.6	29.7	0.0
Sesame Snaps with Coconut, Anglo-Dal*	1 Pack/30g	155	8.8	517	9.7	52.9	29.5	0.0
Sesame Snaps, Anglo-Dal*	1 Pack/30g	157	8.8	522	12.2	49.4	29.4	0.0
Special K, Chocolate Chip, Kellogg's*	1 Bar/22g	90	1.6	401	9.0	76.0	7.0	1.5
Special K, Mint Chocolate, Bliss, Special K, Kellogg's*	1 Bar/22g	88	2.2	401	4.5	74.0	10.0	3.5
Special K, Raspberry & Chocolate, Bliss, Kellogg's*	1 Bar/22g	89	2.2	403	4.0	75.0	10.0	4.0
Special K, Red Berry, Kellogg's*	1 Bar/23g	90	1.2	383	8.0	77.0	5.0	2.0
Strawberry, Fruit Bakes, Go Ahead, McVitie's*	1 Bar/35g	131	3.0	375	3.5	72.0	8.5	4.0
Strawberry, Fruit, Sweet Vine, Aldi*	1 Bar/20g	67	0.8	334	1.2	73.0	3.9	1.7
Strawberry, Shapers, Boots*	1 Bar/22g	75	2.4	343	2.5	77.0	11.0	0.9
Totally Chocolatey, Rice Krispies Squares, Kellogg's*	1 Bar/36g	156	5.3	439	4.5	72.0	15.0	1.5
Tracker, Chocolate Chip, Mars*	1 Bar/37g	178	8.7	480	6.8	58.0	23.6	3.8
Tracker, Roasted Nut, Mars*	1 Bar/26g	127	6.6	489	8.1	55.0	25.3	4.9
Trail, Big Berries, Alpen*	1 Bar/48g	180	2.7	376	6.0	73.0	5.7	4.3
Wafer Biscuit, Milk Chocolate Coated, Value, Tesco*	1 Bar/24g	126	6.7	526	6.9	61.4	28.1	1.7
Wafer, Chocolate Flavour Crisp, Carbolite*	1 Bar/25g	120	8.7	482	8.5	52.3	34.8	2.0
White Chocolate & Hazelnuts, Porridge Oat, Stoats*	1 Bar/85g	398	26.8	468	10.1	64.8	31.5	8.0

BASA

	Measure INFO/WEIGHT	KCAL	FAT	KCAL	PROT	CARB	FAT	FIBRE
Fillets, Lemon & Herb Tempura Battered, Gastro, Youngs*	1 Fillet/151g	279	14.0	185	14.2	10.6	9.3	1.1
Fillets, Lime, Chilli & Coriander, Dusted, Gastro, Youngs*	1 Fillet/152g	288	13.9	189	15.6	11.0	9.1	0.4
Fillets, Sea Salt & Cracked Black Pepper, Gastro, Youngs*	1 Fillet/148g	276	12.2	187	15.8	12.1	8.3	0.6

BASIL

	Measure INFO/WEIGHT	KCAL	FAT	KCAL	PROT	CARB	FAT	FIBRE
Dried, Ground	1 Tsp/1g	4	0.1	251	14.4	43.2	4.0	0.0
Fresh, Average	1 Tbsp/5g	2	0.0	40	3.1	5.1	0.8	0.0

BATTER MIX

	Measure INFO/WEIGHT	KCAL	FAT	KCAL	PROT	CARB	FAT	FIBRE
for Yorkshire Puddings & Pancakes, Morrisons*	1 Pudding/30g	43	0.8	143	6.4	23.1	2.8	4.1
for Yorkshire Puddings & Pancakes, Tesco*	1 Serving/17g	34	0.3	200	2.3	43.3	1.5	2.5
for Yorkshire Puddings, Baked, Aunt Bessie's*	1 Pudding/13g	48	1.1	356	9.8	34.0	8.1	2.3
Green's*	1 Bag/125g	296	9.0	237	8.7	34.3	7.2	0.0
Pancake, Sainsbury's*	1 Pancake/63g	96	1.1	152	6.5	27.4	1.8	3.1
Tesco*	1 Pack/130g	467	1.8	359	12.3	74.4	1.4	7.7

	Measure INFO/WEIGHT	per Measure		Nutrition Values per 100g / 100ml				
		KCAL	FAT	KCAL	PROT	CARB	FAT	FIBRE
BAY LEAVES								
Dried, Average	*1 Tsp/0.6g*	*2*	*0.1*	*313*	*7.6*	*48.6*	*8.4*	*0.0*
BEAN SPROUTS								
Mung, Raw, Average	*1oz/28g*	*9*	*0.1*	*31*	*2.9*	*4.0*	*0.5*	*1.5*
Mung, Stir-Fried in Blended Oil, Average	*1 Serving/90g*	*65*	*5.5*	*72*	*1.9*	*2.5*	*6.1*	*0.9*
Raw, Average	*1 Serving/150g*	*55*	*2.6*	*37*	*2.2*	*3.2*	*1.8*	*1.2*
BEANS								
Aduki, Cooked in Unsalted Water, Average	*1 Tbsp/30g*	*37*	*0.1*	*123*	*9.3*	*22.5*	*0.2*	*5.5*
Aduki, Dried, Raw	*1 Tbsp/30g*	*82*	*0.2*	*272*	*19.9*	*50.1*	*0.5*	*11.1*
Baked in Barbeque Sauce, Tesco*	1 Can/220g	198	1.3	90	5.0	13.6	0.6	5.2
Baked, & Pork Sausages, Tesco*	½ Can/210g	231	5.7	110	5.5	15.6	2.7	3.0
Baked, & Sausages in Tomato Sauce, Smart Price, Asda*	½ Can/203g	256	12.2	126	5.0	13.0	6.0	0.0
Baked, & Sausages, Asda*	½ Can/203g	211	4.0	104	6.7	13.0	2.0	3.5
Baked, & Sausages, Basics, Sainsbury's*	1 Serving/175g	149	2.6	85	4.8	13.1	1.5	2.6
Baked, & Sausages, Value, Tesco*	½ Can/202g	232	7.1	115	5.6	15.0	3.5	2.8
Baked, & Veggie Sausages, in Tomato Sauce, Asda*	½ Can/210g	204	4.0	97	7.4	12.5	1.9	8.4
Baked, Barbecue, Beanz, Heinz*	1 Can/390g	343	0.8	88	4.9	14.6	0.2	3.8
Baked, Curried, Average	**½ Can/210g**	**203**	**1.9**	**96**	**4.8**	**17.2**	**0.9**	**3.6**
Baked, Curry, Beanz, Heinz*	1 Can/200g	218	3.2	109	4.8	17.0	1.6	4.0
Baked, Fiery Chilli, in Tomato & Chilli Sauce, Heinz*	1 Serving/100g	91	0.3	91	4.9	15.1	0.3	3.8
Baked, Five, in Tomato Sauce, Heinz*	1 Can/415g	361	0.8	87	5.4	13.6	0.2	4.3
Baked, in Tomato Sauce, Average	**1 Can/400g**	**318**	**1.6**	**80**	**4.6**	**13.9**	**0.4**	**3.7**
Baked, in Tomato Sauce, Reduced Sugar & Salt	**½ Can/210g**	**159**	**0.7**	**76**	**4.6**	**13.6**	**0.3**	**3.8**
Baked, Sweet Chilli, Mean, Beanz, Heinz*	½ Can/195g	142	0.6	73	4.5	13.0	0.3	3.6
Baked, with HP Sauce, Beanz, Heinz*	½ Can/208g	158	0.6	76	4.8	13.7	0.3	3.9
Baked, with Sausages, Branston, Crosse & Blackwell*	½ Can/202g	233	6.5	115	6.9	12.2	3.2	5.0
Baked, with Veggie Sausages in Tomato Sauce, Tesco*	1 Can/395g	375	8.7	95	7.4	8.7	2.2	3.5
Black, Cooked, Average	**1 Cup/172g**	**227**	**0.9**	**132**	**8.8**	**23.7**	**0.5**	**8.7**
Blackeye, Canned, Average	**1 Can/172g**	**206**	**1.3**	**120**	**8.4**	**19.8**	**0.8**	**3.3**
Blackeye, Dried, Raw	**1oz/28g**	**87**	**0.4**	**311**	**23.5**	**54.1**	**1.6**	**8.2**
Borlotti, Canned, Average	**1oz/28g**	**29**	**0.1**	**103**	**7.6**	**16.9**	**0.5**	**4.7**
Borlotti, Dried, Raw, Average	**1 Serving/100g**	**335**	**1.2**	**335**	**23.0**	**60.0**	**1.2**	**24.7**
Broad, Canned, Drained, Average	**1 Can/195g**	**136**	**1.1**	**70**	**6.9**	**9.2**	**0.6**	**6.8**
Broad, Crispy, Wasabi Flavoured, Khao Shong*	1 Serving/30g	116	3.0	386	17.0	57.0	10.0	7.0
Broad, Dried, Raw, Average	**1oz/28g**	**69**	**0.6**	**245**	**26.1**	**32.5**	**2.1**	**27.6**
Broad, Frozen, Average	**1 Serving/80g**	**63**	**0.6**	**79**	**7.6**	**10.8**	**0.7**	**5.3**
Broad, Weighed with Pod, Raw, Average	**1oz/28g**	**4**	**0.1**	**14**	**1.3**	**1.7**	**0.2**	**1.4**
Butter, Canned, Drained, Average	**1oz/28g**	**23**	**0.1**	**81**	**6.0**	**12.8**	**0.5**	**4.3**
Butter, Dried, Boiled, Average	**1oz/28g**	**30**	**0.2**	**106**	**7.2**	**18.6**	**0.6**	**5.2**
Butter, Dried, Raw, Average	**1oz/28g**	**81**	**0.5**	**290**	**19.1**	**52.9**	**1.7**	**16.0**
Cannellini, Canned, Drained, Average	**1 Portion/80g**	**75**	**0.4**	**94**	**8.7**	**15.0**	**0.5**	**5.7**
Chilli, Canned, Average	**1 Can/420g**	**381**	**3.1**	**91**	**5.2**	**15.8**	**0.7**	**4.4**
Edamame, Sainsbury's*	1 Serving/150g	212	9.6	141	12.3	6.8	6.4	4.2
Fajita Beanz, Heinz*	½ Can/196g	155	1.6	79	4.0	11.7	0.8	4.5
Flageolet, Canned, Average	**1 Can/265g**	**235**	**1.6**	**89**	**6.8**	**14.0**	**0.6**	**3.5**
Flageolet, Dried, LL, Waitrose*	1 Serving/50g	125	3.1	250	30.4	19.8	6.2	40.4
French, Boiled, Average	**1 Serving/150g**	**38**	**0.0**	**25**	**2.3**	**3.8**	**0.0**	**3.7**
French, Canned, Average	**1oz/28g**	**5**	**0.1**	**17**	**1.3**	**2.7**	**0.2**	**1.9**
French, Raw	*1oz/28g*	*6*	*0.1*	*20*	*1.6*	*2.7*	*0.4*	*1.8*
Green, Cut, Average	**1oz/28g**	**7**	**0.1**	**24**	**1.7**	**3.6**	**0.2**	**2.7**
Green, Fine, Average	**1 Serving/75g**	**18**	**0.3**	**24**	**1.8**	**3.2**	**0.4**	**2.9**
Green, Sliced, Average	**1oz/28g**	**6**	**0.1**	**23**	**1.9**	**3.5**	**0.2**	**2.1**
Green, Sliced, Frozen, Average	**1 Serving/50g**	**13**	**0.0**	**26**	**1.8**	**4.4**	**0.1**	**4.1**
Green, Whole, Average	**1oz/28g**	**6**	**0.1**	**22**	**1.6**	**3.0**	**0.4**	**1.7**

	Measure INFO/WEIGHT	per Measure		Nutrition Values per 100g / 100ml				
		KCAL	FAT	KCAL	PROT	CARB	FAT	FIBRE

BEANS

	Measure INFO/WEIGHT	KCAL	FAT	KCAL	PROT	CARB	FAT	FIBRE
Haricot, Canned, Average	1 Can/400g	77	0.5	77	6.2	10.7	0.5	5.9
Haricot, Dried, Boiled in Unsalted Water	1oz/28g	27	0.1	95	6.6	17.2	0.5	6.1
Kidney, Curried, Rajmah, Sohna *	½ Can/225g	217	1.1	97	3.7	17.6	0.5	1.4
Kidney, Red, Canned, Drained, Average	½ Can/120g	115	0.7	96	7.4	20.7	0.5	5.5
Kidney, Red, Dried, Boiled in Unsalted Water	1oz/28g	29	0.1	103	8.4	17.4	0.5	6.7
Kidney, Red, Dried, Raw	1oz/28g	74	0.4	266	22.1	44.1	1.4	15.7
Kidney, Red, in Chilli Sauce, Sainsbury's*	1 Can/420g	365	1.7	87	5.3	15.6	0.4	4.5
Kidney, Red, in Chilli Sauce, Waitrose*	½ Can/201g	175	0.8	87	5.5	15.3	0.4	3.2
Mexican Style, Mix, Tinned, Asda*	1 Serving/81g	71	0.6	88	8.7	11.8	0.7	10.4
Mix, Great Fire Dragon, Graze*	1 Pack/25g	123	7.0	491	15.0	48.1	28.1	2.5
Mixed, Canned, Average	1 Can/300g	300	3.5	100	6.8	15.6	1.2	4.1
Mixed, Spicy, Average	1 Serving/140g	108	0.7	78	4.8	13.4	0.5	3.9
Mung, Whole, Dried, Boiled in Unsalted Water	1oz/28g	25	0.1	91	7.6	15.3	0.4	3.0
Mung, Whole, Dried, Raw	1oz/28g	78	0.3	279	23.9	46.3	1.1	10.0
Pinto, Dried, Boiled in Unsalted Water	1oz/28g	38	0.2	137	8.9	23.9	0.7	0.0
Pinto, Dried, Raw	1oz/28g	92	0.4	327	21.1	57.1	1.6	14.0
Refried, Average	1 Serving/215g	162	1.5	76	4.6	12.7	0.7	1.8
Runner, Average	1 Serving/80g	15	0.3	19	1.3	2.8	0.4	2.2
Soya, Dried, Average	1oz/28g	104	5.1	370	34.2	15.4	18.3	19.6
Soya, Dried, Boiled in Unsalted Water	1oz/28g	39	2.0	141	14.0	5.1	7.3	6.1
Soya, Shelled, Frozen, Raw, Average	1 Serving/80g	99	4.3	124	12.2	6.9	5.3	4.4
Tuscan Beanz, Heinz*	½ Can/195g	178	3.3	91	4.9	12.0	1.7	4.1
Wasabi, Mix, Whitworths*	1 Serving/25g	108	3.4	430	30.9	40.1	13.7	10.7
White, Campo Largo, Lidl*	½ Jar/200g	180	1.0	90	7.1	11.2	0.5	0.0

BEEF

	Measure INFO/WEIGHT	KCAL	FAT	KCAL	PROT	CARB	FAT	FIBRE
Brisket, Boiled, Lean	1 Serving/100g	225	11.0	225	31.4	0.0	11.0	0.0
Brisket, Boiled, Lean & Fat	1 Serving/100g	268	17.4	268	27.8	0.0	17.4	0.0
Brisket, Braised, Lean	1 Serving/100g	280	17.4	280	29.0	0.0	17.4	0.0
Brisket, Raw, Lean	1oz/28g	39	1.7	139	21.1	0.0	6.1	0.0
Brisket, Raw, Lean & Fat	1oz/28g	60	4.4	216	18.2	0.0	15.8	0.0
Cooked, Sliced, From Supermarket, Average	1 Slice/35g	47	1.2	135	23.6	2.0	3.5	0.5
Escalope, Healthy Range, Average	1 Serving/170g	233	6.7	137	24.2	1.2	4.0	0.4
Flank, Pot-Roasted, Lean	1oz/28g	71	3.9	253	31.8	0.0	14.0	0.0
Flank, Pot-Roasted, Lean & Fat	1oz/28g	85	6.1	303	26.6	0.0	21.9	0.0
Flank, Raw, Lean	1oz/28g	49	2.6	175	22.7	0.0	9.3	0.0
Flank, Raw, Lean & Fat	1oz/28g	74	5.8	266	19.7	0.0	20.8	0.0
for Casserole, Lean, Diced, Average	1oz/28g	35	1.1	126	23.0	0.0	3.8	0.0
Fore Rib, Lean & Fat, Average	1oz/28g	40	1.8	144	21.7	0.0	6.2	0.2
Fore Rib, Raw, Lean	1oz/28g	41	1.8	145	21.5	0.0	6.5	0.0
Fore Rib, Roasted, Lean	1oz/28g	66	3.2	236	33.3	0.0	11.4	0.0
Fore Rib, Roasted, Lean & Fat	1oz/28g	84	5.7	300	29.1	0.0	20.4	0.0
Grill Steak, Average	1 Steak/170g	501	39.5	295	19.3	2.1	23.2	0.1
Grill Steak, Peppered, Average	1 Serving/172g	419	24.4	244	23.6	5.2	14.2	0.3
Joint, for Roasting, Average	1oz/28g	38	1.0	134	24.5	1.4	3.4	0.2
Joint, Sirloin, Roasted, Lean	1oz/28g	53	1.8	188	32.4	0.0	6.5	0.0
Joint, Sirloin, Roasted, Lean & Fat	1oz/28g	65	3.5	233	29.8	0.0	12.6	0.0
Mince, Cooked, Average	1 Serving/75g	214	15.3	286	24.0	0.0	20.3	0.0
Mince, Extra Lean, Raw, Average	1 Serving/100g	124	5.0	124	21.2	0.1	5.0	0.0
Mince, Extra Lean, Stewed	1oz/28g	50	2.4	177	24.7	0.0	8.7	0.0
Mince, Lean, Raw, Average	1oz/28g	48	2.8	172	20.8	0.0	10.0	0.1
Mince, Raw, Average	1oz/28g	68	5.1	242	19.6	0.2	18.1	0.0
Mince, Raw, Frozen, Average	1 Serving/100g	176	10.0	176	20.4	0.0	10.0	0.0
Mince, Steak, Extra Lean, Average	1oz/28g	37	1.6	131	20.5	0.4	5.6	0.0

	Measure INFO/WEIGHT	per Measure KCAL	FAT	Nutrition Values per 100g / 100ml KCAL	PROT	CARB	FAT	FIBRE
BEEF								
Mince, Steak, Raw, Average	1 Serving/125g	318	25.0	254	17.2	0.0	20.0	0.0
Mince, Stewed	1oz/28g	59	3.8	209	21.8	0.0	13.5	0.0
Peppered, Sliced, Average	1 Slice/20g	26	1.1	129	18.2	1.3	5.6	1.0
Potted, Binghams*	1 Serving/30g	76	6.6	254	13.8	1.0	22.0	0.6
Roast, Sliced, Average	1 Slice/35g	48	1.3	136	26.1	0.4	3.6	0.2
Salt, Average	1 Serving/70g	80	1.7	114	21.7	1.0	2.5	0.1
Salted, Dried, Raw	1oz/28g	70	0.4	250	55.4	0.0	1.5	0.0
Silverside, Pot-Roasted, Lean	1oz/28g	54	1.8	193	34.0	0.0	6.3	0.0
Silverside, Pot-Roasted, Lean & Fat	1oz/28g	69	3.8	247	31.0	0.0	13.7	0.0
Silverside, Raw, Lean	1oz/28g	38	1.2	134	23.8	0.0	4.3	0.0
Silverside, Raw, Lean & Fat	1oz/28g	60	4.1	213	20.2	0.0	14.7	0.0
Silverside, Salted, Boiled, Lean	1oz/28g	52	1.9	184	30.4	0.0	6.9	0.0
Silverside, Salted, Boiled, Lean & Fat	1oz/28g	63	3.5	224	27.9	0.0	12.5	0.0
Silverside, Salted, Raw, Lean	1oz/28g	39	2.0	140	19.2	0.0	7.0	0.0
Silverside, Salted, Raw, Lean & Fat	1oz/28g	64	5.0	227	16.3	0.0	18.0	0.0
Steak, 8oz Rump & Chips	1 Serving/466g	870	41.1	187	10.7	16.2	8.8	0.0
Steak, Braising, Braised, Lean	1oz/28g	63	2.7	225	34.4	0.0	9.7	0.0
Steak, Braising, Braised, Lean & Fat	1oz/28g	69	3.6	246	32.9	0.0	12.7	0.0
Steak, Braising, Lean, Raw, Average	1oz/28g	40	1.4	144	24.8	0.0	5.0	0.0
Steak, Braising, Raw, Lean & Fat	1oz/28g	44	2.4	158	20.5	0.0	8.5	0.0
Steak, Economy, Average	1oz/28g	53	2.4	190	26.9	1.2	8.7	0.4
Steak, Fillet, Cooked, Average	1oz/28g	54	2.4	191	28.6	0.0	8.5	0.0
Steak, Fillet, Lean, Average	1oz/28g	42	2.0	150	21.0	0.0	7.3	0.0
Steak, Fillet, Lean, Cooked, Average	1oz/28g	52	2.2	186	28.6	0.0	8.0	0.0
Steak, Frying, Average	1 Steak/110g	128	2.7	116	23.7	0.0	2.5	0.0
Steak, Rump, Cooked, Average	1oz/28g	69	4.0	246	29.1	0.5	14.1	0.0
Steak, Rump, Grilled, Rare, Lean	1 Steak/227g	381	15.6	168	26.5	0.0	6.9	0.0
Steak, Rump, Lean, Cooked, Average	1oz/28g	50	1.7	179	31.0	0.0	6.1	0.0
Steak, Rump, Raw, Lean & Fat	1oz/28g	49	2.8	174	20.7	0.0	10.1	0.0
Steak, Rump, Raw, Lean, Average	1 Steak/175g	219	7.2	125	22.0	0.0	4.1	0.0
Steak, Sirloin, Fried, Rare, Lean	1oz/28g	53	2.3	189	28.8	0.0	8.2	0.0
Steak, Sirloin, Fried, Rare, Lean & Fat	1oz/28g	65	3.9	231	26.5	0.0	13.9	0.0
Steak, Sirloin, Grilled, Medium-Rare, Lean	1oz/28g	49	2.2	176	26.6	0.0	7.7	0.0
Steak, Sirloin, Grilled, Medium-Rare, Lean & Fat	1oz/28g	59	3.5	211	24.6	0.0	12.5	0.0
Steak, Sirloin, Grilled, Rare, Lean	1oz/28g	46	1.9	166	26.4	0.0	6.7	0.0
Steak, Sirloin, Grilled, Rare, Lean & Fat	1oz/28g	60	3.6	216	25.1	0.0	12.8	0.0
Steak, Sirloin, Grilled, Well-Done, Lean	1oz/28g	63	2.8	225	33.9	0.0	9.9	0.0
Steak, Sirloin, Grilled, Well-Done, Lean & Fat	1oz/28g	71	4.0	254	31.5	0.0	14.3	0.0
Steak, Sirloin, Raw, Lean & Fat	1oz/28g	56	3.6	201	21.6	0.0	12.7	0.0
Steak, Sirloin, Raw, Lean, Average	1 Steak/150g	202	6.8	135	23.5	0.0	4.5	0.0
Stewed Steak, Average	1 Serving/220g	258	10.1	117	15.8	3.3	4.6	0.0
Stewing Steak, Lean & Fat, Raw, Average	1 Serving/100g	136	4.3	136	24.2	0.1	4.3	0.1
Stewing Steak, Raw, Lean	1oz/28g	34	1.0	122	22.6	0.0	3.5	0.0
Stewing Steak, Stewed, Lean	1oz/28g	52	1.8	185	32.0	0.0	6.3	0.0
Stewing Steak, Stewed, Lean & Fat	1oz/28g	57	2.7	203	29.2	0.0	9.6	0.0
Stir Fry Strips, Raw, Average	1 Serving/125g	149	3.8	119	23.0	0.0	3.0	0.2
Topside, Lean & Fat, Raw, Average	1oz/28g	55	3.6	198	20.4	0.0	12.9	0.0
Topside, Raw, Lean	1oz/28g	32	0.8	116	23.0	0.0	2.7	0.0
Wafer Thin Sliced, Cooked, Average	1 Slice/10g	13	0.3	129	24.5	0.5	3.2	0.2
BEEF &								
Black Bean, Sizzling, Oriental Express*	1 Pack/400g	420	8.4	105	7.2	14.0	2.1	2.1
Onions with Gravy, Minced, Lean, Sainsbury's*	1 Sm Can/198g	285	13.9	144	17.0	3.1	7.0	0.2
Onions, Minced, Asda*	½ Can/196g	314	19.6	160	13.0	4.6	10.0	0.1

	Measure INFO/WEIGHT	per Measure		Nutrition Values per 100g / 100ml				
		KCAL	FAT	KCAL	PROT	CARB	FAT	FIBRE
BEEF BOURGUIGNON								
Finest, Tesco*	½ Pack/300g	247	7.8	82	9.9	4.8	2.6	0.5
BEEF BRAISED								
& New Potatoes, GFY, Asda*	1 Pack/448g	242	6.3	54	8.1	2.2	1.4	3.1
in Ale with Mash & Baby Onions, COU, M&S*	1 Pack/400g	380	9.2	95	7.4	11.0	2.3	1.4
Steak & Mash, Tastes of Home, M Kitchen, Morrisons*	1 Meal/250g	209	6.0	87	6.4	9.1	2.5	1.1
Steak, & Cabbage, COU, M&S*	1 Pack/380g	323	9.9	85	8.3	6.7	2.6	1.9
Tender, Pub Specials, Birds Eye*	1 Pack/450g	243	3.6	54	5.5	6.1	0.8	1.8
BEEF CANTONESE								
Sainsbury's*	½ Pack/175g	200	2.3	114	5.5	20.1	1.3	0.5
BEEF CHILLI								
Crispy, Cantonese, Chilled, Sainsbury's*	1 Pack/250g	682	38.8	273	11.4	22.1	15.5	1.9
Crispy, Tesco*	1 Pack/250g	472	17.2	189	10.8	21.0	6.9	0.5
BEEF DINNER								
Roast with Trimmings	1 Dinner/840g	1310	63.0	156	6.1	17.7	7.5	2.3
Roast, Sainsbury's*	1 Pack/400g	356	6.8	89	6.5	12.0	1.7	1.9
BEEF IN								
Ale, Diet Chef Ltd*	1 Meal/300g	201	3.6	67	8.2	6.0	1.2	2.1
Black Bean Sauce, Chinese, Tesco*	1 Pack/400g	396	12.4	99	9.1	8.7	3.1	0.5
Black Bean Sauce, M&S*	1 Pack/350g	402	22.4	115	8.9	5.7	6.4	1.1
Black Bean with Egg Noodles, M&S*	1 Pack/400g	460	6.0	115	8.6	16.7	1.5	1.8
Black Pepper Sauce & Egg Fried Rice, Tesco*	1 Pack/451g	622	24.8	138	7.0	15.2	5.5	1.2
Gravy, Roast, Birds Eye*	1 Pack/227g	177	3.9	78	13.4	2.2	1.7	0.0
Gravy, Sliced, Iceland*	1 Pack/200g	172	3.2	86	12.1	5.9	1.6	0.3
Gravy, Sliced, Sainsbury's*	1 Serving/125g	100	2.2	80	13.5	2.6	1.8	0.2
Madeira & Mushroom Gravy, Sliced, Finest, Tesco*	1 Pack/400g	536	24.8	134	15.2	4.3	6.2	1.0
Red Onion Gravy, with Veg Crush, Slimming World, Iceland*	1 Pack/550g	297	2.8	54	7.1	4.2	0.5	2.1
Rich Ale Gravy, Slow Cooked Brisket, COU, M&S*	1 Pack/350g	242	6.7	69	8.4	3.7	1.9	1.6
BEEF RAGU								
with Rigatoni Pasta, Chianti, Balanced for You, M&S*	1 Pack/400g	476	14.4	119	9.3	11.5	3.6	1.5
BEEF SZECHUAN								
Sizzling Hot Spicy, Oriental Express*	1 Pack/400g	380	7.6	95	6.4	13.2	1.9	2.0
BEEF WELLINGTON								
Average	*1 Serving/200g*	*530*	*33.3*	*265*	*12.4*	*17.0*	*16.6*	*1.0*
ES, Asda*	1 Serving/218g	605	37.1	277	11.0	20.0	17.0	0.9
BEEF WITH								
Black Bean Sauce, Chilli, Sainsbury's*	1 Pack/300g	336	14.4	112	8.7	8.6	4.8	1.0
Black Bean Sauce, Rice Bowl, Uncle Ben's*	1 Pack/350g	368	4.9	105	5.6	17.4	1.4	0.0
Diane Sauce, Rump Steak, Tesco*	1 Steak/165g	182	8.1	110	15.1	1.1	4.9	0.3
Onion & Gravy, Minced, Princes*	1 Serving/200g	342	24.4	171	9.9	5.5	12.2	0.0
Onions & Gravy, Minced, Tesco*	1 Can/198g	224	10.1	113	14.0	2.8	5.1	0.8
Onions, Carrots & Rich Gravy, Steak, Braised, COU, M&S*	1 Pack/454g	345	6.8	76	11.0	4.0	1.5	1.2
Peppercorn Sauce, Steak, Fried, Simply Cook, Tesco*	½ Pack/125g	215	9.1	172	24.8	1.7	7.3	0.4
Peppercorn Sauce, Steak, Just Cook, Sainsbury's*	½ Pack/128g	174	7.3	136	17.7	3.4	5.7	1.2
Vegetables & Gravy, Minced, Birds Eye*	1 Pack/178g	155	6.1	87	9.1	5.1	3.4	0.6
BEER								
Ale, Bottled, Old Speckled Hen*	1 Bottle/330ml	124	0.3	38	0.2	1.8	0.1	0.2
Ale, Hopping Hare, Hall & Woodhouse Ltd*	1 Bottle/500ml	189	0.0	38	0.4	3.0	0.0	0.0
Ale, Old Speckled Hen*	1 Pint/568ml	185	0.6	32	0.2	1.6	0.1	0.2
Bitter, Average	*1 Can/440ml*	*141*	*0.0*	*32*	*0.3*	*2.3*	*0.0*	*0.0*
Bitter, Banks, Marstons PLC*	1 Pint/568ml	193	0.1	34	0.3	3.4	0.0	0.0
Bitter, Cask, Draught, London Pride, Fullers*	1 Pint/568ml	201	0.0	35	0.0	0.0	0.0	0.0
Bitter, Draught, Average	*1 Pint/568ml*	*182*	*0.0*	*32*	*0.3*	*2.3*	*0.0*	*0.0*
Bitter, Keg, Average	*1 Pint/568ml*	*176*	*0.0*	*31*	*0.3*	*2.3*	*0.0*	*0.0*

INFO/WEIGHT	Measure	per Measure		Nutrition Values per 100g / 100ml				
		KCAL	FAT	KCAL	PROT	CARB	FAT	FIBRE
BEER								
Bitter, Low Alcohol, Average	*1 Pint/568ml*	*74*	*0.0*	*13*	*0.2*	*2.1*	*0.0*	*0.0*
Bitter, Original, Tetley's*	1 Can/440ml	140	0.0	32	0.2	4.6	0.0	0.0
Bitter, Strong, Broadside, Adnams*	1 Bottle/500ml	285	0.0	57	0.0	0.0	0.0	0.0
Brown Ale, Bottled, Average	*1 Bottle/330ml*	*99*	*0.0*	*30*	*0.3*	*3.0*	*0.0*	*0.0*
Especial, Modelo*	1 Bottle/355ml	145	0.0	41	0.0	1.1	0.0	0.0
Goliath, Ale, Wychwood, Marstons PLC*	1 Bottle/500ml	191	0.0	38	0.4	2.8	0.0	0.0
Guinness* Extra Stout, Bottled	1 Bottle/500ml	215	0.0	43	4.0	0.0	0.0	0.0
Guinness*, Draught	1 Can/440ml	158	0.2	36	0.3	3.0	0.0	0.0
Guinness*, Stout	1 Pint/568ml	205	0.0	36	0.3	3.0	0.0	0.0
Honey Dew, Ale, Fullers*	1 Bottle/500ml	232	0.0	46	0.0	4.6	0.0	0.0
Mackeson, Stout	1 Pint/568ml	205	0.0	36	0.4	4.6	0.0	0.0
Mild, Draught, Average	*1 Pint/568ml*	*136*	*0.0*	*24*	*0.2*	*1.6*	*0.0*	*0.0*
Non Alcoholic, Zero, Cobra*	1 Bottle/330ml	79	0.0	24	0.8	2.0	0.0	0.0
Oak Aged, Innis & Gunn*	1 Bottle/330ml	120	0.0	36	0.0	3.6	0.0	0.0
Old Peculiar Ale, Theakstons*	1 Serving/500ml	250	0.0	50	0.0	4.6	0.0	0.0
Pale Ale, IPA, Greene King*	1 Pint/568ml	157	0.1	28	0.2	1.6	0.0	0.1
Pale Ale, Sierra Nevada*	1 Bottle/350g	175	0.0	50	0.4	4.0	0.0	0.0
Raspberry, Framboise, Lindemans*	1 Serving/355ml	185	0.0	52	0.0	8.8	0.0	0.0
Weissbier, Alcohol Free, Erdinger*	1 Bottle/500ml	125	0.0	25	0.4	5.3	0.0	0.0
Wheat, Tesco*	1 Bottle/500ml	155	0.0	31	0.5	0.4	0.0	0.0
Wychcraft, Ale, Wychwood, Marstons PLC*	1 Bottle/500ml	210	0.0	42	0.3	4.2	0.0	0.0
BEETROOT								
Baby, Pickled, Average	*1 Beetroot/13g*	*5*	*0.0*	*37*	*1.7*	*7.2*	*0.1*	*1.2*
Bunched, TTD, Sainsbury's*	1 Serving/100g	38	0.1	38	1.7	7.6	0.1	0.2
Cooked, Boiled, Drained, Average	*1 Serving/100g*	*44*	*0.2*	*44*	*1.7*	*10.0*	*0.2*	*2.0*
Pickled, in Sweet Vinegar, Average	*1oz/28g*	*16*	*0.0*	*57*	*1.2*	*12.8*	*0.1*	*1.5*
Pickled, in Vinegar, Average	*1 Serving/50g*	*18*	*0.0*	*36*	*1.6*	*7.3*	*0.1*	*1.2*
Raw, Unprepared, Average	*1oz/28g*	*8*	*0.0*	*29*	*1.4*	*5.4*	*0.1*	*1.7*
Rosebud, M&S*	½ Pack/90g	45	0.3	50	1.9	8.9	0.3	3.2
Rosebud, Sweet Chilli Marinated, M&S*	1 Serving/80g	52	0.2	65	1.5	12.3	0.3	3.6
Sweetened Vinegar, Pomegranate & Cumin, Waitrose*	½ Pack/90g	70	0.6	78	1.1	15.8	0.7	1.9
BHAJI								
Aubergine & Potato, Fried in Vegetable Oil, Average	*1oz/28g*	*36*	*2.5*	*130*	*2.0*	*12.0*	*8.8*	*1.7*
Cabbage & Pea, Fried in Vegetable Oil, Average	*1oz/28g*	*50*	*4.1*	*178*	*3.3*	*9.2*	*14.7*	*3.4*
Cauliflower & Paneer, Waitrose*	1 Pack/88g	218	14.7	248	7.6	11.6	16.7	10.1
Cauliflower, Fried in Vegetable Oil, Average	*1oz/28g*	*60*	*5.7*	*214*	*4.0*	*4.0*	*20.5*	*2.0*
Mushroom, Fried in Vegetable Oil, Average	*1oz/28g*	*46*	*4.5*	*166*	*1.7*	*4.4*	*16.1*	*1.3*
Okra, Bangladeshi, Fried in Butter Ghee, Average	*1oz/28g*	*27*	*1.8*	*95*	*2.5*	*7.6*	*6.4*	*3.2*
Onion, Asda*	1 Bhaji/49g	96	4.9	196	6.0	20.0	10.0	2.0
Onion, Indian Starter Selection, M&S*	1 Bhaji/22g	65	5.1	295	5.7	15.8	23.3	2.8
Onion, Indian, Mini, Asda*	1 Bhaji/18g	33	1.8	186	4.9	19.0	10.0	6.0
Onion, Mini Indian Selection, Tesco*	1 Bhaji/23g	40	2.2	172	6.1	15.4	9.5	4.6
Onion, Mini, Asda*	1 Bhaji/35g	63	2.8	179	4.8	22.0	8.0	4.4
Onion, Mini, Tesco*	1 Bhaji/23g	48	1.9	210	7.3	26.7	8.2	1.3
Onion, Sainsbury's*	1 Bhaji/38g	93	5.1	245	6.5	24.7	13.4	6.4
Onion, Tesco*	1 Bhaji/47g	85	4.9	181	5.7	16.2	10.4	4.3
Onion, Waitrose*	1 Bhaji/45g	124	9.4	276	4.7	17.5	20.8	2.5
Potato & Onion, Fried in Vegetable Oil, Average	*1oz/28g*	*45*	*2.8*	*160*	*2.1*	*16.6*	*10.1*	*1.6*
Potato, Spinach & Cauliflower, Fried, Average	*1oz/28g*	*47*	*4.2*	*169*	*2.2*	*7.1*	*15.1*	*1.4*
Spinach & Potato, Fried in Vegetable Oil, Average	*1oz/28g*	*53*	*3.9*	*191*	*3.7*	*13.4*	*14.1*	*2.3*
Spinach, Fried in Vegetable Oil, Average	*1oz/28g*	*23*	*1.9*	*83*	*3.3*	*2.6*	*6.8*	*2.4*
Vegetable from 8 Snack Pack, Takeaway, Tesco*	1 Bhaji/21g	36	1.9	175	6.0	16.8	9.1	4.9

	Measure INFO/WEIGHT	per Measure KCAL	FAT	KCAL	PROT	CARB	FAT	FIBRE
BHUNA								
Chicken Tikka, Tesco*	1 Pack/350g	438	23.4	125	11.3	5.0	6.7	0.9
Chicken, Curry, Tesco*	1 Serving/300g	396	22.8	132	11.4	4.5	7.6	0.5
Chicken, Indian Takeaway, Tesco*	1 Pack/350g	438	27.6	125	8.3	4.6	7.9	2.2
Chicken, with Rice, Ready Meal, Average	*1 Pack/350g*	*444*	*20.8*	*127*	*9.4*	*8.9*	*5.9*	*1.4*
King Prawn, M&S*	1 Pack/350g	262	13.3	75	6.7	3.3	3.8	1.5
King Prawn, Morrisons*	1 Pack/350g	301	20.6	86	6.5	1.8	5.9	0.5
Lamb, & Rice, Sainsbury's*	1 Pack/500g	619	26.5	124	7.4	11.6	5.3	2.0
Prawn, Tandoori, Indian, Sainsbury's*	½ Pack/200g	152	8.0	76	5.5	4.5	4.0	1.7
BIERWURST								
Average	*1 Slice/10g*	*25*	*2.1*	*252*	*14.4*	*1.0*	*21.2*	*0.0*
BILBERRIES								
Fresh, Raw	*1oz/28g*	*8*	*0.1*	*29*	*0.6*	*6.8*	*0.2*	*1.8*
BILTONG								
Average	*1 Serving/25g*	*64*	*1.0*	*256*	*50.0*	*0.0*	*4.0*	*0.0*
BIRYANI								
Chicken Tikka, & Lentil Pilau, Fuller Longer, M&S*	1 Pack/400g	440	11.6	110	9.5	12.0	2.9	2.3
Chicken Tikka, BGTY, Sainsbury's*	1 Pack/400g	316	3.8	84	6.8	10.7	1.0	2.9
Chicken Tikka, Northern Indian, Sainsbury's*	1 Pack/450g	698	25.6	155	9.4	16.5	5.7	1.2
Chicken, Indian, Asda*	1 Pack/450g	778	22.5	173	9.0	23.0	5.0	0.7
Chicken, Ready Meal, Average	*1 Pack/400g*	*521*	*17.1*	*130*	*7.5*	*15.2*	*4.3*	*1.6*
Chicken, Ready Meal, Healthy Range, Average	*1 Pack/400g*	*369*	*5.5*	*92*	*7.4*	*12.6*	*1.4*	*0.9*
Chicken, Tikka, Ready Meal, Average	*1 Pack/400g*	*460*	*11.5*	*115*	*7.3*	*14.8*	*2.9*	*1.5*
Chicken, Weight Watchers*	1 Pack/330g	308	3.7	93	6.2	14.6	1.1	0.6
Lamb, Average	*1 Serving/200g*	*390*	*19.4*	*195*	*7.3*	*20.9*	*9.7*	*0.0*
Lamb, Ready Meal, Average	*1 Pack/400g*	*535*	*18.9*	*134*	*6.0*	*16.6*	*4.7*	*2.2*
Seafood, M&S*	1 Pack/450g	619	25.7	138	7.1	14.4	5.7	1.7
Vegetable with Rice, Patak's*	½ Pack/125g	194	1.9	155	3.6	32.9	1.5	1.2
Vegetable, & Rice, Sainsbury's*	½ Pack/125g	229	5.0	183	4.4	32.4	4.0	0.7
BISCUITS								
Abbey Crunch, McVitie's*	1 Biscuit/9g	43	1.6	477	6.0	72.8	17.9	2.5
Abernethy, Simmers*	1 Biscuit/12g	61	2.7	490	5.7	69.2	21.9	0.0
Ace Milk Chocolate, McVitie's*	1 Biscuit/24g	122	5.9	510	6.1	66.2	24.5	1.6
Aero, Orange, Aero, Nestle*	1 Biscuit/19g	101	5.6	534	6.0	60.6	29.3	1.7
All Butter, Tesco*	1 Biscuit/9g	44	2.1	486	6.3	63.5	23.0	1.9
Almond & Chocolate, Biscotti, TTD, Sainsbury's*	1 Biscuit/30g	132	4.8	440	8.4	65.6	16.0	3.1
Almond Fingers, Tesco*	1 Finger/46g	180	6.8	391	6.2	58.4	14.7	1.0
Almond Thins, Continental, Tesco*	1 Biscuit/3g	15	0.5	450	6.7	72.8	14.7	3.1
Amaretti, Average	*1 Biscuit/5g*	*22*	*0.8*	*434*	*8.1*	*66.4*	*15.4*	*2.8*
Amaretti, Doria*	1 Biscuit/4g	17	0.3	433	6.0	84.8	7.8	0.0
Amaretti, M&S*	1 Biscuit/6g	30	1.1	480	9.6	71.3	17.2	3.8
Amaretti, Sainsbury's*	1 Biscuit/6g	27	0.7	450	6.5	80.5	11.3	1.1
Anzac, Bitesmart*	1 Biscuit/20g	84	4.6	420	5.1	46.8	23.0	0.0
Apple & Cinnamon Thins, Finest, Tesco*	1 Biscuit/5g	22	0.8	470	5.9	71.7	17.5	1.5
Apple & Raisin, Slices, Good & Counted, Asda*	1 Pack/29g	109	1.3	382	6.0	77.0	4.5	4.5
Apple Crumble, Officially Low Fat, Fox's*	1 Biscuit/23g	85	0.6	365	5.4	80.4	2.4	2.5
Arrowroot, Thin, Crawfords*	1 Biscuit/7g	35	1.2	450	6.9	71.4	15.2	2.8
Belgian Chocolate Chip, Walkers Shortbread Ltd*	2 Biscuits/25g	124	6.1	494	5.1	63.3	24.5	2.2
Belgian Chocolate, Selection, Finest, Tesco*	1 Biscuit/10g	52	2.7	515	6.0	62.0	27.0	3.0
Belgian Chocolate, Thins, ES, Asda*	1 Biscuit/9g	44	2.0	503	7.0	67.0	23.0	0.2
Belgian Milk Chocolate, M&S*	1 Biscuit/12g	60	2.5	490	6.2	70.1	20.3	2.5
Bisc & Twix, Master Foods*	1 Bar/27g	140	7.6	520	5.2	61.1	28.3	0.0
Biscotti, Chocolate, Heinz*	1 Biscuit/20g	80	1.7	398	8.5	72.0	8.7	5.8
Blueberry & Vanilla, Oaty, Weight Watchers*	1 Biscuit/19g	86	3.3	452	7.3	62.1	17.6	8.0

BISCUITS

	Measure INFO/WEIGHT	per Measure		Nutrition Values per 100g / 100ml				
		KCAL	FAT	KCAL	PROT	CARB	FAT	FIBRE
Blueberry, Biscuit Moments, Special K, Kellogg's*	2 Biscuits/25g	99	2.3	394	4.5	73.0	9.0	1.5
Bn, Chocolate Flavour, McVitie's*	1 Biscuit/18g	83	3.0	460	6.6	71.0	16.7	2.6
Bn, Strawberry Flavour, McVitie's*	1 Biscuit/18g	71	1.2	395	5.6	78.0	6.8	0.0
Bn, Vanilla Flavour, McVitie's*	1 Biscuit/18g	85	3.0	470	5.9	74.0	16.6	1.2
Bourbon Creams, Asda*	1 Biscuit/14g	67	3.1	482	5.0	66.0	22.0	3.4
Bourbon Creams, Sainsbury's*	1 Biscuit/13g	60	2.4	476	5.7	70.4	19.1	1.7
Bourbon Creams, Tesco*	1 Biscuit/14g	68	3.0	485	5.4	66.2	21.6	3.4
Bourbon Creams, Value, Multipack, Tesco*	1 Biscuit/13g	62	2.9	494	5.9	68.0	22.8	1.7
Bourbon, Average	*1 Biscuit/13g*	*63*	*2.8*	*488*	*5.7*	*68.2*	*21.3*	*2.1*
Bourbon, Trufree*	1 Biscuit/13g	61	2.8	486	7.5	62.6	22.6	1.1
Bournville, Cadbury*	1 Biscuit/16g	85	5.0	520	6.0	54.9	30.7	1.4
Brandy Snap, Askeys*	1 Basket/20g	98	4.3	490	1.9	72.7	21.3	0.0
Brandy Snaps, Average	*1 Biscuit/15g*	*69*	*2.2*	*460*	*2.7*	*79.8*	*14.4*	*0.5*
Breakfast, Average	*4 Biscuits/56g*	*249*	*8.8*	*445*	*11.8*	*61.7*	*15.7*	*7.0*
Breakfast, Coconut & Yoghurt, Sainsburys*	2 Biscuits/46g	203	7.3	437	7.6	62.1	15.7	8.7
Breakfast, Cranberry, Belvita, Nabisco*	1 Biscuits/13g	55	1.7	435	8.3	67.5	13.7	5.7
Breakfast, Forest Fruits, Belvita, Nabisco*	1 Biscuit/13g	60	2.1	460	8.5	67.0	16.0	5.3
Breakfast, Golden Grain, Soft Bakes, Belvita*	1 Biscuit/50g	193	6.0	385	5.9	63.0	12.0	6.7
Breakfast, Honey & Nuts, Belvita, Nabisco*	1 Biscuit/13g	58	2.1	464	8.0	68.0	17.0	3.5
Breakfast, Honey & Yoghurt Crunch, Belvita, Kraft*	2 Biscuits/51g	230	8.1	455	7.5	68.5	16.0	4.0
Breakfast, Muesli, Belvita, Nabisco*	1 Biscuit/13g	59	2.1	455	8.2	67.0	16.0	4.1
Breakfast, Original, All Bran, Kellogg's*	1 Pack/40g	176	8.0	440	8.0	49.0	20.0	16.0
Breakfast, Porridge Oats & Blueberries,,McVitie's*	1 Slice/20g	80	2.1	402	7.3	67.1	10.4	6.5
Breakfast, Porridge Oats, with Oats & Honey, McVitie's*	4 Biscuits/50g	226	7.0	452	9.6	69.5	14.0	4.6
Breakfast, Porridge Oats, with Red Berries,,McVitie's*	4 Biscuits/50g	226	6.9	452	9.6	71.0	13.8	5.1
Breakfast, Red Berries, Soft Bakes, Belvita, Mondelez*	1 Biscuit/50g	191	5.5	380	5.5	65.0	11.0	6.6
Breakfast, Strawberry & Yoghurt, Duo Crunch, Belvita*	1 Biscuit/25g	113	3.8	445	6.9	70.0	15.0	4.3
Breakfast, Yogurt Crunch, Belvita, Nabisco*	2 Biscuits/50g	230	8.6	455	7.6	66.0	17.0	4.0
Butter, Covered in 70% Chocolate, Green & Black's*	1 Biscuit/12g	62	3.5	520	7.1	5.6	29.4	0.1
Butter, Crinkle Crunch, Fox's*	1 Biscuit/11g	50	1.9	460	5.8	69.8	17.5	2.4
Butter, Dark Chocolate, Momento, Aldi*	1 Biscuit/14g	69	3.2	491	6.2	63.5	22.6	4.2
Cadbury Creme Egg, Cadbury*	1 Biscuit/18g	80	3.7	435	5.0	58.3	20.1	1.3
Cafe Noir, McVitie's*	1 Biscuit/9g	39	0.5	420	4.5	87.0	5.5	1.1
Cantucci with Honey, Loyd Grossman*	1 Biscuit/7g	32	1.1	450	9.5	66.3	16.3	0.9
Cantuccini with Almonds, Average	*1 Biscotti/30g*	*130*	*5.0*	*433*	*10.0*	*60.0*	*16.7*	*3.3*
Cantuccini, Sainsbury's*	1 Biscotti/8g	35	1.3	440	10.4	63.1	16.2	4.4
Caramelised, Biscoff, Lotus*	1 Biscuit/8g	38	1.5	484	4.9	72.7	19.0	1.3
Caramels, Milk Chocolate, McVitie's*	1 Biscuit/17g	81	3.6	478	5.6	65.8	21.4	2.3
Cheddars, Real Cheddar Cheese, Jacob's*	1 Biscuit/4g	20	1.2	526	11.0	48.6	32.1	3.0
Cheese Melts, Carr's*	1 Biscuit/4g	20	0.9	483	11.2	57.0	22.5	3.9
Cheese Sandwich, Ritz*	1 Biscuit/9g	50	2.8	530	9.5	55.0	30.2	2.0
Cheese Savouries, Sainsbury's*	1 Serving/50g	268	15.3	536	11.6	53.3	30.6	2.5
Cheese, & Chutney, Delicious, Boots*	1 Pack/134g	290	14.7	217	9.0	19.0	11.0	2.3
Cherry Bakewell, Handfinished, M&S*	1 Biscuit/40g	200	9.7	495	5.9	62.1	24.0	0.5
Choc Chip, Paterson's*	1 Biscuit/17g	79	3.6	474	5.6	64.0	21.6	3.1
Chockas, Original, Fox's*	1 Biscuit/24g	85	1.0	355	1.1	10.4	4.2	0.4
Choco Leibniz, Dark Chocolate, Bahlsen*	1 Biscuit/14g	69	3.6	493	6.8	59.0	26.0	5.1
Choco Leibniz, Milk, Bahlsen*	1 Biscuit/14g	72	3.6	515	7.9	63.4	25.5	2.4
Choco Leibniz, Orange Flavour, Bahlsen*	1 Biscuit/14g	70	3.7	504	7.9	58.5	26.4	0.0
Chocolate & Hazelnut, Quirks, McVitie's*	1 Biscuit/13g	66	3.6	511	5.0	58.4	28.0	2.6
Chocolate Chip & Peanut, Trufree*	1 Biscuit/11g	55	2.6	496	4.0	66.0	24.0	2.0
Chocolate Chip GI, Diet Chef Ltd*	1 Pack/20g	90	3.6	450	7.4	64.4	17.9	6.4
Chocolate Fingers, Milk, Cadbury*	1 Biscuit/6g	31	1.6	515	6.8	60.8	27.1	1.7

BISCUITS

INFO/WEIGHT	Measure	per Measure		Nutrition Values per 100g / 100ml				
		KCAL	FAT	KCAL	PROT	CARB	FAT	FIBRE
Chocolate Fingers, Plain, Cadbury*	1 Biscuit/6g	30	1.6	508	6.2	60.6	26.8	0.0
Chocolate Florentine, M&S*	1 Serving/39g	195	9.7	500	7.4	64.5	24.9	1.7
Chocolate Ginger, Organic, Duchy Originals*	1 Biscuit/12g	64	3.6	518	4.6	59.7	29.0	2.1
Chocolate Kimberley, Jacob's*	1 Biscuit/20g	86	3.4	428	3.9	64.4	17.2	1.1
Chocolate Seville, Thorntons*	1 Biscuit/19g	97	5.3	512	5.7	59.0	28.1	0.0
Chocolate Toffee, Crunch, Moments, McVitie's*	1 Biscuit/17g	89	4.7	520	5.6	62.3	27.6	1.7
Chocolate Viennese, Fox's*	1 Biscuit/16g	85	4.9	530	6.7	56.6	30.7	1.7
Chocolate, Belgian Chocolate, Weight Watchers*	1 Biscuit/18g	87	4.1	481	7.1	61.8	22.8	4.5
Chocolate, Breakaway, Nestle*	1 Bar/19g	99	4.9	511	6.1	63.5	25.2	3.0
Chocolate, Fingers, Average	*1 Biscuit/6g*	*31*	*1.6*	*514*	*6.7*	*61.4*	*26.8*	*1.5*
Christmas Shapes, Assorted, Sainsbury's*	1 Biscuit/15g	77	4.3	525	5.2	59.0	29.8	1.7
Classic, Creams, Fox's*	1 Biscuit/14g	72	3.6	516	4.4	65.2	25.8	1.7
Classic, Milk Chocolate, Fox's*	1 Biscuit/13g	67	3.1	517	6.1	64.9	24.0	1.6
Coconut Crinkle, Sainsbury's*	1 Biscuit/11g	54	2.8	500	6.4	59.6	26.2	3.7
Coconut Crinkles, Fox's*	1 Biscuit/11g	53	2.5	487	5.2	63.8	22.6	3.7
Coconut, Ring, Average	*1 Biscuit/9g*	*44*	*2.0*	*490*	*6.1*	*67.4*	*21.8*	*2.6*
Cookies 'n Cream, Eat Me, Aldi*	1 Biscuit/12g	58	2.1	467	5.4	72.0	17.0	2.9
Cranberry & Sunflower Seed, Oaty, Weight Watchers*	1 Biscuit/19g	87	3.7	457	7.9	58.0	19.3	10.0
Crinkles, Classics, Milk Chocolate, Fox's*	1 Biscuit/14g	67	3.1	487	5.7	65.2	22.7	2.7
Crispy Fruit Slices, Apple, Sultana, Go Ahead, McVitie's*	1 Slice/13g	50	0.9	388	5.4	74.0	7.1	2.9
Crispy Fruit Slices, Forest Fruit, Go Ahead, McVitie's*	1 Slice/13g	49	0.9	380	5.4	73.7	7.0	3.0
Crispy Fruit Slices, Orange, Sultana, Go Ahead, McVitie's*	1 Slice/13g	49	0.9	377	5.7	73.4	6.7	2.9
Crispy Slices, Raspberry, Go Ahead, McVitie's*	1 Slice/13g	50	0.9	385	5.3	74.0	7.0	2.8
Crunch Creams, Double Choc, Fox's*	1 Biscuit/15g	77	3.8	511	4.7	65.0	25.0	2.7
Crunchers, Salted, Savoury, Crackers, Sainsbury's*	1 Cracker/5g	22	1.0	448	6.1	59.4	20.4	1.4
Crunchie, Cadbury*	1 Biscuit/13g	64	3.1	495	4.8	65.7	23.6	0.9
Crunchy Caramel, Tesco*	1 Bar/21g	98	5.2	467	4.6	56.0	25.0	1.4
Crunchy Oats, Breakfast, Belvita, Nabisco*	1 Biscuit/13g	59	2.1	455	8.0	67.0	16.0	5.5
Custard Cream, Gluten & Wheat Free, Lovemore*	1 Biscuit/15g	71	2.5	475	0.0	33.0	16.8	0.0
Custard Creams, 25% Less Fat, Sainsbury's*	1 Biscuit/13g	59	2.2	469	5.8	72.7	17.3	1.3
Custard Creams, Asda*	1 Biscuit/12g	59	2.7	495	5.0	67.0	23.0	2.0
Custard Creams, BGTY, Sainsbury's*	1 Biscuit/12g	56	2.1	473	5.8	72.2	17.9	1.2
Custard Creams, Crawfords*	1 Biscuit/11g	57	2.7	517	5.9	69.2	24.1	1.5
Custard Creams, Everyday Value, Tesco*	1 Biscuit/13g	62	2.6	495	5.6	69.7	20.9	1.7
Custard Creams, Sainsbury's*	1 Biscuit/13g	67	3.0	514	5.5	70.4	23.4	1.6
Custard Creams, Smart Price, Asda*	1 Biscuit/13g	61	2.6	486	6.0	69.0	21.0	1.6
Custard Creams, Tesco*	1 Biscuit/13g	65	2.9	505	5.4	68.3	22.5	1.6
Custard Creams, Trufree*	1 Biscuit/12g	60	2.8	504	8.7	65.0	23.0	1.0
Custard Creams, Value, Tesco*	1 Biscuit/11g	51	1.6	450	7.2	72.5	14.3	3.0
Dark Chocolate Ginger, M&S*	1 Biscuit/21g	105	5.7	505	5.0	58.8	27.6	4.2
Dark Chocolate Gingers, Border*	1 Biscuit/17g	74	3.4	445	4.4	61.4	20.1	2.9
Digestive with Wheatgerm, Hovis*	1 Biscuit/12g	37	2.2	306	6.2	66.8	18.5	5.8
Digestive, 25% Less Fat, Asda*	1 Biscuit/16g	73	2.6	455	7.3	69.8	16.3	2.6
Digestive, 25% Less Fat, Tesco*	1 Biscuit/14g	65	2.3	462	7.3	71.0	16.5	3.8
Digestive, BGTY, Sainsbury's*	1 Biscuit/15g	70	2.6	468	7.4	71.0	17.2	3.8
Digestive, Caramels, Milk Chocolate, McVitie's*	1 Biscuit/17g	81	3.7	478	5.6	65.1	21.7	2.3
Digestive, Caramels, Plain Chocolate, McVitie's*	1 Biscuit/17g	82	3.8	481	5.7	65.5	22.1	2.1
Digestive, Chocolate	1 Biscuit/17g	84	4.1	493	6.8	66.5	24.1	2.2
Digestive, Chocolate Chip, Asda*	1 Biscuit/14g	68	3.2	491	6.0	65.0	23.0	2.9
Digestive, Cracker Selection, Tesco*	1 Biscuit/12g	56	2.3	464	7.1	65.2	19.4	4.3
Digestive, Crawfords*	1 Biscuit/12g	58	2.4	484	7.1	68.8	20.0	3.4
Digestive, Creams, McVitie's*	1 Biscuit/12g	60	2.8	502	5.6	68.2	23.0	2.1
Digestive, Dark Chocolate, McVitie's*	1 Biscuit/17g	83	4.1	495	6.0	60.8	24.2	4.2

BISCUITS

	Measure INFO/WEIGHT	per Measure KCAL	FAT	Nutrition Values per 100g / 100ml KCAL	PROT	CARB	FAT	FIBRE
Digestive, Economy, Sainsbury's*	1 Biscuit/13g	65	3.0	498	6.8	66.3	22.8	3.3
Digestive, Everyday Value, Tesco*	1 Biscuit/16g	80	3.4	490	6.7	66.5	21.0	3.0
Digestive, Gluten & Wheat Free, Lovemore*	1 Biscuit/15g	55	2.7	378	3.4	49.3	18.5	18.4
Digestive, Gluten Free, Barkat*	1 Biscuit/15g	56	2.7	378	3.4	49.3	18.5	18.4
Digestive, High Fibre, Reduced Sugar, M&S*	1 Biscuit/13g	60	2.8	460	6.5	59.3	21.7	9.4
Digestive, Hovis*	1 Biscuit/6g	27	1.1	447	10.2	60.0	18.5	4.4
Digestive, Jacob's*	1 Biscuit/14g	67	3.0	479	6.6	65.7	21.1	3.4
Digestive, Lemon & Ginger, McVitie's*	1 Biscuit/15g	72	3.1	480	6.7	66.7	20.7	2.7
Digestive, Light, McVitie's*	1 Biscuit/15g	66	2.1	444	7.3	69.5	14.4	3.6
Digestive, McVitie's*	1 Biscuit/15g	70	3.2	470	7.2	62.7	21.5	3.6
Digestive, Milk Chocolate, 25% Reduced Fat, McVitie's*	1 Biscuit/17g	78	2.9	459	7.2	68.6	17.3	3.2
Digestive, Milk Chocolate, Basics, Sainsbury's*	1 Biscuit/14g	71	3.4	496	6.5	62.9	23.7	2.9
Digestive, Milk Chocolate, Cadbury*	1 Biscuit/16g	80	3.8	490	7.4	61.3	23.3	3.9
Digestive, Milk Chocolate, GFY, Asda*	1 Biscuit/17g	78	2.9	457	7.0	69.0	17.0	3.2
Digestive, Milk Chocolate, Homewheat, McVitie's*	1 Biscuit/17g	83	4.1	486	6.0	61.5	24.0	4.0
Digestive, Milk Chocolate, M&S*	1 Biscuit/17g	85	4.4	505	6.1	62.2	26.0	2.6
Digestive, Milk Chocolate, McVitie's*	1 Biscuit/17g	84	4.0	488	6.7	62.7	23.4	2.9
Digestive, Milk Chocolate, Mini, McVitie's*	1 Bag/25g	124	6.2	496	6.6	61.9	24.7	2.9
Digestive, Milk Chocolate, Sainsbury's*	1 Biscuit/17g	87	6.3	511	6.9	65.9	36.8	2.5
Digestive, Milk Chocolate, Tesco*	1 Biscuit/17g	85	4.1	498	6.6	62.8	23.9	3.1
Digestive, Milk Chocolate, Trufree*	1 Biscuit/12g	63	3.0	521	4.0	70.0	25.0	2.0
Digestive, Oat, Weight Watchers*	1 Biscuit/11g	50	2.1	457	6.0	66.3	18.6	6.9
Digestive, Organic, Sainsbury's*	1 Biscuit/12g	60	2.9	483	6.6	60.9	23.7	5.8
Digestive, Plain Chocolate, Asda*	1 Biscuit/17g	84	4.0	500	7.0	64.0	24.0	3.2
Digestive, Plain Chocolate, Tesco*	1 Biscuit/17g	85	4.1	499	6.2	63.5	24.4	2.8
Digestive, Plain Chocolate, Value, Tesco*	1 Biscuit/19g	97	4.9	510	6.4	61.5	26.0	2.9
Digestive, Plain, Average	***1 Biscuit/14g***	***67***	***2.9***	***480***	***7.1***	***65.6***	***20.5***	***3.5***
Digestive, Plain, M&S*	1 Biscuit/16g	80	3.9	490	6.5	62.7	23.8	3.3
Digestive, Reduced Fat, McVitie's*	1 Biscuit/15g	70	2.4	467	7.1	72.8	16.3	3.4
Digestive, Reduced Fat, Tesco*	1 Biscuit/16g	70	2.6	453	7.0	69.1	16.6	3.4
Digestive, Smart Price, Asda*	1 Biscuit/14g	67	2.9	465	6.0	65.3	20.0	3.1
Digestive, Sweetmeal, Asda*	1 Biscuit/14g	68	3.1	499	7.0	66.0	23.0	3.5
Digestive, Sweetmeal, Sainsbury's*	1 Biscuit/14g	72	3.3	498	6.0	66.4	23.1	3.3
Digestive, Sweetmeal, Tesco*	1 Biscuit/18g	80	2.6	444	8.4	70.0	14.5	3.1
Digestive, Value, Tesco*	1 Biscuit/15g	74	3.4	490	6.9	64.0	22.4	3.3
Digestive, Whole Wheat, Organic, Dove's Farm*	1 Biscuit/13g	56	2.4	446	5.9	61.6	19.5	7.8
Digestives, Chocolate, Belmont, Aldi*	1 Biscuit/17g	85	4.0	499	6.5	63.3	23.8	2.9
Digestives, Double Chocolate, Mcvitie's*	1 Biscuit/17g	83	4.1	497	6.5	60.9	24.3	3.6
Double Choc Chip, Trufree*	1 Biscuit/11g	58	3.0	523	3.0	67.0	27.0	1.8
Extremely Chocolatey Orange, M&S*	1 Biscuit/24g	120	6.2	510	7.5	59.9	26.5	2.7
Extremely Chocolatey, Dark Chocolate Rounds, M&S*	1 Biscuit/19g	97	5.6	510	6.2	55.7	29.3	6.3
Fig Roll, Tesco*	1 Biscuit/19g	70	1.6	375	4.0	69.3	8.8	3.1
Florentines, Decadent Dark Chocolate, Thomas J Fudge*	1 Florentine/19g	107	7.1	565	8.0	46.8	37.3	0.0
Florentines, Sainsbury's*	1 Florentine/8g	40	2.5	506	10.0	47.2	30.8	7.0
Fruit & Fibre, Breakfast, Belvita, Nabisco*	1 Biscuit/13g	56	2.1	430	7.5	64.0	16.0	7.8
Fruit & Spice Oat, Diet Chef Ltd*	2 Biscuits/20g	85	2.9	425	7.8	65.3	14.7	7.6
Fruit Shortcake, McVitie's*	1 Biscuit/8g	37	1.5	462	5.6	65.9	18.9	3.1
Fruit Shortcake, Sainsbury's*	1 Biscuit/8g	39	1.6	483	5.9	69.6	20.1	2.1
Fruit Shortcake, Tesco*	1 Biscuit/9g	43	1.7	473	5.8	70.1	18.8	1.9
Fruit Slices, Apple, Raisin & Currant, Aldi*	1 Biscuit/15g	57	1.0	379	7.0	72.8	6.4	1.3
Fruity Iced, Blue Parrot Cafe, Sainsbury's*	1 Pack/20g	83	1.4	415	6.0	82.0	7.0	1.1
Fruity Oat, Organic, Dove's Farm*	1 Biscuit/12g	53	2.1	453	7.5	65.1	18.1	5.6
Galettes, Bonne Maman*	1 Serving/90g	460	22.5	511	6.0	65.7	25.0	0.0

B

BISCUITS

Measure INFO/WEIGHT	per Measure KCAL	per Measure FAT	Nutrition Values per 100g / 100ml KCAL	PROT	CARB	FAT	FIBRE

	Measure	per Measure		Nutrition Values per 100g / 100ml			
	INFO/WEIGHT	KCAL	FAT	KCAL	PROT	CARB	FAT	FIBRE
Galettes, Lemon & Poppy Seed, Butter, Bonne Maman*	2 Biscuits/28g	142	7.3	506	6.4	62.0	26.0	2.0
Garibaldi, Asda*	1 Biscuit/10g	39	0.9	375	4.7	68.5	9.1	2.2
Garibaldi, Sainsbury's*	1 Biscuit/9g	35	1.0	389	5.7	67.1	10.9	3.3
Garibaldi, Tesco*	1 Biscuit/10g	40	0.9	400	4.7	74.0	9.1	2.2
Ginger Crinkle Crunch, Fox's*	1 Biscuit/12g	50	1.4	435	4.7	75.3	12.5	1.6
Ginger Crinkle, Sainsbury's*	1 Biscuit/11g	53	2.5	486	6.2	63.8	22.9	2.9
Ginger Crunch Creams, Fox's*	1 Biscuit/14g	73	3.7	518	4.6	64.8	26.7	0.0
Ginger Crunch, Hand Baked, Border*	1 Biscuit/12g	54	2.3	470	4.7	71.4	20.4	0.0
Ginger Crunches, Organic, Against the Grain*	1 Biscuit/15g	71	3.4	474	2.8	65.6	23.0	1.2
Ginger GI, Diet Chef Ltd*	1 Biscuit/20g	87	3.0	435	8.8	65.6	15.2	6.1
Ginger Nuts, CBY, Asda*	1 Biscuit/12g	56	2.0	467	5.1	73.5	16.5	1.8
Ginger Nuts, McVitie's*	1 Biscuit/10g	47	1.7	459	5.5	71.1	16.6	2.3
Ginger Nuts, Milk Chocolate, McVitie's*	1 Biscuit/14g	68	2.8	489	5.8	71.8	19.9	1.5
Ginger Nuts, Tesco*	1 Biscuit/10g	46	1.5	450	5.3	73.2	14.7	2.2
Ginger Nuts, Value, Tesco*	1 Biscuit/12g	55	1.9	460	5.2	74.2	15.8	1.6
Ginger Snap, BGTY, Sainsbury's*	1 Biscuit/12g	51	1.2	427	6.5	78.2	9.8	1.8
Ginger Snap, Fox's*	1 Biscuit/8g	35	1.0	443	4.6	77.1	12.8	1.5
Ginger Snap, Sainsbury's*	1 Biscuit/11g	47	1.6	445	5.3	73.0	14.7	2.2
Ginger Snaps, Trufree*	1 Biscuit/11g	51	1.9	467	2.5	76.0	17.0	1.5
Ginger Thins, Anna's*	1 Biscuit/5g	24	1.0	480	6.0	70.0	20.0	2.0
Ginger Thins, Asda*	1 Biscuit/5g	23	0.8	462	6.0	73.0	16.0	1.9
Ginger, Belgian Dark Chocolate, Thins, Waitrose*	1 Biscuit/10g	48	2.2	481	6.2	61.2	22.5	4.6
Ginger, Traditional, Fox's*	1 Biscuit/8g	33	1.0	404	4.4	70.1	11.7	1.4
Ginger, Value, Morrisons*	1 Biscuit/12g	55	1.9	459	5.3	74.0	15.8	1.7
Gingernut	1 Biscuit/11g	50	1.7	456	5.6	79.1	15.2	1.4
Golden Crunch Creams, Fox's*	1 Biscuit/15g	75	3.8	515	4.7	64.8	26.3	1.2
Golden Crunch, Bronte*	1 Biscuit/15g	69	3.3	474	5.1	62.5	22.6	0.0
Happy Faces, Jacob's*	1 Biscuit/16g	78	3.6	485	4.8	66.1	22.3	1.6
Hazelnut Crispies, Occasions, Sainsbury's*	1 Biscuit/7g	36	1.8	518	6.0	64.3	26.3	0.0
Hazelnut Meringue, Sainsbury's*	1 Biscuit/6g	24	1.4	404	5.0	43.0	23.5	1.1
Hobnobs, Chocolate Creams, McVitie's*	1 Biscuit/12g	60	3.1	503	6.7	60.3	26.1	4.0
Hobnobs, Light, 25% Reduced Fat, McVitie's*	1 Biscuit/14g	62	2.3	435	8.1	64.6	16.1	6.2
Hobnobs, McVitie's*	1 Biscuit/15g	72	3.2	473	7.0	61.8	20.7	5.4
Hobnobs, Milk Chocolate, McVitie's*	1 Biscuit/19g	92	4.5	479	6.8	60.7	23.3	4.5
Hobnobs, Plain Chocolate, McVitie's*	1 Biscuit/16g	81	3.9	498	6.7	63.3	24.3	4.2
Hobnobs, Vanilla Creams, McVitie's*	1 Biscuit/12g	60	3.0	501	6.1	62.3	25.2	3.6
Iced Gems, Jacob's*	1 Serving/30g	118	0.9	393	5.0	86.3	3.1	2.0
Jaffa Cakes, Asda*	1 Cake/12g	43	1.0	368	4.7	67.5	8.8	1.9
Jaffa Cakes, Basics, Sainsbury's*	1 Cake/11g	44	1.1	385	4.6	69.7	9.7	2.5
Jaffa Cakes, Belmont Biscuit Co, Aldi*	1 Cake/13g	52	1.3	400	3.7	72.8	10.2	1.0
Jaffa Cakes, Dark Chocolate, M&S*	1 Cake/11g	45	1.5	395	3.7	64.9	13.2	2.8
Jaffa Cakes, Dark Chocolate, Mini, M&S*	1 Cake/5g	20	0.8	410	3.9	62.8	15.8	1.9
Jaffa Cakes, Lunch Box, McVitie's*	1 Cake/7g	26	0.6	395	4.2	74.3	9.0	1.4
Jaffa Cakes, McVitie's*	1 Cake/12g	45	1.0	374	4.8	70.6	8.0	2.1
Jaffa Cakes, Mini Roll, McVitie's*	1 Cake/30g	108	3.5	407	4.2	66.9	13.3	2.9
Jaffa Cakes, Mini, Asda*	1 Cake/5g	21	0.8	412	3.9	63.0	16.0	1.9
Jaffa Cakes, Mini, Orange Pods, McVitie's*	1 Cake/40g	150	3.4	380	4.3	71.2	8.7	3.5
Jaffa Cakes, Mini, Tesco*	1 Cake/5g	19	0.6	380	4.0	64.0	12.0	2.0
Jaffa Cakes, Plain Chocolate, Sainsbury's*	1 Cake/13g	50	1.1	384	4.4	73.3	8.1	1.3
Jaffa Cakes, Sainsbury's*	1 Cake/11g	41	1.0	373	4.3	69.3	8.8	2.0
Jaffa Cakes, Value, Tesco*	1 Cake/11g	42	1.0	370	4.8	67.6	8.8	1.9
Jam Rings, Crawfords*	1 Biscuit/12g	56	2.1	470	5.5	73.0	17.2	1.9
Jam Sandwich Creams, M&S*	1 Biscuit/17g	80	3.7	485	5.7	64.5	22.6	1.8

BISCUITS

INFO/WEIGHT	Measure	per Measure KCAL	FAT	Nutrition Values per 100g / 100ml KCAL	PROT	CARB	FAT	FIBRE
Jam Sandwich Creams, Sainsbury's*	1 Biscuit/16g	77	3.4	486	5.0	67.0	21.8	1.6
Jammie Dodgers, Minis, Lunchbox, Burton's*	1 Pack/20g	90	2.9	452	5.5	72.7	14.7	2.5
Jammie Dodgers, Original, Burton's*	1 Biscuit/19g	83	3.0	437	5.1	69.5	15.9	1.9
Lebkuchen, Sainsbury's*	1 Biscuit/10g	39	0.8	400	5.7	76.1	8.0	1.3
Lemon Butter, Thins, Sainsbury's*	1 Biscuit/13g	65	3.5	515	5.3	60.7	27.9	2.2
Lemon Curd Sandwich, Fox's*	1 Biscuit/14g	69	3.3	494	4.7	66.2	23.4	1.3
Lemon Puff, Jacob's*	1 Biscuit/13g	69	4.1	533	4.3	58.8	31.2	2.8
Lemon Thins, Sainsbury's*	1 Biscuit/10g	47	1.7	468	5.6	72.3	17.3	1.7
Lemon, All Butter, Half Coated, Finest, Tesco*	1 Biscuit/17g	84	4.5	505	5.6	60.4	26.9	3.6
Lincoln, Sainsbury's*	1 Biscuit/8g	40	1.7	479	7.2	66.1	20.6	2.1
Malt, Basics, Sainsbury's*	1 Biscuit/8g	36	1.2	470	7.1	73.6	15.7	0.0
Malted Milk, Asda*	1 Biscuit/8g	39	1.8	490	7.0	66.0	22.0	2.0
Malted Milk, Average	*1 Biscuit/9g*	*42*	*1.9*	*490*	*7.0*	*65.6*	*22.2*	*1.8*
Malted Milk, Chocolate, Tesco*	1 Biscuit/10g	52	2.5	500	6.7	64.4	24.0	1.9
Malted Milk, Milk Chocolate, Asda*	1 Biscuit/11g	56	2.8	509	7.0	64.0	25.0	1.7
Malted Milk, Sainsbury's*	1 Biscuit/8g	40	1.8	488	7.1	65.5	21.9	2.0
Malted Milk, Tesco*	1 Biscuit/9g	44	1.9	495	6.6	66.8	21.8	2.0
Maple Leaf, M&S*	1 Biscuit/13g	50	1.9	395	5.1	59.8	14.8	2.0
Marie, Crawfords*	1 Biscuit/7g	33	1.1	475	7.5	76.3	15.5	2.3
Melts, Sesame with Chive, Carr's*	1 Biscuit/5g	23	1.2	498	8.2	57.4	26.2	3.5
Mikado, Jacob's*	1 Biscuit/13g	53	1.6	397	4.2	67.7	12.1	2.5
Milk & Cereals, Breakfast, Belvita, Nabisco*	1 Biscuit/13g	56	1.9	445	8.7	69.0	15.0	3.6
Milk Chocolate Digestive, Everyday Value, Tesco*	1 Biscuit/17g	82	3.7	494	7.2	65.4	22.3	1.7
Milk Chocolate, All Butter, M&S*	1 Biscuit/14g	70	3.6	490	7.9	57.4	25.5	1.4
Mini Assortment, M&S*	1 Biscuit/3g	12	0.6	480	6.1	63.9	22.5	2.8
Mint, Viscount*	1 Biscuit/13g	73	3.8	552	5.1	60.6	28.8	1.3
Morning Coffee, Asda*	1 Biscuit/5g	22	0.7	455	8.0	72.0	15.0	2.4
Morning Coffee, Tesco*	1 Biscuit/5g	22	0.7	450	7.6	72.3	14.5	2.4
Nice, Asda*	1 Biscuit/8g	38	1.7	480	6.0	68.0	21.0	2.4
Nice, Average	*1 Biscuit/8g*	*36*	*1.6*	*484*	*6.3*	*67.3*	*21.0*	*2.5*
Nice, Cream, Tesco*	1 Biscuit/13g	65	3.1	510	4.9	67.0	24.0	2.0
Nice, Fox's*	1 Biscuit/9g	39	1.7	450	6.3	62.4	19.4	5.0
Nice, Sainsbury's*	1 Biscuit/8g	40	1.7	486	5.9	68.3	20.9	2.7
Nice, Sainsbury's*	1 Biscuit/8g	39	1.9	490	5.8	63.1	23.8	3.8
Nice, Value, Multipack, Tesco*	1 Biscuit/8g	39	1.7	485	6.5	68.0	20.8	2.4
Nice, Value, Tesco*	1 Biscuit/5g	24	1.1	489	6.9	64.6	22.6	2.4
Oat & Chocolate Chip, Cadbury*	1 Biscuit/17g	80	3.9	485	6.9	60.2	23.9	4.2
Oat & Wholemeal, Crawfords*	1 Biscuit/14g	67	3.0	482	7.7	64.2	21.6	4.8
Oat Crumbles, Border*	1 Biscuit/15g	66	3.1	443	5.3	58.9	20.7	1.8
Oat Crunch, M&S*	1 Biscuit/14g	65	2.7	450	7.8	62.0	18.7	6.1
Oat Digestives, Nairn's*	1 Biscuit/11g	50	2.0	437	12.0	57.8	17.5	7.8
Oat Digestives, TTD, Sainsbury's*	1 Biscuit/13g	56	2.3	448	9.8	56.4	18.5	8.5
Oat, Fruit & Spice, Nairn's*	1 Biscuit/10g	43	1.5	425	7.8	65.3	14.7	7.6
Oat, Mixed Berries, Nairn's*	1 Biscuit/10g	43	1.5	427	7.5	64.8	15.3	7.1
Oat, Stem Ginger, Nairn's*	1 Biscuit/10g	43	1.5	434	8.8	65.6	15.2	6.1
Oaten, Organic, Duchy Originals*	1 Biscuit/16g	71	2.7	441	9.8	62.3	16.9	5.3
Oatie Crumbles, CBY, Asda*	1 Biscuit/14g	68	2.9	483	6.6	65.6	20.6	4.5
Oaties, Oatland, Tesco*	1 Biscuit/15g	70	3.1	470	6.5	64.9	20.5	4.5
Oatmeal Crunch, Jacob's*	1 Biscuit/8g	37	1.5	458	6.8	65.9	18.6	3.6
Oatmeal, Asda*	1 Biscuit/12g	54	2.5	470	6.0	62.0	22.0	6.0
Oaty Thins, Rude Health*	1 Thin/6g	23	0.3	380	11.5	68.5	4.7	8.7
Orange Chocolate, Organic, Duchy Originals*	1 Biscuit/13g	64	3.5	509	5.5	60.0	28.0	3.0
Orange Sultana, Go Ahead, McVitie's*	1 Biscuit/15g	58	1.2	400	5.1	75.7	8.1	3.0

BISCUITS

INFO/WEIGHT	Measure	per Measure KCAL	FAT	Nutrition Values per 100g / 100ml KCAL	PROT	CARB	FAT	FIBRE
Parmesan Cheese, Sainsbury's*	1 Biscuit/3g	18	1.0	553	14.7	56.4	29.9	1.8
Party Rings, Iced, Fox's*	1 Biscuit/6g	29	0.9	459	5.1	75.8	15.0	0.0
Peanut Butter, American Style, Sainsbury's*	1 Biscuit/13g	63	2.9	504	5.2	68.7	23.1	2.2
Petit Beurre, Stella Artois*	1 Biscuit/6g	26	0.9	440	9.0	73.0	15.0	0.0
Pink Wafers, Crawfords*	1 Biscuit/7g	36	1.9	521	2.5	68.6	26.5	1.1
Pink Wafers, Eat Me, Aldi*	1 Biscuit/8g	44	2.6	552	4.2	58.4	32.9	2.9
Pink Wafers, Sainsbury's*	1 Biscuit/8g	36	1.8	486	4.6	64.2	23.4	1.7
Puffin, Chocolate, Asda*	1 Biscuit/25g	133	7.2	533	5.0	63.0	29.0	1.2
Puffin, Orange, Asda*	1 Biscuit/25g	133	7.3	529	5.0	62.0	29.0	2.2
Raspberry & Cream Viennese, Melts, Fox's*	1 Biscuit/16g	84	4.5	521	4.0	62.1	28.1	1.7
Redcurrant Puffs, Eat Well, M&S*	1 Biscuit/7g	32	1.4	470	5.6	67.7	19.8	2.0
Rich Shorties, Asda*	1 Biscuit/10g	50	2.3	486	6.0	66.0	22.0	2.0
Rich Tea, 25% Less Fat, Tesco*	1 Biscuit/10g	44	1.1	435	7.1	77.0	11.0	1.3
Rich Tea, Average	**1 Biscuit/10g**	**45**	**1.5**	**451**	**6.8**	**72.8**	**14.5**	**2.5**
Rich Tea, Basics, Sainsbury's*	1 Biscuit/8g	35	1.2	450	7.1	71.3	15.2	2.9
Rich Tea, Belmont Biscuit Co, Aldi*	1 Biscuit/8g	37	1.2	464	7.4	74.0	15.0	3.2
Rich Tea, CBY, Asda*	1 Biscuit/8g	34	1.0	447	7.2	72.9	13.4	3.0
Rich Tea, Classic, McVitie's*	1 Biscuit/8g	38	1.3	453	7.1	71.2	15.5	2.9
Rich Tea, Essential, Waitrose*	1 Biscuit/8g	36	1.2	452	7.1	71.1	15.2	2.9
Rich Tea, Finger, Essential, Waitrose*	1 Biscuit/5g	22	0.7	450	7.2	72.5	14.3	3.0
Rich Tea, Finger, Tesco*	1 Finger/5g	23	0.7	451	7.4	72.9	14.4	2.3
Rich Tea, Fingers, Morrisons*	1 Finger/4g	22	0.7	550	10.0	90.0	17.5	5.0
Rich Tea, Light, McVitie's*	1 Biscuit/8g	36	0.9	436	7.6	75.3	10.7	3.1
Rich Tea, Low Fat, M&S*	1 Biscuit/9g	40	1.0	435	8.3	76.7	10.5	2.4
Rich Tea, Milk Chocolate Covered, Cadbury*	1 Biscuit/12g	60	2.6	490	6.6	67.6	21.4	0.0
Rich Tea, Milk Chocolate, Sainsbury's*	1 Biscuit/13g	66	3.0	504	6.3	68.5	22.7	2.1
Rich Tea, Sainsbury's*	1 Biscuit/8g	34	1.0	440	7.2	72.7	13.4	3.0
Rich Tea, Tesco*	1 Biscuit/8g	36	1.2	460	7.3	72.4	15.2	2.3
Rich Tea, Tesco*	1 Biscuit/10g	43	1.3	451	7.2	72.8	14.0	2.7
Rich Tea, Value, Tesco*	1 Biscuit/8g	35	1.2	453	7.2	72.4	15.0	2.3
Rocky, Chocolate & Caramel, Fox's*	1 Biscuit/21g	107	4.1	507	6.9	60.3	19.3	15.5
Rocky, Chocolate, Fox's*	1 Biscuit/21g	106	5.4	505	5.7	62.4	25.7	2.4
Rocky, Rounds, Chocolate, Fox's*	1 Biscuit/6g	31	1.7	517	7.2	58.5	28.3	1.6
Savoury, Organic, M&S*	1 Biscuit/7g	28	1.0	395	7.0	58.4	14.6	8.7
Scotch Finger, Arnotts Australia*	1 Biscuit/18g	88	3.9	489	6.6	65.8	21.5	0.0
Scottish Sweet Oatie, Organic, Daylesford Organic*	1 Biscuit/23g	119	7.1	516	6.1	53.9	30.7	4.7
Sea Salt & Black Pepper, for Cheese, TTD, Sainsbury's*	3 Biscuits/20g	93	4.3	484	8.8	60.1	22.4	3.8
Shortcake with Real Milk Chocolate, Cadbury*	1 Biscuit/15g	75	3.5	500	6.3	65.8	23.5	0.0
Shortcake, Asda*	1 Biscuit/14g	73	3.6	518	5.0	66.0	26.0	0.2
Shortcake, Average	**1 Biscuit/11g**	**55**	**3.0**	**501**	**6.3**	**66.1**	**27.1**	**2.1**
Shortcake, Caramel, Average	**1 Biscuit/37g**	**183**	**10.5**	**494**	**4.8**	**54.7**	**28.3**	**0.8**
Shortcake, Caramel, Mini, Finest, Tesco*	1 Biscuit/15g	74	4.2	493	4.3	56.3	27.8	1.0
Shortcake, Caramel, Mini, Thorntons*	1 Biscuit/15g	71	4.6	492	4.8	46.3	31.9	0.6
Shortcake, Caramel, Mr Kipling*	1 Biscuit/36g	182	10.4	506	4.2	57.6	28.8	1.3
Shortcake, Caramel, Squares, M&S*	1 Square/40g	190	9.6	475	5.5	59.7	23.9	1.0
Shortcake, Caramel, Squares, Tesco*	1 Square/54g	274	16.4	507	4.6	54.1	30.4	0.4
Shortcake, Crawfords*	1 Biscuit/10g	52	2.5	504	6.2	63.5	24.4	2.6
Shortcake, Dairy Milk Chocolate, Cadbury*	1 Bar/49g	252	13.5	515	7.5	59.2	27.5	0.0
Shortcake, Dutch, M&S*	1 Biscuit/17g	90	5.1	540	5.4	59.0	30.8	2.5
Shortcake, Fruit, Crawfords*	1 Biscuit/8g	34	1.5	419	5.4	55.9	19.3	2.4
Shortcake, Mini Pack, Paterson's*	1 Biscuit/17g	82	4.2	490	5.5	60.8	25.0	3.2
Shortcake, Ring, Creations, Fox's*	1 Biscuit/20g	105	5.6	515	7.8	59.1	27.4	1.0
Shortcake, Rounds, Value, Tesco*	1 Biscuit/22g	120	7.0	540	5.5	58.8	31.4	2.1

	Measure INFO/WEIGHT	per Measure		Nutrition Values per 100g / 100ml				
		KCAL	FAT	KCAL	PROT	CARB	FAT	FIBRE

BISCUITS

Shortcake, Sainsbury's*	1 Biscuit/11g	53	5.2	479	6.1	65.3	47.2	2.5
Shortcake, Snack, Cadbury*	2 Biscuits/15g	70	3.7	475	7.0	54.5	25.0	1.7
Shortcake, Value, Tesco*	1 Biscuit/10g	49	2.1	486	7.1	66.5	21.2	2.1
Shorties, Cadbury*	1 Biscuit/15g	77	3.6	511	6.5	67.3	24.0	0.0
Shorties, Fruit, Value, Tesco*	1 Serving/10g	46	1.7	457	5.7	69.3	17.4	3.0
Shorties, Rich Highland, Tesco*	1 Biscuit/10g	48	2.2	485	6.1	65.3	21.7	2.6
Shorties, Rich, Tesco*	1 Biscuit/10g	48	2.2	484	6.4	65.6	21.8	2.0
Shorties, Sainsbury's*	1 Biscuit/10g	50	2.2	500	6.4	69.8	21.8	2.0
Speculaas, Large, Hema*	1 Biscuit/23g	106	4.8	459	5.4	61.2	20.8	2.6
Spiced, Whole Wheat, Prodia*	1 Biscuit/5g	17	1.0	339	7.1	41.4	19.4	8.5
Strawberry, Biscuit Moments, Special K, Kellogg's*	2 Biscuits/25g	98	2.0	391	5.0	74.0	8.0	1.5
Strawberry, Cream Tease, McVitie's*	1 Biscuit/19g	97	4.8	510	4.8	65.9	25.2	1.2
Sugar Wafers, Vanilla, Flavoured, Triunfo*	1 Biscuit/10g	53	2.5	511	4.1	70.1	24.3	0.6
Sultana & Cinnamon, Weight Watchers*	1 Biscuit/12g	51	1.7	441	4.3	72.3	15.0	3.0
Tasties, Jam & Cream, Sandwich, Mcvitie's*	1 Biscuit/15g	74	3.4	488	4.8	65.6	22.4	2.2
Taxi, McVitie's*	1 Biscuit/27g	134	6.9	504	4.2	63.3	26.0	0.7
Teddy Bear, Mini, M&S*	1 Biscuit/17g	80	3.8	475	5.4	62.6	22.7	3.2
Toffee Apple Crumbles, Border Biscuits Ltd*	1 Biscuit/18g	77	3.7	427	5.0	56.7	20.4	2.3
Triple Chocolate, Fox's*	1 Biscuit/21g	100	5.2	478	5.7	57.3	25.1	2.5
Twix, Caramel Slice, McVitie's*	1 Slice/29g	142	7.8	491	4.5	57.3	26.8	1.4
Viennese Creams, Raspberry, M&S*	1 Biscuit/17g	90	4.9	520	4.6	60.4	28.6	1.3
Viennese Creams, Strawberry, M&S*	1 Biscuit/17g	80	3.7	485	6.4	63.0	22.2	1.7
Viennese Finger, Mr Kipling*	1 Finger/32g	167	10.2	523	4.3	54.9	31.8	0.0
Viennese Whirl, Chocolate, Border*	1 Biscuit/19g	96	4.3	512	6.5	61.9	23.2	0.0
Viennese Whirl, Fox's*	1 Biscuit/25g	130	7.0	518	6.7	60.1	27.8	0.0
Viennese, Bronte*	1 Biscuit/25g	106	6.2	424	4.4	45.6	24.8	0.0
Viennese, Chocolate, Melts, Fox's*	1 Biscuit/12g	64	3.4	526	6.1	60.5	28.3	2.4
Viennese, Jaffa, M&S*	1 Biscuit/17g	80	3.7	465	5.9	61.1	21.7	0.9
Viennese, Sandwich, Chocolate, M&S*	1 Biscuit/15g	80	4.6	535	7.2	58.0	30.6	1.7
Wafer, Vanilla, Loacker*	1 Pack/45g	231	12.6	514	7.5	58.0	28.0	0.0
Water, Asda*	1 Biscuit/6g	25	0.5	412	10.0	75.0	8.0	3.3
Water, Average	*1 Biscuit/6g*	*24*	*0.7*	*440*	*10.8*	*75.8*	*12.5*	*3.1*
Water, High Bake, Jacob's*	1 Biscuit/5g	22	0.4	414	10.5	76.4	7.4	3.0
Water, High Bake, Sainsbury's*	1 Biscuit/5g	21	0.4	412	9.8	76.3	7.5	3.2
Water, High Baked, Tesco*	1 Biscuit/5g	20	0.4	405	10.1	75.0	7.1	4.2
Water, Table, Large, Carr's*	1 Biscuit/8g	31	0.6	408	9.9	73.1	7.5	4.1
Water, Table, Small, Carr's*	1 Biscuit/3g	14	0.3	406	10.1	80.0	7.6	4.2
Wholemeal Brans, Fox's*	1 Biscuit/20g	90	4.0	451	8.5	58.8	20.2	7.5
Yoghurt Break, Red Cherry, Go Ahead, McVitie's*	1 Slice/18g	72	1.8	407	5.5	73.4	10.1	2.2
Yoghurt Break, Strawberry, Go Ahead, McVitie's*	1 Slice/18g	72	2.0	397	5.9	68.0	11.1	2.1
Yorkie, Nestle*	1 Biscuit/25g	128	6.7	510	6.7	60.4	26.8	1.3

BISON

Raw	*1oz/28g*	*31*	*0.5*	*109*	*21.6*	*0.0*	*1.8*	*0.0*

BITES

Cheese, Mrs Crimble's*	1 Bag/60g	263	8.4	439	17.0	61.0	14.0	1.0

BITTER LEMON

Low Calorie, Tesco*	1 Glass/200ml	6	0.2	3	0.1	0.3	0.1	0.1
Schweppes*	1 Glass/250ml	85	0.0	34	0.0	8.2	0.0	0.0

BLACK GRAM

Urad Gram, Dried, Raw	*1oz/28g*	*77*	*0.4*	*275*	*24.9*	*40.8*	*1.4*	*0.0*

BLACK PUDDING

Average, Uncooked	*1 Serving/40g*	*101*	*6.0*	*252*	*10.2*	*19.0*	*14.9*	*0.6*
VLH Kitchens	1 Serving/40g	105	39.0	262	11.0	20.3	15.6	0.4

	Measure INFO/WEIGHT	per Measure KCAL	FAT	Nutrition Values per 100g / 100ml KCAL	PROT	CARB	FAT	FIBRE
BLACKBERRIES								
Fresh, Raw, Average	1oz/28g	7	0.1	25	0.9	5.1	0.2	3.1
Frozen, Average	1 Serving/80g	37	0.1	46	0.9	9.6	0.2	2.9
in Fruit Juice, Average	½ Can/145g	52	0.3	36	0.6	7.9	0.2	1.3
BLACKCURRANTS								
Fresh, Raw, Fresh	1 Serving/80g	22	0.0	27	0.9	6.5	0.0	3.5
in Fruit Juice, Average	1 Serving/30g	11	0.0	38	0.6	8.6	0.2	2.4
Stewed with Sugar	1oz/28g	16	0.0	58	0.7	15.0	0.0	2.8
Stewed without Sugar	1oz/28g	7	0.0	24	0.8	5.6	0.0	3.1
BLUEBERRIES								
Chocolate Covered, Waitrose*	1 Serving/25g	120	5.6	481	4.0	65.6	22.4	3.0
Dried & Sweetened, Sainsbury's*	1oz/28g	77	0.2	275	1.7	65.7	0.6	11.7
Dried, LL, Waitrose*	1 Serving/30g	107	0.2	358	1.1	80.1	0.8	3.6
Dried, Wholefoods, Tesco*	1 Serving/20g	66	0.2	329	2.0	77.9	1.0	3.2
Frozen, Average	1 Serving/80g	41	0.2	51	0.6	13.8	0.2	4.4
Raw, Average	50 Berries/68g	39	0.2	57	0.7	14.5	0.3	2.4
BOAR								
Wild, Raw, Average	1 Serving/200g	244	6.7	122	21.5	0.0	3.3	0.0
BOILED SWEETS								
Average	1 Sweet/7g	21	0.0	327	0.0	87.1	0.0	0.0
Blackcurrant & Liquorice, Co-Op*	1 Sweet/8g	32	0.4	405	0.9	91.0	5.0	0.0
Cherry Drops, Bassett's*	1 Sweet/5g	18	0.0	390	0.0	98.1	0.0	0.0
Clear Fruits, Sainsbury's*	1 Sweet/7g	26	0.0	372	0.1	92.9	0.0	0.0
Fruit Drops, Co-Op*	1 Sweet/6g	24	0.0	395	0.2	98.0	0.0	0.0
Fruit Sherbets, Assorted, M&S*	1 Sweet/9g	35	0.4	405	0.3	91.6	4.3	0.1
Lockets, Mars*	1 Pack/43g	165	0.0	383	0.0	95.8	0.0	0.0
Mentho-Lyptus, Cherry, Sugar Free, Hall's*	1 Lozenge/4g	8	0.0	234	0.0	62.4	0.0	0.0
Mentho-Lyptus, Extra Strong, Hall's*	1 Lozenge/4g	14	0.0	389	0.0	96.9	0.0	0.0
Pear Drops, Bassett's*	1 Sweet/4g	16	0.0	390	0.0	96.4	0.0	0.0
Soothers, Blackcurrant, Hall's*	1 Lozenge/5g	16	0.0	365	0.0	91.4	0.0	0.0
Soothers, Cherry, Hall's*	1 Pack/45g	165	0.0	365	0.0	91.3	0.0	0.0
Soothers, Strawberry Flavour, Hall's*	1 Sweet/5g	19	0.0	385	0.0	96.0	0.0	0.0
BOK CHOY								
Tesco*	1 Serving/100g	11	0.2	11	1.0	1.4	0.2	1.2
BOLOGNESE								
Al Forno, Weight Watchers*	1 Pack/354g	312	6.7	88	6.6	10.3	1.9	1.8
Meatless, Granose*	1 Pack/400g	400	16.0	100	8.0	8.0	4.0	0.0
Pasta, Goodness, Tesco*	1 Pack/280g	324	8.4	116	7.1	15.1	3.0	1.8
Tagliatelle, Weight Watchers*	1 Serving/300g	300	5.4	100	5.5	15.4	1.8	0.1
BOMBAY MIX								
Average	1oz/28g	141	9.2	503	18.8	35.1	32.9	6.2
BON BONS								
Apple, Lemon & Strawberry, Co-Op*	¼ Bag/50g	202	2.5	405	1.0	88.0	5.0	0.0
Bassett's*	1 Sweet/7g	28	0.5	417	1.1	85.4	7.5	0.0
Lemon, Bassett's*	1 Sweet/7g	30	0.7	425	0.0	83.7	9.8	0.0
Mixed Fruit, Vimto, Tangerine Confectionery Ltd*	1 Sweet/5g	20	0.3	409	0.1	85.8	6.7	0.6
BOOST								
Standard Bar, Cadbury*	1 Bar/49g	250	13.8	515	5.8	58.6	28.5	1.5
Treat Size, Cadbury*	1 Bar/24g	130	7.4	535	5.3	59.6	30.5	0.0
BOUILLABAISSE								
Average	1 Serving/400g	556	38.8	139	11.2	2.0	9.7	0.4
BOUILLON								
Powder, Miso, Marigold*	1 Tsp/5g	12	0.5	248	7.0	34.0	9.3	1.4
Powder, Swiss Vegetable, Green Tub, Marigold*	1 Tsp/5g	12	0.4	243	10.5	29.4	8.1	0.7

B

	Measure INFO/WEIGHT	per Measure KCAL	FAT	Nutrition Values per 100g / 100ml KCAL	PROT	CARB	FAT	FIBRE
BOUNTY								
Dark, Mars*	1 Funsize/29g	142	8.0	488	3.7	55.7	27.6	0.0
Milk, Mars*	1 Funsize/29g	142	7.5	488	3.7	58.5	26.0	0.0
BOVRIL*								
Beef Extract, Drink, Made Up with Water, Bovril*	1 Serving/12g	22	0.1	184	38.9	4.6	1.2	0.0
Chicken Savoury Drink, Bovril*	1 Serving/13g	16	0.2	129	9.7	19.4	1.4	2.1
BRANDY								
37.5% Volume, Average	*1 Pub Shot/35ml*	*72*	*0.0*	*207*	*0.0*	*0.0*	*0.0*	*0.0*
40% Volume, Average	*1 Pub Shot/35ml*	*78*	*0.0*	*224*	*0.0*	*0.0*	*0.0*	*0.0*
Cherry, Average	*1 Pub Shot/35ml*	*89*	*0.0*	*255*	*0.0*	*32.6*	*0.0*	*0.0*
BRAWN								
Average	*1 Serving/100g*	*153*	*11.5*	*153*	*12.4*	*0.0*	*11.5*	*0.0*
BRAZIL NUTS								
Average	*6 Whole/20g*	*136*	*13.7*	*682*	*15.3*	*2.8*	*68.4*	*5.4*
Milk Chocolate, Tesco*	1 Nut/8g	47	3.5	585	9.9	38.0	43.7	1.9
BREAD								
50/50, Wholemeal & White, Medium Sliced, Kingsmill*	1 Slice/40g	94	0.9	235	9.9	41.2	2.3	4.9
Apple Sourdough, Gail's*	1 Slice/50g	118	0.4	236	7.5	43.9	0.7	4.3
Arabic, El Amar Bakery*	1 Serving/110g	318	1.3	289	11.6	57.9	1.2	0.0
Bagel, 4 Everything, Finest, Tesco*	1 Bagel/100g	268	1.8	268	11.1	51.9	1.8	2.5
Bagel, 50/50, Duo, Mini, New York Bakery Co*	1 Bagel/45g	114	1.0	254	10.8	45.2	2.2	5.1
Bagel, Caramelised Onion & Poppy Seed, Tesco*	1 Bagel/85g	221	2.1	260	10.9	47.6	2.5	3.8
Bagel, Cinnamon & Raisin, Morrisons*	1 Bagel/85g	215	1.7	253	7.7	51.1	2.0	4.5
Bagel, Cinnamon & Raisin, New York Bagel Co*	1 Bagel/90g	231	1.0	257	10.1	49.9	1.1	3.6
Bagel, Cinnamon & Raisin, Tesco*	1 Bagel/85g	230	1.4	270	10.4	51.3	1.7	3.8
Bagel, Fruit & Spice, Sainsbury's*	1 Bagel/85g	234	1.8	275	9.7	54.3	2.1	3.8
Bagel, Granary, Bagel Factory*	1 Bagel/100g	288	2.1	288	11.9	57.4	2.1	4.5
Bagel, Mini, Sainsbury's*	1 Bagel/25g	67	0.4	268	11.2	52.4	1.6	2.8
Bagel, Multi Seed, New York Bagel Co*	1 Bagel/90g	244	4.3	271	12.4	41.6	4.8	5.8
Bagel, Multigrain, Sainsbury's*	1 Bagel/113g	293	3.5	259	10.0	49.6	3.1	2.0
Bagel, Onion & Poppy Seed, Average	*1 Bagel/85g*	*225*	*2.8*	*264*	*9.0*	*50.5*	*3.3*	*3.2*
Bagel, Onion, New York Bagel Co*	1 Bagel/85g	222	1.6	261	10.6	50.4	1.9	3.1
Bagel, Onion, Tesco*	1 Bagel/85g	233	2.0	274	10.5	52.4	2.4	1.9
Bagel, Plain	1 Bagel/104g	290	2.0	279	10.6	53.8	1.9	2.9
Bagel, Plain, Asda*	1 Bagel/85g	226	2.0	265	15.0	46.0	2.3	2.9
Bagel, Plain, Average	*1 Bagel/78g*	*202*	*1.5*	*259*	*10.1*	*50.4*	*1.9*	*3.1*
Bagel, Plain, New York Bagel Co*	1 Bagel/90g	230	1.7	255	9.1	50.4	1.9	2.9
Bagel, Plain, So Organic, Sainsbury's*	1 Bagel/85g	216	2.3	254	9.0	48.4	2.7	3.6
Bagel, Plain, Tesco*	1 Bagel/85g	220	1.8	259	9.8	50.2	2.1	1.8
Bagel, Red Onion & Chive, New York Bakery Co.*	1 Bagel/90g	225	1.2	250	10.4	47.2	1.3	3.8
Bagel, Sesame Seed, Essential, Waitrose*	1 Bagel/85g	243	2.7	286	9.6	54.6	3.2	3.6
Bagel, Sesame Seed, GFY, Asda*	1 Bagel/84g	227	2.1	271	11.0	51.0	2.5	2.6
Bagel, Sesame, M&S*	1 Bagel/87g	240	2.8	275	10.2	51.2	3.2	2.1
Bagel, Sesame, New York Bagel Co*	1 Bagel/85g	226	2.6	266	10.3	49.2	3.1	4.0
Bagel, Thins, Plain, New York Bakery Co*	1 Thin/48g	133	0.6	277	9.4	55.8	1.2	2.7
Bagel, Thins, Seeded, Sliced, New York Bakery Co*	1 Thin/45g	129	1.5	286	10.0	52.1	3.4	3.9
Bagel, Thins, Sesame, Warburton's*	1 Thin/50g	130	1.7	260	10.1	46.8	3.4	3.6
Bagel, Wee Soda, Genesis Crafty*	1 Bagel/65g	148	2.5	227	6.9	41.3	3.9	2.9
Bagel, White, Asda*	1 Bagel/86g	227	2.7	264	10.0	49.0	3.1	0.0
Bagel, White, Original, Weight Watchers*	1 Bagel/67g	158	0.5	236	9.5	42.4	0.8	10.7
Bagel, Wholemeal, Average	*1 Bagel/90g*	*235*	*2.7*	*261*	*12.7*	*44.6*	*3.0*	*7.7*
Bagel, Wholemeal, Multiseed, M&S*	1 Bagel/84g	215	5.6	255	13.1	35.4	6.6	8.3
Bagel, Wholemeal, New York Bagel Co*	1 Bagel/90g	223	2.1	248	11.4	41.5	2.3	7.5
Baguette, Budgens*	1 Baguette/125g	335	1.5	268	8.5	55.7	1.2	2.3

BREAD

	Measure INFO/WEIGHT	per Measure KCAL	FAT	Nutrition Values per 100g / 100ml KCAL	PROT	CARB	FAT	FIBRE
Baguette, Crusty Brown, M&S*	½ Baguette/71g	160	1.1	225	9.8	42.7	1.6	6.3
Baguette, French, Tesco*	1 Serving/60g	144	0.7	240	7.8	49.5	1.2	3.4
Baguette, Garlic, Slices, Frozen, CBY, Asda*	1 Slice/26g	92	4.7	355	8.2	38.3	18.1	2.8
Baguette, Granary, Average	**1 Serving/100g**	**250**	**2.8**	**250**	**20.0**	**46.0**	**2.8**	**6.0**
Baguette, Granary, Co-Op*	1 Serving/60g	150	1.5	250	20.0	46.0	2.5	6.0
Baguette, Homebake, Half, Tesco*	1 Serving/75g	217	0.9	289	8.6	49.1	1.2	3.5
Baguette, Part Baked, Classique, Delifrance*	1 Pack/250g	745	3.0	298	9.8	54.8	1.2	2.7
Baguette, Part Baked, Half, Tesco*	½ Baguette/75g	180	0.9	240	7.8	49.5	1.2	3.4
Baguette, Paysanne, Stonebaked, Asda*	1/6 Baguette/46g	119	1.4	259	10.0	48.0	3.0	3.3
Baguette, Ready to Bake, Sainsbury's*	½ Baguette/62g	150	0.8	242	7.8	49.7	1.3	2.8
Baguette, Sourdough, la Brea Bakery*	1 Serving/60g	160	0.4	266	8.8	56.1	0.7	1.8
Baguette, White, Half, Crusty, M&S*	1 Baguette/162g	420	1.8	260	8.4	53.5	1.1	2.3
Baguette, White, Homebake, Tesco*	1 Baguette/150g	434	1.8	289	8.6	59.1	1.2	3.5
Baguette, White, Ready to Bake, Asda*	1 Serving/60g	168	1.1	280	10.0	56.0	1.8	2.6
Baguette, White, Sainsbury's*	1 Serving/50g	132	0.8	263	9.3	53.1	1.5	2.7
Baguette, Wholemeal, Part Baked, Asda*	½ Baguette/75g	176	1.0	235	8.2	47.7	1.3	3.0
Baguette, Wholemeal, Part Baked, Mini, Landgut*	½ Baguette/25g	56	0.2	223	7.5	46.0	1.0	0.0
Banana, with Dates & Hazelnuts, Graze*	1 Slice/19g	59	2.7	309	4.8	38.7	14.4	2.7
Baps, Brown, Large, Asda*	1 Bap/58g	140	0.9	242	10.0	47.0	1.6	0.0
Baps, Brown, Malted Grain, Large, Tesco*	1 Bap/93g	228	3.1	245	9.9	42.7	3.3	5.3
Baps, Cheese Top, Sainsbury's*	1 Bap/75g	218	6.4	291	12.1	41.6	8.5	2.0
Baps, Cheese Topped, Baker's Soft, Tesco*	1 Bap/65g	180	3.7	275	10.2	45.8	5.6	2.2
Baps, Cheese Topped, White, Tesco*	1 Bap/65g	179	3.6	275	10.2	45.8	5.6	0.7
Baps, Floured, M&S*	1 Bap/60g	168	3.7	280	11.5	46.8	6.2	0.5
Baps, Giant Malted, Sainsbury's*	1 Bap/109g	282	5.2	260	8.6	45.7	4.8	5.7
Baps, White Sandwich, Kingsmill*	1 Bap/80g	209	3.2	261	10.1	46.2	4.0	2.2
Baps, White, Average	**1 Bap/65g**	**167**	**2.3**	**257**	**9.5**	**47.0**	**3.5**	**1.9**
Baps, White, Floured, Waitrose*	1 Bap/60g	147	1.2	244	8.0	48.6	2.0	1.1
Baps, White, Giant, Sainsbury's*	1 Bap/86g	235	3.2	273	8.3	51.7	3.7	3.4
Baps, White, Giant, Waitrose*	1 Bap/104g	260	3.7	250	9.5	45.0	3.6	4.8
Baps, White, Large, Tesco*	1 Bap/95g	252	4.3	265	8.7	46.2	4.5	2.4
Baps, White, Sliced, Large, Asda*	1 Bap/58g	148	1.0	255	10.0	50.0	1.7	0.0
Baps, White, Soft, Floured, M&S*	1 Bap/61g	175	3.4	285	11.5	46.6	5.5	2.8
Baps, White, Warburton's*	1 Bap/57g	144	2.5	252	9.8	43.4	4.3	2.7
Baps, Wholemeal, Brace's*	1 Bap/59g	137	2.6	234	10.5	42.5	4.4	4.3
Baps, Wholemeal, Country Oven*	1 Bap/40g	92	1.3	231	9.5	41.0	3.3	4.1
Baps, Wholemeal, Giant, Rathbones*	1 Bap/110g	230	2.1	209	9.4	39.0	1.9	8.0
Baps, Wholemeal, Giant, Sainsbury's*	1 Bap/86g	230	3.5	268	9.7	48.1	4.1	7.7
Baps, Wholemeal, Tesco*	1 Bap/46g	104	2.4	227	9.6	41.4	5.3	5.6
Baps, Wholemeal, Waitrose*	1 Bap/63g	148	3.3	235	11.0	35.9	5.3	7.7
Baton, L'ancienne Olive, Bakery, Morrisons*	1 Serving/100g	291	9.3	291	0.0	2.9	9.3	3.4
Best of Both, Farmhouse, Hovis*	1 Slice/44g	99	1.4	226	9.5	40.0	3.1	4.9
Best of Both, Medium, Hovis*	1 Slice/38g	87	0.8	233	5.2	40.4	2.2	5.2
Best of Both, Thick Sliced, Hovis*	1 Slice/50g	113	0.9	224	9.0	40.4	1.8	5.0
Black Olive, Finest, Tesco*	1 Serving/72g	184	4.6	255	9.7	39.7	6.4	2.9
Blackpool Milk Roll, Warburton's*	1 Slice/18g	47	0.5	254	11.0	45.0	2.8	2.8
Bloomer, Multi Seed, Organic, Sainsbury's*	1 Serving/60g	160	4.1	266	10.9	40.3	6.8	8.8
Bloomer, Multi Seed, Sliced, M&S*	1 Slice/54g	150	3.9	280	10.5	43.6	7.2	3.1
Bloomer, Multiseed, Average	**1 Slice/50g**	**120**	**2.4**	**240**	**11.8**	**37.2**	**4.9**	**7.7**
Bloomer, Multiseed, Finest, Tesco*	1 Slice/50g	145	3.8	290	9.8	40.2	7.6	7.4
Bloomer, Multiseed, TTD, Sainsbury's*	1 Slice/50g	119	1.8	239	12.0	39.7	3.6	8.8
Bloomer, Soft Grain, M&S*	1 Slice/34g	80	0.5	235	9.5	45.5	1.5	3.6
Bloomer, Spelt & Sunflower, Bakery, Tesco*	1 Serving/100g	297	9.7	297	8.5	41.5	9.7	6.3

BREAD

	Measure INFO/WEIGHT	per Measure KCAL	per Measure FAT	Nutrition Values per 100g / 100ml KCAL	PROT	CARB	FAT	FIBRE
Bloomer, White, Sliced, Waitrose*	1 Slice/50g	130	0.9	259	8.5	52.1	1.8	2.6
Bloomer, Wholemeal, Organic, M&S*	1 Slice/50g	110	2.1	220	10.2	35.5	4.2	6.4
Both in One, Village Bakery, Aldi*	1 Slice/40g	95	1.0	237	8.5	43.0	2.5	4.3
Brioche, Burger Buns, Luxury, Specially Selected, Aldi*	1 Bun/50g	159	3.7	317	9.5	52.0	7.3	3.1
Brioche, French Marble, with Vanilla, Bon Appetit, Aldi*	1 Serving/50g	132	3.4	264	6.6	42.6	6.7	1.8
Brioche, Loaf, Butter, Sainsbury's*	1/8 Loaf/50g	174	5.2	347	8.0	55.0	10.5	2.2
Brioche, Rolls, Chocolate Chip, Tesco*	1 Serving/35g	131	5.6	374	8.6	49.1	16.0	6.0
Brown Bap, Large, G H Sheldon*	1 Bap/64g	169	4.3	264	5.3	47.5	6.7	4.0
Brown, Ciabatta, Rolls, Gluten Free, Dietary Specials*	1 Roll/50g	137	4.0	274	5.8	36.9	8.1	8.9
Brown, Danish, Sliced, Weight Watchers*	1 Slice/20g	48	0.4	233	9.9	40.7	1.8	7.6
Brown, Danish, Weight Watchers*	1 Slice/20g	47	0.4	235	9.8	40.7	2.0	7.4
Brown, Deli Sub, Roll, Asda*	1 Roll/60g	142	1.9	236	0.0	35.0	3.2	0.0
Brown, Farmhouse, Linwoods*	1 Slice/25g	56	0.4	225	7.3	44.4	1.7	5.8
Brown, Gluten & Wheat Free, Sliced	1 Slice/25g	56	1.3	224	3.4	41.0	5.2	9.4
Brown, Gluten Free, Genius *	1 Slice/35g	97	4.7	277	6.7	42.2	13.3	9.5
Brown, Granary Malted, thick Sliced, Waitrose*	1 Slice/40g	95	0.9	238	9.4	44.8	2.3	5.1
Brown, High Fibre, Ormo*	1 Slice/24g	57	0.6	239	9.2	42.9	2.6	7.5
Brown, Honey & Oat Bran, Vogel*	1 Serving/100g	220	4.5	220	7.9	39.2	4.5	5.7
Brown, Kingsmill Gold, Seeds & Oats, Kingsmill*	1 Slice/45g	126	4.4	280	12.2	35.6	9.8	4.9
Brown, Malted, Average	*1 Thin Slice/25g*	*60*	*0.6*	*242*	*9.4*	*45.5*	*2.4*	*4.2*
Brown, Malted, Farmhouse Gold, Morrisons*	1 Slice/38g	94	0.5	248	8.2	49.6	1.4	3.0
Brown, Medium Slice, Smart Price, Asda*	1 Slice/37g	77	0.6	210	8.0	41.0	1.6	6.0
Brown, Medium Sliced	*1 Slice/34g*	*74*	*0.7*	*218*	*8.5*	*44.3*	*2.0*	*3.5*
Brown, Medium Sliced, Bettabuy, Morrisons*	1 Slice/31g	66	0.4	212	8.6	42.0	1.3	3.6
Brown, Medium Sliced, Premium, Warburton's*	1 Slice/24g	59	0.9	249	10.5	43.2	3.7	4.3
Brown, Medium Sliced, Sainsbury's*	1 Slice/36g	81	0.7	225	8.2	43.8	1.9	3.9
Brown, Medium Sliced, Tesco*	1 Slice/36g	78	0.8	218	8.0	41.6	2.2	4.5
Brown, Mixed Grain, Original, Vogel*	1 Slice/45g	102	0.6	227	9.8	47.1	1.2	6.4
Brown, Multi Grain, Wheat Free, Gluten Free	1 Slice/33g	76	1.7	229	5.1	40.8	5.1	5.6
Brown, Sainsbury's*	1 Slice/34g	81	0.7	239	8.4	46.8	2.1	4.2
Brown, Sandwich Bread, Gluten Free, Udi's*	1 Slice/37g	79	1.1	216	5.2	39.2	2.9	6.3
Brown, Sliced, By Brennans, Weight Watchers*	1 Slice/20g	51	0.4	257	9.5	45.4	2.1	6.8
Brown, Sliced, Free From, Tesco*	1 Slice/45g	121	3.7	268	5.4	43.2	8.2	3.6
Brown, Soda, M&S*	1 Slice/40g	92	1.4	229	9.2	43.6	3.6	4.9
Brown, Sunflower & Barley, Vogel*	1 Slice/42g	100	1.9	239	9.4	40.3	4.5	6.7
Brown, Thick Slice, Tesco*	1 Slice/50g	110	1.2	219	10.3	38.9	2.5	5.3
Brown, Thick, Warburton's*	1 Slice/38g	80	0.7	211	9.4	39.2	1.8	6.2
Brown, Thin Sliced, Sainsbury's*	1 Slice/29g	65	0.5	225	8.2	43.8	1.9	3.9
Brown, Toasted, Medium Sliced, Average	*1 Slice/24g*	*65*	*0.5*	*272*	*10.4*	*56.5*	*2.1*	*4.5*
Brown, Toastie, Thick Sliced, Kingsmill*	1 Slice/44g	101	1.4	230	9.5	40.5	3.3	4.7
Brown, Very Dark, Albert Heijn*	1 Slice/35g	84	1.4	240	12.0	35.0	4.0	7.4
Brown, Wholemeal, Healthy Choice, Warburton's*	1 Slice/40g	98	1.0	244	10.4	40.7	2.5	6.5
Bruschettine, Italian, Toasted, Crosta & Mollica*	1 Portion/11g	41	1.9	382	10.1	66.2	17.6	0.0
Buns, Burger, American Style, Sainsbury's*	1 Bun/50g	131	2.1	261	10.5	45.6	4.1	3.6
Buns, Burger, Cheese & Onion Topped, Finest, Tesco*	1 Serving/105g	309	10.0	294	10.2	41.9	9.5	2.8
Buns, Burger, Giant, Sainsbury's*	1 Bun/95g	249	4.9	262	8.7	45.2	5.2	2.9
Buns, Burger, M&S*	1 Bun/58g	162	3.3	280	10.1	45.7	5.7	2.5
Buns, Burger, Sainsbury's*	1 Bun/56g	154	2.9	275	9.2	47.8	5.2	4.1
Buns, Burger, Sesame, American Style, Sainsbury's*	1 Bun/60g	162	3.8	270	7.3	46.2	6.3	2.2
Buns, Burger, Sesame, Sliced, Tesco*	1 Bun/60g	168	4.0	280	7.9	47.3	6.6	2.1
Buns, White, Burger, Waitrose*	1 Serving/64g	169	2.5	264	10.0	47.2	3.9	2.7
Buns, White, Stay Fresh, Tesco*	1 Bun/56g	152	3.7	271	7.5	45.5	6.6	0.0
Burger Buns, Warburton's*	1 Roll/60g	147	3.9	245	9.0	37.5	6.5	2.0

B

BREAD

	Measure INFO/WEIGHT	per Measure KCAL	FAT	Nutrition Values per 100g / 100ml KCAL	PROT	CARB	FAT	FIBRE
Carrot & Pumpkin, Speciality, Asda*	1 Serving/100g	247	3.4	247	10.3	41.9	3.4	3.6
Challah, Average	*1 Slice/50g*	*143*	*3.6*	*286*	*8.9*	*53.6*	*7.1*	*3.6*
Cheese & Garlic, Pizza Style, Sainsbury's*	¼ Bread/63g	199	8.1	318	10.7	39.7	13.0	2.2
Cheese & Garlic, Stonebaked, Morrisons*	¼ Bread/69g	228	9.9	331	10.9	39.5	14.4	1.9
Cheese & Onion, Tear & Share, Sainsbury's*	¼ Bread/71g	202	6.6	285	9.8	40.6	9.3	1.9
Cheese & Onion, Toastie, Warburton's*	1 Slice/42g	120	5.8	286	7.5	33.1	13.7	0.0
Cheese & Tomato, Tear & Share, Sainsbury's*	¼ Bread/72g	211	9.5	293	8.0	35.7	13.2	1.5
Cheese, Morrisons*	1 Serving/96g	297	13.6	311	9.9	35.9	14.2	3.0
Cheese, Onion & Garlic, Tear & Share, Waitrose*	¼ Bread/112g	326	14.6	290	9.4	33.9	13.0	2.1
Cheese, Tear & Share, Tesco*	¼ Loaf/73g	225	7.8	310	8.8	44.0	10.7	0.8
Cholla, Average	*1/10 Loaf/154g*	*421*	*14.3*	*274*	*6.9*	*40.8*	*9.3*	*1.0*
Ciabatta Stick, Organic, M&S*	1 Stick/140g	315	2.0	225	8.9	48.5	1.4	4.2
Ciabatta, Black Olive, Part Baked, Sainsbury's*	¼ Ciabatta/67g	172	2.5	257	8.8	46.8	3.8	2.4
Ciabatta, Finest, Tesco*	1/6 Ciabatta/45g	124	2.7	275	10.4	44.8	5.9	2.7
Ciabatta, Green Olive, Tesco*	¼ Ciabatta/70g	155	3.1	222	7.4	38.2	4.4	1.9
Ciabatta, Half, M&S*	1 Ciabatta/135g	354	5.5	262	10.3	48.1	4.1	2.1
Ciabatta, Half, Organic, Sainsbury's*	½ Ciabatta/63g	152	0.6	241	9.1	48.7	1.0	2.3
Ciabatta, Half, Part Baked, TTD, Sainsbury's*	¼ Pack/67g	173	3.3	257	8.6	44.6	4.9	3.5
Ciabatta, Half, Tesco*	1 Ciabatta/135g	351	4.7	260	8.9	47.7	3.5	2.2
Ciabatta, Italian Style, Waitrose*	1 Ciabatta/89g	231	1.2	260	10.7	51.2	1.4	2.2
Ciabatta, Organic, Tesco*	1/3 Ciabatta/100g	240	3.6	240	8.7	43.2	3.6	2.4
Ciabatta, Part Baked, Half, Sainsbury's*	½ Ciabbatta/67g	174	2.5	260	8.9	47.7	3.7	2.2
Ciabatta, Plain, Half, Two, Waitrose*	1 Roll/80g	248	5.8	310	10.0	51.3	7.2	2.2
Ciabatta, Plain, Tesco*	¼ Ciabatta/73g	174	2.8	240	9.8	41.5	3.9	2.4
Ciabatta, Ready to Bake, M&S*	1 Serving/150g	393	6.1	262	10.3	48.1	4.1	2.1
Ciabatta, Square, Bake at Home, Part Baked, Asda*	1 Roll/60g	157	2.1	262	8.4	49.1	3.5	2.1
Ciabatta, Sun Dried Tomato & Basil, Tesco*	¼ Ciabatta/75g	193	4.3	257	8.9	42.4	5.7	2.4
Ciabatta, Tomato & Basil, GFY, Asda*	1 Serving/55g	143	1.2	260	9.0	51.0	2.2	0.0
Ciabatta, Tomato & Mozzarella, Iceland*	1 Ciabatta/150g	374	15.2	249	10.0	29.6	10.1	3.3
Ciabatta, TTD, Sainsbury's*	¼ Pack/68g	185	4.0	274	10.4	44.8	5.9	2.7
Cinnamon Swirl, Asda*	1 Serving/25g	87	3.2	349	6.0	52.0	13.0	1.6
Cottage Loaf, Stonebaked, Asda*	1 Serving/67g	155	0.9	232	10.0	45.0	1.3	3.2
Crostini, Olive Oil, TTD, Sainsbury's*	1 Roll/4g	16	0.3	409	11.4	72.2	8.3	3.3
Danish, Lighter, White, Warburton's*	1 Slice/26g	63	0.3	238	10.5	45.8	1.2	2.6
Danish, White, Medium Sliced, Tesco*	1 Slice/20g	47	0.3	234	9.4	45.4	1.7	3.3
Danish, White, Thick Sliced, Tesco*	1 Slice/24g	60	0.6	250	9.7	47.4	2.3	2.9
Farl, Irish Soda, Irwin's Bakery*	1 Farl/150g	334	5.1	223	4.0	44.0	3.4	2.3
Farmhouse with Oatmeal, Batch, Finest, Tesco*	1 Slice/44g	110	1.4	240	9.8	43.2	3.1	5.2
Farmhouse, Batch, Multiseed, LL, Waitrose*	1 Slice/50g	130	3.5	259	9.9	39.2	7.0	7.2
Farmhouse, Poppy Seed, Crusty, Loaf, M&S*	1 Slice/40g	104	1.3	260	9.4	47.6	3.3	2.3
Farmhouse, Wholemeal, Average	*1 Slice/43g*	*94*	*1.4*	*219*	*10.7*	*36.2*	*3.3*	*7.3*
Ficelle, Mixed Olive, Waitrose*	1/5 Stick/50g	133	1.4	267	7.5	51.1	2.8	3.4
Fig & Hazelnut, Loaf, M&S*	1 Serving/100g	285	8.2	285	11.0	38.9	8.2	5.4
Focaccia, Harissa Peperonata, Bun, Bake at Home, M&S*	1 Bun/114g	282	8.3	247	7.9	35.8	7.3	3.2
Focaccia, Roast Cherry Tomato & Olive, GFY, Asda*	½ Pack/148g	350	6.0	237	9.0	41.0	4.1	2.8
Focaccia, Roasted Onion & Cheese, M&S*	1 Serving/89g	240	4.1	270	10.4	45.7	4.6	2.8
French	1.5" Slice/45g	110	0.0	244	8.9	53.3	0.0	2.2
French Stick, Average	*1 Serving/60g*	*147*	*0.2*	*245*	*8.7*	*52.2*	*0.4*	*2.1*
French, Sliced, Parisian*	2 Slices/39g	100	1.0	256	5.1	48.7	2.6	0.0
Fruit & Cinnamon Loaf, Finest, Tesco*	1 Slice/37g	134	4.9	363	6.4	54.6	13.2	1.5
Fruit Loaf, Apple & Cinnamon, Soreen*	1 Serving/10g	31	0.4	307	6.9	60.5	4.2	0.0
Fruit Loaf, Apple, M&S*	1 Slice/39g	100	0.6	255	8.5	51.9	1.5	3.3
Fruit Loaf, Banana, Soreen*	1 Slice/25g	78	1.0	313	6.6	61.2	4.1	2.6

BREAD

	Measure INFO/WEIGHT	per Measure KCAL	FAT	Nutrition Values per 100g / 100ml KCAL	PROT	CARB	FAT	FIBRE
Fruit Loaf, Cinnamon & Raisin, Soreen*	1/8 Loaf/25g	77	1.0	308	7.7	54.1	4.0	4.1
Fruit Loaf, Fruity Five, Snack Pack, Soreen*	1 Pack/61g	200	5.5	329	7.1	54.9	9.0	2.7
Fruit Loaf, Luxury, Christmas, Soreen*	1 Serving/28g	85	0.6	303	4.5	66.6	2.1	0.0
Fruit Loaf, Plum, Lincolnshire, Soreen*	1 Slice/25g	65	0.8	261	8.4	49.3	3.4	2.1
Fruit Loaf, Sliced, Asda*	1 Serving/36g	101	1.5	279	8.2	50.4	4.2	3.6
Fruit Loaf, Sliced, Sainsbury's*	1 Slice/40g	104	1.4	260	8.9	47.9	3.6	2.4
Fruit Loaf, Sliced, Tesco*	1 Slice/36g	100	1.8	278	6.9	51.2	5.1	3.7
Fruit Loaf, Sultana & Cherry, Sainsbury's*	1 Slice/50g	178	6.1	357	2.7	59.0	12.2	1.7
Fruit, Loaf, Banana, Lunchbox, Soreen*	1 Bar/30g	100	1.3	332	8.2	63.3	4.4	2.9
Fruit, Loaf, Toasted, Cafe Instore, Asda*	1 Slice/33g	89	1.2	269	8.0	51.0	3.7	2.9
Fruit, Raisin Swirl, Sun-Maid*	1 Slice/33g	95	1.9	287	8.3	50.4	5.8	2.6
Fruited, Malt Loaf, Weight Watchers*	1 Serving/23g	68	0.4	294	8.9	60.2	1.9	3.6
Garlic & Cheese, Slices, Tesco*	1 Slice/31g	118	5.2	380	11.7	43.9	16.8	2.0
Garlic & Gruyere, Fougasse, TTD, Sainsbury's*	¼ Bread/76g	219	6.8	288	9.5	42.6	8.9	2.9
Garlic & Herb, Ciabatta, GFY, Asda*	¼ Ciabatta/60g	137	1.4	230	8.8	43.2	2.4	1.0
Garlic & Herb, Flatbread, Tear & Share, Sainsbury's*	¼ Bread/68g	201	6.3	297	10.9	42.5	9.3	3.7
Garlic & Herb, Tear & Share, CBY, Asda*	¼ Portion/63g	185	6.7	295	9.2	39.0	10.7	2.7
Garlic with Cheese, Asda*	1 Slice/34g	130	6.1	382	11.0	44.0	18.0	0.0
Garlic, & Cheese, Tesco*	1 Serving/143g	490	24.0	343	9.4	38.5	16.8	2.0
Garlic, & Herb, Giant Feast, Sainsbury's*	1 Serving/50g	158	6.4	317	8.0	42.1	12.9	2.6
Garlic, & Herb, Tear & Share, Tesco*	1 Serving/73g	218	9.2	300	6.3	40.0	12.7	1.7
Garlic, & Parsley, Tesco*	1 Loaf/230g	699	26.7	304	9.0	41.0	11.6	2.7
Garlic, & Tomato, Pizza, Italiano, Tesco*	½ Bread/140g	405	15.1	289	7.5	40.5	10.8	2.5
Garlic, Average	*1 Serving/100g*	*327*	*13.8*	*327*	*8.1*	*43.7*	*13.8*	*1.4*
Garlic, Baguette, 25% Less Fat, Tesco*	1 Serving/100g	292	11.3	292	7.0	40.7	11.3	1.8
Garlic, Baguette, 50% Less Fat, Asda*	¼ Baguette/43g	123	3.0	287	10.0	46.0	7.0	2.5
Garlic, Baguette, Average	*1 Slice/20g*	*66*	*2.8*	*330*	*7.8*	*43.1*	*14.2*	*1.8*
Garlic, Baguette, Extra Strong, Italiano, Tesco*	¼ Baguette/53g	178	8.7	340	7.9	39.8	16.6	2.8
Garlic, Baguette, Extra Strong, Sainsbury's*	½ Baguette/85g	278	12.6	327	8.4	40.0	14.8	3.4
Garlic, Baguette, GFY, Asda*	¼ Baguette/43g	106	2.7	249	8.1	39.9	6.3	2.1
Garlic, Baguette, Good Choice, Iceland*	1/3 Baguette/54g	158	4.6	292	8.7	45.1	8.5	2.9
Garlic, Baguette, Italian, Asda*	¼ Baguette/48g	173	9.5	364	7.0	39.0	20.0	3.4
Garlic, Baguette, Italiano, Tesco*	¼ Baguette/53g	186	9.9	355	6.9	39.2	18.8	2.4
Garlic, Baguette, Light Choices, Tesco*	¼ Baguette/52g	130	2.9	250	7.0	42.2	5.5	2.4
Garlic, Baguette, Morrisons*	½ Baguette/95g	295	14.2	311	6.3	37.8	15.0	1.5
Garlic, Baguette, Reduced Fat, Average	*¼ Baguette/40g*	*102*	*2.6*	*256*	*7.9*	*41.6*	*6.4*	*2.6*
Garlic, Baguette, Reduced Fat, Waitrose*	½ Baguette/85g	230	6.8	270	8.1	41.5	8.0	2.7
Garlic, Baguette, Sainsbury's*	½ Baguette/85g	342	16.3	403	8.9	48.6	19.2	2.3
Garlic, Baguette, Slices, Tesco*	1 Serving/60g	187	9.2	312	9.8	33.8	15.3	1.7
Garlic, Baguette, Value, Tesco*	½ Baguette/85g	270	11.1	318	8.1	42.0	13.1	2.3
Garlic, Baguette, Waitrose*	½ Baguette/85g	290	15.2	341	7.1	37.8	17.9	0.0
Garlic, Baguette, White, Homebake, Tesco*	1/3 Baguette/55g	160	5.5	290	7.0	43.1	10.0	1.9
Garlic, Baguette, with Cheese, HL, Tesco*	1 Serving/50g	114	1.1	229	9.4	43.0	2.2	2.1
Garlic, Ciabatta, & Herb Butter, Sainsbury's*	½ Ciabatta/105g	345	16.3	329	8.5	38.8	15.5	0.0
Garlic, Ciabatta, BGTY, Sainsbury's*	½ Ciabatta/105g	306	13.0	291	8.7	36.2	12.4	2.7
Garlic, Ciabatta, Finest, Tesco*	1 Serving/65g	205	8.9	316	8.1	40.1	13.7	2.4
Garlic, Ciabatta, Italian, Sainsbury's*	1 Serving/145g	454	17.1	313	10.0	41.6	11.8	2.9
Garlic, Ciabatta, Italiano, Tesco*	1 Ciabatta/65g	211	9.4	324	7.7	40.9	14.4	2.2
Garlic, Ciabatta, Mini, Italiano, Tesco*	½ Ciabatta/47g	150	6.9	320	8.2	38.5	14.6	2.8
Garlic, Flatbread, Tesco*	1 Serving/83g	249	8.6	302	6.7	45.3	10.4	3.0
Garlic, Focaccia, & Onion, GFY, Asda*	¼ Focaccia/55g	150	2.2	272	12.0	47.0	4.0	0.0
Garlic, Focaccia, & Rosemary, Sainsbury's*	¼ Focaccia/75g	219	7.4	292	8.0	43.0	9.8	2.8
Garlic, Foccacia, & Rosemary, Tesco*	¼ Loaf/73g	193	4.9	266	9.0	42.1	6.8	3.7

BREAD

	Measure INFO/WEIGHT	per Measure KCAL	FAT	Nutrition Values per 100g / 100ml KCAL	PROT	CARB	FAT	FIBRE
Garlic, Italian Style Stone Baked, Morrisons*	½ Pack/115g	420	22.0	365	7.9	40.4	19.1	1.9
Garlic, Reduced Fat, Waitrose*	1 Pack/170g	551	18.7	324	6.9	49.4	11.0	0.9
Garlic, Slices, 50 % Less Fat, Asda*	1 Slice/29g	75	1.1	262	7.9	47.1	3.9	3.2
Garlic, Slices, Asda*	1 Slice/27g	88	3.3	328	8.0	46.2	12.4	2.8
Garlic, Slices, BGTY, Sainsbury's*	1 Slice/27g	82	2.2	305	9.4	48.9	8.0	2.9
Garlic, Slices, Chilled, Sainsbury's*	1 Pack/368g	1369	60.0	372	9.1	47.3	16.3	3.2
Garlic, Slices, HL, Tesco*	1 Slice/52g	131	2.2	251	8.6	44.6	4.2	2.6
Garlic, Slices, Italian, Chilled, Tesco*	1 Slice/27g	110	6.0	415	6.2	46.8	22.4	2.7
Garlic, Slices, Light Choices, Tesco*	1 Slice/30g	75	1.7	250	7.3	42.3	5.7	2.9
Garlic, Slices, Light Choices, Tesco*	1 Slice/30g	75	1.7	250	7.3	42.3	5.7	2.9
Garlic, Slices, Morrisons*	1 Slice/30g	82	2.7	272	7.3	40.2	9.1	2.6
Garlic, Stonebaked, M&S*	1 Loaf/85g	264	10.1	310	9.3	41.4	11.9	3.1
Garlic, to Share, M&S*	¼ Loaf/82g	230	10.7	280	6.5	33.2	13.0	1.3
Gluten Free, Burger Buns, Wellfoods*	1 Bun/95g	226	3.6	238	1.5	49.2	3.8	1.2
Gluten Free, Rolls, Wellfoods*	1 Roll/70g	157	1.5	224	1.9	48.8	2.2	1.5
Granary Rolls, Homebake, Hovis*	1 Roll/75g	194	1.6	259	10.2	47.7	2.2	3.6
Granary White, Hovis*	1 Slice/44g	102	1.5	233	9.7	40.8	3.5	5.6
Granary, Average	**1 Med Slice/35g**	**85**	**1.0**	**242**	**9.8**	**44.0**	**2.8**	**4.8**
Granary, Baps, Large, Asda*	1 Bap/64g	143	1.4	224	10.0	41.0	2.2	4.3
Granary, Country, Multiseeded, Hovis*	1 Slice/44g	96	1.3	218	11.1	37.0	2.9	6.5
Granary, M&S*	1 Slice/30g	75	0.9	250	9.5	46.4	3.1	3.2
Granary, Malted, Medium Brown, Asda*	1 Slice/35g	81	0.9	231	9.0	43.0	2.6	3.3
Granary, Original, Thin Sliced, Hovis*	1 Slice/33g	84	0.8	256	10.6	46.4	2.4	3.7
Granary, Original, Thick Sliced, Hovis*	1 Slice/44g	112	1.0	256	10.3	46.4	2.4	3.7
Granary, Seeded, Sunflower, Hovis*	1 Slice/44g	119	2.5	271	10.1	44.9	5.7	2.9
Granary, Thick Slice, COU, M&S*	1 Slice/25g	60	0.6	240	10.5	44.1	2.2	6.0
Granary, Waitrose*	1 Slice/40g	88	1.0	220	9.4	39.9	2.5	4.3
Granary, White, Seeded, Medium Sliced, Hovis*	1 Slice/44g	109	1.8	248	10.9	41.7	4.2	3.8
Granary, Wholemeal, Average	**1 Med Slice/35g**	**80**	**0.9**	**228**	**10.8**	**38.4**	**2.6**	**6.6**
Granary, Wholemeal, Hovis*	1 Slice/44g	104	1.1	237	10.6	39.8	2.4	6.8
Granary, Wholemeal, Seeded, Medium Sliced, Hovis*	1 Slice/44g	104	1.1	237	10.6	39.8	2.4	6.8
Half Wheat Rye, The Polish Bakery, Tesco*	1 Slice/40g	93	0.6	233	5.7	51.1	1.5	6.6
Heyford Sliced Bloomer, Waitrose*	1 Slice/50g	104	1.6	208	10.1	35.0	3.1	6.6
High Bran, Loaf, M&S*	2 Slices/62g	143	2.4	230	13.1	31.7	3.9	7.7
Hot Cross Bun, Loaf, Warburton's*	1 Slice/35g	94	1.3	269	8.3	50.4	3.7	2.9
Irish Barm Brack, Tesco*	1 Serving/75g	232	5.2	310	16.0	47.6	6.9	3.0
Irish Brown Soda, Tesco*	1 Serving/50g	110	1.9	219	9.2	36.2	3.8	6.4
Irish Brown, Soda, Sainsbury's*	1 Serving/100g	208	3.0	208	8.8	36.4	3.0	5.3
Irish Cottage Wheaten, Tesco*	1 Serving/40g	79	0.8	198	9.1	35.4	1.9	6.1
Irish Sliced Fruit Soda, Irwin's Bakery*	2 Slices/80g	218	4.2	273	2.4	53.8	5.3	2.5
Juvela*	1 Slice/25g	60	0.8	240	3.3	50.0	3.0	1.7
Khobez, Flatbread, White, Dina Foods Ltd*	1 Bread/56g	158	0.6	282	10.5	57.5	1.1	3.0
Low GI, Multiseed, Percy Ingle*	1 Med Slice/35g	99	3.1	283	0.0	0.0	8.9	6.0
Malt Loaf, Chocolate, Soreen*	1 Serving/100g	334	6.3	334	8.0	58.7	6.3	5.1
Malt Loaf, Family, Asda*	1 Serving/20g	54	0.3	270	8.0	56.0	1.5	5.0
Malt Loaf, Fruity, Sliced, Soreen*	1 Slice/33g	101	0.7	303	7.6	62.1	2.2	3.8
Malt Loaf, Original, Low Fat, Soreen*	1 Slice/22g	63	0.4	288	7.5	60.0	1.6	2.0
Malted Brown, Slice, BGTY, Sainsbury's*	1 Slice/22g	53	0.6	239	12.1	41.4	2.8	5.8
Malted Brown, Thick Sliced, Organic, Tesco*	1 Slice/44g	111	0.9	249	8.9	48.8	2.0	3.5
Malted Danish, Weight Watchers*	1 Slice/20g	49	0.3	241	12.3	44.5	1.7	4.3
Malted Grain, Co-Op*	1 Slice/43g	99	0.9	230	8.0	46.0	2.0	3.0
Malted Grain, Good As Gold, Kingsmill*	1 Slice/47g	114	1.2	243	9.5	45.4	2.6	4.2
Malted Wheatgrain, Roberts Bakery*	1 Slice/30g	80	1.0	265	11.0	48.0	3.3	3.6

	Measure INFO/WEIGHT	per Measure		Nutrition Values per 100g / 100ml				
		KCAL	FAT	KCAL	PROT	CARB	FAT	FIBRE
BREAD								
Malted, & Seeded, Batch, Organic, Waitrose*	1 Slice/50g	118	2.0	236	10.9	39.5	3.9	6.2
Malted, Danish, Sliced, Weight Watchers*	1 Slice/20g	51	0.3	249	11.8	45.1	1.5	4.2
Malted, Wheat Loaf, Crusty, Finest, Tesco*	1 Slice/50g	115	0.8	230	9.8	44.2	1.5	4.4
Mediterranean Olive, Waitrose*	1 Slice/30g	82	2.8	273	7.4	40.1	9.2	4.9
Milk Roll, Warburton's*	1 Slice/18g	46	0.5	253	11.0	45.1	2.7	2.7
Mixed Seed, Organic, Duchy Originals*	1 Slice/43g	114	3.4	269	10.9	39.1	8.1	5.3
Multi Seeded Loaf, Gluten & Wheat Free, Lovemore*	1 Serving/35g	102	4.3	291	0.0	3.0	12.3	0.0
Multigrain, Batch, Finest, Tesco*	1 Slice/50g	117	1.4	235	10.8	40.4	2.9	5.5
Multigrain, Brennans*	1 Slice/40g	110	1.3	275	8.8	48.0	3.3	6.3
Multigrain, Brown, Farmhouse Baker's, M&S*	1 Slice/51g	115	2.8	225	13.0	31.2	5.4	5.1
Multigrain, Crusty, Finest, Tesco*	1 Slice/40g	98	1.4	245	9.0	44.7	3.4	5.0
Multigrain, Sliced, Fresh & Easy*	1 Slice/40g	110	1.0	275	10.0	52.5	2.5	5.0
Multigrain, Soft Batch, Sainsbury's*	1 Slice/44g	106	2.9	242	11.3	34.5	6.5	5.6
Multigrain, Sub Rolls, Asda*	1 Sub/150g	357	6.3	238	0.0	0.0	4.2	0.0
Multigrain, Tesco*	1 Slice/31g	66	1.0	214	11.1	36.8	3.2	8.9
Multigrain, Thick Sliced, Tesco*	1 Slice/50g	112	1.2	225	8.4	42.2	2.5	3.9
Multiseed Farmhouse Batch, Finest, Tesco*	1 Slice/44g	108	1.9	245	9.9	40.4	4.4	7.5
Multiseed, Farmhouse, Finest, Tesco*	1 Slice/50g	135	3.8	270	12.5	37.0	7.7	5.8
Naan, Asda*	1 Naan/130g	308	2.3	237	7.7	47.4	1.8	2.2
Naan, Average	**1 Naan/130g**	**344**	**5.6**	**264**	**8.3**	**48.5**	**4.3**	**2.0**
Naan, Bombay Brassiere, Sainsbury's*	1 Naan/140g	372	4.3	266	9.8	49.6	3.1	2.9
Naan, Chilli & Mango, Finest, Tesco*	½ Naan/90g	230	5.1	255	8.4	41.9	5.7	3.2
Naan, Garlic & Coriander, Large, TTD, Sainsbury's*	¼ Pack/70g	194	3.8	277	9.4	47.7	5.4	2.2
Naan, Garlic & Coriander, M&S*	1 Naan/150g	375	2.1	250	9.8	50.1	1.4	2.0
Naan, Garlic & Coriander, Mild, Patak's*	1 Naan/140g	452	15.1	323	9.0	47.5	10.8	0.0
Naan, Garlic & Coriander, Mini, Asda*	1 Naan/110g	320	12.5	291	6.9	40.2	11.4	2.5
Naan, Garlic & Coriander, Mini, Finest, Tesco*	1 Naan/50g	160	6.8	320	6.7	42.4	13.5	0.8
Naan, Garlic & Coriander, Mini, Sainsbury's*	1 Naan/50g	140	2.0	280	8.2	51.2	4.1	2.6
Naan, Garlic & Coriander, Mini, Sharwood's*	1 Naan/40g	114	3.0	285	7.5	45.5	7.5	3.4
Naan, Garlic & Coriander, Mini, Tesco*	1 Naan/65g	185	5.0	285	7.6	45.6	7.7	2.6
Naan, Garlic & Coriander, Mini, Weight Watchers*	1 Naan/40g	100	1.0	250	9.3	47.6	2.5	4.2
Naan, Garlic & Coriander, Sainsbury's*	1 Serving/130g	373	10.0	287	8.7	45.8	7.7	2.4
Naan, Garlic & Coriander, Tesco*	½ Naan/83g	235	6.4	285	7.6	45.6	7.7	2.6
Naan, Garlic & Coriander, TTD, Sainsbury's*	1 Serving/70g	215	8.1	307	7.0	43.9	11.5	2.9
Naan, Garlic & Coriander, Weight Watchers*	1 Naan/60g	155	2.6	259	8.9	46.0	4.3	3.4
Naan, Light Choices, Tesco*	1 Naan/71g	181	1.6	255	7.5	50.7	2.2	2.3
Naan, Mini, Light Choices, Tesco*	1 Naan/65g	150	1.8	230	8.1	42.5	2.8	2.9
Naan, Onion & Mint, M&S*	½ Naan/135g	351	11.7	260	8.9	35.8	8.7	2.5
Naan, Peshwari, Apple & Coconut, Mini, Sharwood's*	1 Naan/40g	112	2.7	281	6.9	46.6	6.7	3.1
Naan, Peshwari, Finest, Tesco*	1 Naan/130g	338	7.3	260	8.6	43.7	5.6	4.9
Naan, Peshwari, Mega, Asda*	1 Naan/220g	680	26.4	309	7.1	43.1	12.0	2.7
Naan, Peshwari, Sharwood's*	1 Naan/130g	334	6.9	257	7.2	45.1	5.3	2.5
Naan, Peshwari, Tesco*	1 Naan/215g	684	26.7	318	7.5	48.9	12.4	4.8
Naan, Plain, Average	**1 Naan/160g**	**437**	**10.5**	**273**	**8.0**	**45.7**	**6.5**	**2.1**
Naan, Plain, Large, Sainsbury's*	½ Naan/70g	191	4.6	273	7.1	46.2	6.6	3.0
Naan, Plain, Mega, Indian Takeaway, Asda*	1 Naan/222g	572	8.4	258	7.0	49.0	3.8	2.5
Naan, Plain, Mini, Asda*	1 Naan/58g	156	2.7	269	8.0	49.0	4.6	2.3
Naan, Plain, Mini, BGTY, Sainsbury's*	1 Naan/50g	113	1.1	226	8.2	43.2	2.2	3.3
Naan, Plain, Mini, Weight Watchers*	1 Naan/44g	108	1.1	245	9.1	46.5	2.5	4.9
Naan, Plain, Sharwood's*	1 Naan/120g	326	8.9	272	8.5	42.9	7.4	2.4
Naan, Plain, Tesco*	1 Naan/150g	392	6.9	261	8.4	46.4	4.6	2.3
Naan, Plain, Value, Tesco*	1 Naan/135g	363	9.7	269	8.1	42.9	7.2	1.6
Naan, Take Away, Tesco*	1 Naan/39g	97	1.3	248	8.7	45.6	3.4	1.7

BREAD

	Measure INFO/WEIGHT	per Measure KCAL	per Measure FAT	Nutrition Values per 100g / 100ml KCAL	PROT	CARB	FAT	FIBRE
Naan, Tandoori Baked, Waitrose*	1 Naan/140g	372	4.3	266	9.8	49.6	3.1	2.9
Oatmeal, Loaf, Greggs*	1 Serving/80g	190	2.0	238	10.0	38.8	2.5	0.0
Oatmeal, Sliced Loaf, Tesco*	1 Slice/50g	111	1.7	222	7.4	40.5	3.4	2.8
Olive, Waitrose*	1 Slice/28g	86	3.0	306	9.0	43.6	10.6	2.0
Pain Au Raisin, M&S*	1 Pain/74g	215	9.5	290	5.3	38.7	12.8	1.2
Pane Pugliese, Italian, Toasting, Crosta & Mollica*	1 Slice/69g	184	0.8	267	8.6	55.5	1.2	0.2
Pave, Walnut, Sainsbury's*	1 Serving/50g	140	4.8	280	9.0	40.0	9.5	3.5
Petit Pain, Homebake, Mini, Tesco*	1 Roll/50g	120	0.6	240	7.8	48.5	1.2	3.4
Petit Pain, Organic, Tesco*	1 Roll/100g	235	0.8	235	7.8	49.1	0.8	1.2
Petit Pain, Part Bake, Weight Watchers*	1 Roll/50g	111	0.4	223	6.8	43.5	0.9	6.8
Petits Pains, Mini, Homebake, Tesco*	1 Roll/45g	110	0.6	245	7.8	49.7	1.3	2.5
Pitta, 159, Pride Valley*	1 Pitta/63g	159	1.2	252	10.1	51.2	1.9	2.6
Pitta, Bakersfield*	1 Pitta/67g	167	0.7	250	7.0	52.0	1.0	1.5
Pitta, Brown, Organic, Waitrose*	1 Pitta/53g	124	0.5	234	8.5	43.9	1.0	7.4
Pitta, Free From, Sainsbury's*	1 Pitta/65g	164	2.5	252	4.1	50.0	3.9	2.9
Pitta, Garlic & Coriander, Asda*	1 Pitta/55g	116	0.5	212	7.0	44.0	0.9	1.8
Pitta, Garlic & Herb, Tesco*	1 Pitta/60g	134	1.2	223	9.6	44.6	2.0	3.0
Pitta, Garlic, Morrisons*	1 Pitta/60g	149	1.1	249	9.7	51.1	1.8	0.0
Pitta, Multi Seed & Cereal, The Food Doctor*	1 Pitta/70g	157	1.9	224	10.1	39.9	2.7	10.2
Pitta, Organic, Tesco*	1 Pitta/60g	124	0.8	206	8.3	40.2	1.4	5.7
Pitta, Pockets, Pride Valley*	1 Pitta/63g	151	0.6	239	9.3	48.4	0.9	3.2
Pitta, Pockets, Sainsbury's*	1 Pitta/75g	188	0.8	250	8.5	52.0	1.0	3.5
Pitta, Seeded, HL, Tesco*	1 Pitta/60g	153	3.6	255	10.8	39.4	6.0	12.8
Pitta, White Picnic, Waitrose*	1 Pitta/30g	75	0.4	249	10.3	49.3	1.2	3.5
Pitta, White, Average	*1 Pitta/75g*	*191*	*1.1*	*255*	*9.2*	*50.8*	*1.5*	*2.7*
Pitta, White, Basics, Sainsbury's*	1 Pitta/48g	124	0.6	261	8.8	52.7	1.2	2.0
Pitta, White, Free From, Tesco*	1 Pitta/55g	140	1.2	255	6.5	52.6	2.1	5.5
Pitta, White, Greek Style, Asda*	1 Pitta/50g	126	1.0	253	8.0	51.0	1.9	0.0
Pitta, White, Large, Tesco*	1 Pitta/90g	252	1.9	280	9.8	55.1	2.1	3.4
Pitta, White, M&S*	1 Pitta/61g	146	1.2	240	9.3	46.9	2.0	3.6
Pitta, White, Mini, Sainsbury's*	1 Pitta/20g	54	0.2	268	8.8	54.6	1.2	2.0
Pitta, White, Mini, Tesco*	1 Pitta/30g	84	0.6	280	9.8	55.1	2.1	3.4
Pitta, White, Organic, Sainsbury's*	1 Pitta/59g	150	0.6	254	10.3	50.7	1.1	2.5
Pitta, White, Sainsbury's*	1 Pitta/60g	161	0.8	269	9.0	54.1	1.3	2.5
Pitta, White, Speciality Breads, Waitrose*	1 Pitta/60g	149	0.7	249	10.3	49.3	1.2	3.5
Pitta, White, Tesco*	1 Pitta/60g	170	1.3	283	9.8	55.2	2.2	3.3
Pitta, White, Weight Watchers*	1 Pitta/45g	106	0.3	238	8.7	45.9	0.7	6.7
Pitta, Wholemeal, Acropolis, Lidl*	1 Pitta/57g	136	0.9	238	12.0	44.0	1.6	6.0
Pitta, Wholemeal, Asda*	1 Pitta/56g	133	0.9	238	12.0	44.0	1.6	6.0
Pitta, Wholemeal, Average	*1 Pitta/64g*	*154*	*1.1*	*241*	*11.0*	*45.8*	*1.7*	*6.4*
Pitta, Wholemeal, Essential, Waitrose*	1 Pitta/60g	145	0.5	242	12.4	46.0	0.9	6.0
Pitta, Wholemeal, Healthy Eating, Co-Op*	1 Pitta/63g	135	1.3	215	12.0	37.0	2.0	9.0
Pitta, Wholemeal, Hollyl& Bakery*	1 Pitta/20g	48	0.3	242	13.1	43.7	1.6	6.0
Pitta, Wholemeal, M&S*	1 Pitta/60g	155	1.6	255	10.0	45.0	2.6	5.5
Pitta, Wholemeal, Mini, M&S*	1 Pitta/18g	44	0.4	247	10.3	45.8	2.5	5.6
Pitta, Wholemeal, Mini, Organic, Newbury Phillips*	1 Pitta/100g	144	1.7	144	10.3	50.8	1.7	6.4
Pitta, Wholemeal, Mini, Tesco*	1 Pitta/30g	76	0.5	255	11.8	48.2	1.7	4.2
Pitta, Wholemeal, Sainsbury's*	1 Pitta/60g	154	1.0	257	9.8	47.8	1.7	5.8
Pitta, Wholemeal, Tesco*	1 Pitta/63g	151	0.8	240	9.5	44.5	1.2	6.4
Pitta, Wholemeal, Waitrose*	1 Pitta/60g	145	0.5	242	12.4	46.0	0.9	3.1
Pitta, Wholemeal, Weight Watchers*	1 Pitta/46g	106	0.6	229	8.7	44.5	1.2	7.6
Potato & Rosemary, M&S*	1 Serving/40g	108	2.7	270	9.4	42.2	6.8	2.3
Potato Farls, Irish, Rankin Selection, Irwin's Bakery*	1 Farl/60g	110	2.2	184	2.3	34.4	3.6	2.5

BREAD

INFO/WEIGHT	Measure	per Measure		Nutrition Values per 100g / 100ml				
		KCAL	FAT	KCAL	PROT	CARB	FAT	FIBRE
Potato Farls, M&S*	1 Farl/55g	79	0.2	144	4.2	33.8	0.4	4.7
Potato Farls, Sunblest*	1 Farl/100g	156	0.9	156	3.8	33.2	0.9	1.9
Pumpernickel, Average	*1 Slice/50g*	*96*	*0.6*	*191*	*5.5*	*37.9*	*1.1*	*7.8*
Pumpernickel, Organic, Bavarian Pumpernickel*	1 Slice/50g	90	0.5	180	6.0	38.0	1.0	10.0
Pumpernickel, Rye, Kelderman*	1 Slice/50g	92	0.5	185	6.0	38.0	1.0	0.0
Raisin & Pumpkin Seed, Organic, Tesco*	1 Slice/30g	76	1.7	253	9.7	40.6	5.8	3.8
Raisin Loaf with Cinnamon, Warburton's*	1 Slice/36g	96	1.3	267	7.2	51.1	3.7	3.2
Roasted Onion, M&S*	1 Slice/50g	125	1.6	250	9.0	46.7	3.3	2.1
Rolls, American Style Deli, Tesco*	1 Roll/65g	162	2.2	249	7.8	46.8	3.4	1.6
Rolls, Batched Sandwich, Warburton's*	1 Roll/60g	148	2.5	246	9.6	42.7	4.1	0.0
Rolls, Best of Both, Hovis*	1 Roll/62g	148	2.9	239	9.8	39.7	4.6	5.0
Rolls, Brioche	1 Roll/53g	191	7.5	361	8.8	50.1	14.1	1.5
Rolls, Brioche, Average	*1 Roll/49g*	*177*	*6.9*	*361*	*8.8*	*50.1*	*14.1*	*1.5*
Rolls, Brioche, Butter, Tesco*	1 Roll/35g	124	4.0	355	8.8	53.3	11.4	2.0
Rolls, Brioche, Continental Classics*	1 Roll/35g	122	3.3	349	8.2	58.3	9.3	0.0
Rolls, Brioche, La Boulangere, Lidl*	1 Roll/35g	122	3.6	350	8.2	55.5	10.2	1.8
Rolls, Brioche, Milk Chocolate Chip, CBY, Asda*	1 Roll/25g	91	3.6	363	8.0	50.0	14.5	1.8
Rolls, Brioche, Plain Chocolate Chip, Sainsbury's*	1 Roll/35g	131	5.6	374	8.5	49.0	16.0	5.9
Rolls, Brioche, Sainsbury's*	1 Roll/32g	116	3.7	362	8.5	56.0	11.5	3.6
Rolls, Brioche, Tesco*	1 Roll/26g	92	2.9	349	8.5	54.0	11.0	0.0
Rolls, Brown, Crusty	*1 Roll/50g*	*128*	*1.4*	*255*	*10.3*	*50.4*	*2.8*	*3.5*
Rolls, Brown, Free From, Tesco*	1 Roll/65g	174	5.3	268	5.4	43.2	8.2	3.6
Rolls, Brown, Large, Asda*	1 Roll/57g	138	0.9	242	10.0	47.0	1.6	0.0
Rolls, Brown, M&S*	1 Roll/105g	242	6.4	230	9.2	37.3	6.1	4.4
Rolls, Brown, Malted Grain, Tesco*	1 Roll/58g	144	1.9	248	8.7	46.2	3.2	1.9
Rolls, Brown, Mini, M&S*	1 Roll/33g	80	2.5	245	9.8	35.5	7.6	3.8
Rolls, Brown, Morning, Farmfoods*	1 Roll/50g	134	1.8	269	12.0	47.0	3.7	4.2
Rolls, Brown, Old Fashioned, Waitrose*	1 Roll/63g	152	2.6	241	9.6	41.3	4.1	4.7
Rolls, Brown, Seeded, Organic, Sainsbury's*	1 Roll/70g	166	3.2	237	9.9	39.1	4.6	6.5
Rolls, Brown, Snack, Allinson*	1 Roll/44g	119	2.9	270	10.8	41.6	6.7	5.6
Rolls, Brown, Soft, Average	*1 Roll/50g*	*134*	*1.9*	*268*	*10.0*	*51.8*	*3.8*	*3.5*
Rolls, Brown, Soft, Organic, Sainsbury's*	1 Roll/70g	166	3.2	237	9.9	39.1	4.6	6.6
Rolls, Brown, Soft, Tesco*	1 Roll/50g	118	1.8	235	9.0	41.6	3.6	4.5
Rolls, Cheese Topped, Sandwich Rolls, Warburton's*	1 Roll/62g	168	4.0	270	12.1	40.7	6.5	2.6
Rolls, Cheese Topped, Village Green*	1 Roll/56g	159	4.1	284	13.1	41.2	7.4	4.8
Rolls, Ciabatta, Cheese Topped, Mini, Finest, Tesco*	1 Roll/30g	85	2.4	282	11.5	40.9	8.1	3.8
Rolls, Ciabatta, M&S*	1 Roll/80g	210	3.3	262	10.3	48.1	4.1	2.1
Rolls, Ciabatta, Mini, Finest, Tesco*	1 Roll/30g	89	2.0	297	9.9	49.1	6.8	4.1
Rolls, Ciabatta, Sun Dried Tomato, Mini, Finest, Tesco*	1 Roll/30g	79	1.9	262	8.7	42.3	6.4	2.6
Rolls, Ciabatta, Tesco*	1 Roll/80g	208	2.5	260	8.6	48.2	3.1	3.3
Rolls, Corn Topped, Greggs*	1 Roll/76g	190	2.5	250	9.9	44.7	3.3	0.0
Rolls, Country Grain, Mini, M&S*	1 Roll/31g	85	3.0	275	10.2	38.9	9.7	3.8
Rolls, Crisp, Original, Organic, Kallo*	1 Roll/9g	34	0.5	390	11.0	74.0	5.6	3.0
Rolls, Crusty, Booths*	1 Roll/50g	124	0.6	247	8.7	50.3	1.2	2.6
Rolls, Crusty, French, M&S*	1 Roll/65g	159	0.8	245	8.1	50.5	1.2	3.3
Rolls, Crusty, Part-Baked, Budgens*	1 Roll/50g	148	0.7	296	9.4	61.4	1.4	2.5
Rolls, Finger, Morrisons*	1 Roll/46g	119	0.8	259	10.7	50.0	1.8	2.3
Rolls, Finger, White, Sainsbury's*	1 Roll/40g	96	1.0	240	9.0	45.2	2.6	3.2
Rolls, Focaccia, Tesco*	1 Roll/75g	226	7.0	302	8.7	45.6	9.4	3.8
Rolls, Gluten Free, Antoinette Savill*	1 Roll/70g	157	1.5	224	1.9	48.8	2.2	1.5
Rolls, Granary, Average	*1 Roll/70g*	*176*	*2.7*	*251*	*9.6*	*45.2*	*3.9*	*3.3*
Rolls, Granary, Bakers Premium, Tesco*	1 Roll/65g	158	0.8	243	9.9	47.8	1.3	2.3
Rolls, Granary, Mini, Tesco*	1 Roll/34g	92	2.2	271	10.0	43.5	6.5	3.8

BREAD

INFO/WEIGHT	Measure	per Measure		Nutrition Values per 100g / 100ml				
		KCAL	FAT	KCAL	PROT	CARB	FAT	FIBRE
Rolls, Granary, Original, Hovis*	1 Roll/70g	180	2.9	257	10.7	44.3	4.1	5.3
Rolls, Granary, Waitrose*	1 Roll/59g	160	3.8	271	10.0	47.2	6.4	3.8
Rolls, Green Olive, M&S*	1 Roll/75g	210	4.5	280	11.2	44.0	6.0	1.8
Rolls, Heyford Wholemeal, Soft & Grainy, Waitrose*	1 Roll/75g	164	1.3	219	11.2	36.7	1.7	5.8
Rolls, Hot Dog, Sliced, Asda*	1 Roll/84g	197	2.8	234	7.0	44.0	3.3	0.0
Rolls, Hot Dog, Tesco*	1 Roll/85g	200	2.8	235	7.3	44.0	3.3	1.9
Rolls, Hot Dog, Value, Tesco*	1 Roll/40g	93	0.8	232	8.7	45.0	1.9	2.2
Rolls, Hot Dog, Warburton's*	1 Roll/60g	137	2.8	228	8.7	37.8	4.7	1.7
Rolls, Malted Grain, Sainsbury's*	1 Roll/68g	190	2.9	280	8.7	51.6	4.3	4.2
Rolls, Malted, Whole Grain Rolls, Batched, Soft, M&S*	1 Roll/80g	180	3.6	225	7.8	38.5	4.5	3.1
Rolls, Mini Submarine, M&S*	1 Roll/23g	63	1.1	275	11.4	47.7	4.9	1.1
Rolls, Morning, Tesco*	1 Roll/48g	117	1.2	243	10.4	44.8	2.5	4.7
Rolls, Multi Seed, Free From, Free From, Tesco*	1 Roll/70g	214	8.3	305	5.4	44.2	11.8	6.3
Rolls, Multigrain, Pain Rustique, Finest, Tesco*	1 Roll/60g	162	4.3	270	12.7	38.4	7.1	9.6
Rolls, Multigrain, Torpedo, Sainsbury's*	1 Roll/112g	328	7.5	293	10.5	47.7	6.7	6.3
Rolls, Oatmeal, Ploughmans, GFY, Asda*	1 Roll/72g	181	3.2	252	10.0	43.0	4.4	3.9
Rolls, Oatmeal, Soft, M&S*	1 Roll/83g	224	3.9	270	12.3	43.4	4.7	3.4
Rolls, Panini, Sainsbury's*	1 Roll/90g	249	5.6	276	11.0	44.1	6.2	3.0
Rolls, Panini, White, Tesco*	1 Roll/75g	210	4.6	280	10.1	45.2	6.1	2.7
Rolls, Part Baked, Mini, Tesco*	1 Roll/50g	120	0.6	240	7.8	49.5	1.2	3.4
Rolls, Poppy Seeded Knot, Waitrose*	1 Roll/60g	169	3.2	282	10.3	48.3	5.3	2.2
Rolls, Pumpkin Seed, Lidl*	1 Roll/80g	271	9.0	339	15.0	42.5	11.2	3.8
Rolls, Scottish Morning, Morrisons*	1 Roll/60g	157	1.3	261	11.3	51.4	2.2	2.4
Rolls, Seeded, Deli, Rowan Hill Bakery, Lidl*	1 Roll/75g	221	5.6	295	11.0	43.0	7.5	5.7
Rolls, Seeded, Mixed Mini Loaf Pack, M&S*	1 Roll/76g	220	7.3	290	10.6	39.7	9.6	4.0
Rolls, Seeded, Oval Bite, Gregg's *	1 Roll/79g	220	4.5	278	10.1	44.3	5.7	0.0
Rolls, Snack, Mini, Tesco*	1 Roll/35g	95	2.1	271	19.0	43.0	6.0	4.0
Rolls, Soft, Wholemeal, Finger, M&S*	1 Roll/66g	145	1.3	220	12.6	38.0	2.0	5.8
Rolls, Sub, Seeded, Greggs*	1 Roll/97g	270	4.0	278	11.3	46.9	4.1	0.0
Rolls, Sun Dried Tomato, Homebake, Tesco*	1 Roll/50g	123	1.5	246	11.3	44.0	3.0	0.0
Rolls, Sunflower Seed, Toasting, Good & Hot*	1 Roll/65g	162	3.2	250	8.5	41.0	5.0	8.0
Rolls, Tiger, Crusty, Baked by Us, Morrisons*	1 Roll/63g	143	1.8	227	6.3	46.0	2.9	2.5
Rolls, Triple Seeded, Genius *	1 Roll/75g	242	9.8	322	5.6	38.0	13.0	7.1
Rolls, White, 50/50, Soft, Kingsmill*	1 Roll/63g	154	2.4	245	9.3	41.2	3.8	4.4
Rolls, White, BGTY, Sainsbury's*	1 Roll/50g	114	0.5	227	9.1	45.3	1.0	3.0
Rolls, White, Cheese Topped, Asda*	1 Roll/46g	121	2.0	264	10.0	46.0	4.4	2.0
Rolls, White, Cheese Topped, Sainsbury's*	1 Roll/75g	218	6.4	291	12.1	41.6	8.5	2.0
Rolls, White, Chunky, Hovis*	1 Roll/73g	173	2.4	237	9.4	41.7	3.3	2.5
Rolls, White, Crusty, Average	*1 Roll/50g*	*140*	*1.2*	*280*	*10.9*	*57.6*	*2.3*	*1.5*
Rolls, White, Crusty, Home Bake, Tesco*	1 Roll/69g	185	1.0	270	9.3	54.2	1.4	2.9
Rolls, White, Crusty, Morning, M&S*	1 Roll/65g	176	0.8	270	8.8	53.8	1.3	2.7
Rolls, White, Finger, Smart Price, Asda*	1 Roll/50g	121	0.8	242	9.0	48.0	1.6	2.1
Rolls, White, Finger, Tesco*	1 Roll/68g	170	2.4	250	8.5	45.8	3.5	2.1
Rolls, White, Finger, Value, Tesco*	1 Roll/50g	116	1.0	232	8.7	45.0	1.9	2.2
Rolls, White, Floured, Batch, Tesco*	1 Roll/76g	193	2.5	254	8.8	47.3	3.3	2.2
Rolls, White, Floured, Warburton's*	1 Roll/50g	124	1.9	247	9.8	43.3	3.8	2.7
Rolls, White, Floury Batch, Sainsbury's*	1 Roll/68g	168	1.9	247	8.3	47.2	2.8	2.2
Rolls, White, Hot Dog, Jumbo, Sainsbury's*	1 Roll/85g	239	5.2	281	7.5	49.1	6.1	2.9
Rolls, White, Hot Dog, Tesco*	1 Roll/65g	169	2.4	260	9.6	46.1	3.7	3.2
Rolls, White, Large, Sliced, Warburton's*	1 Roll/89g	230	4.0	258	10.1	44.4	4.5	2.7
Rolls, White, Mini, Submarine, M&S*	1 Roll/30g	86	1.5	285	11.4	47.7	4.9	1.1
Rolls, White, Morning, Co-Op*	1 Roll/47g	134	1.4	285	12.0	53.0	3.0	2.0
Rolls, White, Old Fashioned, Waitrose*	1 Roll/64g	176	2.9	275	8.8	49.8	4.5	2.8

BREAD

INFO/WEIGHT	Measure	per Measure		Nutrition Values per 100g / 100ml				
		KCAL	FAT	KCAL	PROT	CARB	FAT	FIBRE
Rolls, White, Organic, Sainsbury's*	1 Roll/65g	170	2.0	262	8.7	49.9	3.0	1.0
Rolls, White, Ploughman's, Sainsbury's*	1 Roll/65g	185	2.5	285	8.6	54.1	3.8	2.3
Rolls, White, Premium Soft, Rathbones*	1 Roll/65g	190	3.9	293	9.3	50.3	6.0	2.7
Rolls, White, Premium, Brown Hill Bakery*	1 Roll/74g	206	2.2	279	11.0	51.5	3.0	2.3
Rolls, White, Premium, Hovis*	1 Roll/70g	180	3.1	257	9.5	44.8	4.4	3.0
Rolls, White, Sandwich, Large, Warburton's*	1 Roll/88g	224	3.5	254	10.2	44.3	4.0	2.5
Rolls, White, Sandwich, Regular, Warburton's*	1 Roll/58g	143	2.5	249	9.7	42.6	4.4	2.4
Rolls, White, Scottish, Tesco*	1 Roll/48g	117	1.2	243	10.4	44.8	2.5	4.7
Rolls, White, Seeded, Sainsbury's*	1 Roll/80g	217	4.7	271	10.9	43.4	5.9	4.8
Rolls, White, Seeded, Soft, M&S*	1 Roll/75g	214	4.3	285	11.7	46.2	5.7	2.8
Rolls, White, Snack, Sainsbury's*	1 Roll/67g	159	0.7	237	7.9	49.2	1.0	2.3
Rolls, White, Soft, Average	**1 Sm Roll/45g**	**114**	**1.5**	**253**	**9.2**	**46.5**	**3.3**	**2.2**
Rolls, White, Soft, Dietary Specials*	1 Roll/75g	130	2.9	172	2.2	29.8	3.8	4.7
Rolls, White, Soft, Farmhouse, TTD, Sainsbury's*	1 Slice/47g	111	0.8	235	8.1	45.4	1.7	2.9
Rolls, White, Soft, Farmhouse, Warburton's*	1 Roll/59g	148	2.6	250	9.7	43.0	4.4	2.5
Rolls, White, Soft, Hovis*	1 Roll/70g	180	3.1	257	9.5	44.8	4.4	3.0
Rolls, White, Soft, Kingsmill*	1 Roll/62g	156	1.7	252	8.9	46.7	2.8	2.4
Rolls, White, Soft, M&S*	1 Roll/60g	150	1.9	250	10.3	45.2	3.1	2.7
Rolls, White, Soft, Morrisons*	1 Roll/42g	100	0.8	238	9.1	46.4	1.9	2.4
Rolls, White, Soft, Tesco*	1 Roll/72g	175	1.8	243	7.6	46.7	2.5	2.8
Rolls, White, Split, Asda*	1 Roll/45g	113	1.5	251	10.0	45.0	3.4	2.8
Rolls, White, Sub, Tesco*	1 Roll/100g	258	4.0	258	11.1	44.4	4.0	2.8
Rolls, White, Submarine, M&S*	1 Roll/109g	300	5.4	275	11.0	47.0	5.0	1.0
Rolls, White, Tesco*	1 Roll/30g	79	0.7	262	9.7	50.5	2.3	2.9
Rolls, White, Tesco*	1 Roll/65g	180	2.5	277	8.7	52.0	3.8	2.7
Rolls, White, Warburton's*	1 Roll/57g	141	2.4	248	9.7	42.8	4.2	0.0
Rolls, Wholemeal	**1 Roll/45g**	**108**	**1.3**	**241**	**9.0**	**48.3**	**2.9**	**5.9**
Rolls, Wholemeal, Asda*	1 Roll/58g	130	1.6	225	11.0	39.0	2.8	6.0
Rolls, Wholemeal, Deli, Tesco*	1 Roll/65g	156	3.1	240	9.0	40.2	4.8	5.7
Rolls, Wholemeal, Floury Batch, Sainsbury's*	1 Roll/68g	152	2.3	223	9.9	37.8	3.4	6.5
Rolls, Wholemeal, Golden, Hovis*	1 Roll/50g	112	2.0	223	10.5	36.5	3.9	6.8
Rolls, Wholemeal, HL, Tesco*	1 Roll/68g	155	1.4	230	10.4	41.3	2.1	6.6
Rolls, Wholemeal, Kingsmill*	1 Roll/68g	167	2.7	245	10.7	41.5	4.0	5.1
Rolls, Wholemeal, Mini, Assorted, Waitrose*	1 Roll/35g	86	2.1	244	9.7	37.9	6.0	7.3
Rolls, Wholemeal, Morrisons*	1 Roll/67g	155	2.7	231	10.2	38.6	4.0	6.3
Rolls, Wholemeal, Oat Topped, Deli, Tesco*	1 Roll/65g	170	3.5	260	10.9	38.3	5.3	6.7
Rolls, Wholemeal, Oat Topped, Tesco*	1 Roll/65g	166	2.9	255	11.3	42.2	4.5	5.1
Rolls, Wholemeal, Old Fashioned, Waitrose*	1 Roll/57g	135	2.7	236	11.1	37.2	4.8	6.6
Rolls, Wholemeal, Organic, Sainsbury's*	1 Roll/66g	152	1.8	230	10.7	41.0	2.7	6.6
Rolls, Wholemeal, Sainsbury's*	1 Roll/65g	153	2.1	236	10.7	40.8	3.3	7.4
Rolls, Wholemeal, Seeded, The Country Miller, Waitrose*	1 Roll/75g	190	7.7	255	13.6	26.9	10.3	7.6
Rolls, Wholemeal, Sliced, Hovis*	1 Roll/60g	150	3.5	250	10.6	38.7	5.9	6.8
Rolls, Wholemeal, Soft, Average	**1 Roll/65g**	**151**	**2.7**	**233**	**10.8**	**37.3**	**4.1**	**6.3**
Rolls, Wholemeal, Soft, Sainsbury's*	1 Roll/60g	133	2.0	221	9.9	37.8	3.4	6.5
Rolls, Wholemeal, Soft, Seeded, Sainsbury's*	1 Roll/75g	193	5.6	257	11.8	35.6	7.4	6.2
Rolls, Wholemeal, Submarine, Tesco*	1 Roll/100g	221	3.1	221	9.3	39.0	3.1	5.2
Rolls, Wholemeal, Submarine, Warburton's*	1 Roll/94g	231	4.1	246	10.9	40.6	4.4	6.3
Rolls, Wholemeal, Sunflower & Honey, Sainsbury's*	1 Roll/85g	225	4.3	265	9.2	45.4	5.1	4.5
Rolls, Wholemeal, Tasty, Great Everyday, Kingsmill*	1 Roll/68g	158	2.6	232	10.6	38.8	3.8	6.5
Rolls, Wholemeal, Warburton's*	1 Roll/58g	124	2.1	214	10.2	35.1	3.7	6.6
Rosemary, Olive Oil, Round, la Brea Bakery*	1 Serving/100g	250	3.5	250	7.0	47.5	3.5	1.6
Roti, Tesco*	1 Bread/95g	256	5.2	269	8.4	46.4	5.5	3.2
Rye with Sunflower Seeds, Organic, Schneider Brot*	1 Slice/72g	138	2.6	191	6.2	33.4	3.6	7.9

BREAD

INFO/WEIGHT	per Measure KCAL	FAT	Nutrition Values per 100g / 100ml KCAL	PROT	CARB	FAT	FIBRE
Rye with Sunflower Seeds, Organic, Sunnyvale*	1 Slice/25g	50	1.6	198	5.1	30.3	6.3	7.9
Rye, Average	*1 Slice/25g*	*55*	*0.4*	*219*	*8.3*	*45.8*	*1.7*	*4.4*
Rye, Dark, Sliced, Trianon*	1 Slice/41g	74	0.6	180	6.5	35.0	1.5	0.0
Rye, German Style, Bolletje*	1 Slice/60g	114	1.2	190	6.0	35.0	2.0	9.5
Rye, German Style, Kelderman*	1 Slice/64g	122	1.3	190	6.0	35.0	2.0	9.5
Rye, German Style, Loaf, Bakery in Store, M&S*	2 Slices/50g	112	0.6	225	9.5	40.8	1.1	6.3
Rye, Organic with Coriander, Village Bakery*	1 Thin Slice/30g	63	0.8	209	4.9	49.9	2.7	8.5
Rye, Organic, Waitrose*	1 Serving/100g	207	1.2	207	6.4	42.7	1.2	5.1
Rye, with Seeds, Organic, The Village Bakery Melmerby*	1 Slice/42g	80	1.0	190	6.9	35.6	2.3	9.4
Sandwich Thins, 50/50, Kingsmill*	1 Thin/37g	99	1.0	266	10.6	46.2	2.8	5.2
Sandwich Thins, White, CBY, Asda*	1 Thin/55g	141	2.2	257	9.3	44.3	4.0	3.1
Sandwich Thins, White, Kingsmill*	1 Thin/40g	99	1.0	248	9.4	45.6	2.5	2.9
Sandwich Thins, Wholemeal, Kingsmill*	1 Thin/41g	98	1.2	240	10.3	39.8	3.0	6.1
Seeded, Batch, Finest, Tesco*	1 Slice/65g	168	4.0	259	9.3	41.8	6.1	6.1
Seeded, Farmhouse, Loaf, ES, Asda*	1 Slice/44g	92	0.5	207	11.0	38.0	1.2	8.0
Seeded, Medium Sliced, Average	*1 Slice/44g*	*116*	*2.9*	*262*	*11.3*	*38.6*	*6.5*	*5.6*
Seeded, Rye, Loaf, la Brea Bakery*	1 Slice/55g	120	0.6	218	7.0	42.5	1.0	5.7
Seriously Seeded, Gold, Kingsmill*	1 Slice/50g	136	3.4	272	10.9	41.6	6.9	6.4
Sesame Seed, la Brea Bakery*	1 Slice/35g	85	0.8	244	8.8	47.1	2.3	2.0
Soda	*1oz/28g*	*72*	*0.7*	*258*	*7.7*	*54.6*	*2.5*	*2.1*
Soda Farls, M&S*	1 Farl/110g	267	3.0	243	9.6	50.1	2.7	2.3
Soda Farls, Tesco*	1 Farl/142g	325	4.5	229	7.1	42.2	3.2	2.6
Soda, Fruit, M&S*	1 Slice/40g	105	1.9	260	5.9	51.3	4.6	2.5
Soda, M&S*	1 Slice/40g	82	0.6	205	8.7	39.2	1.6	4.2
Softgrain, Mighty White*	1 Slice/36g	81	0.5	224	7.2	45.5	1.5	3.7
Sourdough, Average	*1 Med Slice/50g*	*144*	*0.9*	*289*	*11.8*	*56.4*	*1.8*	*2.4*
Soya & Linseed, Vogel*	1 Slice/42g	95	2.1	227	11.7	34.1	4.9	6.8
Sprouted Grain, Ezekiel *	1 Slice/34g	80	0.5	235	11.8	44.1	1.5	0.9
Square Wraps, White, Warburton's*	1 Wrap/65g	159	2.9	245	12.5	38.6	4.5	2.2
Sunflower & Honey, M&S*	1 Serving/67g	206	9.0	308	12.9	34.0	13.4	5.6
Sunflower & Honey, Organic, Cranks*	1 Slice/30g	64	0.9	215	11.6	37.2	3.0	8.3
Sunflower & Pumpkin Seed, Batched, Organic, Tesco*	1 Slice/30g	73	2.2	243	11.0	33.1	7.4	5.2
Sunflower & Pumpkin Seed, So Organic, Sainsbury's*	1 Slice/30g	76	1.6	254	11.4	40.0	5.4	12.9
Sunflower, Multi-Grain, Allinson*	1 Slice/47g	113	2.2	240	9.8	39.6	4.7	3.9
Tasty, Wholemeal, Thick, Kingsmill*	1 Slice/44g	105	1.7	239	10.5	37.7	3.8	6.2
Ten Seed, Organic, The Village Bakery*	1 Slice/25g	66	1.4	263	9.0	43.8	5.7	3.8
The Really Seeded One, Kingsmill*	1 Slice/44g	118	3.2	268	10.4	37.3	7.3	5.5
The White, Toastie, LBU, Co-Op*	1 Slice/50g	120	1.2	240	7.9	45.4	2.4	2.6
Three Cheese to Share, Morrisons*	1 Serving/100g	263	4.2	263	9.9	46.5	4.2	2.1
Three Grain, Organic, Schneider Brot*	1 Slice/72g	142	1.6	199	5.3	34.5	2.3	9.3
Tiger Loaf, Tesco*	1 Slice/40g	96	0.8	239	8.7	46.6	2.0	2.6
Toaster, White, Rathbones*	1 Slice/38g	92	0.5	243	9.1	48.6	1.3	2.3
Tomato & Chilli, BGTY, Sainsbury's*	¼ Bread/65g	155	3.1	238	11.9	36.9	4.7	2.8
Tomato & Garlic, Flatbread, Sainsbury's*	1/3 Bread/73g	191	4.9	261	8.4	41.7	6.7	3.4
Tomato & Garlic, Italian Style, Morrisons*	½ Pack/155g	355	12.4	229	5.8	33.4	8.0	2.5
Tomato & Herb, Tear & Share, Tesco*	¼ Pack/73g	164	3.2	226	6.3	40.2	4.4	2.1
Veda Malt, St Michael*	1 Serving/45g	99	0.5	219	7.1	45.3	1.1	2.2
Walnut, Waitrose*	1/8 Loaf/50g	170	7.6	339	10.0	40.6	15.2	5.9
Wheat	*1 Slice/25g*	*65*	*1.0*	*260*	*9.1*	*47.2*	*4.1*	*4.3*
Wheat, Tasty, Kingsmill*	1 Serving/38g	84	1.3	221	10.1	37.6	3.4	6.8
Wheaten, Big Slice	1 Slice/65g	139	1.7	214	7.5	40.2	2.6	3.6
Wheaten, Loaf, Sliced, Genesis*	1 Slice/40g	86	1.0	214	7.5	40.2	2.6	3.6
Wheaten, M&S*	1 Slice/33g	74	1.2	225	9.3	42.9	3.5	3.9

BREAD

Food	Measure INFO/WEIGHT	per Measure KCAL	per Measure FAT	KCAL	PROT	CARB	FAT	FIBRE
Wheaten, Sliced, Healthy, Irwin's Bakery*	1 Slice/40g	76	0.8	190	9.0	40.5	1.9	6.2
Wheatgerm, Hovis, Soft, Sliced, M&S*	1 Slice/23g	50	0.7	220	10.1	38.5	3.0	4.6
White, Average	*1 Thick Slice/40g*	*94*	*0.8*	*235*	*8.4*	*49.3*	*1.9*	*1.5*
White, Batch Loaf, ES, Asda*	1 Slice/47g	109	0.9	233	9.0	45.0	1.9	2.2
White, Batch, Warburton's*	1 Slice/42g	98	0.9	233	9.8	43.6	2.1	2.7
White, Bloomer, Loaf, Greggs*	1 Serving/56g	138	1.0	247	10.2	46.2	1.7	3.0
White, Ciabatta, Roll, Gluten Free, Dietary Specials*	1 Roll/50g	106	0.9	213	4.1	40.9	1.8	8.3
White, Classic, Medium Sliced, Hovis*	1 Slice/38g	91	0.9	240	11.4	40.3	2.3	2.5
White, Classic, Thick Sliced, Hovis*	1 Slice/50g	120	2.2	240	9.2	40.5	4.5	3.1
White, Commercially Prepared, Average	*1oz/28g*	*74*	*0.9*	*266*	*7.6*	*50.6*	*3.3*	*2.4*
White, Commercially Prepared, Toasted, Average	*1oz/28g*	*82*	*1.1*	*293*	*9.0*	*54.4*	*4.0*	*2.5*
White, Crusty, Fresh, Finest, Tesco*	1 Slice/52g	130	1.0	250	8.6	48.5	1.9	2.4
White, Crusty, Hovis*	1 Slice/44g	103	1.0	233	8.8	44.3	2.2	2.1
White, Crusty, Sliced Loaf, Tesco*	1 Slice/50g	116	1.0	233	7.4	46.0	2.1	2.0
White, Danish Style, Thick Sliced, Light, Tesco*	1 Slice/22g	55	0.6	255	9.4	47.3	2.9	2.7
White, Danish, Sliced, Weight Watchers*	1 Slice/21g	50	0.3	243	9.8	46.5	1.3	2.9
White, Danish, Soft & Light, Thick Cut, Asda*	1 Slice/26g	60	0.4	230	9.0	45.0	1.6	2.1
White, Extra Thick Sliced, Kingsmill*	1 Slice/58g	135	1.4	232	8.8	43.8	2.4	2.8
White, Farmhouse Crusty, M&S*	1 Slice/34g	82	0.7	240	8.9	46.6	2.2	3.0
White, Farmhouse, Seeded, Waitrose*	1 Serving/75g	192	4.1	256	10.8	40.9	5.5	5.6
White, Farmhouse, Thick, Hovis*	1 Slice/44g	103	1.0	234	8.7	44.6	2.3	2.4
White, Fibre, Morrisons*	1 Slice/40g	96	0.7	240	8.0	44.6	1.7	0.3
White, Fried in Blended Oil	*1 Slice/28g*	*141*	*9.0*	*503*	*7.9*	*48.5*	*32.2*	*1.6*
White, Gluten & Wheat Free, Free From, Sainsbury's*	1 Slice/33g	75	2.8	227	1.9	35.5	8.6	1.0
White, Gold Seeded, Kingsmill*	1 Slice/44g	108	2.5	245	9.7	38.8	5.7	3.5
White, Loaf, Crusty, Premium, Warburton's*	1 Slice/31g	76	0.7	249	10.6	46.5	2.3	2.6
White, Loaf, Danish, Asda*	1 Serving/23g	53	0.5	236	9.0	45.0	2.2	2.0
White, Medium Sliced, Asda*	1 Slice/37g	80	0.6	218	8.0	43.0	1.5	3.3
White, Medium Sliced, Average	*1 Slice/39g*	*93*	*0.6*	*238*	*7.5*	*48.5*	*1.6*	*1.8*
White, Medium Sliced, Basics, Sainsbury's*	1 Slice/36g	83	0.5	231	8.0	46.4	1.5	2.1
White, Medium Sliced, Brace's*	1 Slice/32g	75	0.4	235	9.5	46.6	1.2	2.6
White, Medium Sliced, Great Everyday, Kingsmill*	1 Slice/40g	93	0.8	232	9.0	44.6	2.0	2.7
White, Medium Sliced, Mother's Pride*	1 Slice/36g	82	0.6	229	8.0	45.6	1.6	3.0
White, Medium Sliced, Sainsbury's*	1 Slice/36g	78	0.7	216	8.7	41.1	1.9	7.1
White, Medium Sliced, Smart Price, Asda*	1 Slice/36g	81	0.5	226	7.0	46.0	1.5	2.8
White, Medium Sliced, Stay Fresh, Tesco*	1 Slice/36g	88	0.7	250	8.9	47.7	2.0	2.9
White, Medium Sliced, Superlife, Morrisons*	1 Slice/30g	79	1.2	263	9.6	47.4	3.9	2.5
White, Medium Sliced, Tesco*	1 Slice/36g	86	0.5	240	8.2	47.8	1.5	3.0
White, Medium Sliced, Value, Tesco*	1 Slice/36g	81	0.4	225	7.9	46.1	1.0	2.1
White, Medium Sliced, Warburton's*	1 Slice/40g	94	0.8	234	9.9	43.8	2.0	2.6
White, Medium VLH Kitchens	1 Serving/30g	72	6.3	241	8.4	49.3	1.9	1.5
White, Mega Thick, Roberts Bakery*	1 Slice/66g	154	1.2	233	8.3	46.2	1.8	2.2
White, Organic, Sainsbury's*	1 Slice/36g	84	0.6	234	8.9	45.5	1.8	2.3
White, Plain, Scottish, Sunblest*	1 Slice/57g	133	1.5	233	10.1	42.3	2.6	2.8
White, Premium Farmhouse, Lidl*	1 Slice/44g	99	0.7	225	7.4	45.4	1.5	2.5
White, Sandwich Thins, Warburton's*	1 Thin/42g	100	1.0	239	9.2	47.1	2.5	3.8
White, Sandwich, Bakery, Sainsbury's*	1 Slice/50g	121	0.3	242	10.3	49.0	0.6	2.9
White, Scottish Plain, Mother's Pride*	1 Med Slice/50g	114	0.8	227	8.7	44.6	1.5	3.0
White, Seeded, Batch, Loaf, Truly Irresistible, Co-Op*	1 Slice/47g	129	3.4	275	11.6	41.1	7.2	4.3
White, Sliced, Roberts Bakery*	1 Slice/35g	87	0.7	249	10.0	48.0	2.1	2.5
White, Small Loaf, Classic, Hovis*	1 Slice/33g	75	0.8	228	11.4	40.3	2.3	6.5
White, Soft Batch, Sliced, Sainsbury's*	1 Slice/44g	102	0.8	232	8.2	45.4	1.9	2.3
White, Soft Crusty, M&S*	1 Slice/25g	64	0.6	256	9.3	49.0	2.5	2.4

BREAD

	Measure INFO/WEIGHT	per Measure KCAL	FAT	Nutrition Values per 100g / 100ml KCAL	PROT	CARB	FAT	FIBRE
White, Soft, Batch Loaf, Sliced, Tesco*	1 Slice/50g	116	1.0	233	7.5	46.1	2.1	2.1
White, Soft, Burger, Thins, Kingsmill*	1 Thin/44g	112	1.1	254	9.1	47.0	2.6	3.0
White, Soft, Farmhouse, M&S*	1 Slice/25g	60	0.8	239	9.8	42.6	3.3	2.5
White, Soft, Gold, Kingsmill*	1 Slice/47g	112	1.5	239	8.2	44.5	3.1	2.7
White, Soft, Hovis*	1 Slice/40g	94	0.9	234	8.7	44.6	2.3	2.4
White, Soft, M&S*	1 Slice/47g	105	0.8	225	7.3	46.1	1.7	2.4
White, Soft, Milk Roll, Warburton's*	1 Slice/18g	46	0.5	251	10.8	45.3	3.0	2.8
White, Soft, Sliced, Hovis*	1 Thin Slice/25g	58	0.6	234	8.7	44.6	2.3	2.4
White, Sourdough, Country, Oval, la Brea Bakery*	1 Slice/60g	143	0.4	239	8.8	49.4	0.6	1.6
White, Square, Medium Sliced, Hovis*	1 Slice/40g	92	0.8	231	8.5	44.7	2.0	2.6
White, Square, Thick Sliced, Hovis*	1 Slice/50g	116	1.0	231	8.5	44.7	2.0	2.6
White, Super Toastie, Warburton's*	1 Slice/57g	134	1.0	235	10.1	44.6	1.8	2.7
White, Thick Sliced, Bakers Gold, Asda*	1 Slice/44g	101	0.8	229	8.0	45.0	1.9	2.3
White, Thick Sliced, Brace's*	1 Slice/38g	90	0.5	235	9.5	46.6	1.2	2.6
White, Thick Sliced, Budgens*	1 Slice/40g	89	0.5	223	7.4	45.3	1.3	2.5
White, Thick Sliced, Healthy, Warburton's*	1 Slice/38g	84	0.7	222	10.3	41.2	1.8	4.1
White, Thick Sliced, M&S*	1 Slice/42g	96	0.5	228	7.3	46.7	1.3	2.8
White, Thick Sliced, Organic, Tesco*	1 Slice/44g	108	0.9	245	8.5	46.8	2.1	3.1
White, Thick Sliced, Sainsbury's*	1 Slice/44g	95	0.8	216	8.7	41.1	1.9	7.1
White, Thick Sliced, Square Cut, Asda*	1 Slice/44g	101	0.7	230	8.0	46.0	1.5	2.1
White, Thick Sliced, Super Toastie, Morrisons*	1 Slice/50g	128	1.5	257	8.7	48.9	3.0	2.1
White, Thick Sliced, Tesco*	1 Slice/44g	106	0.7	240	8.2	47.8	1.5	3.0
White, Thick Sliced, Warburton's*	1 Slice/28g	65	0.6	233	9.8	43.6	2.1	2.7
White, Thick Sliced, Warburton's, Weight Watchers*	1 Slice/29g	69	0.2	237	10.4	48.6	0.8	2.0
White, Thick, So Organic, Sainsbury's*	1 Slice/44g	102	1.0	231	8.2	44.6	2.2	3.1
White, Thick, Super Soft, M&S*	1 Slice/48g	115	1.2	240	8.7	45.3	2.6	2.5
White, Thick, Toastie, 800g Loaf, Warburton's*	1 Slice/47g	111	0.9	234	9.9	43.9	1.9	2.5
White, Thin Sliced, Sainsbury's*	1 Slice/29g	66	0.4	228	7.1	46.4	1.5	2.8
White, Thin Sliced, Tesco*	1 Slice/30g	68	0.4	228	9.5	44.5	1.3	3.4
White, Toasted, Average	*1 Slice/33g*	*87*	*0.5*	*265*	*9.3*	*57.1*	*1.6*	*1.8*
White, Toastie, Thick Cut, Hovis*	1 Slice/50g	115	1.0	230	8.5	44.8	2.0	2.5
White, Toastie, Thick, Love to Toast, Kingsmill*	1 Slice/50g	116	1.0	232	9.0	44.6	2.0	2.7
White, Weight Watchers*	1 Serving/5g	12	0.1	246	12.3	45.1	1.6	3.3
White, Whole, Kingsmill*	1 Slice/38g	87	1.0	230	9.0	42.9	2.5	3.4
White, Wholesome, Loaf, Sainsbury's*	1 Slice/36g	81	0.7	224	9.4	42.5	1.8	4.4
Whole Grain & Rye, Schneider Brot*	1 Slice/50g	98	0.6	197	5.9	36.6	1.2	8.2
Whole Grain, Batch, Finest, Tesco*	1 Slice/44g	112	1.2	254	9.8	47.7	2.7	4.2
Whole Grain, Brennans*	1 Slice/39g	79	0.6	203	9.0	40.0	1.5	4.9
Whole Wheat, Harvest	1 Slice/42g	90	1.0	214	7.1	45.2	2.4	7.1
Wholegrain, Medium Sliced, Irish Pride*	1 Slice/38g	90	0.8	237	9.2	46.6	2.1	7.6
Wholegrain, Soft, M&S*	1 Slice/51g	115	2.8	225	13.0	31.2	5.4	8.2
Wholegrain, Thick Sliced, Average	*1 Slice/44g*	*117*	*1.9*	*265*	*13.4*	*43.3*	*4.2*	*7.4*
Wholegrain, Thick Sliced, Toasted, Average	*1 Slice/40g*	*117*	*1.9*	*288*	*14.5*	*47.1*	*4.6*	*8.1*
Wholemeal & Oat, Loaf, Vogel*	1 Slice/42g	86	0.6	205	8.7	34.3	1.5	9.7
Wholemeal Loaf, British Farmers, Hovis*	1 Slice/47g	108	1.3	229	10.0	37.9	2.8	6.8
Wholemeal Oatbran, Sliced, Tesco*	1 Slice/45g	90	0.7	200	10.1	35.3	1.6	7.4
Wholemeal, & Oat Flakes, Gold, Kingsmill*	1 Slice/47g	103	1.6	220	10.0	37.3	3.4	7.0
Wholemeal, 7 Seed Sensation, Hovis*	1 Slice/44g	109	2.5	249	11.9	31.4	5.6	12.4
Wholemeal, 7 Seeded, Irwin's Bakery*	1 Slice/38g	90	2.0	237	9.5	33.4	5.2	9.4
Wholemeal, American Sandwich, Harry's*	1 Slice/43g	110	2.1	259	9.0	45.0	5.0	5.0
Wholemeal, Average	*1 Thick Slice/40g*	*88*	*1.0*	*215*	*9.2*	*41.6*	*2.5*	*5.8*
Wholemeal, Baker`s Soft, Medium, Tesco*	1 Slice/40g	94	1.1	235	10.8	37.8	2.8	6.9
Wholemeal, Batch, Organic, Waitrose*	1 Slice/40g	88	1.0	219	10.0	38.8	2.6	7.2

	Measure INFO/WEIGHT	per Measure		Nutrition Values per 100g / 100ml				
		KCAL	FAT	KCAL	PROT	CARB	FAT	FIBRE

BREAD

Wholemeal, BGTY, Sainsbury's*	1 Slice/20g	41	0.2	207	12.6	36.8	1.0	7.3
Wholemeal, Brennans*	1 Slice/33g	78	1.4	236	11.2	38.4	4.2	7.7
Wholemeal, Brown, Medium Sliced, 400g, Hovis*	1 Slice/29g	64	0.8	221	10.0	37.8	2.8	6.8
Wholemeal, COU, M&S*	1 Slice/21g	45	0.5	213	13.6	33.7	2.6	7.0
Wholemeal, Crusty, Finest, Tesco*	1 Slice/50g	103	0.8	206	10.8	37.0	1.7	6.9
Wholemeal, Danish, Warburton's*	1 Slice/25g	57	0.6	229	13.3	38.5	2.4	7.2
Wholemeal, Farmhouse Batch, Sliced, LL, Waitrose*	1 Slice/48g	102	1.2	212	10.4	36.2	2.6	7.6
Wholemeal, Farmhouse, Hovis*	1 Slice/44g	91	1.0	207	11.0	36.0	2.2	7.1
Wholemeal, Golden Wheat, Kingsmill*	1 Slice/44g	97	1.3	221	10.9	37.8	2.9	6.0
Wholemeal, Light, Irish Pride*	1 Slice/28g	68	0.4	241	13.3	44.1	1.3	4.5
Wholemeal, Little Brown Loaf, Unsliced, Hovis*	1 Slice/40g	86	1.1	216	10.0	37.8	2.7	6.8
Wholemeal, Loaf, Sliced, Medium, 800g, Hovis*	1 Slice/40g	88	1.1	221	10.0	37.8	2.7	6.8
Wholemeal, Loaf, Sliced, Thick, 800g, Hovis*	1 Slice/50g	115	1.4	229	10.0	37.8	2.7	6.8
Wholemeal, Medium Sliced, Baked by Us, Morrisons*	1 Slice/32g	69	0.4	216	9.6	38.0	1.4	6.5
Wholemeal, Medium Sliced, Great Everyday, Kingsmill*	1 Slice/40g	91	1.5	227	10.5	37.7	3.8	6.2
Wholemeal, Medium Sliced, Little Big Loaf, Kingsmill*	1 Slice/39g	93	1.5	239	10.5	37.7	3.8	6.2
Wholemeal, Medium Sliced, M&S*	1 Slice/40g	80	1.2	200	10.5	32.7	3.1	6.7
Wholemeal, Medium Sliced, Organic, Tesco*	1 Slice/27g	55	0.7	209	9.2	37.2	2.8	6.0
Wholemeal, Medium Sliced, Roberts Bakery*	1 Slice/37g	86	0.6	233	10.9	38.1	1.5	6.6
Wholemeal, Medium Sliced, Sainsbury's*	1 Slice/36g	77	0.9	214	10.3	37.8	2.4	7.4
Wholemeal, Medium Sliced, The Village Bakery*	1 Slice/33g	69	0.7	209	9.8	38.0	2.0	6.0
Wholemeal, Medium Sliced, Waitrose*	1 Slice/36g	76	0.9	213	10.1	37.6	2.4	7.0
Wholemeal, Medium, 800g Loaf, Warburton's*	1 Slice/40g	93	1.0	231	10.2	39.6	2.5	6.5
Wholemeal, Multi Seeded, TTD, Sainsbury's*	1 Slice/47g	110	3.4	234	11.7	30.7	7.2	8.1
Wholemeal, Multigrain, Sliced, Finest, Tesco*	1 Slice/50g	123	2.0	246	10.1	42.1	4.1	6.5
Wholemeal, Multigrain, Soft Batch, Sainsbury's*	1 Slice/44g	106	2.9	242	11.3	34.5	6.5	5.6
Wholemeal, Multiseed, Organic, Sainsbury's*	1 Slice/26g	75	2.5	289	13.8	36.6	9.7	6.0
Wholemeal, Oat Topped, TTD, Sainsbury's*	1 Slice/47g	109	1.3	232	10.0	38.5	2.8	0.3
Wholemeal, Organic, 400g Loaf, Warburton's*	1 Slice/28g	63	0.9	223	10.3	37.9	3.2	6.7
Wholemeal, Organic, Hovis*	1 Slice/44g	92	1.3	209	10.2	35.6	2.9	7.6
Wholemeal, Premium, Medium Slice, M&S*	1 Slice/33g	65	1.0	200	10.5	32.9	3.1	6.7
Wholemeal, Premium, Thick Slice, M&S*	1 Slice/50g	95	1.5	190	9.8	30.8	3.0	6.4
Wholemeal, Rolls, Mini Loaves, Hovis*	1 Loaf/70g	175	4.1	250	10.6	38.7	5.9	6.8
Wholemeal, Rustic, Tin, Tesco*	1 Slice/37g	92	1.3	249	12.2	44.0	3.5	3.1
Wholemeal, Sandwich Loaf, Brennans*	1 Slice/40g	88	0.7	221	9.8	38.5	1.7	8.0
Wholemeal, Sandwich Thins, Good Inside, Hovis*	1 Thin/45g	114	2.3	254	11.1	37.5	5.2	7.1
Wholemeal, Seeded Batch Loaf, Truly Irresistible, Co-Op*	1 Slice/47g	115	1.9	245	11.5	36.2	4.0	6.6
Wholemeal, Sliced, Medium, Tesco*	1 Slice/36g	79	0.8	220	11.0	39.1	2.2	6.6
Wholemeal, Soft Crusty, M&S*	1 Slice/25g	58	0.8	230	11.4	39.1	3.1	6.5
Wholemeal, Square Cut, Thick Sliced, Asda*	1 Slice/44g	91	1.0	208	10.0	37.0	2.2	6.0
Wholemeal, Stoneground, 800g Loaf, Warburton's*	1 Slice/45g	95	1.2	210	10.4	35.8	2.6	6.8
Wholemeal, Stoneground, Organic, Waitrose*	1 Sm Slice/25g	57	0.9	228	10.8	38.2	3.6	7.1
Wholemeal, Stoneground, Thick Slice, LL, Waitrose*	1 Slice/40g	86	1.1	214	10.1	36.5	2.8	7.9
Wholemeal, Stoneground, Thick Sliced, Sainsbury's*	1 Slice/44g	92	0.8	210	10.2	37.9	1.9	7.8
Wholemeal, Supersoft, Eat Well, M&S*	1 Slice/33g	81	1.1	245	10.9	40.0	3.3	6.7
Wholemeal, Tasty, Medium, Kingsmill*	1 Slice/40g	96	1.5	239	10.5	37.7	3.8	6.2
Wholemeal, Thick Slice, Brennans*	1 Slice/27g	69	0.6	257	9.2	45.4	2.1	6.8
Wholemeal, Thick Sliced, Great Everyday, Kingsmill*	1 Slice/44g	100	1.7	227	10.5	37.7	3.8	6.2
Wholemeal, Thick Sliced, Healthy Living, Co-Op*	1 Slice/44g	95	0.9	215	11.0	38.0	2.0	7.0
Wholemeal, Thick Sliced, Sainsbury's*	1 Slice/48g	102	1.2	213	10.1	37.4	2.6	8.5
Wholemeal, Thick Sliced, Tesco*	1 Slice/40g	96	1.1	240	9.5	40.9	2.7	6.8
Wholemeal, Thick Sliced, Waitrose*	1 Slice/44g	94	1.1	213	10.1	37.6	2.4	7.0
Wholemeal, Thick Sliced, with Mustard Seed, Lozzas	1 Slice/26g	56	0.7	215	13.6	33.7	2.6	7.0

	Measure INFO/WEIGHT	per Measure KCAL	FAT	Nutrition Values per 100g / 100ml KCAL	PROT	CARB	FAT	FIBRE
BREAD								
Wholemeal, Toasted, Average	*1 Med Slice/26g*	*58*	*0.6*	*224*	*8.6*	*42.3*	*2.2*	*5.8*
Wholemeal, Toastie, 800g Loaf, Warburton's*	1 Slice/45g	101	1.1	224	9.7	39.3	2.4	6.6
Wholemeal, Unsliced, Organic, Dove's Farm*	1 Med Slice/35g	77	0.9	221	11.4	37.9	2.6	8.3
Wholewheat, No Crusts, Harry's*	1 Slice/25g	58	1.1	233	8.0	40.0	4.5	5.5
Wrap, Tortilla, BGTY, Sainsbury's*	1 Tortilla/50g	136	1.4	271	7.9	53.7	2.7	1.9
Wrap, Tortillas, 8 Pack, Asda*	1 Tortilla/50g	143	3.0	286	8.0	50.0	6.0	1.9
Wrap, Tortillas, Flour, Soft, Old El Paso*	1 Tortilla/41g	123	2.1	299	8.5	53.7	5.2	1.9
Wrap, Tortillas, Large, Essential, Waitrose*	1 Tortilla/64g	190	3.7	297	7.2	52.5	5.8	3.1
Wrap, Tortillas, Plain, Ready to Eat, Sunnyhills, Aldi*	1 Wrap/64g	181	2.2	283	7.1	54.5	3.4	3.0
Wrap, Tortillas, Tomato & Herb, Tesco*	1 Serving/63g	165	3.5	262	7.9	45.1	5.5	2.1
Wrap, Tortillas, Whole & White, Mini, Kids, Sainsbury's*	1 Tortilla/26g	67	1.4	258	9.2	42.9	5.5	6.2
Wrap, Tortillas, Wholemeal, Discovery*	1 Wrap/40g	109	3.3	273	9.2	40.4	8.3	6.4
Wraps, Chapatis, Plain, Original, Patak's*	1 Chapati/42g	115	3.2	273	9.4	48.8	7.5	0.0
Wraps, Mediterranean Herb, Rowan Hill Bakery, Lidl*	1 Wrap/64g	178	2.2	278	7.3	53.0	3.5	2.5
Wraps, Plain, Tortillas, HL, Tesco*	1 Wrap/67g	188	1.9	280	8.5	54.2	2.8	3.3
Wraps, Plain, Tortillas, Tesco*	1 Tortilla/64g	192	3.8	300	8.4	52.2	5.9	2.7
Wraps, Tortillas, Plain, Sainsbury's*	1 Wrap/64g	182	2.9	285	7.8	51.2	4.5	4.3
Wraps, Tortillas, White, M&S*	1 Tortilla/64g	170	2.4	265	7.9	49.0	3.8	1.6
BREAD & BUTTER PUDDING								
Average	*1 Serving/250g*	*400*	*19.5*	*160*	*6.2*	*17.5*	*7.8*	*0.3*
BGTY, Sainsbury's*	1 Serving/125g	126	2.9	101	6.3	13.4	2.3	5.4
Finest, Tesco*	1 Serving/153g	379	22.0	248	4.9	24.6	14.4	0.9
Individual, M&S*	1 Pudding/130g	280	16.4	215	4.4	21.4	12.6	0.5
Low Fat, Individual, BGTY, Sainsbury's*	1 Pack/125g	125	2.9	100	6.3	13.4	2.3	5.4
Sainsbury's*	½ Pudding/115g	223	11.2	194	4.8	21.9	9.7	0.4
BREAD MIX								
Brown, Sunflower, Sainsbury's*	1 Serving/60g	151	3.7	251	10.0	38.9	6.1	4.0
Crusty White, Made Up, Tesco*	1 Slice/126g	316	2.3	251	9.4	49.3	1.8	2.5
Focaccia, Garlic & Herb, Asda*	1 Serving/125g	385	10.0	308	11.0	48.0	8.0	3.3
Multiseed, Baked, Sainsbury's*	1 Slice/44g	112	4.3	252	10.8	30.5	9.6	6.8
Parmesan & Sun Dried Tomato, Made Up, Wrights*	1 Slice/45g	103	0.6	229	9.3	46.0	1.3	2.4
White Loaf, Asda*	1 Slice/60g	150	0.9	250	10.0	49.0	1.5	3.1
Wholemeal, Hovis*	1 Serving/65g	148	3.1	227	10.0	35.8	4.8	6.8
Wholemeal, Made Up, M&S*	1 Loaf/600g	1410	14.4	235	11.0	42.0	2.4	5.3
BREADCRUMBS								
Average	*1oz/28g*	*98*	*0.5*	*350*	*10.8*	*74.8*	*1.9*	*2.6*
BREADFRUIT								
Raw	*1oz/28g*	*19*	*0.1*	*67*	*0.9*	*16.4*	*0.2*	*0.0*
BREADSTICKS								
Asda*	1 Serving/5g	21	0.4	412	12.0	73.0	8.0	2.9
Bruschetta, Olive & Rosemary, Graze*	1 Punnet/29g	138	7.5	480	13.4	53.0	26.0	4.1
Grissini, Italian, Sainsbury's*	1 Breadstick/5g	20	0.4	408	11.6	72.9	7.8	2.9
Grissini, Thin with Olive Oil, Forno Bianco*	1 Stick/5g	21	0.4	420	11.0	77.0	7.5	0.0
Grissini, Waitrose*	1 Breadstick/6g	25	0.4	397	12.0	72.5	6.2	3.1
Italian Original, Tesco*	1 Stick/6g	23	0.4	410	11.6	72.9	7.8	2.9
Mini, Sainsbury's*	4 Breadsticks/5g	20	0.4	404	15.6	68.7	7.4	4.8
Olive Oil & Rosemary, Finest, Tesco*	2 Sticks/10g	42	1.2	427	13.9	64.4	12.6	4.1
Olive, Italian, Finest, Tesco*	1 Stick/40g	170	5.4	424	10.5	65.0	13.6	4.8
Original, Organic, Kallo*	1 Breadstick/6g	24	0.5	393	11.8	69.5	7.6	4.7
Plain, You Count, LL, Waitrose*	1 Breadstick/5g	17	0.1	349	13.4	70.1	1.7	5.6
Sesame Seed Grissini, Sainsbury's*	1 Breadstick/5g	21	0.6	419	12.7	65.5	11.8	3.2
BREAKFAST CEREAL								
Advantage, Weetabix*	1 Serving/30g	105	0.7	350	10.2	72.0	2.4	9.0

BREAKFAST CEREAL

	Measure INFO/WEIGHT	per Measure KCAL	FAT	Nutrition Values per 100g / 100ml KCAL	PROT	CARB	FAT	FIBRE
All Bran, Asda*	1 Serving/40g	110	1.4	276	15.0	46.0	3.5	27.0
All Bran, Bran Flakes, & Fruit, Kellogg's*	1 Serving/40g	143	2.4	358	8.0	68.0	6.0	9.0
All Bran, Bran Flakes, Kellogg's*	1 Serving/30g	107	0.6	356	11.0	66.0	2.0	15.0
All Bran, Fruit 'n' Fibre, Kellogg's*	1 Serving/30g	114	1.8	380	8.0	69.0	6.0	9.0
All Bran, Fruitful, Kellogg's*	1 Serving/40g	136	3.0	340	12.5	57.5	7.5	0.0
All Bran, Golden Crunch, Kellogg's*	1 Serving/45g	182	5.0	405	8.0	62.0	11.0	13.0
All Bran, High Fibre, Morrisons*	1 Serving/40g	109	1.4	272	14.8	45.5	3.5	27.0
All Bran, Original, High Fibre, Kellogg's*	1 Serving/40g	134	1.4	334	14.0	48.0	3.5	27.0
Almond, Oats & More, Nestle*	1 Serving/30g	119	2.7	398	10.7	68.7	8.9	5.5
Almond, Pecan & Cashew Muesli, Kellogg's*	1 Serving/45g	188	6.3	418	11.0	62.0	14.0	8.0
Alpen*, Crunchy Bran*	1 Serving/40g	120	1.9	299	11.8	52.3	4.7	24.8
Amaranth, Flakes, Organic, Gillian McKeith*	1 Serving/50g	198	2.0	396	10.0	80.0	4.0	3.0
Apple & Cinnamon Flakes, M&S*	1 Serving/30g	111	0.6	370	6.0	82.7	1.9	3.4
Apple & Cinnamon, Crisp, Sainsbury's*	1 Serving/50g	216	7.4	433	6.2	69.1	14.7	3.4
Apple & Cinnamon, Quaker Oats*	1 Sachet/38g	136	2.1	358	8.0	68.0	5.5	2.5
Apricot Wheats, Whole Grain, Tesco*	1 Serving/40g	130	0.6	326	7.6	70.6	1.4	8.0
Balance, Sainsbury's*	1 Serving/30g	111	0.4	370	11.4	77.7	1.5	3.2
Banana & Toffee Crisp, Mornflake*	1 Serving/30g	133	4.8	443	5.7	68.8	16.1	5.4
Banana, Papaya & Honey Oat, Crunchy, Waitrose*	1 Serving/40g	170	4.8	426	9.6	69.8	12.0	5.5
Benefit Flakes, Original, Harvest Morn, Aldi*	1 Serving/40g	154	0.5	384	12.0	80.0	1.3	2.2
Berry Granola, Rude Health*	1 Serving/40g	178	6.4	446	10.0	61.0	16.0	7.0
Bircher Muesli, LL, Waitrose*	1 Serving/45g	153	3.5	341	8.8	57.7	7.7	6.8
Biscuit, Baked with Golden Syrup, Weetabix*	2 Biscuits/44g	158	0.8	363	10.3	72.0	1.9	8.2
Blueberry Wheats, Tesco*	1 Serving/50g	165	0.8	330	7.5	71.6	1.5	8.5
Bran Flakes, Asda*	1 Serving/47g	157	1.5	333	11.0	65.0	3.2	14.0
Bran Flakes, Kellogg's*	1 Serving/50g	163	1.0	326	10.0	67.0	2.0	15.0
Bran Flakes, Organic, Sainsbury's*	1 Serving/30g	100	0.7	332	10.2	67.4	2.4	14.1
Bran Flakes, Sainsbury's*	1 Serving/30g	100	0.8	333	10.3	67.5	2.5	14.3
Bran Flakes, Sultana Bran, Kellogg's*	1 Serving/40g	138	0.8	344	8.0	67.0	2.0	13.0
Bran Flakes, Sultana, Dry, Sainsbury's*	1 Serving/30g	98	0.6	325	8.3	68.6	1.9	12.1
Bran Flakes, Wholegrain, Sainsbury's*	1 Serving/30g	110	0.6	365	10.5	69.4	2.0	13.8
Bran, Natural, Sainsbury's*	1 Serving/30g	64	1.5	212	14.7	27.0	5.0	36.0
Cheerios, Chocolate, Dry, Nestle*	1 Serving/30g	115	1.0	384	8.0	73.4	3.5	2.2
Cheerios, Honey Nut, Nestle*	1 Serving/30g	112	1.1	374	7.0	78.3	3.7	5.2
Cheerios, Honey, Nestle*	1 Serving/50g	184	1.4	369	6.6	79.2	2.8	5.8
Cheerios, Nestle*	1 Serving/30g	114	1.1	381	8.6	74.5	3.8	7.1
Choc & Nut Crisp, Tesco*	1 Serving/40g	185	8.0	462	8.3	62.5	19.9	4.8
Choco Flakes, Kellogg's*	1 Serving/30g	114	0.9	380	5.0	84.0	3.0	2.5
Choco Hoops, Tesco*	1 Serving/30g	116	1.2	385	7.5	75.0	4.0	8.0
Choco Snaps, Asda*	1 Serving/30g	115	0.7	382	5.0	85.0	2.4	1.9
Chocolate Crisp, Minis, Weetabix*	1 Serving/36g	134	1.9	371	9.0	71.7	5.3	8.5
Chocolate Rice, Puffed, Average	*1 Serving/30g*	*117*	*1.2*	*389*	*5.7*	*81.0*	*4.1*	*3.2*
Chocolate, Granola, Diet Chef Ltd*	1 Serving/40g	195	11.5	488	10.7	45.0	28.7	13.0
Cinnamon Grahams, Nestle*	1 Serving/40g	164	3.9	411	4.7	76.1	9.8	4.2
Clusters, Nestle*	1 Serving/30g	111	1.4	371	9.3	72.6	4.8	7.4
Coco Pops, Crunchers, Kellogg's*	1 Serving/30g	114	1.0	380	7.0	81.0	3.5	3.0
Coco Pops, Kellogg's*	1 Serving/30g	116	0.8	387	5.0	85.0	2.5	2.0
Coco Shreddies with 125ml Semi Skimmed Milk, Nestle*	1 Serving/40g	210	2.7	525	18.0	90.2	6.7	8.7
Coco Snaps, Value, Tesco*	1 Serving/30g	117	0.7	390	7.0	84.1	2.4	2.4
Cookie Crunch, Nestle*	1 Serving/40g	154	1.1	385	4.6	85.3	2.8	1.8
Corn Flakes with 125ml Semi Skimmed Milk, Kellogg's*	1 Serving/30g	170	2.5	567	20.0	106.7	8.3	3.0
Corn Flakes, Asda*	1 Serving/30g	111	0.2	370	7.0	84.0	0.7	3.0
Corn Flakes, Honey Nut, Average	*1 Serving/30g*	*118*	*1.3*	*393*	*7.0*	*81.4*	*4.3*	*2.4*

BREAKFAST CEREAL

	Measure INFO/WEIGHT	per Measure KCAL	FAT	Nutrition Values per 100g / 100ml KCAL	PROT	CARB	FAT	FIBRE
Corn Flakes, Honey Nut, Harvest Home, Nestle*	1 Serving/30g	118	1.3	392	7.4	81.1	4.2	2.5
Corn Flakes, Kellogg's*	1 Serving/30g	113	0.3	378	7.0	84.0	0.9	3.0
Corn Flakes, Organic, Lima*	1 Serving/50g	178	0.5	355	8.3	77.7	1.0	6.4
Corn Flakes, Organic, Whole Earth*	1 Serving/40g	154	0.4	386	8.6	84.2	1.0	3.0
Corn Flakes, Sainsbury's*	1 Serving/25g	93	0.2	371	7.3	83.8	0.7	3.0
Corn Flakes, Tesco*	1 Serving/25g	93	0.2	371	7.3	83.8	0.7	3.0
Corn Flakes, Value, Tesco*	1 Serving/30g	111	0.4	370	7.3	82.4	1.2	3.5
Country Crisp with Real Raspberries, Jordans*	1 Serving/50g	214	7.9	429	7.5	64.1	15.8	7.1
Country Crisp with Real Strawberries, Jordans*	1 Serving/50g	214	7.8	428	7.5	64.1	15.7	7.1
Country Crisp, Four Nut Combo, Jordans*	1 Serving/50g	240	12.4	480	8.9	55.4	24.7	6.9
Cranberry Wheats, Tesco*	1 Serving/50g	160	0.8	320	7.6	72.0	1.5	8.0
Cranberry Wheats, Whole Grain, Sainsbury's*	1 Serving/50g	162	0.7	325	7.3	70.9	1.4	7.7
Crispy Rice & Wheat Flakes, Asda*	1 Serving/50g	185	0.8	370	11.0	78.0	1.5	3.2
Crunchy Bran Muesli, Diet Chef Ltd*	1 Serving/40g	164	3.8	409	8.1	68.4	9.5	8.9
Crunchy Bran, Weetabix*	1 Serving/40g	140	1.4	350	11.9	57.6	3.6	20.0
Crunchy Nut, Clusters, Honey & Nut, Kellogg's*	1 Serving/40g	161	2.0	402	6.0	82.0	5.0	2.5
Crunchy Nut, Clusters, Milk Chocolate Curls, Kellogg's*	1 Serving/40g	183	7.2	458	6.0	66.0	18.0	4.0
Crunchy Nut, Corn Flakes, Kellogg's*	1 Serving/30g	118	1.2	392	6.0	83.0	4.0	2.5
Crunchy Nut, Oat Granola, with Chocolate, Kellogg's*	1 Serving/45g	224	11.2	497	8.0	57.0	25.0	6.0
Crunchy Oat with Raisins, Almonds & Fruit, Tesco*	1 Serving/50g	202	6.3	403	8.5	63.8	12.6	6.6
Crunchy Oat with Tropical Fruits, Tesco*	1 Serving/35g	146	4.8	417	7.8	65.3	13.8	6.1
Crunchy Oat, Golden Sun, Lidl*	1 Serving/50g	206	6.4	411	8.6	65.0	12.9	6.2
Curiously Cinnamon, Nestle*	1 Serving/30g	124	3.0	412	4.9	75.9	9.9	4.1
Fibre Flakes, Gluten Free, Organic, Dove's Farm*	1 Serving/30g	105	0.4	351	7.1	69.7	1.5	15.0
Fitnesse & Fruits, Nestle*	1 Serving/40g	148	0.4	370	6.6	83.4	1.1	3.4
Flakes & Clusters, Tesco*	1 Serving/50g	220	8.5	440	11.2	55.4	17.0	10.5
Flakes & Grains, Exotic Fruit, BGTY, Sainsbury's*	1 Serving/30g	113	1.5	377	6.8	76.4	4.9	5.9
Frosted Flakes, Tesco*	1 Serving/30g	112	0.1	374	4.9	87.8	0.4	2.4
Frosted Wheats, Kellogg's*	1 Serving/30g	104	0.6	346	10.0	72.0	2.0	9.0
Frosties, Kellogg's*	1 Serving/30g	112	0.2	375	4.5	87.0	0.6	2.0
Fruit & Fibre, Asda*	1 Serving/40g	146	2.6	366	8.2	68.4	6.6	8.5
Fruit & Fibre, Flakes, Waitrose*	1 Serving/40g	143	2.5	357	8.2	67.2	6.2	9.9
Fruit & Fibre, Harvest Morn, Aldi*	1 Serving/30g	105	1.5	349	8.5	67.6	4.9	10.1
Fruit & Fibre, Lidl*	1 Serving/25g	91	1.2	363	8.8	70.9	4.9	8.0
Fruit & Fibre, Morrisons*	1 Serving/30g	110	2.2	366	8.8	66.5	7.2	8.5
Fruit & Fibre, Organic, Sainsbury's*	1 Serving/40g	147	1.6	367	10.0	72.4	4.1	7.8
Fruit & Fibre, Value, Tesco*	1 Serving/40g	144	2.2	359	11.4	65.7	5.6	8.0
Fruit & Fibre, Whole Grain, Sainsbury's*	1 Serving/30g	108	1.8	361	8.1	68.7	6.0	8.9
Fruit & Nut Crisp, Minis, Weetabix*	1 Serving/40g	144	1.8	359	9.3	70.0	4.6	8.9
Fruit 'n' Fibre, Kellogg's*	1 Serving/40g	152	2.4	380	8.0	69.0	6.0	9.0
Fruit, Nuts & Flakes, M&S*	1 Serving/30g	117	2.6	391	9.1	69.6	8.5	3.5
Golden Grahams, Nestle*	1 Serving/30g	112	0.9	375	6.0	81.0	3.0	3.4
Golden Honey Puffs, Tesco*	1 Serving/30g	115	0.4	382	6.6	86.3	1.2	3.0
Golden Nuggets, Nestle*	1 Serving/40g	152	0.3	381	6.2	87.4	0.7	1.5
Golden Puffs, Sainsbury's*	1 Serving/28g	107	0.3	383	6.6	86.3	1.2	3.0
Granola	1 Serving/45g	194	8.7	430	17.5	48.8	19.4	16.8
Granola & Strawberries with Bio Yoghurt, Rumblers*	1 Pot/168g	267	9.7	159	4.3	22.4	5.8	1.1
Granola, Chocolate, Dorset Cereals*	1 Serving/40g	206	12.0	515	8.8	47.2	30.0	10.5
Granola, Crunchy Nut Glorious Oat, Kellogg's*	1 Serving/45g	212	9.4	470	7.0	61.0	21.0	4.5
Granola, Crunchy Oat, Tropical Fruit, Harvest Morn, Aldi*	1 Serving/40g	174	5.2	436	9.4	66.0	13.0	7.4
Granola, Honey, Dorset Cereals*	1 Serving/40g	204	12.0	511	13.0	44.0	30.0	7.4
Granola, Low Fat, Home Farm*	1 Serving/55g	180	3.0	328	7.3	69.0	5.4	9.0
Granola, Multigrain Nutty, Good & Balanced, Asda*	1 Serving/40g	162	6.0	406	9.9	54.0	15.0	7.6

BREAKFAST CEREAL

	Measure INFO/WEIGHT	per Measure KCAL	FAT	Nutrition Values per 100g / 100ml KCAL	PROT	CARB	FAT	FIBRE
Granola, Nut, Simply Nut, Dorset Cereals*	1 Serving/40g	200	10.8	500	11.0	48.0	27.0	8.3
Granola, Oat Clusters, Apple & Cinnamon, Quaker Oats*	1 Pack/48g	193	3.8	403	8.0	70.2	8.0	9.4
Granola, Oat, Simply Oat, Dorset Cereals*	1 Serving/40g	177	6.8	443	8.8	60.0	17.0	7.4
Granola, Original, Diet Chef Ltd*	1 Pack/50g	248	14.6	496	10.9	46.2	29.3	10.6
Granola, Original, Lizi's, The GoodCarb Food Company*	1 Serving/50g	248	14.6	496	10.9	46.2	29.3	10.6
Granola, Pecan & Brazil Nut, Wholesome, Quaker Oats*	1 Serving/45g	189	5.0	420	11.1	61.8	11.1	13.2
Granola, Pink Apple & Cinnamon, Diet Chef Ltd*	1 Pack/40g	193	10.7	483	10.1	49.3	26.8	11.2
Granola, Quaker Oats*	1 Serving/48g	210	7.0	438	10.4	72.9	14.6	6.2
Granola, Seed & Nut, The Natural Low Carb store*	1 Serving/30g	151	11.5	504	19.4	5.4	38.4	29.9
Granola, Summer Fruits, Pomegranate Infused, M&S*	1 Serving/50g	200	6.4	400	8.6	63.2	12.7	5.8
Granola, Super Fruity, Jordan's*	1 Serving/45g	194	5.6	431	9.5	66.6	12.4	7.5
Granola, Superfoods, Jordans*	1 Serving/50g	208	6.7	415	9.0	64.7	13.4	8.6
Granola, Treacle & Pecan, Diet Chef Ltd*	1 Pack/40g	196	11.3	490	9.7	47.6	28.3	11.3
Grape Nuts, Kraft*	1 Serving/45g	158	0.9	350	10.9	81.9	2.0	11.9
Harvest Crunch, Nut, Quaker Oats*	1 Serving/40g	184	7.8	459	8.0	62.5	19.5	6.0
Harvest Crunch, Soft Juicy Raisins, Quaker Oats*	1 Serving/50g	221	8.0	442	6.0	67.0	16.0	4.0
High Bran, CBY, Asda*	1 Serving/40g	136	1.5	341	13.6	49.5	3.8	27.1
High Fibre Bran, Sainsbury's*	1 Serving/40g	134	1.5	335	14.3	48.4	3.7	25.4
High Fruit Muesli, BGTY, Sainsbury's*	1 Serving/50g	164	1.0	328	6.7	71.0	1.9	6.6
Honey & Nut Crisp, Mini, Weetabix*	1 Serving/40g	150	0.8	375	9.4	75.1	2.0	9.3
Honey Cheerios with 125ml Semi Skimmed Milk, Nestle*	1 Serving/30g	174	2.9	580	21.0	99.7	9.7	5.7
Honey Loops, Kellogg's*	1 Serving/30g	110	0.9	367	8.0	77.0	3.0	6.0
Honey Numbers, Harvest Morn, Aldi*	1 Serving/30g	114	1.0	379	6.9	78.7	3.3	3.3
Honey Raisin & Almond, Crunchy, Waitrose*	1 Serving/40g	170	4.8	425	10.5	68.8	12.0	5.7
Honey, Oats & More, Nestle*	1 Serving/30g	114	1.6	379	9.7	73.1	5.3	5.9
Hoops, Multigrain, Asda*	1 Serving/30g	113	1.2	376	6.5	78.4	4.0	4.6
Hoops, Multigrain, Tesco*	1 Serving/30g	112	1.1	375	6.5	78.6	3.8	4.6
Hot Oat, Aldi*	1 Serving/40g	142	3.3	356	11.6	58.8	8.3	8.9
Hot Oats, Instant, Tesco*	1 Serving/30g	108	2.6	360	11.8	58.4	8.7	7.9
Just Right, Kellogg's*	1 Serving/40g	145	1.2	362	7.0	77.0	3.0	4.5
Krave, Chocolate & Hazelnut, Kellogg's*	1 Serving/30g	132	4.8	440	8.0	66.0	16.0	4.0
Lion, Nestle*	1 Serving/40g	166	3.1	415	7.2	76.9	7.7	4.3
Luxury Muesli, Diet Chef Ltd*	1 Pack/40g	166	4.7	414	10.6	61.0	11.8	10.9
Malted Wheaties, CBY, Asda*	1 Serving/40g	146	0.8	366	10.3	72.7	1.9	8.2
Malted Wheats, Waitrose*	1 Serving/32g	110	0.6	343	9.7	71.7	1.9	9.9
Malties, Sainsbury's*	1 Serving/40g	137	1.2	343	10.0	69.2	2.9	10.0
Malty Flakes, Tesco*	1 Serving/40g	148	0.6	371	11.0	78.4	1.5	4.3
Maple & Pecan Crisp, Sainsbury's*	1 Serving/50g	226	9.8	452	7.9	61.3	19.5	5.4
Maple & Pecan Crisp, Tesco*	1 Serving/50g	215	7.6	430	10.5	62.5	15.2	10.2
Maple & Pecan, Crisp, Asda*	1 Serving/30g	135	5.7	451	8.0	62.0	19.0	6.0
Millet Rice Oatbran Flakes, Nature's Path*	1 Serving/56g	204	3.2	365	11.3	67.0	5.8	10.0
Mini Wheats, Original, Frosted, Kellogg's*	1 Serving/54g	190	1.0	352	9.3	83.3	1.8	11.1
Mini Wheats, Sainsbury's*	1 Serving/45g	157	1.0	348	11.8	69.9	2.3	11.8
Minibix, Weetabix*	1 Serving/40g	134	1.5	335	8.8	71.2	3.8	8.1
Muesli, Basics, Sainsbury's*	1 Serving/50g	178	2.6	355	11.2	61.5	5.1	9.2
Muesli, Berries & Cherries, Dorset Cereals*	1 Serving/70g	225	1.5	321	6.5	68.8	2.2	6.3
Muesli, Carb Control, Tesco*	1 Serving/35g	154	9.3	439	25.0	25.0	26.6	13.8
Muesli, COU, M&S*	1 Serving/60g	201	1.5	335	7.6	70.2	2.5	8.1
Muesli, Creamy Tropical Fruit, Finest, Tesco*	1 Serving/80g	283	4.5	354	7.2	68.8	5.6	6.9
Muesli, Crunchy, Organic, Sainsbury's*	1 Serving/40g	168	5.8	420	10.6	62.0	14.4	9.2
Muesli, De Luxe, No Added Salt or Sugar, Sainsbury's*	1 Serving/40g	161	5.6	403	11.9	57.6	13.9	8.4
Muesli, Fruit & Nut, COU, M&S*	1 Serving/40g	128	1.1	320	7.4	74.5	2.8	7.4
Muesli, Fruit & Nut, Jordans*	1 Serving/50g	180	4.7	361	8.0	61.2	9.4	7.5

	Measure INFO/WEIGHT	per Measure		Nutrition Values per 100g / 100ml				
		KCAL	FAT	KCAL	PROT	CARB	FAT	FIBRE
BREAKFAST CEREAL								
Muesli, Fruit & Nut, Luxury, Co-Op*	1 Serving/40g	150	4.0	375	8.0	64.0	10.0	6.0
Muesli, Fruit & Nut, Luxury, Lidl*	1 Serving/57g	205	5.6	360	8.0	60.0	9.8	7.5
Muesli, Fruit & Nut, Luxury, Sainsbury's*	1 Serving/50g	178	4.6	355	10.3	57.9	9.1	11.3
Muesli, Fruit & Nut, M&S*	1 Serving/40g	128	1.1	320	7.4	74.5	2.8	7.4
Muesli, Fruit & Nut, Organic, M&S*	1 Serving/50g	166	3.0	333	8.2	61.6	6.0	7.6
Muesli, Fruit & Nut, Sainsbury's*	1 Serving/30g	114	3.1	379	9.5	58.7	10.3	6.9
Muesli, Fruit & Nut, Tesco*	1 Serving/50g	190	5.6	380	8.4	60.3	11.3	5.3
Muesli, Fruit & Seeds, Organic, Pertwood Farm*	1 Serving/50g	164	3.4	328	11.4	55.5	6.7	12.6
Muesli, Fruit Nut & Seed, Organic, Dorset Cereals*	1 Serving/70g	251	6.9	358	10.8	56.6	9.8	8.4
Muesli, Fruit, Nuts & Seeds, Dorset Cereals*	1 Serving/70g	265	8.0	379	10.6	58.4	11.4	6.1
Muesli, Fruit, Waitrose*	1 Serving/30g	101	1.4	338	7.2	66.8	4.7	6.8
Muesli, Luxury Fruit, Harvest Morn, Aldi*	1 Serving/50g	158	1.6	315	6.8	64.5	3.3	6.9
Muesli, Luxury, Finest, Tesco*	1 Serving/50g	197	6.6	394	8.3	60.8	13.1	5.4
Muesli, Natural, No Added Sugar or Salt, Jordans*	1 Serving/45g	161	2.2	357	9.5	63.7	5.0	9.7
Muesli, No Added Sugar Or Salt, Organic, Jordans*	1 Serving/50g	175	4.4	350	9.2	58.4	8.8	9.3
Muesli, No Added Sugar, Waitrose*	1 Serving/40g	146	2.5	364	12.0	64.9	6.3	6.7
Muesli, Organic, Waitrose*	1 Serving/50g	188	0.8	375	10.3	59.6	1.6	8.3
Muesli, Original, Holland & Barrett*	1 Serving/30g	105	2.5	351	11.1	61.2	8.4	7.1
Muesli, Really Nutty, Dorset Cereals*	1 Serving/70g	253	6.1	362	9.8	61.1	8.7	6.3
Muesli, Simply Delicious, Dorset Cereals*	1 Serving/45g	160	3.3	356	9.9	58.1	7.4	8.9
Muesli, Simply Fruity, As Sold, Dorset Cereals*	1 Serving/45g	152	1.1	337	7.3	68.0	2.4	6.8
Muesli, Simply Sumptuous, Luxury Fruit, Lidl*	1 Serving/45g	154	1.5	343	6.5	68.7	3.3	6.2
Muesli, Special, Jordans*	1 Serving/50g	183	5.4	366	7.9	59.5	10.7	8.5
Muesli, Super Berry, Jordans*	1 Serving/50g	174	3.8	348	9.0	60.8	7.6	8.1
Muesli, Super High Fibre, Dorset Cereals*	1 Serving/70g	250	6.6	357	8.0	60.1	9.4	8.4
Muesli, Swiss Style with Fruit, Tesco*	1 Serving/40g	144	2.1	360	10.4	67.4	5.3	7.4
Muesli, Swiss Style, Aldi*	1 Serving/50g	180	3.2	359	9.8	65.3	6.5	8.3
Muesli, Swiss Style, Bettabuy, Morrisons*	1 Serving/50g	170	2.5	340	11.0	62.8	5.0	9.4
Muesli, Swiss Style, Co-Op*	1 Serving/40g	148	2.4	370	11.0	67.0	6.0	6.0
Muesli, Swiss Style, No Added Salt Or Sugar, Tesco*	1 Serving/50g	182	3.2	364	11.0	61.0	6.4	9.6
Muesli, Swiss Style, No Added Sugar Or Salt, Asda*	1 Serving/50g	182	3.5	363	11.0	64.0	7.0	8.0
Muesli, Swiss Style, Smart Price, Asda*	1 Serving/60g	222	3.6	370	9.0	70.0	6.0	10.0
Muesli, The Ultimate, Organic, Rude Health*	1 Serving/50g	163	4.5	326	10.8	50.5	9.0	12.3
Muesli, Toasted, Gluten Free, Buckwheat, Eat Natural*	1 Serving/50g	230	11.4	461	11.7	53.2	22.8	2.0
Muesli, Tropical, Sainsbury's*	1 Serving/50g	182	3.4	365	6.5	69.4	6.8	6.4
Muesli, Tropical, Tesco*	1 Serving/50g	173	2.4	346	7.8	68.2	4.7	9.1
Muesli, Unsweetened, M&S*	1 Serving/40g	129	1.1	322	8.1	68.0	2.7	9.4
Muesli, Value, Tesco*	1 Serving/50g	177	2.6	354	10.3	60.9	5.2	11.3
Muesli, Whole Wheat, No Added Sugar & Salt, Tesco*	1 Serving/40g	154	5.0	386	9.5	59.1	12.4	7.4
Muesli, Wholesome, Fruit Nut & Seed, LL, Waitrose*	1 Serving/45g	159	6.7	392	12.2	48.5	16.6	8.0
Multigrain Boulders, Tesco*	1 Serving/30g	112	0.4	375	8.2	82.3	1.3	3.6
Multigrain Flakes with Fruit & Nuts, Aldi*	1 Serving/30g	108	0.7	360	7.5	77.1	2.4	4.5
Multigrain Flakes, with Fruit, Tesco*	1 Serving/30g	147	0.9	367	7.2	77.3	2.2	4.7
Multigrain, Fitnesse, Nestle*	1 Serving/30g	109	0.4	363	8.0	79.8	1.3	5.1
Multigrain, Hoops, Average	*1 Serving/30g*	*112*	*1.1*	*374*	*6.6*	*77.4*	*3.6*	*6.1*
Oat Bran, Hodgson Mill*	1 Serving/40g	48	1.2	120	6.0	23.0	3.0	6.0
Oat Crunchy, Blueberry & Cranberry, Waitrose*	1 Serving/60g	259	9.1	432	8.0	65.9	15.2	8.5
Oat Granola, Quaker Oats*	1 Serving/50g	206	4.4	411	8.6	73.0	8.8	5.2
Oat Meal, Medium, Heart's Content, Mornflake*	1 Serving/30g	108	2.4	359	11.0	60.4	8.1	8.5
Oat, Crunchy, Sainsbury's*	1 Serving/50g	226	10.2	453	8.2	59.3	20.3	6.6
Oatbran & Oatgerm, Prewett's*	1 Serving/30g	104	2.9	345	14.8	49.7	9.7	15.2
Oatbran 100%, Mornflake*	1 Serving/40g	146	3.8	364	13.4	47.3	9.4	18.2
Oatbran Flakes, Original, Mornflake*	1 Serving/40g	149	2.1	372	11.9	63.2	5.2	12.4

BREAKFAST CEREAL

	Measure INFO/WEIGHT	per Measure KCAL	FAT	Nutrition Values per 100g / 100ml KCAL	PROT	CARB	FAT	FIBRE
Oatbran Sprinkles, Mornflake*	1 Serving/40g	146	3.8	364	13.4	47.3	9.4	18.2
Oatbran, Original Pure, Mornflake*	1 Serving/30g	104	2.9	345	14.8	49.7	9.7	15.2
Oatibix, Flakes, Weetabix*	1 Serving/50g	190	2.8	381	9.5	73.2	5.6	3.5
Oatibix, Original, Bitesize, Weetabix*	1 Serving/36g	133	2.4	370	10.6	66.5	6.8	10.1
Oatibix, Weetabix*	2 Biscuits/48g	189	3.8	394	12.5	64.3	8.0	7.3
Oatmeal, Instant, Heart to Heart, Kashi*	1 Serving/43g	150	2.0	349	7.0	76.7	4.6	9.3
Oatmeal, Quick Oats, Dry, Quaker Oats*	1 Serving/30g	114	2.0	380	14.0	66.7	6.7	10.0
Oatmeal, Raw	*1oz/28g*	*112*	*2.4*	*401*	*12.4*	*72.8*	*8.7*	*6.8*
Oatmeal, Scottish, Hamlyns of Scotland*	1 Portion/40g	157	3.7	392	11.2	66.0	9.2	7.1
Oats, Ginger Bread, Bench Press, Instant, Oomf*	1 Pot/75g	296	3.4	395	28.3	57.1	4.5	6.7
Oats, Jumbo, Organic, Waitrose*	1 Serving/50g	180	4.0	361	11.0	61.1	8.1	7.8
Oats, Pure, Free From, Sainsbury's*	1 Serving/40g	164	3.2	410	14.9	64.0	8.0	11.0
Oats, Superfast, Mornflake*	1 Serving/40g	144	3.2	359	11.0	60.4	8.1	8.5
Oats, Tesco*	1 Serving/40g	142	3.2	356	11.0	60.0	8.0	8.0
Oats, Wholegrain, Organic, Quaker Oats*	1 Serving/25g	89	2.0	356	11.0	60.0	8.0	9.0
Organic, Weetabix*	2 Biscuits/38g	134	0.7	358	11.5	68.6	2.0	10.0
Original, Crunchy, Raisins & Almonds, Jordans*	1 Serving/50g	204	6.4	407	8.7	64.0	12.9	6.6
Perfekt, Granola, Ultimate, Organic, GranoVita*	1 Serving/40g	190	6.6	474	13.3	40.6	16.4	11.8
Porage Oats, Old Fashioned, Dry, Scotts*	1 Serving/40g	142	3.2	355	11.0	60.0	8.0	9.0
Porage Oats, Original, Dry, Scotts*	1 Serving/40g	142	3.2	356	11.0	60.0	8.0	9.0
Porage Oats, Original, So-Easy, Dry, Scotts*	1 Serving/30g	109	2.6	364	11.0	60.0	8.5	9.0
Porage Oats, Syrup Swirl, So-Easy, Dry, Scotts*	1 Sachet/37g	135	2.2	366	8.0	70.0	6.0	6.5
Porridge 5 Grain, 5 Seed, Rude Health*	1 Serving/50g	176	4.1	351	12.2	57.1	8.2	12.4
Porridge Oats, & Bran, Co-Op*	1 Serving/40g	141	2.8	353	12.5	60.0	7.0	12.0
Porridge Oats, Co-Op*	1 Serving/40g	144	3.2	360	12.0	61.0	8.0	9.0
Porridge Oats, Dry Weight, Value, Tesco*	1 Serving/50g	180	4.0	359	11.0	60.4	8.1	8.5
Porridge Oats, Mornflake*	1 Serving/50g	180	4.0	359	11.0	60.4	8.1	8.5
Porridge Oats, Organic, Tesco*	1 Serving/28g	100	2.3	358	11.0	60.4	8.1	8.5
Porridge Oats, Original, Dry, Quaker Oats*	1 Serving/45g	160	3.6	356	11.0	60.0	8.0	4.0
Porridge Oats, Original, Paw Ridge, Quaker Oats*	1 Sachet/25g	89	2.0	356	11.0	60.0	8.0	9.0
Porridge Oats, Rolled, Tesco*	1 Serving/50g	180	4.0	359	11.0	60.4	8.1	8.5
Porridge Oats, Scottish, Organic, Sainsbury's*	1 Serving/45g	172	2.2	383	10.0	74.4	5.0	7.9
Porridge Oats, Scottish, Tesco*	1 Serving/50g	180	4.0	359	11.0	60.4	8.1	8.5
Porridge Oats, with Bran, Scottish, Sainsbury's*	1 Serving/50g	190	2.5	380	9.6	74.1	5.0	10.3
Porridge Oats, with Wheatbran, Essential, Waitrose*	1 Serving/50g	168	3.8	336	11.2	55.8	7.6	13.0
Porridge, Apple & Cinnamon, Express, Sainsbury's*	1 Sachet/36g	138	2.1	383	8.6	70.3	5.9	7.2
Porridge, Apple & Cinnamon, Variety Box, Graze*	1 Bag/67g	240	3.4	356	8.0	68.0	5.0	10.0
Porridge, Apple & Pear, Variety Box, Graze*	1 Bag/63g	226	3.7	359	9.4	65.0	5.9	11.0
Porridge, Apple, Sultana & Cinnamon, M&S*	1 Sachet/40g	144	3.0	360	10.3	62.3	7.5	8.6
Porridge, Banana, Ready Brek, Weetabix*	1 Serving/40g	146	2.6	365	8.9	68.0	6.4	6.7
Porridge, Berry Burst, Oat So Simple, Quaker Oats*	1 Serving/39g	144	2.3	370	8.0	70.0	6.0	6.5
Porridge, Caramel, Pot, Oat So Simple, Quaker Oats*	1 Pot/57g	208	3.2	365	10.5	67.7	5.6	6.3
Porridge, Chocolate, Ready Brek, Weetabix*	1 Serving/30g	114	2.4	380	10.0	63.6	8.0	7.0
Porridge, Country Honey, Oat So Simple, Quaker Oats*	1 Serving/36g	134	2.3	373	8.5	69.0	6.5	6.0
Porridge, Free From, Sainsbury's*	1 Serving/50g	174	1.5	348	8.6	72.0	3.0	3.4
Porridge, Fruit & Nut, Fruity, Dorset Cereals*	1 Serving/70g	242	5.6	346	9.4	59.0	8.0	8.2
Porridge, Golden Honey, Oatibix, Weetabix*	1 Serving/40g	145	2.6	363	9.2	66.7	6.6	7.0
Porridge, Golden Syrup, Oat So Simple, Quaker Oats*	1 Sachet/36g	137	2.2	380	8.4	68.7	6.2	6.8
Porridge, Honey & Vanilla, Oat So Simple, Quaker Oats*	1 Pot/57g	213	2.9	374	15.1	64.1	5.1	5.5
Porridge, Multigrain, Jordans*	1 Serving/40g	134	2.2	335	10.4	60.9	5.5	10.0
Porridge, Oats, Dry, Smart Price, Asda*	1 Serving/50g	186	4.0	372	11.0	60.0	8.0	8.0
Porridge, Oats, Golden Syrup, Sainsbury's*	1 Sachet/39g	143	2.1	367	6.3	73.6	5.3	6.7
Porridge, Original, As Sold, Moma Foods*	1 Pot/70g	257	4.2	367	15.6	59.0	6.0	7.6

BREAKFAST CEREAL

INFO/WEIGHT	Measure	per Measure KCAL	FAT	Nutrition Values per 100g / 100ml KCAL	PROT	CARB	FAT	FIBRE
Porridge, Original, Diet Chef Ltd*	1 Sachet/40g	157	2.5	392	12.0	67.0	6.3	9.8
Porridge, Original, Dry, Oat So Simple, Quaker Oats*	1 Serving/27g	100	2.1	370	11.0	58.9	7.7	10.5
Porridge, Original, Express, Sachet, Sainsbury's*	1 Pack/27g	100	2.2	370	11.0	58.0	8.0	10.8
Porridge, Original, Ready Brek, Weetabix*	1 Serving/40g	149	3.5	373	11.7	57.9	8.7	7.9
Porridge, Original, Simply, Sachet, Asda*	1 Sachet/27g	96	2.2	356	11.0	60.0	8.0	8.0
Porridge, Plain, Instant, Quaker Oats*	1 Serving/34g	124	2.9	364	11.0	60.0	8.5	9.0
Porridge, Rice & Buckwheat, Free From, Sainsbury's*	1 Serving/50g	179	0.4	358	6.8	81.1	0.7	1.4
Porridge, Strawberry, Diet Chef Ltd*	1 Serving/40g	159	3.1	398	11.2	65.9	7.7	10.6
Porridge, Superfoods, Jordans*	1 Serving/40g	145	3.6	362	10.4	59.8	9.0	8.3
Porridge, Vanilla & Banana, Diet Chef Ltd*	1 Pack/40g	151	2.2	378	10.7	70.6	5.6	9.8
Porridge, with Apple & Cinnamon, Diet Chef Ltd*	1 Pack/40g	150	1.9	375	8.9	69.5	4.7	9.0
Porridge, with Cocao Nib, Diet Chef Ltd*	1 Pack/40g	164	3.5	410	10.9	67.3	8.8	9.5
Protein Crunch, Chocolate, As Sold, Weetabix*	1 Serving/30g	114	1.0	379	20.0	64.0	3.2	7.0
Puffed Rice, Average	*1 Serving/30g*	*115*	*0.8*	*382*	*7.1*	*82.2*	*2.8*	*3.0*
Puffed Rice, Honey, Organic, Kallo*	1 Serving/25g	98	0.9	392	5.0	85.0	3.5	2.1
Puffed Rice, Organic, Natural, Kallo*	1 Serving/25g	92	0.5	370	7.0	81.0	2.0	3.0
Puffed Wheat, Quaker Oats*	1 Serving/15g	49	0.2	328	15.3	62.4	1.3	5.6
Puffed Wheat, Tesco*	1 Serving/28g	104	0.9	373	13.9	72.2	3.2	5.7
Raisin Wheats, Kellogg's*	1 Serving/30g	99	0.6	330	9.0	70.0	2.0	8.0
Raisin Wheats, Sainsbury's*	1 Serving/50g	166	0.8	332	8.2	71.5	1.5	8.0
Raisin, Bran Flakes, Asda*	1 Serving/50g	166	1.5	331	7.0	69.0	3.0	10.0
Raisin, Oats & More, Nestle*	1 Serving/30g	112	1.4	373	8.9	73.7	4.7	5.8
Red Berries, Special K, Kellogg's*	1 Serving/30g	112	0.4	374	14.0	76.0	1.5	3.0
Red Berry, & Almond, Luxury Crunch, Jordans*	1 Serving/40g	176	7.4	441	8.2	60.5	18.5	6.6
Rice Krispies, Kellogg's*	1 Serving/30g	115	0.3	383	6.0	87.0	1.0	1.0
Rice Krispies, Multi-Grain, Shapes, Kellogg's*	1 Serving/30g	111	0.8	370	8.0	77.0	2.5	8.0
Rice Pops, Organic, Dove's Farm*	1 Serving/30g	107	0.2	357	6.8	86.1	0.8	2.0
Rice Pops, Sainsbury's*	1 Serving/25g	98	0.4	391	6.7	87.1	1.4	1.7
Rice Snaps, Asda*	1 Serving/28g	105	0.4	376	7.0	84.0	1.3	1.5
Rice Snaps, Everyday Value, Tesco*	1 Serving/30g	115	0.3	380	7.5	84.5	0.9	1.4
Ricicles, Kellogg's*	1 Serving/30g	114	0.2	381	4.5	89.0	0.8	0.8
Right Balance, Morrisons*	1 Serving/50g	181	1.1	362	6.9	78.6	2.2	5.3
Shredded Wheat, Average	*2 Biscuits/45g*	*157*	*0.8*	*348*	*9.0*	*77.0*	*1.8*	*10.0*
Shredded Wheat, Bitesize, Nestle*	1 Serving/40g	148	0.9	369	11.8	69.6	2.2	11.8
Shredded Wheat, Fruitful, No Added Salt, Nestle*	1 Serving/40g	142	2.0	354	8.3	68.7	5.1	8.9
Shredded Wheat, Honey Nut, Nestle*	1 Serving/40g	151	2.6	378	11.2	68.8	6.5	9.4
Shreddies, Coco Orange Flavoured, Nestle*	1 Serving/40g	150	0.8	374	8.5	76.2	2.0	8.6
Shreddies, Coco, Nestle*	1 Serving/45g	161	0.9	358	8.4	76.5	2.0	8.6
Shreddies, Frosted, Nestle*	1 Serving/45g	164	0.7	365	7.4	80.7	1.5	6.4
Shreddies, Honey, Nestle*	1 Serving/45g	169	0.7	375	8.2	78.1	1.5	8.1
Shreddies, Malt Wheats, Tesco*	1 Serving/45g	169	0.9	375	10.3	73.8	2.0	8.2
Shreddies, Nestle*	1 Serving/45g	186	1.0	371	10.0	73.7	1.9	9.9
Special Flakes, Tesco*	1 Serving/20g	74	0.3	371	11.0	78.4	1.5	4.3
Special Flakes, with Red Berries, Crownfield, Lidl*	1 Serving/30g	113	0.5	377	6.5	81.0	1.6	6.4
Special K, Bliss, Creamy Berry Crunch, Kellogg's*	1 Serving/30g	114	0.8	379	13.0	76.0	2.5	2.5
Special K, Bliss, Strawberry & Chocolate, Kellogg's*	1 Serving/30g	115	0.9	383	13.0	76.0	3.0	2.5
Special K, Choco, Kellogg's*	1 Serving/40g	160	2.8	400	14.0	70.0	7.0	3.5
Special K, Kellogg's*	1 Serving/30g	114	0.4	379	14.0	76.0	1.5	2.5
Special K, Oats & Honey, Kellogg's*	1 Serving/30g	114	0.9	381	9.0	77.0	3.0	5.0
Special K, Peach & Apricot, Kellogg's*	1 Serving/30g	112	0.3	373	14.0	77.0	1.0	2.5
Special K, Purple Berries, Kellogg's*	1 Serving/30g	112	0.3	374	13.0	77.0	1.0	3.5
Special K, Yoghurty, Kellogg's*	1 Serving/30g	115	0.9	383	14.0	75.0	3.0	2.5
Start, Kellogg's*	1 Serving/30g	117	1.0	390	8.0	79.0	3.5	5.0

	Measure INFO/WEIGHT	per Measure KCAL	FAT	Nutrition Values per 100g / 100ml KCAL	PROT	CARB	FAT	FIBRE
BREAKFAST CEREAL								
Strawberry & Almond Crunch, M&S*	1 Serving/40g	186	7.4	465	8.0	66.0	18.6	4.9
Strawberry Crisp, Asda*	1 Serving/45g	194	7.0	431	8.1	64.7	15.5	5.9
Strawberry, Alpen*	1 Serving/40g	144	1.9	359	9.4	69.5	4.8	7.9
Sugar Puffs, Quaker Oats*	1 Serving/30g	114	0.5	379	5.3	85.8	1.6	3.7
Sultana Bran, Co-Op*	1 Serving/40g	130	1.2	325	9.0	66.0	3.0	11.0
Sultana Bran, HL, Tesco*	1 Serving/30g	98	0.6	325	8.2	68.0	1.9	12.0
Sultana Bran, Morrisons*	1 Serving/30g	98	0.9	325	8.8	65.8	3.0	11.4
Sultana Bran, Waitrose*	1 Serving/30g	97	0.6	324	8.2	68.6	1.9	11.6
Vitality, with Red Fruit, Asda*	1 Serving/30g	110	0.5	366	11.0	77.0	1.6	3.8
Weet Bix, Sanitarium*	2 Biscuits/30g	106	0.4	352	12.0	67.0	1.4	10.5
Weetabix, Banana, Weetabix*	1 Serving/44g	157	0.9	357	10.0	70.4	2.0	9.8
Weetabix, Chocolate, Weetabix*	2 Biscuits/45g	166	1.8	368	10.1	67.9	4.0	10.0
Weetaflakes, Weetabix*	1 Serving/30g	102	0.4	340	8.9	72.9	1.4	11.0
Weetos, Chocolate, Weetabix*	1 Serving/30g	113	1.5	378	8.4	75.1	4.9	5.8
Wheat Biscuits, Average	**2 Biscuits/38g**	**130**	**0.8**	**347**	**11.7**	**68.4**	**2.2**	**9.9**
Wheat Bisks, Banana, Mini, Asda*	1 Serving/50g	190	2.7	380	9.7	73.1	5.4	7.4
Wheat Bisks, Harvest Morn, Aldi*	2 Biscuits/38g	136	0.8	358	11.5	68.6	2.0	10.0
Wheat Flakes, Malted, Toasted, Suma*	1 Serving/75g	260	1.4	346	10.3	72.0	1.9	10.4
Wholegrain Hoops, Goldenvale, Aldi*	1 Serving/30g	111	0.8	371	6.9	74.0	2.6	10.7
Wholegrain, Apricot, Wheats, Sainsbury's*	1 Serving/50g	160	0.8	320	7.9	71.6	1.5	8.2
Wholegrain, Fruit & Fibre, Sainsbury's*	1 Serving/30g	109	1.8	363	8.1	69.1	6.0	8.9
Wholegrain, Mini Wheats, Sainsbury's*	1 Serving/40g	144	0.7	359	11.8	68.2	1.8	11.2
Wholegrain, Minis, Weetabix*	1 Serving/40g	149	0.8	372	10.2	73.2	2.0	10.0
Wholegrain, Sultana Bran, Sainsbury's*	1 Serving/30g	98	0.6	325	8.3	68.6	1.9	12.1
Yoghurt & Raspberry, Crisp, Sainsbury's*	1 Serving/45g	191	6.7	424	7.5	65.2	14.8	6.4
BRESAOLA								
Della Valtellina, Air Dried Beef, Deluxe, Lidl*	1 Pack/80g	130	2.4	163	33.5	0.5	3.0	0.0
Della Valtellina, Sainsbury's*	1 Slice/14g	23	0.4	163	34.7	0.1	2.6	0.1
Finest, Tesco*	1 Serving/35g	64	1.4	182	36.0	0.5	4.0	0.0
BROCCOLI								
& Cauliflower, Crowns, TTD, Sainsbury's*	1 Serving/100g	33	0.9	33	4.4	1.8	0.9	2.6
& Cauliflower, Floret Mix, Fresh, Tesco*	1 Serving/80g	27	0.7	34	3.9	2.5	0.9	2.7
& Cauliflower, Floret Mix, Iceland*	1 Serving/100g	26	0.7	26	2.6	2.2	0.7	2.4
Bellaverde, TTD, Sainsbury's*	1 Serving/100g	33	0.9	33	4.4	1.8	0.9	2.6
Chinese, Kai Lan, Cooked	1 Serving/80g	18	0.6	22	1.4	3.8	0.7	2.5
Green, Boiled, Average	*1 Serving/80g*	*19*	*0.6*	*24*	*3.1*	*1.1*	*0.8*	*2.3*
Green, Raw, Average	*1 Serving/80g*	*24*	*0.7*	*30*	*3.7*	*1.6*	*0.8*	*2.5*
Purple Sprouting, Boiled, Average	*1 Serving/80g*	*15*	*0.5*	*19*	*2.1*	*1.3*	*0.6*	*2.3*
Purple Sprouting, Raw	*1oz/28g*	*10*	*0.3*	*35*	*3.9*	*2.6*	*1.1*	*3.5*
Steamed, Average	*1 Serving/100g*	*24*	*0.8*	*24*	*3.1*	*1.1*	*0.8*	*2.3*
Tenderstem, Average	*1oz/28g*	*10*	*0.2*	*35*	*4.1*	*2.9*	*0.6*	*2.3*
BROWNIES								
Average	*1 Brownie/60g*	*243*	*10.1*	*405*	*4.6*	*0.0*	*16.8*	*0.0*
Chocolate & Pecan, Gu*	1 Brownie/40g	188	11.6	471	7.2	47.6	29.1	2.5
Chocolate Orange, Organic, The Village Bakery*	1 Brownie/30g	126	6.7	421	5.0	50.5	22.2	0.9
Chocolate, Average	*1 Serving/100g*	*446*	*22.3*	*446*	*5.9*	*55.6*	*22.3*	*2.2*
Chocolate, Bites, Mini, Weight Watchers*	1 Brownie/9g	29	0.5	325	5.3	63.7	5.5	2.2
Chocolate, Chewy, M&S*	1 Brownie/29g	130	6.0	455	6.5	59.8	21.1	2.0
Chocolate, Chunky, Belgian, M&S*	1 Brownie/55g	242	11.2	440	6.2	57.7	20.3	2.5
Chocolate, Fudgy, M&S*	1 Brownie/87g	400	21.9	460	4.8	56.9	25.2	3.0
Chocolate, Mini Bites, Asda*	1 Brownie/15g	62	3.0	420	5.0	55.0	20.0	1.4
Chocolate, Sainsbury's*	1 Brownie/60g	265	13.6	442	4.6	55.0	22.6	1.6
Chocolate, Slices, M&S*	1 Brownie/36g	158	8.7	440	5.3	51.1	24.1	1.3

B

	Measure INFO/WEIGHT	per Measure		Nutrition Values per 100g / 100ml				
		KCAL	FAT	KCAL	PROT	CARB	FAT	FIBRE
BROWNIES								
Chocolate, Tray Bake, Tesco*	1 Brownie/37g	155	6.8	420	5.5	57.1	18.4	5.7
Chocolate, Waitrose*	1 Brownie/45g	192	8.9	426	6.3	55.6	19.8	2.7
Chocolate, Weight Watchers*	1 Brownie/47g	143	1.8	304	4.8	62.5	3.8	3.2
Chocolate, Wheat & Gluten Free, Mrs Crimble's*	1 Slice/48g	180	9.6	379	4.2	47.9	20.3	1.5
Double Chocolate Iced, Otis Spunkmeyer*	1 Brownie/57g	250	6.8	439	3.5	61.4	12.0	1.8
Double Chocolate, Mini Bites, Sainsbury's*	1 Brownie/15g	49	2.5	326	5.8	38.9	16.4	1.6
Praline, Mini, Finest, Tesco*	1 Brownie/12g	59	3.1	492	4.2	60.0	25.8	0.8
The Graze Brownie, Graze*	1 Portion/30g	110	5.4	368	7.1	50.5	17.9	3.8
BRUSCHETTA								
Cheese & Tomato, Asda*	1 Bruschetta/38g	68	1.7	180	8.6	26.0	4.6	2.9
Pane Italia*	1 Serving/75g	367	18.8	489	12.4	53.6	25.1	1.4
Red Pepper & Onion, Brunchetta, Golden Vale*	1 Pack/90g	266	17.1	296	14.6	17.0	19.0	1.3
Toasted, Olive Oil & Sea Salt, Tesco*	1 Serving/30g	126	4.6	420	11.5	58.7	15.5	4.5
BRUSSELS SPROUTS								
Boiled, Average	*1 Serving/80g*	*27*	*1.0*	*33*	*3.0*	*3.0*	*1.2*	*3.3*
Button, Raw, Average	*1 Serving/80g*	*28*	*1.0*	*36*	*3.3*	*2.8*	*1.3*	*3.0*
Canned, Drained	*1oz/28g*	*5*	*0.2*	*17*	*1.6*	*1.5*	*0.6*	*1.6*
Raw, Average	*1 Serving/80g*	*28*	*0.8*	*35*	*3.3*	*3.1*	*1.0*	*2.9*
Steamed, Average	*1 Serving/100g*	*35*	*1.3*	*35*	*3.1*	*3.2*	*1.3*	*3.5*
BUBBLE & SQUEAK								
Fried in Vegetable Oil	1oz/28g	35	2.5	124	1.4	9.8	9.1	1.5
Tesco*	½ Pack/325g	292	12.7	90	1.6	11.3	3.9	0.9
Waitrose*	½ Pack/225g	166	5.2	74	1.4	11.9	2.3	2.2
BUCKWHEAT								
Average	*1oz/28g*	*102*	*0.4*	*364*	*8.1*	*84.9*	*1.5*	*2.1*
BULGAR WHEAT								
Dry Weight, Average	*1oz/28g*	*99*	*0.5*	*353*	*9.7*	*76.3*	*1.7*	*8.0*
with Chick Peas, & Quinoa, Ready to Eat, Sainsbury's*	½ Pack/125g	239	4.1	191	7.7	30.0	3.3	4.7
BUNS								
Bath, M&S*	1 Bun/71g	217	5.7	305	8.3	49.8	8.0	1.9
Belgian, Asda*	1 Bun/133g	464	19.9	350	4.8	49.0	15.0	2.2
Belgian, Co-Op*	1 Bun/118g	413	15.3	350	5.0	54.0	13.0	2.0
Belgian, Iced, CBY, Asda*	1 Bun/115g	375	6.8	327	6.1	62.3	5.9	2.9
Belgian, Sainsbury's*	1 Bun/110g	398	11.3	362	6.1	61.3	10.3	1.9
Belgian, Tesco*	1 Bun/123g	438	15.7	356	5.2	54.9	12.8	2.2
Chelsea	1 Bun/78g	285	10.8	366	7.8	56.1	13.8	1.7
Chelsea, Sainsbury's*	1 Bun/85g	239	4.4	281	6.9	51.6	5.2	2.9
Chelsea, Tesco*	1 Bun/85g	269	6.5	316	7.9	53.9	7.6	2.3
Choux, Caramel, Asda*	1 Bun/189g	745	51.0	394	4.3	33.5	27.0	1.3
Choux, Custard, M&S*	1 Bun/85g	234	18.7	275	4.2	15.0	22.0	0.3
Choux, Fresh Cream, Tesco*	1 Bun/95g	340	23.7	358	4.9	28.5	24.9	0.9
Currant	1 Bun/60g	178	4.5	296	7.6	52.7	7.5	0.0
Currant, Sainsbury's*	1 Bun/72g	197	3.7	274	7.0	50.0	5.1	2.8
Fingers, Sticky, Iced, CBY, Asda*	1 Finger/40g	132	2.4	330	7.1	62.0	5.9	2.7
Fruit, Waitrose*	1 Bun/54g	155	2.3	287	8.1	54.0	4.3	1.6
Hot Cross	1 Bun/50g	156	3.5	312	7.4	58.5	7.0	1.7
Hot Cross, 25% Reduced Fat, Asda*	1 Bun/61g	153	1.4	253	9.0	49.0	2.3	3.0
Hot Cross, Apple & Cinnamon, Large, Finest, Tesco*	1 Bun/117g	342	8.2	292	7.3	49.9	7.0	3.6
Hot Cross, Asda*	1 Bun/60g	190	3.8	317	10.0	55.0	6.3	3.3
Hot Cross, BGTY, Sainsbury's*	1 Bun/70g	187	1.9	267	6.3	52.7	2.7	3.5
Hot Cross, Chocolate, Coles*	1 Bun/86g	296	9.0	344	7.0	53.4	10.5	0.0
Hot Cross, Classics, M&S*	1 Bun/65g	159	1.2	245	8.5	49.1	1.8	2.2
Hot Cross, Co-Op*	1 Bun/60g	165	3.6	275	8.0	47.0	6.0	3.0

	Measure INFO/WEIGHT	per Measure KCAL	FAT	Nutrition Values per 100g / 100ml KCAL	PROT	CARB	FAT	FIBRE
BUNS								
Hot Cross, Extra Spicy, M&S*	1 Bun/76g	175	1.4	230	8.6	44.1	1.9	4.2
Hot Cross, Finest, Tesco*	1 Bun/75g	210	4.0	280	7.8	49.5	5.4	2.8
Hot Cross, Golden Wholemeal, Sainsbury's*	1 Bun/65g	180	4.0	277	9.9	45.4	6.2	4.3
Hot Cross, HE, Tesco*	1 Bun/60g	155	1.5	258	8.6	50.3	2.5	2.6
Hot Cross, HL, Tesco*	1 Bun/70g	176	1.9	251	6.7	50.3	2.7	2.6
Hot Cross, Less Than 3% Fat, M&S*	1 Bun/70g	175	1.3	250	8.1	49.8	1.8	2.2
Hot Cross, Luxury, M&S*	1 Bun/79g	201	3.2	255	8.6	46.2	4.0	2.1
Hot Cross, Luxury, Rowan Hill Bakery, Lidl*	1 Bun/75g	204	3.5	272	8.3	47.0	4.7	4.0
Hot Cross, Mini, M&S*	1 Bun/41g	110	1.4	265	7.8	51.4	3.4	3.7
Hot Cross, Morrisons*	1 Bun/72g	178	1.4	247	7.4	49.9	2.0	3.3
Hot Cross, Tesco*	1 Bun/70g	186	1.9	265	7.4	51.8	2.7	3.6
Hot Cross, TTD, Sainsbury's*	1 Bun/75g	200	4.2	267	7.2	47.0	5.6	3.8
Hot Cross, White, Kingsmill*	1 Bun/70g	186	2.4	266	8.7	48.0	3.5	3.6
Hot Cross, White, Sainsbury's*	1 Bun/70g	199	3.4	284	7.9	50.6	4.8	3.4
Hot Cross, White, Waitrose*	1 Bun/68g	174	2.1	258	8.1	49.5	3.1	3.9
Hot Cross, Wholemeal, Asda*	1 Bun/70g	182	4.2	262	9.0	43.0	6.0	6.0
Hot Cross, Wholemeal, Organic, Tesco*	1 Bun/55g	140	2.7	254	7.6	44.8	4.9	4.5
Hot Cross, Wholemeal, Waitrose*	1 Bun/64g	177	4.3	276	8.8	45.2	6.7	4.9
Iced Finger, Tesco*	1 Bun/41g	115	1.4	280	7.1	54.7	3.4	2.9
Iced Lemon, Tesco*	1 Bun/48g	156	4.2	325	5.2	56.5	8.7	1.9
Iced, Filled with Raspberry Jam, M&S*	1 Bun/48g	155	3.2	320	6.4	58.9	6.6	1.9
Iced, Finger, Average	**1 Bun/40g**	**130**	**3.1**	**325**	**7.2**	**57.0**	**7.7**	**2.3**
Iced, Spiced Fruit, M&S*	1 Bun/90g	270	3.3	300	7.0	60.3	3.7	1.5
Iced, Tesco*	1 Bun/35g	117	3.4	334	7.0	54.8	9.6	2.5
Marlborough, M&S*	1 Bun/71g	215	6.3	305	6.2	43.4	8.9	2.2
Vanilla Iced, Soft, M&S*	1 Bun/39g	125	3.1	320	7.6	54.9	8.0	2.9
BURGERS								
Beef, & Caramelised Red Onion, Steak, TTD, Sainsbury's*	1 Burger/133g	287	15.3	216	20.2	7.8	11.5	0.5
Beef, & Mature Cheddar, Asda*	1 Burger/80g	178	10.0	223	21.5	6.2	12.5	0.5
Beef, & Onion, Grilled, Asda*	1 Burger/81g	201	11.5	248	23.1	6.9	14.2	0.5
Beef, 100%, Average	**1 Burger/52g**	**148**	**11.6**	**286**	**20.5**	**0.6**	**22.3**	**0.1**
Beef, 100%, Birds Eye*	1 Burger/41g	120	10.2	292	17.3	0.0	24.8	0.0
Beef, 100%, Half Pounders, Sainsbury's*	1 Burger/148g	462	33.1	313	26.0	1.7	22.4	0.2
Beef, 100%, Organic, Waitrose*	1 Burger/57g	140	9.6	247	23.6	0.0	16.9	0.0
Beef, 100%, Pure, Ross*	1 Burger/56g	128	9.6	229	17.1	1.4	17.1	0.0
Beef, 100%, Quarter Pounders, Aldi*	1 Burger/114g	320	23.3	282	24.3	0.1	20.5	1.3
Beef, 100%, Sainsbury's*	1 Burger/44g	133	10.4	302	21.4	0.9	23.6	0.9
Beef, Aberdeen Angus, Asda*	1 Burger/112g	249	13.3	222	22.2	6.7	11.8	0.9
Beef, Aberdeen Angus, Fresh, Waitrose*	1 Burger/113g	269	21.0	238	16.4	1.2	18.6	0.0
Beef, Aberdeen Angus, Gourmet, Finest, Tesco*	1 Burger/118g	225	13.4	190	18.9	2.0	11.3	1.0
Beef, Aberdeen Angus, M&S*	1 Burger/142g	298	18.9	210	18.3	4.1	13.3	0.1
Beef, Asda*	1 Burger/114g	304	18.6	267	26.8	3.2	16.3	0.7
Beef, BGTY, Sainsbury's*	1 Burger/110g	177	6.0	161	20.8	7.1	5.5	1.1
Beef, British, Grilled, Finest, Tesco*	1 Burger/95g	185	11.8	195	17.2	3.3	12.4	0.9
Beef, British, Organic, Waitrose*	1 Burger/85g	226	16.6	266	19.0	3.5	19.5	1.0
Beef, British, Waitrose*	1 Burger/113g	279	21.0	247	18.6	1.2	18.6	0.0
Beef, Chargrill, Tesco*	1 Burger/114g	246	18.4	217	17.0	0.8	16.2	2.5
Beef, Economy, Value, Tesco*	1 Burger/41g	105	5.9	255	21.6	8.5	14.5	0.3
Beef, Flame Grilled, Feasters*	1 Burger/58g	164	13.5	282	19.3	2.6	23.2	0.0
Beef, in a Bun, HE, Tesco*	1 Pack/189g	282	2.5	149	13.6	20.7	1.3	2.1
Beef, Morrisons*	1 Burger/57g	169	14.3	298	12.3	5.5	25.2	0.6
Beef, Organic, M&S*	1 Burger/110g	239	17.6	217	18.2	0.0	16.0	0.2
Beef, Original, & Best, Birds Eye*	1 Burger/46g	115	8.9	252	14.1	5.1	19.5	0.4

BURGERS

Measure INFO/WEIGHT	per Measure KCAL	per Measure FAT	Nutrition Values per 100g / 100ml KCAL	PROT	CARB	FAT	FIBRE
Beef, Original, with Onion, Grilled, Birds Eye*	1 Burger/38g	110	9.5	287	13.4	2.6	24.8	0.3
Beef, Quarter Pounder, Chilled, Morrisons*	1 Burger/115g	228	13.9	198	17.2	4.4	12.1	0.2
Beef, Quarter Pounders, BGTY, Sainsbury's*	1 Burger/114g	188	9.3	166	16.9	6.1	8.2	1.0
Beef, Quarter Pounders, Farmfoods*	1 Burger/113g	289	22.1	256	14.4	5.4	19.6	0.1
Beef, Quarter Pounders, Flame Grilled, Rustlers*	1 Burger/190g	557	28.7	293	14.9	24.3	15.1	0.0
Beef, Quarter Pounders, Flame Grilled, Tesco*	1 Burger/88g	246	20.4	280	13.1	4.8	23.2	0.8
Beef, Quarter Pounders, Jalapeno, Signature, Morrisons*	1 Burger/97g	205	9.9	212	20.8	8.7	10.2	0.8
Beef, Quarter Pounders, Steak Country, Lidl*	1 Burger/68g	188	15.1	276	16.3	2.4	22.2	0.1
Beef, Quarter Pounders, with Onion, BGTY, Sainsbury's*	1 Burger/83g	171	7.8	205	26.6	3.8	9.3	0.9
Beef, Quarter Pounders, with Onion, Birds Eye*	1 Burger/114g	286	22.1	252	14.1	5.1	19.5	0.4
Beef, Quarter Pounders, with Onion, Cooked, Birds Eye*	1 Burger/100g	230	16.0	230	16.0	5.9	16.0	0.4
Beef, Sainsbury's*	1 Burger/57g	152	9.1	267	29.6	1.3	15.9	1.5
Beef, Scotch, Quarter Pounders, Sainsbury's*	1 Burger/114g	255	15.4	225	22.2	3.5	13.6	0.5
Beef, Scotch, Quarter Pounders, The Best, Morrisons*	1 Burger/97g	223	13.9	230	21.0	4.0	14.3	0.5
Beef, Scotch, Ultimate, TTD, Sainsbury's*	1 Burger/119g	265	15.8	223	25.3	0.5	13.3	1.0
Beef, Simply Seasoned, TTD, Sainsbury's*	1 Burger/110g	298	25.0	271	15.3	18.1	22.7	0.5
Beef, Smoked Garlic, Steak, Finest, Tesco*	1 Burger/80g	178	12.6	223	18.0	2.0	15.8	0.5
Beef, Steak & Sunblush Tomato, TTD, Sainsbury's*	1 Burger/127g	279	15.9	220	21.7	5.0	12.5	0.6
Beef, Steak, British, Cooked, TTD, Sainsbury's*	1 Burger/93g	191	11.9	205	21.0	1.5	12.8	0.5
Beef, Steak, British, Tesco*	1 Burger/80g	184	10.9	230	24.8	2.2	13.6	0.1
Beef, Steak, Full of Flavour, Finest, Tesco*	1 Burger/86g	200	12.6	233	22.6	2.3	14.6	0.5
Beef, Steak, Ultimate, TTD, Sainsbury's*	1 Burger/136g	355	24.1	261	25.3	0.1	17.7	0.5
Beef, Wagyu, Specially Selected, Aldi*	1 Burger/150g	420	30.0	280	19.0	5.1	20.0	0.5
Beef, with Cheese Melt, COOK!, M&S*	1 Burger/182g	400	28.9	220	17.9	1.3	15.9	1.2
Beef, with Fresh Garden Herbs, TTD, Sainsbury's*	1 Burger/142g	280	14.8	197	21.5	4.4	10.4	1.3
Beef, with Herbs, Finest, Tesco*	1 Burger/105g	200	11.8	190	17.3	4.5	11.2	0.7
Beef, with Jalapeno Chilli, Finest, Tesco*	1 Burger/205g	379	22.3	185	17.0	3.4	10.9	0.4
Beef, with West Country Cheddar, TTD, Sainsbury's*	1 Burger/112g	252	13.7	225	26.4	2.3	12.2	0.0
Cheeseburger	1 Serving/275g	706	29.0	257	13.7	25.6	10.6	1.8
Cheeseburger, American, Tesco*	1 Burger/275g	660	26.3	240	13.6	24.9	9.6	1.6
Cheeseburger, Bacon with Bun, Chargrilled, Tesco*	1 Burger/265g	726	42.1	274	13.0	19.6	15.9	1.0
Chicken Crunch & Fries, M&S*	1 Pack/425g	915	47.6	215	8.8	20.8	11.2	2.1
Chicken with Sesame Seed Bun, Breaded, Tesco*	1 Burger/205g	588	32.2	287	10.2	26.2	15.7	2.9
Chicken, Average	*1 Burger/46g*	*111*	*5.6*	*242*	*14.9*	*18.7*	*12.1*	*1.0*
Chicken, Breaded, Value, Tesco*	1 Burger/57g	165	10.8	290	10.5	19.2	19.0	1.4
Chicken, Fillets, Cajun, Birds Eye*	1 Burger/92g	128	4.3	140	20.1	4.8	4.7	0.2
Chicken, Fresh, Non Coated, Waitrose*	1 Burger/100g	141	4.0	141	16.0	10.4	4.0	0.9
Chicken, Golden Breadcrumbs, Frozen, Birds Eye*	1 Burger/56g	130	6.9	232	13.8	16.4	12.4	0.3
Chicken, Quarter Pounders, Birds Eye*	1 Burger/117g	280	16.1	239	13.5	15.2	13.8	0.6
Chicken, Sainsbury's*	1 Burger/46g	115	7.0	247	15.6	12.2	15.1	1.3
Chicken, Southern Fried, Sainsbury's*	1 Burger/52g	154	10.3	297	12.6	17.2	19.8	1.3
Chilli, Quarter Pounders, Asda*	1 Burger/88g	221	14.0	252	25.0	2.0	16.0	0.0
Lamb, Minted, Average	*1 Burger/56g*	*125*	*7.4*	*223*	*20.6*	*5.5*	*13.2*	*0.2*
Lamb, Minted, Quarter Pounders, Asda*	1 Burger/114g	241	14.0	212	19.2	6.1	12.3	0.0
Lamb, Quarter Pounder, Average	*1 Burger/113g*	*283*	*19.3*	*250*	*17.4*	*5.2*	*17.1*	*0.8*
Lamb, Quarter Pounders, Asda*	1 Burger/85g	213	13.9	251	20.9	5.2	16.3	0.9
Lamb, Waitrose*	1 Burger/67g	99	4.7	148	15.7	5.4	7.0	0.9
Mushroom & Spinach, Cooked, Love Veg, Sainsbury's*	1 Burger/76g	192	11.0	254	5.2	22.7	14.6	5.6
Ostrich, Quarter Pounder, Oslinc*	1 Burger/113g	132	1.5	117	22.9	3.5	1.3	1.1
Pork & Apple, Grilled, Finest, Tesco*	1 Burger/88g	251	18.4	285	14.3	9.6	20.9	1.2
Pork & Apple, Quarter Pounder, Grilled, Asda*	1 Burger/80g	147	6.4	184	23.9	4.1	8.0	0.5
Pork, Free Range, Waitrose*	1 Burger/115g	306	19.9	266	19.3	7.7	17.3	1.0
Pork, Quarter Pounders, Birds Eye*	1 Burger/122g	292	23.2	239	13.9	3.2	19.0	0.2

	Measure INFO/WEIGHT	per Measure KCAL	FAT	Nutrition Values per 100g / 100ml KCAL	PROT	CARB	FAT	FIBRE
BURGERS								
Quarter Pounder with Cheese & Buns, Sainsbury's*	1 Burger/198g	471	22.8	238	15.6	19.1	11.5	1.4
Quarter Pounder with Cheese, Flame Grilled, Feasters*	1 Burger/200g	550	19.8	275	17.2	22.1	9.9	0.9
Quarter Pounders, Iceland*	1 Burger/83g	253	18.8	305	20.4	5.1	22.6	0.6
Salmon, Quarter Pounders, Tesco*	1 Burger/114g	145	2.7	128	15.9	10.6	2.4	1.2
Spicy Bean, in Herby Nacho Crumb, Morrisons*	1 Burger/102g	185	8.1	181	5.2	19.5	7.9	5.5
Spicy Bean, Sainsbury's*	1 Burger/110g	262	13.5	240	5.0	27.1	12.4	2.0
Steak, Peppered, M&S*	1 Burger/114g	310	24.4	272	18.8	0.8	21.4	0.7
Steak, Rump, The Grill, M&S*	1 Burger/169g	330	20.6	195	18.7	2.6	12.2	1.1
Turkey, Crispy Crumb, Bernard Matthews*	1 Burger/60g	158	9.5	263	12.6	17.5	15.8	1.8
Venison, As Sold, Tesco*	1 Burger/113g	149	4.0	132	19.3	5.5	3.5	0.5
Venison, Grilled, Tesco*	1 Burger/96g	149	4.0	155	22.8	6.2	4.2	0.5
Venison, Lightly Seasoned, As Consumed, Waitrose*	1 Burger/95g	159	6.2	168	23.8	3.3	6.6	0.1
Venison, M&S*	1 Burger/90g	121	5.0	134	17.8	2.8	5.6	0.5
Venison, TTD, Sainsbury's*	1 Burger/150g	224	6.3	149	20.4	6.5	4.2	3.2
BURGERS VEGETARIAN								
Aubergine & Feta, Aromatic & Minty, Waitrose*	1 Burger/105g	238	12.9	235	5.2	22.3	12.7	5.3
Bean, Tesco*	1 Burger/90g	192	10.9	213	4.4	21.6	12.1	5.0
Chilli Bean, Crisp & Spicy, Frozen, Cooked, Waitrose*	1 Burger/95g	226	8.3	238	5.8	31.0	8.7	6.1
Crisp & Golden Vegetable, Quarter Pounders, Waitrose*	1 Burger/113g	236	8.8	209	4.8	28.2	7.8	3.4
Meat Free, Asda*	1 Burger/60g	138	6.0	230	24.0	11.0	10.0	0.3
Meat Free, Sainsbury's*	1 Burger/57g	86	2.8	151	22.0	4.4	5.0	3.4
Meat Free, Sainsbury's*	1 Burger/57g	92	4.2	161	19.6	3.9	7.4	4.8
Meat Free, Spicy, Bean & Nacho, Cooked, Asda*	1 Burger/113g	247	9.6	218	5.3	27.7	8.5	4.7
Mexican Style, Bean, Meat Free, Tesco*	1 Burger/106g	238	10.9	225	6.2	22.7	10.3	8.3
Mozzarella ¼ Pound, Linda McCartney*	1 Burger/114g	233	15.5	205	16.5	7.7	13.6	3.3
Mushroom, Meat Free, Tesco*	1 Burger/87g	151	9.4	173	3.6	15.3	10.8	3.7
Peri Peri, Frozen, Linda McCartney*	1 Burger/113g	251	9.7	222	20.8	14.7	8.6	4.1
Quarter Pounder, Average	*1 Burger/113g*	*210*	*9.8*	*186*	*9.1*	*17.7*	*8.6*	*3.2*
Quarter Pounders, Beef Style, Sainsbury's*	1 Burger/114g	216	10.8	190	20.0	6.0	9.5	2.5
Quarter Pounders, Linda McCartney*	1 Burger/114g	187	11.3	165	14.4	4.4	10.0	4.2
Spicy Bean, Average	*1 Burger/56g*	*125*	*6.8*	*223*	*5.6*	*24.3*	*12.2*	*4.8*
Spicy Bean, BGTY, Sainsbury's*	1 Burger/85g	123	2.3	145	6.9	23.3	2.7	3.1
Spicy Bean, Cauldron Foods*	1 Burger/88g	203	9.8	232	5.4	27.4	11.2	6.2
Spicy Bean, Linda McCartney*	1 Burger/85g	190	9.5	223	4.3	26.2	11.2	2.9
Spicy Bean, Quarter Pounder, Dalepak*	1 Burger/115g	237	12.5	206	4.6	22.3	10.9	2.6
Tesco*	1 Burger/56g	92	4.5	164	16.0	7.0	8.0	2.5
Traditional, Fry's Special Vegetarian*	1 Burger/75g	175	9.0	233	19.2	13.0	12.0	0.2
Vegeburger, Retail, Grilled	1oz/28g	55	3.1	196	16.6	8.0	11.1	4.2
Vegetable, Average	*1 Burger/56g*	*100*	*4.5*	*179*	*4.4*	*22.4*	*8.0*	*2.3*
Vegetable, Organic, Goodlife*	1 Burger/67g	114	3.9	170	3.2	26.3	5.8	2.6
Vegetable, Organic, Tesco*	1 Burger/90g	108	3.9	120	2.6	17.6	4.3	2.1
Vegetable, Quarter Pounders, Crunchy, Birds Eye*	1 Burger/114g	240	11.6	211	4.8	24.9	10.2	1.8
Vegetable, Quarter Pounders, Tesco*	1 Burger/108g	227	13.1	211	4.4	20.8	12.2	2.7
Vegetable, Spicy, Asda*	1 Burger/56g	108	6.2	193	3.4	20.0	11.0	0.0
BURRITO								
Beef	1 Serving/225g	430	19.0	191	9.6	18.7	8.5	2.2
Beef, Chilli, Cooked, World Cafe, Waitrose*	½ Pack/87g	169	5.5	195	8.8	24.4	6.3	2.5
BUTTER								
Brandy, Average	*1 Serving/10g*	*56*	*3.8*	*556*	*0.2*	*46.2*	*38.4*	*0.1*
Clarified, Cook's Range, Lurpak*	1 Serving/100g	898	99.8	898	0.0	0.0	99.8	0.0
Coconut, Artisana*	2 Tbsp/32g	186	18.0	574	6.2	21.6	55.5	15.4
Creamery, Average	*1 Serving/10g*	*74*	*8.1*	*736*	*0.5*	*0.4*	*81.4*	*0.0*
Fresh, Average	*1 Thin Spread/7g*	*51*	*5.7*	*735*	*0.6*	*0.4*	*81.3*	*0.0*

B

	Measure INFO/WEIGHT	per Measure KCAL	FAT	Nutrition Values per 100g / 100ml KCAL	PROT	CARB	FAT	FIBRE
BUTTER								
Goats, St Helen's Farm*	1 Serving/10g	79	8.8	794	0.5	0.0	88.0	0.0
Granules, Butter Buds*	1 Tsp/1g	5	0.1	368	1.8	77.9	6.5	2.3
Reduced Fat, Fresh, Average	*1 Thin Spread/7g*	*26*	*2.8*	*368*	*2.3*	*1.2*	*39.4*	*0.2*
Salted, Average	*1 Thin Spread/7g*	*51*	*5.7*	*729*	*0.4*	*0.3*	*81.1*	*0.0*
Spreadable, Fresh, Average	*1 Thin Spread/7g*	*51*	*5.7*	*730*	*0.4*	*0.3*	*80.8*	*0.0*
Spreadable, Reduced Fat, Average	*1 Thin Spread/7g*	*38*	*4.2*	*540*	*0.5*	*0.5*	*60.0*	*0.0*
with Crushed Garlic, Lurpak*	1 Serving/10g	70	7.5	700	1.0	4.0	75.0	0.0
BUTTERMILK								
Average	*1 Mug/400ml*	*177*	*1.3*	*44*	*4.2*	*5.9*	*0.3*	*0.0*
BUTTONS								
Chocolate, Giant, Dairy Milk, Cadbury*	1 Button/3g	15	0.9	525	7.7	56.7	29.9	0.7
Milk Chocolate, Asda*	1 Bag/70g	368	21.0	526	7.0	57.0	30.0	1.5
Milk Chocolate, M&S*	1 Pack/75g	375	19.0	500	8.6	59.8	25.3	1.9
Milk Chocolate, Tesco*	1 Bag/70g	359	19.3	513	7.1	59.1	27.6	2.1
White Chocolate, Dairy Milk, Cadbury*	1 Pack/32g	174	9.5	540	4.7	63.0	29.5	0.0
White Chocolate, Milkybar, Nestle*	1 Bag/30g	164	9.5	546	7.5	58.1	31.6	0.0

	Measure INFO/WEIGHT	per Measure KCAL	FAT	Nutrition Values per 100g / 100ml KCAL	PROT	CARB	FAT	FIBRE
CABBAGE								
& Leek, Crunchy Mix, Ready to Cook, Sainsbury's*	1 Serving/125g	34	0.6	27	1.9	3.7	0.5	2.6
& Leek, Ready Sliced, Sainsbury's*	1 Pack/240g	53	1.2	22	1.1	2.2	0.5	2.1
& Leek, Sliced, Tesco*	1/3 Pack/100g	32	0.6	32	2.1	3.4	0.6	2.6
Boiled, Average	**1 Serving/90g**	**14**	**0.3**	**15**	**1.0**	**2.2**	**0.3**	**1.7**
Creamed, Cooked, Sainsbury's*	½ Pack/150g	95	6.8	67	2.0	2.6	4.8	2.5
Greens, Trimmed, Average	**1oz/28g**	**8**	**0.1**	**28**	**2.9**	**3.0**	**0.5**	**3.4**
Medley, Red, Spring & Savoy, Sainsbury's*	½ Pack/80g	26	0.5	32	2.0	3.4	0.6	2.3
Medley, Washed, Ready to Cook, Tesco*	1 Pack/200g	60	1.2	30	2.3	3.7	0.6	2.8
Raw, Average	**1 Serving/100g**	**21**	**0.4**	**21**	**1.3**	**3.2**	**0.4**	**1.8**
Red, & Beetroot, Mash Direct*	1 Serving/88g	67	2.1	76	1.2	12.4	2.4	2.6
Red, Average	**1 Serving/90g**	**19**	**0.2**	**21**	**1.0**	**3.7**	**0.3**	**2.2**
Red, Braised with Red Wine, M&S*	½ Pack/150g	180	7.2	120	1.4	17.1	4.8	1.0
Red, Pickled, Average	**1 Serving/100g**	**26**	**0.2**	**26**	**0.9**	**4.6**	**0.2**	**1.6**
Red, Spiced, Steamer, Sainsbury's*	½ Pack/150g	105	3.3	70	1.0	10.5	2.2	2.9
Red, with Apple, Finest, Tesco*	½ Pack/150g	177	8.8	118	1.6	14.7	5.9	4.6
Red, with Apples, Onions & Redcurrant Jelly, M&S*	½ Pack/150g	112	3.3	75	0.9	12.4	2.2	2.0
Red, with Bramley Apple, Aunt Bessie's*	1 Serving/125g	72	1.1	58	0.9	10.0	0.9	2.7
Red, with Bramley Apple, Braised, Sainsbury's*	½ Pack/150g	146	7.2	97	0.9	12.6	4.8	1.7
Savoy, Boiled in Salted Water, Average	**1 Serving/90g**	**15**	**0.4**	**17**	**1.1**	**2.2**	**0.5**	**2.0**
Savoy, Raw, Average	**1 Serving/90g**	**24**	**0.4**	**27**	**2.1**	**3.9**	**0.5**	**3.1**
Spring Greens, Boiled, Average	**1 Serving/80g**	**16**	**0.6**	**20**	**1.9**	**1.6**	**0.7**	**2.6**
Spring Greens, Raw, Average	**1 Serving/80g**	**22**	**0.7**	**28**	**2.5**	**2.6**	**0.8**	**2.9**
Steamed, Average	**1 Serving/100g**	**15**	**0.3**	**15**	**1.0**	**2.2**	**0.3**	**1.7**
Sweetheart, Raw	**1 Serving/100g**	**26**	**0.6**	**26**	**2.1**	**3.2**	**0.6**	**2.8**
White, Raw, Average	**1oz/28g**	**8**	**0.1**	**27**	**1.4**	**5.0**	**0.2**	**2.1**
CAKE								
Alabama Chocolate Fudge, Farmfoods*	1/6 Cake/61g	201	5.9	329	4.7	55.7	9.7	2.7
Alabama Chocolate Fudge, Morrisons*	1/6 Cake/58g	195	6.4	337	4.5	55.1	11.0	2.3
Almond Flavoured Rounds, Country Garden Cakes*	1 Cake/45g	183	6.7	403	4.3	62.4	14.7	2.3
Almond Slices, Mr Kipling*	1 Slice/33g	131	4.6	403	6.3	63.4	14.0	2.0
Almond Slices, Sainsbury's*	1 Serving/27g	120	7.1	444	5.9	45.9	26.3	1.5
Angel Slices, Mr Kipling*	1 Slice/33g	145	6.1	431	3.0	63.4	18.2	0.6
Angel Slices, Snap Packs, Mr Kipling*	1 Slice/34g	148	6.6	417	2.7	60.1	18.5	0.6
Angel, Average	**1 Slice/44g**	**175**	**7.9**	**397**	**4.2**	**54.9**	**17.9**	**0.8**
Angel, Sainsbury's*	1/8 Cake/41g	171	8.1	417	4.1	55.7	19.8	0.8
Apple & Blackcurrant, Crumble, Graze*	1 Punnet/33g	121	7.5	365	6.1	34.5	22.7	3.1
Apple Bakes, Go Ahead, McVitie's*	1 Cake/35g	126	2.7	361	2.6	70.0	7.8	2.0
Apple Slice, Delightful, Mr Kipling*	1 Slice/29g	92	1.1	317	4.4	66.2	3.9	1.3
Apple, Bramley, & Blackberry Crumble, M&S*	1/8 Cake/56g	221	10.0	395	4.4	54.1	17.9	1.5
Apple, Home Style, M&S*	1 Cake/54g	189	7.9	350	5.3	49.4	14.7	1.5
Apricot & Apple, Trimlyne*	1 Cake/50g	134	1.4	267	4.3	58.4	2.7	1.9
Bakewell Slice, Weight Watchers*	1 Slice/26g	84	0.6	324	3.7	71.0	2.4	2.0
Bakewell Slices, Mr Kipling*	1 Slice/36g	163	7.3	454	4.2	63.4	20.4	1.2
Bakewell, Lemon, Average	**1 Cake/42g**	**173**	**6.4**	**411**	**3.7**	**64.6**	**15.2**	**1.3**
Bakewell, The Handmade Flapjack Company*	1 Cake/75g	311	17.1	415	4.5	47.4	22.8	0.0
Banana Loaf, Waitrose*	1 Slice/70g	236	7.5	337	5.0	55.2	10.7	1.7
Banana, Iced, Waitrose*	1/6 Cake/55g	190	5.9	345	4.2	58.0	10.7	2.7
Banana, Organic, Loaf, Respect Organics*	¼ Pack/65g	254	13.6	391	3.9	48.6	21.0	1.5
Banana, with An Afternoon Tea Infusion, Graze*	1 Punnet/18g	55	2.5	307	5.0	39.0	14.0	3.0
Banoffee Slices, Dessert Classics, Mr Kipling*	1 Slice/34g	140	6.2	414	2.9	59.0	18.4	0.6
Bara Brith, Tan Y Castell*	1 Serving/100g	261	1.0	261	4.0	58.8	1.0	1.5
Battenberg, Asda*	1 Slice/25g	104	3.0	418	6.0	71.1	12.2	0.8
Battenberg, Mini, Mr Kipling*	1 Cake/33g	134	3.4	410	4.2	74.2	10.4	1.2

CAKE

INFO/WEIGHT	Measure	per Measure KCAL	per Measure FAT	Nutrition Values per 100g / 100ml KCAL	PROT	CARB	FAT	FIBRE
Battenberg, Mr Kipling*	1 Serving/38g	161	4.6	421	5.0	73.3	12.0	1.6
Belgian Chocolate, Waitrose*	1 Slice/47g	223	12.6	474	4.8	53.1	26.9	1.9
Birthday Present, Tesco*	1 Serving/79g	347	13.9	439	3.5	66.6	17.6	0.4
Birthday, M&S*	1 Serving/60g	240	7.1	400	2.3	70.9	11.9	0.8
Bites, Caramel, Mr Kipling*	1 Bite/14g	68	3.8	492	5.9	55.3	27.4	0.8
Bites, Chocolate Roll, Mini, Tesco*	1 Bite/18g	78	3.6	435	6.0	58.0	19.8	1.9
Bites, Coconut, Sainsbury's*	1 Bite/80g	339	16.9	424	5.3	53.0	21.2	4.2
Blackcurrant Delice, Specially Selected, Aldi*	1/6 Cake/74g	152	6.9	206	2.6	28.0	9.3	0.8
Brilliant Banana Bread, Graze*	1 Cake/23g	72	3.6	312	5.2	40.4	15.6	3.0
Butterfly, Mr Kipling*	1 Cake/29g	114	6.4	392	4.4	43.4	22.2	0.6
Caramel Shortbread, Devondale*	1 Cake/75g	356	18.6	474	3.0	57.0	24.8	0.8
Caramel Shortbread, Tray Bake, Kate's Cakes Ltd*	1 Serving/100g	471	27.3	471	3.0	53.3	27.3	1.2
Caramel Shortcake Slices, McVitie's*	1 Slice/32g	146	7.7	463	4.3	56.5	24.4	1.6
Caramel Slice, M&S*	1 Slice/64g	304	16.1	475	4.9	60.4	25.2	2.6
Caramel, Milk Chocolate, Holly Lane*	1 Cake/25g	110	5.1	441	6.9	57.6	20.3	1.1
Carrot & Orange, ES, Asda*	1/6 Cake/65g	240	11.7	369	4.7	47.0	18.0	0.9
Carrot & Orange, Finest, Tesco*	1/8 Cake/50g	205	10.2	410	4.6	51.2	20.5	2.1
Carrot & Orange, Waitrose*	1/6 Cake/47g	164	7.4	350	5.3	46.8	15.7	1.8
Carrot & Pecan, M&S*	1 Slice/90g	330	14.6	365	6.4	48.7	16.2	2.3
Carrot & Walnut, Layered, Asda*	1 Serving/42g	172	8.0	409	4.6	55.0	19.0	1.0
Carrot & Walnut, Mini Classics, Mr Kipling*	1 Cake/39g	172	9.8	440	4.5	48.6	25.2	1.0
Carrot Slices, Less Than 3% Fat, BGTY, Sainsbury's*	1 Slice/30g	94	0.8	313	3.4	68.7	2.7	2.4
Carrot Slices, Weight Watchers*	1 Slice/27g	84	0.2	311	2.8	73.0	0.8	0.9
Carrot, Average	*1 Slice/56g*	*211*	*10.4*	*377*	*4.6*	*47.6*	*18.6*	*1.4*
Carrot, Handmade, Delicious, Boots*	1 Slice/75g	292	13.5	389	4.1	53.0	18.0	1.4
Carrot, Iced, Tesco*	1 Serving/61g	246	12.0	404	3.1	53.7	19.6	1.6
Carrot, Mini, Weight Watchers*	1 Cake/31g	120	3.3	388	3.7	68.9	10.8	2.7
Carrot, Organic, Respect Organics*	1 Slice/45g	179	10.1	398	3.1	47.4	22.4	1.5
Carrot, Slices, Asda*	1 Slice/80g	302	13.2	377	3.4	53.8	16.5	1.7
Carrot, Slices, Eat Smart, Morrisons*	1 Cake/27g	84	0.6	312	3.0	70.0	2.2	2.3
Carrot, Slices, Inspirations, Mr Kipling*	1 Slice/34g	139	6.3	411	3.5	57.7	18.5	1.3
Carrot, Square, Margaret's Country Kitchen*	1 Cake/80g	307	13.5	384	3.6	54.4	16.9	2.4
Celebration, Sainsbury's*	1/12 Cake/100g	265	9.2	265	2.1	43.6	9.2	0.3
Cherry & Almond, Slices, Free From, Sainsbury's*	1 Slice/33g	144	7.9	442	6.5	48.7	24.3	1.0
Cherry Bakewell, Co-Op*	1 Cake/47g	205	8.0	435	3.7	67.2	16.9	1.8
Cherry Bakewell, Gluten Free, Bakers Delight*	1 Cake/50g	211	8.2	422	2.9	66.1	16.3	0.4
Cherry Bakewell, M&S*	1 Cake/44g	185	7.8	420	4.5	61.7	17.7	1.0
Cherry Bakewell, Mini, Sainsbury's*	1 Cake/27g	101	3.3	370	3.4	62.2	12.0	0.4
Cherry Bakewell, Smart Price, Asda*	1 Cake/38g	157	6.8	413	2.7	60.0	18.0	2.6
Cherry Bakewells, Delightful, Mr Kipling*	1 Cake/45g	176	5.8	390	3.9	66.4	12.9	1.2
Cherry Bakewells, Mr Kipling*	1 Cake/45g	193	8.3	428	3.9	61.3	18.5	1.4
Cherry, Asda*	1 Slice/37g	131	4.5	351	4.7	56.0	12.0	0.6
Cherry, M&S*	1 Serving/75g	285	9.5	380	5.0	60.6	12.7	0.8
Chewy Rice Pop & Chocolate, Dove's Farm*	1 Bar/35g	156	7.1	447	3.9	69.9	20.2	2.3
Chocolate	1oz/28g	128	7.4	456	7.4	50.4	26.4	1.7
Chocolate & Caramel Tiffin Bites, Gu*	1 Tiffin/35g	168	9.9	480	3.8	51.9	28.3	2.8
Chocolate & Madeira, Marble Loaf, M&S*	1/6 Cake/88g	380	20.4	430	5.0	50.0	23.1	1.0
Chocolate & Orange Rolls, M&S*	1 Cake/60g	228	17.0	380	3.6	27.0	28.4	1.3
Chocolate & Sweetest, Beetroot, Battle Bakehouse*	1/6 Cake/49g	185	8.7	379	5.2	48.6	17.9	4.0
Chocolate Brownie, Fudge, Entenmann's*	1/8 Cake/55g	168	2.4	306	4.0	62.7	4.4	1.5
Chocolate Brownie, Gluten & Wheat Free, Lovemore*	1 Slice/36g	127	4.6	352	3.7	56.1	12.8	0.2
Chocolate Brownie, Tray Bake, Kate's Cakes Ltd*	1 Serving/100g	435	22.0	435	5.7	51.5	22.0	3.3
Chocolate Button, Cakes for the Connoisseur*	1 Cake/30g	145	9.8	485	5.2	42.1	32.8	2.3

CAKE	Measure INFO/WEIGHT	per Measure KCAL	per Measure FAT	Nutrition Values per 100g / 100ml KCAL	PROT	CARB	FAT	FIBRE
Chocolate Chip, Co-Op*	1/6 Cake/63g	275	16.9	440	5.0	44.0	27.0	0.5
Chocolate Crunch, Tray Bake, Kate's Cakes Ltd*	1 Serving/80g	400	23.0	500	4.8	53.4	28.8	3.7
Chocolate Fudge	1 Serving/110g	415	19.1	377	4.4	50.4	17.4	1.4
Chocolate Fudge Slice, Waitrose*	1 Slice/60g	230	9.7	383	4.7	54.6	16.2	1.5
Chocolate Fudge, Belgian, TTD, Sainsbury's*	1 Slice/66g	278	14.3	423	4.4	52.5	21.7	2.5
Chocolate Fudge, Classics, M&S*	1 Serving/71g	195	7.5	275	2.8	42.8	10.6	1.1
Chocolate Fudge, Sainsbury's*	1/8 Cake/98g	402	21.9	410	5.5	47.3	22.3	1.9
Chocolate Fudge, Tray bake, Kate's Cakes Ltd*	1 Serving/100g	360	16.9	360	4.8	46.8	16.9	1.1
Chocolate Heaven, ES, Asda*	1/6 Cake/66g	255	13.1	388	4.0	48.0	20.0	1.0
Chocolate Indulgence, Finest, Tesco*	1 Slice/51g	207	9.1	405	4.8	55.9	17.9	1.2
Chocolate Orange, Sponge, Asda*	1 Serving/70g	298	18.2	425	4.9	42.9	26.0	3.0
Chocolate Party, M&S*	1 Serving/61g	240	12.6	395	4.6	46.9	20.8	1.1
Chocolate Rice Crispy, Knightsbridge, Lidl*	1 Cake/24g	88	4.2	368	3.9	48.7	17.5	0.1
Chocolate Roll, Sainsbury's*	1 Slice/50g	210	10.2	420	5.0	54.0	20.4	3.3
Chocolate Slices, Mr Kipling*	1 Slice/33g	132	6.7	406	5.6	50.4	20.6	2.7
Chocolate Sponge, Less Than 5% Fat, Asda*	1 Sponge/110g	198	4.2	180	4.4	32.0	3.8	1.1
Chocolate Sponge, Morrisons*	1 Serving/59g	179	7.6	303	4.4	42.5	12.8	0.7
Chocolate Sponge, Tesco*	1 Serving/37g	129	3.6	358	5.1	60.8	10.1	1.7
Chocolate Tiffin, Devondale*	1 Cake/100g	513	27.0	513	2.8	54.0	27.0	1.7
Chocolate Truffle, ES, Asda*	1 Serving/103g	402	26.8	390	5.0	34.0	26.0	1.8
Chocolate Truffle, Mini, Finest, Tesco*	1 Cake/28g	125	6.6	448	5.9	52.9	23.7	0.3
Chocolate Victoria Sponge, Co-Op*	1 Slice/61g	201	9.8	330	5.0	42.0	16.0	1.0
Chocolate with Butter Icing, Average	***1oz/28g***	***135***	***8.3***	***481***	***5.7***	***50.9***	***29.7***	***0.0***
Chocolate, Birthday, Tesco*	1 Serving/54g	229	13.2	425	5.9	45.5	24.4	2.1
Chocolate, Caterpillar, Tesco*	1 Serving/53g	248	13.2	468	5.7	55.3	24.9	1.1
Chocolate, Cup, Mini, Weight Watchers*	1 Cake/17g	72	3.6	422	6.1	52.0	21.1	1.8
Chocolate, Fudge, The Cake Shop*	1 Cake/37g	178	10.8	480	3.7	50.5	29.2	1.3
Chocolate, Happy Birthday, Tesco*	1 Serving/58g	241	13.2	415	4.7	46.9	22.7	2.9
Chocolate, Iced, Tesco*	1 Serving/40g	158	6.3	395	4.7	58.5	15.8	1.8
Chocolate, Individual with Mini Eggs, Cadbury*	1 Cake/26g	119	6.1	455	4.6	57.5	23.1	1.3
Chocolate, Large, Happy Birthday, Tesco*	1/18 Cake/63g	249	12.2	396	6.2	49.3	19.3	1.8
Chocolate, Loaf, Moist, McVitie's*	1 Slice/30g	119	6.1	398	4.8	49.0	20.3	1.9
Chocolate, Morrisons*	1 Serving/32g	159	10.2	505	5.3	48.0	32.4	1.2
Chocolate, Party, Tesco*	1 Slice/62g	244	13.1	394	4.6	46.3	21.2	0.9
Chocolate, Sainsbury's*	1 Serving/30g	118	5.6	395	4.1	52.6	18.5	1.3
Chocolate, Smarties, Celebration, Large, Nestle*	1/16 Cake/71g	308	17.4	432	5.4	48.9	24.4	1.2
Chocolate, The Handmade Flapjack Company*	1 Cake/75g	303	16.2	404	12.5	39.8	21.6	0.0
Chocolate, Thorntons*	1 Serving/87g	408	25.1	469	5.2	47.1	28.8	0.6
Chocolate, Triple Layer, Celebration, Tesco*	1/24 of cake/79g	345	18.8	430	5.0	47.7	23.4	2.8
Chocolate, White Button, Asda*	1 Cake/30g	117	6.3	390	5.0	44.0	21.0	2.0
Chorley, Asda*	1 Cake/60g	269	12.6	449	6.0	59.0	21.0	2.2
Christmas Slices, Mr Kipling*	1 Slice/43g	157	3.8	361	3.0	67.0	8.7	1.4
Christmas, Connoisseur, M&S*	1 Slice/60g	216	5.5	360	4.1	64.7	9.2	3.3
Christmas, Gluten Free, Costa*	1 Portion/98g	403	12.0	411	3.9	70.3	12.2	1.2
Christmas, Iced Rich Fruit, Finest, Tesco*	1 Serving/100g	345	7.7	345	3.1	65.3	7.7	3.7
Christmas, Iced, Slices, Tesco*	1 Slice/45g	168	4.4	369	2.9	67.6	9.6	1.2
Christmas, Rich Fruit, All Iced, Sainsbury's*	1/16 Cake/85g	307	7.6	361	4.0	66.4	8.9	1.5
Christmas, Rich Fruit, Organic, Tesco*	1 Serving/76g	282	7.6	374	3.9	67.1	10.0	2.0
Christmas, Rich Fruit, Tesco*	1 Serving/75g	256	5.6	342	3.9	64.3	7.4	3.1
Christmas, Royal Iced, Waitrose*	1/6 Cake/75g	270	4.6	360	3.7	71.3	6.2	2.0
Classic Lemon Drizzle, M&S*	1/6 Cake/68g	253	10.3	375	4.7	55.0	15.3	0.6
Coconut	1 Slice/70g	304	16.7	434	6.7	51.2	23.8	2.5
Coconut & Raspberry, M&S*	1 Serving/52g	231	13.9	445	5.0	45.5	26.8	2.3

	INFO/WEIGHT	per Measure KCAL	FAT	Nutrition Values per 100g / 100ml KCAL	PROT	CARB	FAT	FIBRE

CAKE

	INFO/WEIGHT	KCAL	FAT	KCAL	PROT	CARB	FAT	FIBRE
Coconut Snowball, Bobby's*	1 Cake/18g	80	4.0	436	2.2	57.3	22.1	0.0
Coconut Snowballs, Tunnock's*	1 Cake/30g	134	6.2	446	4.2	56.7	20.8	3.6
Coconut Sponge, Memory Lane*	1/6 Cake/42g	172	7.5	406	4.1	57.1	17.6	1.5
Coconut Sponge, Mini Classics, Mr Kipling*	1 Cake/38g	155	8.7	409	3.7	47.0	22.9	0.9
Coffee & Walnut Slices, HE, Tesco*	1 Slice/23g	69	0.5	301	4.4	65.7	2.3	2.8
Coffee Sponge Roll, M&S*	1/6 Roll/42g	160	7.4	385	3.1	53.1	17.8	1.4
Coffee, Iced, M&S*	1 Slice/33g	135	6.5	410	4.4	54.5	19.6	1.6
Coffee, TTD, Sainsbury's*	1 Slice/68g	294	16.4	430	4.3	49.1	24.0	2.6
Colin the Caterpillar, M&S*	1 Slice/60g	234	12.8	390	5.3	57.2	21.3	1.3
Corn Flake, Chocolate, Mini Bites, Tesco*	1 Bite/14g	62	2.5	446	7.1	64.1	17.9	5.9
Cornflake, Average	**1 Cake/18g**	**83**	**3.7**	**464**	**5.2**	**64.6**	**20.4**	**2.0**
Cornflake, Chocolate Clusters, Asda*	1 Cake/14g	64	2.6	460	8.2	65.2	18.5	2.7
Cream Oysters, M&S*	1 Cake/72g	227	15.3	315	3.6	27.5	21.2	3.0
Cream Slices, M&S*	1 Slice/80g	310	18.3	387	2.3	45.7	22.9	0.6
Crispy Chocolate Clusters, Mini, Tesco*	1 Cluster/8g	37	1.5	470	7.0	67.8	18.7	2.5
Date & Walnut Loaf, Sainsbury's*	1/10 Slice/40g	148	8.2	371	6.7	40.1	20.4	1.0
Date, Linda Kearns*	1 Serving/100g	269	16.8	269	12.7	24.4	16.8	4.4
Double Chocolate Ganache, M&S*	1/12 Cake/61g	281	16.8	460	5.9	46.1	27.6	2.5
Eccles, All Butter, M&S*	1 Cake/86g	345	14.8	400	4.5	57.4	17.2	3.2
Eccles, Fresh Baked	**1 Cake/45g**	**171**	**7.6**	**381**	**4.3**	**56.3**	**17.0**	**1.5**
Fairy, Average	**1 Cake/23g**	**96**	**4.6**	**416**	**5.1**	**53.0**	**20.2**	**1.5**
Fairy, Holly Lane*	1 Cake/26g	118	6.7	460	3.7	52.5	26.1	3.5
Fairy, Iced, Average	**1 Cake/23g**	**91**	**3.4**	**394**	**4.2**	**60.8**	**14.8**	**0.9**
Fairy, Lemon Iced, Average	**1 Cake/23g**	**90**	**3.1**	**393**	**4.4**	**63.2**	**13.6**	**1.1**
Fairy, Plain, Average	**1 Cake/23g**	**95**	**4.6**	**413**	**5.5**	**51.1**	**20.2**	**1.5**
Fairy, Smart Price, Asda*	1 Cake/15g	66	3.3	438	6.0	54.0	22.0	1.0
Fairy, Strawberry Iced, Tesco*	1 Cake/24g	94	3.2	392	4.9	62.9	13.4	1.4
Fairy, Vanilla Iced, Average, Tesco*	1 Cake/23g	89	2.8	388	4.4	65.1	12.2	1.2
Flake, Cadbury*	1 Cake/20g	90	4.5	445	6.3	54.5	22.3	0.0
Fondant Fancies, Lemon, Waitrose*	1 Cake/40g	176	7.1	441	2.5	67.9	17.7	0.6
Fondant Fancies, Sainsbury's*	1 Cake/27g	95	2.4	353	2.4	65.7	9.0	0.4
Fondant, Dark Chocolate, Graze*	1 Pack/40g	157	5.8	393	3.5	66.2	14.5	0.0
Fondants with Chocolate, Mini, Delhaize*	1 Cake Mini/20g	88	6.2	440	4.6	36.3	30.8	3.8
French Fancies, Average	**1 Cake/27g**	**100**	**2.5**	**371**	**2.7**	**69.6**	**9.1**	**0.8**
French Fancies, Lemon, Mr Kipling*	1 Cake/28g	106	2.7	378	2.5	69.9	9.8	0.5
French Fancies, M&S*	1 Cake/25g	91	2.0	365	2.7	70.6	8.1	1.3
French Fancies, Mr Kipling*	1 Cake/28g	106	2.8	378	2.6	69.7	9.9	0.6
French Fancies, Strawberry, Mr Kipling*	1 Cake/28g	106	2.7	379	2.5	70.6	9.6	0.4
Fruit & Nut Cluster, TTD, Sainsbury's*	1 Slice/62g	239	9.2	383	5.7	56.8	14.8	4.2
Fruit Cake with Marzipan & Icing, Asda*	1/12 Slice/76g	280	6.8	369	3.9	68.0	9.0	0.0
Fruit Slices, Rich, Iced, Finest, Tesco*	1 Slice/41g	152	3.4	370	3.2	69.4	8.3	2.1
Fruit, Iced, Smart Price, Asda*	1 Serving/100g	371	8.2	371	4.0	70.2	8.2	3.0
Fruit, Luxury, Fully Iced Slice, The Best, Morrisons*	1 Serving/50g	178	3.8	356	3.7	66.6	7.6	3.1
Fruit, Parisienne, Rich, Finest, Tesco*	1 Serving/69g	262	9.7	380	4.7	55.2	14.1	1.9
Fruit, Plain, Average	**1 Slice/90g**	**319**	**11.6**	**354**	**5.1**	**57.9**	**12.9**	**0.0**
Fruit, Rich, Average	**1 Slice/70g**	**225**	**8.8**	**322**	**4.9**	**50.7**	**12.5**	**1.7**
Fruit, Rich, Iced	1 Slice/70g	249	8.0	356	4.1	62.7	11.4	1.7
Fruit, Rich, M&S*	1 Serving/50g	158	3.2	315	3.1	60.9	6.5	4.3
Fruit, Slices, Gluten & Wheat Free, Lovemore*	1 Slice/40g	122	3.8	304	2.3	51.1	9.4	1.5
Fruit, Slices, Value, Tesco*	1 Slice/23g	84	4.0	372	4.0	48.7	17.7	1.3
Genoa, Tesco*	1 Serving/44g	150	3.9	340	3.7	59.1	8.8	3.1
Ginger Drizzle, Iced, Co-Op*	1/6 Cake/65g	226	7.7	350	3.0	58.0	12.0	1.0
Glitzy Bag, Birthday, Tesco*	1 Serving/81g	314	6.9	388	2.1	75.9	8.5	0.6

CAKE

INFO/WEIGHT	Measure	per Measure KCAL	per Measure FAT	Nutrition per 100g/100ml KCAL	PROT	CARB	FAT	FIBRE
Granola Square, M&S*	1 Square/72g	330	18.1	464	7.9	49.3	25.5	5.0
Happy Birthday, Sainsbury's*	1 Slice/50g	207	8.0	414	2.8	64.5	16.1	0.6
Hot Chocolate Fudge, Sainsbury's*	1/8 Cake/91g	343	15.6	376	5.1	50.3	17.1	3.5
Iced Madeira, Sainsbury's*	1/8 Cake/47g	182	6.6	388	3.6	61.6	14.1	0.7
Jamaica Ginger, McVitie's*	1 Cake/291g	1056	30.6	363	3.7	63.4	10.5	1.6
La Madeleine, Bonne Maman*	1 Cake/25g	112	6.8	449	6.4	44.0	27.0	2.3
Lardy, Warings The Bakers*	1 Slice/120g	379	14.8	316	0.0	48.0	12.3	0.0
Lemon & Orange, Finest, Tesco*	1 Serving/53g	216	10.7	410	4.5	52.4	20.3	1.1
Lemon Bakewell, Mr Kipling*	1 Cake/43g	185	7.4	430	3.6	64.4	17.3	1.0
Lemon Buttercream & Lemon Curd, The Cake Shop*	1 Cake/28g	124	7.8	444	3.5	43.4	27.8	0.6
Lemon Drizzle Cake, Asda*	1 Serving/50g	150	6.0	299	2.8	45.0	12.0	0.4
Lemon Drizzle Slices, Light Choices, Tesco*	1 Slice/23g	67	0.5	290	4.8	62.7	2.0	2.8
Lemon Drizzle, M&S*	1/6 Cake/63g	230	8.8	365	4.2	55.8	13.9	1.4
Lemon Drizzle, Tray Bake, Kate's Cakes Ltd*	1 Serving/100g	324	14.4	324	4.5	44.2	14.4	1.1
Lemon Madeira, Half Moon, Dan Cake*	1 Slice/50g	215	10.0	430	3.5	59.0	20.0	0.0
Lemon Slices, Low Fat, Weight Watchers*	1 Slice/26g	79	0.5	303	3.1	68.1	2.0	2.2
Lemon Slices, Mr Kipling*	1 Slice/27g	109	4.5	405	4.1	59.4	16.7	0.7
Lemon, Average	*1 Slice/81g*	*320*	*14.5*	*396*	*4.1*	*54.8*	*18.0*	*0.6*
Lemon, Half Moon, Bobby's*	1/6 Cake/60g	244	11.0	406	4.1	55.7	18.4	0.0
Lemon, Loaf, M&S*	1 Slice/47g	190	8.8	400	2.1	55.8	18.6	0.6
Lemon, Mini, Weight Watchers*	1 Cake/27g	90	3.0	333	3.7	66.7	11.1	11.1
Leo the Lion, Birthday, Asda*	1 Slice/81g	325	12.9	402	2.6	62.0	16.0	0.5
Loaf, Golden Syrup Drizzle, Kate's Cakes Ltd*	1 Serving/100g	383	18.7	383	5.2	48.4	18.7	1.2
Luxury Chocolate Fudge, Kate's Cakes Ltd*	1 Serving/100g	415	20.8	415	5.1	50.4	20.8	2.8
Madeira	1 Slice/40g	157	6.8	393	5.4	58.4	16.9	0.9
Madeira, All Butter, Sainsbury's*	1 Serving/30g	116	5.9	388	5.2	47.4	19.7	0.8
Madeira, Cherry, Tesco*	1/4 Cake/100g	342	11.2	342	4.3	55.9	11.2	2.6
Madeira, Iced, Tesco*	1/16 Cake/56g	218	6.8	389	2.6	67.2	12.2	0.4
Madeira, Lemon Iced, Co-Op*	1 Cake/290g	1131	52.2	390	4.0	53.0	18.0	0.6
Madeira, Lemon Iced, Tesco*	1 Slice/30g	122	5.2	407	4.5	57.8	17.5	0.9
Madeira, Lightly Fruited, Yorkshire Baking Company*	1 Portion/54g	261	12.7	484	6.3	60.3	23.5	1.3
Madeira, Party, Sainsbury's*	1 Slice/75g	321	15.2	427	4.1	56.8	20.2	1.1
Madeira, Tesco*	1 Serving/50g	197	7.8	394	5.5	57.9	15.6	1.2
Manor House, Mr Kipling*	1 Serving/69g	277	13.8	400	5.3	49.7	20.0	1.4
Marble, Tesco*	1/8 Cake/45g	184	8.4	410	4.4	55.9	18.7	1.5
Melting Double Chocolate, Hot, Cadbury*	1 Cake/50g	225	10.6	445	5.6	57.3	20.9	2.4
Mini Log, Chocolate, Free From, Sainsbury's*	1 Slice/45g	202	10.8	450	5.6	51.0	24.0	3.0
Mini Rolls, Blackforest, Weight Watchers*	1 Cake/24g	89	3.4	374	5.3	58.9	14.2	4.4
Mini Rolls, Cadbury*	1 Roll/27g	120	6.1	445	4.4	56.4	22.5	1.3
Mini Rolls, Chocolate, Average	*1 Cake/27g*	*122*	*6.2*	*453*	*4.8*	*56.9*	*22.9*	*0.9*
Mini Rolls, Chocolate, Tesco*	1 Roll/29g	135	6.7	465	5.5	58.1	23.1	1.3
Mini Rolls, Cola, Chocolate, Cadbury*	1 Roll/27g	115	6.1	435	4.8	50.4	23.1	2.3
Mini Rolls, Jaffa, Average	*1 Cake/29g*	*111*	*3.3*	*382*	*3.5*	*67.2*	*11.2*	*1.4*
Mini Rolls, Jam, Average	*1 Cake/29g*	*115*	*4.5*	*395*	*3.8*	*59.8*	*15.6*	*1.8*
Mini Rolls, Jammy Strawberry, Cadbury*	1 Cake/29g	119	4.8	411	4.9	59.8	16.5	0.5
Mini Rolls, Juicy Orange, Cadbury*	1 Cake/28g	110	4.7	390	5.0	55.0	16.8	0.0
Mini Rolls, Milk Chocolate, Cadbury*	1 Roll/27g	120	6.0	445	4.4	56.5	22.2	0.0
Mini Rolls, Raspberry Ripple,Cadbury*	1 Roll/29g	126	5.7	435	4.5	59.0	19.6	1.4
Orange Marmalade Loaf, Aldi*	1 Slice/33g	88	0.7	267	4.5	57.4	2.2	1.8
Orange Marmalade, M&S*	1 Slice/50g	195	9.2	390	3.6	53.2	18.3	1.8
Panettone, Average	*1 Portion/90g*	*345*	*15.3*	*383*	*8.0*	*52.0*	*17.0*	*0.0*
Panettone, Luxury, Christmas, Tesco*	1 Serving/83g	307	11.6	370	7.0	53.5	14.0	2.5
Party, Asda*	1 Serving/57g	238	9.0	421	2.3	67.0	16.0	0.4

CAKE

INFO/WEIGHT	Measure	per Measure		Nutrition Values per 100g / 100ml				
		KCAL	FAT	KCAL	PROT	CARB	FAT	FIBRE
Perfect Pumpkin & Ginger, Graze*	1 Punnet/34g	101	5.1	298	6.1	38.6	15.0	4.0
Piece of Cake, Birthday, M&S*	1 Serving/85g	395	24.4	465	4.3	39.7	28.7	0.9
Raisin, Tesco*	1 Cake/38g	158	7.6	417	5.6	53.8	19.9	1.4
Raspberry Flavour Sponge, Value, Tesco*	1 Slice/39g	130	4.6	334	3.4	53.4	11.9	0.7
Rich Fruit Slices, Free From, Sainsbury's*	1 Slice/40g	144	5.0	361	4.5	57.4	12.6	3.7
Rich Fruit, Iced, Finest, Tesco*	1 Slice/57g	191	4.7	335	3.6	61.2	8.3	4.4
Rock	1 Sm Cake/40g	158	6.6	396	5.4	60.5	16.4	1.5
Rock, Tesco*	1 Serving/87g	311	8.4	357	7.4	60.1	9.7	1.6
Seriously Chocolatey, Belgian Choc Ganache, Sainsbury's*	1 Slice/84g	383	21.2	454	4.1	51.3	25.1	3.2
Shrek Birthday, Tesco*	1/16 Cake/72g	248	8.8	344	3.3	64.0	12.2	0.5
Slice, Caramel, Kate's Cakes Ltd*	1 Serving/100g	520	29.7	520	9.5	52.1	29.7	1.5
Slices, Carrot & Orange, Light Choices, Tesco*	1 Slice/30g	93	0.7	310	3.2	68.5	2.2	1.9
Snowballs, Tesco*	1 Snowball/18g	79	4.0	432	2.5	55.8	22.1	5.4
Spicy Apple, Tray Bake, Kate's Cakes Ltd*	1 Serving/100g	363	20.6	363	4.4	40.0	20.6	2.4
Sponge	1 Slice/53g	243	13.9	459	6.4	52.4	26.3	0.9
Sponge Roll, Chocolate, M&S*	¼ Cake/66g	251	12.1	380	3.9	50.5	18.4	1.8
Sponge with Butter Icing	1 Slice/65g	318	19.9	490	4.5	52.4	30.6	0.6
Sponge, Fresh Cream & Strawberry, Asda*	1/12 Cake/60g	170	6.0	284	4.6	44.0	10.0	1.1
Sponge, Iced, M&S*	1 Serving/100g	400	17.0	400	3.4	58.4	17.0	1.3
Sponge, Jam Filled	1 Slice/65g	196	3.2	302	4.2	64.2	4.9	1.8
Stem Ginger, Mrs Crimble's*	1 Slice/48g	158	1.1	329	2.7	73.3	2.2	2.7
Stollen, Bites, Finest, Tesco*	1 Piece/22g	81	3.2	370	6.5	52.7	14.4	4.4
Stollen, Marzipan Butter, Mini, Favorina, Lidl*	1 Stollen/18g	87	4.3	483	9.9	55.9	24.0	0.0
Stollen, Marzipan, Marzipan, Finest, Favorina, Lidl*	1 Slice/50g	206	9.3	412	6.2	53.4	18.6	0.0
Stollen, Rich Fruit, Brandy Laced, Christmas, Finest, Tesco*	1 Slice/70g	248	8.2	355	5.6	56.4	11.7	3.1
Stollen, Slices, Average	**1 Slice/42g**	**160**	**6.3**	**381**	**5.5**	**55.8**	**15.0**	**3.1**
Strawberry Sponge Roll, M&S*	1/6 Cake/49g	160	4.6	330	2.8	58.0	9.5	0.8
Sultana & Cherry, Tesco*	1 Cake/37g	124	4.0	334	4.7	54.4	10.8	2.5
Sultana, Apple & Cranberry, 99% Fat Free, Trimlyne*	1/6 Cake/67g	130	0.6	195	4.6	45.5	0.9	3.3
Sultana, Fair Trade, Co-Op*	1/8 Cake/45g	155	4.0	345	5.0	60.0	9.0	1.0
Super Carrot, Graze*	1 Punnet/31g	102	4.9	330	4.1	46.5	15.7	3.5
Swiss Roll, Average	**1oz/28g**	**77**	**1.2**	**276**	**7.2**	**55.5**	**4.4**	**0.8**
Swiss Roll, Chocolate Flavour, Value, Tesco*	1 Slice/20g	79	3.9	394	5.5	49.2	19.5	1.4
Swiss Roll, Chocolate, Lyons*	1 Serving/50g	190	9.6	379	4.3	47.0	19.3	0.9
Swiss Roll, Chocolate, M&S*	1 Serving/46g	168	11.1	365	4.6	32.6	24.2	1.2
Swiss Roll, Chocolate, Morrisons*	1/6 Roll/26g	103	4.9	401	4.4	56.4	18.9	3.1
Swiss Roll, Chocolate, Value, Tesco*	1 Serving/20g	81	3.7	404	5.0	54.1	18.7	2.1
Swiss Roll, Raspberry & Vanilla, Morrisons*	1 Serving/28g	98	2.7	350	4.2	61.8	9.5	0.0
Swiss Roll, Raspberry Jam, Mr Kipling*	1/6 Cake/52g	184	5.3	355	2.8	63.0	10.2	1.0
Swiss Roll, Raspberry, Lyons*	1 Roll/175g	485	2.4	277	5.2	60.6	1.4	0.0
Syrup & Ginger, Tesco*	1 Serving/32g	134	7.0	420	4.5	51.4	21.8	0.7
Tiffin, Chocolate, Sainsbury's*	1 Cake/61g	184	11.6	301	2.7	29.8	19.0	1.3
Toffee & Pecan Slices, M&S*	1 Slice/36g	160	8.5	445	4.7	54.0	23.7	1.3
Toffee Apple, McVitie's*	1 Slice/29g	104	3.2	354	3.5	60.2	11.0	1.5
Toffee, Iced, Tesco*	1 Serving/35g	132	5.2	376	3.3	57.2	14.9	1.6
Toffee, Thorntons*	1/6 Cake/70g	302	16.8	431	4.6	49.2	24.0	0.8
Trifle Bakewells, Mr Kipling*	1 Tart/45g	193	8.0	423	3.7	62.2	17.5	1.1
Triple Chocolate Roll, Cadbury*	1 Serving/40g	165	6.7	410	4.3	60.1	16.6	1.5
Turkish Delight, Fry's*	1 Cake/26g	96	2.8	371	4.5	62.4	10.8	0.5
Vanilla Sponge, Fresh Cream, Sainsbury's*	1 Slice/50g	152	5.1	304	7.5	45.6	10.2	0.4
Victoria Sandwich, Average	**1 Slice/68g**	**267**	**12.9**	**392**	**4.4**	**50.9**	**19.0**	**1.0**
Victoria Sponge, Free From, Finest, Tesco*	1 Slice/60g	234	9.7	389	3.3	57.4	16.1	0.8
Victoria Sponge, Fresh Cream, Value, Tesco*	1 Serving/50g	168	8.7	337	4.4	40.7	17.4	0.6

	Measure INFO/WEIGHT	per Measure KCAL	per Measure FAT	Nutrition Values per 100g / 100ml KCAL	PROT	CARB	FAT	FIBRE
CAKE								
Victoria Sponge, Kate's Cakes Ltd*	1 Serving/100g	410	19.7	410	4.0	52.8	19.7	0.9
Victoria Sponge, Lemon, Co-Op*	1 Slice/42g	151	8.0	360	4.0	44.0	19.0	0.7
Victoria Sponge, Mini, Bobby's*	1 Cake/35g	164	9.6	469	4.0	51.3	27.5	0.2
Victoria Sponge, Mini, Mr Kipling*	1 Cake/36g	152	6.9	420	3.9	58.5	19.0	0.8
Victoria, Sponge, TTD, Sainsbury's*	1 Slice/57g	229	11.0	401	5.0	51.8	19.3	1.4
Viennese Whirl, Average	*1 Cake/28g*	*131*	*6.9*	*467*	*4.1*	*56.7*	*24.8*	*1.1*
Viennese Whirl, Lemon, Mr Kipling*	1 Cake/28g	115	4.5	409	4.2	62.2	15.9	0.7
Viennese Whirl, Mr Kipling*	1 Cake/28g	145	8.5	514	3.8	56.2	30.2	1.3
Walnut, Sandwich, Sainsbury's*	1/8 Cake/48g	182	8.3	379	5.4	53.8	17.3	1.3
Wedding, Rich Fruit, with Cognac, Iced, Sainsbury's*	1 Slice/55g	212	5.5	385	3.8	68.9	10.0	2.0
Welsh, Average	*1oz/28g*	*121*	*5.5*	*431*	*5.6*	*61.8*	*19.6*	*1.5*
CAKE BAR								
Boost, Cadbury*	1 Bar/40g	190	10.8	475	5.3	52.8	26.9	1.1
Caramel, Weight Watchers*	1 Bar/23g	89	3.0	381	5.3	56.2	12.8	9.9
Carrot with Cheese Cream Icing, Kate's Cakes Ltd*	1 Serving/100g	345	15.6	345	3.3	48.3	15.6	1.5
Carrot, Gu*	1 Slice/38g	135	6.6	354	1.4	17.2	17.5	0.9
Carrot, Tesco*	1 Bar/68g	239	12.6	351	4.7	41.4	18.5	2.4
Chocolate Chip, Average	*1 Cake/28g*	*428*	*21.6*	*428*	*6.3*	*51.9*	*21.6*	*1.6*
Chocolate Chip, Mr Kipling*	1 Bar/32g	151	8.4	472	5.3	53.5	26.3	1.2
Chocolate Chip, Value, Tesco*	1 Cake/28g	115	5.5	410	6.3	52.2	19.5	1.7
Chocolate, Average	*1 Cake/28g*	*125*	*6.2*	*446*	*5.6*	*56.3*	*22.1*	*1.9*
Chocolate, Snack Cakes, Penguin, McVitie's*	1 Bar/24g	122	7.2	510	4.8	54.6	30.2	1.6
Double Chocolate, Free From, Sainsbury's*	1 Cake/50g	196	7.9	391	4.2	58.2	15.7	1.0
Double Chocolate, Free From, Tesco*	1 Serving/45g	190	9.1	425	4.2	55.6	20.3	4.1
Flake, Cadbury*	1 Cake/22g	97	5.1	442	6.5	51.8	23.3	0.5
Fudge, Cadbury*	1 Pack/52g	220	9.2	420	5.7	60.3	17.6	0.0
Golden Syrup, McVitie's*	1 Cake/33g	127	4.8	385	3.6	60.2	14.4	1.2
Jaffa Cakes, Spooky, McVitie's*	1 Bar/25g	96	3.5	390	3.2	62.1	14.2	2.7
Jaffa, McVitie's*	1 Bar/25g	94	3.5	385	3.2	61.1	14.2	2.4
Jamaica Ginger, McVitie's*	1 Cake/33g	128	4.9	388	3.5	60.2	14.7	1.2
Milk Chocolate Orange, Sandwich Bar, Lyons*	1 Bar/28g	142	8.0	516	5.0	62.0	29.0	0.0
Milk Chocolate, Cadbury*	1 Bar/35g	150	7.6	430	5.6	53.3	21.7	1.2
Milky Way, McVitie's*	1 Cake/26g	124	6.2	476	5.1	58.5	23.6	1.2
CAKE MIX								
Cheesecake, Tesco*	1 Serving/76g	199	7.9	262	4.1	38.0	10.4	1.6
Classic Vanilla, Sponge, Gluten Free, Hale & Hearty*	1 Serving/100g	368	1.0	368	2.7	87.1	1.0	1.2
Sponge, Value, Tesco*	1 Slice/55g	181	4.8	329	4.6	57.9	8.8	1.4
CALLALOO								
Leaves, Raw, Unprepared	*1 Cup/28g*	*6*	*0.1*	*23*	*2.5*	*4.0*	*0.3*	*0.0*
CALZONE								
Ham & Gruyere, Asda*	1 Serving/280g	661	22.4	236	10.0	31.0	8.0	2.7
Ham & Mushroom, Waitrose*	½ Pizza/145g	362	13.5	250	10.0	31.6	9.3	1.6
Speciale, Ristorante, Dr Oetker*	½ Pizza/145g	378	23.2	261	11.5	22.1	16.0	0.0
Three Cheese, Waitrose*	1 Pizza/265g	747	31.8	282	10.4	33.0	12.0	1.4
CANAPES								
Aegean Tomato, Finest, Tesco*	1 Canape/15g	45	2.2	300	7.2	34.3	14.7	2.1
Caponata, Puff Pastry, Occasions, Sainsbury's*	1 Square/12g	30	1.9	249	4.1	22.9	15.7	2.1
Salmon & Dill, Finest, Tesco*	1 Canape/15g	47	2.4	315	9.2	32.7	16.1	1.9
Smoked Salmon, Youngs*	1 Canape/10g	21	1.5	210	15.9	2.0	15.2	0.7
CANNELLONI								
Beef & Red Wine, Waitrose*	½ Pack/170g	355	16.0	209	17.5	13.8	9.4	1.0
Beef, Italian, Sainsbury's*	1 Pack/400g	498	26.2	124	5.9	10.5	6.6	1.6
Beef, Italian, Tesco*	1 Pack/400g	520	26.8	130	5.3	11.6	6.7	0.9

C

	Measure INFO/WEIGHT	per Measure		Nutrition Values per 100g / 100ml				
		KCAL	FAT	KCAL	PROT	CARB	FAT	FIBRE
CANNELLONI								
Beef, Ready Meal	1 Serving/335g	501	21.8	149	8.4	14.1	6.5	1.4
Chicken & Pesto, Italian, Sainsbury's*	1 Pack/450g	675	33.8	150	6.1	14.4	7.5	1.1
Mediterranean Vegetable, Waitrose*	1 Serving/170g	330	15.3	194	9.7	18.7	9.0	1.9
Mushroom, Italian, Sainsbury's*	1 Pack/450g	598	31.0	133	5.2	12.5	6.9	0.5
Spinach & Cheese, Finest, Tesco*	1 Pack/350g	532	31.8	152	5.4	12.1	9.1	1.5
Spinach & Ricotta, Charlie Bigham's*	½ Pack/330g	489	30.4	148	5.9	10.5	9.2	0.7
Spinach & Ricotta, Fresh, Ready Meal, Average	**1 Serving/300g**	**393**	**22.0**	**131**	**5.0**	**10.8**	**7.4**	**1.2**
Spinach & Ricotta, Italian Style, Co-Op*	1 Pack/450g	540	27.0	120	5.0	12.0	6.0	2.0
Spinach & Ricotta, Ready Meal, Average	**1 Serving/300g**	**426**	**22.0**	**142**	**5.6**	**13.3**	**7.3**	**1.4**
Tubes, Dry, Average	**1oz/28g**	**101**	**1.0**	**361**	**12.5**	**69.1**	**3.6**	**1.2**
CAPERS								
Caperberries, Spanish, Waitrose*	1 Serving/55g	9	0.3	17	1.1	2.1	0.5	2.5
Capucines, Sainsbury's*	1 Tsp/6g	1	0.0	14	1.4	1.3	0.3	2.2
in Brine, Tesco*	1 Tsp/2g	1	0.0	29	2.4	3.5	0.6	2.7
in Vinegar, Average	**1 Tsp/5g**	**2**	**0.0**	**34**	**1.7**	**3.0**	**0.6**	**0.0**
CARAMAC								
Nestle*	1 Bar/30g	174	11.0	571	5.9	55.5	36.1	0.0
CARAMBOLA								
Average	**1oz/28g**	**9**	**0.1**	**31**	**0.5**	**7.1**	**0.3**	**1.3**
CARAWAY								
Seeds, Schwartz*	1 Pack/38g	170	8.1	448	23.3	40.9	21.2	0.0
CARDAMOM								
Black, Ground, Average	**1 Tsp/2g**	**6**	**0.1**	**311**	**10.8**	**68.5**	**6.7**	**28.0**
CAROB POWDER								
Average	**1 Tsp/2g**	**3**	**0.0**	**159**	**4.9**	**37.0**	**0.1**	**0.0**
CARROT & SWEDE								
Diced, for Mashing, Average	**½ Pack/250g**	**58**	**0.7**	**23**	**0.6**	**4.7**	**0.3**	**1.9**
Mash, From Supermarket, Average	**1 Serving/150g**	**138**	**7.5**	**92**	**1.3**	**10.4**	**5.0**	**1.3**
CARROTS								
& Peas, Sainsbury's*	1 Serving/200g	100	1.0	50	3.3	8.3	0.5	3.8
Baby, Canned, Average	**1 Can/195g**	**40**	**0.5**	**21**	**0.5**	**4.2**	**0.3**	**2.1**
Baby, Fresh, Average	**1 Serving/80g**	**28**	**0.1**	**35**	**0.6**	**8.2**	**0.1**	**2.9**
Batons & Sliced Runner Beans, Sainsbury's*	1 Serving/200g	40	1.0	20	1.0	3.2	0.5	3.2
Batons, Fresh, Average	**½ Pack/150g**	**41**	**0.4**	**28**	**0.6**	**5.7**	**0.3**	**2.6**
Boiled, Average	**1oz/28g**	**6**	**0.1**	**22**	**0.6**	**4.4**	**0.4**	**2.3**
Canned, Average	**1oz/28g**	**6**	**0.1**	**20**	**0.5**	**4.0**	**0.2**	**1.9**
Chantenay, Steamer, Sainsbury's*	½ Pack/125g	60	2.1	48	0.5	7.7	1.7	2.2
Raw, Scrubbed, Average	**1 Serving/80g**	**24**	**0.4**	**30**	**0.7**	**6.0**	**0.5**	**2.4**
Roasting, with Honey & Ginger Glaze, Aunt Bessie's*	1 Serving/133g	80	4.1	60	0.7	6.1	3.1	2.5
Sliced, Canned, Average	**1 Serving/180g**	**36**	**0.2**	**20**	**0.7**	**4.1**	**0.1**	**1.5**
Sliced, Fresh, Average	**1 Serving/60g**	**17**	**0.2**	**28**	**0.7**	**5.7**	**0.3**	**2.0**
Whole, Raw, Peeled, Average	**1 Carrot/75g**	**21**	**0.2**	**29**	**0.6**	**6.4**	**0.3**	**2.2**
with Parsley & English Butter, M&S*	½ Pack/100g	65	3.9	65	0.6	7.1	3.9	2.4
CASHEW NUTS								
BBQ, Graze*	1 Pack/26g	142	10.8	546	13.9	37.0	41.7	0.0
Cracking Black Pepper, Graze*	1 Punnet/36g	216	16.6	600	19.0	26.0	46.0	4.0
Plain, Average	**½ Pack/25g**	**146**	**12.2**	**584**	**15.7**	**18.8**	**48.9**	**3.4**
Roasted & Salted, Average	**1 Serving/50g**	**306**	**25.6**	**612**	**18.8**	**19.6**	**51.1**	**3.1**
Salt & Pepper, Morrisons*	1 Pack/100g	595	46.3	595	20.9	20.4	46.3	6.6
CASSAVA								
Baked, Average	**1oz/28g**	**43**	**0.1**	**155**	**0.7**	**40.1**	**0.2**	**1.7**
Boiled in Unsalted Water, Average	**1oz/28g**	**36**	**0.1**	**130**	**0.5**	**33.5**	**0.2**	**1.4**
Gari, Average	**1oz/28g**	**100**	**0.1**	**358**	**1.3**	**92.9**	**0.5**	**0.0**

CASEROLE	Measure INFO/WEIGHT	per Measure KCAL	FAT	Nutrition Values per 100g / 100ml KCAL	PROT	CARB	FAT	FIBRE
CASSEROLE								
Bean & Lentil, Morrisons*	1 Can/410g	287	1.6	70	4.1	12.5	0.4	0.0
Bean Cassoulet, Organic, Free & Easy*	1 Tin/400g	256	1.2	64	3.4	11.9	0.3	2.3
Beef	1 Serving/336g	490	23.0	146	16.3	4.6	6.8	0.6
Beef & Ale, Finest, Tesco*	½ Pack/300g	234	4.2	78	11.5	5.0	1.4	1.1
Beef & Red Wine, BGTY, Sainsbury's*	1 Pack/300g	192	1.8	64	8.0	6.7	0.6	0.9
Beef & Red Wine, Fuller Longer, M&S*	1 Pack/420g	355	11.7	85	7.2	6.9	2.8	1.7
Beef & Red Wine, You Count, LL, Waitrose*	1 Pack/381g	297	5.2	78	6.5	9.5	1.4	0.9
Beef with Dumplings, GFY, Asda*	1 Pack/400g	416	8.8	104	11.0	10.0	2.2	0.9
Beef, & Ale, Average	*1 Serving/300g*	*251*	*6.8*	*84*	*9.4*	*6.5*	*2.2*	*1.3*
Beef, & Red Wine, Average	*1 Serving/350g*	*290*	*7.3*	*83*	*7.2*	*8.2*	*2.1*	*1.5*
Beef, Mini Favourites, M&S*	1 Pack/200g	210	8.4	105	7.1	9.3	4.2	1.4
Beef, with Dumplings, Ready Meal, Average	*1 Serving/350g*	*464*	*21.1*	*132*	*9.5*	*10.1*	*6.0*	*1.5*
Chicken & Asparagus in White Wine, Tesco*	½ Pack/300g	444	23.7	148	11.5	7.7	7.9	0.8
Chicken & Red Wine, Duchy Originals*	½ Pack/175g	187	7.5	107	14.0	5.1	4.3	1.6
Chicken & Tomato, Asda*	¼ Pack/273g	569	41.0	208	16.0	2.2	15.0	0.5
Chicken & White Wine, BGTY, Sainsbury's*	1 Serving/300g	216	6.6	72	7.2	5.9	2.2	1.3
Chicken with Dumplings, M&S*	½ Pack/227g	261	10.0	115	9.7	9.0	4.4	0.9
Chicken, & Vegetable, Ready Meal, Healthy Range	1 Serving/330g	265	11.9	80	4.7	7.6	3.6	1.1
Chicken, & White Wine, Ready Meal, Healthy Range	1 Serving/300g	234	7.4	78	7.7	6.3	2.4	1.2
Chicken, Carrots, Peas & Potatoes, Weight Watchers*	1 Serving/302g	193	4.2	64	4.3	8.6	1.4	0.5
Chicken, Leek & Mushroom, Tesco*	1 Pack/350g	382	22.0	109	4.5	8.6	6.3	1.0
Lamb, Braised, British Classics, Tesco*	1 Pack/350g	332	18.2	95	7.5	4.6	5.2	1.0
Lamb, COU, M&S*	1 Pack/390g	254	6.6	65	5.9	6.7	1.7	1.6
Lamb, Ready Meal, Healthy Range, Average	*1 Serving/220g*	*200*	*7.3*	*91*	*10.5*	*4.9*	*3.3*	*1.0*
Pork & Leek Sausage, 387, Wiltshire Farm Foods*	1 Serving/280g	307	17.3	110	4.6	7.8	6.2	1.0
Pork, Normandy Style, Finest, Tesco*	1 Pack/450g	405	21.6	90	7.6	4.1	4.8	2.3
Rabbit, Average	*1oz/28g*	*29*	*1.4*	*102*	*11.6*	*2.6*	*5.1*	*0.4*
Sausage, & Potato, M&S*	1 Serving/200g	190	11.8	95	3.3	7.5	5.9	0.9
Sausage, CBY, Asda*	1 Pot/400g	240	15.2	60	3.6	1.9	3.8	2.1
Sausage, Pork, Diet Chef Ltd*	1 Pack/300g	303	18.3	101	6.6	4.9	6.1	1.4
Spiced Chickpea & Vegetable, Pegoty Hedge, Abel & Cole*	1 Pack/400g	668	9.2	167	11.6	24.9	2.3	4.0
Steak & Ale, British Classics, Tesco*	1 Serving/100g	93	3.4	93	11.2	4.5	3.4	1.1
Steak & Kidney, Mini, Favourites, M&S*	1 Pack/200g	240	10.8	120	7.9	9.5	5.4	1.5
Steak & Mushroom, Asda*	½ Pack/304g	411	30.4	135	7.0	4.2	10.0	0.3
Vegetable & Lentil, Canned, Granose*	1 Can/400g	272	8.0	68	3.5	9.0	2.0	3.0
Vegetable, Average	*1 Serving/275g*	*77*	*0.8*	*28*	*0.8*	*5.5*	*0.3*	*1.5*
Venison, Scottish Wild, & Beaujolais, Tesco*	1 Pack/425g	366	8.9	86	11.9	4.9	2.1	0.6
CASSEROLE MIX								
Beef & Ale, Colman's*	1 Pack/45g	144	0.9	320	9.2	66.3	2.0	2.3
Beef, Colman's*	1 Pack/40g	123	0.6	308	7.5	66.0	1.5	2.5
Beef, Recipe, Colman's*	1 Pack/42g	142	0.5	338	9.1	13.1	1.1	4.0
Beef, Recipe, Schwartz*	1 Pack/43g	123	0.9	287	7.0	56.6	2.1	6.6
Chicken Chasseur, Asda*	1 Pack/80g	273	0.8	341	9.0	74.0	1.0	1.4
Chicken, Authentic, Schwartz*	1 Pack/36g	131	1.5	363	10.4	70.7	4.3	2.0
Chicken, Recipe, As Sold, Colman's*	1 Pack/40g	131	1.0	328	6.2	68.2	2.6	3.1
Chicken, Traditional, Colman's*	1 Pack/40g	124	0.5	311	5.7	69.4	1.3	1.5
Lamb, Authentic, Schwartz*	1 Pack/35g	116	1.2	332	7.7	68.0	3.3	1.3
Moroccan Lamb, As Sold, Schwartz*	1 Pack/35g	114	0.9	327	5.5	67.4	2.6	5.8
Peppered Beef, Schwartz*	1 Pack/40g	129	2.0	323	7.0	62.9	4.9	7.3
Pork, Colman's*	1 Pack/40g	131	0.6	328	6.7	72.0	1.4	2.8
Sausage & Onion, Colman's*	1 Pack/45g	143	1.2	318	9.6	64.2	2.6	2.6
Sausage, Asda*	¼ Pack/25g	80	1.0	321	6.0	65.0	4.1	3.0
Sausage, Classic, Schwartz*	1 Pack/35g	96	0.9	275	12.4	50.1	2.7	14.9

INFO/WEIGHT	Measure	per Measure		Nutrition Values per 100g / 100ml				
		KCAL	FAT	KCAL	PROT	CARB	FAT	FIBRE
CASSEROLE MIX								
Sausage, Colman's*	1 Pack/40g	144	0.6	361	8.9	77.7	1.6	1.6
Somerset Pork, Schwartz*	1 Pack/36g	115	1.4	320	9.4	61.9	3.8	7.7
Turkey, Colman's*	1 Pack/50g	156	1.0	313	5.9	68.0	1.9	3.5
CATFISH								
Cooked, Steamed, Weighed with Bone, Average	*1 Serving/100g*	*101*	*3.1*	*101*	*18.2*	*0.0*	*3.1*	*0.7*
Raw, Average	*1oz/28g*	*27*	*0.8*	*96*	*17.6*	*0.0*	*2.8*	*0.0*
CAULIFLOWER								
Boiled, Average	*1 Serving/80g*	*22*	*0.7*	*28*	*2.9*	*2.1*	*0.9*	*1.6*
Florets, Peas & Carrots, Frozen, Asda*	1 Serving/100g	37	0.6	37	3.0	5.0	0.6	2.8
Raw, Average	*1 Serving/80g*	*25*	*0.7*	*31*	*3.2*	*2.7*	*0.8*	*1.6*
Steamed, Average	*1 Serving/100g*	*28*	*0.9*	*28*	*2.9*	*2.1*	*0.9*	*1.6*
CAULIFLOWER CHEESE								
& Bacon, Gastropub, M&S*	1 Pack/300g	318	21.0	106	6.3	4.5	7.0	1.0
& Broccoli, Average	*1 Serving/200g*	*127*	*6.4*	*64*	*3.8*	*4.6*	*3.2*	*2.0*
& Broccoli, Sainsbury's*	1 Serving/130g	83	2.1	64	4.8	7.6	1.6	2.7
Asda*	1 Pack/450g	486	36.0	108	4.6	4.3	8.0	1.5
Average	*1 Meal/400g*	*362*	*23.3*	*90*	*4.5*	*4.6*	*5.8*	*1.3*
Basics, Sainsbury's*	1 Pack/300g	180	12.0	60	3.0	3.0	4.0	1.6
BFY, Morrisons*	1 Pack/300g	231	12.3	77	4.5	5.4	4.1	1.2
Eat Smart, Morrisons*	1 Pack/300g	192	6.0	64	4.9	6.7	2.0	1.5
Finest, Tesco*	1 Serving/250g	325	22.2	130	5.7	5.9	8.9	1.2
Florets in a Cheese Sauce, Sainsbury's*	1 Pack/400g	400	26.4	100	4.8	5.4	6.6	0.9
Frozen, Iceland*	1 Serving/200g	190	12.0	95	4.0	5.5	6.0	1.3
Frozen, Tesco*	1 Pack/450g	428	30.2	95	4.2	4.3	6.7	1.3
Grills, Meat Free, Tesco*	1 Grill/91g	160	7.4	175	5.3	20.0	8.1	2.9
Grills, Tesco*	1 Grill/92g	207	10.9	225	6.5	22.2	11.9	4.0
LBU, Co-Op*	1 Serving/150g	120	7.4	80	3.7	4.5	4.9	1.4
M&S*	1 Serving/150g	150	9.2	100	5.5	5.9	6.1	1.1
Made with Semi-Skimmed Milk	1oz/28g	28	1.8	100	6.0	5.2	6.4	1.3
Morrisons*	½ Pack/225g	200	14.6	89	3.3	4.4	6.5	1.0
TTD, Sainsbury's*	½ Pack/186g	284	22.5	153	5.8	5.3	12.1	1.0
Waitrose*	1 Pack/450g	328	21.6	73	4.1	3.3	4.8	1.6
with Wexford Mature Cheddar, M&S*	½ Pack/150g	176	11.7	117	6.7	4.3	7.8	1.3
CAVIAR								
Average	*1oz/28g*	*25*	*1.3*	*89*	*11.6*	*0.5*	*4.6*	*0.0*
CELERIAC								
Boiled in Salted Water, Average	*1oz/28g*	*5*	*0.1*	*18*	*0.9*	*1.9*	*0.4*	*3.2*
Raw, Average	*1 Serving/80g*	*17*	*0.3*	*21*	*1.0*	*1.9*	*0.4*	*3.2*
CELERY								
Boiled in Salted Water	*1 Serving/50g*	*4*	*0.2*	*8*	*0.5*	*0.8*	*0.3*	*1.2*
Raw, Trimmed, Average	*1 Stalk/40g*	*3*	*0.1*	*7*	*0.5*	*0.9*	*0.2*	*1.1*
CHAMPAGNE								
Average	*1 Glass/125ml*	*95*	*0.0*	*76*	*0.3*	*1.4*	*0.0*	*0.0*
CHANNA MASALA								
Indian, Sainsbury's*	1 Serving/149g	165	7.3	111	4.2	12.4	4.9	3.3
M&S*	1 Pack/225g	360	23.7	160	5.6	11.2	10.5	8.2
Waitrose*	1 Pack/300g	300	18.3	100	3.7	7.4	6.1	7.9
CHAPATIS								
Brown Wheat Flour, Waitrose*	1 Chapati/42g	128	3.4	305	8.6	49.4	8.0	4.6
Elephant Atta*	1 Chapati/45g	129	2.9	287	7.5	53.1	6.4	3.2
Indian Style, Asda*	1 Chapati/43g	95	0.4	221	8.0	45.0	1.0	2.9
Made with Fat	1 Chapati/60g	197	7.7	328	8.1	48.3	12.8	0.0
Made without Fat	1 Chapati/55g	111	0.6	202	7.3	43.7	1.0	0.0

	Measure INFO/WEIGHT	per Measure KCAL	FAT	Nutrition Values per 100g / 100ml KCAL	PROT	CARB	FAT	FIBRE
CHAPATIS								
Morrisons*	1 Chapati/40g	108	2.8	269	8.6	49.8	6.9	0.0
Wholemeal, Patak's*	1 Chapati/42g	130	4.0	310	11.2	44.9	9.5	9.0
CHARD								
Average	*1 Serving/80g*	*15*	*0.2*	*19*	*1.4*	*3.3*	*0.2*	*0.8*
Swiss, Boiled in Unsalted Water	*1oz/28g*	*6*	*0.0*	*20*	*1.9*	*4.1*	*0.1*	*2.1*
Swiss, Raw	*1oz/28g*	*5*	*0.1*	*17*	*1.7*	*3.4*	*0.2*	*1.5*
CHEDDARS								
Baked, Mini, Cheese & Ham Flavour, McVitie's*	1 Bag/30g	160	8.9	534	11.0	55.5	29.8	2.0
Baked, Mini, Original, Cheddar Cheese, Jacob's*	1 Bag/25g	129	7.4	516	10.7	50.3	29.5	2.5
McVitie's*	1 Cracker/4g	20	1.2	526	10.9	47.2	31.9	2.9
Mini, Average	*1 Bag/26g*	*134*	*7.8*	*516*	*11.2*	*50.8*	*29.9*	*2.4*
CHEESE								
Babybel, Cheddar Variety, Mini, Fromageries Bel*	1 Cheese/20g	75	6.2	375	24.0	0.0	31.0	0.0
Babybel, Emmental, Fromageries Bel*	1 Serving/20g	63	4.9	316	23.0	1.0	24.5	0.0
Babybel, Goat's Variety, Mini, Fromageries Bel*	1 Cheese/20g	65	5.4	327	21.0	0.0	27.0	0.0
Babybel, Gouda Variety, Mini, Fromageries Bel*	1 Cheese/20g	68	5.6	340	22.0	0.0	28.0	0.0
Babybel, Light, Mini, Fromageries Bel*	1 Babybel/20g	42	2.4	208	25.0	0.0	12.0	0.0
Babybel, Original, Mini, Fromageries Bel*	1 Cheese/20g	61	4.8	304	22.0	0.1	24.0	0.0
Bavarian, Smoked with Ham, Sainsbury's*	1 Serving/30g	89	7.2	298	19.4	0.8	24.1	0.0
Bavarian, Smoked, Slices, Asda*	1 Slice/18g	50	4.1	277	17.0	0.4	23.0	0.0
Bites, Quattro Formaggi, Specially Selected, Aldi*	½ Pack/35g	185	10.5	528	20.0	44.0	30.0	3.1
Bleu D' Auvergne, Sainsbury's*	1 Serving/25g	84	6.6	335	22.0	2.0	26.5	0.0
Blue, Basics, Sainsbury's*	1 Serving/100g	410	35.0	410	23.7	0.1	35.0	0.0
Blue, Castello, Soft, Castello*	¼ Pack/38g	162	15.6	432	14.0	0.5	41.5	0.0
Blue, French, CBY, Asda*	1 Serving/30g	90	7.4	301	20.0	0.0	24.5	0.0
Blue, Saint Agur*	1 Serving/30g	109	9.9	363	16.0	0.2	33.0	0.0
Brie, Average	*1 Serving/25g*	*74*	*6.0*	*296*	*19.7*	*0.3*	*24.0*	*0.0*
Brie, Reduced Fat, Average	*1 Serving/50g*	*99*	*5.7*	*198*	*23.0*	*0.8*	*11.4*	*0.0*
Caerphilly, Average	*1 Serving/50g*	*187*	*15.6*	*374*	*23.0*	*0.1*	*31.3*	*0.0*
Cambazola, Tesco*	1 Serving/30g	128	12.3	425	13.5	0.5	41.0	0.0
Camembert, Average	*1 Serving/50g*	*141*	*11.1*	*283*	*20.5*	*0.1*	*22.2*	*0.0*
Camembert, Breaded, Average	*1 Serving/90g*	*307*	*20.9*	*342*	*16.6*	*14.2*	*23.2*	*0.4*
Cantal, French, Sainsbury's*	1 Serving/30g	106	8.7	353	23.0	0.1	29.0	0.0
Cheddar & Mozzarella, Spicy, Grated, Tesco*	1 Serving/40g	140	10.5	350	26.0	2.5	26.2	0.0
Cheddar with Caramelised Onion, Sainsbury's*	1 Serving/28g	109	8.7	391	22.8	5.1	31.0	0.0
Cheddar with Caramelised Onion, Tesco*	1 Serving/50g	183	14.0	366	21.4	7.1	28.0	0.4
Cheddar with Onion & Chives, Davidson*	1 Serving/25g	100	8.3	400	24.3	0.6	33.3	0.0
Cheddar with Pickled Onion Relish, Christmas, Tesco*	¼ Cheese/50g	191	15.5	382	23.0	2.7	31.0	0.1
Cheddar, Average	*1 Serving/30g*	*123*	*10.3*	*410*	*25.0*	*0.1*	*34.4*	*0.0*
Cheddar, Canadian, Average	*1 Serving/30g*	*123*	*10.3*	*409*	*25.0*	*0.1*	*34.3*	*0.0*
Cheddar, Davidstow, Mature, Average	*1 Serving/28g*	*115*	*9.6*	*410*	*25.0*	*0.1*	*34.4*	*0.0*
Cheddar, Extra Mature, Average	*1 Serving/30g*	*123*	*10.3*	*410*	*25.1*	*0.1*	*34.4*	*0.0*
Cheddar, Grated, Average	*1 Serving/50g*	*206*	*17.2*	*413*	*24.4*	*1.5*	*34.3*	*0.0*
Cheddar, Mature, Average	*1 Serving/30g*	*123*	*10.3*	*410*	*25.0*	*0.1*	*34.4*	*0.0*
Cheddar, Mature, Grated, Average	*1 Serving/28g*	*113*	*9.3*	*404*	*24.7*	*1.6*	*33.2*	*0.0*
Cheddar, Mature, Reduced Fat, Average	*1 Serving/25g*	*68*	*4.2*	*271*	*30.0*	*0.1*	*16.7*	*0.0*
Cheddar, Medium, Average	*1 Serving/30g*	*123*	*10.4*	*411*	*24.9*	*0.2*	*34.5*	*0.0*
Cheddar, Mild, Average	*1 Serving/30g*	*123*	*10.3*	*409*	*25.0*	*0.1*	*34.3*	*0.0*
Cheddar, Reduced Fat, Average	*1 Serving/30g*	*76*	*4.2*	*255*	*32.2*	*0.1*	*14.0*	*0.0*
Cheddar, Scotch Bonnet, Slices, Tesco*	1 Slice/28g	110	9.0	394	20.3	4.8	32.2	1.7
Cheddar, Sharp, Shredded, Sargento*	1 Serving/30g	118	9.6	393	25.0	3.6	32.1	0.0
Cheddar, Smoked, Average	*1 Serving/30g*	*123*	*10.3*	*411*	*25.2*	*0.1*	*34.4*	*0.0*
Cheddar, West Country Farmhouse, Average	*1 Serving/28g*	*115*	*9.6*	*410*	*25.0*	*0.1*	*34.4*	*0.0*

CHEESE

INFO/WEIGHT	Measure	per Measure KCAL	FAT	Nutrition Values per 100g / 100ml KCAL	PROT	CARB	FAT	FIBRE
Cheddar, Wexford, Average	**1 Serving/20g**	**82**	**6.9**	**410**	**25.0**	**0.1**	**34.4**	**0.0**
Chedds, Bricks, Cathedral City, Dairy Crest Ltd*	1 Brick/18g	75	6.3	416	25.4	0.1	34.9	0.0
Chedds, Nibbles, Cathedral City, Dairy Crest Ltd*	1 Mini Bag/16g	67	5.6	416	25.4	0.1	34.9	0.0
Cheshire	**1oz/28g**	**106**	**8.8**	**379**	**24.0**	**0.1**	**31.4**	**0.0**
Cottage, Arla*	1 Serving/25g	22	1.0	90	12.0	2.0	4.0	0.0
Cottage, BFY, Morrisons*	1 Pot/125g	110	1.1	88	13.0	6.9	0.9	0.0
Cottage, Danone*	1 Serving/100g	89	3.9	89	11.2	2.3	3.9	0.0
Cottage, Fat Free, Longley Farm*	½ Pot/125g	79	0.4	63	10.8	3.9	0.3	0.0
Cottage, Healthy Choice, Nisa Heritage*	1 Pot/227g	175	4.1	77	11.8	3.4	1.8	0.3
Cottage, Jocca, Kraft*	1 Serving/50g	54	2.8	109	9.3	5.0	5.5	0.0
Cottage, Less Than 5% Fat, Sainsbury's*	½ Pot/125g	131	5.2	105	12.3	4.4	4.2	0.0
Cottage, Low Fat, 2% Fat, Natural, Average	**1 Serving/75g**	**68**	**1.4**	**90**	**13.7**	**3.6**	**1.9**	**0.0**
Cottage, Natural, COU, M&S*	½ Pot/125g	100	2.2	80	11.9	3.3	1.8	0.3
Cottage, Natural, Healthy Living, Co-Op*	1 Pot/250g	188	5.0	75	10.0	4.0	2.0	0.0
Cottage, Natural, HL, Tesco*	1 Sm Pot/125g	94	1.6	75	10.8	4.7	1.3	0.0
Cottage, Natural, Light Choices, Tesco*	1 Serving/60g	44	0.8	75	10.8	4.7	1.3	0.0
Cottage, Natural, Longley Farm*	1 Pot/250g	260	15.0	104	10.3	2.2	6.0	0.0
Cottage, Natural, Loseley*	½ Tub/100g	115	7.1	115	9.4	2.9	7.1	0.0
Cottage, Natural, Organic, Sainsbury's*	1 Pot/201g	185	3.6	92	12.8	6.3	1.8	0.0
Cottage, Natural, Plain, Average	**1oz/28g**	**27**	**1.1**	**98**	**11.8**	**3.9**	**3.8**	**0.1**
Cottage, Natural, Tesco*	1 Serving/50g	49	1.8	98	12.4	3.2	3.5	0.4
Cottage, Natural, Waitrose*	½ Pot/125g	120	4.4	96	12.4	3.6	3.5	0.4
Cottage, Onion & Chives, Light Choices, Tesco*	1 Serving/60g	51	0.9	85	11.4	4.8	1.5	0.1
Cottage, Pineapple, Light Choices, Tesco*	1 Serving/60g	54	0.8	90	9.8	8.5	1.3	0.4
Cottage, Plain, Average	**1 Tbsp/20g**	**19**	**0.7**	**93**	**12.0**	**3.3**	**3.5**	**0.1**
Cottage, Plain, Reduced Fat, Average	**1oz/28g**	**24**	**0.5**	**85**	**12.3**	**4.4**	**1.9**	**0.1**
Cottage, Value, Tesco*	½ Tub/150g	98	0.8	65	9.5	5.0	0.5	0.0
Cottage, Virtually Fat Free, Average	**1 Tbsp/20g**	**16**	**0.2**	**79**	**13.0**	**4.5**	**1.0**	**0.0**
Cottage, Virtually Fat Free, Longley Farm*	½ Pot/125g	84	0.1	67	13.4	3.0	0.1	0.0
Cottage, West Country, Low Fat 1.5%, Waitrose*	1 Serving/100g	77	1.5	77	11.8	4.4	1.5	0.0
Cottage, West Country, Waitrose*	1 Serving/100g	113	6.1	113	6.1	3.3	6.1	0.0
Cottage, Whole Milk, Natural, Average	**1 Serving/75g**	**77**	**3.4**	**103**	**12.5**	**2.7**	**4.5**	**0.0**
Cottage, with Black Pepper, HE, Tesco*	1 Pot/125g	101	2.2	81	12.1	4.0	1.8	0.0
Cottage, with Chives, Low Fat, Westacre*	1 Pot/100g	81	1.4	81	13.7	3.5	1.4	1.2
Cottage, with Chives, Virtually Fat free, Longley Farm*	½ Pot/125g	88	0.1	70	14.3	2.9	0.1	0.0
Cottage, with Cucumber & Mint, HE, Tesco*	½ Pot/125g	91	2.1	73	10.7	3.8	1.7	0.1
Cottage, with Grilled Pepper & Pesto, Light Choices, Tesco*	1 Portion/60g	45	0.9	75	10.2	4.3	1.5	0.5
Cottage, with Mango & Pineapple, BGTY, Sainsbury's*	½ Pot/125g	112	0.9	90	10.7	10.4	0.7	0.2
Cottage, with Onion & Chive, GFY, Asda*	¼ Tub/75g	50	1.0	66	9.3	3.8	1.4	0.5
Cottage, with Onion & Chive, HL, Tesco*	1 Serving/60g	45	1.0	75	10.0	5.0	1.6	0.5
Cottage, with Onion & Chive, M&S*	¼ Pot/65g	88	5.5	135	10.4	4.0	8.5	0.1
Cottage, with Onion & Chives, Everyday, Value, Tesco*	1 Portion/60g	45	0.9	75	10.2	5.0	1.5	0.5
Cottage, with Pineapple, BGTY, Sainsbury's*	1 Serving/125g	105	0.9	84	10.5	8.9	0.7	0.1
Cottage, with Pineapple, GFY, Asda*	1 Pot/227g	193	2.3	85	9.0	10.0	1.0	0.5
Cottage, with Pineapple, Less Than 5% Fat, Sainsbury's*	½ Pot/125g	122	4.2	98	10.0	6.8	3.4	0.1
Cottage, with Pineapple, NUME, Morrisons*	½ Tub/125g	100	1.6	80	8.7	8.1	1.3	0.5
Cottage, with Sweet Chilli, & Red Pepper, CBY, Asda*	½ Tub/150g	118	2.0	79	9.9	7.1	1.3	0.3
Cottage, with Tomato & Cracked Black Pepper, Asda*	½ Pot/113g	86	2.4	76	10.0	3.1	2.1	1.3
Cream, Average	**1 Portion/30g**	**132**	**14.2**	**439**	**3.1**	**0.0**	**47.4**	**0.0**
Cream, Garlic & Herbs, Light, Boursin*	1 Portion/20g	26	1.8	131	8.0	4.5	9.0	0.0
Cream, Reduced Fat, Average	**1 Serving/20g**	**23**	**1.1**	**117**	**13.0**	**4.0**	**5.3**	**0.1**
Cream, with Onion & Chives, Morrisons*	1 Serving/20g	38	3.0	190	11.0	3.0	15.0	0.0
Cream, with Pineapple, Asda*	1 Serving/40g	77	5.2	193	8.0	11.0	13.0	0.0

CHEESE

INFO/WEIGHT	Measure	per Measure KCAL	FAT	Nutrition Values per 100g / 100ml KCAL	PROT	CARB	FAT	FIBRE
Cream, with Red Peppers & Onion, GFY, Asda*	1 Serving/32g	42	1.9	130	13.0	6.0	6.0	0.0
Creme de Saint Agur, Saint Agur*	1 Serving/10g	28	2.5	285	13.5	2.3	24.7	0.0
Dairylea, Light, Slices, Kraft*	1 Slice/25g	51	2.6	205	17.0	8.6	10.5	0.0
Dairylea, Slices, Kraft*	1 Slice/25g	69	5.1	275	13.0	8.6	20.5	0.0
Danish Blue, Average	*1 Serving/30g*	*106*	*8.7*	*352*	*20.8*	*0.0*	*29.1*	*0.0*
Demi Pont L'eveque, Finest, Tesco*	1 Serving/46g	138	10.6	301	21.1	0.4	23.0	0.0
Dolcelatte, Average	*1 Serving/30g*	*110*	*9.7*	*366*	*17.8*	*0.4*	*32.3*	*0.4*
Double Gloucester with Onion & Chives, Sainsbury's*	1 Serving/30g	110	8.5	365	22.2	5.5	28.2	0.0
Double Gloucester, Average	*1 Serving/30g*	*121*	*10.2*	*404*	*24.5*	*0.1*	*34.0*	*0.0*
Doux De Montagne, Average	*1 Serving/25g*	*88*	*7.1*	*352*	*22.9*	*1.5*	*28.3*	*0.0*
Edam, Average	*1 Serving/10g*	*33*	*2.5*	*326*	*25.3*	*0.0*	*24.9*	*0.0*
Edam, Dutch, Garlic & Herb Wedge, Asda*	1 Serving/60g	197	15.0	329	26.0	0.0	25.0	0.0
Edam, Reduced Fat, Average	*1 Serving/30g*	*69*	*3.3*	*230*	*32.4*	*0.1*	*11.1*	*0.0*
Edam, Slices, Average	*1 Slice/30g*	*96*	*7.2*	*320*	*25.0*	*0.4*	*24.1*	*0.0*
Emmental, Average	*1 Serving/10g*	*37*	*2.8*	*368*	*28.4*	*0.0*	*28.4*	*0.0*
Emmental, Grated, President*	1 Pack/200g	728	56.0	364	28.0	0.0	28.0	0.0
Emmental, Light, Slices, President*	1 Slice/20g	60	3.6	298	34.0	0.0	18.0	0.0
Feta, Average	*1 Serving/30g*	*79*	*6.4*	*262*	*16.3*	*1.0*	*21.5*	*0.0*
Feta, Light, Greek, Salad, 40% Reduced Fat, Attis*	1 Portion/30g	51	3.6	170	20.0	0.6	12.0	0.0
Fondue, Original, Fromalp*	1 Pack/400g	888	68.0	222	15.0	2.5	17.0	0.0
Fondue, Swiss, Easy Cook, Tesco*	¼ Pack/100g	235	17.0	235	15.5	4.0	17.0	0.0
Fondue, Traditionnelle, Co-Op*	1 Serving/100g	409	34.0	409	26.0	0.9	34.0	0.0
Fontina, Average	*1 Serving/28g*	*109*	*9.0*	*389*	*25.0*	*0.0*	*32.1*	*0.0*
for Pizza, Grated	*1 Serving/50g*	*163*	*12.2*	*326*	*25.0*	*1.6*	*24.4*	*0.0*
Goats, Average	*1 Tsp/10g*	*26*	*2.1*	*262*	*13.8*	*3.8*	*21.2*	*0.0*
Goats, Breaded, Bites, Sainsbury's*	1 Bite/25g	84	6.2	337	13.0	15.1	25.0	0.8
Goats, Breaded, Cheese Emporium, Aldi*	1 Portion/25g	78	5.5	312	10.8	17.2	22.0	2.0
Goats, French, Mild, Average	*1 Serving/30g*	*49*	*3.5*	*163*	*11.2*	*3.0*	*11.8*	*0.0*
Goats, Premium, Average	*1 Serving/30g*	*98*	*7.8*	*327*	*20.5*	*0.6*	*26.1*	*0.0*
Goats, Soft, Average	*1 Serving/30g*	*79*	*6.3*	*262*	*16.7*	*1.8*	*20.8*	*0.5*
Goats, Welsh with Herbs, Sainsbury's*	1 Serving/30g	90	7.4	299	15.3	3.6	24.8	0.1
Gorgonzola, Average	*1 Serving/30g*	*100*	*8.1*	*334*	*20.0*	*0.0*	*27.0*	*0.0*
Gouda, Average	*1 Serving/30g*	*113*	*9.4*	*376*	*24.0*	*0.0*	*31.5*	*0.0*
Gran Padano, Reserva, Deluxe, Lidl*	1 Serving/10g	39	2.8	388	33.0	0.0	28.4	0.0
Grana Padano, Italian Cheese, Waitrose*	1 Serving/14g	54	4.0	388	33.0	0.0	28.4	0.0
Gruyere	*1oz/28g*	*115*	*9.3*	*409*	*27.2*	*0.0*	*33.3*	*0.0*
Halloumi, Average	*1 Serving/80g*	*253*	*19.7*	*316*	*20.8*	*1.6*	*24.7*	*0.0*
Halloumi, Light Average	*1 Serving/100g*	*245*	*15.3*	*245*	*24.7*	*1.7*	*15.3*	*0.0*
Havarti, Slices, Tesco*	1 Slice/25g	85	6.5	340	24.0	1.4	26.0	0.0
Healthy Range, Slices, Average	*1 Slice/25g*	*45*	*2.2*	*180*	*19.5*	*5.4*	*9.0*	*0.0*
Italian, Grated, Average	*1 Serving/30g*	*144*	*10.0*	*481*	*44.0*	*1.1*	*33.4*	*0.0*
Jarlsberg, Slices, Average	*1 Slice/15g*	*54*	*4.0*	*360*	*27.0*	*0.0*	*27.0*	*0.0*
Lactose Free, Arla*	1 Serving/30g	103	8.1	344	25.3	1.0	27.0	0.0
Lactose Free, Semi Hard, Lactofree, Arla*	1 Serving/30g	103	8.1	344	25.3	1.0	27.0	0.0
Lancashire	*1oz/28g*	*104*	*8.7*	*373*	*23.3*	*0.1*	*31.0*	*0.0*
Leerdammer, Lighter, Sliced, M&S*	1 Slice/23g	62	3.9	271	29.5	0.1	17.0	0.0
Manchego	*1 Serving/70g*	*340*	*30.8*	*485*	*22.2*	*0.1*	*44.0*	*0.0*
Mascarpone, 25% Less Fat, Sainsbury's*	1 Portion/30g	95	9.0	316	6.7	4.8	30.0	0.0
Mascarpone, Average	*1 Serving/30g*	*131*	*13.1*	*437*	*5.6*	*4.1*	*43.6*	*0.0*
Mature, Half Fat, Average	*1 Serving/25g*	*66*	*3.9*	*265*	*29.9*	*0.4*	*15.6*	*0.1*
Mild, Reduced Fat, Grated, Average	*1 Serving/30g*	*70*	*3.3*	*235*	*31.5*	*2.2*	*11.1*	*0.0*
Monterey Jack, Iga*	1 Serving/28g	110	9.0	393	25.0	0.0	32.1	0.0
Monterey Jack, Shredded, Kraft*	¼ Cup/28g	101	8.1	360	22.0	3.6	28.8	0.0

C

C

CHEESE

	Measure INFO/WEIGHT	per Measure KCAL	FAT	Nutrition Values per 100g / 100ml KCAL	PROT	CARB	FAT	FIBRE
Morbier, Sainsbury's*	1 Serving/10g	33	2.4	330	28.0	0.1	24.2	0.0
Mozzarella, Average	*½ Ball/63g*	*172*	*12.9*	*275*	*21.2*	*1.2*	*20.6*	*0.0*
Mozzarella, Reduced Fat, Average	*½ Ball/63g*	*115*	*6.4*	*184*	*21.2*	*1.0*	*10.2*	*0.0*
Mozzarella, Sticks, Breaded, The Cheese Emporium, Aldi*	1 Stick/25g	80	4.8	320	14.0	23.0	19.0	1.0
Neufchâtel, Soft, Average	*1 Serving/30g*	*76*	*6.9*	*253*	*9.0*	*3.6*	*23.0*	*0.0*
Ossau-Iraty, Average	*1 Serving/30g*	*120*	*10.2*	*400*	*22.3*	*0.2*	*34.0*	*0.0*
Parlick Fell, Hard, Sheeps, Sainsbury's*	1 Serving/30g	109	9.1	364	22.6	0.0	30.4	0.0
Parmesan, Average	*1 Tbsp/10g*	*40*	*2.9*	*401*	*35.2*	*0.0*	*29.4*	*0.0*
Pecorino, Italian, Tesco*	1 Serving/30g	119	9.9	397	22.0	0.0	33.0	0.0
Piccante Gorgonzola, TTD, Sainsbury's*	1 Serving/30g	108	9.0	359	22.1	0.5	29.8	0.1
Poivre, Boursin*	1oz/28g	116	11.8	414	7.0	2.0	42.0	0.0
Quark, Average	*1 Serving/20g*	*13*	*0.0*	*66*	*11.9*	*4.0*	*0.2*	*0.0*
Raclette, Richsmonts*	1 Slice/28g	100	8.0	357	25.0	0.0	28.6	0.0
Reblochon	*1 Serving/30g*	*95*	*8.0*	*318*	*19.7*	*0.0*	*26.6*	*0.0*
Red Leicester, Average	*1 Serving/30g*	*120*	*10.1*	*400*	*23.8*	*0.1*	*33.7*	*0.0*
Red Leicester, Reduced Fat, Average	*1 Serving/30g*	*78*	*4.6*	*261*	*30.2*	*0.1*	*15.4*	*0.0*
Ricotta, Average	*1 Serving/50g*	*67*	*4.8*	*134*	*9.3*	*2.9*	*9.5*	*0.0*
Roquefort, Average	*1oz/28g*	*105*	*9.2*	*375*	*19.7*	*0.0*	*32.9*	*0.0*
Roule, French, Sainsbury's*	1 Serving/30g	96	9.2	321	8.5	3.0	30.5	0.0
Sage Derby	*1oz/28g*	*113*	*9.5*	*402*	*24.2*	*0.1*	*33.9*	*0.0*
Shropshire, Blue, Average	*1 Serving/50g*	*196*	*17.1*	*391*	*21.0*	*0.0*	*34.2*	*0.0*
Slices, Average	*1 Slice/23g*	*82*	*6.6*	*358*	*24.0*	*0.8*	*28.6*	*0.0*
Slices, Cheddar with Mexican Spices & Jalapeno, Tesco*	1 Slice/28g	105	8.4	375	22.7	2.5	30.1	0.8
Slices, Leerdammer*	1 Slice/20g	71	5.5	356	27.0	0.1	27.5	0.0
Slices, Light Choices, Tesco*	1 Slice/20g	37	2.1	185	19.8	4.0	10.6	0.0
Slices, Morrisons*	1 Slice/20g	39	2.0	196	21.0	5.4	10.0	0.0
Slices, Red Leicester, Tesco*	1 Slice/30g	120	10.1	400	23.7	0.0	33.7	0.0
Slices, Smoked with Ham, Aldi*	1 Slice/21g	66	5.2	313	21.0	1.0	25.0	0.1
Soft, & Smooth, Extra Light, HL, Tesco*	1 Serving/30g	39	1.8	130	14.2	3.7	6.0	0.0
Soft, 40% Less Fat, Lighter, M&S*	1 Serving/30g	48	3.3	159	11.0	4.3	10.9	0.5
Soft, Black Pepper, Light, Sainsbury's*	½ Pack/100g	205	16.5	205	11.0	3.0	16.5	0.0
Soft, Extra Light, Average	*1 Serving/20g*	*25*	*1.2*	*125*	*14.3*	*3.6*	*5.9*	*0.1*
Soft, Extra Light, Simply, M&S*	1 Serving/30g	32	1.0	107	12.3	7.1	3.3	0.0
Soft, Fruit & Rum Halo, Discover*	1 Serving/25g	104	8.5	414	8.6	11.7	34.1	0.0
Soft, Full Fat, Average	*1 Serving/50g*	*156*	*15.2*	*312*	*8.2*	*1.7*	*30.3*	*0.0*
Soft, Full Fat, Original, Lactose Free, Kraft*	1 Serving/30g	84	8.2	280	4.5	2.7	27.5	0.3
Soft, Garlic & Herb, Extra Light, Light Choices, Tesco*	1 Serving/38g	49	2.4	130	12.3	5.1	6.3	0.3
Soft, Garlic & Herb, Roulade, M&S*	1 Portion/100g	295	27.3	295	7.8	4.1	27.3	1.3
Soft, Garlic & Herbs, Full Fat, Deli, Boursin*	1 Serving/28g	84	8.3	299	3.5	5.0	29.5	0.0
Soft, Garlic & Herbs, Lighter, Asda*	½ Pack/100g	106	4.4	106	11.8	4.3	4.4	0.1
Soft, Garlic & Herbs, Medium Fat, Westacre*	1 Serving/30g	56	4.8	188	8.0	3.0	16.0	0.1
Soft, Herbs & Garlic, Sensations, Philadelphia, Kraft*	1 Serving/30g	78	7.2	260	6.4	3.3	24.0	0.3
Soft, Light, Average	*1 Tbsp/30g*	*54*	*3.9*	*179*	*12.1*	*3.2*	*13.1*	*0.0*
Soft, Low Fat, Linessa, Lidl*	1 Serving/50g	30	0.1	61	11.0	3.9	0.2	1.4
Soft, Medium Fat, Average	*1 Serving/30g*	*62*	*5.4*	*207*	*8.4*	*3.0*	*17.9*	*0.0*
Soft, Onion & Chives, Lighter, Asda*	1 Serving/30g	32	1.3	105	11.6	4.5	4.3	0.2
Soft, Original, Whipped, Sensations, Philadelphia, Kraft*	1 Serving/30g	80	7.5	265	6.5	2.6	25.0	0.1
Soft, Philadelphia, Basil, Light, Philadelphia*	1 Serving/35g	51	3.7	146	8.0	4.0	10.5	0.5
Soft, Philadelphia, Blue, Philadelphia*	1 Serving/28g	76	7.1	270	6.8	3.4	25.5	0.2
Soft, Philadelphia, Cadbury Chocolate, Mini, Philadelphia*	1 Mini Tub/30g	86	4.0	287	6.5	34.0	13.3	1.7
Soft, Philadelphia, Cadbury Chocolate, Philadelphia*	1 Serving/30g	86	3.9	285	6.5	34.0	13.0	1.7
Soft, Philadelphia, Chives, Light, Philadelphia*	1 Serving/30g	48	3.6	160	8.3	4.3	12.0	0.7
Soft, Philadelphia, Cracked Pepper, Mini, Philadelphia*	1 Tub/35g	56	4.6	161	7.7	2.5	13.0	0.4

CHEESE	Measure INFO/WEIGHT	per Measure KCAL	per Measure FAT	Nutrition Values per 100g / 100ml KCAL	PROT	CARB	FAT	FIBRE
Soft, Philadelphia, Extra Light, Mini Tubs, Philadelphia*	1 Tub/35g	38	1.8	108	11.0	4.2	5.0	0.6
Soft, Philadelphia, Extra Light, Philadelphia*	1 Serving/30g	33	1.4	110	11.7	5.0	4.7	0.3
Soft, Philadelphia, Garlic & Herb, Light, Philadelphia*	1 Serving/30g	45	3.2	149	7.3	5.4	10.5	0.5
Soft, Philadelphia, Grilled Peppers, Light, Philadelphia*	1 Portion/30g	44	3.2	147	7.0	5.4	10.5	0.7
Soft, Philadelphia, Light, Mini Tubs, Philadelphia*	1 Tub/35g	55	4.0	158	8.7	4.0	11.5	0.4
Soft, Philadelphia, Light, Philadelphia*	1 Serving/30g	47	3.5	157	8.7	4.0	11.7	0.3
Soft, Philadelphia, Original, Full Fat, Philadelphia*	1 Serving/30g	70	6.4	235	5.5	4.0	21.5	0.2
Soft, Pineapple Halo, Discover*	1 Serving/25g	101	8.2	404	7.2	16.6	32.6	1.2
Soft, Roasted Onion & Chive, Low Fat, Weight Watchers*	¼ Pack/50g	46	1.4	92	12.4	4.5	2.7	2.5
Soft, Sun Dried Tomato & Basil, Light, Philadelphia*	1/8 Pack/25g	39	2.8	157	8.3	4.8	11.0	0.4
Soft, White, Lactofree, Arla*	1 Serving/30g	59	5.0	197	8.6	3.0	16.5	0.0
Soft, with Garlic & Herbs, Light, Sainsbury's*	2 Servings/100g	157	11.4	157	10.6	3.1	11.4	0.0
Soft, with Pineapple, Creamy, Asda*	1 Serving/32g	62	4.2	193	8.0	11.0	13.0	0.0
Soya	*1oz/28g*	*89*	*7.6*	*319*	*18.3*	*0.0*	*27.3*	*0.0*
Stilton, Average	*1 Serving/30g*	*123*	*10.6*	*410*	*22.4*	*0.1*	*35.5*	*0.0*
Stilton, Blue, Average	*1 Serving/30g*	*124*	*10.7*	*412*	*22.8*	*0.1*	*35.7*	*0.0*
Stilton, White with Cranberries, Tesco*	1 Serving/50g	184	14.8	368	15.8	9.5	29.7	0.7
Stilton, White with Mango & Ginger, Tesco*	1/3 Pack/65g	228	14.0	350	13.1	25.8	21.6	0.6
Stilton, White, Average	*1oz/28g*	*101*	*8.8*	*362*	*19.9*	*0.1*	*31.3*	*0.0*
Taleggio D.o.p., Finest, Tesco*	1 Serving/30g	89	7.5	297	18.0	0.0	25.0	0.0
Triangles, Light, Creamy Swiss, The Laughing Cow *	1 Triangle/18g	25	1.2	143	13.7	6.8	6.8	0.0
Twisted, Cheestrings*	1 String/20g	61	4.5	305	23.0	2.5	22.5	0.0
Wedge, Leerdammer*	1 Serving/30g	107	8.3	357	27.0	0.0	27.7	0.0
Wedges, Camembert, Breaded, Morrisons*	1 Wedge/25g	88	5.6	352	15.1	22.9	22.2	2.0
Wensleydale, & Ginger, Truckle, Morrisons*	1 Truckle/90g	330	23.7	367	18.0	14.0	26.3	1.1
Wensleydale, Average	*1 Serving/25g*	*92*	*7.8*	*369*	*22.4*	*0.1*	*31.0*	*0.0*
Wensleydale, Cranberry & Mustard, Lozzas	1 Block/50g	179	13.9	359	20.7	6.4	27.8	0.0
Wensleydale, with Blueberries, M&S*	1 Portion/30g	111	7.9	370	18.7	13.4	26.4	0.9
Wensleydale, with Cranberries, Sainsbury's*	1 Serving/50g	180	13.9	359	20.7	6.4	27.8	0.0
Wensleydale, with Mango & Ginger, Waitrose*	1 Portion/30g	109	6.6	363	13.5	27.1	21.9	1.7
CHEESE ALTERNATIVE								
Cheezly, Cheddar Style, Garlic & Herb, The Redwood Co*	1 Serving/25g	62	4.4	249	3.6	19.4	17.4	0.0
Mozzarella, Slices, Dairy Free	1 Slice/19g	80	6.0	420	10.5	10.5	31.5	0.0
Vegetarian, Average	*1 Serving/30g*	*110*	*8.4*	*368*	*28.2*	*0.0*	*28.1*	*0.0*
CHEESE ON TOAST								
Average	*1 Slice/130g*	*494*	*34.2*	*380*	*13.8*	*23.8*	*26.3*	*0.7*
CHEESE PUFFS								
Average	*1 Bag/25g*	*129*	*7.4*	*517*	*7.8*	*54.8*	*29.5*	*1.5*
Cheeky, Tesco*	1 Bag/20g	108	7.0	542	6.7	50.2	34.9	0.0
Morrisons*	1 Bag/25g	136	8.7	542	6.7	50.2	34.9	1.1
Sainsbury's*	1 Pack/100g	530	32.0	530	9.1	51.4	32.0	1.9
Shapers, Boots*	1 Bag/16g	80	3.8	500	7.1	64.0	24.0	0.9
Value, Tesco*	1 Pack/16g	84	4.6	525	6.2	60.0	28.8	0.6
CHEESE SINGLES								
50% Less Fat, Asda*	1 Slice/20g	38	2.0	190	19.0	6.0	10.0	0.0
American, 2% Milk, Kraft*	1 Slice/19g	45	3.0	237	21.0	5.3	15.8	0.0
Half Fat, Co-Op*	1 Slice/20g	47	2.4	235	25.0	7.0	12.0	0.0
Kraft*	1 Single/20g	52	3.7	260	13.5	7.6	18.5	0.0
Light Choices, Tesco*	1 Slice/20g	37	2.0	185	19.8	4.0	10.0	0.0
CHEESE SPREAD								
60% Less Fat, Asda*	1 Serving/30g	52	2.7	174	16.0	7.3	9.0	0.0
Asda*	1 Serving/33g	92	7.9	280	9.0	7.0	24.0	0.0
Average	*1 Serving/30g*	*76*	*6.4*	*254*	*9.4*	*5.9*	*21.4*	*0.1*

	INFO/WEIGHT	KCAL	FAT	KCAL	PROT	CARB	FAT	FIBRE
CHEESE SPREAD								
BGTY, Sainsbury's*	1 Serving/25g	28	1.4	111	11.0	4.3	5.5	0.4
Cheese & Ham, Primula*	1 Serving/20g	40	3.0	200	12.3	3.1	15.0	4.9
Cream, Light, Sainsbury's*	1 Serving/50g	94	7.8	187	7.8	4.1	15.5	0.3
Creamery, Light, Sainsbury's*	1 Serving/25g	46	3.8	185	9.0	3.5	15.0	0.0
Dairylea, Light, Tub, Kraft*	1 Serving/30g	47	2.2	158	16.5	5.2	7.2	0.0
Dairylea, Tub, Kraft*	1 Serving/25g	60	4.9	240	11.0	5.3	19.5	0.0
Light, Primula*	1 Serving/20g	30	1.8	149	15.2	3.0	8.9	3.6
Low Fat, Weight Watchers*	1 Serving/50g	56	1.4	112	18.1	3.4	2.9	1.2
Plain, Original, Primula*	1 Serving/25g	49	3.8	196	12.8	4.1	15.2	5.9
Soft, Low Fat, M&S*	1 Pack/100g	111	4.5	111	13.0	4.2	4.5	0.3
Squeeze, Light, Laughing Cow, Fromageries Bel*	1 Portion/30g	42	2.1	139	12.0	7.0	7.0	5.0
Squeeze, Original, Laughing Cow, Fromageries Bel*	1 Portion/30g	71	6.0	236	9.0	5.0	20.0	0.0
with Chives, Primula*	1 Serving/30g	57	4.3	190	12.5	2.9	14.2	4.5
with Garlic & Herb, Soft, Free From, Sainsbury's*	1 Serving/30g	91	9.0	302	2.5	5.5	30.0	0.1
with Prawn, Primula*	1 Squeeze/25g	48	3.6	190	12.5	3.3	14.4	3.6
CHEESE STRAWS								
& Bacon, Party, Tesco*	1 Straw/13g	40	2.6	321	10.5	23.8	20.4	2.1
Cheddar, M&S*	1 Straw/11g	59	3.8	535	14.9	40.1	34.9	2.4
Cheese Twists, Tesco*	1 Serving/20g	99	5.6	494	14.0	46.4	28.0	4.2
Homemade or Bakery, Average	*1 Straw/41g*	*173*	*12.6*	*422*	*12.0*	*24.2*	*30.7*	*0.7*
Mature Cheddar, Puffed, Thomas J Fudge*	1 Straw/10g	53	3.2	532	12.3	46.8	31.9	0.0
Selection, Sainsbury's*	1 Straw/7g	41	2.9	558	16.6	34.5	39.3	2.8
CHEESE TRIANGLES								
Average	*1 Triangle/14g*	*33*	*2.2*	*238*	*10.3*	*14.2*	*15.6*	*0.2*
Dairylea, Light, Kraft*	1 Triangle/18g	36	2.2	205	15.5	6.3	12.5	0.0
Extra Light, The Laughing Cow, Fromageries Bel*	1 Triangle/18g	20	0.5	116	15.0	6.5	3.0	0.0
Light Choices, Tesco*	1 Triangle/18g	30	1.2	170	17.5	8.5	7.0	0.0
Light, Cheddar, The Laughing Cow, Fromageries Bel*	1 Triangle/16g	25	1.4	159	13.5	6.0	9.0	0.0
Original, The Laughing Cow, Fromageries Bel*	1 Triangle/18g	42	3.3	239	11.0	6.0	19.0	0.0
Reduced Fat, Average	*1 Triangle/18g*	*27*	*1.2*	*154*	*15.4*	*7.0*	*7.0*	*0.0*
CHEESE TWISTS								
All Butter, M&S*	1 Pack/125g	625	33.4	500	14.2	50.2	26.7	3.2
Asda*	1 Twist/8g	42	2.4	500	14.0	48.0	28.0	5.0
Gruyere & Poppy Seed, Truly Irresistible, Co-Op*	1 Twist/8g	42	2.4	520	13.2	48.8	30.1	2.5
Gruyere & Poppy Seed, TTD, Sainsbury's*	1 Serving/8g	41	2.3	509	13.7	50.5	28.0	2.6
Parmesan, All Butter, TTD, Sainsbury's*	1 Serving/8g	38	2.0	487	13.8	51.0	25.3	2.8
Pre Packed, Average	*1 Twist/8g*	*41*	*2.2*	*515*	*13.7*	*47.9*	*27.7*	*2.3*
CHEESECAKE								
After Noon, Mango & Passionfruit, 3 Pack, Gu*	1 Portion/45g	155	11.3	345	3.4	26.5	25.2	0.4
American Red White & Blueberry, Sainsbury's*	1/6 Cake/83g	264	15.4	318	3.8	35.1	18.5	0.4
Apple & Cinnamon, Baked, M&S*	1 Serving/116g	390	22.0	335	3.7	39.7	18.9	2.1
Apricot, Co-Op*	1 Cake/100g	230	11.0	230	4.0	29.0	11.0	0.9
Apricot, HL, Tesco*	1 Pot/100g	179	2.3	179	4.9	34.7	2.3	1.6
Autumn Berry, Waitrose*	1 Slice/92g	316	20.3	343	4.4	31.5	22.1	2.0
Average	*1 Slice/115g*	*490*	*40.8*	*426*	*3.7*	*24.6*	*35.5*	*0.4*
Belgian Chocolate, M&S*	1 Slice/100g	385	23.9	385	5.3	39.2	23.9	2.5
Blackcurrant Devonshire, McVitie's*	1/6 Cake/67g	193	11.5	288	3.8	29.7	17.1	1.7
Blackcurrant, Average	*1 Serving/90g*	*237*	*11.9*	*263*	*3.6*	*32.3*	*13.2*	*2.4*
Blackcurrant, Sainsbury's*	1 Serving/100g	238	9.3	238	3.9	34.6	9.3	1.3
Blackcurrant, VLH Kitchens	1 Serving/120g	341	13.7	285	3.4	32.0	16.4	0.9
Blueberry & Lemon Flavour Wedges, Sainsbury's*	1 Serving/80g	262	16.9	327	5.1	29.2	21.1	1.2
Blueberry & Vanilla, TTD, Sainsbury's*	1 Serving/95g	353	24.8	372	5.4	28.9	26.1	2.1
Cherry, Healthy Range, Average	*1 Serving/90g*	*172*	*3.0*	*191*	*3.7*	*36.4*	*3.3*	*1.1*

CHEESECAKE

	Measure INFO/WEIGHT	per Measure KCAL	FAT	Nutrition Values per 100g / 100ml KCAL	PROT	CARB	FAT	FIBRE
Chocolate & Hazelnut, Sara Lee*	1 Serving/65g	224	13.9	345	6.5	31.2	21.4	1.2
Chocolate & Irish Cream Liqueur, Tesco*	1 Serving/93g	385	28.0	414	5.0	30.7	30.1	0.8
Chocolate & Vanilla, Gu*	1 Pot/90g	379	27.1	421	4.1	34.6	30.1	1.6
Chocolate & Vanilla, Reduced Fat, M&S*	1 Serving/114g	319	13.7	280	7.0	37.9	12.0	1.5
Chocolate & Vanilla, Tesco*	1 Serving/90g	330	19.4	365	5.2	37.1	21.5	1.6
Chocolate Truffle, HL, Tesco*	1 Slice/96g	250	13.2	260	10.3	23.7	13.8	6.5
Chocolate, Average	*1 Serving/75g*	*265*	*15.7*	*353*	*5.7*	*35.6*	*20.9*	*1.9*
Chocolate, Tesco*	1 Serving/91g	317	17.4	348	6.2	37.8	19.1	1.5
Chocolate, Weight Watchers*	1 Cake/95g	143	3.8	151	7.5	20.7	4.0	0.7
Citrus, Good Choice, Mini, Iceland*	1 Cake/111g	198	4.7	178	3.5	31.6	4.2	0.4
Commercially Prepared	1/6 Cake/80g	257	18.0	321	5.5	25.5	22.5	0.4
Creamy Vanilla, New York, Slices, Tesco*	1 Slice/106g	371	26.7	350	4.6	25.9	25.2	2.2
Devonshire Strawberry, McVitie's*	1/6 Cake/66g	192	10.7	291	4.4	31.8	16.2	3.6
Double Chocolate Wedge, Sainsbury's*	1 Serving/75g	327	24.8	436	5.7	29.0	33.0	1.7
Fruit, Average	*1 Serving/75g*	*207*	*10.9*	*276*	*5.3*	*32.3*	*14.5*	*1.6*
Fudge, Tesco*	1 Serving/102g	384	23.6	376	4.6	37.5	23.1	0.5
Indulgent with Liqueur, Average	*1 Serving/90g*	*366*	*23.4*	*406*	*5.0*	*38.2*	*26.0*	*0.8*
Lemon Creamy & Light, M&S*	1/6 Cake/68g	236	13.8	350	3.5	32.3	20.4	0.4
Lemon Meringue, Tesco*	1 Slice/94g	352	25.0	375	3.8	30.1	26.6	0.3
Lemon Swirl, Individual, Sainsbury's*	1 Pot/125g	380	23.0	304	3.0	31.1	18.4	0.9
Lemon Swirl, Sainsbury's*	1/6 Cake/95g	350	21.0	369	4.8	37.2	22.1	1.0
Lemon, Asda*	1 Slice/90g	319	21.2	354	4.3	31.2	23.5	1.1
Lemon, Average	*1 Serving/90g*	*307*	*19.5*	*341*	*4.1*	*33.0*	*21.6*	*1.8*
Lemon, Sainsbury's*	1 Serving/180g	650	37.1	361	4.0	39.9	20.6	1.3
Lemon, Tesco*	1 Slice/93g	315	21.0	339	5.2	28.6	22.6	0.3
Lemon, Value, Tesco*	1 Serving/79g	221	11.8	281	4.3	32.2	15.0	4.2
Mandarin, Morrisons*	1 Serving/135g	335	16.9	248	3.8	32.2	12.5	0.8
Milk Chocolate, Belgian, Specially Selected, Aldi*	1/6 Cake/93g	386	25.1	415	5.8	37.0	27.0	1.6
Millionaires, Belgian Chocolate, Pot, Bistro, Morrisons*	1 Pot/128g	469	27.2	366	2.8	40.4	21.2	1.4
Raspberry & Mascarpone, Best, Morrisons*	1 Cake/84g	257	14.0	306	3.9	34.8	16.7	1.0
Raspberry & Strawberry, M&S*	1 Slice/105g	340	21.1	325	3.9	33.4	20.2	1.2
Raspberry Passionfruit, Specially Selected, Aldi*	1/6 Cake/83g	257	16.6	310	4.1	28.0	20.0	1.1
Raspberry Rapture, Slices, Tesco*	1 Slice/110g	341	20.4	310	4.2	30.8	18.5	1.8
Raspberry Ripple, Sainsbury's*	1 Portion/95g	348	21.3	366	4.7	36.0	22.4	0.8
Raspberry Swirl, Heinz*	1 Serving/100g	266	14.5	266	3.9	30.1	14.5	2.8
Raspberry, Light Choices, Tesco*	1 Cake/95g	185	4.1	195	4.3	34.7	4.3	1.3
Raspberry, M&S*	1 Slice/105g	331	21.5	315	5.0	32.2	20.5	1.0
Rhubarb Crumble, Sainsbury's*	1 Serving/114g	268	10.6	235	3.1	34.8	9.3	2.4
Sticky Toffee, Tesco*	1 Slice/66g	248	16.0	375	4.0	35.3	24.2	0.5
Strawberries & Cream, Finest, Tesco*	1 Serving/104g	325	22.4	312	4.3	25.3	21.5	0.5
Strawberry Swirl, CBY, Asda*	1 Serving/100g	329	15.9	329	4.5	41.5	15.9	1.0
Strawberry, Finest, Tesco*	1 Slice/113g	383	25.1	339	4.8	30.1	22.2	0.9
Strawberry, Fresh, M&S*	¼ Cake/125g	300	19.2	240	2.8	23.1	15.4	1.1
Strawberry, Tesco*	1 Serving/100g	254	12.0	254	3.9	32.5	12.0	0.0
Summerfruit, GFY, Asda*	1/6 Cake/92g	175	3.8	191	3.7	34.5	4.2	1.4
Toffee & Pecan, Wedge, Sainsbury's*	1 Serving/75g	296	21.8	395	5.4	28.1	29.0	3.1
Toffee Swirl, CBY, Asda*	1 Serving/100g	334	16.1	334	5.5	41.4	16.1	0.9
Toffee, American Style, Asda*	1 Serving/75g	269	15.8	359	4.5	38.0	21.0	3.8
Toffee, Mini, Asda*	1 Cake/20g	57	2.4	286	4.6	40.0	12.0	2.1
Toffee, Morrisons*	1 Serving/100g	341	17.4	341	5.5	40.4	17.4	0.0
Toffee, Tesco*	1 Serving/100g	265	12.9	265	4.3	33.1	12.9	0.8
Vanilla	1 Serving/100g	395	26.2	395	5.3	42.8	26.2	1.1
Vanilla Chocolate, Baked, Slice, Sainsbury's*	1 Slice/90g	349	23.0	388	5.7	33.8	25.6	2.7

	Measure INFO/WEIGHT	per Measure KCAL	FAT	Nutrition Values per 100g / 100ml KCAL	PROT	CARB	FAT	FIBRE
CHEESECAKE								
Vanilla, Tesco*	1 Serving/115g	417	28.4	363	5.7	29.4	24.7	0.6
CHERRIES								
Black in Syrup, Average	*1 Serving/242g*	*160*	*0.0*	*66*	*0.6*	*16.0*	*0.0*	*0.7*
Black, Fresh, Average	*1 Serving/80g*	*41*	*0.1*	*51*	*0.9*	*11.5*	*0.1*	*1.6*
Black, in Kirsch, Drained, Opies*	1 Jar/250g	155	0.5	62	0.5	15.0	0.2	1.1
Dried, LL, Waitrose*	1 Portion/10g	35	0.1	348	0.2	84.3	1.1	2.1
Dried, Sainsbury's*	1 Tbsp/14g	45	0.2	319	3.8	72.4	1.5	6.2
Dried, Wholefoods, Tesco*	1 Serving/25g	86	0.2	345	1.9	81.6	0.8	4.6
Glace, Average	*1oz/28g*	*79*	*0.0*	*280*	*0.4*	*71.2*	*0.2*	*1.1*
Picota, Average	*1 Serving/80g*	*42*	*0.1*	*52*	*0.9*	*11.4*	*0.1*	*1.2*
Raw, Average	*1oz/28g*	*14*	*0.0*	*49*	*0.9*	*11.2*	*0.1*	*1.4*
Stewed with Sugar, Average	*1oz/28g*	*23*	*0.0*	*82*	*0.7*	*21.0*	*0.1*	*0.7*
Stewed without Sugar, Average	*1oz/28g*	*12*	*0.0*	*42*	*0.8*	*10.1*	*0.1*	*0.8*
CHERRYADE								
Sugar Free, Tesco*	1 Glass/200ml	2	0.0	1	0.0	0.0	0.0	0.0
CHESTNUTS								
Roasted, Peeled, Average	*1 Nut/10g*	*17*	*0.3*	*170*	*2.0*	*36.6*	*2.7*	*4.1*
CHEWING GUM								
Airwaves, Sugar Free, Wrigleys*	1 Pack/15g	23	0.0	155	0.0	62.0	0.0	0.0
Extra, Cool Breeze, Wrigleys*	1 Piece/2g	3	0.0	153	0.0	64.0	0.0	0.0
Extra, Peppermint, Sugar Free, Wrigleys*	1 Piece/2g	3	0.0	155	0.0	39.0	0.0	0.0
Spearmint, Extra, Wrigleys*	1 Piece/1g	1	0.0	143	0.0	64.3	0.0	0.0
Splash, Raspberry & Peach, Trident*	1 Piece/2g	4	0.0	180	1.6	68.5	0.5	0.0
CHICK PEAS								
Bombay Firecracker Flavour, Dry Roasted, Garbanzo*	1 Bag/65g	88	1.3	135	10.2	23.8	2.0	7.4
Canned, Drained, Average	*1 Can/240g*	*276*	*6.0*	*115*	*7.4*	*15.2*	*2.5*	*4.6*
Dried, Average	*1 Serving/100g*	*319*	*5.4*	*319*	*21.7*	*47.4*	*5.4*	*8.0*
Dried, Boiled, Average	*1 Serving/75g*	*85*	*1.7*	*114*	*7.3*	*16.4*	*2.2*	*2.6*
in Water, Canned, Average	*1 Can/250g*	*282*	*6.6*	*113*	*7.2*	*15.3*	*2.6*	*4.8*
Thai Sweet Chilli Flavour, Dry Roasted, Garbanzo*	1 Bag/65g	88	1.3	135	10.2	23.8	2.0	7.4
Tomato, Garlic & Herb, Dry Roasted, Garbanzo*	1 Pack/65g	88	1.3	135	10.2	23.8	2.0	7.4
CHICKEN								
Bites, Hot & Spicy, Fridge Raiders, Mattessons*	1 Bag/60g	131	7.3	218	21.1	5.4	12.2	1.1
Bites, Hot & Spicy, Tesco*	1 Pack/110g	143	1.8	130	18.9	9.6	1.6	2.5
Bites, Piri Piri, Fridge Raiders, Mattessons*	1 Bag/60g	122	7.0	203	19.5	4.9	11.6	0.7
Bites, Southern Fried, Fridge Raiders, Mattessons*	1 Bag/60g	133	8.5	221	18.8	4.2	14.2	0.8
Bites, Southern Fried, Tesco*	1 Pack/300g	720	33.3	240	18.1	16.9	11.1	2.1
Bites, Tikka Flavour, Fridge Raiders, Mattessons*	1 Bag/60g	110	6.2	184	19.9	2.0	10.4	1.3
Bites, Tikka, Average	*1 Serving/50g*	*96*	*5.3*	*193*	*20.7*	*3.8*	*10.5*	*1.9*
Breast, Chargrilled, Premium, Average	*1 Piece/10g*	*20*	*1.1*	*197*	*21.6*	*1.5*	*11.2*	*0.3*
Breast, Chargrilled, Sliced, Average	*1 Slice/19g*	*24*	*0.5*	*124*	*24.4*	*0.5*	*2.7*	*0.4*
Breast, Diced, Average	*1 Serving/188g*	*242*	*4.4*	*129*	*26.9*	*0.1*	*2.4*	*0.1*
Breast, Fillets, Breaded, Average	*1 Fillet/112g*	*246*	*11.6*	*220*	*17.6*	*14.0*	*10.4*	*1.3*
Breast, Fillets, Breaded, Lemon & Pepper, Average	*1 Fillet/89g*	*133*	*2.0*	*150*	*22.0*	*10.1*	*2.3*	*1.3*
Breast, Fillets, Cajun, Average	*1 Fillet/93g*	*124*	*2.6*	*134*	*23.6*	*3.5*	*2.8*	*0.3*
Breast, Fillets, Chargrilled, Average	*1 Serving/100g*	*120*	*1.1*	*120*	*27.3*	*0.3*	*1.1*	*0.3*
Breast, Fillets, Korma Style, Average	*1 Serving/100g*	*132*	*2.8*	*132*	*27.4*	*0.8*	*2.8*	*0.6*
Breast, Fillets, Lime & Coriander, Just Add, M&S*	1 Pack/140g	182	2.4	130	26.1	2.7	1.7	0.1
Breast, Fillets, Mexican Style, Ready to Eat, Asda*	½ Pack/100g	147	1.5	147	27.8	5.5	1.5	0.1
Breast, Fillets, Mini, Raw, Average	*1oz/28g*	*34*	*0.4*	*121*	*26.9*	*0.2*	*1.5*	*0.1*
Breast, Fillets, Organic, Average	*1 Serving/150g*	*153*	*1.1*	*102*	*24.0*	*0.0*	*0.8*	*0.0*
Breast, Fillets, Skin On, Free Range, TTD, Sainsbury's*	1 Fillet/162g	235	7.6	145	25.7	0.0	4.7	0.0
Breast, Fillets, Skinless & Boneless, Raw, Average	*1 Breast/100g*	*129*	*2.0*	*129*	*27.7*	*0.0*	*2.0*	*0.0*

CHICKEN

Measure INFO/WEIGHT		per Measure KCAL	FAT	Nutrition Values per 100g / 100ml KCAL	PROT	CARB	FAT	FIBRE

	Measure INFO/WEIGHT	per Measure KCAL	FAT	KCAL	PROT	CARB	FAT	FIBRE
Breast, Fillets, Skinless & Boneless, Raw, HL, Tesco*	1 Fillet/125g	136	2.1	109	23.5	0.0	1.7	0.0
Breast, Grilled, Average	*1 Breast/130g*	*174*	*2.8*	*134*	*29.0*	*0.1*	*2.2*	*0.0*
Breast, Joint, Sage & Onion Stuffing, CBY, Asda*	1 Serving/150g	213	6.9	142	21.1	3.7	4.6	0.5
Breast, Meat & Skin, Raw, Average	*1 Serving/145g*	*249*	*13.4*	*172*	*20.8*	*0.0*	*9.2*	*0.0*
Breast, Meat & Skin, Weighed with Bone, Raw, Average	*1oz/28g*	*39*	*2.1*	*138*	*16.7*	*0.0*	*7.4*	*0.0*
Breast, Meat Only, Fried	*50g*	*68*	*1.7*	*137*	*24.4*	*0.4*	*3.4*	*0.0*
Breast, Mini Roasts, Ready to Cook, Aldi*	½ Pack/238g	352	14.5	148	20.0	3.0	6.1	0.8
Breast, Nacho, Fresh Tastes, Asda*	½ Pack/159g	243	9.9	153	18.2	6.0	6.2	1.9
Breast, Pieces, BBQ, Sainsbury's*	½ Pack/70g	93	0.8	132	23.8	6.3	1.2	0.5
Breast, Pieces, Tikka, Average	*1 Serving/100g*	*154*	*3.4*	*154*	*28.2*	*2.8*	*3.4*	*0.4*
Breast, Pieces, with Lemon, Garlic & Herbs, Waitrose*	½ Pack/65g	94	1.8	144	29.6	0.1	2.8	0.2
Breast, Piri Piri, Oven Baked, Braemoor, Lidl*	1 Breast/166g	249	9.3	150	24.3	0.3	5.6	0.0
Breast, Roast, Sliced, From Supermarket, Average	*1 Slice/13g*	*17*	*0.4*	*139*	*25.0*	*1.8*	*3.5*	*0.2*
Breast, Roast, without Skin, Average	*1oz/28g*	*41*	*1.3*	*146*	*24.8*	*1.0*	*4.6*	*0.2*
Breast, Roll, Average	*1 Slice/10g*	*17*	*1.0*	*167*	*16.1*	*3.2*	*10.0*	*0.2*
Breast, Short Sliced, Mexican, Sainsbury's*	1 Pack/130g	177	2.9	136	26.4	2.5	2.2	0.1
Breast, Sliced, Mexican Style, Cooked, Asda*	1 Pack/234g	307	5.1	131	25.5	4.3	2.2	0.1
Breast, Slices, Chargrill Style, Asda*	1 Slice/28g	31	0.6	112	22.7	0.8	2.0	0.0
Breast, Slices, Maple, Dulano, Lidl*	1 Slice/9g	10	0.2	111	20.0	3.0	2.0	0.5
Breast, Smoked, Sliced, Average	*1 Slice/20g*	*22*	*0.5*	*110*	*20.7*	*0.9*	*2.6*	*0.1*
Breast, Strips, Raw, Average	*1 Serving/280g*	*358*	*5.7*	*128*	*27.1*	*0.4*	*2.0*	*0.3*
Breast, Strips, with Garlic & Rosemary, Sainsbury's*	1 Serving/58g	87	2.9	150	25.9	0.3	5.0	0.0
Breast, Tandoori Style, Average	*1 Serving/180g*	*237*	*6.8*	*132*	*22.3*	*2.3*	*3.8*	*1.0*
Breast, Thai Style Mrinade, Chargrilled, GFY, Asda*	½ Pack/178g	178	5.3	100	17.0	1.3	3.0	0.5
Breast, Tikka, Sliced, Average	*1oz/28g*	*34*	*0.5*	*120*	*24.9*	*2.0*	*1.7*	*0.6*
Breast, with Piri Piri Marinade, Simply Cook, Tesco*	½ Pack/150g	235	9.0	157	23.8	1.9	6.0	0.1
Breast, with Piri Piri Marinade, Simply Cook, Tesco*	1 Breast/190g	266	11.4	140	19.7	1.0	6.0	0.1
Breast, with Pork, Lemon & Herb Stuffing, Joint, Waitrose*	½ Pack/250g	418	18.0	167	23.2	2.4	7.2	0.0
Breast, Wrapped in Bacon, with Cheese Sauce, Aldi*	1 Breast/178g	292	11.9	164	25.0	0.5	6.7	0.6
Breton, Charlie Bigham's*	½ Pack/300g	474	32.0	157	14.1	0.8	10.6	0.0
Chargrills, Garlic, Weight Before Cooking, Birds Eye*	1 Chargrill/95g	190	10.7	200	20.3	4.2	11.3	0.1
Chargrills, Original, Weight Before Cooking, Birds Eye*	1 Chargrill/95g	156	8.6	164	17.5	3.2	9.0	0.1
Chargrills, Weight After Cooking, Baked, Birds Eye*	1 Chargrill/90g	160	8.7	178	18.9	3.4	9.7	0.1
Cordon Bleu, Breast, Fillets, Sainsbury's*	1 Serving/150g	304	14.3	203	17.5	11.5	9.5	1.6
Cordon Bleu, Waitrose*	1 Serving/160g	325	15.4	203	20.1	9.1	9.6	2.4
Coronation, Filler, CBY, Asda*	1 Portion/50g	120	8.4	240	12.4	91.0	16.8	1.5
Dippers, Crispy, Average	*5 Dippers/93g*	*231*	*14.3*	*249*	*13.2*	*14.4*	*15.4*	*0.6*
Drumsticks, & Thighs, Garlic & Herb, Sainsbury's*	1 Serving/120g	184	10.7	153	16.6	1.5	8.9	0.1
Drumsticks, BBQ Flavour, Average	*1 Serving/200g*	*348*	*16.0*	*174*	*22.6*	*3.1*	*8.0*	*0.4*
Drumsticks, Breaded, Fried, Average	*1oz/28g*	*66*	*3.9*	*237*	*18.7*	*9.4*	*13.9*	*0.6*
Drumsticks, Chinese Style, Average	*1 Drumstick/100g*	*178*	*8.1*	*178*	*22.6*	*3.6*	*8.1*	*0.7*
Drumsticks, Free Range, TTD, Sainsbury's*	1 Piece/67g	126	6.7	188	24.4	0.0	10.0	0.0
Drumsticks, Meat & Skin, Weighed with Bone, Raw	*1 Drumstick/133g*	*188*	*11.0*	*141*	*15.7*	*0.1*	*8.3*	*0.0*
Drumsticks, Meat, no Skin, with Bone, Roast, Average	*1 Serving/100g*	*116*	*5.5*	*116*	*16.0*	*0.3*	*5.5*	*0.1*
Drumsticks, Meat, Weighed with Bone, Raw, Average	*1 Drumstick/122g*	*159*	*9.3*	*130*	*14.4*	*0.1*	*7.6*	*0.0*
Drumsticks, Southern Fried, Sainsbury's*	1 Serving/87g	190	8.6	218	20.8	11.2	9.9	0.7
Drumsticks, with Skin, Average	*1 Piece/125g*	*268*	*16.6*	*215*	*22.1*	*1.8*	*13.3*	*0.3*
Escalope, Breaded, Average	*1 Escalope/128g*	*361*	*21.6*	*282*	*13.4*	*19.1*	*16.9*	*0.7*
Escalope, Lemon & Herb, Waitrose*	1 Serving/200g	242	6.4	121	22.0	1.0	3.2	0.6
Escalope, Plain, Breast, Average	*1 Serving/100g*	*110*	*2.2*	*110*	*22.3*	*0.7*	*2.2*	*0.5*
Fillets, Battered, Average	*1 Fillet/90g*	*199*	*10.4*	*221*	*16.1*	*13.3*	*11.5*	*0.5*
Fillets, Breaded, Average	*1 Piece/98g*	*214*	*10.5*	*219*	*14.2*	*15.9*	*10.7*	*1.9*
Fillets, Breaded, Mini, Cooked, Goodness, Tesco*	1 Fillet/58g	130	4.4	224	18.4	18.4	7.6	1.0

CHICKEN

INFO/WEIGHT	Measure	per Measure KCAL	FAT	Nutrition Values per 100g / 100ml KCAL	PROT	CARB	FAT	FIBRE
Fillets, Chilli & Mango, Tesco*	1 Serving/100g	130	0.7	130	27.1	3.7	0.7	1.0
Fillets, Coronation, BGTY, Sainsbury's*	1 Fillet/100g	136	2.6	136	27.1	2.4	2.6	1.0
Fillets, Green Thai, Marinated, Mini, LL, Waitrose*	½ Pack/138g	153	3.3	111	21.2	1.2	2.4	0.6
Fillets, Lime & Coriander, Mini, Average	*1 Fillet/42g*	*49*	*0.5*	*118*	*24.3*	*2.6*	*1.3*	*0.6*
Fillets, Piri Piri Style, Mini, Ready to Eat, Tesco*	1 Pack/190g	256	2.1	135	22.7	7.6	1.1	0.8
Fillets, Roast, Sweet Chilli, Mini, British, Waitrose*	½ Pack/88g	119	0.9	136	23.5	8.0	1.0	0.5
Fillets, Sweet Chilli & Lime, Mini, M&S*	1 Serving/50g	78	1.1	155	28.3	5.1	2.2	0.0
Fillets, Tandoori Style, Mini, Average	*1 Serving/100g*	*128*	*2.0*	*128*	*24.7*	*2.6*	*2.0*	*0.4*
Fillets, Thigh, TTD, Sainsbury's*	1 Piece/60g	96	3.5	160	26.8	0.0	5.9	0.0
Fillets, Tikka, Average	*1 Serving/100g*	*141*	*5.0*	*141*	*22.4*	*1.7*	*5.0*	*1.1*
Fillets, Tikka, Mini, Average	*1oz/28g*	*35*	*0.6*	*124*	*25.1*	*1.3*	*2.2*	*1.2*
Firecracker, & Rice, Asian Fusion, Waitrose*	1 Pack/350g	483	6.3	138	7.0	22.8	1.8	1.5
Fricassee, Diet Chef Ltd*	1 Pack/300g	345	18.3	115	8.3	6.6	6.1	0.9
Garlic & Herb, Ready to Cook, COOK!, M&S*	½ Pack/130g	157	4.4	121	22.2	0.3	3.4	0.5
Ginger & Chilli, Ready to Cook, M&S*	½ Pack/166g	204	5.5	123	21.4	1.7	3.3	0.2
Goujons, Breaded, Average	*1 Serving/114g*	*293*	*17.1*	*258*	*15.8*	*15.2*	*15.0*	*1.0*
Goujons, Breaded, Tesco*	3 Goujons/83g	235	14.7	285	14.1	15.2	17.8	2.1
Goujons, Breast, Fresh, Average	*1oz/28g*	*36*	*0.5*	*127*	*28.0*	*0.0*	*1.6*	*0.0*
Green Thai, Meal For One, CBY, Asda*	1 Pot/350g	332	6.3	95	5.6	13.5	1.8	1.2
Honey Roast, Sliced, Average	*1 Slice/13g*	*15*	*0.3*	*117*	*21.6*	*2.2*	*2.4*	*0.1*
Hunter's, Asda*	½ Pack/190g	348	14.1	183	19.1	10.1	7.4	0.0
Jamaican Jerk, Bowl, Bol*	1 Bowl/380g	403	10.3	106	6.9	11.6	2.7	4.0
Leg or Thigh, Hot & Spicy, Average	*1oz/28g*	*50*	*3.0*	*179*	*19.4*	*1.0*	*10.8*	*0.4*
Leg Portion, Roast, weighed with Bone, without Skin	1 Portion/114g	175	11.0	153	30.9	0.0	9.6	0.0
Leg Portion, Roasted Dry, with Skin, without Bone	*1 Portion/120g*	*188*	*11.8*	*156*	*16.7*	*0.2*	*9.8*	*0.2*
Leg, Meat Only, Raw, Average	*1oz/28g*	*34*	*1.1*	*120*	*20.1*	*0.0*	*3.8*	*0.0*
Leg, Meat Only, Raw, Weighed with Skin & Bone	*1oz/28g*	*21*	*0.7*	*76*	*12.8*	*0.0*	*2.4*	*0.0*
Leg, Meat Only, Stewed with Bone & Skin, Average	*1oz/28g*	*31*	*1.4*	*111*	*15.8*	*0.0*	*4.8*	*0.0*
Leg, with Skin, Raw, Average	*1oz/28g*	*48*	*2.9*	*172*	*19.1*	*0.0*	*10.4*	*0.0*
Leg, with Skin, Roasted, Weighed with Bone, Average	*1oz/28g*	*47*	*3.3*	*166*	*15.3*	*0.1*	*11.6*	*0.0*
Lemon & Pepper, Pasta, Heated, Finest, Tesco*	1 Pack/355g	385	8.2	108	9.0	12.3	2.3	1.4
Light Meat, Raw	*1oz/28g*	*30*	*0.3*	*106*	*24.0*	*0.0*	*1.1*	*0.0*
Light Meat, Roasted	*1oz/28g*	*43*	*1.0*	*153*	*30.2*	*0.0*	*3.6*	*0.0*
Meat & Skin Portions, Deep Fried, Average	*1oz/28g*	*73*	*4.7*	*259*	*26.9*	*0.0*	*16.8*	*0.0*
Meat & Skin, Roasted, Average	*1oz/28g*	*60*	*3.9*	*216*	*22.6*	*0.0*	*14.0*	*0.0*
Meat, Roasted, Average	*1oz/28g*	*50*	*2.1*	*177*	*27.3*	*0.0*	*7.5*	*0.0*
Mexican Chilli, Sliced, Eat Well, M&S*	1 Pack/130g	169	3.4	130	25.9	0.8	2.6	0.5
Mexican with a Bean & Sweetcorn Salad, COU, M&S*	1 Pack/330g	307	5.9	93	10.6	5.5	1.8	7.3
Mince, Average	*1oz/28g*	*39*	*1.7*	*140*	*20.9*	*0.1*	*6.0*	*0.2*
Nuggets, Battered, Average	*1 Nugget/20g*	*50*	*2.9*	*251*	*13.5*	*16.9*	*14.4*	*0.9*
Nuggets, Breaded, Average	*1 Nugget/14g*	*37*	*2.0*	*263*	*14.8*	*19.8*	*13.8*	*1.9*
Nuggets, Breaded, Oven Baked, Birds Eye*	5 Nuggets/99g	255	12.8	256	12.0	22.6	12.9	0.0
Peri Peri, Chargrill, Birds Eye*	1 Serving/92g	157	8.5	171	16.9	5.2	9.2	0.3
Pieces, Barbeque, Chunky, Ready to Eat, Tesco*	1 Pack/200g	290	4.0	145	25.4	5.3	2.0	0.5
Pieces, Garlic, Crunchy, Birds Eye*	1 Piece/99g	259	15.0	262	14.4	16.9	15.2	0.9
Piri Piri, & Seasoned Wedges, Easy to Cook, Waitrose*	½ Pack/336g	527	29.5	157	9.6	9.7	8.8	0.5
Pops, Southern Fried, Frozen, Tesco*	1 Pack/225g	518	25.9	230	13.1	18.1	11.5	1.9
Roll, Value, Tesco*	1 Slice/13g	30	2.2	223	15.4	3.9	16.2	0.1
Shashlik, Patak's*	1 Serving/250g	203	3.6	81	12.4	4.4	1.4	0.0
Skewers, Marinated, Asda*	1 Skewer/35g	50	0.4	142	24.9	8.0	1.2	0.9
Skewers, Sticky Sweet Soy Marinade, Mini, M&S*	½ Pack/124g	155	1.4	125	20.7	7.6	1.1	0.3
Skewers, Tandoori, Six, M Kitchen, Morrisons*	½ Pack/90g	158	5.0	175	28.9	2.0	5.6	0.5
Skewers, with Chorizo, Charlie Bigham's*	1 Skewer/95g	129	6.5	136	17.1	1.5	6.9	0.5

		per Measure		Nutrition Values per 100g / 100ml				
	INFO/WEIGHT	KCAL	FAT	KCAL	PROT	CARB	FAT	FIBRE

CHICKEN

		per Measure		Nutrition Values per 100g / 100ml				
Skewers, Yakitori, M&S*	1 Box/65g	125	4.5	192	20.9	11.2	6.9	0.6
Skin, Dry, Roasted or Grilled, Average	*1 Serving/100g*	*501*	*46.1*	*501*	*21.5*	*0.0*	*46.1*	*0.0*
Sliced, Cooked, Average	*1 Slice/15g*	*18*	*0.4*	*118*	*22.4*	*1.6*	*2.4*	*0.1*
Spanish Style & Patatas Bravas, Weight Watchers*	1 Pack/400g	347	9.6	87	5.1	10.5	2.4	1.4
Spatchcock, Garlic & Herb, LBU, Co-Op*	¼ Pack/192g	403	27.3	210	18.4	1.8	14.2	0.4
Spatchcock, Piri Piri, Cooked, Tesco*	¼ Chicken/155g	353	19.2	228	28.2	0.4	12.4	1.0
Spatchcock, Piri Piri, Raw, As Sold, Tesco*	¼ Chicken/300g	606	42.6	202	17.6	0.6	14.2	0.9
Spatchcock, Poussin, Sainsbury's*	1 Serving/122g	168	6.6	138	21.1	0.1	5.4	0.2
Spatchcock, Salt & Cracked Pepper, Sainsbury's*	1 Serving/122g	168	6.6	138	21.1	0.1	5.4	0.2
Spicy, Fried, Sainsbury's*	1 Serving/150g	414	24.9	276	28.8	2.9	16.6	2.1
Steaks, Average	*1 Serving/100g*	*205*	*9.4*	*205*	*21.1*	*9.0*	*9.4*	*0.7*
Steaks, Garlic & Herb, Tesco*	1 Serving/138g	354	23.2	257	14.1	12.2	16.9	1.7
Strips, Mexican, Sliced, M&S*	½ Pack/70g	77	0.4	110	24.3	2.3	0.6	0.5
Thai Green, Steamed, HE, Tesco*	1 Pack/321g	309	6.1	96	6.5	12.6	1.9	1.3
Thigh, Fillets, Tesco*	1 Serving/100g	165	9.8	165	18.3	0.0	9.8	0.0
Thigh, Meat & Skin, Casseroled, Average	*1oz/28g*	*65*	*4.6*	*233*	*21.5*	*0.0*	*16.3*	*0.0*
Thigh, Meat & Skin, Raw, Average	*1 Serving/100g*	*218*	*14.7*	*218*	*21.4*	*0.0*	*14.7*	*0.0*
Thigh, Meat & Skin, Weighed with Bone, Raw, Average	*1 Serving/100g*	*186*	*14.1*	*186*	*13.8*	*0.2*	*14.1*	*0.0*
Thigh, Meat Only, Diced, Casseroled	*1oz/28g*	*50*	*2.4*	*180*	*25.6*	*0.0*	*8.6*	*0.0*
Thigh, Meat Only, Raw, Average	*1 Thigh/90g*	*113*	*4.9*	*126*	*19.4*	*0.0*	*5.4*	*0.0*
Thigh, Roast, Average	*1 Serving/100g*	*238*	*15.6*	*238*	*23.8*	*0.4*	*15.6*	*0.0*
Tikka, Steaks, Cooked, Butchers Selection, Asda*	1 Serving/100g	160	3.7	160	29.7	1.8	3.7	0.1
Wafer Thin, Average	*1 Slice/10g*	*12*	*0.4*	*120*	*19.0*	*2.8*	*3.6*	*0.2*
Whole, Roast, Average	*1oz/28g*	*37*	*2.4*	*133*	*13.4*	*0.9*	*8.4*	*0.1*
Whole, Roasted, Brown Sugar Marinade, Tesco*	1 Serving/100g	195	11.3	195	22.1	0.1	11.3	0.1
Wing Quarter, Meat Only, Casseroled	*1oz/28g*	*46*	*1.8*	*164*	*26.9*	*0.0*	*6.3*	*0.0*
Wing, Breaded, Fried, Average	*1oz/28g*	*77*	*4.8*	*273*	*17.1*	*13.0*	*17.2*	*0.4*
Wing, Meat & Skin, Cooked, Average	*1oz/28g*	*67*	*4.4*	*241*	*23.3*	*1.9*	*15.6*	*0.3*
Wings, BBQ Flavour, Average	*1oz/28g*	*61*	*3.5*	*220*	*20.3*	*6.6*	*12.4*	*0.6*
Wings, Chinese Style, Average	*1oz/28g*	*72*	*4.3*	*256*	*24.2*	*5.1*	*15.5*	*0.6*
Wings, Hickory Smoke Flavour, Nibbles, Sainsbury's*	1 Wing/100g	245	15.3	245	23.5	3.5	15.3	0.5
Wings, Hot & Spicy, Average	*1oz/28g*	*65*	*3.8*	*231*	*21.8*	*5.2*	*13.6*	*0.8*
Wings, Meat & Skin, Raw, Average	*1oz/28g*	*52*	*3.3*	*184*	*19.0*	*0.5*	*11.8*	*0.2*
Zaatar, Ilumi*	1 Pack/275g	327	4.9	119	9.8	15.0	1.8	0.0

CHICKEN

		per Measure		Nutrition Values per 100g / 100ml				
Dijonnaise, Cooked, TTD, Sainsbury's*	1 Pack/380g	524	16.3	138	9.2	14.2	4.3	3.2

CHICKEN &

		per Measure		Nutrition Values per 100g / 100ml				
Bacon Parcels, Finest, Tesco*	1 Pack/233g	379	21.6	163	16.1	3.7	9.3	0.5
Balsamic Roasted Pepper Pasta, M&S*	1 Pack/310g	418	11.5	135	7.8	17.2	3.7	1.7
Black Bean Noodles, Sainsbury's*	1 Serving/130g	155	0.9	119	4.3	23.9	0.7	0.8
Black Bean with Noodles, Tesco*	1 Pack/475g	470	7.6	99	7.6	13.6	1.6	0.2
Black Bean, Chinese Takeaway, Tesco*	1 Serving/200g	190	6.6	95	8.3	8.0	3.3	0.5
Black Bean, Chinese, Tesco*	1 Pack/350g	382	17.2	109	8.9	7.4	4.9	0.7
Black Bean, Egg Fried Rice, Ready Meal, Average	*1 Serving/400g*	*390*	*6.1*	*97*	*6.5*	*14.5*	*1.5*	*0.8*
Butternut Squash, Curry Pot, Weight Watchers*	1 Pot/250g	232	3.5	93	6.6	12.5	1.4	1.6
Cashew Nuts, Chinese, Cantonese, Sainsbury's*	½ Pack/175g	172	8.8	98	8.4	4.9	5.0	1.3
Cashew Nuts, Chinese, Ready Meal, Average	*1 Serving/400g*	*497*	*24.0*	*124*	*9.2*	*7.5*	*6.0*	*1.2*
Cashew Nuts, Chinese, Tesco*	1 Pack/350g	378	19.6	108	9.5	4.9	5.6	0.6
Chargrilled Vegetable Roll, HL, Tesco*	1 Pack/221g	336	6.0	152	10.1	21.8	2.7	2.3
Chorizo Paella, Go Cook, Asda*	½ Pack/475g	591	10.5	124	10.2	15.9	2.2	2.6
Fries, Southern Fried, Sainsbury's*	½ Pack/250g	562	21.7	225	10.5	26.2	8.7	0.8
Gravy, COU, M&S*	1 Pack/300g	216	3.9	72	7.2	7.8	1.3	1.6
Herb Pasta with Lemon, HL, Tesco*	1 Pack/400g	520	8.0	130	8.2	18.8	2.0	1.6

	Measure INFO/WEIGHT	per Measure KCAL	FAT	Nutrition Values per 100g / 100ml KCAL	PROT	CARB	FAT	FIBRE
CHICKEN &								
King Prawn Special Fried Rice, Finest, Tesco*	1 Pack/450g	734	32.0	163	7.7	17.0	7.1	0.7
King Prawn, Yaki Udon, Sainsbury's*	1 Pack/380g	505	17.5	133	7.4	13.7	4.6	3.8
Mushroom in White Wine Sauce, GFY, Asda*	1 Pack/400g	272	7.2	68	6.0	7.0	1.8	1.2
Mushroom with Rice, Egg Fried, Average	*1 Serving/400g*	*421*	*10.1*	*105*	*6.3*	*14.4*	*2.5*	*0.8*
Mushroom, Chinese, Iceland*	1 Pack/400g	276	9.2	69	8.2	3.8	2.3	0.4
Mushroom, Chinese, Sainsbury's*	½ Pack/175g	116	3.5	66	7.6	4.4	2.0	0.9
Mushroom, Chinese, Tesco*	1 Pack/460g	474	12.9	103	5.7	13.8	2.8	1.0
Mushroom, with Puff Pastry, 134, Oakhouse Foods Ltd*	1 Meal/400g	516	23.2	129	7.9	11.1	5.8	1.3
Noodles, Chinese Style, HE, Tesco*	1 Pack/370g	422	6.3	114	8.5	15.9	1.7	1.5
Peppers in a Black Bean Sauce, M&S*	1 Pack/320g	256	4.8	80	9.4	7.3	1.5	1.2
Peppers, M&S*	1 Serving/240g	264	10.8	110	14.7	2.3	4.5	0.6
Pineapple, Chilled, Tesco*	1 Pack/350g	364	8.4	104	9.6	11.1	2.4	5.5
Roasted Potatoes, Spanish, Charlie Bigham's*	½ Pack/387g	441	20.9	114	7.1	10.0	5.4	0.0
Stuffing, Roast, HL, Tesco*	1 Serving/17g	19	0.2	111	23.3	1.3	1.4	0.2
Tomato Saag with Pilau Rice, BGTY, Sainsbury's*	1 Pack/400g	404	4.0	101	7.3	15.6	1.0	1.0
CHICKEN ALFREDO								
Average	*1 Pack/400g*	*416*	*10.0*	*104*	*12.2*	*8.2*	*2.5*	*0.8*
CHICKEN ARRABBIATA								
Bistro, Waitrose*	½ Pack/175g	156	5.2	89	12.9	2.5	3.0	0.5
Easy Steam, HL, Tesco*	1 Pack/400g	284	3.2	71	8.4	7.6	0.8	1.2
GFY, Asda*	1 Pack/448g	394	3.1	88	5.2	15.1	0.7	1.1
Meal for One, M&S*	1 Pack/400g	528	20.8	132	7.9	12.5	5.2	1.9
CHICKEN BANG BANG								
Waitrose*	1 Pack/350g	368	17.2	105	9.4	5.9	4.9	1.2
CHICKEN BUTTER								
with Rice, Average	*1 Serving/400g*	*561*	*27.6*	*140*	*10.6*	*8.9*	*6.9*	*1.4*
CHICKEN CAJUN								
Breast, Chargrilled, Iceland*	1 Serving/80g	114	1.5	142	27.4	3.9	1.9	0.0
Breast, Morrisons*	½ Pack/180g	328	16.9	182	16.6	7.7	9.4	2.0
HE, Tesco*	1 Pack/365g	412	4.7	113	7.9	17.3	1.3	0.7
CHICKEN CANTONESE								
Breast, Fillets, Sainsbury's*	1 Serving/154g	168	2.3	109	20.3	3.6	1.5	0.6
Honey, Sesame, Sainsbury's*	1/3 Pack/135g	116	3.6	86	9.8	5.5	2.7	0.8
CHICKEN CARIBBEAN								
Fruity with Rice & Peas, New, BGTY, Sainsbury's*	1 Pack/400g	352	3.6	88	6.9	13.1	0.9	2.2
Style, Breasts, COU, M&S*	1 Serving/205g	205	3.1	100	14.6	7.3	1.5	1.3
with Rice & Beans, One Pot, Cook*	1 Pot/300g	387	19.2	129	6.7	7.4	6.4	7.4
CHICKEN CHASSEUR								
Average	*1 Serving/400g*	*363*	*9.2*	*91*	*12.2*	*4.9*	*2.3*	*0.9*
Breast Fillets, Morrisons*	1 Pack/380g	384	11.4	101	15.7	2.9	3.0	0.8
Finest, Tesco*	½ Pack/200g	200	6.4	100	14.3	2.4	3.2	1.1
Mix, Colman's*	1 Pack/38g	120	0.4	316	8.6	68.2	1.0	3.7
CHICKEN CHILLI								
Sweet & Egg Fried Rice, HL, Tesco*	1 Serving/450g	446	8.1	99	5.7	15.0	1.8	0.4
Sweet with Noodles, Frozen, HL, Tesco*	1 Pack/369g	340	5.1	92	6.8	13.1	1.4	1.0
Sweet, CBY, Asda*	½ Pack/170g	253	6.8	149	19.1	8.9	4.0	0.7
Sweet, Just Cook, Sainsbury's*	½ Pack/191g	200	1.3	105	15.2	9.4	0.7	0.5
Sweet, Pieces, Morrisons*	1 Pack/200g	282	5.0	141	25.5	4.1	2.5	0.5
Sweet, with Noodles, Ready Meal, Average	*1 Serving/400g*	*404*	*5.8*	*101*	*6.5*	*15.5*	*1.4*	*1.4*
CHICKEN CHINESE								
& Prawns, Sizzler, House Special, Tesco*	1 Serving/450g	684	23.4	152	7.5	18.8	5.2	1.2
Balls, M&S*	1 Ball/16g	45	2.2	280	10.8	29.2	13.6	2.1
Battered with Plum Sauce, Tesco*	1 Pack/350g	648	20.3	185	6.7	26.5	5.8	0.8

	Measure INFO/WEIGHT	per Measure		Nutrition Values per 100g / 100ml				
		KCAL	FAT	KCAL	PROT	CARB	FAT	FIBRE
CHICKEN CHINESE								
Crispy Aromatic, Half, Tesco*	1 Serving/233g	524	24.2	225	16.3	16.7	10.4	1.2
Fillets, with Sweet Chilli Sauce, Tesco*	1 Serving/350g	592	22.0	169	8.8	19.2	6.3	0.7
Stir Fry, Morrisons*	1 Serving/319g	341	5.4	107	5.7	17.0	1.7	1.5
Style & Noodles, HE, Tesco*	1 Pack/370g	278	4.1	75	6.9	9.4	1.1	0.7
with Ginger & Spring Onion, Tesco*	1 Serving/350g	299	10.1	85	7.6	7.3	2.9	0.6
CHICKEN CORONATION								
M&S*	1 Serving/200g	420	26.4	210	12.6	10.6	13.2	1.3
CHICKEN DINNER								
Breast with Pork, Sage & Onion Stuffing, Tesco*	1 Serving/180g	277	14.8	154	19.4	0.7	8.2	0.5
Kershaws*	1 Pack/350g	210	3.5	60	4.3	8.4	1.0	1.2
Roast, Microwaved, Fresh Tastes, Asda*	1 Serving/400g	339	7.2	85	7.2	8.9	1.8	2.1
Roast, with Mash, Green Beans & Carrots, CBY, Asda*	1 Dinner/400g	280	6.8	70	6.4	6.2	1.7	2.2
CHICKEN EN CROUTE								
Charlie Bigham's*	½ Pack/230g	568	36.8	247	11.1	14.1	16.0	0.6
Creamy Bacon, Cheese & Leek Sauce, Easy, Waitrose*	½ Pack/177g	479	29.8	270	11.9	17.4	16.8	2.8
Just Cook, Sainsbury's*	1 Serving/180g	481	27.2	267	16.8	15.9	15.1	0.4
with Cheddar & Ham, CBY, Asda*	½ Pack/209g	568	33.4	272	16.0	15.1	16.0	1.7
CHICKEN IN								
Barbeque Sauce, Breasts, COU, M&S*	1 Pack/350g	420	6.7	120	8.5	20.6	1.9	0.6
BBQ Sauce, Breast, Sainsbury's*	1 Serving/170g	199	1.2	117	14.5	13.1	0.7	1.3
BBQ Sauce, Chargrilled, Breast, GFY, Asda*	1 Serving/166g	214	6.1	129	19.0	5.0	3.7	1.0
Black Bean Sauce with Rice, Asda*	1 Pack/400g	500	7.6	125	7.0	20.0	1.9	0.6
Black Bean Sauce, Chinese Takeaway, Iceland*	1 Pack/400g	348	12.8	87	9.3	5.3	3.2	0.7
Black Bean Sauce, Sainsbury's*	1 Pack/465g	484	7.9	104	5.0	17.3	1.7	0.3
Broccoli & Mushroom with Rice, HE, Tesco*	1 Pack/400g	440	4.8	110	7.5	17.1	1.2	0.7
Cabernet Sauvignon Wine, Finest, Tesco*	½ Pack/192g	213	6.1	111	14.7	5.6	3.2	0.6
Cheese & Bacon, Wrapped, Breast, Tesco*	1 Serving/300g	474	23.4	158	20.7	1.2	7.8	0.5
Cider, West Country, & Wholegrain Mustard, LBU, Co-Op*	½ Pack/380g	570	29.6	150	16.1	3.2	7.8	0.3
Creamy Mushroom Sauce, Weight Watchers*	1 Pack/330g	343	9.6	104	7.0	12.5	2.9	0.6
Creamy Mustard Sauce, GFY, Asda*	1 Pack/400g	468	9.2	117	6.0	18.0	2.3	0.4
Creamy Tikka Style Sauce, Tesco*	1 Breast/190g	215	10.4	113	15.1	0.7	5.5	0.8
Garlic & Cream Sauce, Breast Fillets, Morrisons*	1 Serving/180g	262	15.8	146	14.9	1.8	8.8	0.6
Garlic & Herbs, Breast, Sainsbury's*	1 Serving/200g	316	5.2	158	28.3	5.4	2.6	0.1
Ginger & Chilli with Veg Noodles, COU, M&S*	1 Pack/400g	300	2.4	75	6.4	10.7	0.6	1.1
Hot Ginger Sauce with Thai Sticky Rice, Sainsbury's*	1 Pack/450g	603	20.7	134	6.8	16.3	4.6	0.5
Hunter's BBQ Sauce, Asda*	½ Pack/190g	348	14.1	183	19.1	10.3	7.4	0.0
Lemon & Garlic Marinade, Thighs, Go Cook, Asda*	½ Pack/265g	493	30.2	186	19.7	1.2	11.4	0.8
Lemon Sauce with Rice, Sainsbury's*	1 Pack/450g	513	6.8	114	8.1	17.0	1.5	0.7
Light Batter, Bites, Captain Birds Eye, Birds Eye*	1 Piece/15g	32	1.9	210	18.6	5.8	12.5	0.2
Madeira Sauce with Mushrooms, Finest, Tesco*	½ Pack/200g	210	8.3	105	13.8	3.0	4.2	1.0
Mexican Salsa, Tesco*	1 Pack/320g	368	8.6	115	19.5	3.1	2.7	0.6
Mexican Style Sauce, Tesco*	1 Serving/180g	128	1.4	71	13.3	2.6	0.8	0.7
Mushroom & Red Wine Sauce, Breast Fillets, Morrisons*	1 Serving/177g	184	4.4	104	15.7	4.6	2.5	0.7
Oyster Sauce with Mushrooms, Tesco*	1 Pack/350g	189	3.2	54	8.0	3.5	0.9	0.8
Pesto Style Dressing, Asda*	1 Serving/150g	210	10.0	140	18.7	1.3	6.7	0.0
Red Wine Sauce, Buttery Mash, Carrots & Peas, M&S*	1 Pack/400g	340	11.2	85	7.4	6.2	2.8	2.7
Smoky Barbecue Sauce, Breast, Fresh Tastes, Asda*	1 Breast/160g	258	6.2	161	21.9	9.6	3.9	0.9
Smoky Barbeque Sauce, Tesco*	1 Serving/185g	229	3.9	124	16.3	9.9	2.1	1.0
Smoky BBQ Marinade, Breast, Fillets, Mini, CBY, Asda*	3 Fillets/150g	144	1.5	96	18.5	3.3	1.0	0.0
Sundried Tomato & Basil, Breast, Fillets, M&S*	½ Pack/110g	165	4.5	150	22.5	4.7	4.1	1.1
Sweet Chilli Marinade, Breast Slices, Breast, Sainsbury's*	1/6 Pack/50g	69	0.8	138	26.4	4.4	1.5	0.7
Sweet Chilli Sauce, Breast, Fresh Tastes, Asda*	½ Pack/180g	288	9.0	160	18.4	10.3	5.0	0.5
Tomato & Basil Sauce, Breast, GFY, Asda*	1 Pack/392g	447	13.3	114	12.0	9.0	3.4	1.5

	Measure INFO/WEIGHT	per Measure KCAL	per Measure FAT	Nutrition Values per 100g / 100ml KCAL	PROT	CARB	FAT	FIBRE
CHICKEN IN								
Tomato & Basil Sauce, Oven Baked, Asda*	½ Pack/143g	153	3.0	107	19.3	2.3	2.1	0.7
Tomato & Herb Sauce, Breasts, Tesco*	½ Pack/173g	155	2.4	90	15.0	3.6	1.4	0.5
White Sauce, Canned, Asda*	½ Can/400g	644	44.0	161	12.0	3.5	11.0	0.0
White Wine & Tarragon Sauce, Waitrose*	½ Pack/225g	281	17.3	125	10.7	3.1	7.7	0.3
White Wine Sauce, with Leeks, Breasts, Finest, Tesco*	½ Pack/200g	234	9.0	117	15.9	3.0	4.5	0.4
White Wine Sauce, with Pasta, LowLow*	1 Pack/320g	330	6.7	103	5.8	14.4	2.1	1.7
White Wine, Tagliatelle & Green Beans, Weight Watchers*	1 Pack/380g	331	9.1	87	5.4	10.3	2.4	1.4
CHICKEN KATSU								
Curry, City Kitchen, Tesco*	1 Pack/385g	465	13.2	121	6.0	16.3	3.4	1.3
CHICKEN KIEV								
Breast, Hand Filled, Birds Eye*	1 Kiev/172g	330	17.2	192	15.5	9.9	10.0	2.0
Cheese & Ham Sauce, Inspirations, Birds Eye*	1 Breast/124g	294	14.9	237	13.0	19.0	12.0	0.7
Cooked, M Kitchen, Fresh Ideas, Morrisons*	1 Kiev/145g	359	20.8	248	17.5	12.0	14.4	0.9
COU, M&S*	1 Kiev/150g	188	2.7	125	15.8	10.8	1.8	0.5
Creamy Peppercorn, Tesco*	1 Kiev/132g	290	17.3	220	13.1	12.1	13.1	0.6
Fillets, Whole, Frozen, Cooked, Birds Eye*	1 Portion/150g	300	16.0	200	14.7	11.3	10.7	1.4
Finest, Tesco*	1 Kiev/217g	380	12.8	175	21.9	8.3	5.9	0.5
Garlic & Herb Sauce, Inspirations, Birds Eye*	1 Breast/125g	305	16.5	244	12.2	18.8	13.2	0.7
Garlic & Herb, Reduced Fat, Sainsbury's*	1 Kiev/142g	317	18.0	223	15.1	12.1	12.7	0.6
Garlic & Herb, Sainsbury's*	1 Kiev/134g	319	19.6	239	15.0	11.7	14.7	1.3
Garlic & Parsley Butter, Breaded, British, Waitrose*	1 Kiev/156g	410	27.0	263	15.0	11.5	17.3	0.8
Garlic & Parsley, BGTY, Sainsbury's*	1 Kiev/126g	289	15.3	229	14.0	15.9	12.1	1.1
Garlic & Parsley, Sainsbury's*	1 Kiev/120g	365	25.6	304	11.1	17.1	21.3	0.8
Garlic Butter, Frozen,, Tesco*	1 Kiev/126g	340	22.6	270	13.1	14.0	17.9	0.0
Garlic Butter, HL, Tesco*	1 Kiev/143g	285	16.4	200	14.3	9.9	11.5	0.6
Garlic, 25% Reduced Fat, Tesco*	1 Kiev/130g	299	18.6	230	13.7	11.5	14.3	0.7
Garlic, Ashfield Farm, Aldi*	1 Kiev/131g	363	25.9	277	9.5	13.8	19.8	2.9
Garlic, Creamy, Tesco*	1 Kiev/153g	323	17.6	211	12.6	13.5	11.5	1.7
Garlic, M&S*	1 Kiev/150g	370	24.8	247	15.6	8.2	16.5	2.9
Garlic, Morrisons*	1 Kiev/122g	289	19.2	237	14.3	9.8	15.7	0.0
Garlic, Whole Breast, Asda*	1 Pack/290g	638	38.0	220	15.2	10.4	13.1	0.0
Good Choice, Iceland*	1 Kiev/120g	366	27.2	305	12.7	12.6	22.7	0.8
Ham & Cheese, Tesco*	1 Kiev/143g	307	18.6	215	14.4	9.3	13.0	1.3
in Crispy Breadcrumbs, Sainsbury's*	1 Kiev/117g	310	22.4	266	12.8	10.6	19.2	1.1
Maitre Jean Pierre, Lidl*	1 Kiev/140g	385	26.7	275	13.3	12.7	19.1	0.8
Morrisons*	1 Kiev/134g	304	17.4	227	16.1	11.5	13.0	1.0
Tomato & Mozzarella, Tesco*	1 Kiev/143g	285	17.4	200	13.4	9.0	12.2	1.4
CHICKEN LEMON								
Battered, Cantonese, Sainsbury's*	1 Pack/350g	560	19.6	160	10.7	16.6	5.6	0.9
Battered, Chinese Meal for Two, Tesco*	½ Serving/175g	294	13.0	168	6.6	18.8	7.4	2.0
Chinese, Tesco*	1 Serving/350g	564	11.2	161	7.0	26.0	3.2	0.3
Tesco*	½ Pack/175g	214	7.4	122	11.0	10.1	4.2	0.6
CHICKEN MOROCCAN								
Style with Spicy Cous Cous, BGTY, Sainsbury's*	1 Serving/225g	304	3.8	135	9.2	20.6	1.7	0.0
Style, Sainsbury's*	½ Pack/269g	334	7.0	124	14.7	10.4	2.6	3.1
with Bulgur Wheat, Good & Balanced, Asda*	1 Pack/375g	365	3.4	98	7.4	13.3	0.9	3.4
CHICKEN PASANDA								
M&S*	½ Pack/150g	240	16.4	160	11.3	3.8	10.9	1.3
Sainsbury's*	1 Serving/200g	368	24.8	184	14.7	3.4	12.4	2.3
CHICKEN PIRI PIRI								
& Rice, HE, Tesco*	1 Pack/395g	395	7.9	100	8.2	12.0	2.0	1.7
Breast, Fillets, Mini, Tesco*	½ Pack/100g	135	1.1	135	22.7	7.6	1.1	0.0
GFY, Asda*	1 Pack/400g	406	2.8	102	5.8	18.0	0.7	1.4

INFO/WEIGHT	Measure	per Measure		Nutrition Values per 100g / 100ml				
		KCAL	FAT	KCAL	PROT	CARB	FAT	FIBRE
CHICKEN PIRI PIRI								
M&S*	1 Pack/300g	420	23.1	140	10.0	7.3	7.7	1.3
Sainsbury's*	½ Pack/200g	248	10.8	124	14.0	4.8	5.4	0.5
with Rice, BGTY, Sainsbury's*	1 Serving/399g	395	4.4	99	10.3	11.9	1.1	1.6
CHICKEN PROVENCALE								
M&S*	1 Pack/430g	366	11.6	85	13.2	2.3	2.7	0.6
CHICKEN ROLL								
with Pork, Sage & Onion Stuffing, Value, Tesco*	1 Roll/125g	166	8.9	133	9.4	7.8	7.1	0.5
CHICKEN TANDOORI								
Fresh Tastes, Asda*	1 Pack/400g	356	5.6	89	6.4	12.7	1.4	2.1
Masala, Indian, Tesco*	1 Serving/350g	430	25.9	123	10.2	4.0	7.4	1.8
Masala, Sainsbury's*	1 Pack/400g	536	27.2	134	13.2	5.0	6.8	0.5
Steam Meal, As Consumed, Simply Bistro, Aldi*	1 Pack/400g	317	7.5	80	5.5	9.3	1.9	2.1
Tesco*	1 Serving/175g	198	8.6	113	10.6	6.7	4.9	1.0
CHICKEN TERIYAKI								
& Noodles, Asda*	½ Pack/340g	445	8.8	131	9.0	18.0	2.6	0.9
Asda*	1 Pack/360g	299	5.0	83	9.1	8.6	1.4	0.8
Japanese with Ramen Noodles, Sainsbury's*	1 Pack/450g	482	9.4	107	6.5	15.5	2.1	0.8
CHICKEN TIKKA								
& Coriander Rice, Weight Watchers*	1 Pack/400g	348	2.4	87	6.2	14.3	0.6	1.6
& Lemon Rice, Deli Meal, M&S*	1 Pack/360g	342	7.2	95	9.8	10.2	2.0	0.7
Creamy, Breast, Tesco*	1 Breast/190g	215	10.4	113	15.1	0.7	5.5	0.8
with Basmati Rice, Weight Watchers*	1 Pack/380g	342	6.5	90	6.6	11.8	1.7	1.1
CHICKEN VINDALOO								
Average	*1 Serving/410g*	*787*	*51.2*	*192*	*18.5*	*2.6*	*12.5*	*0.3*
Sainsbury's*	1 Pack/400g	460	16.8	115	14.6	4.8	4.2	0.6
Waitrose*	1 Pack/340g	398	18.4	117	10.6	6.4	5.4	1.6
CHICKEN WITH								
5 Spice, Vegetables & Vietnamese Dressing, COU, M&S*	1 Pack/275g	138	4.4	50	5.0	4.0	1.6	2.3
a Sea Salt & Black Pepper Crust, Breasts, Asda*	1 Serving/154g	186	4.3	121	19.0	5.0	2.8	0.0
a Sticky Honey & Chilli Sauce, Breast, Asda*	1 Serving/175g	247	5.6	141	20.0	8.0	3.2	0.0
Basil Pesto & Parmesan Crust, Breast, COOK!, M&S*	½ Pack/150g	240	11.0	160	20.9	1.8	7.3	0.8
Black Bean Sauce, Green Peppers & Rice, Farmfoods*	1 Meal/324g	408	12.6	126	5.5	17.1	3.9	0.4
Broccoli & Pesto Pasta, BGTY, Sainsbury's*	1 Pack/301g	328	5.1	109	10.3	13.2	1.7	2.5
Butternut Squash Rice, Reggae Reggae, Levi Roots*	1 Pack/450g	495	13.5	110	5.8	14.0	3.0	1.1
Caesar Melt & Prosciutto, Breast, M&S*	1 Pack/375g	488	18.8	130	19.6	1.3	5.0	1.0
Cheddar & Bacon Filling, Breast, Just Cook, Sainsbury's*	1 Serving/180g	346	14.6	192	23.2	6.5	8.1	0.1
Cheese & Bacon, Tesco*	½ Pack/175g	262	11.9	150	18.9	2.6	6.8	0.4
Cheese, Leek & Ham, Breast, Fresh Tastes, Asda*	1 Pack/430g	658	30.5	153	18.9	3.4	7.1	0.7
Chorizo & Manchego Cheese, Breasts, M&S*	½ Pack/178g	222	8.9	125	18.3	1.7	5.0	0.6
Garlic & Chilli Balti, Tesco*	1 Pack/400g	320	7.6	80	11.0	4.4	1.9	0.8
Garlic Mushrooms, Asda*	1 Serving/320g	342	16.0	107	13.8	1.8	5.0	2.2
Garlic Mushrooms, Breast, Simply Cook, Tesco*	½ Pack/125g	170	6.6	136	22.0	0.1	5.3	0.1
Garlic Mushrooms, Breast, Tesco*	1 Breast/125g	149	5.9	119	19.0	0.2	4.7	0.1
Gruyere Cheese & Parma Ham, Breast, COOK!, M&S*	1 Breast/194g	349	21.3	180	18.0	2.5	11.0	0.9
Hoisin Sauce, Ooodles of Noodles, Oriental Express*	1 Pack/425g	400	9.4	94	5.3	13.2	2.2	1.7
Honey & Mustard Sauce, Breasts, Simply Cook, Tesco*	½ Pack/219g	230	1.3	105	16.3	8.0	0.6	0.3
Leek & Bacon, Creamy Sauce, Simply Bistro, Aldi*	1 Pack/400g	348	10.8	87	7.5	7.3	2.7	2.1
Leek & Bacon, M&S*	½ Pack/183g	239	12.8	131	15.3	1.2	7.0	0.9
Lyonnaise Potatoes, M&S*	½ Pack/260g	286	8.1	110	12.6	8.0	3.1	0.9
Manchego & Sun Dried Tomato Filling, Tesco*	½ Pack/225g	325	10.5	144	24.3	1.0	4.7	0.5
Mango, Lime & Coriander, Asda*	1 Pack/400g	416	6.0	104	6.6	15.9	1.5	1.4
Mozzarella & Pancetta, Breast, Finest, Tesco*	½ Pack/225g	326	14.0	145	14.4	7.9	6.2	1.1
Mozzarella & Pesto Melt, Breasts, COOK!, M&S*	½ Pack/165g	206	10.2	125	16.4	1.3	6.2	0.7

CHICKEN WITH	Measure INFO/WEIGHT	per Measure KCAL	per Measure FAT	Nutrition Values per 100g / 100ml KCAL	PROT	CARB	FAT	FIBRE
Mushroom & Bacon, Fillets, M&S*	½ Pack/188g	225	11.2	120	15.5	0.5	6.0	1.7
Mushroom Risotto, M&S*	1 Pack/400g	480	11.6	120	6.9	16.7	2.9	0.8
Pesto & Linguine Pasta, Meal, SteamFresh, Birds Eye*	1 Pack/400g	440	16.0	110	8.5	10.0	4.0	1.3
Plum Tomatoes & Basil, Breast, Birds Eye*	1 Serving/172g	200	8.1	116	13.3	5.0	4.7	0.6
Pork Stuffing, Breast, Roast, M&S*	1 Serving/100g	165	6.5	165	24.1	3.0	6.5	0.0
Potato Wedges, Tomato & Basil, Weight Watchers*	1 Pack/330g	254	6.6	77	4.7	9.2	2.0	1.6
Rice 'n' Peas, Sainsbury's*	1 Pack/300g	489	18.3	163	12.5	14.4	6.1	2.1
Rice, Jamaican Jerk, Healthier Choice, Co-Op*	1 Pack/406g	365	9.3	90	7.8	9.8	2.3	3.4
Sage & Onion Stuffing, Breast, Roast, Sliced, M&S*	1 Slice/17g	27	1.1	165	24.1	3.0	6.5	0.0
Spirelli, Steam Meal, Tesco*	1 Serving/400g	400	10.8	100	6.6	12.0	2.7	1.2
Spring Vegetables, Chargrilled, COU, M&S*	1 Pack/414g	290	3.7	70	8.8	7.3	0.9	1.8
Stilton & Port Sauce, Breasts, Finest, Tesco*	1 Serving/400g	668	34.4	167	18.5	3.9	8.6	0.7
Stuffing, TTD, Sainsbury's*	1 Slice/34g	50	2.0	148	22.7	1.3	5.8	0.9
Sweet Chilli & Garlic, Chinese, Asda*	1 Serving/400g	436	2.4	109	8.0	18.0	0.6	2.1
Sweet Chilli Sauce & Egg Fried Rice, Tesco*	1 Pack/380g	494	10.3	130	7.5	18.2	2.7	1.3
Tomato & Basil Sauce, HL, Tesco*	1 Breast/200g	154	2.4	77	12.0	3.9	1.2	1.2
Vegetables, Curried, Plumrose*	1 Serving/196g	253	16.1	129	5.8	8.0	8.2	0.0
CHICORY								
Fresh, Raw, Average	**1 Head/150g**	**30**	**0.9**	**20**	**0.6**	**2.8**	**0.6**	**0.9**
CHILLI								
& Potato Wedges, Sainsbury's*	1 Pack/371g	393	15.2	106	7.2	10.1	4.1	2.2
& Rice, GFY, Asda*	1 Pack/400g	352	1.6	88	5.0	16.0	0.4	1.8
& Rice, Morrisons*	1 Serving/500g	630	15.5	126	5.7	18.9	3.1	1.1
& Wedges, GFY, Asda*	1 Pack/400g	364	10.0	91	7.0	10.1	2.5	2.5
Beef & Mushrooms, GFY, Asda*	1 Pack/400g	364	6.0	91	9.1	10.2	1.5	1.2
Beef with Rice, GFY, Asda*	1 Serving/402g	354	6.0	88	4.7	14.0	1.5	0.9
Beef with Rice, Sainsbury's*	1 Serving/300g	360	5.1	120	5.6	20.6	1.7	1.1
Beef, Asda*	½ Pack/200g	190	7.8	95	7.0	8.0	3.9	1.2
Con Carne & Rice, Everyday, Value, Tesco*	1 Pack/400g	455	11.1	115	5.0	15.5	2.8	3.3
Con Carne, & Mexican Rice, Charlie Bigham's*	½ Pack/430g	563	22.8	131	6.0	14.7	5.3	0.0
Con Carne, & Rice, BGTY, Sainsbury's*	1 Pack/400g	376	7.2	94	4.9	13.4	1.8	2.2
Con Carne, Asda*	1 Can/392g	376	13.7	96	7.0	9.0	3.5	0.0
Con Carne, Beef, Look What We Found*	1 Pack/270g	194	7.6	72	7.8	2.9	2.8	2.3
Con Carne, Canned, El Tequito, Lidl*	1 Serving/320g	365	10.2	114	7.1	14.0	3.2	0.5
Con Carne, Canned, Sainsbury's*	½ Can/200g	162	4.2	81	6.6	8.9	2.1	2.5
Con Carne, Canned, Tesco*	½ Can/200g	220	11.4	110	7.8	6.4	5.7	4.7
Con Carne, Classic, Canned, Stagg*	½ Can/200g	260	10.0	130	7.0	13.0	5.0	4.5
Con Carne, Cooked, BGTY, Sainsbury's*	1 Pack/400g	356	6.8	94	4.9	13.4	1.8	2.2
Con Carne, Diet Chef Ltd*	1 Pack/300g	333	13.5	111	7.3	10.4	4.5	2.1
Con Carne, Dynamite Hot, Stagg*	1 Serving/250g	310	15.5	124	7.6	9.6	6.2	2.5
Con Carne, From Restaurant, Average	**1 Serving/253g**	**256**	**8.3**	**101**	**9.7**	**8.7**	**3.3**	**0.0**
Con Carne, Homepride*	1 Can/390g	234	2.3	60	2.5	11.2	0.6	1.5
Con Carne, M&S*	1 Pack/285g	285	10.5	100	8.7	7.4	3.7	2.0
Con Carne, Recipe Mix, Colman's*	1 Pack/50g	158	1.2	316	10.4	62.9	2.5	6.8
Con Carne, with Long Grain Rice, COU, M&S*	1 Pack/400g	388	7.6	97	5.0	13.9	1.9	2.1
Con Carne, with Rice, Morrisons*	1 Pack/400g	328	5.2	82	5.3	12.2	1.3	1.4
Con Carne, with Rice, Weight Watchers*	1 Pack/300g	279	4.2	93	4.6	15.1	1.4	1.1
Diced Beef, with Rice, 672, Wiltshire Farm Foods*	1 Portion/380g	328	9.2	86	5.5	10.0	2.4	1.6
Mexican, with Long Grain Rice, Rice Time, Uncle Ben's*	1 Pot/300g	339	3.0	113	2.5	22.8	1.0	1.3
Minced Beef with Rice, Mini, CBY, Asda*	1 Pack/250g	308	9.8	123	5.3	15.8	3.9	1.7
Mixed Vegetable, Tesco*	1 Pack/400g	352	11.6	88	3.9	11.0	2.9	3.2
Steak & Coriander Rice, Taste Mexico, M&S*	1 Pack/400g	532	15.2	133	7.1	16.4	3.8	2.4
Three Bean, Diet Chef Ltd*	1 Pack/300g	195	2.7	65	4.0	10.3	0.9	3.6

	Measure INFO/WEIGHT	per Measure		Nutrition Values per 100g / 100ml				
		KCAL	FAT	KCAL	PROT	CARB	FAT	FIBRE
CHILLI								
Vegetable	1oz/28g	16	0.2	57	3.0	10.8	0.6	2.6
Vegetable & Rice, BGTY, Sainsbury's*	1 Pack/450g	410	5.0	91	3.5	16.7	1.1	3.5
Vegetable Garden, Stagg*	1 Can/410g	254	2.0	62	3.6	10.8	0.5	2.3
Vegetable, Canned, Heated, Asda*	½ Can/200g	158	1.0	79	3.2	14.1	0.5	2.5
Vegetable, Canned, Sainsbury's*	1 Can/400g	230	1.6	58	3.1	10.4	0.4	3.2
Vegetable, Diet Chef Ltd*	1 Pack/300g	258	4.8	86	3.4	14.5	1.6	4.4
Vegetable, Retail	1oz/28g	20	0.6	70	4.0	9.4	2.1	0.0
CHINESE LEAF								
Fresh, Raw, Average	***1oz/28g***	***4***	***0.1***	***14***	***1.5***	***1.5***	***0.2***	***1.7***
CHIPS								
& Curry Sauce, Tesco*	1 Serving/400g	440	20.0	110	2.1	14.1	5.0	1.0
American Style, Oven, Co-Op*	1 Serving/150g	255	9.0	170	2.0	26.0	6.0	3.0
American Style, Oven, Sainsbury's*	1 Serving/165g	314	13.7	190	5.4	23.6	8.3	1.3
American Style, Thin, Oven, Tesco*	1 Serving/125g	210	8.1	168	2.7	24.6	6.5	2.1
British Classics, HL, Tesco*	½ Pack/200g	250	1.6	125	2.6	26.9	0.8	1.3
Chunky Oven, Harry Ramsden's*	1 Serving/150g	184	5.4	123	2.8	19.9	3.6	1.6
Chunky, Baked, Organic, M&S*	1 Serving/100g	150	3.7	150	1.7	27.1	3.7	2.2
Chunky, British, Oven, Frozen, Cooked, Finest, Tesco*	1 Serving/125g	240	5.1	192	2.3	35.1	4.1	2.7
Chunky, COU, M&S*	1 Serving/150g	158	2.4	105	2.1	20.5	1.6	2.3
Chunky, Crisp & Golden, Waitrose*	½ Pack/225g	259	7.0	115	2.1	17.7	3.1	3.9
Chunky, Fresh, Chilled, Finest, Tesco*	1 Pack/450g	608	18.0	135	2.1	22.3	4.0	2.7
Chunky, Gastropub, M&S*	1 Pack/400g	520	12.4	130	2.6	22.4	3.1	2.3
Chunky, Ready to Bake, M&S*	1 Serving/200g	310	8.4	155	2.2	26.8	4.2	2.0
Crinkle Cut, Frozen, Fried in Corn Oil	1oz/28g	81	4.7	290	3.6	33.4	16.7	2.2
Crinkle Cut, M&S*	1 Serving/150g	270	8.1	180	3.3	29.5	5.4	2.4
Crinkle Cut, Oven Baked, Aunt Bessie's*	1 Serving/100g	206	9.2	206	2.9	28.0	9.2	3.2
Crinkle Cut, Oven, Asda*	1 Serving/100g	134	3.8	134	2.0	23.0	3.8	8.0
Family Fries, Oven, Tesco*	1 Serving/125g	164	4.6	131	2.0	22.4	3.7	1.8
Fat with Fluffy Centres, M&S*	1 Serving/200g	210	9.0	105	1.6	14.2	4.5	1.8
Fine Cut, Frozen, Fried in Blended Oil	1oz/28g	102	6.0	364	4.5	41.2	21.3	2.4
Fine Cut, Frozen, Fried in Corn Oil	1oz/28g	102	6.0	364	4.5	41.2	21.3	2.7
Fried, Average	***1 Serving/130g***	***266***	***10.9***	***204***	***3.2***	***29.6***	***8.4***	***1.2***
Fried, Chip Shop, Average	***1 Serving/100g***	***239***	***12.4***	***239***	***3.2***	***30.5***	***12.4***	***2.2***
Frozen, Crinkle Cut, Aunt Bessie's*	1 Serving/100g	163	7.3	163	3.1	21.3	7.3	2.2
Frying, Cooked in Sunflower Oil, Value, Tesco*	1 Portion/125g	172	4.9	138	2.5	23.1	3.9	1.6
Frying, Crinkle Cut, Tesco*	1 Serving/125g	161	4.1	129	2.6	22.2	3.3	1.9
Homefries, Chunky, Weighed Baked, McCain*	1 Serving/100g	153	3.1	153	3.2	28.0	3.1	2.3
Homefries, Chunky, Weighed Frozen, McCain*	1 Serving/100g	123	2.5	123	2.5	22.6	2.5	1.6
Homefries, Crinkle Cut, Weighed Baked, McCain*	1 Serving/100g	176	5.0	176	2.6	30.1	5.0	2.3
Homefries, Crinkle Cut, Weighed Frozen, McCain*	1 Serving/100g	142	5.1	142	1.9	22.2	5.1	1.3
Homefries, Straight Cut, Weighed Baked, McCain*	1 Serving/100g	181	6.2	181	3.1	28.1	6.2	2.4
Homefries, Straight Cut, Weighed Frozen, McCain*	1 Serving/100g	134	4.6	134	2.2	21.0	4.6	1.7
Homefries, Thin & Crispy, Weighed Frozen, McCain*	1 Serving/100g	143	4.1	143	2.6	24.0	4.1	1.5
Homemade, Actify, 1000g Potatoes, 3ml Oil, Actifry*	1 Portion/250g	197	1.2	79	1.9	16.9	0.5	1.2
Homemade, Fried in Blended Oil, Average	***1oz/28g***	***53***	***1.9***	***189***	***3.9***	***30.1***	***6.7***	***2.2***
Homemade, Fried in Corn Oil, Average	***1oz/28g***	***53***	***1.9***	***189***	***3.9***	***30.1***	***6.7***	***2.2***
Homemade, Fried in Dripping, Average	***1oz/28g***	***53***	***1.9***	***189***	***3.9***	***30.1***	***6.7***	***2.2***
Homestyle Oven, Sainsbury's*	1 Serving/125g	206	5.4	165	2.4	29.2	4.3	2.1
Homestyle, Frozen, Aunt Bessie's*	1 Serving/200g	292	8.0	146	2.4	24.0	4.0	1.7
Homestyle, Oven Cooked, Aunt Bessie's*	1 Serving/100g	191	7.8	191	3.1	27.0	7.8	2.9
Homestyle, Oven, Straight Cut,Tesco*	1 Serving/125g	251	10.6	201	3.0	26.2	8.5	3.5
Lattices, with a Lightly Spiced Coating, Sainsbury's*	1 Serving/125g	305	13.8	244	3.8	32.0	11.0	3.3
Micro Chips, Crinkle Cut, Cooked, McCain*	1 Pack/100g	166	4.2	166	2.9	28.9	4.2	2.4

C

CHIPS

	Measure INFO/WEIGHT	KCAL	FAT	KCAL	PROT	CARB	FAT	FIBRE
Micro Chips, Straight Cut, Cooked, McCain*	1 Pack/100g	163	4.8	163	2.3	27.7	4.8	2.0
Microwave, Cooked	1oz/28g	62	2.7	221	3.6	32.1	9.6	2.9
Oven, 5% Fat, Frozen, McCain*	1 Serving/200g	238	6.0	119	1.9	21.0	3.0	1.6
Oven, Champion*	1 Pack/133g	210	6.0	158	2.5	27.0	4.5	0.0
Oven, Chunky, ES, Asda*	1 Serving/125g	238	7.0	190	3.4	31.5	5.6	3.2
Oven, Chunky, Ross*	1 Serving/100g	177	6.5	177	3.1	26.6	6.5	3.9
Oven, Chunky, TTD, Sainsbury's*	1 Serving/166g	250	5.3	151	2.0	28.6	3.2	2.3
Oven, Cooked, Value, Tesco*	1 Serving/125g	308	9.8	246	4.5	39.5	7.8	2.9
Oven, Cooked, Weight Watchers*	1 Serving/100g	150	3.0	150	2.8	33.7	3.0	5.9
Oven, Crinkle Cut, 5% Fat, Weighed Baked, McCain*	1 Serving/100g	163	4.3	163	3.1	27.9	4.3	3.0
Oven, Crinkle Cut, 5% Fat, Weighed Frozen, McCain*	1 Serving/100g	134	3.6	134	2.4	23.2	3.6	2.4
Oven, Crinkle Cut, Frozen, Essential, Waitrose*	1 Serving/165g	225	6.4	136	2.7	22.6	3.9	1.7
Oven, Crinkle Cut, Sainsbury's*	1 Serving/165g	297	9.1	180	3.3	29.5	5.5	2.4
Oven, Frozen, Baked	1 Serving/80g	130	3.4	162	3.2	29.8	4.2	2.0
Oven, Frozen, Basics, Sainsbury's*	1 Serving/165g	249	8.1	151	3.0	23.6	4.9	2.9
Oven, Frozen, BGTY, Sainsbury's*	1 Serving/165g	226	4.6	137	2.9	25.0	2.8	2.7
Oven, Frozen, Value, Tesco*	1 Serving/125g	189	5.7	151	2.8	24.7	4.6	1.9
Oven, Homefries, McCain*	1 Serving/100g	134	4.6	134	2.2	21.0	4.6	1.7
Oven, Morrisons*	1 Serving/100g	134	3.9	134	2.4	22.2	3.9	0.0
Oven, Organic, Waitrose*	1 Serving/165g	233	6.3	141	1.5	25.1	3.8	1.6
Oven, Original, McCain*	1 Serving/100g	158	3.8	158	2.5	28.5	3.8	2.3
Oven, Original, Straight Cut, 5% Fat, Cooked, McCain*	1 Serving/100g	158	3.8	158	3.8	28.5	3.8	2.3
Oven, Original, Straight Cut, 5% Fat, Frozen, McCain*	1 Serving/100g	138	4.0	138	2.5	26.2	4.0	1.9
Oven, Steak Cut, Asda*	1 Serving/100g	153	4.1	153	2.0	27.0	4.1	2.5
Oven, Steak Cut, Sainsbury's*	1 Serving/165g	266	7.8	161	2.6	27.1	4.7	2.8
Oven, Steak Cut, Waitrose*	1 Serving/165g	218	5.6	132	2.7	22.7	3.4	1.7
Oven, Steakhouse, Frozen, Tesco*	1 Serving/125g	165	4.2	132	2.7	22.7	3.4	1.7
Oven, Straight Cut, 5% Fat, Sainsbury's*	1 Serving/165g	280	8.1	170	3.4	28.0	4.9	2.5
Oven, Straight Cut, Asda*	1 Serving/100g	199	5.0	199	3.5	35.0	5.0	3.0
Oven, Straight Cut, BFY, Morrisons*	1 Serving/165g	249	5.8	151	2.8	27.1	3.5	2.1
Oven, Straight Cut, Frozen Weight, HL, Tesco*	1 Serving/125g	132	2.4	106	2.1	20.0	1.9	2.3
Oven, Straight Cut, Iceland*	1 Serving/100g	197	6.2	197	3.6	31.6	6.2	2.3
Oven, Straight Cut, Reduced Fat, Tesco*	1 Serving/100g	127	3.0	127	2.3	22.7	3.0	2.1
Oven, Straight Cut, Waitrose*	1 Serving/165g	219	6.1	133	2.0	23.0	3.7	1.7
Oven, Sweet Potato, Cooked, Tesco*	¼ Pack/125g	180	7.1	145	2.5	18.2	5.7	3.7
Oven, Thin & Crispy, Tesco*	1 Portion/100g	205	4.9	205	2.7	37.6	4.9	5.8
Oven, Thin Cut, American Style, Asda*	1 Serving/100g	240	10.0	240	3.4	34.0	10.0	3.0
Oven, Thin Fries, Morrisons*	1 Serving/100g	161	6.1	161	2.9	23.6	6.1	1.2
Potato, Lights, Reduced Fat, Lay's*	1 Serving/25g	118	5.5	470	7.5	60.0	22.0	5.0
Roasted Root Vegetable, Cooked, Tesco*	½ Pack/250g	198	7.5	79	1.1	10.3	3.0	3.1
Rustic, TTD, Sainsbury's*	½ Pack/122g	176	2.9	144	2.8	27.9	2.4	2.8
Steak Cut, Oven, Tesco*	1 Serving/165g	233	6.4	141	2.0	24.4	3.9	2.0
Straight Cut, Frozen, Fried in Blended Oil	1oz/28g	76	3.8	273	4.1	36.0	13.5	2.4
Straight Cut, Frozen, Fried in Corn Oil	1oz/28g	76	3.8	273	4.1	36.0	13.5	2.4
Straight Cut, Oven, BGTY, Sainsbury's*	1 Portion/165g	226	3.5	137	2.7	26.8	2.1	4.1
The Big Chip, Frozen, Tesco*	1 Serving/200g	220	4.8	110	1.8	20.3	2.4	2.1
Thick Cut, Frozen, Fried in Corn Oil, Average	*1oz/28g*	*66*	*2.9*	*234*	*3.6*	*34.0*	*10.2*	*2.4*
Three Way Cook, Skinny, Co-Op*	1 Serving/100g	175	7.0	175	2.0	26.0	7.0	3.0
with Gravy, Mayflower*	1 Box/330g	403	19.2	122	1.8	15.8	5.8	1.4

CHIVES

	Measure INFO/WEIGHT	KCAL	FAT	KCAL	PROT	CARB	FAT	FIBRE
Fresh, Average	*1 Tsp/2g*	*0*	*0.0*	*23*	*2.8*	*1.7*	*0.6*	*1.9*

CHOC ICES

	Measure INFO/WEIGHT	KCAL	FAT	KCAL	PROT	CARB	FAT	FIBRE
Chocolate, Dark, Seriously Creamy, Waitrose*	1 Ice/82g	195	12.9	238	2.6	21.6	15.7	1.7

	Measure INFO/WEIGHT	per Measure KCAL	FAT	Nutrition Values per 100g / 100ml KCAL	PROT	CARB	FAT	FIBRE
CHOC ICES								
Chocolate, Real Milk, Sainsbury's*	1 Ice/48g	151	9.5	312	3.5	30.3	19.7	0.8
Mini Mix, Eis Stern*	1 Ice/39g	129	8.9	334	4.2	29.0	23.0	0.0
Neapolitan Chocolate, Co-Op*	1 Ice/62g	120	8.2	194	2.0	16.9	13.2	0.4
Smart Price, Asda*	1 Ice/31g	81	5.9	262	2.8	20.0	19.0	0.0
CHOCOLATE								
Advent Calendar, Dairy Milk, Cadbury*	1 Chocolate/4g	22	1.3	525	7.5	56.6	30.1	0.7
Advent Calendar, Sainsbury's*	1 Chocolate/4g	20	1.2	557	7.2	52.7	34.3	2.1
Advent Calendar, The Snowman, M&S*	1 Chocolate/4g	21	1.2	550	6.6	60.4	31.0	0.0
Alpine Milk, Milka*	1 Serving/25g	132	7.4	530	6.6	58.5	29.5	1.8
Bar, Animal, Nestle*	1 Bar/19g	97	5.0	513	5.8	63.6	26.1	0.0
Bar, Bliss, Hazelnut Truffle, Cadbury*	1 Serving/100g	565	37.9	565	7.2	47.7	37.9	2.6
Bar, Chocolate Cream, Fry's*	1 Piece/10g	42	1.3	415	2.8	70.8	13.2	1.2
Bar, Cookies & Cream, Hello, Lindt*	1 Square/10g	56	3.7	565	7.0	52.0	37.0	0.0
Bar, Dark with Ginger, Thorntons*	1 Bar/90g	495	35.1	550	8.0	39.0	39.0	0.0
Bar, Dark, Thorntons*	1 Sm Bar/48g	250	17.7	521	7.3	39.9	36.9	10.9
Bar, Extra Dark, 60% Cocoa, Lindor, Lindt*	1 Bar/150g	900	73.5	600	5.0	35.0	49.0	2.0
Bar, Hazel Nut & Cashew, Dairy Milk, Cadbury*	3 Chunks/18g	96	6.0	540	8.8	50.6	33.5	1.8
Bar, Milk, Thorntons*	1 Sm Bar/50g	269	16.0	538	7.5	54.8	32.0	1.0
Bar, Strawberries & Creme, Dairy Milk, Cadbury*	1 Chunk/5g	28	1.8	560	5.7	53.5	35.5	0.5
Bar, Truffle, M&S*	1 Bar/35g	168	11.4	480	5.9	41.7	32.5	8.3
Bar, Truffle, Orange, M&S*	1 Bar/33g	177	10.5	535	6.6	55.6	31.9	1.4
Bar, Twisted, Creme Egg, Cadbury*	1 Bar/45g	210	9.4	465	5.2	64.6	20.8	0.5
Bar, Very Peculiar, Milk with Marmite Flavour, Marmite*	4 Squares/13g	70	4.2	540	6.9	54.9	32.1	2.0
Bar, Viennese, Continental, Thorntons*	1 Bar/38g	206	13.0	542	4.2	54.0	34.2	0.8
Bars, Alpini, Continental, Thorntons*	1 Bar/36g	192	11.4	538	6.9	55.3	32.0	2.7
Bars, Bubbles, Galaxy, Mars*	1 Bar/31g	172	10.6	555	6.5	54.7	34.2	1.5
Bars, Chocolate, Cherry, Lindt*	1 Bar/100g	470	22.8	470	4.5	61.7	22.8	0.0
Bars, Chocolate, Strawberry, Lindt*	1 Bar/100g	470	22.8	470	4.5	61.6	22.8	0.0
Bars, Chocoletti, Stracciatella, Lindt*	1 Bar/6g	32	2.3	590	7.7	49.0	41.0	0.0
Bars, Milk Chocolate, Galaxy, Mars*	1 Bar/46g	250	15.0	544	6.6	56.3	32.5	1.5
Bars, Milk Chocolate, Gold, Lindt*	1 Bar/300g	1605	92.9	535	6.6	58.7	31.0	0.0
Bars, Milk Chocolate, Hazelnut, Gold, Lindt*	1 Bar/300g	1665	108.2	555	7.9	50.7	36.1	0.0
Bars, Milk Chocolate, Hazelnut, Lindt*	1 Bar/100g	570	38.8	570	8.5	47.0	38.8	0.0
Bars, Milk Chocolate, Lindt*	1 Bar/100g	535	31.0	535	6.6	57.6	31.0	0.0
Bars, Milk Chocolate, Raisin & Hazelnut, Gold, Lindt*	1 Bar/300g	1590	94.8	530	6.8	54.7	31.6	0.0
Beans, Coffee, Dark, Solid, M&S*	1 Serving/10g	53	3.8	532	4.7	42.4	37.6	11.6
Bear, Lindt*	1 Bear/11g	60	3.6	572	7.5	57.7	34.6	0.0
Belgian Milk, TTD, Sainsbury's*	1 Piece/10g	55	3.5	549	9.6	48.3	35.3	2.0
Belgian, Milk, Mini Eggs, M&S*	1 Egg/8g	43	2.5	535	7.0	55.8	31.7	2.7
Blueberry Intense, Excellence, Lindt*	1 Serving/40g	200	12.4	500	6.0	50.0	31.0	0.0
Bubbly Santa, M&S*	1 Santa/23g	124	7.3	540	7.0	55.8	31.7	2.7
Bubbly, Dairy Milk, Cadbury*	1 Bar/35g	185	10.5	525	7.7	56.9	29.7	0.7
Bunny, Easter, Mars*	1 Bunny/29g	155	9.2	535	6.2	56.2	31.7	0.0
Bunny, Lindt*	1 Bunny/11g	60	3.6	572	7.5	57.5	34.6	0.0
Buttons, Dairy Milk, Cadbury*	1 Pack/32g	170	9.7	525	7.7	56.7	29.9	0.7
Cappuccino, Nestle*	1 Serving/20g	109	6.6	545	6.1	56.0	32.9	0.0
Caramel, Chunk, Dairy Milk, Cadbury*	1 Chunk/33g	158	7.6	480	5.0	63.0	23.0	0.0
Caramel, Dairy Milk, Cadbury*	1 Bar/45g	215	10.4	480	4.9	62.8	23.2	0.4
Chocolat Noir, Lindt*	1/6 Bar/17g	87	5.4	510	6.0	50.0	32.0	0.0
Chomp, Cadbury*	1 Bar/24g	112	4.8	465	3.3	67.9	20.0	0.2
Christmas Tree Decoration, Average	**1 Chocolate/12g**	**63**	**3.6**	**522**	**7.6**	**56.4**	**29.9**	**0.4**
Christmas Tree Decoration, Cadbury*	1 Piece/12g	60	3.4	525	7.6	56.2	29.9	0.0
Christmas Tree Decorations, Caramel, Dairy Milk, Cadbury*	1 Chocolate/11g	53	2.8	485	5.6	59.7	25.1	0.0

C

CHOCOLATE

	Measure INFO/WEIGHT	per Measure KCAL	FAT	Nutrition Values per 100g / 100ml KCAL	PROT	CARB	FAT	FIBRE
Chunk Bar, Dairy Milk, Cadbury*	1 Chunk/7g	35	2.0	525	7.5	57.0	29.8	0.1
Chunky Hazelnut Bar, M&S*	1 Bar/52g	293	19.4	563	8.8	48.1	37.3	1.7
Coconut, White, Excellence, Lindt*	1 Square/10g	61	4.4	610	6.0	48.0	44.0	0.0
Coins, Milk, Sainsbury's*	1 Coin/5g	26	1.4	502	5.5	58.8	27.1	2.5
Crispello Double Choc, Cadbury*	1 Peice/10g	55	3.5	560	7.0	51.0	36.0	1.9
Crispies, Dairy Milk, Cadbury*	1 Bar/49g	250	13.4	510	7.6	58.6	27.4	0.0
Dairy Milk with Oreo, Dairy Milk, Cadbury*	3 Chunks/15g	85	5.4	560	6.1	53.5	35.5	0.7
Dairy Milk, Cadbury*	1 Bar/45g	240	13.8	530	7.5	56.5	30.5	0.7
Dairy Milk, Toffee Popcorn, Dairy Milk, Cadbury*	1 Bar/150g	765	39.8	510	7.0	59.5	26.5	1.7
Dark with a Soft Mint Centre, Organic, Green & Black's*	1 Bar/100g	478	27.3	478	7.4	50.5	27.3	8.6
Dark with Chilli, Thorntons*	4 Squares/20g	107	7.9	533	7.2	36.3	39.5	10.4
Dark with Crystallised Ginger, Green & Black's*	150g	752	43.6	501	6.8	53.0	29.1	9.6
Dark with Hazelnuts & Currant, Green & Black's*	1 Bar/100g	513	33.5	513	7.6	45.4	33.5	9.2
Dark with Orange & Spices, Maya Gold, Green & Black's*	1 Sm Bar/35g	184	11.8	526	7.3	48.2	33.8	8.2
Dark, 60%, Amazonas, Lidl*	1 Square/13g	75	5.2	574	5.7	44.0	40.0	7.5
Dark, 70% Cocoa Solids, Extra Fine, Lindt*	1 Square/10g	54	4.1	537	8.0	33.0	41.0	0.0
Dark, 70% Cocoa Solids, Organic, Green & Black's*	1 Sm Bar/35g	193	14.4	551	9.3	36.0	41.1	11.5
Dark, 70% Cocoa Solids, Organic, Morrisons*	½ Bar/50g	266	20.6	531	7.9	31.6	41.1	11.0
Dark, 75% Cacao, Rausch*	1 Row/31g	163	12.9	522	8.8	28.5	41.1	15.0
Dark, 85% Cocoa, Excellence, Lindt*	1 Serving/40g	212	18.4	530	11.0	19.0	46.0	0.0
Dark, 85% Cocoa, TTD, Sainsbury's*	1 Serving/25g	142	12.8	569	9.7	17.0	51.4	14.1
Dark, 99% Cocoa, Excellence, Lindt*	1 Serving/25g	142	12.5	567	13.0	8.0	50.0	8.0
Dark, Belgian, ES, Asda*	2 Squares/20g	102	8.0	508	11.0	26.0	40.0	16.0
Dark, Bittersweet with Cherries, Green & Black's*	1 Bar/100g	477	28.2	477	7.9	48.0	28.2	8.7
Dark, Chilli, Excellence, Lindt*	1 Serving/40g	202	12.8	506	5.4	49.0	32.0	0.0
Dark, Classic, Bourneville, Cadbury*	4 Squares/25g	125	6.8	505	4.7	58.8	27.3	2.0
Dark, Co-Op*	1 Bar/50g	252	14.5	505	4.0	57.0	29.0	6.0
Dark, Ecuador, 70%, with Raspberry, J D Gross, Lidl*	1 Square/13g	70	5.2	541	7.2	33.3	39.7	0.0
Dark, Espresso with Coffee, Organic, Green & Black's*	1 Bar/150g	824	62.4	549	9.8	33.8	41.6	11.7
Dark, Fair Trade, Co-Op*	1 Bar/45g	214	13.0	475	4.0	49.0	29.0	6.0
Dark, Finest, 85% Cocoa, Moser Roth, Aldi*	1 Bar/25g	152	12.8	608	11.0	18.0	51.0	15.0
Dark, Mint, Intense, Lindt*	1 Square/10g	53	3.2	529	5.0	51.0	32.0	0.0
Dark, Orange & Almond, Moser Roth, Aldi*	1 Serving/25g	133	8.0	532	5.9	51.0	32.0	7.9
Dark, Orange with Slivered Almonds, Excellence, Lindt*	1 Square/10g	50	3.1	500	6.0	49.0	31.0	0.0
Dark, Plain, Average	**1oz/28g**	**143**	**7.8**	**510**	**5.0**	**63.5**	**28.0**	**2.5**
Dark, Plain, Rich, Co-Op*	1 Bar/200g	1010	58.0	505	4.0	57.0	29.0	6.0
Dark, Raw Organic, Loving Earth*	1 Serving/20g	99	7.9	495	9.3	46.4	39.5	0.0
Dark, Rich, Tesco*	1 Serving/20g	98	6.1	491	5.8	60.0	30.4	11.5
Dark, Smooth, Bar, Galaxy, Mars*	1 Bar/125g	651	42.0	521	6.2	48.0	33.6	9.3
Dark, Smooth, No Added Sugar, Sainsbury's*	1 Piece/10g	53	4.2	529	8.2	34.3	42.2	11.0
Dark, Whole Nut, Tesco*	1 Serving/13g	67	4.5	539	6.1	48.3	35.7	6.5
Diet, Ritter Sport*	1 Square/6g	25	1.8	412	6.0	44.0	30.0	0.0
Drops, Plain, Asda*	1 Serving/100g	489	29.0	489	7.0	50.0	29.0	10.0
Egg, Caramel, Cadbury*	1 Egg/39g	187	9.5	480	4.0	60.0	24.5	0.4
Eggs, Milk, Raspberry, Favorina, Lidl*	1 Egg/19g	86	3.6	453	4.1	64.3	19.1	0.0
Elves, Magical, with Popping Candy, Cadbury*	1 Elf/15g	77	4.2	515	6.9	60.0	27.7	0.0
Ferrero Rocher, Ferrero*	1 Chocolate/13g	75	5.3	603	8.2	44.4	42.7	0.0
Freddo, Caramel, Dairy Milk, Cadbury*	1 Freddo/19g	93	4.7	490	5.5	60.5	24.8	0.5
Freddo, Dairy Milk, Cadbury*	1 Freddo/18g	95	5.4	530	7.5	57.0	29.8	0.7
Fruit & Nut, Belgian, Waitrose*	1 Serving/50g	254	14.6	508	8.6	54.6	29.2	3.4
Fruit & Nut, Dark, Tesco*	4 Squares/25g	124	7.0	494	5.8	54.8	27.9	6.5
Ginger, Traidcraft*	1 Bar/50g	212	7.4	424	3.9	68.2	14.8	0.0
Golden Biscuit Crunch, Dairy Milk, Cadbury*	4 Chunks/25g	135	8.2	545	6.2	55.5	33.0	0.8

CHOCOLATE

	Measure INFO/WEIGHT	per Measure		Nutrition Values per 100g / 100ml				
		KCAL	FAT	KCAL	PROT	CARB	FAT	FIBRE
Golf Balls, Milk Chocolate, Lindt*	1 Pack/110g	619	39.5	563	6.5	53.6	35.9	0.0
Hazelnut & Walnut, Dark, Organic, Seeds of Change*	1 Bar/100g	559	41.7	559	8.4	37.5	41.7	9.2
Kinder Maxi, Ferrero*	1 Bar/21g	116	7.1	550	10.0	51.0	34.0	0.0
Kinder Surprise, Ferrero*	1 Egg/20g	110	7.0	550	10.0	50.0	35.0	0.0
Kinder, Bueno Bar, Milk, Ferrero*	1 Bar/22g	123	8.0	575	9.2	49.5	37.3	2.0
Kinder, Bueno, Bar, White, Ferrero*	1 Piece/20g	111	7.0	571	8.8	52.6	35.9	1.0
Kinder, Riegel, Ferrero*	1 Bar/21g	117	7.1	558	10.0	53.0	34.0	0.0
Kitten, Milk Chocolate, Lindt*	1 Kitten/11g	60	3.6	572	7.5	57.7	34.6	0.0
Lait Intense, Experiences, Cote D'or*	3 Squares/100g	575	40.0	575	7.2	44.5	40.0	5.0
Light & Whippy, Bite Sized, Sainsbury's*	1 Bar/15g	66	2.4	439	3.3	69.7	16.3	0.1
Little Bars, Dairy Milk, Cadbury*	1 Bar/21g	110	6.3	530	7.7	56.6	30.1	0.7
Matchmakers, Mint, Nestle*	1 Stick/4g	20	0.8	477	4.3	69.7	20.1	0.9
Milk for Baking, Value, Tesco*	½ Bar/50g	265	14.5	530	6.7	60.0	29.0	2.2
Milk with Honey & Almond Nougat, Swiss, Toblerone*	1 Piece/8g	42	2.4	525	5.4	59.0	29.5	2.2
Milk with Peanut Butter Filling, Ghirardelli*	1 Serving/45g	250	17.0	556	8.9	48.9	37.8	2.2
Milk with Raisins & Hazelnuts, Green & Black's*	1 Bar/100g	556	36.9	556	9.2	46.8	36.9	3.2
Milk with Whole Almonds, Organic, Green & Black's*	1 Bar/100g	578	42.2	578	11.8	37.7	42.2	5.2
Milk, a Darker Shade of Milk Chocolate, Green & Black's*	1 Sm Bar/35g	183	10.4	523	9.9	54.0	29.7	3.7
Milk, Average	*1oz/28g*	*146*	*8.6*	*520*	*7.7*	*56.9*	*30.7*	*0.8*
Milk, Bars, M&S*	1 Bar/40g	214	12.8	535	7.8	54.0	32.0	1.9
Milk, Biscuit Sticks, Mikado, Kraft*	1 Stick/2g	11	0.5	475	7.8	67.0	19.8	3.1
Milk, Creamy, Organic, Green & Black's*	6 Pieces/20g	110	7.0	560	9.1	50.3	35.5	1.6
Milk, Extra Creamy, Excellence, Lindt*	1 Bar/100g	560	37.1	560	6.0	51.1	37.1	0.0
Milk, Extra Fine, Swiss, M&S*	1 Serving/25g	141	9.2	565	7.2	50.9	36.7	2.3
Milk, Fair Trade, Tesco*	1 Serving/45g	236	13.3	524	7.6	56.7	29.6	2.0
Milk, Figures, Hollow, Dairyfine, Aldi*	1 Serving/11g	58	3.2	523	5.5	59.9	29.0	3.1
Milk, Giant Buttons, M&S*	1 Button/8g	44	2.7	550	7.1	52.3	34.2	0.4
Milk, Lindor, Lindt*	1 Square/11g	68	5.2	615	4.7	43.0	47.0	0.0
Milk, Ryelands*	4 Squares/29g	155	8.2	520	7.3	60.7	27.6	1.7
Milk, Sainsbury's*	4 Squares/25g	133	7.7	533	9.2	54.6	30.8	2.2
Milk, Smart Price, Asda*	1 Square/6g	32	1.9	536	8.0	54.0	32.0	1.8
Milk, Swiss, Diabetic with Fruit & Nuts, Boots*	½ Bar/21g	97	6.7	462	7.0	55.0	32.0	2.7
Milk, Swiss, Finest, Tesco*	2 Squares/20g	112	7.0	558	8.5	50.6	35.2	2.3
Milk, Tesco*	1 Serving/25g	133	7.7	533	9.5	54.7	30.7	2.2
Milk, Value, Tesco*	1/6 Bar/16g	83	4.5	520	6.8	60.0	28.0	2.3
Milk, Whole Nut, Tesco*	1 Serving/25g	129	8.4	517	8.7	53.4	33.8	9.0
Milk, with Crunchy Butterscotch, Green & Black's*	1 Bar/100g	555	34.5	555	8.8	50.5	34.5	2.7
Milky Bar, Giant Buttons, Mars*	1 Sweet/2g	11	0.6	546	7.5	57.7	31.6	0.0
Mini Eggs, Cadbury*	1 Egg/3g	16	0.7	495	4.6	69.5	21.5	1.3
Mini Eggs, Caramel, Cadbury*	1 Mini Egg/11g	55	2.9	485	5.7	59.0	25.7	0.4
Mini Eggs, Lindor, Lindt*	3 Eggs/15g	92	6.8	611	5.4	45.0	45.0	0.0
Mini, Toblerone*	1 Serving/6g	32	1.8	525	5.6	57.5	30.0	3.5
Mint Creme, Sainsbury's*	1 Serving/20g	93	4.9	467	2.8	62.7	24.5	2.1
Mint Crisps, M&S*	1 Mint/8g	40	2.4	494	5.4	54.8	29.6	3.1
Mistletoe Kisses, Mars*	1 Pack/42g	209	11.5	498	5.3	57.0	27.3	0.0
Mountain Bar, Swiss, M&S*	1 Bar/100g	555	35.3	555	6.5	55.2	35.3	0.2
Natural Orange, Excellence, Lindt*	1 Bar/100g	560	37.0	560	7.0	50.0	37.0	0.0
Natural Vanilla, Excellence, Lindt*	1 Bar/100g	590	40.0	590	6.0	51.0	40.0	0.0
Nibs, Raw, Cacao, Organic, Navitas Naturals*	1 Serving/28g	130	12.0	464	14.3	35.7	42.9	32.1
NutRageous, Reese's, Hershey*	1 Bar/51g	260	16.0	510	11.8	54.9	31.4	3.9
Nutty Nougat, Bite Sized, Sainsbury's*	1 Bar/23g	111	5.5	481	7.6	59.0	23.8	0.6
Old Jamaica, Bournville, Cadbury*	4 Chunks/23g	107	5.4	465	4.2	59.6	23.4	2.0
Orange, Bar, Terry's*	1 Bar/40g	210	11.7	530	7.3	58.0	29.5	2.1

CHOCOLATE

	Measure INFO/WEIGHT	per Measure KCAL	FAT	Nutrition Values per 100g / 100ml KCAL	PROT	CARB	FAT	FIBRE
Orange, Crunchball, Terry's*	1 Segment/9g	45	2.4	520	6.9	59.8	28.1	2.0
Orange, Dark, Terry's*	1 Segment/9g	45	2.6	511	4.3	57.0	29.3	6.2
Orange, Fair Trade, Divine Foods*	4 Squares/17g	92	5.4	541	6.5	57.7	31.5	0.0
Orange, Milk, Mini Segments, Minis, Terry's*	1 Segment/4g	21	1.1	525	5.4	60.5	28.5	2.1
Orange, Milk, Terry's*	1 Orange/175g	931	51.6	532	7.4	57.8	29.5	2.1
Orange, Sainsbury's*	4 Squares/19g	100	5.8	531	9.2	54.3	30.7	2.2
Orange, Segsations, Terry's*	1 Segsation/8g	43	2.3	520	6.9	58.5	28.5	2.8
Peanut Butter Cup, Big Cup, Reese's, Hershey*	1 Cup/39g	210	12.0	538	10.3	53.8	30.8	2.6
Peanut Butter Cup, Miniature, Reese's, Hershey*	1 Cup/9g	44	2.6	500	9.1	59.1	29.6	2.3
Peanut Butter Cup, Reese's, Hershey*	1 Cup/21g	105	6.5	500	11.9	57.1	31.0	5.9
Peppermint Cream, Fry's*	1 Bar/51g	217	7.9	425	2.6	68.8	15.4	0.0
Peppermint Patty, Hershey*	3 Patties/41g	160	3.0	390	2.4	80.5	7.3	0.0
Peppermint, Ritter Sport*	1 Bar/100g	483	26.0	483	3.0	60.0	26.0	0.0
Plain with Hazelnuts, Tesco*	4 Squares/25g	135	8.9	539	6.1	48.3	35.7	6.5
Plain, 72% Cocoa Solids, Finest, Tesco*	1 Square/10g	60	4.4	603	7.7	44.0	44.0	3.7
Plain, Belgian, Organic, Waitrose*	1 Bar/100g	505	37.6	505	9.6	32.0	37.6	5.6
Plain, Continental, Waitrose*	1 Square/4g	23	1.8	558	7.7	32.9	44.0	5.9
Plain, Dark, Fruit & Nut, Rich, Sainsbury's*	4 Squares/25g	122	7.0	489	5.2	53.9	27.9	5.7
Plain, Whole Nut, Belgian, Waitrose*	4 Squares/25g	135	9.5	540	6.3	45.4	38.0	7.8
Planets, Mars*	1 Pack/37g	178	8.3	481	4.9	65.4	22.4	0.0
Praline, M&S*	1 Bar/34g	185	12.0	545	7.3	49.6	35.2	3.1
Probiotic, Bar, Ohso*	1 Bar/14g	72	5.0	514	5.0	47.0	36.0	15.5
Puddles, Hazelnut Flavour Filling, Dairy Milk, Cadbury*	¼ Bar/23g	114	6.2	505	6.3	57.0	27.5	0.9
Rafaello, Roche, Ferrero*	1 Sweet/10g	60	4.7	600	9.7	35.4	46.6	0.0
Reese's Pieces, Bite Size, Minis, Hershey*	11 Pieces/39g	200	12.0	513	7.7	59.0	30.8	2.6
Reese's, Fast Break, Candy Bar, Hershey*	1 Bar/56g	260	12.0	464	8.9	62.5	21.4	3.6
Reindeer, Lindt*	1 Reindeer/107g	588	35.3	550	7.2	55.0	33.0	0.0
Rocky Road, Clusters, Tesco*	1 Serving/32g	160	9.5	500	7.1	51.0	29.7	6.7
Shortcake, Snack Shots, Cadbury*	½ Bag/50g	260	14.0	520	5.8	60.4	27.9	2.0
Smooth Praline, Choceur, Aldi*	1 Square/5g	27	1.6	544	7.8	52.0	33.0	3.9
Snack Bar, Kinder*	1 Bar/21g	116	7.1	554	10.0	52.0	34.0	0.0
Snack Size, Dairy Milk, Cadbury*	1 Bar/30g	159	9.0	530	7.8	57.1	29.9	0.0
Snickers, More Nuts, Snickers*	1 Bar/58g	299	17.3	515	10.1	52.8	29.8	0.0
Snowman, Mousse, Dairy Milk, Cadbury*	1 Snowman/29g	162	10.2	560	6.7	54.5	35.0	0.4
Speckled Eggs, M&S*	1 Egg/6g	25	1.0	440	6.6	63.1	18.2	1.5
Teddy Bear, Milk Chocolate, Thorntons*	1 Teddy/250g	1358	83.8	543	7.6	52.6	33.5	1.0
Toffifee, Storck*	1 Sweet/8g	43	2.4	516	5.9	58.5	28.7	0.0
Turkish Delight, Large Bar, Dairy Milk, Cadbury*	1 Square/8g	35	1.6	470	5.6	63.2	21.4	0.5
Twirl, Bites, Cadbury*	1 Bite/2g	11	0.6	530	7.7	56.5	30.3	0.8
Whips, Double Chocolate, M&S*	1 Whip/29g	140	7.3	485	6.6	57.8	25.3	1.0
White with Honey & Almond Nougat, Toblerone*	1 Serving/25g	132	7.2	530	6.2	60.5	29.0	0.2
White with Strawberries, Divine*	1 Piece/3g	16	0.9	534	7.6	59.9	29.3	0.1
White, Average	*1oz/28g*	*148*	*8.7*	*529*	*8.0*	*58.3*	*30.9*	*0.0*
White, Creamy Vanilla, Green & Black's*	1 Sm Bar/35g	201	12.8	573	7.4	53.5	36.6	0.1
White, Creamy, Tesco*	1 Serving/25g	139	8.7	557	5.1	55.7	34.9	3.3
White, Crispy, Fair Trade, Co-Op*	½ Bar/50g	278	17.5	555	9.0	51.0	35.0	0.1
White, Nestle*	4 Pieces/40g	220	13.0	550	7.5	55.0	32.5	0.0
White, Smart Price, Asda*	1 Serving/25g	137	8.2	549	7.0	56.0	33.0	0.0
White, Value, Tesco*	1 Serving/10g	55	3.1	548	4.7	62.0	31.2	0.0
Whole Nut, Dairy Milk, Cadbury*	1 Bar/49g	270	17.4	550	8.9	49.5	35.4	1.7
Wispa, Bitsa Wispa, Cadbury*	¼ Bag/43g	238	14.7	550	7.3	53.0	34.0	0.9
with Creme Egg, Dairy Milk, Cadbury*	1 Bar/45g	210	9.3	470	5.2	64.8	20.9	0.5
with Crunchie Bits, Dairy Milk, Cadbury*	1 Bar/200g	1000	48.8	500	6.2	63.3	24.4	0.0

	Measure INFO/WEIGHT	per Measure		Nutrition Values per 100g / 100ml				
		KCAL	FAT	KCAL	PROT	CARB	FAT	FIBRE
CHOCOLATE								
with Shortcake Biscuit, Dairy Milk, Cadbury*	1 Square/6g	31	1.7	520	7.5	59.0	28.0	0.0
CHOCOLATE NUTS								
Almonds, Dark Chocolate Covered, Bolero*	2 Almonds/3g	15	1.0	510	2.6	48.8	33.5	0.0
Peanuts, Assorted, Thorntons*	1 Bag/140g	785	57.1	561	13.8	34.8	40.8	3.6
Peanuts, Belgian Coated, M&S*	1 Serving/20g	109	7.6	545	14.7	35.6	38.0	5.8
Peanuts, Milk, Tesco*	1 Bag/227g	1221	86.0	538	17.5	31.8	37.9	4.4
CHOCOLATE RAISINS								
Assorted, Thorntons*	1 Bag/140g	601	27.6	429	4.2	58.8	19.7	2.9
Bonds Sweetstars*	1 Serving/28g	109	4.5	391	4.7	57.0	16.0	0.0
Californian, Tesco*	½ Bag/57g	268	11.7	472	5.2	66.2	20.7	1.3
Coated, Californian, M&S*	1 Bag/130g	520	19.1	400	4.3	63.2	14.7	1.9
Co-Op*	½ Pack/50g	205	7.5	410	4.0	64.0	15.0	1.0
Milk Chocolate Coated, Average	**1 Serving/50g**	**207**	**7.7**	**415**	**4.4**	**64.6**	**15.4**	**2.0**
Milk, Asda*	1 Serving/28g	120	4.2	430	5.1	66.4	15.1	4.2
Milk, Co-Op*	½ Bag/100g	420	17.0	420	5.0	63.0	17.0	6.0
CHOCOLATE SPREAD								
& Caramel, CBY, Asda*	1 Serving/100g	564	34.7	564	2.5	60.1	34.7	0.8
Average	**1 Tsp/12g**	**68**	**4.5**	**569**	**4.1**	**57.1**	**37.6**	**0.0**
Hazelnut, Nutella, Ferrero*	1oz/28g	149	8.7	533	6.6	56.4	31.0	3.5
with Nuts	**1 Tsp/12g**	**66**	**4.0**	**549**	**6.2**	**60.5**	**33.0**	**0.8**
CHOCOLATES								
All Gold, Dark, Terry's*	1 Serving/30g	152	8.7	505	4.0	57.5	29.0	4.3
All Gold, Milk, Terry's*	1 Serving/30g	158	9.2	525	4.8	58.0	30.5	1.5
Almond Marzipan, Milk Chocolate, Thorntons*	1 Chocolate/13g	60	2.9	464	6.6	59.4	22.6	5.6
Alpini, Thorntons*	1 Chocolate/13g	70	4.2	538	7.0	54.6	32.3	2.3
Bittermint, Bendicks*	1 Mint/18g	80	3.0	440	4.3	68.9	16.3	2.4
Brandy Liqueurs, Asda*	1 Chocolate/8g	34	1.4	409	4.0	60.0	17.0	0.8
Cappuccino from Continental Selection, Thorntons*	1 Chocolate/13g	70	4.7	538	5.9	48.5	36.2	0.8
Caramels, Sainsbury's*	1 Sweet/12g	57	2.6	490	3.5	69.0	22.2	0.2
Celebrations, Mars*	1 Sweet/8g	40	2.0	497	5.6	61.7	25.0	1.7
Cherry Liqueur, M&S*	1 Chocolate/13g	55	2.6	435	3.2	50.6	20.2	4.1
Classic Collection, Thorntons*	1 Chocolate/12g	58	2.8	472	4.3	62.7	22.8	2.4
Coconut, Lindor, Lindt*	1 Ball/13g	79	6.0	632	5.4	42.0	48.0	0.0
Coffee Cream, Average	**1 Chocolate/12g**	**54**	**2.0**	**446**	**3.3**	**70.4**	**17.0**	**2.4**
Coffee Creme, Dark, Thorntons*	1 Chocolate/13g	52	1.4	400	3.0	71.5	10.8	0.8
Coffee Creme, Milk, Thorntons*	1 Chocolate/13g	52	1.3	400	2.8	74.6	10.0	0.8
Continental, Belgian, Thorntons*	1 Chocolate/13g	67	3.9	514	5.8	53.5	30.3	2.9
Continental, Thorntons*	1 Chocolate/15g	76	4.4	506	5.6	54.5	29.3	2.7
Country Caramel, Milk, Thorntons*	1 Chocolate/9g	45	2.4	500	4.6	62.2	26.7	0.0
Dairy Box, Milk, Nestle*	1 Piece/11g	50	2.1	456	4.4	65.9	19.4	0.7
Dark, Elegant, Elizabeth Shaw*	1 Chocolate/8g	38	1.8	469	2.9	62.5	23.1	0.0
Dark, Rose & Violet Creams	1 Chocolate/13g	55	1.6	422	2.2	76.1	12.5	1.7
Dark, Swiss Thins, Lindt*	1 Pack/125g	681	46.2	545	4.8	49.2	37.0	0.0
Eclipse, Truffle, Plain, Dark, Montezuma*	1 Truffle/16g	93	8.5	581	0.6	21.9	53.1	0.0
Filled, Average	**1 Chocolate/13g**	**58**	**2.8**	**447**	**4.9**	**62.9**	**21.3**	**1.3**
Heroes, Cadbury*	1 Sweet/8g	38	1.8	480	4.8	65.1	22.4	0.4
Italian Collection, Amaretto, M&S*	1 Chocolate/13g	60	3.1	480	4.4	59.7	25.1	2.3
Italian Collection, Favourites, M&S*	1 Chocolate/14g	74	4.7	530	5.7	50.4	33.7	1.6
Liqueur, Barrels, Cointreau	1 Chocolate/10g	44	1.8	435	3.5	57.0	18.0	0.0
Milk Tray, Cadbury*	1 Chocolate/9g	47	2.4	495	4.7	61.5	25.8	0.7
Milk, Mini Eggs, Green & Black's*	1 Mini Egg/8g	42	2.7	562	8.6	48.3	35.5	3.8
Milk, Swiss Thins, Lindt*	1 Pack/125g	688	43.3	550	5.8	53.6	34.6	0.0
Mini Eggs, with Soft White Truffle Centre, M&S*	1 Egg/6g	33	2.0	550	6.5	56.3	33.9	1.4

CHOCOLATES

	Measure INFO/WEIGHT	per Measure KCAL	FAT	Nutrition Values per 100g / 100ml KCAL	PROT	CARB	FAT	FIBRE
Mint Creams, Dark, Smooth & Fragrant, Waitrose*	1 Sweet/10g	42	0.9	410	3.0	77.9	9.1	2.4
Mint Crisp, Bendicks*	1 Mint/8g	38	2.3	494	5.2	55.0	29.9	0.0
Mint Crisp, Dark, Elizabeth Shaw*	1 Chocolate/6g	27	1.2	458	1.9	68.0	20.7	0.0
Mint Crisp, Milk, Elizabeth Shaw*	1 Chocolate/6g	30	1.3	493	4.0	70.9	21.4	0.0
Mint Crisp, Thorntons*	1 Chocolate/7g	34	2.2	486	7.7	40.0	31.4	4.3
Mints, After Eight, Dark, Nestle*	1 Sweet/7g	32	0.9	461	5.0	63.0	12.9	2.0
Mints, After Eight, Straws, Nestle*	1 Sweet/5g	24	1.4	526	5.1	56.6	31.0	4.0
Misshapes, Assorted, Cadbury*	1 Chocolate/8g	41	2.3	515	5.2	57.5	29.1	0.0
Moments, Thorntons*	1 Chocolate/7g	37	2.0	511	5.4	59.9	27.8	1.9
Orange Cream, Average	***1 Chocolate/12g***	***53***	***2.0***	***440***	***3.2***	***69.3***	***16.7***	***0.0***
Orange Crisp, Elizabeth Shaw*	1 Chocolate/6g	29	1.3	478	2.9	68.2	21.5	0.0
Peppermint Cream, Average	***1 Chocolate/12g***	***50***	***1.4***	***418***	***1.9***	***76.4***	***11.4***	***1.6***
Praline, Coffee, Thorntons*	1 Chocolate/7g	37	2.4	529	7.0	47.1	34.3	2.9
Praline, Hazelnut, Thorntons*	1 Chocolate/5g	27	1.8	540	7.0	48.0	36.0	4.0
Praline, Marzipan, Thorntons*	1 Chocolate/14g	63	3.0	450	5.9	58.6	21.4	2.1
Praline, Roast Hazelnut, Thorntons*	1 Chocolate/13g	70	4.4	538	6.0	51.5	33.8	3.1
Quality Street, Nestle*	1 Sweet/9g	44	1.9	470	3.5	67.3	20.5	1.5
Roses, Cadbury*	1 Chocolate/9g	41	1.9	480	3.3	66.0	22.5	1.3
Sea Shells, Belgian, Guylian*	1 Shell/11g	62	3.8	550	7.6	52.0	34.0	0.0
Seashells, Belgian, Woolworths*	1 Box/63g	346	19.6	550	5.5	52.9	31.1	0.0
Seashells, Milk & White, Belgian, Waitrose*	1 Serving/15g	77	4.6	511	5.0	53.1	31.0	2.8
Strawberries & Cream, Thorntons*	1 Chocolate/12g	64	3.9	533	5.1	54.2	32.5	0.8
Swiss Tradition, De Luxe, Lindt*	1 Pack/250g	1388	90.7	555	6.3	51.9	36.3	0.0
Swiss Tradition, Mixed, Lindt*	1 Pack/392g	2215	149.4	565	6.1	49.8	38.1	0.0
Truffle Filled, Swiss, Balls, Finest, Tesco*	3 Balls/37g	240	19.0	640	5.0	40.7	50.8	1.5
Truffle Hearts, Baileys*	1 Chocolate/15g	76	4.3	506	5.2	52.6	28.9	1.3
Truffle, Belgian, Flaked, Tesco*	1 Truffle/14g	80	5.4	575	4.4	52.7	38.5	2.3
Truffle, Brandy, Thorntons*	1 Chocolate/14g	68	3.8	486	6.1	52.1	27.1	0.7
Truffle, Caramel, Thorntons*	1 Chocolate/14g	67	3.6	479	4.2	57.9	25.7	2.1
Truffle, Champagne, Premier, Thorntons*	1 Chocolate/17g	88	5.6	518	6.9	45.3	32.9	2.4
Truffle, Cherry, Thorntons*	1 Chocolate/14g	58	3.0	414	4.2	50.7	21.4	1.4
Truffle, Dark, Balls, Lindor, Lindt*	1 Ball/12g	76	6.2	630	3.4	38.5	51.4	0.0
Truffle, French Cocoa Dusted, Sainsbury's*	1 Truffle/10g	57	4.5	570	4.0	37.0	45.0	0.0
Truffle, Hazelnut, Balls, Lindor, Lindt*	1 Ball/12g	76	6.1	632	5.0	39.1	50.6	0.0
Truffle, Lemon, White, Thorntons*	1 Chocolate/14g	63	3.5	450	4.6	64.3	25.0	0.7
Truffle, Milk Chocolate, Balls, Lindor, Lindt*	1 Ball/12g	73	6.0	611	5.6	41.7	50.0	2.8
Truffle, Rum, Thorntons*	1 Chocolate/13g	63	3.2	485	4.8	58.5	24.6	4.8
Truffle, Seville, Thorntons*	1 Chocolate/14g	76	4.7	543	7.1	53.6	33.6	1.4
Truffle, Thorntons*	1 Chocolate/7g	33	1.9	471	6.0	48.6	27.1	1.4
Truffle, Vanilla, Thorntons*	1 Chocolate/13g	64	3.5	492	4.8	57.7	26.9	1.5
Truffle, Viennese, Dark, Thorntons*	1 Chocolate/10g	53	3.6	530	5.9	47.0	36.0	3.0
Truffle, Viennese, Milk, Thorntons*	1 Chocolate/10g	56	3.6	560	4.9	54.0	36.0	0.0
Truffle, White Chocolate, Balls, Lindor, Lindt*	1 Ball/12g	78	6.2	649	5.2	40.2	51.9	0.0
Truffles, Belgian Milk, Waitrose*	1 Truffle/14g	74	4.8	525	5.8	52.9	34.1	1.2
Truffles, Mini Milk Chocolate Balls, Lindor, Lindt*	3 Balls/15g	90	7.0	600	6.7	40.0	46.7	0.0
Truffles, Rum, Average	***1 Truffle/11g***	***57***	***3.7***	***521***	***6.1***	***49.7***	***33.7***	***1.9***
Twilight, Dark with Mint, Terry's*	1 Chocolate/6g	33	1.9	530	3.1	59.5	30.5	4.2
Valentine, Thorntons*	1 Chocolate/11g	60	3.8	542	5.7	52.0	34.5	2.1
Winter Selection, Thorntons*	1 Chocolate/10g	51	3.1	506	6.2	51.3	30.6	3.8

CHOP SUEY

Chicken with Noodles, Sainsbury's*	1 Pack/300g	300	7.5	100	5.7	13.6	2.5	1.2
Vegetable, M&S*	½ Pack/150g	90	6.1	60	2.0	3.1	4.1	2.9

	Measure INFO/WEIGHT	per Measure KCAL	FAT	Nutrition Values per 100g / 100ml KCAL	PROT	CARB	FAT	FIBRE
CHOW MEIN								
Beef, Ready Meal, Average	*1 Serving/400g*	*422*	*12.2*	*106*	*6.0*	*13.4*	*3.0*	*1.0*
Beef, Sainsbury's*	1 Pack/450g	500	11.2	111	6.6	15.5	2.5	0.8
Cantonese Vegetable Stir Fry, Sainsbury's*	¼ Pack/100g	85	3.8	85	2.2	10.6	3.8	1.2
Chicken & Vegetable, Fuller Longer, M&S*	1 Pack/380g	266	4.9	70	6.3	8.7	1.3	2.1
Chicken with Vegetable Spring Roll, Oriental Express*	1 Pack/300g	213	1.8	71	5.5	12.4	0.6	1.9
Chicken, Ainsley Harriott*	1 Serving/250g	447	11.8	179	14.0	21.2	4.7	2.0
Chicken, CBY, Asda*	1 Pack/400g	312	2.8	78	8.3	9.2	0.7	0.9
Chicken, Chinese Takeaway, Sainsbury's*	1 Pack/316g	338	8.5	107	9.1	11.6	2.7	0.7
Chicken, Chinese Takeaway, Tesco*	1 Serving/350g	294	8.4	84	8.1	7.5	2.4	1.1
Chicken, Chinese, CBY, Asda*	1 Pack/400g	479	20.4	120	6.7	11.0	5.1	1.5
Chicken, Chinese, Pot, My Goodness, Sainsbury's*	1 Pot/350g	287	4.9	82	4.2	12.0	1.4	2.0
Chicken, COOK!, M&S*	1 Pack/375g	356	7.9	95	7.9	10.5	2.1	1.7
Chicken, COU, M&S*	1 Pack/200g	170	5.4	85	5.9	9.5	2.7	1.4
Chicken, Less Than 3% Fat, BGTY, Sainsbury's*	1 Pack/400g	358	9.1	94	6.5	10.3	2.4	2.8
Chicken, Light Choices, Tesco*	1 Pack/400g	380	4.0	95	8.1	12.6	1.0	1.7
Chicken, Morrisons*	1 Pack/400g	368	9.2	92	5.8	13.0	2.3	1.1
Chicken, Ready Meal, Average	*1 Serving/400g*	*375*	*9.4*	*94*	*6.5*	*11.5*	*2.4*	*1.2*
Chicken, Ready Meal, Healthy Range, Average	*1 Serving/400g*	*329*	*8.5*	*82*	*5.9*	*9.9*	*2.1*	*1.3*
Chicken, Sainsbury's*	1 Pack/450g	558	21.2	124	6.5	12.6	4.7	2.6
Chicken, Waitrose*	1 Serving/400g	384	11.6	96	6.0	11.4	2.9	1.3
Seafood, M&S*	1 Pack/350g	354	10.9	101	6.9	10.6	3.1	1.5
Special, COU, M&S*	1 Pack/400g	400	15.2	100	6.6	10.3	3.8	1.4
Special, Ready Meal, Average	*1 Serving/400g*	*383*	*9.7*	*96*	*6.5*	*12.1*	*2.4*	*1.0*
Vegetable, Ready Meal, Average	*1 Serving/400g*	*337*	*6.7*	*84*	*4.2*	*12.8*	*1.7*	*2.0*
CHRISTMAS PUDDING								
Alcohol Free, 450g, Sainsbury's*	1 Serving/114g	330	3.5	290	2.7	61.3	3.1	3.2
Average	*1oz/28g*	*81*	*2.7*	*291*	*4.6*	*49.5*	*9.7*	*1.3*
Individual, Sainsbury's*	1 Pudding/100g	293	4.7	293	1.8	59.3	4.7	3.4
Luxury, Tesco*	¼ Pudding/114g	346	11.0	305	3.7	50.8	9.7	1.3
Matured, Finest, Tesco*	1 Serving/100g	353	13.4	353	4.6	51.4	13.4	2.0
Nut Free & Alcohol Free, HE, Tesco*	1 Serving/100g	258	2.7	258	2.8	55.6	2.7	4.3
Rich Fruit, Tesco*	1 Serving/114g	331	6.7	290	2.4	55.0	5.9	0.0
Sticky Toffee, Tesco*	¼ Pudding/114g	372	7.3	326	2.5	64.5	6.4	0.8
Ultimate, Finest, Tesco*	1 Serving/100g	285	7.0	285	3.7	51.6	7.0	4.7
Vintage, M&S*	1/8 Pudding/113g	335	6.4	295	2.6	59.8	5.6	1.4
VLH Kitchens	1 Serving/114g	310	2.2	272	3.1	59.3	2.5	4.6
CHUTNEY								
Albert's Victorian, Baxters*	1 Serving/25g	40	0.1	159	1.1	37.9	0.3	1.5
Apple & Pear, TTD, Sainsbury's*	1 Serving/20g	38	0.2	190	0.6	45.2	0.8	1.7
Apple & Walnut, Waitrose*	1 Serving/20g	49	0.5	243	12.0	53.8	2.6	3.8
Apple, Tomato & Sultana, Tesco*	1 Serving/50g	88	0.1	176	1.1	42.4	0.2	1.3
Apricot, Sharwood's*	1 Tsp/16g	21	0.0	131	0.6	32.0	0.1	2.3
Bengal Spice Mango, Sharwood's*	1 Tsp/5g	12	0.0	236	0.5	58.0	0.2	1.2
Caramelised Onion, Sainsbury's*	1 Serving/25g	28	0.4	111	1.1	23.5	1.4	1.1
Caramelised Onion, TTD, Sainsbury's*	1 Serving/20g	31	0.1	157	0.8	37.3	0.5	2.1
Caramelised Red Onion, Loyd Grossman*	1 Serving/10g	11	0.0	111	0.5	27.2	0.0	0.5
Cheese Board, Cottage Delight Ltd*	1 Tbsp/15g	42	0.5	277	1.0	46.6	3.1	0.0
Cranberry & Caramelised Red Onion, Baxters*	1 Serving/20g	31	0.0	154	0.3	38.0	0.1	0.3
Fruit, Spiced, Baxters*	1 Tsp/16g	23	0.0	143	6.0	34.8	0.1	0.0
Lime & Chilli, Geeta's*	1 Serving/25g	69	0.4	277	2.0	64.0	1.4	1.9
Mango & Chilli, Geeta's*	1 Serving/30g	74	0.0	246	0.5	60.7	0.1	0.2
Mango with Hint of Chilli & Ginger, Waitrose*	1 Serving/20g	52	0.0	259	0.5	64.2	0.0	0.7
Mango, Green Label, Sharwood's*	1 Tsp/10g	24	0.0	241	0.3	59.7	0.1	0.9

INFO/WEIGHT	Measure	per Measure KCAL	FAT	Nutrition Values per 100g / 100ml KCAL	PROT	CARB	FAT	FIBRE
CHUTNEY								
Mango, Hot & Spicy, Waitrose*	1 Serving/20g	46	0.1	230	0.6	51.6	0.3	1.8
Mango, Hot, Patak's*	1 Jar/340g	877	0.7	258	0.4	67.1	0.2	0.7
Mango, Indian Takeaway, Asda*	1 Pack/70g	145	0.1	207	0.3	50.9	0.2	1.0
Mango, Premium, Geeta's*	1 Serving/50g	126	0.1	253	0.8	62.0	0.2	0.8
Mango, Spicy, Sainsbury's*	1 Tbsp/15g	24	0.1	160	0.7	37.0	0.7	1.3
Mango, Sweet	**1 Heaped Tsp/16g**	**30**	**0.0**	**189**	**0.7**	**48.3**	**0.1**	**0.0**
Mango, Tesco*	1 Serving/20g	45	0.0	224	0.4	55.5	0.1	1.3
Mango, Waitrose*	1 Serving/20g	43	0.3	215	1.0	49.0	1.5	2.0
Mixed Fruit	**1 Heaped Tsp/16g**	**25**	**0.0**	**155**	**0.6**	**39.7**	**0.0**	**0.0**
Peach, Spicy, Waitrose*	1 Serving/20g	43	0.3	215	1.0	49.0	1.5	1.5
Ploughman's Plum, The English Provender Co.*	1 Tsp/10g	16	0.0	160	1.3	38.1	0.2	1.6
Sweet Mango, Patak's*	1 Tbsp/15g	39	0.0	259	0.3	67.4	0.1	0.7
Sweet Tomato & Chilli, The English Provender Co.*	1 Tea Spoon/10g	19	0.0	189	0.9	46.0	0.2	1.7
Tomato	**1 Heaped Tsp/16g**	**20**	**0.0**	**128**	**1.2**	**31.0**	**0.2**	**1.3**
Tomato & Chilli, Specially Selected, Aldi*	1 Tbsp/15g	21	0.1	138	12.0	32.0	0.5	1.3
Tomato & Red Pepper, Baxters*	1 Jar/312g	512	1.2	164	2.0	38.0	0.4	1.5
Tomato, Baxters*	1 Tsp/12g	18	0.0	152	1.1	35.9	0.4	1.0
Tomato, Waitrose*	1 Pot/100g	195	0.3	195	1.3	46.8	0.3	0.0
CIDER								
Berry, Irish, Magner's*	1 Bottle/500ml	215	0.0	43	0.0	4.3	0.0	0.0
Cyder, Organic, Aspall*	1 Serving/200ml	120	0.2	60	0.1	3.1	0.1	0.0
Cyder, Perronelle's Blush, Aspall*	1 Serving/200ml	122	0.2	61	0.1	5.4	0.1	0.5
Cyder, Premier Cru, Aspall*	1 Serving/200ml	120	0.0	60	0.1	3.1	0.0	0.0
Cyder, Suffolk, Medium, Aspall*	1 Serving/200ml	134	0.0	67	0.1	4.4	0.0	0.0
Dry, Average	**1 Pint/568ml**	**205**	**0.0**	**36**	**0.0**	**2.6**	**0.0**	**0.0**
Dry, Strongbow*	1 Bottle/375ml	161	0.0	43	0.0	3.4	0.0	0.0
Gold, Thatchers*	1 Bottle/500ml	230	0.0	46	0.0	4.5	0.0	0.0
Light, Bulmers*	1 Can/500ml	140	0.0	28	0.0	0.8	0.0	0.0
Low Alcohol	**1 Pint/568ml**	**97**	**0.0**	**17**	**0.0**	**3.6**	**0.0**	**0.0**
Low Alcohol, Sainsbury's*	1 Serving/200ml	62	0.0	31	0.0	6.4	0.0	0.0
Low Carb, Stowford*	1 Bottle/500ml	140	0.0	28	0.0	0.2	0.0	0.0
Magner's*	½ Pint/284ml	105	0.0	37	0.0	2.0	0.0	0.0
Organic, Westons*	1 Serving/200ml	96	0.0	48	0.0	3.1	0.0	0.0
Original, Bulmers*	1 Serving/250ml	105	0.0	42	0.0	4.0	0.0	0.0
Original, Gaymers*	1 Bottle/330ml	148	0.0	45	0.0	4.7	0.0	0.0
Pear, Average	**1 Serving/200ml**	**86**	**0.0**	**43**	**0.0**	**3.6**	**0.0**	**0.0**
Pear, Bulmers*	1 Serving/200ml	86	0.0	43	0.0	3.6	0.0	0.0
Pear, Magner's*	1 Bottle/568ml	179	0.0	32	0.0	0.0	0.0	0.0
Pear, Non Alcoholic, Kopparberg*	1 Bottle/500ml	170	0.5	34	0.0	8.4	0.1	0.0
Scrumpy, Average	**1 Serving/200ml**	**93**	**0.0**	**46**	**0.0**	**2.3**	**0.0**	**0.0**
Scrumpy, Westons*	1 Serving/200ml	94	0.0	47	0.0	1.8	0.0	0.0
Sweet, Average	**1 Pint/568ml**	**239**	**0.0**	**42**	**0.0**	**4.3**	**0.0**	**0.0**
Vintage	**1 Pint/568ml**	**574**	**0.0**	**101**	**0.0**	**7.3**	**0.0**	**0.0**
CINNAMON								
Ground, Average	**1 Tsp/3g**	**8**	**0.1**	**261**	**3.9**	**55.5**	**3.2**	**0.0**
CLAMS								
in Brine, Average	**1oz/28g**	**22**	**0.2**	**79**	**16.0**	**2.4**	**0.6**	**0.0**
Raw, Average	**20 Sm/180g**	**133**	**1.7**	**74**	**12.8**	**2.6**	**1.0**	**0.0**
CLEMENTINES								
Easy Peel, Value, Tesco*	2 Clementine/142g	55	0.1	39	0.9	8.6	0.1	1.3
Raw, Weighed with Peel, Average	**1 Med/61g**	**22**	**0.1**	**35**	**0.6**	**9.0**	**0.1**	**1.3**
Raw, Weighed without Peel, Average	**1 Med/46g**	**22**	**0.1**	**47**	**0.8**	**12.0**	**0.2**	**1.7**
Sweet, TTD, Sainsbury's*	1 Serving/100g	37	0.1	37	0.9	8.7	0.1	1.2

	Measure INFO/WEIGHT	per Measure KCAL	FAT	Nutrition Values per 100g / 100ml KCAL	PROT	CARB	FAT	FIBRE
COCKLES								
Boiled	*1 Cockle/4g*	*2*	*0.0*	*53*	*12.0*	*0.0*	*0.6*	*0.0*
Bottled in Vinegar, Drained	*1oz/28g*	*8*	*0.1*	*28*	*6.3*	*0.0*	*0.3*	*0.0*
COCKTAIL								
Alcoholic, Juice Based, Average	*1 Glass/200ml*	*464*	*29.2*	*232*	*6.4*	*18.7*	*14.6*	*1.4*
Bloody Mary, Average	*1 Glass/250ml*	*86*	*0.0*	*42*	*0.0*	*2.3*	*0.0*	*0.6*
Bucks Fizz, Premixed, M&S*	1 Glass/250ml	152	0.0	61	0.0	9.0	0.0	0.0
Cosmopolitan, Canned, M&S*	1 Serving/200ml	456	0.0	228	0.0	22.0	0.0	0.0
Daiquiri, Strawberry, Frozen, Average	*1 Glass/250ml*	*132*	*0.0*	*53*	*0.0*	*14.1*	*0.0*	*0.0*
Grenadine, Orange Juice, Pineapple Juice	1 Serving/200ml	158	0.3	79	0.5	19.2	0.1	0.2
Long Island Iced Tea, Average	*1 Glass/250ml*	*282*	*0.0*	*113*	*0.0*	*13.6*	*0.0*	*0.0*
Mai Tai, Average	*1 Serving/200ml*	*209*	*0.1*	*105*	*0.2*	*13.9*	*0.1*	*0.1*
Pina Colada	1 Glass/250ml	592	20.0	237	1.0	28.0	8.0	0.0
COCOA								
Nibs, Naturya*	1 Serving/10g	58	5.0	578	13.0	18.2	50.3	13.4
COCOA POWDER								
Cadbury*	1 Tbsp/16g	52	3.3	322	23.1	10.5	20.8	0.0
Dry, Unsweetened, Average	*1 Tbsp/5g*	*11*	*0.7*	*229*	*19.6*	*54.3*	*13.7*	*33.2*
Organic, Green & Black's*	1 Tsp/4g	16	0.8	405	22.0	19.0	21.0	27.0
COCONUT								
Chips, Caramel, Navitas Naturals*	1 Pack/57g	377	31.4	662	6.3	35.0	55.0	14.0
Chips, Organic, Infinity Foods*	1 Serving/100g	604	62.0	604	5.6	6.4	62.0	13.7
Creamed, Average	*1oz/28g*	*186*	*19.2*	*666*	*6.0*	*6.7*	*68.4*	*7.0*
Desiccated, Average	*1oz/28g*	*169*	*17.4*	*604*	*5.6*	*6.4*	*62.0*	*13.7*
Fresh, Flesh Only, Average	*1oz/28g*	*69*	*7.1*	*246*	*2.2*	*2.6*	*25.2*	*5.1*
Ice, Average	*1oz/28g*	*104*	*3.6*	*371*	*1.7*	*66.7*	*12.7*	*2.6*
Milk, Average	*1 Can/400ml*	*698*	*69.7*	*174*	*1.4*	*2.9*	*17.4*	*2.9*
Milk, Cuisine, Alpro*	1 Serving/40g	40	3.5	100	1.2	2.3	8.8	0.0
Milk, Half Fat, Waitrose*	½ Can/135ml	92	8.1	68	0.7	2.7	6.0	0.0
Milk, KTC*	1 Can/400g	776	73.2	194	0.9	1.2	18.3	0.0
Milk, Lighter, Sainsbury's*	¼ Can/100ml	75	6.5	75	0.9	2.9	6.5	0.5
Milk, Organic, Tesco*	1/8 Can/49g	85	8.3	175	1.8	2.7	17.0	1.3
Milk, Reduced Fat, Amoy*	1 Tin/400ml	440	44.0	110	1.0	2.0	11.0	1.0
Milk, Reduced Fat, Average	*1 Serving/100g*	*104*	*10.0*	*104*	*1.0*	*2.4*	*10.0*	*0.4*
Milk, Reduced Fat, Canned, Essential, Waitrose*	1 Can/400ml	244	24.0	61	0.0	1.8	6.0	0.0
Water with Pineapple, Vita Coco*	1 Carton/330ml	82	0.0	25	0.0	6.0	0.0	0.0
Water, Pret Pure, Pret a Manger*	1 Serving/330ml	63	0.0	19	0.0	4.8	0.0	0.0
COD								
Bake, with Crab & Potato, Finest, Tesco*	1 Pack/364g	312	10.9	86	6.9	7.3	3.0	1.0
Baked, Average	*1oz/28g*	*27*	*0.3*	*96*	*21.4*	*0.0*	*1.2*	*0.0*
Beer Battered, Crispy, Finest, Tesco*	1 Portion/250g	575	35.0	230	12.0	13.4	14.0	1.3
Bites & Chips, 573, Wiltshire Farm Foods*	1 Portion/310g	433	12.1	140	6.2	19.0	3.9	0.0
Dried, Salted, Average	*1oz/28g*	*82*	*0.7*	*290*	*62.8*	*0.0*	*2.4*	*0.0*
Dried, Salted, Boiled, Average	*1oz/28g*	*32*	*0.2*	*115*	*27.0*	*0.0*	*0.7*	*0.0*
Fillets, Battered, Average	*1 Fillet/125g*	*219*	*10.2*	*176*	*12.6*	*13.0*	*8.2*	*1.0*
Fillets, Battered, Harry Ramsdens, Birds Eye*	1 Fillet/122g	310	18.8	254	11.4	17.2	15.4	0.6
Fillets, Battered, Large, Frozen, Chip Shop, Youngs*	1 Fillet/120g	269	17.5	224	10.4	12.7	14.6	2.6
Fillets, Breaded, Average	*1 Fillet/125g*	*258*	*12.2*	*206*	*13.0*	*16.7*	*9.8*	*1.0*
Fillets, Breaded, BGTY, Sainsbury's*	1 Fillet/110g	172	2.5	156	16.6	16.4	2.3	1.9
Fillets, Breaded, Chunky, Average	*1 Piece/135g*	*204*	*8.0*	*151*	*13.7*	*10.9*	*5.9*	*1.4*
Fillets, Breaded, Chunky, Prime, HL, Tesco*	1 Fillet/125g	162	3.1	130	12.9	12.8	2.5	0.7
Fillets, Breaded, Light, Healthy Range, Average	*1 Fillet/135g*	*209*	*6.9*	*154*	*13.6*	*13.3*	*5.1*	*1.2*
Fillets, Chunky, Average	*1 Fillet/198g*	*267*	*7.3*	*135*	*17.1*	*8.2*	*3.7*	*0.8*
Fillets, Freshly Breaded, Waitrose*	1 Fillet/220g	409	20.0	186	9.1	11.5	9.1	0.8

	Measure INFO/WEIGHT	per Measure KCAL	FAT	Nutrition Values per 100g / 100ml KCAL	PROT	CARB	FAT	FIBRE
COD								
Fillets, Lemon & Black Pepper, Inspirations, Birds Eye*	1 Portion/113g	231	11.3	204	14.0	14.0	10.0	0.8
Fillets, Lightly Dusted Seeded, Gastro, Youngs*	1 Fillet/106g	209	10.1	198	14.4	13.1	9.6	0.6
Fillets, Lightly Dusted, Garlic & Herb Crumb, Birds Eye*	1 Fillet/113g	240	12.0	212	14.2	14.2	10.6	0.8
Fillets, Olive Oil, Rosemary & Tomato, Birds Eye*	1 Fillet/140g	190	10.9	131	14.9	0.9	7.5	0.0
Fillets, Portions, Large, Battered, Morrisons*	1 Fillet/118g	219	11.9	186	9.6	14.1	10.1	1.3
Fillets, Skinless & Boneless, Raw, Average	**1 Fillet/140g**	**137**	**2.4**	**98**	**17.8**	**0.0**	**1.8**	**0.4**
Fillets, Smoked, Average	**1 Serving/150g**	**152**	**2.4**	**101**	**21.6**	**0.0**	**1.6**	**0.0**
Fillets, Strips, in Sweet Chilli, Crispy Crumb, Youngs*	½ Pack/121g	282	12.2	233	13.0	21.8	10.1	1.4
Fillets, with Cheddar Cheese & Chive Sauce, Tesco*	1 Pack/400g	520	22.0	130	14.3	4.4	5.5	0.6
Fillets, with Tomato & Basil Sauce, Simply Bake, Tesco*	1 Fillet/142g	170	8.1	120	15.2	1.8	5.7	0.1
Fillets,Beer Battered, Gastro, Youngs*	1 Fillet/119g	232	10.7	195	13.6	14.4	9.0	1.1
Loin, Skinless, TTD, Sainsbury's*	1 Serving/100g	83	0.9	83	18.6	0.0	0.9	0.0
Loins, Average	**1 Serving/145g**	**116**	**1.2**	**80**	**17.9**	**0.1**	**0.8**	**0.2**
Loins, Beer Battered, TTD, Sainsbury's*	1 Fillet/93g	182	10.8	196	14.4	8.5	11.6	2.7
Loins, in Sundried Tomato & Garlic Sauce, Gastro, Youngs*	1 Serving/134g	135	4.9	101	16.1	0.7	3.7	0.4
Loins, Steaks, Skinless & Boneless, TTD, Sainsbury's*	1 Steak/100g	105	0.4	105	25.2	0.1	0.4	0.1
Loins, with a Sicilian Lemon & Herb Sauce, Gastro, Youngs*	1 Bag/135g	126	4.1	93	16.2	0.1	3.0	0.4
Mornay, Nutritionally Balanced, M&S*	1 Pack/400g	320	10.4	80	6.8	7.2	2.6	1.6
Mornay, Sainsbury's*	1 Serving/180g	277	16.9	154	15.2	2.2	9.4	0.9
Poached, Average	**1oz/28g**	**26**	**0.3**	**94**	**20.9**	**0.0**	**1.1**	**0.0**
Smoked, Raw, Average	**1oz/28g**	**22**	**0.2**	**78**	**18.1**	**0.0**	**0.6**	**0.0**
Spinach & Cheese, Gratin, Gastro, Youngs*	1 Pack/325g	475	23.1	146	7.4	12.3	7.1	1.4
Steaks, Battered, Chip Shop Style, Average	**1 Serving/150g**	**321**	**18.0**	**214**	**12.5**	**14.3**	**12.0**	**1.1**
Steamed, Average	**1oz/28g**	**23**	**0.3**	**83**	**18.6**	**0.0**	**0.9**	**0.0**
COD & CHIPS								
& Peas, 240, Oakhouse Foods Ltd*	1 Meal/300g	510	18.6	170	6.4	22.3	6.2	2.2
Asda*	1 Serving/280g	450	14.0	161	8.0	21.0	5.0	1.1
Chunky, M&S*	1 Serving/340g	510	20.4	150	6.5	17.5	6.0	1.5
COD IN								
a Sweet Red Pepper Sauce, Fillets, GFY, Asda*	½ Pack/170g	143	2.7	84	15.0	2.3	1.6	0.1
Butter Sauce, Sainsbury's*	1 Serving/170g	224	15.3	132	10.6	2.0	9.0	0.1
Butter Sauce, Steaks, Birds Eye*	1 Pack/170g	185	9.4	109	9.8	5.0	5.5	0.1
Butter Sauce, Steaks, Frozen, Asda*	1 Pouch/152g	163	4.0	107	16.0	5.0	2.6	0.8
Butter Sauce, Steaks, Morrisons*	1 Steak/170g	153	5.6	90	10.9	4.1	3.3	0.4
Butter Sauce, Steaks, Youngs*	1 Pack/139g	107	3.2	77	9.7	4.1	2.3	0.4
Butter Sauce, Tesco*	1 Pack/150g	123	5.4	82	9.4	2.9	3.6	0.5
Cheese Sauce, Steaks, Birds Eye*	1 Pack/182g	175	6.4	96	10.9	5.2	3.5	0.1
Mushroom Sauce, BGTY, Sainsbury's*	1 Serving/170g	112	2.9	66	9.9	2.8	1.7	0.1
Parsley Sauce, Frozen, M&S*	1 Pack/184g	156	7.2	85	11.1	1.9	3.9	1.0
Parsley Sauce, Pre Packed, Average	**1 Serving/150g**	**123**	**4.7**	**82**	**10.1**	**3.3**	**3.1**	**0.5**
Parsley Sauce, Steaks, Birds Eye*	1 Steak/172g	155	4.8	90	10.5	5.6	2.8	0.1
COD MEDITERRANEAN								
Style, Fillets, GFY, Asda*	1 Pack/397g	274	9.9	69	9.0	2.5	2.5	0.9
COD WITH								
Fish Pesto, Fillets, COOK!, M&S*	½ Pack/165g	210	5.1	127	16.4	8.4	3.1	4.2
Roasted Vegetables, M&S*	1 Serving/280g	238	10.6	85	8.0	4.9	3.8	1.7
Salsa & Rosemary Potatoes, BGTY, Sainsbury's*	1 Pack/450g	356	4.0	79	4.7	13.1	0.9	1.6
Tomato Sauce, Fillets, Asda*	1 Serving/181g	210	10.9	116	13.0	2.6	6.0	2.3
COFFEE								
& Chicory, Breakfast Drink, Ricore, Nestle*	1 Tsp/5g	7	0.0	141	2.7	9.1	0.0	45.3
Azera, Barista Style Instant, Nescafe*	1 Serving/200ml	2	0.0	1	0.1	0.0	0.0	0.0
Black, Average	**1 Mug/270ml**	**5**	**0.0**	**2**	**0.2**	**0.3**	**0.0**	**0.0**
Cafe Caramel, Cafe Range, Nescafe*	1 Sachet/17g	72	2.4	423	9.2	64.6	14.1	1.3

COFFEE

INFO/WEIGHT	Measure	per Measure KCAL	FAT	Nutrition Values per 100g / 100ml KCAL	PROT	CARB	FAT	FIBRE
Cafe Hazelnut, Nescafe*	1 Sachet/17g	73	2.4	428	9.3	66.0	14.1	0.0
Cafe Irish Cream, Cafe Range, Nescafe*	1 Sachet/23g	98	3.2	425	8.2	65.2	14.1	1.2
Cafe Latte, Dry, Douwe Egberts*	1 Serving/12g	58	2.6	480	10.0	60.0	22.0	0.0
Cafe Latte, Instant, Made Up, Maxwell House*	1 Serving/13g	53	1.7	424	6.4	68.0	13.6	0.0
Cafe Mocha, Cafe Range, Nescafe*	1 Sachet/22g	92	2.9	418	8.5	66.6	13.1	0.0
Cafe Vanilla, Latte, Cafe Range, Nescafe*	1 Sachet/19g	73	1.6	395	9.2	68.3	8.5	4.1
Cappuccino Ice, Made Up, Dolce Gusto, Nescafe*	1 Serving/240ml	111	2.8	46	1.8	7.2	1.2	0.2
Cappuccino, Cafe Mocha, Dry, Maxwell House*	1 Serving/23g	100	2.5	434	4.3	78.2	10.8	0.0
Cappuccino, Cappio, Kenco*	1 Sachet/18g	79	1.9	439	11.7	73.9	10.6	0.6
Cappuccino, Caramel, Full Fat Milk, Medio, Costa*	1 Medio/363ml	243	10.9	67	3.0	7.2	3.0	0.0
Cappuccino, Decaff, Instant, Made Up, Nescafe*	1 Mug/200ml	68	2.3	34	1.0	5.0	1.2	0.0
Cappuccino, Decaff, Nescafe*	1 Sachet/16g	68	2.3	428	11.6	62.6	14.6	0.0
Cappuccino, Decaff, Unsweetened, Nescafe*	1 Sachet/16g	70	3.1	437	14.5	51.2	19.4	4.3
Cappuccino, Dry, Maxwell House*	1 Mug/15g	52	1.4	350	12.0	64.0	9.6	0.4
Cappuccino, Dry, Waitrose*	1 Sachet/13g	58	2.3	439	15.1	56.0	17.2	4.4
Cappuccino, Iced, Cowbelle, Aldi*	1 Serving/250ml	169	4.5	68	3.3	9.6	1.8	0.3
Cappuccino, Instant, Aldi*	1 Sachet/13g	49	1.7	393	12.5	55.1	13.6	0.0
Cappuccino, Instant, Asda*	1 Sachet/15g	60	2.3	399	13.0	53.0	15.2	0.9
Cappuccino, Instant, Made Up, Maxwell House*	1 Serving/280g	123	5.3	44	0.6	5.8	1.9	0.0
Cappuccino, Italian, Nescafe*	1 Cup/150ml	60	2.9	40	1.2	4.4	1.9	0.0
Cappuccino, M&S*	1 Serving/164g	66	2.6	40	1.5	4.4	1.6	0.0
Cappuccino, Made Up, Dolce Gusto, Nescafe*	1 Serving/240ml	84	3.7	35	1.6	4.0	1.5	0.3
Cappuccino, Original, Sachets, Nescafe*	1 Sachet/18g	80	3.1	444	11.7	60.3	17.4	0.0
Cappuccino, Semi Skimmed Milk, Average	***1 Serving/200ml***	***63***	***2.3***	***31***	***2.2***	***3.2***	***1.2***	***0.0***
Cappuccino, Unsweetened Taste, Maxwell House*	1 Serving/15g	65	2.9	434	17.4	47.6	19.3	0.3
Cappuccino, Unsweetened, Nescafe*	1 Sachet/16g	74	3.8	464	15.0	47.3	23.8	0.0
Chococino, Made Up, Dolce Gusto, Nescafe*	1 Serving/210g	147	5.4	70	2.3	9.4	2.6	0.7
Compliment*	1 Serving/14ml	20	1.8	143	1.4	6.4	12.9	0.0
Dandelion, Symingtons*	1 Rounded Tsp/6g	19	0.0	320	2.8	79.3	0.0	0.0
Double Choca Mocha, Cafe Range, Nescafe*	1 Sachet/23g	94	2.5	408	9.2	68.0	11.0	2.8
Espresso, Instant, Nescafe*	1 Tsp/2g	2	0.0	118	7.8	3.1	0.2	34.1
Espresso, Made Up, Dolce Gusto, Nescafe*	1 Serving/60ml	1	0.1	2	0.1	0.0	0.2	0.3
Gold Blend, Decafefinated, Nescafe*	1 Tsp/5g	3	0.0	63	7.0	9.0	0.2	27.0
Gold Blend, Nescafe*	1 Cup 200ml/5g	3	0.0	63	7.0	9.0	0.2	27.0
Infusion, Average with Semi-Skimmed Milk	***1 Cup/220ml***	***15***	***0.4***	***7***	***0.6***	***0.7***	***0.2***	***0.0***
Infusion, Average with Single Cream	***1 Cup/220ml***	***31***	***2.6***	***14***	***0.4***	***0.3***	***1.2***	***0.0***
Infusion, Average with Whole Milk	***1 Cup/220ml***	***15***	***0.9***	***7***	***0.5***	***0.5***	***0.4***	***0.0***
Instant, Alta Rica, Nescafe*	1 Tsp/2g	2	0.0	98	13.8	10.0	0.3	21.0
Instant, Decaffeinated, Nescafe*	1 Tsp/2g	2	0.0	101	14.9	10.0	0.2	8.4
Instant, Made with Skimmed Milk	1 Serving/270ml	15	0.0	6	0.6	0.8	0.0	0.0
Instant, Made with Water & Semi-Skimmed Milk	1 Serving/350ml	24	1.4	7	0.4	0.5	0.4	0.0
Instant, Original, Nescafe*	1 Tsp/2g	1	0.0	63	7.0	9.0	0.2	27.0
Instant, with Skimmed Milk, Costa Rican, Kenco*	1 Mug/300ml	17	0.1	6	0.6	0.8	0.0	0.0
Latte Macchiato, Made Up, Dolce Gusto, Nescafe*	1 Serving/220g	89	4.2	40	2.0	4.1	1.9	0.3
Latte, Cafe, M&S*	1 Serving/190g	142	5.3	75	4.3	8.3	2.8	0.0
Latte, Macchiato, Tassimo*	1 Cup/275ml	135	7.7	49	2.3	3.6	2.8	0.0
Latte, Nescafe*	1 Sachet/22g	110	6.3	498	14.5	45.7	28.5	0.0
Latte, No Sugar, in Cup, From Machine, Kenco*	1 Cup/4g	17	0.9	400	7.6	44.0	22.0	0.0
Latte, Skinny, Nescafe*	1 Sachet/20g	72	1.1	359	24.1	54.3	5.3	1.1
Mocha Chocolate Frappuccino, Bottle, Starbucks*	1 Bottle/250ml	160	3.0	64	2.9	10.0	1.2	0.0
Mocha, Made Up, Dolce Gusto, Nescafe*	1 Serving/210g	117	5.1	56	2.4	6.1	2.4	0.6
Skinny Cappuccino, Made Up, Dolce Gusto, Nescafe*	1 Mug/15g	49	0.1	337	33.3	48.8	0.9	2.3

	Measure INFO/WEIGHT	per Measure KCAL	FAT	Nutrition Values per 100g / 100ml KCAL	PROT	CARB	FAT	FIBRE
COFFEE SUBSTITUTE								
Bambu, Vogel*	1 Tsp/3g	10	0.0	320	3.5	75.3	0.5	0.0
COFFEE WHITENER								
Light, Tesco*	1 Tsp/3g	13	0.4	429	0.9	77.7	12.7	0.0
Original, Coffee Mate, Nestle*	1 Tsp/4g	19	1.2	547	2.4	56.7	34.4	0.0
Tesco*	1 Tsp/3g	16	0.9	533	1.2	61.3	31.4	0.0
Virtually Fat Free, Coffee Mate, Nestle*	1 Tsp/5g	10	0.2	200	1.0	42.0	3.0	0.0
COGNAC								
40% Volume	**1 Pub Shot/35ml**	**78**	**0.0**	**222**	**0.0**	**0.0**	**0.0**	**0.0**
COLA								
Average	**1 Can/330ml**	**135**	**0.0**	**41**	**0.0**	**10.9**	**0.0**	**0.0**
Coke with Lemon, Diet, Coca-Cola*	1 Can/330ml	5	0.0	1	0.0	0.0	0.0	0.0
Coke, Cherry, Coca-Cola*	1 Bottle/500ml	225	0.0	45	0.0	11.2	0.0	0.0
Coke, Cherry, Zero, Coca-Cola*	1 Can/330ml	1	0.0	0	0.0	0.0	0.0	0.0
Coke, Coca-Cola*	1 Can/330ml	142	0.0	43	0.0	10.7	0.0	0.0
Coke, Diet with Cherry, Coca-Cola*	1 Bottle/500ml	5	0.0	1	0.0	0.0	0.0	0.0
Coke, Diet, Caffeine Free, Coca-Cola*	1 Can/330ml	1	0.0	0	0.0	0.1	0.0	0.0
Coke, Diet, Coca-Cola*	1 Can/330ml	1	0.0	0	0.0	0.0	0.0	0.0
Coke, Vanilla, Coca-Cola*	1 Bottle/500ml	215	0.0	43	0.0	10.7	0.0	0.0
Curiosity, Fentiman's*	1 Bottle/275ml	129	0.0	47	0.1	11.6	0.0	0.0
Diet, Asda*	1 Serving/200ml	0	0.0	0	0.0	0.0	0.0	0.0
Diet, Average	**1 Serving/200ml**	**1**	**0.0**	**1**	**0.0**	**0.0**	**0.0**	**0.0**
Diet, Basics, Sainsbury's*	1 Glass/250ml	3	0.0	1	0.0	0.2	0.0	0.0
Diet, Classic, Sainsbury's*	1 Can/330ml	1	0.0	0	0.0	0.0	0.0	0.0
Diet, Just, Asda*	1 Bottle/250ml	0	0.0	0	0.0	0.0	0.0	0.0
Diet, M&S*	1 Can/330ml	3	0.0	1	0.0	0.3	0.0	0.0
Diet, Morrisons*	1 Glass/250ml	2	0.0	1	0.0	0.0	0.0	0.0
Diet, Pepsi*	1 Can/330ml	1	0.0	0	0.0	0.0	0.0	0.0
Diet, Tesco*	1 Glass/200ml	2	0.2	1	0.1	0.1	0.1	0.0
Max, Pepsi*	1 Can/330ml	1	0.0	0	0.0	0.0	0.0	0.0
Pepsi*	1 Can/330ml	135	0.0	41	0.0	11.0	0.0	0.0
Tesco*	1 Can/330ml	145	0.0	44	0.0	10.8	0.0	0.0
Twist, Light, Pepsi*	1 Bottle/500ml	4	0.0	1	0.0	0.1	0.0	0.0
Zero, Caffeine Free, Coca-Cola*	1 Glass/200ml	0	0.0	0	0.0	0.0	0.0	0.0
Zero, Coca-Cola*	1 Can/330ml	2	0.0	0	0.0	0.0	0.0	0.0
COLESLAW								
20% Less Fat, Asda*	1 Serving/100g	88	6.0	88	1.5	7.0	6.0	1.7
99% Fat Free, Kraft*	1 Serving/40ml	50	0.4	126	1.0	28.9	1.0	0.0
Aldi*	1 Serving/100g	206	18.7	206	0.8	8.6	18.7	0.0
Apple, Raisin & Walnut, TTD, Sainsbury's*	2 Heap Tbsp/75g	212	19.6	283	2.3	8.0	26.2	2.8
Asda*	1 Serving/100g	190	18.0	190	1.0	6.0	18.0	1.4
Basics, Sainsbury's*	1 Serving/25g	27	2.4	107	1.0	3.7	9.8	1.6
Budgens*	1 Serving/50g	103	9.0	206	1.2	9.5	18.1	2.0
Cheese, Asda*	1 Serving/100g	242	22.0	242	4.8	6.3	22.0	1.6
Cheese, Co-Op*	1 Serving/125g	344	31.2	275	6.0	6.0	25.0	1.0
Cheese, Deli Style, Waitrose*	¼ Tub/75g	247	24.3	330	3.8	5.1	32.5	0.9
Cheese, M&S*	1 Serving/57g	185	19.1	325	4.2	2.0	33.5	1.7
Cheese, Sainsbury's*	1 Serving/75g	184	16.8	246	3.8	6.5	22.4	1.4
Cheese, Supreme, Waitrose*	¼ Pack/88g	197	18.2	225	4.5	5.0	20.8	1.2
Cheese, TTD, Sainsbury's*	¼ Pot/75g	213	20.4	284	5.0	4.7	27.2	2.7
Cheese, West Country Cheddar, TTD, Sainsbury's*	1 Tub/300g	852	81.6	284	5.0	4.7	27.2	2.7
Coronation, Sainsbury's*	¼ Pot/75g	145	11.6	193	1.0	11.4	15.5	1.9
COU, M&S*	½ Pack/125g	75	3.4	60	1.3	7.4	2.7	1.7
Creamy, Asda*	1 Serving/25g	62	6.0	248	0.9	7.0	24.0	1.8

INFO/WEIGHT	Measure	per Measure		Nutrition Values per 100g / 100ml				
		KCAL	FAT	KCAL	PROT	CARB	FAT	FIBRE
COLESLAW								
Creamy, GFY, Asda*	1 Serving/100g	163	14.9	163	0.7	6.5	14.9	0.8
Creamy, Light Choices, Tesco*	1/3 Pot/100g	105	8.8	105	1.2	4.9	8.8	1.6
Creamy, Morrisons*	1 Serving/40g	111	11.1	277	1.1	5.5	27.7	1.3
Creamy, Tesco*	1 Serving/75g	142	13.4	190	1.0	5.5	17.8	1.5
Crunchy, Premium, Millcroft*	1 Pack/400g	756	69.6	189	0.9	7.3	17.4	1.5
Deli Style, BGTY, Sainsbury's*	1 Serving/75g	75	5.6	100	1.1	6.2	7.5	1.7
Deli Style, M&S*	1 Serving/50g	110	10.6	220	1.0	4.8	21.2	1.9
Deli Style, Sainsbury's*	½ Pot/150g	267	25.5	178	0.8	5.4	17.0	1.5
Essential, Waitrose*	¼ Pot/75g	206	20.4	275	1.1	5.8	27.2	1.1
Finest, Tesco*	1 Serving/51g	145	15.0	285	0.8	4.1	29.4	1.3
Fruity, Asda*	½ Pot/125g	101	6.1	81	1.3	8.0	4.9	1.7
Fruity, M&S*	1 Serving/63g	151	14.3	240	1.1	8.3	22.7	3.1
Half Fat, Waitrose*	1 Serving/100g	38	2.7	38	0.6	2.9	2.7	1.2
Iceland*	1 Serving/110g	112	8.2	102	0.7	7.8	7.5	1.6
Jalapeno, Sainsbury's*	1 Serving/75g	142	13.4	190	0.9	5.6	17.9	1.6
Less Than 5% Fat, Side Salad, M&S*	1 Serving/80g	44	3.4	55	1.0	3.4	4.2	3.9
Light, Reduced Fat, Morrisons*	1 Serving/30g	38	3.1	125	0.8	7.4	10.2	0.0
Luxury, Asda*	1 Serving/50g	108	10.5	217	0.9	6.0	21.0	0.0
Luxury, Lidl*	1 Serving/50g	102	9.7	203	0.9	5.9	19.4	0.0
Luxury, Morrisons*	1 Serving/50g	136	13.5	273	1.2	6.4	27.0	0.0
Mango & Chilli, Sainsbury's*	1 Serving/75g	97	7.7	129	0.9	7.2	10.3	1.8
Piri Piri, Sainsbury's*	½ Tub/70g	113	9.9	162	1.1	6.6	14.2	1.8
Prawn, CBY, Asda*	1 Pot/280g	490	43.1	175	2.2	6.8	15.4	1.8
Premium, Co-Op*	1 Serving/50g	160	17.0	320	1.0	3.0	34.0	2.0
Reduced Calorie, Budgens*	½ Pot/125g	124	8.6	99	1.0	8.3	6.9	2.3
Reduced Calorie, Iceland*	1 Serving/50g	51	3.8	102	0.7	7.8	7.5	1.6
Reduced Fat, Asda*	1 Pot/250g	218	15.8	87	1.5	6.0	6.3	1.6
Reduced Fat, Average	**1 Tbsp/20g**	**23**	**1.9**	**113**	**1.0**	**6.4**	**9.3**	**2.0**
Reduced Fat, Co-Op*	1 Serving/50g	45	3.5	90	0.9	6.0	7.0	2.0
Reduced Fat, Creamy, Morrisons*	1 Portion/100g	163	14.5	163	1.3	7.2	14.5	1.7
Reduced Fat, Essential, Waitrose*	1/6 Tub/50g	65	5.1	130	1.2	8.3	10.2	1.6
Reduced Fat, Healthy Living, Co-Op*	1 Serving/50g	48	3.5	95	0.8	8.0	7.0	2.0
Reduced Fat, M&S*	½ Tub/112g	230	22.4	205	1.1	5.4	20.0	2.8
Tesco*	1 Serving/50g	79	7.2	158	2.2	5.2	14.3	1.6
Three Cheese, Finest, Tesco*	1/3 Pack/100g	255	22.7	255	6.4	5.8	22.7	1.1
TTD, Sainsbury's*	¼ Pot/75g	179	17.2	238	1.2	6.0	22.9	1.6
with 60% Less Fat, GFY, Asda*	1 Serving/41g	36	2.5	88	1.5	7.0	6.0	1.7
with Reduced Calorie Dressing, Retail	1 Serving/40g	27	1.8	67	0.9	6.1	4.5	1.4
COLESLAW MIX								
Average	**1oz/28g**	**8**	**0.2**	**30**	**0.8**	**4.9**	**0.8**	**2.0**
COLEY								
Portions, Raw, Average	**1 Serving/92g**	**65**	**0.6**	**71**	**15.9**	**0.0**	**0.6**	**0.0**
Steamed, Average	**1oz/28g**	**29**	**0.4**	**105**	**23.3**	**0.0**	**1.3**	**0.0**
CONCHIGLIE								
Cooked, Average	**1 Serving/185g**	**247**	**1.6**	**134**	**4.8**	**26.6**	**0.8**	**0.6**
Dry Weight, Average	**1 Serving/100g**	**352**	**1.7**	**352**	**12.5**	**71.6**	**1.7**	**2.6**
Shells, Dry, Average	**1 Serving/100g**	**346**	**1.5**	**346**	**12.3**	**70.4**	**1.5**	**3.0**
Whole Wheat, Dry Weight, Average	**1 Serving/75g**	**237**	**1.5**	**316**	**12.6**	**62.0**	**2.0**	**10.7**
CONCHIGLIONI								
Dry, Waitrose*	1 Serving/75g	256	1.0	341	12.5	69.8	1.3	3.7
CONSERVE								
Apricot, Average	**1 Tbsp/15g**	**37**	**0.0**	**244**	**0.5**	**59.3**	**0.2**	**1.5**
Apricot, Reduced Sugar, Streamline*	1 Tbsp/20g	37	0.0	184	0.5	45.0	0.2	0.0

C

CONSERVE

Apricot, TTD, Sainsbury's*	1 Tbsp/15g	43	0.0	285	0.4	70.5	0.1	0.5
Blackcurrant, Average	*1 Tbsp/15g*	*37*	*0.0*	*245*	*0.6*	*60.0*	*0.1*	*1.9*
Morello Cherry, Waitrose*	1 Tbsp/15g	39	0.0	258	0.4	64.2	0.0	1.4
Plum, TTD, Sainsbury's*	1 Tbsp/15g	44	0.0	295	0.3	73.1	0.1	0.5
Raspberry, Average	*1 Tbsp/15g*	*37*	*0.1*	*249*	*0.6*	*61.0*	*0.3*	*1.3*
Raspberry, TTD, Sainsbury's*	1 Serving/15g	43	0.0	290	0.7	71.5	0.1	0.5
Red Cherry, TTD, Sainsbury's*	1 Tbsp/15g	43	0.0	283	0.4	70.2	0.1	0.5
Rhubarb & Ginger, M&S*	1 Tbsp/15g	29	0.0	194	0.3	47.9	0.1	1.0
Strawberry, Average	*1 Tbsp/15g*	*37*	*0.0*	*250*	*0.4*	*61.6*	*0.1*	*0.5*
Strawberry, TTD, Sainsbury's*	1 Tbsp/15g	43	0.0	287	0.4	71.1	0.1	0.5

CONSOMME

Average	*1oz/28g*	*3*	*0.0*	*12*	*2.9*	*0.1*	*0.0*	*0.0*
Beef, Luxury, with Sherry, Baxters*	1 Can/415g	62	0.0	15	2.7	1.0	0.0	0.0

COOKIES

All Butter, Almond, Italian Style, M&S*	1 Cookie/23g	120	6.4	515	6.7	59.4	27.6	3.6
All Butter, Ginger Bread, M&S*	1 Cookie/23g	102	5.0	445	4.3	57.5	21.8	2.4
All Butter, Italian Style Sorrento Lemon, M&S*	1 Cookie/24g	120	6.4	500	4.9	60.4	26.7	2.1
All Butter, Melting Moment, M&S*	1 Cookie/23g	110	6.4	470	4.5	51.5	27.5	3.4
All Butter, Sultana, TTD, Sainsbury's*	1 Cookie/17g	79	3.8	476	5.4	62.7	22.6	2.0
Almond, Ose*	1 Cookie/10g	46	1.4	456	8.4	74.0	14.0	0.0
Apple Crumble, M&S*	1 Cookie/26g	90	0.5	345	4.6	76.8	2.0	2.9
Apple Pie, The Biscuit Collection*	1 Cookie/19g	90	4.2	474	3.9	65.0	22.1	0.0
Belgian Chocolate, Quadruple, All Butter, Deluxe, Lidl*	1 Cookie/26g	126	6.2	485	6.4	59.7	23.9	2.8
Belgian Dark Chocolate & Ginger, Truly Irresistible, Co-Op*	1 Cookie/26g	122	5.0	470	2.7	70.7	19.2	2.1
Big Milk Chocolate Chunk, Cookie Coach*	1 Cookie/35g	174	8.8	497	6.2	61.4	25.1	0.0
Bites, Weight Watchers*	1 Pack/21g	97	4.0	464	5.8	67.0	19.2	4.3
Brazil Nut, Prewett's*	1 Cookie/50g	122	7.4	244	2.6	25.2	14.8	1.0
Butter & Sultana, Sainsbury's*	1 Cookie/13g	61	2.6	473	4.5	68.4	20.1	1.6
Cherry Bakewell, COU, M&S*	1 Cookie/25g	90	0.6	355	6.0	77.2	2.5	3.4
Choc Chip & Coconut, Maryland*	1 Cookie/10g	55	2.5	512	5.1	62.9	23.7	0.0
Choc Chip & Hazelnut, Maryland*	1 Cookie/11g	55	2.7	513	6.3	65.3	25.0	0.0
Choc Chip, Bronte*	1 Cookie/17g	79	3.6	474	5.8	64.0	21.6	0.0
Choc Chip, Cadbury*	1 Cookie/11g	55	2.8	503	5.9	62.2	25.6	0.0
Choc Chip, Giant, Paterson's*	1 Cookie/60g	296	15.2	493	0.1	61.3	25.3	3.2
Choc Chip, Lyons*	1 Cookie/11g	57	2.7	499	5.2	68.3	23.4	1.7
Choc Chip, Maryland*	1 Cookie/11g	56	2.6	511	6.2	68.0	23.9	1.3
Choc Chip, Sainsbury's*	1 Cookie/11g	55	2.6	508	6.2	67.0	23.9	1.3
Choc Chunk & Hazelnut, Co-Op*	1 Cookie/17g	89	5.3	525	6.0	56.0	31.0	3.0
Choc Chunk, Fabulous Bakin' Boys*	1 Cookie/60g	270	12.6	450	5.0	59.0	21.0	3.0
Choc Chunk, Finest, Tesco*	1 Cookie/80g	355	14.1	445	5.7	65.3	17.7	1.8
Chocolate & Nut, Organic, Evernat*	1 Cookie/69g	337	15.6	489	7.2	64.1	22.6	0.0
Chocolate & Orange, COU, M&S*	1 Cookie/26g	90	0.7	350	5.7	77.2	2.6	3.2
Chocolate Chip & Hazelnut, ES, Asda*	1 Cookie/25g	130	8.1	516	6.0	51.0	32.0	2.5
Chocolate Chip, Asda*	1 Cookie/12g	57	2.9	497	5.0	63.0	25.0	2.6
Chocolate Chip, Average	*1 Cookie/10g*	*49*	*2.5*	*489*	*5.5*	*64.1*	*24.7*	*2.9*
Chocolate Chip, BGTY, Sainsbury's*	1 Cookie/17g	72	2.0	428	4.5	75.6	11.9	2.5
Chocolate Chip, Chips Ahoy*	1 Cookie/11g	55	2.8	500	6.0	65.0	25.0	3.0
Chocolate Chip, Co-Op*	1 Cookie/11g	55	2.6	500	5.0	65.0	24.0	1.0
Chocolate Chip, Gluten & Wheat Free, Lovemore*	1 Cookie/17g	81	4.5	483	3.8	57.8	26.8	3.5
Chocolate Chip, Gluten Free, Organic, Dove's Farm*	1 Cookie/17g	77	3.1	451	4.3	66.9	18.5	0.0
Chocolate Chip, Handbaked, Border*	1 Cookie/15g	72	3.4	480	5.9	67.4	22.6	0.0
Chocolate Chip, Lyons*	1 Cookie/12g	56	2.5	483	5.6	66.5	21.6	1.7
Chocolate Chip, M&S*	1 Cookie/12g	59	3.0	495	5.7	62.1	24.8	2.7

COOKIES

	Measure INFO/WEIGHT	per Measure KCAL	FAT	Nutrition Values per 100g / 100ml KCAL	PROT	CARB	FAT	FIBRE
Chocolate Chip, McVitie's*	1 Cookie/11g	54	2.8	496	5.8	60.2	25.8	3.0
Chocolate Chip, Mini, McVitie's*	1 Bag/40g	196	9.2	491	5.5	65.1	23.1	2.8
Chocolate Chip, Mini, Tesco*	1 Bag/30g	148	7.1	493	5.4	64.6	23.7	1.7
Chocolate Chip, Morrisons*	1 Cookie/10g	52	2.5	502	5.0	66.2	24.1	1.3
Chocolate Chip, Organic, Sainsbury's*	1 Cookie/17g	89	4.9	530	5.0	61.8	29.2	0.3
Chocolate Chip, Organic, Tesco*	1 Cookie/17g	88	4.7	520	4.0	63.3	27.4	2.8
Chocolate Chip, Tesco*	1 Cookie/11g	56	2.7	510	5.2	67.2	24.1	1.6
Chocolate Chip, Value, Tesco*	1 Cookie/11g	56	2.9	512	4.8	64.8	26.0	1.6
Chocolate Chip, Weight Watchers*	1 Cookie/11g	49	1.9	443	7.6	65.4	17.2	4.6
Chocolate Chunk & Hazelnut, TTD, Sainsbury's*	1 Cookie/17g	88	5.2	528	6.5	54.8	31.4	2.8
Chocolate Chunk, All Butter, COU, M&S*	1 Cookie/24g	110	4.3	460	5.7	69.1	17.9	2.3
Chocolate Chunk, All Butter, M&S*	1 Cookie/24g	120	6.0	500	5.2	62.4	25.2	2.9
Chocolate Chunk, Cadbury*	1 Cookie/22g	119	6.9	540	6.5	58.0	31.2	0.0
Chocolate Chunk, Devondale*	1 Cookie/65g	308	16.3	474	4.6	59.2	25.1	2.8
Chocolate Fruit & Nut, ES, Asda*	1 Cookie/25g	125	7.1	509	6.0	56.0	29.0	2.0
Chocolate, Belgian, ES, Asda*	1 Cookie/26g	138	8.0	535	6.0	58.0	31.0	2.0
Chocolate, Milk, Free From, Tesco*	1 Cookie/20g	100	6.1	500	5.6	50.4	30.7	4.1
Chocolate, Soft, American Style, Budgens*	1 Cookie/50g	216	9.3	431	5.1	60.8	18.6	2.2
Chocolate, Triple, Half Coated, Finest, Tesco*	1 Cookie/25g	131	7.3	525	5.7	58.7	29.3	2.3
Chunkie Extremely Chocolatey, Fox's*	1 Cookie/26g	130	6.8	506	6.2	61.0	26.3	2.6
Coconut & Raspberry, Gluten Free, Sainsbury's*	1 Cookie/20g	102	5.9	511	5.9	56.0	29.3	6.7
Cranberry & Orange, Finest, Tesco*	1 Cookie/26g	125	5.8	490	4.1	67.4	22.6	3.2
Danish Butter, Tesco*	1 Cookie/26g	133	6.6	516	4.7	66.7	25.6	1.3
Dark Chocolate Chunk & Ginger, The Best, Morrisons*	1 Cookie/25g	126	6.4	503	4.6	63.7	25.5	2.8
Dark Treacle, Weight Watchers*	1 Cookie/11g	49	1.7	423	5.2	66.7	15.1	1.7
Double Choc Chip, Giant, Paterson's*	1 Cookie/60g	293	15.2	489	0.3	61.3	25.3	3.7
Double Choc Chip, Mini, M&S*	1 Cookie/22g	108	5.2	490	5.3	63.6	23.7	1.8
Double Choc Chip, Tesco*	1 Cookie/11g	55	2.7	500	4.2	65.3	24.7	3.0
Double Choc Chip, Weight Watchers*	1 Cookie/11g	49	1.9	443	7.6	65.4	17.2	4.6
Double Choc, Maryland*	1 Cookie/10g	51	2.6	510	5.2	64.4	25.7	0.0
Double Chocolate & Walnut, Soft, Tesco*	1 Cookie/25g	116	6.4	463	5.8	52.1	25.7	4.7
Double Chocolate Chip, Co-Op*	1 Cookie/17g	87	4.6	510	5.0	63.0	27.0	2.0
Double Chocolate Chip, Organic, Waitrose*	1 Cookie/18g	96	5.6	535	5.1	58.6	31.0	1.9
Fortune, Average	*1 Cookie/8g*	*30*	*0.2*	*378*	*4.2*	*84.0*	*2.7*	*1.6*
Fruit & Oat, Soft, Diet Chef Ltd*	1 Cookie/45g	198	8.8	439	4.8	58.8	19.6	4.0
Fruit, Giant, Cookie Coach*	1 Cookie/60g	280	13.2	466	4.9	62.0	22.0	0.0
Fruity Shrewsbury, Giant, Paterson's*	1 Cookie/60g	298	15.2	496	4.8	62.6	25.4	1.7
Fudge Brownie, Maryland*	1 Cookie/11g	56	2.8	510	5.8	63.0	25.0	0.0
Ginger & Choc Chip, BGTY, Sainsbury's*	1 Cookie/17g	69	3.2	415	5.8	55.3	19.0	12.1
Ginger, Gluten Free, Barkat*	1 Cookie/17g	85	4.4	501	3.2	63.8	25.9	0.0
Ginger, Low Fat, M&S*	1 Cookie/23g	82	1.0	358	5.1	74.9	4.3	2.4
Jaffa, Tesco*	1 Cookie/42g	175	5.9	417	4.8	66.9	14.0	1.9
Lemon Zest, Gluten Free, Organic, Dove's Farm*	1 Cookie/17g	80	3.1	473	3.3	73.7	18.3	0.0
Milk Chocolate Chunk, Average	*1 Cookie/25g*	*129*	*6.9*	*515*	*6.6*	*60.0*	*27.6*	*1.6*
Milk Chocolate Chunk, Greggs*	1 Cookie/75g	380	20.3	506	7.0	58.5	27.0	2.8
Milk Chocolate, Classic, Millie's Cookies*	1 Cookie/45g	190	10.2	422	5.1	49.3	22.7	1.3
Oat & Raisin, Gluten Free, Prewett's*	1 Cookie18g	80	2.7	442	6.2	63.0	15.0	5.1
Oat & Raisin, Health Matters*	1 Cookie/8g	33	0.7	414	7.0	76.6	8.8	3.3
Oat & Treacle, TTD, Sainsbury's*	1 Cookie/25g	121	5.9	482	5.7	61.8	23.6	3.7
Oat, Giant Jumbo, Paterson's*	1 Cookie/60g	299	16.2	499	0.4	58.4	27.0	3.2
Oatflake & Raisin, Waitrose*	1 Cookie/17g	80	3.8	469	5.8	61.7	22.1	4.7
Oatmeal, Chocolate Chip, Chewy, Dad's*	1 Cookie/15g	70	3.0	467	6.7	66.7	20.0	3.3
Oreo, Mini, Oreo*	1 Pack/25g	120	4.8	480	4.8	70.0	19.2	2.4

	Measure INFO/WEIGHT	per Measure KCAL	FAT	Nutrition Values per 100g / 100ml KCAL	PROT	CARB	FAT	FIBRE
COOKIES								
Oreo, Nabisco*	1 Cookie/11g	52	2.3	471	5.9	70.6	20.6	2.9
Quadruple Chocolate, TTD, Sainsbury's*	1 Cookie/20g	104	5.7	518	6.2	59.8	28.2	1.6
Raisin & Cinnamon, Low Fat, M&S*	1 Cookie/22g	78	0.9	355	6.2	73.0	4.1	3.2
Rolo, Nestle*	1 Cookie/39g	178	7.4	456	5.4	64.8	19.0	2.2
Stem Ginger, Aldi*	1 Cookie/13g	58	2.4	463	3.6	68.5	19.4	0.0
Stem Ginger, Deluxe, Lidl*	1 Cookie/17g	80	3.6	468	5.1	62.0	21.0	5.4
Stem Ginger, Free From, Sainsbury's*	1 Cookie/17g	84	4.8	489	6.5	58.0	28.0	6.8
Stem Ginger, Less Than 5% Fat, M&S*	1 Cookie/22g	79	0.9	360	6.2	73.9	4.3	3.0
Stem Ginger, Reduced Fat, Waitrose*	1 Cookie/17g	75	2.7	448	4.5	71.0	16.2	1.6
Stem Ginger, Tesco*	1 Cookie/20g	98	4.8	489	4.2	64.0	24.0	2.0
Stem Ginger, TTD, Sainsbury's*	1 Cookie/17g	79	3.7	476	5.2	64.3	22.0	2.3
Sultana, All Butter, Reduced Fat, M&S*	1 Cookie/17g	70	2.4	420	4.9	68.6	14.2	2.6
Sultana, Deluxe, Lidl*	1 Cookie/17g	77	3.2	453	5.3	64.7	18.8	2.9
Sultana, Soft & Chewy, Sainsbury's*	1 Cookie/25g	104	3.5	414	4.4	67.8	13.9	2.5
Toffee, Weight Watchers*	2 Cookies/152g	686	27.4	451	6.8	61.7	18.0	7.5
Treacle & Oat, All Butter, Finest, Tesco*	1 Cookie/20g	100	5.0	500	4.8	62.9	25.0	2.1
Triple Chocolate Chunk, Bakery, Finest, Tesco*	1 Cookie/80g	360	15.9	450	7.4	59.2	19.9	2.1
Triple Chocolate Chunk, Greggs*	1 Cookie/75g	374	20.3	498	6.5	56.0	27.0	4.2
White Chocolate & Raspberry, Finest, Tesco*	1 Cookie/76g	304	9.6	400	5.2	66.3	12.6	2.4
White Chocolate & Raspberry, McVitie's*	1 Cookie/17g	87	4.4	512	4.7	64.1	25.9	1.8
White Chocolate, Asda*	1 Cookie/54g	256	11.9	474	5.0	64.0	22.0	2.1
White Chocolate, Chunk, Average	*1 Cookie/25g*	*124*	*6.2*	*498*	*5.5*	*62.8*	*24.8*	*1.0*
White Chocolate, Maryland*	1 Cookie/10g	51	2.5	512	5.7	64.0	25.0	0.0
White Chocolate, TTD, Sainsbury's*	1 Cookie/25g	126	6.4	504	5.5	62.5	25.8	1.2
COQ AU VIN								
Diet Chef Ltd*	1 Pack/300g	285	13.2	95	7.7	6.1	4.4	2.2
Finest, Tesco*	1 Serving/273g	251	9.8	92	14.3	0.7	3.6	1.8
CORDIAL								
Elderflower, Made Up, Bottle Green*	1 Glass/200ml	46	0.0	23	0.0	5.6	0.0	0.0
Elderflower, Undiluted, Waitrose*	1 Serving/20ml	22	0.0	110	0.0	27.5	0.0	0.0
Lemon & Lime, High Juice, M&S*	1 Glass/250ml	75	0.0	30	0.0	7.0	0.0	0.0
Lime Juice, Concentrated	1 Serving/20ml	22	0.0	112	0.1	29.8	0.0	0.0
Lime Juice, Diluted	1 Glass/250ml	55	0.0	22	0.0	6.0	0.0	0.0
Lime Juice, Waitrose*	1 Serving/20ml	21	0.0	104	10.0	23.7	0.0	0.0
Lime, Juice, Diluted, Rose's*	1 Serving/50ml	12	0.0	24	0.0	5.7	0.0	0.0
Lime, Sainsbury's*	1 Serving/50ml	14	0.0	27	0.0	6.2	0.0	0.0
Lime, Tesco*	1 Pint/74ml	8	0.0	11	0.2	0.5	0.0	0.0
Pomegranate & Elderflower, Bottle Green*	1 fl oz/30ml	9	0.0	30	0.0	7.0	0.0	0.0
CORIANDER								
Leaves, Dried, Average	*1oz/28g*	*78*	*1.3*	*279*	*21.8*	*41.7*	*4.8*	*0.0*
Leaves, Fresh, Average	*1 Bunch/20g*	*5*	*0.1*	*23*	*2.1*	*3.7*	*0.5*	*2.8*
Seeds, Ground, Schwartz*	1 Tsp/5g	22	0.9	446	14.2	54.9	18.8	0.0
CORN								
Baby, & Mange Tout, Eat Fresh, Tesco*	1 Serving/100g	31	0.2	31	2.9	3.3	0.2	2.1
Baby, Average	*1 Serving/80g*	*21*	*0.3*	*26*	*2.5*	*3.1*	*0.4*	*1.7*
Baby, Canned, Drained, Average	*1 Serving/80g*	*18*	*0.3*	*23*	*2.9*	*2.0*	*0.4*	*1.5*
Cobs, Boiled, Weighed with Cob, Average	*1 Ear/200g*	*78*	*1.7*	*39*	*1.5*	*6.8*	*0.8*	*0.4*
Creamed Style, Green Giant*	1 Can/418g	238	2.1	57	1.2	11.9	0.5	3.0
Nuts, Roasted, Kraft*	1 Serving/28g	120	4.5	429	10.7	71.4	16.1	7.1
CORN CAKES								
Organic, Kallo*	1 Cake/5g	16	0.2	340	12.7	74.3	4.1	11.2
Slightly Salted, Mrs Crimble's*	1 Pack/28g	104	0.9	380	7.9	80.0	3.4	5.4

Measure INFO/WEIGHT		per Measure		Nutrition Values per 100g / 100ml				
		KCAL	FAT	KCAL	PROT	CARB	FAT	FIBRE
CORNED BEEF								
Average	**1 Slice/35g**	**75**	**4.3**	**214**	**25.9**	**0.7**	**12.2**	**0.0**
Lean, Healthy Range, Average	**1 Slice/30g**	**57**	**2.6**	**191**	**27.0**	**1.0**	**8.7**	**0.0**
Morrisons*	1 Can/340g	738	42.5	217	25.0	1.0	12.5	0.0
Sliced, Morrisons*	1 Slice/31g	63	3.2	203	26.0	1.3	10.3	0.0
Sliced, Premium, Average	**1 Slice/31g**	**69**	**3.9**	**222**	**26.6**	**0.5**	**12.6**	**0.0**
CORNFLOUR								
Average	**1 Tsp/5g**	**18**	**0.1**	**355**	**0.6**	**86.9**	**1.2**	**0.1**
COURGETTE								
Fried, Average	**1oz/28g**	**18**	**1.3**	**63**	**2.6**	**2.6**	**4.8**	**1.2**
Raw, Average	**1 Courgette/224g**	**40**	**0.9**	**18**	**1.8**	**1.8**	**0.4**	**0.9**
COUS COUS								
& Chargrilled Vegetables, M&S*	1 Serving/200g	200	3.0	100	3.9	17.3	1.5	1.6
Chargrilled Red & Yellow Pepper, Tesco*	1 Pack/200g	212	3.6	106	4.6	17.8	1.8	0.5
Chargrilled Vegetable, Morrisons*	1 Serving/225g	227	5.4	101	3.3	16.5	2.4	1.3
Chargrilled Vegetables & Olive Oil, Delphi*	½ Pot/75g	105	2.9	140	3.8	22.5	3.9	1.9
Citrus Kick, Cooked, Ainsley Harriott*	1 Serving/130g	182	1.6	140	4.3	27.9	1.2	2.4
Citrus Kick, Dry, Ainsley Harriott*	½ Sachet/50g	184	1.2	368	11.6	77.0	2.4	9.2
Cooked, Average	**1 Tbsp/15g**	**24**	**0.3**	**158**	**4.3**	**31.4**	**1.9**	**1.3**
Coriander & Lemon, As Consumed, Sainsbury's*	½ Pack/140g	195	1.0	139	4.8	27.5	0.7	1.9
Coriander & Lemon, Made Up per Instructions, Asda*	1 Pack Dry/110g	378	3.5	128	5.1	24.2	1.2	2.5
Coriander & Lemon, Morrisons*	1 Serving/100g	159	3.4	159	4.4	27.7	3.4	1.4
Dry, Average	**1 Serving/50g**	**178**	**0.7**	**356**	**13.7**	**72.8**	**1.5**	**2.6**
Garlic & Coriander, Dry, Waitrose*	1 Serving/70g	235	2.5	336	11.7	64.2	3.6	6.2
Giant, Tesco*	1 Pack/220g	350	14.4	160	4.1	20.7	6.6	1.2
Harissa Style Savoury, Sainsbury's*	1 Serving/260g	434	12.0	167	4.7	26.8	4.6	1.3
Hot & Spicy Flavour, Dry, Amazing Grains, Haldane's*	1 Serving/50g	182	2.1	365	12.5	67.0	4.2	3.1
Lemon & Coriander, Cooked, Tesco*	1 Serving/137g	207	3.3	151	4.0	28.3	2.4	2.0
Lemon & Coriander, Dry, Tesco*	1 Pack/110g	375	3.0	341	11.0	68.2	2.7	6.1
Mediterranean Style, Cooked, Tesco*	1 Serving/146g	215	3.8	147	4.4	26.5	2.6	1.3
Mediterranean Style, Dry, Tesco*	1 Pack/110g	368	3.3	335	11.9	65.1	3.0	5.6
Mediterranean Tomato, GFY, Asda*	½ Pack/141g	192	1.3	136	5.0	27.0	0.9	1.7
Moroccan Medley, Ainsley Harriott*	½ Sachet/130g	178	2.0	137	5.4	25.4	1.5	2.2
Moroccan Style, Cooked, Sainsbury's*	½ Pack/140g	200	1.1	143	6.2	26.4	0.8	2.5
Moroccan Style, Finest, Tesco*	1 Tub/225g	292	5.6	130	4.3	22.6	2.5	3.7
Moroccan Style, Fruity, M&S*	1 Serving/200g	370	5.4	185	3.4	36.7	2.7	3.4
Moroccan Style, Spiced, Meadow Fresh, Lidl*	1 Pack/280g	456	14.8	163	3.0	25.0	5.3	1.6
Moroccan Style, TTD, Sainsbury's*	1 Pot/200g	364	7.2	182	4.4	30.3	3.6	5.5
Moroccan, Co-Op*	1 Pack/110g	155	1.8	141	4.8	26.0	1.6	1.6
Morrisons*	1 Serving/100g	126	1.2	126	5.5	23.2	1.2	3.5
Plain, Dry Weight, Tesco*	1 Serving/50g	182	0.6	365	15.1	73.1	1.1	0.8
Roasted Vegetable, Cooked, Ainsley Harriott*	1 Serving/130g	180	2.0	138	5.6	25.5	1.5	2.6
Roasted Vegetable, Dry, Ainsley Harriott*	½ Sachet/50g	180	2.0	360	14.6	66.4	4.0	6.8
Roasted Vegetable, Snack Salad Pot, HL, Tesco*	1 Pack/60g	213	2.4	355	15.1	64.6	4.0	4.2
Roasted Vegetables, Waitrose*	1 Serving/200g	328	13.2	164	3.9	22.0	6.6	0.9
Spice Fusion, Lyttos*	1 Serving/100g	134	1.5	134	4.3	23.9	1.5	3.4
Spice Sensation, Dry, Ainsley Harriott*	½ Sachet/50g	166	1.2	332	11.6	66.2	2.4	9.2
Sundried Tomato & Garlic, Made Up, Ainsley Harriott*	½ Pack/162g	244	2.3	151	5.5	27.9	1.4	2.2
Tangy Tomato, Cooked, Ainsley Harriott*	1 Serving/133g	166	0.8	125	4.6	25.3	0.6	3.3
Tomato & Basil, Made Up, Tesco*	1 Serving/200g	348	16.6	174	3.9	21.0	8.3	3.4
Tomato & Onion, Dry Weight, Waitrose*	1 Pack/110g	376	4.0	342	12.6	64.9	3.6	5.1
Wholewheat, Tesco*	1 Serving/50g	178	1.0	355	12.0	72.0	2.0	5.0
with Sun Dried Tomato, CBY, Asda*	1 Pack/310g	515	12.1	166	4.6	26.2	3.9	4.0

C

CRAB

	Measure INFO/WEIGHT	per Measure KCAL	FAT	Nutrition Values per 100g / 100ml KCAL	PROT	CARB	FAT	FIBRE
Blue, Soft Shelled, Raw, Average	*1 Crab/84g*	*73*	*0.9*	*87*	*18.1*	*0.0*	*1.1*	*0.0*
Boiled, Meat Only, Average	*1 Tbsp/40g*	*51*	*2.2*	*128*	*19.5*	*0.0*	*5.5*	*0.0*
Cocktail, Waitrose*	1 Serving/100g	217	17.6	217	10.8	3.8	17.6	0.4
Cornish 50/50, Seafood & Eat It*	1 Pot/100g	144	5.8	144	21.6	1.2	5.8	0.5
Cornish Potted, Seafood & Eat It*	1 Pack/100g	235	17.5	235	15.0	5.1	17.5	0.8
Dressed, Average	*1 Can/43g*	*66*	*3.4*	*154*	*16.8*	*4.1*	*7.9*	*0.2*
Meat in Brine, Average	*½ Can/60g*	*41*	*0.2*	*69*	*15.6*	*0.8*	*0.4*	*0.1*
Meat, Raw, Average	*1oz/28g*	*28*	*0.2*	*100*	*20.8*	*2.8*	*0.6*	*0.0*
White Cornish, Seafood & Eat It*	1 Pack/100g	81	0.5	81	19.0	0.1	0.5	0.0
White Meat, Scottish, Sainsburys*	½ Pot/50g	46	0.4	91	19.0	1.4	0.9	0.5
White Meat, See Food & Eat It*	1 Pack/100g	81	0.5	81	19.0	0.1	0.5	0.0

CRAB CAKES

Goan, M&S*	1 Pack/190g	228	7.6	120	8.0	12.9	4.0	1.8
Iceland*	1 Serving/18g	52	3.2	288	7.2	25.6	18.0	1.3
Shetl& Isles, Dressed, TTD, Sainsbury's*	1 Crab/75g	130	8.3	174	12.4	6.0	11.1	0.5
Tesco*	1 Serving/130g	281	16.0	216	11.0	15.4	12.3	1.1
Thai, TTD, Sainsbury's*	½ Pack/106g	201	9.5	189	9.5	17.8	8.9	1.4

CRAB STICKS

Average	*1 Stick/15g*	*14*	*0.0*	*94*	*9.1*	*13.9*	*0.3*	*0.0*

CRACKERBREAD

Original, Ryvita*	1 Slice/5g	19	0.1	378	10.8	75.0	2.8	4.8
Rice, Asda*	1 Slice/5g	19	0.1	374	9.1	79.4	2.2	1.9
Sainsbury's*	1 Slice/5g	19	0.2	380	10.0	80.0	4.0	2.0
Wholegrain, Ryvita*	1 Slice/6g	20	0.2	360	12.4	68.7	3.9	9.8

CRACKERS

Bath Oliver, Jacob's*	1 Cracker/12g	52	1.6	432	9.6	67.6	13.7	2.6
Bean Mix, Habas Tapas, Graze*	1 Punnet/30g	131	3.8	438	11.7	68.9	12.8	1.5
Black Olive, M&S*	1 Cracker/4g	20	1.0	485	8.3	59.4	23.5	4.3
Black Pepper for Cheese, Ryvita*	1 Cracker/7g	27	0.2	384	13.2	72.9	2.9	6.8
Brooklyn Bites, Graze*	1 Punnet/29g	157	11.3	541	4.1	33.0	39.0	4.0
Butter Puff, Sainsbury's*	1 Cracker/10g	54	2.7	523	10.4	60.7	26.5	2.5
Cheese Thins, Asda*	1 Cracker/4g	21	1.3	532	12.0	49.0	32.0	0.0
Cheese Thins, Cheddar, The Planet Snack Co*	1 Serving/30g	153	8.8	509	11.5	50.1	29.2	2.1
Cheese, Cheddar, Crispies, TTD, Sainsbury's*	1 Thin/4g	21	1.5	576	14.2	39.0	40.4	2.2
Cheese, Oat Bakes, Nairn's*	1 Bag/30g	130	4.7	432	15.0	57.4	15.8	1.3
Cheese, Ritz*	1 Cracker/4g	17	0.9	486	10.1	55.9	24.7	2.2
Chives, Jacob's*	1 Cracker/6g	28	1.0	457	9.5	67.5	16.5	2.7
Choice Grain, Jacob's*	1 Cracker/8g	32	1.1	427	9.0	65.5	14.3	5.4
Corn Thins, 97% Fat Free, Real Foods*	1 Cracker/6g	23	0.2	378	10.2	81.7	3.0	8.6
Corn Thins, Real Foods*	1 Cracker/6g	22	0.2	378	10.2	81.7	3.0	8.6
Cream, Aldi*	1 Cracker/8g	36	1.2	456	9.1	71.7	14.7	3.0
Cream, Asda*	1 Cracker/8g	35	1.2	443	10.0	67.0	15.0	0.0
Cream, Average	*1 Cracker/7g*	*31*	*1.1*	*440*	*9.5*	*68.3*	*16.3*	*2.2*
Cream, BGTY, Sainsbury's*	1 Cracker/8g	32	0.6	400	10.9	71.7	7.7	3.1
Cream, Choice Grain, Jacob's*	1 Cracker/7g	30	0.9	400	10.9	64.5	11.8	7.0
Cream, Jacob's*	1 Cracker/8g	34	1.1	431	10.0	67.5	13.5	3.8
Cream, Light, Jacob's*	1 Cracker/8g	31	0.5	388	10.6	72.2	6.3	4.1
Cream, Morrisons*	1 Cracker/8g	36	1.2	446	9.6	68.5	14.8	2.7
Cream, Reduced Fat, Tesco*	1 Cracker/8g	31	0.5	406	10.9	74.4	7.2	2.8
Cream, Roasted Onion, Jacob's*	1 Cracker/8g	35	1.2	441	10.2	66.8	14.8	2.9
Cream, Sainsbury's*	1 Cracker/8g	35	1.3	422	9.5	66.7	15.2	2.8
Cream, Tesco*	1 Cracker/8g	34	1.2	447	9.0	69.0	15.0	3.0
Crispy Cheese, M&S*	1 Cracker/4g	20	1.0	470	9.4	58.1	22.1	3.0

	Measure INFO/WEIGHT	per Measure KCAL	FAT	Nutrition Values per 100g / 100ml KCAL	PROT	CARB	FAT	FIBRE
CRACKERS								
Cruskits, Arnotts*	2 Cruskits/12g	40	0.2	331	9.0	63.7	1.5	0.0
El Picante, Graze*	1 Punnet/25g	126	6.7	506	15.0	49.0	27.0	6.0
Extra Wheatgerm, Hovis*	1 Cracker/6g	27	1.1	447	10.2	60.0	18.5	4.4
Garlic, CBY, Asda*	2 Crackers/12g	58	2.6	483	7.0	63.3	21.5	4.2
Harvest Grain, Sainsbury's*	1 Cracker/6g	27	1.1	458	8.5	64.5	18.4	4.1
Herb & Onion, 99% Fat Free, Rakusen's*	1 Cracker/5g	18	0.0	360	9.1	82.6	1.0	3.9
Herb & Spice, Jacob's*	1 Cracker/6g	27	1.0	457	9.5	67.5	16.5	2.7
High Fibre, Dietary Specials*	1 Cracker/6g	23	0.6	391	2.1	60.0	11.0	17.0
Japanese Beef Teriyaki, Sensations, Walkers*	1 Serving/24g	118	6.3	490	1.4	62.0	26.0	3.5
Krackawheat, McVitie's*	1 Cracker/7g	33	1.4	446	9.7	60.0	18.6	5.8
Lightly Salted, Italian, Jacob's*	1 Cracker/6g	26	0.8	429	10.3	67.6	13.0	2.9
Mediterranean, Jacob's*	1 Cracker/6g	27	1.0	450	9.7	66.5	16.1	2.7
Mix, Yaki Soba, Graze*	1 Punnet/32g	159	9.3	498	24.0	36.0	29.0	6.0
Mixed Seed, Multi Grain, Asda*	1 Cracker/6g	28	1.1	445	11.0	62.0	17.0	4.4
Multi-grain, Aldi, Savour Bakes, Aldi*	1 Cracker/5g	20	0.8	404	8.3	55.0	16.8	5.1
Multigrain, Corn Thins, Real Foods*	1 Cracker/6g	23	0.2	388	10.9	71.0	3.7	10.3
Multigrain, Morrisons*	10 Crackers/20g	76	2.2	379	8.8	61.3	11.0	5.1
Multigrain, Tesco*	1 Cracker/6g	27	1.1	458	8.5	64.5	18.4	4.1
Oat & Wheat, Weight Watchers*	4 Crackers/20g	74	0.5	370	10.5	75.0	2.5	4.0
Peanut, Wasabi, Graze*	1 Pack/26g	125	5.6	479	15.2	53.8	21.4	5.4
Peking Spare Rib & 5 Spice, Oriental, Sensations, Walkers*	1 Bag/24g	116	6.2	485	1.3	62.0	26.0	3.5
Poppy & Sesame Seed, Sainsbury's*	1 Cracker/4g	21	1.1	530	9.6	58.9	28.4	3.4
Ritz, Mini, Kraft*	1 Bag/25g	126	6.0	504	7.9	63.0	24.0	2.0
Ritz, Original, Jacob's*	1 Cracker/3g	17	1.0	509	6.9	55.6	28.8	2.0
Salt & Black Pepper, Jacob's*	1 Cracker/6g	27	1.0	457	9.5	67.5	16.5	2.7
Salt & Pepper, Sainsbury's*	1 Cracker/6g	27	1.2	485	7.3	64.5	21.3	3.0
Salted, Ritz, Nabisco*	1 Cracker/3g	17	0.9	493	7.0	57.5	26.1	2.9
Selection, Finest, Tesco*	1 Serving/30g	136	4.3	452	9.6	71.0	14.4	0.0
Sesame & Poppy Thins, Tesco*	1 Cracker/4g	20	1.0	485	9.9	57.6	23.5	4.4
Sweet Chilli, Oat Bakes, Nairn's*	1 Bag/30g	128	4.0	426	8.1	68.4	13.3	7.2
Sweet Chilli, Thins, Savours, Jacob's*	1 Cracker/4g	21	0.9	472	8.0	62.3	21.2	3.6
Tarallini with Fennel Seeds, Crosta & Mollica*	1 Cracker/4g	21	0.9	529	8.2	67.5	22.0	4.2
Thai Spicy Vegetable, Sainsbury's*	1 Pack/50g	231	10.4	462	7.2	61.5	20.8	2.6
The British Barbecue, Graze*	1 Punnet/23g	117	7.4	508	17.4	36.8	32.2	7.4
Tuc, Cheese Sandwich, Jacob's*	1 Cracker/14g	72	4.3	531	8.4	53.8	31.4	0.0
Tuc, Jacob's*	1 Cracker/5g	25	1.4	517	7.7	56.4	28.6	2.1
Unsalted, Tops, Premium Plus, Impress*	1 Cracker/3g	13	0.3	448	10.3	75.9	10.3	0.0
Waterthins, Wafers, Philemon*	1 Crackers/2g	7	0.1	392	10.6	77.9	3.6	5.0
Wheaten, M&S*	1 Cracker/4g	20	0.9	450	10.2	57.0	20.2	5.0
Whole Wheat, 100%, Oven Baked, Master Choice*	1 Cracker/4g	17	0.4	429	10.0	75.0	9.6	12.1
Wholemeal, Tesco*	1 Cracker/7g	29	1.0	414	9.4	60.6	14.9	10.4
CRANBERRIES								
& Raisins, Dried, Sweetened, Ocean Spray*	1 Serving/50g	163	0.2	326	0.1	80.3	0.5	4.6
Dried, Fruit bag, The Foodie Market, Aldi*	1 Serving/50g	172	0.7	343	0.3	80.1	1.3	4.7
Dried, Sweetened, Average	*1 Serving/10g*	*34*	*0.1*	*335*	*0.3*	*81.1*	*0.8*	*4.4*
Dried, Wholesome, LL, Waitrose*	¼ Pack/25g	92	0.2	370	0.3	86.8	0.8	4.6
Fresh, Raw, Average	*1oz/28g*	*4*	*0.0*	*15*	*0.4*	*3.4*	*0.1*	*3.0*
CRAYFISH								
Raw	*1oz/28g*	*19*	*0.2*	*67*	*14.9*	*0.0*	*0.8*	*0.0*
Tails in Brine, Luxury, The Big Prawn Co*	½ Tub/90g	46	0.6	51	10.1	1.0	0.7	0.0
CREAM								
Aerosol, Average	*1oz/28g*	*87*	*8.7*	*309*	*1.8*	*6.2*	*30.9*	*0.0*
Aerosol, Reduced Fat, Average	*1 Serving/55ml*	*33*	*3.0*	*60*	*0.6*	*2.0*	*5.4*	*0.0*

C

	Measure INFO/WEIGHT	per Measure KCAL	FAT	Nutrition Values per 100g / 100ml KCAL	PROT	CARB	FAT	FIBRE
CREAM								
Brandy, Really Thick, Finest, Tesco*	½ Pot/125ml	579	49.5	463	1.3	19.7	39.6	0.0
Brandy, Really Thick, Tesco*	1 Pot/250ml	1162	98.2	465	1.4	21.3	39.3	0.0
Chantilly, TTD, Sainsbury's*	2 Tbsp/30g	136	14.0	455	1.4	6.9	46.8	0.0
Clotted, Fresh, Average	*1 Serving/28g*	*162*	*17.5*	*579*	*1.6*	*2.3*	*62.7*	*0.0*
Clotted, TTD, Sainsbury's*	1 Serving/30g	176	19.0	587	1.6	2.2	63.5	0.0
Double, Average	*1 Tbsp/15ml*	*68*	*7.3*	*452*	*1.6*	*2.4*	*48.4*	*0.0*
Double, Reduced Fat, Average	*1 Serving/30g*	*73*	*7.0*	*243*	*2.7*	*5.6*	*23.3*	*0.1*
Extra Thick, 99% Real Dairy Cream, Anchor*	1 Serving/13g	51	5.4	409	1.7	3.9	43.0	0.0
Extra Thick, Reduced Fat, Weight Watchers*	1 Serving/30g	42	3.4	140	2.5	6.7	11.5	0.8
Extra Thick, with Baileys, Baileys*	1 fl oz/30ml	129	11.6	431	1.5	13.4	38.6	0.0
Oat Alternative, Dairy Free, Oatly*	1 Carton/250ml	375	32.5	150	1.0	6.0	13.0	0.8
Single, Average	*1 Tbsp/15ml*	*28*	*2.7*	*188*	*2.6*	*3.9*	*18.0*	*0.1*
Single, Extra Thick, Average	*1 Serving/38ml*	*72*	*6.9*	*192*	*2.7*	*4.1*	*18.4*	*0.0*
Sour, Avonmore*	1 Tub/200ml	440	50.0	220	2.4	4.0	25.0	0.5
Sour, Eat Smart, Morrisons*	2 Tbsps/30g	37	2.7	124	3.9	7.0	9.0	0.0
Soured, Fresh, Average	*1 Tsp/5ml*	*10*	*0.9*	*191*	*2.7*	*3.9*	*18.4*	*0.0*
Soured, Reduced Fat, Average	*1 Tsp/5ml*	*6*	*0.4*	*119*	*5.2*	*6.7*	*8.6*	*0.4*
Soya, Dairy Free, Alternative to Single Cream, Alpro*	1 Serving/30g	52	5.2	174	2.0	1.6	17.3	0.4
Thick, Sterilised, Average	*1 Tbsp/15ml*	*35*	*3.5*	*233*	*2.6*	*3.6*	*23.1*	*0.0*
Uht, Double, Average	*1 Tbsp/15g*	*41*	*3.9*	*274*	*2.2*	*7.4*	*26.3*	*0.0*
Uht, Reduced Fat, Average	*1 Serving/25ml*	*16*	*1.4*	*62*	*0.6*	*2.2*	*5.6*	*0.0*
Uht, Single, Average	*1 Tbsp/15ml*	*29*	*2.8*	*194*	*2.6*	*4.0*	*18.8*	*0.0*
Whipping, Average	*1 Tbsp/15ml*	*52*	*5.5*	*348*	*2.1*	*3.2*	*36.4*	*0.0*
CREAM SODA								
Diet, Sainsbury's*	1 Serving/250ml	2	0.0	1	0.0	0.0	0.0	0.0
No Added Sugar, Sainsbury's*	1 Can/330ml	2	0.3	0	0.1	0.1	0.1	0.1
Shapers, Boots*	1 Bottle/300ml	3	0.0	1	0.0	0.0	0.0	0.0
Traditional Style, Tesco*	1 Can/330ml	139	0.0	42	0.0	10.4	0.0	0.0
CREME BRULEE								
Average	*1 Serving/100g*	*313*	*26.0*	*313*	*3.8*	*15.7*	*26.0*	*0.2*
Gastropub, M&S*	1 Brulee/84g	285	24.6	340	3.1	15.7	29.3	0.7
M&S*	1 Pot/100g	360	32.6	360	3.3	13.0	32.6	0.0
Reduced Fat, M&S*	1 Serving/89g	186	13.1	210	4.9	14.2	14.8	0.5
CREME CARAMEL								
Asda*	1 Pot/100g	113	2.6	113	2.4	20.0	2.6	0.0
Average	*1 Serving/128g*	*140*	*2.8*	*109*	*3.0*	*20.6*	*2.2*	*0.0*
Carmelle, Green's*	1 Pack/70g	82	2.8	117	3.0	17.0	4.0	0.0
Tesco*	1 Pot/100g	115	1.6	115	2.8	21.8	1.6	0.0
CREME EGG								
Cadbury*	1 Egg/40g	177	6.0	440	3.2	73.0	15.0	0.4
Minis, Cadbury*	1 Egg/12g	50	1.9	435	4.2	67.0	16.5	0.5
CREME FRAICHE								
Average	*1 Pot/295g*	*1067*	*112.2*	*362*	*2.2*	*2.6*	*38.0*	*0.0*
Half Fat, Average	*1 Tbsp/15g*	*27*	*2.4*	*181*	*3.1*	*5.5*	*16.2*	*0.0*
Lighter, Sainsbury's*	¼ Pot/75ml	122	11.2	163	2.7	4.4	15.0	0.5
Low Fat, Average	*1 Tbsp/30ml*	*43*	*3.6*	*143*	*3.3*	*5.6*	*12.1*	*0.1*
Low Fat, Weight Watchers*	1 Tbsp/20g	15	0.5	76	5.1	7.7	2.7	0.5
Reduced Fat, Cowbelle, Aldi*	1 Serving/30ml	49	4.5	163	2.7	4.4	15.0	0.5
TTD, Sainsbury's*	1 Tbsp/30g	114	12.0	381	2.4	2.9	40.0	0.0
CREPES								
Chocolate Filled, Tesco*	1 Crepe/32g	140	5.8	438	5.9	62.5	18.1	1.6
Mushroom, M&S*	1 Pack/186g	195	4.5	105	5.7	17.1	2.4	2.5

	Measure	per Measure		Nutrition Values per 100g / 100ml				
	INFO/WEIGHT	KCAL	FAT	KCAL	PROT	CARB	FAT	FIBRE
CRISPBAKES								
Cheese & Onion, Cooked, Dalepak*	1 Bake/86g	192	8.8	223	4.9	26.9	10.2	1.7
Cheese & Onion, M&S*	1 Bake/114g	285	18.5	250	6.4	19.4	16.2	1.7
Cheese & Onion, Tesco*	1 Bake/109g	275	17.2	252	7.9	19.6	15.8	2.1
Cheese, Spring Onion & Chive, Sainsbury's*	1 Bake/114g	287	16.8	253	7.1	24.5	14.8	1.7
Dutch, Asda*	1 Bake/8g	31	0.3	388	14.7	74.9	3.3	4.2
Dutch, Co-Op*	1 Bake/10g	38	0.4	375	16.0	69.6	3.5	6.5
Dutch, HL, Tesco*	1 Bake/8g	30	0.2	385	14.7	74.9	2.7	4.2
Dutch, Sainsbury's*	1 Bake/10g	38	0.5	392	14.5	72.3	5.0	5.8
Ham Hock, Cheese & Leek, British, Sainsbury's*	1 Bake/150g	317	15.5	211	10.9	17.9	10.3	1.7
Minced Beef, M&S*	1 Bake/113g	226	12.3	200	10.0	15.6	10.9	1.5
Vegetable, M&S*	1 Bake/114g	200	10.3	175	2.5	19.2	9.0	2.6
Vegetable, Sainsbury's*	1 Bake/114g	246	13.0	216	2.0	26.2	11.4	2.0
CRISPBREAD								
3 Seed, Classic, Gourmet, Dr Karg*	1 Bread/25g	108	4.9	430	16.5	46.6	19.7	10.9
3 Seed, Organic, Gourmet	1 Bread/25g	101	4.7	405	15.8	48.8	18.8	14.6
Corn Thins, Sesame, Real Foods*	1 Thin/6g	23	0.2	384	10.7	69.9	3.4	10.2
Corn, Orgran*	1 Bread/5g	18	0.1	360	7.5	83.0	1.8	3.0
Cracked Black Pepper, Ryvita*	1 Slice/11g	38	0.2	344	8.8	66.6	1.6	14.5
Cream Cheese & Chives, Minis, Ryvita*	1 Pack/30g	114	2.3	380	8.7	75.7	7.7	13.0
Crisp 'n' Light, Wasa*	1 Bread/7g	24	0.1	360	12.0	73.0	2.2	5.3
Dark Rye, Ryvita*	1 Bread/10g	34	0.1	342	8.5	66.5	1.2	15.2
Emmental Cheese & Pumpkin Seed, Organic, Dr Karg*	1 Bread/25g	114	5.2	456	19.6	41.1	20.9	12.4
Fibre Plus, Wholegrain with Sesame, Wasa*	1 Bread/10g	35	0.7	350	13.0	47.0	7.0	24.0
Fruit Crunch, Ryvita*	1 Slice/15g	54	0.8	358	8.3	61.8	5.4	14.9
Gluten Free	1 Serving/8g	25	0.1	331	6.4	72.9	1.5	0.0
Hint of Chilli, Ryvita*	1 Slice/12g	42	0.2	349	8.6	66.6	1.9	16.8
Mini, Sesame & Linseed, Dr Karg*	1 Bread/3g	13	0.4	424	12.1	57.6	12.1	9.1
Mixed Grain, Jacobs*	1 Cracker/10g	41	1.3	436	9.1	66.7	13.9	4.2
Multigrain, Ryvita*	1 Slice/11g	41	0.8	370	11.2	56.0	7.2	18.3
Original Rye, Thin, Finn Crisp*	1 Slice/6g	22	0.2	339	10.0	59.0	2.6	20.0
Original Rye, Wasa*	1 Bread/11g	35	0.2	315	9.0	67.0	1.4	14.0
Original, Ryvita*	1 Bread/10g	35	0.2	350	8.5	66.9	1.7	16.5
Provita*	1 Bread/6g	26	0.6	416	12.5	68.4	9.9	0.0
Pumpkin Seeds & Oats, Ryvita*	1 Slice/13g	46	0.9	370	11.2	56.0	7.2	18.3
Rosemary & Apricot, Toasts, M&S*	1 Toast/8g	34	1.4	434	12.3	54.3	17.8	3.7
Rustikal, Wasa*	1 Bread/15g	51	0.2	340	9.0	6.4	1.5	16.0
Salt & Vinegar, Minis, Ryvita*	1 Pack/24g	90	1.9	376	8.2	74.0	7.8	11.4
Scan Bran, Slimming World*	1 Slice/10g	31	0.5	310	14.9	29.0	5.3	42.1
Seeded, Spelt, Organic, Dr Karg*	1 Bread/25g	108	4.5	430	17.2	44.4	18.0	11.2
Sesame, Ryvita*	1 Bread/10g	37	0.7	373	10.5	58.3	7.0	17.5
Sesame, Savour Bakes, Aldi*	1 Bread/9g	33	0.5	366	12.3	57.2	5.2	20.6
Spelt, Cheese, Sunflower Seeds, Organic, Dr Karg*	1 Bread/25g	103	4.5	411	19.2	42.8	18.1	10.4
Spelt, Muesli, Organic, Dr Karg*	1 Bread/25g	94	2.8	375	14.2	54.4	11.2	10.6
Spelt, Sesame, Sunflower, Amisa*	1 Bread/29g	85	4.3	297	11.7	28.5	15.1	5.0
Sport, Wasa*	1 Bread/15g	46	0.2	310	9.0	64.0	1.5	16.0
Sunflower Seeds & Oats, Ryvita*	1 Bread/12g	46	1.1	384	9.7	58.4	9.0	15.3
Sweet Chilli, Minis, Ryvita*	1 Pack/24g	90	1.8	376	8.5	75.9	7.4	10.3
Sweet Onion, Ryvita*	1 Bread/12g	43	0.2	356	9.0	70.6	1.4	12.6
Thin Crisps, Original Taste, Finn Crisp*	1 Bread/6g	20	0.2	320	11.0	63.0	2.4	19.0
Wholemeal Rye, Organic, Kallo*	1 Bread/10g	31	0.2	314	9.7	65.0	1.7	15.4
Wholemeal, Organic, Allinson*	1 Bread/5g	17	0.1	336	14.2	66.0	1.7	12.2

C

CRISPS

	Measure INFO/WEIGHT	per Measure KCAL	FAT	Nutrition Values per 100g / 100ml KCAL	PROT	CARB	FAT	FIBRE
Argentinean Flame Grilled Steak, Walkers*	1 Bag/35g	182	11.3	520	6.5	50.7	32.4	4.2
Bacon & Cheddar, Baked, Walkers*	1 Pack/38g	149	3.2	397	6.5	73.7	8.5	4.7
Bacon Crispies, Sainsbury's*	1 Bag/25g	117	5.7	468	19.9	45.8	22.8	4.8
Bacon Flavour Rashers, BGTY, Sainsbury's*	1 Pack/10g	34	0.2	340	10.8	70.3	1.6	3.5
Bacon Rashers, Blazin, Tesco*	1 Bag/25g	121	6.6	485	16.5	45.7	26.3	3.8
Bacon Rashers, COU, M&S*	1 Pack/20g	72	0.6	360	9.4	77.5	2.9	3.5
Bacon Rashers, Iceland*	1 Bag/75g	330	13.2	440	8.3	61.9	17.6	2.9
Bacon Rashers, Snackrite, Aldi*	1 Bag/18g	89	4.3	496	5.6	63.0	24.0	1.7
Bacon Rice Bites, Asda*	1 Bag/30g	136	4.8	452	7.0	70.0	16.0	0.4
Bacon Sizzler, Ridge Cut, McCoys*	1 Bag/32g	165	9.7	516	7.1	53.6	30.3	3.9
Bacon, Shapers, Boots*	1 Bag/23g	99	3.4	431	8.0	66.0	15.0	3.0
Bacon, Sizzler, Ridged, Snackrite, Aldi*	1 Pack/30g	148	7.5	493	7.2	57.9	25.1	3.2
Bacon, Webs, Monster Munch*	1 Pack/15g	74	3.4	497	6.5	65.2	23.1	1.6
Baked Bean Flavour, Walkers*	1 Bag/35g	184	11.6	525	6.5	50.0	33.0	4.0
Baked, Average	**1 Bag/25g**	**93**	**1.5**	**374**	**6.5**	**73.5**	**5.9**	**5.8**
Baked, Ready Salted, Walkers*	1 Pack/38g	146	3.0	390	6.0	74.0	8.0	5.5
Baked, Sour Cream & Chive, Walkers*	1 Pack/38g	148	3.2	395	7.0	73.0	8.5	5.0
Barbecue Beef, Select, Tesco*	1 Pack/25g	134	8.7	536	6.4	49.2	34.8	4.4
Barbecue, Handcooked, Tesco*	1 Bag/40g	187	10.0	468	6.6	53.8	25.1	5.2
Barbecue, Savoury Snacks, Weight Watchers*	1 Pack/22g	81	1.9	366	18.6	61.0	8.7	6.1
Barbecue, Snack Rite*	1 Bag/25g	131	8.3	524	5.1	51.3	33.2	0.0
Barbecue, Sunseed Oil, Walkers*	1 Pack/33g	171	10.7	525	6.5	50.0	33.0	4.0
Beef & Onion Flavour, Average	**1 Bag/25g**	**131**	**8.3**	**524**	**6.5**	**50.0**	**33.1**	**4.3**
Beef & Onion, Tayto*	1 Bag/35g	184	11.9	526	7.6	47.3	34.0	4.5
Beef & Onion, Walkers*	1 Bag/33g	171	10.7	525	6.5	50.0	33.0	4.0
Beef, Space Raiders, KP Snacks*	1 Pack/13g	64	2.9	495	6.5	65.3	22.8	1.0
Beef, Squares, Walkers*	1 Bag/25g	105	4.5	420	6.0	59.0	18.0	4.6
Buffalo Mozzarella Tomato & Basil, Kettle Chips*	1 Serving/50g	238	12.8	476	6.7	54.4	25.7	4.9
Butter & Chive, COU, M&S*	1 Bag/26g	95	0.5	365	7.7	77.3	1.9	4.6
Canadian Ham Flavour, Seabrook*	1 Pack/30g	159	9.8	531	5.7	50.9	32.7	5.1
Chargrilled Chicken Crinkles, Shapers, Boots*	1 Bag/20g	96	4.8	482	6.6	60.0	24.0	4.0
Chargrilled Chicken, Ridge Cut, McCoys*	1 Pack/32g	167	10.0	521	7.0	52.9	31.3	4.0
Chargrilled Steak, Max, Walkers*	1 Bag/55g	289	18.2	525	6.5	50.0	33.0	4.0
Cheddar & Onion, Crinkles, Walkers*	1 Pack/28g	150	9.3	538	6.0	51.5	33.3	3.5
Cheddar & Onion, Ridge Cut, McCoys*	1 Bag/32g	165	9.8	516	7.0	53.2	30.6	3.9
Cheddar & Red Onion Chutney, Sensations, Walkers*	1 Bag/40g	198	11.2	495	6.5	54.0	28.0	4.5
Cheddar & Sour Cream, Extra Crunchy, Walkers*	1 Serving/30g	143	6.8	476	6.6	59.1	22.6	4.7
Cheddar & Spring Onion, 35% Less Fat, Sainsbury's*	1 Pack/20g	93	4.2	463	6.3	62.4	20.9	0.9
Cheddar Cheese & Bacon, Temptingly, Walkers*	1 Pack/32g	169	10.0	520	6.2	52.3	30.9	4.2
Cheese & Chives, Walkers*	1 Bag/33g	172	10.7	530	6.5	50.0	33.0	4.1
Cheese & Onion Flavour, Asda*	1 Bag/25g	130	7.8	519	5.6	53.6	31.4	3.7
Cheese & Onion Rings, Crunchy, Shapers, Boots*	1 Bag/15g	56	0.4	374	5.9	81.0	2.9	2.0
Cheese & Onion, Baked, Walkers*	1 Sm Bag/25g	99	2.1	396	6.5	73.8	8.3	4.7
Cheese & Onion, BGTY, Sainsbury's*	1 Bag/25g	120	6.2	479	7.0	57.0	24.8	5.7
Cheese & Onion, Crinkle Cut, Low Fat, Waitrose*	1 Bag/25g	122	5.8	490	7.7	62.6	23.2	4.7
Cheese & Onion, Crinkle Cut, Reduced Fat, Linessa, Lidl*	1 Pack/25g	116	5.2	463	6.9	60.4	20.6	4.0
Cheese & Onion, Crinkle, Seabrook*	1 Pack/32g	170	10.5	536	5.9	51.1	33.1	5.2
Cheese & Onion, GFY, Asda*	1 Pack/26g	122	5.7	470	7.0	61.0	22.0	4.2
Cheese & Onion, Golden Wonder*	1 Bag/25g	129	7.9	516	5.8	52.4	31.5	3.8
Cheese & Onion, KP Snacks*	1 Bag/25g	134	8.7	534	6.6	48.7	34.8	4.8
Cheese & Onion, Lights, Walkers*	1 Sm Bag/24g	113	5.0	470	7.5	62.0	21.0	5.0
Cheese & Onion, M&S*	1 Bag/25g	134	8.9	535	5.5	48.8	35.5	5.0
Cheese & Onion, Max, Walkers*	1 Pack/50g	262	16.0	525	6.8	52.0	32.0	5.2

CRISPS

INFO/WEIGHT	Measure	per Measure		Nutrition Values per 100g / 100ml				
		KCAL	FAT	KCAL	PROT	CARB	FAT	FIBRE
Cheese & Onion, Pom Bear, Intersnack Ltd*	1 Bag/19g	95	5.3	498	3.8	58.1	27.8	3.2
Cheese & Onion, Sainsbury's*	1 Bag/25g	132	8.7	527	4.6	48.8	34.8	3.9
Cheese & Onion, Snack Rite*	1 Pack/25g	132	8.4	527	5.3	51.3	33.4	0.0
Cheese & Onion, Squares, Walkers*	1 Bag/25g	108	4.5	430	6.5	61.0	18.0	5.5
Cheese & Onion, Sunseed Oil, Walkers*	1 Bag/33g	171	10.7	525	7.0	50.0	33.0	4.0
Cheese & Onion, Tesco*	1 Pack/25g	135	8.0	535	5.4	54.8	31.8	3.2
Cheese & Red Onion, Extra Crunchy, Walkers*	1 Serving/30g	140	6.3	468	6.8	60.6	20.9	4.9
Cheese Curls, Morrisons*	1 Bag/17g	95	6.1	557	3.1	54.8	35.6	2.6
Cheese Curls, Shapers, Boots*	1 Pack/14g	68	3.8	489	4.5	57.0	27.0	2.7
Cheese Curls, Sprinters*	1 Bag/14g	68	3.8	483	4.1	56.4	26.8	0.0
Cheese Curls, Tesco*	1 Bag/14g	75	4.5	520	4.5	54.4	31.1	1.9
Cheese Curls, Weight Watchers*	1 Pack/20g	78	1.7	392	5.0	73.8	8.6	3.4
Cheese Heads, Walkers*	1 Bag/27g	128	6.0	475	10.8	58.0	22.3	2.8
Cheese Moments, Smiths*	1 Pack/28g	148	9.2	530	8.0	50.0	33.0	2.0
Cheese Puffs, Weight Watchers*	1 Pack/18g	80	1.9	444	7.8	77.2	10.6	3.3
Cheese Tasters, M&S*	1 Sm Bag/30g	154	8.8	515	8.1	55.0	29.3	1.7
Cheeses with Onion, Soulmates, Kettle Chips*	1 Pack/40g	195	11.6	488	7.7	50.2	29.0	5.4
Cheesy Curls, Tesco*	1 Pack/17g	90	5.4	530	3.5	56.0	32.0	1.9
Cheesy Puffs, Co-Op*	1 Bag/60g	321	20.4	535	3.0	54.0	34.0	2.0
Cheshire Cheese, Red Wine & Cranberry, Kettle Chips*	1 Serving/30g	154	8.8	512	8.0	51.6	29.3	5.4
Chicken, Oven Roasted with Lemon & Thyme, Walkers*	1 Bag/40g	200	11.2	500	6.5	55.0	28.0	4.5
Chilli & Lemon, Walkers*	1 Pack/25g	131	8.2	525	6.3	51.0	33.0	3.8
Cider Vinegar & Sea Salt, Tyrrells*	1 Pack/40g	192	9.8	481	7.2	60.1	24.6	2.4
Corn Snacks, Crispy, Bugles*	1 Bag/20g	102	5.6	508	4.8	60.7	28.0	1.4
Cream Cheese & Chive, Waffles, Spar*	1 Pack/27g	132	6.8	488	4.2	60.7	25.3	1.3
Cream Cheese & Onion, Crisp & Thin, Ritz*	1 Serving/30g	135	4.8	450	5.7	68.0	16.0	5.1
Crunchy Sticks, Ready Salted, M&S*	1 Pack/75g	398	24.8	530	5.6	52.2	33.0	3.8
Crunchy Sticks, Salt & Vinegar, Sainsbury's*	1 Bag/25g	118	6.1	474	5.9	58.0	24.3	2.4
Crunchy Sticks, Salt & Vinegar, Tesco*	1 Serving/25g	118	6.1	470	6.9	55.7	24.4	2.7
Crunchy Sticks, Salt & Vinegar, Value, Tesco*	1 Bag/22g	113	5.9	512	5.7	62.1	26.8	0.7
Crushed Natural Sea Salt, Darling Spuds*	1 Bag/40g	195	12.0	488	5.6	53.4	30.0	4.5
D'lites, Cheddar & Red Onion Bites, The Real Crisp Co.*	1 Pack/20g	83	2.0	414	2.1	78.8	10.0	2.7
Double Gloucester & Red Onion, Kettle Chips*	1 Serving/40g	188	9.9	471	6.6	55.5	24.7	4.8
Extra Crunchy, Salt & Malt Vinegar, Walkers*	1 Pack/30g	139	6.2	463	6.6	59.9	20.8	4.8
Flame Grilled Steak, Ridge Cut, McCoys*	1 Bag/32g	165	9.8	516	7.0	53.0	30.7	4.0
Flamed Grilled Steak, Deep Ridge, Walkers*	1 Pack/28g	144	8.4	515	6.4	52.6	30.1	4.3
Four Cheese & Red Onion, Sensations, Walkers*	1 Bag/40g	194	10.8	485	6.5	54.0	27.0	4.5
Guinness, Burts*	1 Bag/40g	206	11.5	514	5.1	58.6	28.8	2.5
Ham & Mustard, Salty Dog*	1 Pack/40g	192	10.8	480	7.5	54.5	27.1	4.2
Hand Cooked, Honey Roast Ham, Finest, Tesco*	1 Serving/25g	130	7.3	515	5.1	58.6	28.8	2.5
Honey & BBQ, Wholgrain, Snacks, M&S*	1 Serving/30g	146	7.5	485	7.8	57.6	24.9	5.2
Honey Roast Gammon & English Mustard, Sainsbury's*	1 Serving/50g	236	12.4	472	7.2	55.0	24.8	5.0
Hoops, Ready Salted, Weight Watchers*	1 Bag/20g	73	0.3	365	3.4	82.7	1.4	4.1
Hot Jalapeño Chilli, Hand Cooked, Finest, Tesco*	1 Serving/25g	130	7.2	519	5.1	58.6	28.8	2.5
Kale, Pret a Manger*	1 Pack/25g	105	6.6	420	14.4	30.8	26.4	17.2
Lamb & Mint, Slow Roasted, Sensations, Walkers*	1 Bag/35g	170	9.4	485	6.5	54.0	27.0	4.5
Lentil Tubes, Smokey Bacon, M&S*	1 Pack/22g	87	1.8	394	11.4	67.3	8.0	3.7
Lightly Salted, Baked, COU, M&S*	1 Bag/25g	88	0.6	350	8.5	76.4	2.3	5.7
Lightly Salted, Crinkle Cut, Low Fat, Waitrose*	1 Pack/35g	163	8.0	466	5.2	60.1	22.8	5.1
Lightly Salted, Handcooked, Finest, Tesco*	1 Bag/40g	206	11.5	515	5.1	58.6	28.8	2.5
Lightly Salted, Kettle Chips*	1 Serving/50g	255	15.2	510	5.9	50.5	30.3	5.6
Lightly Salted, Potato Bakes, Weight Watchers*	1 Pack/20g	78	1.8	392	5.0	72.0	9.0	5.0
Lightly Salted, Reduced Fat, Crinkles, Eat Well, M&S*	1 Pack/30g	140	6.6	460	6.7	59.4	21.8	4.5

CRISPS

	Measure INFO/WEIGHT	per Measure KCAL	FAT	Nutrition Values per 100g / 100ml KCAL	PROT	CARB	FAT	FIBRE
Lightly Sea Salted, Hand Cooked, English, Tyrrells*	1 Pack/25g	125	6.4	501	5.9	49.0	25.4	5.3
Lightly Sea Salted, Potato Chips, Hand Fried, Burts*	¼ Bag/50g	252	13.8	504	6.4	57.4	27.7	0.0
Lime & Thai Spices, Gently Infused, Sensations, Walkers*	1 Pack/40g	200	11.6	500	6.5	54.0	29.0	4.0
Mango & Chilli, Baked, Walkers*	1 Pack/38g	147	3.0	392	6.4	74.0	8.0	4.8
Mango Chilli, Kettle Chips*	1 Serving/40g	190	9.6	475	6.3	53.9	24.0	6.1
Marmite*	1 Pack/25g	130	7.7	519	6.2	52.6	30.7	3.7
Marmite, Sunseed, Walkers*	1 Bag/33g	169	10.7	520	6.5	49.0	33.0	4.0
Mature Cheddar & Chive, Kettle Chips*	1 Serving/50g	239	12.7	478	8.1	54.4	25.4	5.0
Mature Cheddar & Chive, Tyrrells*	1 Bag/40g	194	10.0	485	8.4	58.7	25.1	2.4
Mature Cheddar & Onion, Deep Ridge, Walkers*	1 Pack/28g	145	8.6	518	6.4	51.8	30.7	4.3
Mature Cheddar & Red Onion, Deluxe, Lidl*	1 Pack/25g	121	6.2	483	7.4	54.6	25.0	5.0
Mature Cheddar, Hand Fried, Potato Chips, Burts*	1 Serving/40g	202	11.1	504	6.4	57.4	27.7	0.0
Mature Cheese & Chives, Potato Chips, Tyrrells*	1 Bag/50g	261	14.0	522	6.1	56.5	27.9	0.0
Mexican Chilli, Ridge Cut, McCoys*	1 Bag/32g	164	9.8	514	6.9	53.0	30.5	4.5
Mexican Lime with a Hint of Chilli, Kettle Chips*	1 Serving/50g	242	13.8	484	5.0	54.1	27.5	5.4
Naked, Tyrrells*	1 Pack/150g	748	41.2	499	7.7	56.5	27.5	0.0
New York Cheddar, Kettle Chips*	1 Bag/50g	242	13.4	483	6.7	53.9	26.7	4.5
Onion Rings, Corn Snacks, Average	**1 Bag/25g**	**122**	**6.1**	**486**	**5.8**	**60.9**	**24.2**	**2.7**
Onion Rings, M&S*	1 Pack/40g	186	8.6	465	5.2	62.1	21.5	4.3
Onion Rings, Tayto*	1 Pack/17g	82	4.1	484	3.0	63.4	24.0	2.4
Onion Rings, Tesco*	1 Serving/30g	148	7.6	495	8.4	57.8	25.5	2.5
Paprika, Max, Walkers*	1 Bag/50g	260	16.0	520	6.5	52.0	31.9	5.1
Pickled Onion, Beastie Bites, Asda*	1 Bag/20g	100	5.2	498	6.0	60.0	26.0	0.0
Pickled Onion, Golden Wonder*	1 Bag/25g	131	8.5	524	5.6	49.0	34.0	2.0
Pickled Onion, Space Raiders, KP Snacks*	1 Bag/13g	64	2.9	495	6.5	65.3	22.8	1.0
Pom Bear, Smoky Bacon, Potato Snack, Intersnack Ltd*	1 Bag/19g	98	5.1	515	3.9	63.8	27.0	0.7
Pom Bear, Zoo, Really Cheesy, Potato Snack	1 Bag/19g	100	5.8	525	3.6	57.0	30.7	3.1
Pom-Bear, Prawn Cocktail, Potato Snack, Intersnack Ltd*	1 Bag/19g	97	5.2	508	3.4	61.6	27.2	1.8
Potato	1oz/28g	148	9.6	530	5.7	53.3	34.2	5.3
Potato Chips, Anglesey Sea Salt, Red Sky*	1 Serving/40g	185	8.7	463	6.8	59.8	21.8	5.0
Potato Chips, Popped, Cheeses & Onion Flavour, M&S*	1 Bag/23g	95	3.2	413	7.4	60.9	13.9	4.4
Potato Rings, Ready Salted, M&S*	1 Serving/75g	375	21.1	500	3.5	58.9	28.1	2.6
Potato Rings, Ready Salted, Sainsbury's*	1 Serving/50g	257	14.2	514	3.2	61.5	28.4	1.8
Potato Squares, Ready Salted, Sainsbury's*	1 Bag/50g	192	8.0	384	6.5	53.8	15.9	7.8
Potato, Baked, COU, M&S*	1 Bag/25g	88	0.6	350	8.5	76.4	2.3	5.7
Potato, Cheddar & Onion, Hand Cooked, Aldi*	1 Pack/150g	753	41.8	502	7.7	54.9	27.9	4.0
Potato, Low Fat	1oz/28g	128	6.0	458	6.6	63.5	21.5	5.9
Potato, Tyrrells*	1 Pack/261g	1362	72.8	522	6.1	56.5	27.9	0.0
Prawn Cocktail Flavour, Seabrook*	1 Bag/30g	163	10.1	544	5.7	49.2	33.7	4.5
Prawn Cocktail, 30% Less Fat, Sainsbury's*	1 Pack/25g	118	5.9	470	6.3	58.9	23.6	5.7
Prawn Cocktail, Crusti Croc, Lidl*	1 Pack/25g	136	8.2	546	5.3	55.1	33.0	3.9
Prawn Cocktail, Golden Wonder*	1 Bag/25g	131	7.7	521	5.3	53.9	30.8	3.5
Prawn Cocktail, Lites, Shapers, Boots*	1 Bag/21g	92	3.8	438	5.1	64.0	18.0	4.1
Prawn Cocktail, Snack Rite*	1 Bag/25g	129	8.3	516	5.0	49.2	33.2	0.0
Prawn Cocktail, Spirals, Shapers, Boots*	1 Bag/15g	73	3.8	489	3.3	61.0	25.0	3.0
Prawn Cocktail, Sunseed Oil, Walkers*	1 Bag/33g	171	10.7	525	6.5	50.0	33.0	4.0
Prawn Cocktail, Tayto*	1 Bag/35g	185	12.3	526	7.5	46.6	35.0	4.5
Prawn Crackers, Tesco*	1 Bag/60g	316	17.5	527	3.2	62.8	29.2	0.8
Prawn, Spirals, Shapers, Boots*	1 Pack/100g	468	22.0	468	3.1	64.0	22.0	2.8
Ready Salted, Average	**1 Bag/25g**	**127**	**7.4**	**508**	**6.1**	**53.4**	**29.7**	**4.0**
Ready Salted, Co-Op*	1 Bag/25g	131	8.5	525	6.0	51.0	34.0	3.0
Ready Salted, Deep Ridge, Walkers*	1 Pack/28g	148	9.0	529	6.4	51.1	32.1	4.6
Ready Salted, Everyday Value, Tesco*	1 Pack/18g	100	6.1	535	5.0	52.8	32.7	3.8

CRISPS

	Measure INFO/WEIGHT	per Measure KCAL	FAT	Nutrition Values per 100g / 100ml KCAL	PROT	CARB	FAT	FIBRE
Ready Salted, Golden Wonder*	1 Bag/25g	135	8.8	539	5.5	49.9	35.3	2.0
Ready Salted, Lidl*	1 Bag/25g	138	9.2	554	4.9	50.3	37.0	0.0
Ready Salted, Lower Fat, Asda*	1 Bag/25g	120	6.2	481	6.0	58.0	25.0	4.8
Ready Salted, M&S*	1 Bag/25g	136	9.2	545	5.6	47.8	36.6	4.9
Ready Salted, Morrisons*	1 Bag/25g	134	8.7	536	4.9	50.9	34.8	4.3
Ready Salted, Potato Chips, Sainsbury's*	¼ Pack/33g	174	10.9	526	5.6	51.7	33.0	3.8
Ready Salted, Potato Chips, Tesco*	1 Bag/25g	132	8.2	526	5.6	51.7	33.0	3.8
Ready Salted, Reduced Fat, Tesco*	1 Pack/25g	114	6.2	456	6.3	52.0	24.7	5.9
Ready Salted, Ridge Cut, McCoys*	1 Bag/49g	257	15.6	524	6.6	52.6	31.9	4.1
Ready Salted, Sainsbury's*	1 Bag/25g	132	8.1	530	5.0	52.5	32.5	3.7
Ready Salted, Smart Price, Asda*	1 Bag/18g	96	5.9	531	5.0	52.6	32.6	3.8
Ready Salted, Squares, M&S*	1 Bag/35g	150	6.3	430	6.8	63.5	18.1	3.9
Ready Salted, Squares, Walkers*	1 Pack/25g	109	4.8	435	6.5	60.0	19.0	6.0
Ready Salted, Sunseed Oil, Walkers*	1 Bag/33g	175	11.1	537	5.9	49.7	34.1	4.2
Ready Salted, Tesco*	1 Bag/25g	140	8.5	545	5.0	55.4	33.2	1.8
Ready Salted, Value, Morrisons*	1 Pack/18g	95	6.0	528	6.7	50.0	33.3	0.6
Red Leicester & Spring Onion, Handcooked, M&S*	1 Pack/40g	194	10.6	485	6.8	55.0	26.4	5.1
Ridge, Thick & Chunky, Ready Salted, Eastmans*	1 Pack/30g	155	9.2	515	5.9	53.5	30.6	4.1
Roast Beef & Mustard, Thick Cut, Brannigans*	1 Bag/40g	203	12.0	507	7.6	51.7	30.0	3.7
Roast Beef, KP Snacks*	1 Bag/25g	134	8.8	534	6.6	47.5	35.3	4.7
Roast Chicken & Sage Flavour, M&S*	1 Bag/25g	135	8.6	540	5.9	50.6	34.6	4.6
Roast Chicken Flavour	1 Bag/25g	130	7.7	519	5.2	53.5	30.8	3.7
Roast Chicken Flavour, Average	***1 Bag/25g***	***132***	***8.6***	***528***	***6.1***	***48.8***	***34.2***	***3.9***
Roast Chicken Flavour, Crinkle, Weight Watchers*	1 Pack/16g	76	3.3	475	5.6	63.1	20.6	6.2
Roast Chicken, Golden Wonder*	1 Bag/25g	130	8.4	522	6.2	48.6	33.6	2.0
Roast Chicken, Select, Tesco*	1 Bag/25g	134	8.8	536	6.6	48.6	35.0	4.4
Roast Chicken, Snack Rite*	1 Bag/25g	132	8.3	526	5.3	51.3	33.3	0.0
Roast Chicken, Sunseed Oil, Walkers*	1 Bag/33g	171	10.7	525	6.5	50.0	33.0	4.0
Roast Pork & Apple Sauce, Select, Tesco*	1 Bag/25g	136	8.8	544	6.5	50.0	35.3	3.7
Roasted Lamb, Moroccan Spices, Sensations, Walkers*	1 Bag/40g	198	11.6	495	6.0	53.0	29.0	4.5
Roasted Peanut Puffs, Ellert*	1 Serving/25g	125	6.0	500	13.0	56.0	24.0	4.1
Salsa with Mesquite, Kettle Chips*	1 Serving/50g	231	12.1	462	5.8	55.2	24.2	5.7
Salt & Black Pepper, Handcooked, M&S*	1 Bag/40g	180	9.2	450	5.7	55.0	22.9	5.2
Salt & Malt Vinegar Flavour, Sainsbury's*	1 Bag/25g	134	8.8	538	4.9	50.3	35.2	2.3
Salt & Malt Vinegar, Deep Ridge, Walkers*	1 Pack/28g	143	8.6	511	6.1	50.7	30.7	4.3
Salt & Malt Vinegar, Hunky Dorys*	1 Serving/30g	141	8.6	469	6.3	49.3	28.7	0.0
Salt & Malt Vinegar, Ridge Cut, McCoys*	1 Bag/32g	165	9.8	515	6.7	53.3	30.6	3.9
Salt & Shake, Walkers*	1 Pack/24g	128	7.8	533	6.2	52.2	32.3	4.4
Salt & Vinegar Chiplets, M&S*	1 Pack/50g	220	9.4	440	5.7	61.3	18.9	4.7
Salt & Vinegar Flavour, Asda*	1 Bag/25g	130	8.5	522	6.0	48.0	34.0	4.2
Salt & Vinegar Flavour, Half Fat, M&S*	1 Bag/40g	168	6.8	420	5.8	61.0	17.0	7.7
Salt & Vinegar Flavour, Sprinters*	1 Bag/25g	133	8.8	532	4.8	49.1	35.2	0.0
Salt & Vinegar Fries, COU, M&S*	1 Bag/25g	85	0.4	340	5.0	80.0	1.6	4.0
Salt & Vinegar in Sunflower Oil, Sainsbury's*	1 Serving/25g	131	8.4	524	5.2	49.7	33.8	3.7
Salt & Vinegar, 30% Less Fat, Sainsbury's*	1 Bag/25g	114	5.4	458	7.2	58.3	21.8	5.1
Salt & Vinegar, Average	***1 Bag/25g***	***130***	***8.2***	***519***	***5.5***	***50.3***	***32.9***	***3.4***
Salt & Vinegar, Baked, Walkers*	1 Pack/38g	150	3.0	400	6.0	73.5	8.1	4.6
Salt & Vinegar, Crinkle Cut, Reduced Fat, Lidl*	1 Pack/25g	116	5.2	464	6.7	60.6	20.8	3.6
Salt & Vinegar, Crinkle Cut, Seabrook*	1 Multi Pack/25g	126	7.2	502	5.9	52.9	28.7	3.9
Salt & Vinegar, Crinkle, M&S*	1 Pack/25g	120	5.9	485	6.5	61.0	24.0	3.5
Salt & Vinegar, Crispy Discs, Shapers, Boots*	1 Bag/21g	92	4.0	439	4.8	63.0	19.0	4.9
Salt & Vinegar, Distinctively, Walkers*	1 Pack/33g	169	10.0	519	5.9	52.6	30.8	4.2
Salt & Vinegar, Everyday Value, Tesco*	1 Bag/18g	95	5.7	530	5.0	54.1	31.7	3.7

CRISPS

INFO/WEIGHT	Measure	per Measure		Nutrition Values per 100g / 100ml				
		KCAL	FAT	KCAL	PROT	CARB	FAT	FIBRE
Salt & Vinegar, Everyday, Co-Op*	1 Bag/17g	77	3.4	455	6.0	62.0	20.0	2.0
Salt & Vinegar, GFY, Asda*	1 Bag/26g	120	5.7	466	6.0	61.0	22.0	4.1
Salt & Vinegar, Golden Lights, Golden Wonder*	1 Bag/21g	94	3.9	446	4.2	65.7	18.5	3.7
Salt & Vinegar, Golden Wonder*	1 Bag/25g	130	8.5	522	5.4	48.5	34.0	2.0
Salt & Vinegar, Lights, Walkers*	1 Bag/28g	133	6.2	475	7.0	62.0	22.0	4.5
Salt & Vinegar, Lower Fat, Asda*	1 Bag/25g	120	6.2	481	5.0	58.0	25.0	4.8
Salt & Vinegar, M&S*	1 Bag/25g	131	8.6	525	5.4	48.8	34.5	4.6
Salt & Vinegar, Morrisons*	1 Bag/25g	129	7.8	515	4.9	53.9	31.1	3.6
Salt & Vinegar, Odd Bites, Savoury Bakes, Aldi*	1 Bag/25g	115	4.0	459	8.6	69.0	16.0	3.4
Salt & Vinegar, Oven Baked, Asda*	1 Bag/25g	95	2.0	380	5.1	72.0	8.0	2.9
Salt & Vinegar, Pom Bear, Intersnack Ltd*	1 Pack/25g	124	6.8	494	3.0	58.8	27.4	2.7
Salt & Vinegar, Rough Cuts, Tayto*	1 Bag/30g	152	9.2	506	4.6	56.8	30.8	0.0
Salt & Vinegar, Sainsbury's*	1 Bag/25g	130	8.8	522	4.1	46.9	35.3	3.9
Salt & Vinegar, Select, Tesco*	1 Bag/25g	132	8.7	529	5.9	47.8	34.9	4.3
Salt & Vinegar, Snack Rite*	1 Bag/25g	127	8.2	508	4.7	48.1	33.0	0.0
Salt & Vinegar, Spirals, Shapers, Boots*	1 Pack/15g	73	3.8	486	3.0	61.0	25.0	3.4
Salt & Vinegar, Squares, Walkers*	1 Bag/28g	121	4.9	441	6.5	61.0	18.0	5.5
Salt & Vinegar, Sunseed Oil, Walkers*	1 Bag/33g	171	10.7	525	6.5	50.0	33.0	4.0
Salt & Vinegar, Tayto*	1 Bag/35g	184	11.9	526	7.6	47.3	34.0	4.5
Salt & Vinegar, Thick Ridged, Snackrite, Aldi*	1 Bag/30g	159	9.3	529	5.8	55.0	31.0	3.4
Salt & Vinegar, Waitrose*	1 Pack/25g	132	8.4	529	6.3	50.5	33.8	4.4
Salt Your Own, Excluding Salt, Aldi*	1 Pack/24g	130	8.1	536	6.0	52.6	33.5	4.5
Salt Your Own, Sainsbury's*	1 Pack/24g	127	7.9	520	5.0	52.2	32.3	3.7
Salt Your Own, Snackrite, Aldi*	1 Pack/24g	130	8.1	536	6.0	52.6	33.5	4.5
Sausage & Tomato Flavour, Golden Wonder*	1 Bag/35g	174	10.6	505	6.1	51.3	30.6	4.5
Scampi, Smiths, Walkers*	1 Bag/27g	134	7.0	496	13.0	52.5	26.0	0.0
Sea Sal & Vinegar, Crisp & Thin, Ritz*	1 Serving/30g	134	4.8	445	5.6	67.0	16.0	5.3
Sea Salt & Balsamic Vinegar, Delux, Lidl*	1 Pack/25g	121	6.3	484	6.0	56.8	25.2	4.4
Sea Salt & Balsamic Vinegar, Kettle Chips*	1 Bag/40g	201	11.4	502	5.4	53.0	28.4	6.1
Sea Salt & Black Pepper, GFY, Asda*	1 Bag/100g	476	24.0	476	6.0	59.0	24.0	6.0
Sea Salt & Black Pepper, Tyrrells*	¼ Pack/38g	182	9.3	480	7.3	59.9	24.5	2.4
Sea Salt & Cider Vinegar, TTD, Sainsbury's*	1/3 Pack/50g	245	14.3	489	5.5	52.7	28.5	6.1
Sea Salt & Cracked Black Pepper, Sensations, Walkers*	1 Bag/40g	196	10.8	490	6.5	55.0	27.0	4.0
Sea Salt & Crushed Black Peppercorn, Deluxe, Lidl*	1 Pack/25g	120	6.1	481	6.2	57.0	24.3	4.9
Sea Salt & Indian Black Pepper, Pipers Crisps*	1 Pack/40g	195	11.6	487	6.6	49.9	29.0	0.0
Sea Salt & Malt Vinegar, Sensations, Walkers*	1 Bag/40g	194	10.8	485	6.5	54.0	27.0	4.5
Sea Salt & Modena Balsamic Vivegar, Darling Spuds*	1 Bag/40g	190	11.4	475	5.4	54.3	28.5	4.2
Sea Salt, Gourmet, TTD, Sainsbury's*	1/3 Pack/50g	249	15.0	498	5.7	51.4	30.0	6.4
Sea Salt, Original, Crinkle Cut, Seabrook*	1 Bag/30g	155	9.3	517	5.7	53.7	31.1	4.2
Sea Salt, Ridge Crisps, Morrisons*	1 Serving/25g	126	6.6	504	6.5	58.8	26.3	2.9
Sea Salted, Furrows, Tyrells *	1 Serving/30g	143	7.2	476	6.2	59.9	23.9	0.0
Shells, Prawn Cocktail, Asda*	1 Bag/18g	90	5.3	501	4.6	54.9	29.2	6.2
Simply Salted, Extra Crunchy, Walkers*	1 Bag/30g	142	6.5	473	6.8	59.8	21.8	5.0
Simply Salted, Lights, Walkers*	1 Bag/24g	113	5.3	470	7.0	61.0	22.0	5.0
Sizzling Beef, Spice, McCoys*	1 Bag/35g	175	10.4	501	6.4	51.7	29.8	4.0
Sizzling King Prawn, Ridge Cut, McCoys*	1 Pack/50g	259	15.2	518	6.6	54.7	30.3	4.0
Smoked Ham & Pickle, Thick Cut, Brannigans*	1 Bag/40g	203	11.9	507	7.0	52.8	29.8	3.8
Smokey Bacon Potato Hoops, COU, M&S*	1 Pack/16g	58	0.4	360	5.6	78.7	2.7	4.5
Smokey Bacon, Budgens*	1 Bag/25g	130	8.2	519	6.2	49.3	33.0	4.8
Smokey Bacon, Select, Tesco*	1 Bag/25g	134	8.7	536	6.4	49.0	34.9	4.3
Smoky Bacon Flavour, Average	**1 Bag/25g**	**132**	**8.4**	**527**	**6.2**	**49.7**	**33.7**	**3.2**
Smoky Bacon, Golden Wonder*	1 Bag/25g	131	8.4	523	5.9	49.1	33.7	2.0
Smoky Bacon, Snack Rite*	1 Bag/25g	131	8.3	525	5.5	51.2	33.1	0.0

CRISPS	Measure INFO/WEIGHT	per Measure KCAL	FAT	Nutrition Values per 100g / 100ml KCAL	PROT	CARB	FAT	FIBRE
Smoky Bacon, Sunseed Oil, Walkers*	1 Bag/35g	183	11.4	530	6.5	51.0	33.0	4.0
Smoky Bacon, Tayto*	1 Bag/35g	184	11.9	526	7.6	47.3	34.0	4.5
Snaps, Spicy Tomato Flavour, Walkers*	1 Bag/13g	61	3.2	508	1.5	65.5	26.8	0.0
Snax, Tayto*	1 Pack/17g	82	3.7	483	2.4	70.0	21.5	1.6
Sour Cream & Black Pepper, Multigrain, Snackrite, Aldi*	1 Pack/25g	112	3.8	449	7.2	70.0	15.0	1.6
Sour Cream & Chilli Lentil Curls, M&S*	1 Pack/60g	243	5.2	405	13.6	65.3	8.7	4.3
Sour Cream & Chive Baked Potato, COU, M&S*	1 Pack/24g	84	0.7	350	7.5	73.2	2.8	7.9
Sour Cream & Chive Crispy Discs, Shapers, Boots*	1 Bag/21g	94	4.0	448	5.7	61.9	19.0	4.3
Sour Cream & Chive Flavour, Average	*1 Bag/25g*	*127*	*7.7*	*508*	*6.8*	*50.7*	*30.9*	*4.6*
Sour Cream & Chive, Crinkle, Reduced Fat, M&S*	1 Bag/40g	178	8.2	445	5.6	58.8	20.6	5.6
Sour Cream & Chive, Lights, Walkers*	1 Bag/24g	114	5.3	475	7.5	62.0	22.0	5.0
Sour Cream & Chive, Potato Bakes, Weight Watchers*	1 Bag/20g	83	1.8	417	3.8	80.7	8.8	3.6
Sour Cream & Chive, Potato Bites, BGTY, Sainsbury's*	1 Pack/20g	73	0.6	365	7.2	77.8	2.8	3.9
Sour Cream & Onion, Golden Lights, Golden Wonder*	1 Bag/21g	93	3.8	442	4.1	66.0	17.9	4.4
Spicy Chilli, Sunseed, Walkers*	1 Pack/35g	183	11.4	530	6.5	51.0	33.0	4.0
Spring Onion Flavour, Tayto*	1 Bag/35g	184	11.9	526	7.6	47.3	34.0	4.5
Steak & Onion, Walkers*	1 Pack/33g	169	10.7	520	6.5	49.0	33.0	4.0
Sun Bites, Lightly Sea Salted, Wholegrain, Walkers*	1 Bag/25g	120	5.4	481	7.5	60.7	21.7	6.6
Sunbites, Cheddar & Caramelised Onion, Walkers*	1 Bag/25g	120	5.4	480	7.6	60.8	21.6	6.4
Sweet Chill, Mexican, Phileas Fogg*	1 Bag/38g	193	11.0	507	6.7	54.8	29.0	4.2
Sweet Chilli & Red Pepper, Potato Chips, Tyrrells*	¼ Pack/37g	180	9.2	481	7.9	59.7	24.5	2.4
Sweet Chilli & Red Peppers, Fusion, Tayto*	1 Bag/28g	140	8.3	500	4.9	52.2	29.8	4.6
Sweet Chilli Flavour, Average	*1 Bag/25g*	*115*	*5.6*	*461*	*5.1*	*59.9*	*22.6*	*4.6*
Sweet Chilli, Baked Potato, COU, M&S*	1 Bag/26g	91	0.7	350	7.6	73.9	2.8	8.5
Sweet Chilli, Cracker, Special K, Kellogg's*	21 Crisps/23g	94	2.1	409	5.0	73.0	9.0	8.0
Sweet Chilli, Crinkle Cut, Weight Watchers*	1 Sm Bag/20g	94	4.1	470	5.6	62.9	20.6	5.8
Sweet Chilli, Hand Cooked, Asda*	1 Pack/25g	120	7.1	479	5.7	54.5	28.3	4.5
Sweet Potato, Lightly Salted, Baked, Kettle Chips*	1 Serving/20g	82	2.7	409	6.3	60.0	13.4	11.6
Sweet Red Chilli, Crisp & Thin, Ritz*	1 Serving/30g	135	4.8	450	6.1	68.0	16.0	5.3
T Bone Steak, Roysters*	1 Pack/28g	148	9.0	530	5.2	55.3	32.0	3.0
Tangy Sweet Chilli, Delight Bites, Snackrite, Aldi*	1 Pack/25g	111	4.2	445	6.6	66.0	17.0	2.3
Tangy Toms, Red Mill*	1 Bag/15g	76	4.1	507	6.0	60.0	27.3	0.7
Thai Bites, Mild, Jacob's*	1 Bag/25g	93	0.8	373	6.9	79.0	3.3	1.0
Thai Curry & Coriander, Tyrrells*	1 Pack/50g	261	14.0	522	6.1	56.5	27.9	5.4
Thai Sweet Chicken, Ridge Cut, McCoys*	1 Bag/50g	257	15.0	514	7.0	54.0	30.0	4.1
Thai Sweet Chilli Flavour, Velvet Crunch, King*	1 Pack/20g	81	1.9	404	1.6	77.5	9.7	2.0
Thai Sweet Chilli, Sensations, Walkers*	1 Bag/40g	194	10.4	485	6.0	57.0	26.0	4.2
Tomato & Herb, Shapers, Boots*	1 Bag/20g	94	4.2	468	3.7	66.0	21.0	3.9
Tomato Ketchup Flavour, Golden Wonder*	1 Bag/25g	135	8.0	521	5.1	54.0	30.8	3.6
Tortillas, Nacho Cheese Flavour, Weight Watchers*	1 Pack/18g	78	2.9	433	6.1	66.7	16.1	3.9
Traditional, Hand Cooked, Finest, Tesco*	1 Bag/150g	708	39.2	472	6.4	52.9	26.1	5.1
Twirls, Salt & Vinegar, Tesco*	1 Bag/80g	349	14.0	436	3.9	65.8	17.5	2.4
Vegetable, Average	*1 Bag/25g*	*118*	*7.4*	*470*	*4.1*	*46.5*	*29.6*	*12.1*
Vegetable, Crunchy, Asda*	½ Bag/50g	251	12.0	502	1.4	70.0	24.0	6.0
Vegetable, Finest, Tesco*	1 Serving/50g	203	12.8	406	5.0	39.0	25.5	14.6
Vegetable, TTD, Sainsbury's*	½ Pack/52g	254	17.9	490	4.8	39.9	34.5	12.8
Vegetable, Waitrose*	1 Pack/100g	490	35.2	490	4.7	38.5	35.2	13.0
Waffles, Bacon Flavour, BGTY, Sainsbury's*	1 Serving/12g	41	0.2	345	6.4	79.7	1.4	2.9
Wheat Crunchies, Golden Wonder*	1 Pack/35g	172	8.7	491	11.1	55.9	24.8	0.0
Wheat Crunchies, Salt & Vinegar, Golden Wonder*	1 Bag/34g	165	8.5	484	10.5	54.5	24.9	2.8
Wheat Crunchies, Worcester Sauce, Golden Wonder*	1 Bag/35g	172	8.9	492	9.3	56.4	25.5	3.9
Wild Paprika Flavour, Croky*	1 Pack/45g	234	13.0	521	6.0	58.0	29.0	0.0
Worcester Sauce Flavour, Hunky Dorys*	1 Bag/45g	211	12.9	469	6.3	49.3	28.7	0.0

INFO/WEIGHT	Measure	per Measure KCAL	FAT	Nutrition Values per 100g / 100ml KCAL	PROT	CARB	FAT	FIBRE
CRISPS								
Worcester Sauce, Sunseed Oil, Walkers*	1 Bag/33g	168	9.9	516	6.2	52.0	30.5	4.3
CRISPY PANCAKE								
Beef Bolognese, Findus*	1 Pancake/65g	104	2.6	160	6.5	25.0	4.0	1.0
Chicken, Bacon & Sweetcorn, Findus*	1 Pancake/63g	101	2.5	160	5.5	26.0	4.0	1.1
Minced Beef, As Consumed, Findus*	1 Pancake/115g	90	1.4	78	2.9	12.8	1.2	0.9
Three Cheese, As Consumed, Findus*	2 Pancakes/107g	183	3.6	171	6.5	28.0	3.4	1.4
CROISSANT								
All Butter, BGTY, Sainsbury's*	1 Croissant/44g	151	6.5	343	9.3	42.7	14.8	1.8
All Butter, Budgens*	1 Croissant/45g	185	11.1	412	7.9	39.7	24.6	3.3
All Butter, Finest, Tesco*	1 Croissant/77g	328	18.2	426	8.6	44.9	23.6	1.9
All Butter, M&S*	1 Croissant/54g	222	12.8	415	7.4	45.2	23.8	1.6
All Butter, Mini, Sainsbury's*	1 Croissant/30g	126	7.0	420	8.1	42.9	23.4	2.6
All Butter, Mini, Tesco*	1 Croissant/35g	150	8.2	430	9.3	45.2	23.5	2.0
All Butter, Reduced Fat, Tesco*	1 Croissant/52g	164	5.5	315	7.5	47.4	10.6	1.8
All Butter, Sainsbury's*	1 Croissant/44g	188	10.8	428	9.2	42.6	24.5	1.2
All Butter, Tesco*	1 Croissant/48g	192	10.4	400	8.5	41.7	21.6	2.6
Asda*	1 Croissant/47g	190	9.9	405	9.0	45.0	21.0	0.0
Average	**1 Croissant/50g**	**180**	**10.2**	**360**	**8.3**	**38.3**	**20.3**	**1.6**
Butter, Asda*	1 Croissant/46g	191	11.0	416	8.0	42.0	24.0	1.9
Butter, GFY, Asda*	1 Croissant/44g	153	7.0	352	6.0	46.0	16.0	2.0
Butter, Morrisons*	1 Croissant/44g	196	12.5	446	9.3	38.2	28.4	2.0
Cheese & Ham, Delice de France*	1 Croissant/91g	225	12.3	247	7.0	24.4	13.5	2.5
Cheese & Ham, Mini, Waitrose*	1 Croissant/17g	64	4.1	383	13.2	28.1	24.6	3.0
Flaky Pastry with a Plain Chocolate Filling, Tesco*	1 Croissant/78g	318	19.0	408	6.5	41.0	24.3	2.0
French Butter, You Count, LL, Waitrose*	1 Croissant/44g	168	7.4	382	9.8	46.4	16.8	3.1
Low Fat, M&S*	1 Croissant/45g	180	9.1	400	8.2	46.0	20.2	1.8
Mini, Lidl*	1 Croissant/30g	112	5.0	373	7.8	48.0	16.6	0.0
Reduced Fat, Asda*	1 Croissant/44g	159	6.5	361	9.7	47.2	14.8	2.0
Reduced Fat, Sainsbury's*	1 Croissant/44g	173	7.7	393	9.8	49.2	17.5	2.2
TTD, Sainsbury's*	1 Croissant/70g	289	16.1	413	8.1	43.4	23.0	2.5
Wholesome, Sainsbury's*	1 Croissant/44g	192	12.1	436	8.8	38.3	27.5	4.0
with Egg, Cheese & Ham from Restaurant, Average	**1 Croissant/152g**	**474**	**33.6**	**312**	**12.4**	**15.9**	**22.1**	**0.0**
CROQUETTES								
Morrisons*	1 Serving/150g	231	8.1	154	3.3	23.1	5.4	1.1
Potato & Parsnip, Finest, Tesco*	2 Croquettes/74g	155	7.3	210	6.0	23.2	9.9	3.9
Potato, Asda*	3 Croquettes/81g	144	5.7	177	2.0	26.5	7.0	2.2
Potato, Birds Eye*	1 Croquette/29g	44	1.7	152	2.6	22.6	5.7	1.2
Potato, Cheese & Onion, Mash Direct*	2 Croquettes/100g	214	10.0	214	3.7	26.1	10.0	2.3
Potato, Chunky, Aunt Bessie's*	1 Serving/41g	62	2.5	152	2.3	23.9	6.1	1.8
Potato, Crispy, Chilled, Sainsbury's*	3 Croquettes/125g	245	11.5	196	2.5	25.7	9.2	1.9
Potato, Fried in Blended Oil, Average	**1 Croquette/80g**	**171**	**10.5**	**214**	**3.7**	**21.6**	**13.1**	**1.3**
Potato, M&S*	1 Croquette/41g	68	3.6	165	2.4	19.3	8.8	2.2
Potato, Sainsbury's*	½ Pack/110g	227	10.9	223	3.3	27.1	10.7	2.8
Potato, Waitrose*	1 Croquette/30g	47	2.4	157	3.0	17.9	8.1	1.5
Sweet Potato, Moroccan Style, Heated, Sainsburys*	1 Croquette/40g	91	4.2	228	5.9	25.1	10.4	5.3
Vegetable, Sainsbury's*	1 Serving/175g	392	20.8	224	5.8	23.3	11.9	2.2
CROSTINI								
with Goats Cheese & Red Onion Chutney, Waitrose*	1 Crostini/17g	47	1.3	274	9.1	33.5	7.8	3.1
with Oregano, Crosta & Mollica*	1 Pack/150g	726	21.2	484	11.7	74.2	14.1	6.4
CROUTONS								
Fresh, M&S*	1 Serving/10g	53	3.3	530	11.4	50.0	32.8	3.2
Garlic, Waitrose*	1 Serving/40g	209	12.0	522	10.8	52.1	30.0	2.7
Herb & Garlic, La Rochelle*	¼ Pack/18g	106	7.2	587	6.9	49.8	40.0	2.1

C

	Measure INFO/WEIGHT	per Measure KCAL	FAT	Nutrition Values per 100g / 100ml KCAL	PROT	CARB	FAT	FIBRE
CROUTONS								
Herb, Sainsbury's*	1 Serving/15g	64	1.7	429	13.4	68.2	11.4	2.8
Italian Salad, Sainsbury's*	1 Pack/40g	204	10.0	510	8.5	62.7	25.0	2.5
Lightly Sea Salted, Asda*	1 Serving/20g	83	1.9	414	12.9	69.7	9.3	4.3
Prepacked, Average	**1 Serving/15g**	**74**	**3.6**	**495**	**10.8**	**58.7**	**24.0**	**2.6**
Sun Dried Tomato, Sainsbury's*	¼ Pack/15g	75	3.8	497	11.7	55.2	25.5	2.5
CRUDITES								
Selection, Prepared, M&S*	1 Serving/250g	75	1.0	30	1.4	5.8	0.4	2.0
Vegetable Sticks, Average	**1 Serving/100g**	**24**	**0.2**	**24**	**0.7**	**4.5**	**0.2**	**1.9**
CRUMBLE								
Almond & Apricot, Devondale*	1 Cake/80g	314	13.2	392	3.6	57.0	16.5	9.8
Apple & Blackberry, Asda*	1 Serving/175g	427	15.8	244	2.7	38.0	9.0	1.2
Apple & Blackberry, M&S*	1 Serving/135g	398	15.1	295	3.5	44.9	11.2	1.6
Apple & Blackberry, Sainsbury's*	1 Serving/110g	232	6.2	211	3.0	37.1	5.6	2.1
Apple & Blackberry, Tesco*	1 Crumble/335g	737	32.2	220	2.8	30.7	9.6	2.0
Apple & Custard, Asda*	1 Serving/125g	250	8.8	200	2.3	32.0	7.0	0.0
Apple with Custard, Green's*	1 Serving/79g	171	5.3	216	1.9	37.0	6.7	1.2
Apple with Custard, Individual, Sainsbury's*	1 Pudding/120g	286	13.9	238	2.0	31.4	11.6	2.4
Apple with Sultanas, Weight Watchers*	1 Dessert/110g	196	4.3	178	1.4	34.2	3.9	1.3
Apple, Average	**1 Serving/240g**	**497**	**12.0**	**207**	**0.9**	**40.5**	**5.0**	**1.1**
Apple, Basics, Sainsbury's*	¼ Crumble/125g	235	4.9	188	1.7	36.5	3.9	1.2
Apple, Fresh, Chilled, Tesco*	¼ Pack/150g	368	13.4	245	2.8	38.0	8.9	1.4
Apple, Sainsbury's*	1 Crumble/565g	1034	32.8	183	2.3	30.5	5.8	2.9
Apple, Waitrose*	1 Serving/125g	310	2.9	248	2.2	54.5	2.3	1.2
Bramley Apple & Blackberry, BGTY, Sainsbury's*	1 Crumble/120g	196	2.9	163	1.7	32.3	2.4	2.9
Bramley Apple, M&S*	1 Serving/149g	387	13.7	260	4.3	40.3	9.2	1.1
Fruit	1 Portion/170g	337	11.7	198	2.0	34.0	6.9	1.7
Fruit with Custard	1 Serving/270g	463	17.6	171	2.4	27.0	6.5	1.3
Fruit, Wholemeal	1oz/28g	54	2.0	193	2.6	31.7	7.1	2.7
Gooseberry, M&S*	1 Serving/133g	379	14.2	285	3.5	43.3	10.7	1.7
Rhubarb with Custard, Sainsbury's*	1 Serving/120g	288	13.9	240	2.4	31.4	11.6	2.3
Rhubarb, Asda*	½ Crumble/200g	460	24.0	230	2.4	28.0	12.0	5.0
Rhubarb, Average	**1 Portion/150g**	**330**	**11.1**	**220**	**2.7**	**35.5**	**7.4**	**1.9**
Rhubarb, M&S*	1 Serving/133g	366	13.2	275	3.4	42.6	9.9	1.4
Rhubarb, Sainsbury's*	1 Serving/50g	112	2.8	224	3.1	40.4	5.6	1.8
Rhubarb, Tesco*	1/6 Crumble/117g	228	9.7	195	2.8	27.3	8.3	1.7
CRUMBLE MIX								
Luxury, Tesco*	¼ Pack/55g	243	9.0	441	5.7	67.9	16.3	3.2
Topping, Morrisons*	1 Serving/40g	179	6.6	448	5.4	69.5	16.5	2.8
Topping, Sainsbury's*	1 Serving/47g	188	9.2	401	5.9	50.3	19.6	5.3
CRUMPETS								
Asda*	1 Crumpet/45g	85	0.4	188	6.0	39.0	0.9	2.1
Basics, Sainsbury's*	1 Crumpet/35g	69	0.4	198	5.9	41.0	1.1	1.6
Co-Op*	1 Crumpet/40g	70	0.3	175	7.0	35.0	0.7	2.0
Essential, Waitrose*	1 Crumpet/52g	94	0.6	182	6.5	35.1	1.1	2.6
Everyday, Value, Tesco*	1 Crumpet/40g	75	0.4	190	6.0	37.5	0.9	2.9
Fruit from Bakery, Tesco*	1 Crumpet/73g	161	1.7	220	6.2	43.2	2.3	1.1
Gluten, Wheat & Milk Free, Free From, Livwell*	1 Crumpet/55g	83	1.7	151	3.6	26.9	3.1	2.0
Less Than 2% Fat, M&S*	1 Crumpet/61g	116	0.8	190	8.0	36.9	1.3	2.1
Morrisons*	1 Crumpet/40g	70	0.3	174	6.6	35.3	0.7	1.8
Mother's Pride*	1 Crumpet/43g	80	0.4	185	5.6	38.3	1.0	2.3
Perfectly Balanced, Waitrose*	1 Crumpet/55g	94	0.2	171	6.1	36.1	0.3	4.4
Premium, Sainsbury's*	1 Crumpet/50g	96	0.7	191	6.1	38.6	1.4	1.7
Rowan Hill Bakery, Lidl*	1 Crumpet/44g	78	0.5	178	5.5	34.5	1.2	0.0

C

	Measure INFO/WEIGHT	per Measure KCAL	FAT	Nutrition Values per 100g / 100ml KCAL	PROT	CARB	FAT	FIBRE
CRUMPETS								
Sainsbury's*	1 Crumpet/46g	92	0.6	199	6.0	39.7	1.3	2.4
Scottish, Nick Nairn's*	1 Serving/100g	186	9.6	186	5.3	43.0	9.6	1.5
Smart Price, Asda*	1 Crumpet/36g	67	0.3	188	6.0	39.0	0.9	2.1
Square, Tesco*	1 Crumpet/60g	101	0.5	168	6.3	33.8	0.8	2.7
Thins, Kingsmill*	1 Thin/27g	54	0.3	199	6.9	39.3	1.1	2.3
Toasted, Average	*1 Crumpet/40g*	*80*	*0.4*	*199*	*6.7*	*43.4*	*1.0*	*2.0*
Toasted, Tesco*	1 Crumpet/65g	120	0.6	185	5.2	37.9	0.9	3.7
TTD, Sainsbury's*	1 Crumpet/65g	124	1.0	191	5.9	38.5	1.5	2.3
Waitrose*	1 Crumpet/62g	116	0.7	188	6.3	37.9	1.2	2.1
Warburton's*	1 Crumpet/55g	98	0.4	178	5.6	36.1	0.7	2.3
CRUNCHIE								
Cadbury*	1 Bar/40g	185	7.5	465	4.0	69.5	18.9	0.5
Treat Size, Cadbury*	1 Bar/17g	80	3.1	470	4.0	71.5	18.4	0.0
CUCUMBER								
Average	*1 Serving/80g*	*8*	*0.1*	*10*	*0.7*	*1.5*	*0.1*	*0.6*
Sweet, Sandwich Slices, Mrs Elswood*	¼ Jar/78g	32	0.2	41	0.6	9.3	0.2	0.0
CUMIN								
Seeds, Ground, Schwartz*	1 Tsp/5g	22	1.2	446	19.0	40.3	23.2	0.0
Seeds, Whole, Average	*1 Tsp/2g*	*8*	*0.5*	*375*	*17.8*	*44.2*	*22.7*	*10.5*
CUPCAKES								
Assorted, Sainsbury's*	1 Cake/38g	130	2.3	341	2.2	69.3	6.1	0.4
Carrot, Average	*1 Cake/40g*	*157*	*8.6*	*392*	*3.6*	*45.4*	*21.6*	*0.6*
Chocolate, Average	*1 Cake/40g*	*159*	*6.4*	*398*	*3.5*	*59.9*	*16.0*	*1.2*
Chocolate, Fabulous Bakin' Boys*	1 Cupcake/34g	152	8.1	448	4.0	54.0	24.0	1.0
Cookies & Cream, Secret Chocolate Centre, Tesco*	1 Cupcake/69g	335	20.0	485	2.7	52.2	29.0	1.0
Iced Cupcake, Gluten & Wheat Free, Lovemore*	1 Cake/33g	138	6.3	418	2.1	54.5	19.0	0.4
Lemon, Average	*1 Cake/40g*	*184*	*10.1*	*461*	*3.0*	*55.5*	*25.3*	*1.1*
Lemon, COU, M&S*	1 Cupcake/43g	130	0.9	305	3.3	68.1	2.1	2.0
Lemon, Mini, Weight Watchers*	1 Cupcake/17g	56	0.8	333	2.4	63.3	4.9	12.1
Mini, Jack O' Lantern, Vanilla Iced, The Cookieman Ltd*	1 Cake/25g	105	3.8	419	2.4	66.8	15.3	2.0
CURACAO								
Average	*1 Pub Shot/35ml*	*109*	*0.0*	*311*	*0.0*	*28.3*	*0.0*	*0.0*
CURLY WURLY								
Cadbury*	1 Bar/26g	115	4.5	442	3.5	69.2	17.3	0.8
CURRANTS								
Average	*1oz/28g*	*75*	*0.1*	*267*	*2.3*	*67.8*	*0.4*	*1.9*
CURRY								
& Chips, Curry Sauce, Chipped Potatoes, Kershaws*	1 Serving/330g	391	8.2	118	10.0	14.0	2.5	2.0
Aubergine	1oz/28g	33	2.8	118	1.4	6.2	10.1	1.5
Beef with Rice, Asda*	1 Pack/406g	548	15.8	135	6.0	19.0	3.9	1.2
Beef with Rice, Morrisons*	1 Serving/400g	480	20.0	120	6.0	12.6	5.0	0.6
Beef with Rice, Tesco*	1 Pack/400g	595	18.0	149	2.8	23.1	4.5	1.9
Beef, Hot, Canned, M&S*	1 Can/425g	446	21.7	105	12.2	2.8	5.1	1.0
Beef, Sainsbury's*	1 Serving/400g	552	32.8	138	10.7	5.4	8.2	0.9
Beef, Thai, Finest, Tesco*	1 Serving/500g	770	29.0	154	9.0	16.5	5.8	1.2
Blackeye Bean, Gujerati	1oz/28g	36	1.2	127	7.2	16.1	4.4	2.8
Bombay Butternut Squash, Veg Pot, Innocent*	1 Pot/380g	296	4.2	78	2.6	12.5	1.1	4.1
Cabbage	1oz/28g	23	1.4	82	1.9	8.1	5.0	2.1
Cauliflower & Chickpea, Lovely Vegetables, M&S*	1 Serving/390g	351	13.6	90	2.9	11.2	3.5	3.7
Cauliflower & Potato	1oz/28g	17	0.7	59	3.4	6.6	2.4	1.8
Cauliflower & Spinach, 695, Wiltshire Farm Foods*	1 Portion/430g	399	9.0	93	3.0	15.0	2.1	1.2
Chana Dahl, Curry Special*	1 Pack/350g	434	22.8	124	6.0	10.5	6.5	5.9
Chick Pea, Whole, Average	*1oz/28g*	*50*	*2.1*	*179*	*9.6*	*21.3*	*7.5*	*4.5*

CURRY

	Measure INFO/WEIGHT	per Measure KCAL	FAT	Nutrition Values per 100g / 100ml KCAL	PROT	CARB	FAT	FIBRE
Chick Pea, Whole, Basic, Average	**1oz/28g**	**30**	**1.0**	**108**	**6.0**	**14.2**	**3.6**	**3.3**
Chicken & Vegetable, Big Eat, Heinz*	1 Pot/350g	392	18.2	112	5.4	10.9	5.2	4.3
Chicken with Potatoes, Diet Chef Ltd*	1 Pack/300g	291	13.2	97	7.5	6.9	4.4	2.8
Chicken with Rice, Average	**1 Serving/400g**	**465**	**11.0**	**116**	**5.1**	**17.8**	**2.8**	**0.8**
Chicken with Rice, Fruity, HL, Tesco*	1 Pack/450g	495	5.4	110	6.5	18.2	1.2	1.2
Chicken, Asda*	1 Can/200g	210	10.0	105	10.0	5.0	5.0	0.0
Chicken, Chinese with Rice, Ready Meal, Average	**1 Serving/450g**	**490**	**11.5**	**109**	**7.2**	**14.1**	**2.6**	**1.3**
Chicken, Garlic, Indian, Waitrose*	1 Pack/350g	458	23.1	131	12.6	4.5	6.6	1.4
Chicken, Green Thai Style & Sticky Rice, Asda*	1 Pack/450g	585	10.8	130	7.0	20.0	2.4	0.1
Chicken, Green Thai, BGTY, Sainsbury's*	1 Pack/400g	316	10.4	79	10.6	3.4	2.6	1.9
Chicken, Green Thai, Birds Eye*	1 Pack/450g	536	19.8	119	4.7	15.2	4.4	0.3
Chicken, Green Thai, Breasts, Finest, Tesco*	1 Serving/200g	292	16.0	146	16.5	2.0	8.0	0.7
Chicken, Green Thai, Charlie Bigham's*	½ Pack/300g	402	26.7	134	9.9	3.6	8.9	0.8
Chicken, Green Thai, Jasmine Rice, Weight Watchers*	1 Pack/320g	291	3.2	91	6.1	14.3	1.0	0.5
Chicken, Hot, Can, Tesco*	1 Can/418g	514	26.3	123	9.7	6.9	6.3	0.9
Chicken, Kashmiri, Waitrose*	1 Serving/400g	640	36.4	160	14.5	5.0	9.1	0.6
Chicken, Malaysian, Finest, Tesco*	1 Pack/375g	375	8.3	100	7.4	12.2	2.2	0.8
Chicken, Medium Hot, M&S*	1 Serving/200g	310	14.2	155	7.8	14.3	7.1	0.8
Chicken, Mild, BGTY, Sainsbury's*	1 Serving/200g	184	5.2	92	10.0	7.2	2.6	0.5
Chicken, Red Thai with Jasmine Rice, Weight Watchers*	1 Pack/400g	344	3.2	86	6.5	12.9	0.8	0.8
Chicken, Red Thai with Rice, Tesco*	1 Serving/475g	746	32.3	157	7.2	16.8	6.8	1.1
Chicken, Red Thai, & Fragrant Rice, Charlie Bigham's*	½ Pack/418g	602	28.4	144	6.7	14.0	6.8	0.0
Chicken, Red Thai, Asda*	1 Pack/360g	461	27.7	128	9.1	5.5	7.7	1.0
Chicken, Red Thai, COU, M&S*	1 Pack/400g	420	9.2	105	7.1	13.4	2.3	1.4
Chicken, Red Thai, Tesco*	1 Serving/175g	215	11.6	123	10.5	5.5	6.6	1.4
Chicken, Rendang, Sainsbury's*	1 Pack/350g	690	53.6	197	9.6	5.1	15.3	1.7
Chicken, Thai Green, Nutritionally Balanced, M&S*	1 Pack/400g	400	5.2	100	9.2	12.4	1.3	1.4
Chicken, Thai Mango, Sainsbury's*	½ Pack/200g	288	17.8	144	11.2	4.8	8.9	1.9
Chicken, Thai, & Basmati Rice, Stir Your Senses, Birds Eye*	1 Pack/350g	360	10.1	101	5.1	12.8	2.8	1.5
Chicken, Thai, Green, Jasmine Rice, Ready Meal	**1 Serving/450g**	**520**	**17.2**	**116**	**7.7**	**12.6**	**3.8**	**1.1**
Chicken, Thai, Green, No Rice, Average	**1 Serving/200g**	**174**	**7.0**	**87**	**8.2**	**5.0**	**3.5**	**1.4**
Chicken, Thai, Red, & Rice, Ready Meal, Healthy Range	1 Serving/400g	400	7.8	100	6.4	14.0	2.0	1.0
Chicken, Thai, Red, No Rice, Average	**1 Serving/200g**	**194**	**6.9**	**97**	**7.2**	**9.0**	**3.4**	**1.4**
Chicken, Thai, Red, Sticky Rice, Ready Meal, Average	**1 Serving/450g**	**527**	**15.7**	**117**	**6.7**	**14.2**	**3.5**	**1.7**
Chicken, Yellow Thai Style, HL, Tesco*	1 Pack/450g	504	12.2	112	9.3	12.6	2.7	0.5
Chinese Chicken, Morrisons*	1 Pack/340g	347	15.6	102	10.3	5.0	4.6	0.8
Courgette & Potato	1oz/28g	24	1.5	86	1.9	8.7	5.2	1.2
Fish & Vegetable, Bangladeshi, Average	**1oz/28g**	**33**	**2.4**	**117**	**9.1**	**1.4**	**8.4**	**0.5**
Fish, Bangladeshi, Average	**1oz/28g**	**35**	**2.2**	**124**	**12.2**	**1.5**	**7.9**	**0.3**
Fish, Red Thai, Waitrose*	1 Pack/500g	275	11.0	55	5.2	3.7	2.2	1.0
Indian Daal, Tasty Veg Pot, Innocent*	1 Pot/380g	319	9.9	84	2.8	9.7	2.6	5.3
King Prawn Malay, Waitrose*	1 Pack/350g	364	19.2	104	6.6	7.1	5.5	0.9
King Prawn, Coconut & Lime, Sainsbury's*	½ Pack/351g	207	8.8	59	3.7	5.4	2.5	1.0
King Prawn, Goan, M&S*	1 Pack/400g	680	44.4	170	5.1	11.6	11.1	1.5
King Prawn, Malay with Rice, Sainsbury's*	1 Pack/400g	608	20.4	152	5.0	21.5	5.1	1.4
King Prawn, Red Thai, City Kitchen, Tesco*	1 Pack/385g	460	14.4	119	4.5	16.7	3.7	1.0
Lamb & Potato, 385, Wiltshire Farm Foods*	1 Serving/210g	334	23.0	159	8.9	6.2	11.0	1.7
Lamb, Hot, M&S*	½ Can/213g	320	19.6	150	14.9	6.0	9.2	2.3
Masala, Indian, Veg Pot, Innocent*	1 Pot/380g	331	10.3	87	2.9	11.6	2.7	3.6
Matar Paneer, Peas & Cheese, Ashoka*	½ Pack/150g	183	10.0	122	5.3	10.0	6.7	2.0
Medium, with Long Grain Rice, Rice Time, Uncle Ben's*	1 Pot/300g	396	9.0	132	2.3	23.2	3.0	1.2
Monkfish, & King Prawn, Gastropub, M&S*	½ Pack/285g	270	15.3	95	8.5	2.3	5.4	1.4
Mushroom & Pea, Masala, Indian, Sainsbury's*	1 Pack/300g	264	14.7	88	3.3	5.2	4.9	5.1

INFO/WEIGHT	Measure	per Measure		Nutrition Values per 100g / 100ml				
		KCAL	FAT	KCAL	PROT	CARB	FAT	FIBRE
CURRY								
Potato & Pea	1oz/28g	26	1.1	92	2.9	13.0	3.8	2.4
Prawn with Rice, Asda*	1 Pack/400g	420	10.4	105	3.5	17.0	2.6	1.1
Prawn with Rice, Frozen, Sainsbury's*	1 Pack/400g	552	7.6	138	3.9	26.4	1.9	2.1
Prawn, Red Thai, Sainsbury's*	1 Pack/300g	546	39.6	182	6.3	9.4	13.2	1.7
Red Kidney Bean, Punjabi	1oz/28g	30	1.6	106	4.7	10.1	5.6	3.8
Red Thai with Rice, Finest, Tesco*	1 Pack/500g	660	15.5	132	8.0	17.8	3.1	0.6
Red Thai, Vegetarian, Tesco*	1 Pack/429ml	588	21.9	137	5.4	17.3	5.1	1.6
Salmon, Green, Waitrose*	1 Pack/401g	581	40.5	145	9.1	4.5	10.1	2.7
Spicy Paneer, Lovely Vegetables, M&S*	1 Pot/300g	330	12.0	110	4.3	11.9	4.0	4.0
Sweet Potato & Cauli, Quinoa, Rice Pot, Pret a Manger*	1 Pot/320g	432	16.2	135	3.3	19.0	5.1	0.5
Thai Chicken, Diet Chef Ltd*	1 Pouch/300g	288	9.3	96	9.1	8.0	3.1	0.5
Thai Green, Chicken Breast, Cooked, Tesco*	½ Pack/165g	206	6.3	125	20.5	1.7	3.8	1.0
Thai Red, Chicken with Rice, Pod Foods*	1 Serving/500g	649	23.6	130	7.4	14.5	4.7	0.9
Vegetable in Sweet Sauce, Average	*1 Serving/330g*	*162*	*6.9*	*49*	*1.4*	*6.7*	*2.1*	*1.3*
Vegetable with Rice, Healthy Range, Average	*1 Serving/400g*	*351*	*4.6*	*88*	*2.3*	*16.8*	*1.1*	*1.9*
Vegetable with Rice, Ready Meal, Average	*1 Serving/330g*	*337*	*9.9*	*102*	*3.3*	*16.4*	*3.0*	*0.0*
Vegetable with Yoghurt, Average	*1oz/28g*	*17*	*1.1*	*62*	*2.6*	*4.6*	*4.1*	*1.4*
Vegetable, Asda*	1 Pack/350g	329	21.0	94	1.9	8.0	6.0	1.9
Vegetable, Canned, Sainsbury's*	½ Can/200g	200	12.2	100	1.4	9.8	6.1	1.8
Vegetable, Diet Chef Ltd*	1 Pack/300g	153	3.6	51	2.0	8.0	1.2	2.1
Vegetable, Frozen, Mixed Vegetables, Average	*1oz/28g*	*25*	*1.7*	*88*	*2.5*	*6.9*	*6.1*	*0.0*
Vegetable, Indian, Canned, Tesco*	1 Can/400g	320	18.0	80	2.0	6.7	4.5	1.1
Vegetable, Indian, Sainsbury's*	½ Pack/200g	206	14.6	103	2.5	6.8	7.3	4.6
Vegetable, Light Choices, Tesco*	1 Pack/350g	350	4.2	100	2.3	19.4	1.2	1.5
Vegetable, Medium, Tesco*	1 Pack/350g	326	21.7	93	2.3	7.1	6.2	1.9
Vegetable, Pakistani, Average	*1oz/28g*	*17*	*0.7*	*60*	*2.2*	*8.7*	*2.6*	*2.2*
Vegetable, Takeaway, Average	*1 Serving/330g*	*346*	*24.4*	*105*	*2.5*	*7.6*	*7.4*	*0.0*
Vegetable, Yellow Thai, Sainsbury's*	1 Pack/400g	624	48.8	156	2.2	9.4	12.2	1.1
CURRY LEAVES								
Fresh	*1oz/28g*	*23*	*0.3*	*81*	*6.6*	*11.0*	*1.1*	*0.0*
CURRY PASTE								
Balti, Asda*	1 Tube/100g	164	9.8	164	4.2	11.6	9.8	6.3
Balti, Sharwood's*	¼ Pack/73g	328	28.7	453	5.0	19.2	39.6	3.1
Balti, Tomato & Coriander, Original, Patak's*	1 Tbsp/15g	58	5.1	388	4.0	14.6	34.0	3.7
Green Thai, Average	*1 Tsp/5g*	*6*	*0.4*	*128*	*2.1*	*11.7*	*7.9*	*3.1*
Jalfrezi, Patak's*	1 Serving/30g	96	8.1	320	3.7	14.2	26.9	5.6
Madras, Cumin & Chilli, Hot, Patak's*	¼ Jar/70g	202	18.1	289	4.7	7.6	25.9	10.8
Mild, Coriander & Cumin, Original, Patak's*	1 Serving/35g	99	8.6	283	4.8	9.1	24.6	10.7
Mild, Sharwood's*	1oz/28g	78	6.0	279	3.6	17.7	21.5	3.4
Red, Thai, Average	*1 Tsp/5g*	*7*	*0.5*	*132*	*2.3*	*9.5*	*9.1*	*3.0*
Rogan Josh, Tomato & Paprika, Patak's*	1 Serving/30g	119	11.0	397	4.1	12.7	36.7	5.9
Tandoori, Tamarind & Ginger, Patak's*	1 Serving/30g	33	0.5	110	3.1	20.4	1.8	2.6
Tikka Masala, Coriander & Lemon, Medium, Patak's*	1 Serving/30g	111	9.5	369	3.8	16.9	31.8	2.9
Tikka Masala, Spice, Patak's*	1 Tbsp/15g	46	3.4	305	3.4	17.8	22.8	5.6
Tikka, Asda*	½ Tube/50g	118	8.5	235	4.5	16.1	17.0	1.6
Tom Yum, Thai Taste*	1 Tsp/13g	35	2.0	269	5.4	30.8	15.4	7.7
Yellow Thai, Tesco*	1 Tbsp/15g	15	0.6	100	1.9	13.6	4.1	4.9
Yellow, Thai, Barts*	1 Serving/30g	84	3.8	281	2.7	30.4	12.8	8.3
CURRY POWDER								
Average	*1 Tsp/2g*	*6*	*0.3*	*325*	*12.7*	*41.8*	*13.8*	*0.0*
CUSTARD								
Banana Flavour, Ambrosia*	1 Sm Pot/135g	139	3.9	103	2.9	16.1	2.9	0.0
Chocolate Flavour, Ambrosia*	1 Pot/150g	177	4.4	118	3.0	20.0	2.9	0.7

	Measure INFO/WEIGHT	per Measure KCAL	FAT	Nutrition Values per 100g / 100ml KCAL	PROT	CARB	FAT	FIBRE
CUSTARD								
Chocolate Flavour, Pot, Average	**1 Pot/125g**	**138**	**3.4**	**111**	**3.1**	**18.2**	**2.7**	**0.6**
Low Fat, Average	**1/3 Pot/141g**	**116**	**1.6**	**82**	**2.9**	**15.0**	**1.2**	**0.0**
Powder	**1 Tsp/5g**	**18**	**0.0**	**354**	**0.6**	**92.0**	**0.7**	**0.1**
Ready to Eat, Chocolate, Tesco*	1 Pot/150g	150	3.4	100	3.2	16.2	2.3	0.3
Ready to Serve, Aldi*	¼ Pot/125g	152	7.2	122	2.7	15.0	5.8	0.0
Ready to Serve, Average	**1 Serving/50g**	**59**	**2.3**	**118**	**3.3**	**16.1**	**4.6**	**0.2**
Ready to Serve, Canned, Everyday Value, Tesco*	½ Can/192g	133	1.3	69	2.8	12.9	0.7	0.0
Vanilla Bean, Dollop*	1 Dollop/100g	127	3.0	127	20.2	27.7	3.0	0.0
Vanilla Flavour, Pot, Average	**1 Pot/125g**	**128**	**3.5**	**102**	**2.8**	**16.4**	**2.8**	**0.0**
Vanilla with Apple Crunch, Ambrosia*	1 Pack/193g	276	8.7	143	3.4	22.4	4.5	0.8
Vanilla, Low Fat, Fresh, Waitrose*	1/5 Pot/100g	104	2.4	104	3.5	17.1	2.4	0.0
Vanilla, Madagascan, Simply Creamy, Fresh, Waitrose*	1/5 Pot/100g	208	14.4	208	3.4	16.3	14.4	1.1
Vanilla, TTD, Sainsbury's*	1 Pot/150g	312	23.2	208	2.5	14.7	15.5	0.1
CUSTARD APPLE								
Cherimoya, Weighed without Skin & Seeds, Average	**1 Cherimoya/312g**	**234**	**2.1**	**75**	**1.6**	**17.7**	**0.7**	**3.0**
CUTLETS								
Nut, Goodlife*	1 Cutlet/88g	283	19.4	322	9.1	21.8	22.0	3.4
Nut, Meat Free, Tesco*	1 Cutlet/70g	240	16.2	340	8.0	22.7	23.0	3.8
Nut, Retail, Grilled, Average	**1 Cutlet/90g**	**191**	**11.7**	**212**	**5.1**	**19.9**	**13.0**	**1.8**
Vegetable & Nut, Asda*	1 Cutlet/88g	296	20.3	335	10.0	22.0	23.0	4.6
CUTTLEFISH								
Raw	**1oz/28g**	**16**	**0.2**	**56**	**12.7**	**0.0**	**0.6**	**0.0**

C

	Measure INFO/WEIGHT	per Measure KCAL	FAT	Nutrition Values per 100g / 100ml KCAL	PROT	CARB	FAT	FIBRE
DAB								
Raw	*1oz/28g*	*21*	*0.3*	*74*	*15.7*	*0.0*	*1.2*	*0.0*
DAIM								
Mondelez*	1 Bar/28g	148	8.7	530	2.9	59.0	31.0	1.2
DAIRYLEA DUNKERS								
Baked Crisps, Dairylea, Kraft*	1 Pack/45g	101	4.0	225	9.2	26.0	9.0	1.1
Jumbo Munch, Dairylea, Kraft*	1 Serving/50g	150	9.2	300	7.2	26.5	18.5	1.2
with Jumbo Tubes, Kraft*	1 Pack/43g	108	5.1	255	9.1	27.0	12.0	0.9
with Ritz Crackers, Dairylea, Kraft*	1 Tub/46g	122	6.2	265	9.5	25.0	13.5	1.4
DAMSONS								
Raw, Weighed with Stones, Average	*1oz/28g*	*9*	*0.0*	*31*	*0.4*	*7.7*	*0.0*	*1.4*
Raw, Weighed without Stones, Average	*1oz/28g*	*11*	*0.0*	*38*	*0.5*	*9.6*	*0.0*	*1.8*
DANDELION & BURDOCK								
Fermented, Botanical, Fentiman's*	1 Bottle/275ml	130	0.0	47	0.0	11.6	0.0	0.0
Original, Ben Shaws*	1 Can/440ml	128	0.0	29	0.0	7.0	0.0	0.0
Sparkling, Diet, Morrisons*	1 Glass/200ml	2	0.0	1	0.0	0.3	0.0	0.0
DANISH PASTRY								
Apple & Cinnamon, Danish Twist, Entenmann's*	1 Serving/52g	150	1.0	288	5.6	62.0	1.9	1.5
Apple & Sultana, Tesco*	1 Pastry/72g	293	16.4	407	5.4	45.0	22.8	1.4
Apple Danish, Bakery, Waitrose*	1 Pastry/123g	400	22.2	325	5.1	35.7	18.0	2.4
Apple, Iceland*	¼ Pastry/95g	223	5.0	235	5.3	41.5	5.3	2.3
Average	*1 Pastry/110g*	*411*	*19.4*	*374*	*5.8*	*51.3*	*17.6*	*1.6*
Custard, Bar, Sara Lee*	¼ Bar/100g	228	6.4	228	6.6	36.1	6.4	0.8
Fruit Filled, Average	*1 Pastry/94g*	*335*	*15.9*	*356*	*5.1*	*47.9*	*17.0*	*0.0*
Pecan, M&S*	1 Serving/67g	287	17.4	428	6.2	45.0	26.0	1.3
Toasted Pecan, Danish Twist, Entenmann's*	1 Slice/48g	171	7.6	351	7.0	47.2	15.6	1.4
DATES								
Bite Size, Snack Pack, Whitworths*	1 Pack/35g	119	0.6	340	2.0	74.7	1.8	8.2
Deglet Nour, LL, Waitrose*	1 Portion/50g	144	0.1	287	3.3	68.0	0.2	8.0
Dried, Average	*1 Date/20g*	*53*	*0.1*	*266*	*2.8*	*64.1*	*0.4*	*4.1*
Dried, Medjool, Average	*1 Date/20g*	*56*	*0.1*	*279*	*2.2*	*69.3*	*0.3*	*4.3*
Fresh, Raw, Yellow, Average	*1 Date/20g*	*21*	*0.0*	*107*	*1.3*	*27.1*	*0.1*	*1.5*
Halawi, Tesco*	6 Dates/60g	165	0.1	275	2.3	65.5	0.2	4.3
Medjool, LL, Waitrose*	1 Date/20g	58	0.0	291	3.3	68.0	0.2	6.7
Medjool, Stuffed with Walnuts, Tesco*	2 Dates/40g	98	2.3	245	4.4	44.0	5.7	3.4
Medjool, TTD, Sainsbury's*	1 Serving/50g	148	0.0	296	1.9	72.0	0.1	6.7
Milk Chocolate Coated, Julian Graves*	1 Pack/200g	768	22.6	384	4.5	66.0	11.3	2.6
Organic, Medjool, Pitted, LL, Waitrose*	1 Date/18g	52	0.0	292	3.3	68.0	0.2	6.7
Pitted, Organic, Able & Cole*	1 Date/8g	13	0.0	158	2.1	36.5	0.4	0.0
Soft, Dried, Whitworths*	1 Serving/25g	85	0.4	340	2.0	74.7	1.8	8.2
Sweet & Sticky, Delicious, Boots*	1 Pack/50g	148	0.1	295	3.3	68.0	0.2	4.0
DELI FILLER								
Cheese & Onion, Essential, Waitrose*	1 Pot/170g	692	64.8	407	10.8	4.5	38.1	1.5
Cheese & Onion, Sainsbury's*	1 Pack/170g	673	62.7	396	10.8	4.8	36.9	0.9
Chicken & Bacon, Co-Op*	1 Pack/200g	420	29.6	210	17.6	1.0	14.8	2.6
Prawn & Mayonnaise, M&S*	1 Serving/60g	150	13.8	250	11.3	1.0	23.0	0.5
Prawn Cocktail, Eat Well, M&S*	½ Pot/85g	119	7.3	140	9.1	6.4	8.6	0.6
Smoked Salmon & Soft Cheese, M&S*	1 Serving/85g	207	17.3	244	11.7	3.3	20.4	0.5
DELIGHT								
Butterscotch Flavour, No Added Sugar, Tesco*	1 Pack/49g	225	10.0	460	4.8	63.3	20.5	0.0
DESSERT								
After Dark, Black Forest, Gateaux, Gu*	1 Pot/85g	258	18.5	303	3.0	24.7	21.8	1.3
After Eight, Dark Chocolate & Mint, Nestle*	1 Pot/70g	125	4.9	178	4.2	25.3	7.0	0.0
Almond, Naturgreen*	1 Serving/130g	143	6.2	110	2.3	14.5	4.8	0.2

DESSERT

	INFO/WEIGHT	KCAL	FAT	KCAL	PROT	CARB	FAT	FIBRE
Apple Crumble, Sainsbury's*	1 Pot/136g	291	10.5	214	3.2	33.0	7.7	2.7
Baked Lemon, COU, M&S*	1 Serving/100g	140	2.5	140	6.8	22.0	2.5	0.8
Banana Split	1 Serving/175g	368	25.5	210	2.2	18.0	14.6	0.2
Banoffee, Frozen, HL, Tesco*	1 Serving/60g	92	1.6	153	2.5	29.9	2.6	0.6
Banoffee, Sainsbury's*	1 Pot/140g	360	19.1	257	2.7	30.9	13.6	1.3
Banoffee, Weight Watchers*	1 Dessert/81g	170	3.6	210	4.9	37.7	4.4	1.4
Black Forest, Tesco*	1 Pot/100g	287	14.4	287	3.5	35.8	14.4	2.4
Blueberry Muffin, Tesco*	1 Pot/91g	265	18.7	291	2.0	24.5	20.6	3.0
Buttons, Milk Chocolate, Cadbury*	1 Pot/100g	280	14.9	280	6.2	30.8	14.9	0.0
Caramel Crunch, Weight Watchers*	1 Serving/89g	174	2.6	196	4.6	37.9	2.9	1.7
Caramel Flavour, Soya, Dairy Free, Organic, Provamel*	1 Pot/125g	125	2.2	100	3.0	17.8	1.8	0.5
Caramel, Delights, Shape, Danone*	1 Pot/110g	109	2.5	99	3.3	16.3	2.3	0.1
Caramel, Pots of Joy, Dairy Milk, Cadbury*	1 Pot/70g	150	7.3	215	2.5	27.1	10.5	0.1
Cheeky & Saucy Little Pots Au Chocolat, Gu*	1 Pot/45g	199	16.6	443	3.3	24.1	36.9	2.3
Chocolate Banoffee, Gu*	1 Pot/85g	325	21.5	382	3.9	35.0	25.3	1.0
Chocolate Brownie, M&S*	¼ Pack/144g	610	39.5	425	4.7	39.6	27.5	1.0
Chocolate Buttons, Cadbury*	1 Pack/100g	275	14.5	275	5.0	30.5	14.5	0.0
Chocolate Creme, King Frais, Lidl*	1 Pot/125g	131	3.6	105	2.6	17.0	2.9	0.0
Chocolate Duetto, Weight Watchers*	1 Pot/85g	99	2.4	117	4.4	18.4	2.8	0.0
Chocolate Fudge Brownie, Tesco*	1 Pot/125g	374	16.6	299	4.6	40.2	13.3	1.3
Chocolate Fudge, Pot, Fabulous, Thorntons*	1 Pot/65g	168	10.4	258	5.5	22.7	16.0	0.0
Chocolate Hazelnut, Charolait, Aldi*	1 Serving/200g	270	11.0	135	3.3	18.1	5.5	0.0
Chocolate Honeycomb Crisp, COU, M&S*	1 Serving/71g	110	2.1	155	4.6	27.6	2.9	1.0
Chocolate Mint Torte, Weight Watchers*	1 Dessert/88g	174	4.1	198	4.7	34.3	4.7	5.2
Chocolate Mousse Cake, Weight Watchers*	1 Dessert/75g	148	2.2	198	5.9	37.1	2.9	1.0
Chocolate Muffin, COU, M&S*	1 Pot/110g	154	2.8	140	6.1	26.1	2.5	1.5
Chocolate Muffin, Light Choices, Tesco*	1 Pot/108g	140	2.4	130	4.3	22.6	2.2	1.3
Chocolate Muffin, Tesco*	1 Serving/104g	354	21.2	340	3.5	35.5	20.4	2.1
Chocolate Muffin, Waitrose*	1 Serving/110g	138	3.0	126	5.2	20.0	2.7	0.4
Chocolate Orange, Pots of Joy, Terry's*	1 Pot/70g	150	7.3	215	3.7	26.0	10.5	0.1
Chocolate Toffee, Weight Watchers*	1 Dessert/89g	177	4.0	197	4.3	34.9	4.5	2.2
Chocolate, & Chocolate Coated Balls, Pud Corner, Muller*	1 Pot/85g	149	5.4	176	4.0	26.4	6.4	0.0
Chocolate, & White Chocolate Flakes, Pud Corner, Muller*	1 Pot/85g	147	5.0	173	3.7	27.0	5.9	0.0
Chocolate, Delights, Shape, Danone*	1 Pot/110g	109	2.4	99	3.3	16.3	2.2	0.6
Chocolate, Everyday Value, Tesco*	1 Pot/100g	121	4.0	121	2.7	18.4	4.0	0.4
Chocolate, Frappe, Skinny, COU, M&S*	1 Pot/100g	116	2.6	116	6.2	16.9	2.6	0.5
Chocolate, Weight Watchers*	1 Serving/82g	145	2.5	177	5.2	32.3	3.0	2.9
Coffee Escape, Pots of Joy, Roses, Cadbury*	1 Pot/71g	146	7.1	205	3.5	24.4	10.0	0.5
Creme Au Chocolat, Bonne Maman*	1 Pot/100g	182	9.4	182	5.0	19.0	9.4	0.0
Creme Caramel, Sainsbury's*	1 Pot/100g	116	1.6	116	2.6	22.9	1.6	0.0
Custard with Caramel, Layers, Ambrosia*	1 Pot/161g	183	4.7	114	2.5	19.6	2.9	0.0
Dairy Milk, Pots of Joy, Cadbury*	1 Pot/70g	158	8.2	225	4.2	25.6	11.7	0.1
Double Chocolate Brownie, Weight Watchers*	1 Pot/86g	167	3.3	194	5.1	33.7	3.8	2.4
Flake, Milk Chocolate, Cadbury*	1 Pot/90g	216	11.3	240	4.4	26.6	12.6	0.0
Fudge, Pot, Fabulous, Thortons*	1 Pot/65g	177	10.8	272	4.9	25.8	16.6	0.0
Fudge, Scottish, Handmade, EAT*	1 Serving/45g	194	4.1	431	1.5	85.8	9.0	0.6
Gulabjam Indian, Waitrose*	1 Pot/180g	479	15.5	266	4.8	42.9	8.6	0.6
Jaffa Cake, COU, M&S*	1 Serving/120g	138	3.1	115	2.4	20.1	2.6	1.0
Key Lime Pie	1 Serving/125g	431	25.0	344	4.1	37.9	20.0	1.4
Lemon Mousse Cake, Weight Watchers*	1 Serving/90g	130	2.4	144	3.2	26.7	2.7	0.5
Lemoncello, Italian, Co-Op*	1 Pot/90g	266	14.4	295	3.0	34.0	16.0	0.1
Mandarin, COU, M&S*	1 Serving/150g	195	5.7	130	1.0	22.0	3.8	0.1
Millionaire's Shortbread, M&S*	1 Dessert/120g	440	27.8	365	3.2	35.5	23.1	1.0

DESSERT	Measure INFO/WEIGHT	per Measure KCAL	FAT	Nutrition Values per 100g / 100ml KCAL	PROT	CARB	FAT	FIBRE
Mississippi Mud Pie	1 Serving/125g	480	32.0	384	5.3	33.1	25.6	1.8
Mix, Chocolate, Basics, Sainsbury's*	1 Serving/100g	92	3.3	92	4.0	11.5	3.3	0.5
Pineapple & Passionfruit, M&S*	1 Pot/100g	130	3.8	130	0.8	21.7	3.8	0.3
Raspberry Frappe, Skinny, COU, M&S*	1 Pot/94g	114	2.1	121	3.1	22.0	2.2	0.5
Raspberry Royale, Essential, Waitrose*	1 Pot/150g	216	10.6	144	1.1	18.9	7.1	0.5
Rich Chocolate, Weight Watchers*	1 Pot/70g	62	1.7	89	3.5	13.4	2.4	1.4
Rolo, Nestle*	1 Pot/70g	170	8.3	243	3.3	30.8	11.9	0.5
Serious Chocolate Orange & Grand Marnier, Waitrose*	1/8 Portion/50g	130	5.2	260	4.7	36.0	10.5	1.4
Snowy Delight, Pots of Joy, Dairy Milk, Cadbury*	1 Pot/70g	156	7.0	223	4.8	28.5	10.0	0.5
Strawberries & Cream, BFY, Morrisons*	1 Serving/200g	244	2.2	122	2.2	26.0	1.1	0.1
Tiramisu	1 Serving/150g	420	20.8	280	4.4	34.0	13.9	0.8
Toffee Banana Crunch, Farmfoods*	1/6 Dessert/82g	219	9.3	267	2.6	38.5	11.4	0.7
Toffee Fudge, Pot, Fabulous, Thorntons*	1 Pot/65g	178	10.5	274	4.8	27.3	16.1	0.0
Toffee Muffin, COU, M&S*	1 Serving/100g	180	2.2	180	3.7	35.8	2.2	0.3
Toffee with Biscuit Pieces, Iced, Weight Watchers*	1 Pot/57g	93	2.7	163	2.7	26.2	4.8	0.2
Toffee, & Chocolate Biscuit Balls, Pud Corner, Muller*	1 Pot/85g	132	5.7	156	3.1	21.3	6.7	0.0
Trifle, Chocolate, Cadbury*	1 Pot/90g	234	13.8	260	4.8	22.5	15.3	0.0
Triple Chocolate Layered, BGTY, Sainsbury's*	1 Pot/105g	147	2.9	140	4.2	24.4	2.8	0.5
Triple Chocolate, Delice, Sainsbury's*	1 Serving/105g	399	27.4	380	3.8	32.4	26.1	0.7
Twix Mix, Twin Pot, Mars*	1 Pot/120g	212	10.5	177	2.5	22.0	8.8	0.0
Vanilla & Caramel, Little Desserts, Petits Filous, Yoplait*	1 Pot/50g	75	2.6	150	4.7	21.0	5.3	0.2
Vanilla & Chocolate Twist, Desira, Aldi*	1 Pack/150g	182	7.2	121	0.0	15.0	4.8	0.0
Vanilla & Raspberry Swirl, Weight Watchers*	1 Serving/100ml	81	2.2	81	1.5	13.3	2.2	0.2
Vanilla Creme, with Raspberries, Bonne Maman*	1 Pot/90g	158	9.0	175	1.7	19.0	10.0	1.1
Vanilla Flavour, Soya, Dairy Free, Organic, Provamel*	1 Pot/125g	105	2.2	84	3.2	13.4	1.8	0.5
White Buttons, Pots of Joy, Cadbury*	1 Pot/70g	158	6.6	225	4.8	30.4	9.4	0.0
Zabaglione	1 Serving/100g	278	18.3	278	3.6	24.3	18.3	2.3
DHAL								
Black Gram, Average	**1oz/28g**	**21**	**1.0**	**74**	**4.2**	**7.0**	**3.4**	**1.7**
Chick Pea	1oz/28g	42	1.7	149	7.4	17.7	6.1	3.8
Chick Pea, Asda*	1 Serving/400g	404	12.0	101	4.5	14.0	3.0	3.0
Chick Pea, Canned, Asda*	½ Can/194g	198	6.2	102	4.3	14.0	3.2	2.9
Chick Pea, Sainsbury's*	½ Can/200g	432	18.2	216	10.8	22.7	9.1	7.1
Chickpea, Mazadar*	1 Tin/400g	360	11.2	90	4.5	11.6	2.8	4.5
Lentil, Patak's*	1 Can/283g	156	2.8	55	2.8	9.3	1.0	1.0
Lentil, Red Masoor & Tomato with Butter, Average	**1oz/28g**	**26**	**1.4**	**94**	**4.0**	**9.7**	**4.9**	**0.9**
Lentil, Red Masoor & Vegetable, Average	**1oz/28g**	**31**	**1.1**	**110**	**5.8**	**14.7**	**3.8**	**1.8**
Lentil, Red Masoor with Vegetable Oil, Average	**1oz/28g**	**48**	**2.2**	**172**	**7.6**	**19.2**	**7.9**	**1.8**
Lentil, Red Masoor, Punjabi, Average	**1oz/28g**	**39**	**1.3**	**139**	**7.2**	**19.2**	**4.6**	**2.0**
Lentil, Red Masoorl & Mung Bean, Average	**1oz/28g**	**32**	**1.9**	**114**	**4.8**	**9.9**	**6.7**	**1.6**
Lentil, Red, Way to Five, Sainsbury's*	½ Pack/273g	254	4.1	93	5.5	14.4	1.5	1.4
Lentil, Tesco*	1 Serving/200g	248	13.2	124	5.1	10.6	6.6	2.5
Makhani, Curry Collection, Veetee*	1 Pack/300g	306	17.4	102	4.2	11.1	5.8	2.8
Mung Bean, Bengali	1oz/28g	20	0.9	73	4.2	7.4	3.3	1.7
Mung Beans, Dried, Boiled in Unsalted Water	1oz/28g	26	0.1	92	7.8	15.3	0.4	0.0
Split Peas, Yellow, Chana, Asda*	1 Serving/275g	300	19.2	109	2.6	9.0	7.0	1.8
Tadkha, Rich & Golden, Waitrose*	½ Pack/150g	172	8.3	114	6.0	10.9	5.5	5.5
Tarka, Asda*	½ Pack/150g	216	12.0	144	6.0	12.0	8.0	6.0
DHANSAK								
Chicken with Bagara Rice, Waitrose*	1 Pack/450g	549	8.1	122	8.2	18.2	1.8	1.2
Vegetable, Sainsbury's*	1 Serving/200g	148	5.6	74	3.1	8.9	2.8	2.8
DILL								
Dried, Average	**1 Tsp/1g**	**3**	**0.0**	**253**	**19.9**	**42.2**	**4.4**	**13.6**

	Measure INFO/WEIGHT	per Measure KCAL	per Measure FAT	Nutrition Values per 100g / 100ml KCAL	PROT	CARB	FAT	FIBRE
DILL								
Fresh, Average	*1 Tbsp/3g*	*1*	*0.0*	*25*	*3.7*	*0.9*	*0.8*	*2.5*
DIP								
Aubergine, Fresh, Waitrose*	1 Serving/85g	159	12.8	187	2.5	10.5	15.0	1.7
Beetroot & Sesame, Sainsbury's*	¼ Pot/45g	65	3.7	145	4.2	11.8	8.3	3.1
Blue Cheese, Fresh, Sainsbury's*	1/5 Pot/34g	115	11.7	337	3.6	3.1	34.5	0.1
Cajun Red Pepper, Sainsbury's*	1 Serving/50g	25	0.9	50	1.4	7.0	1.8	1.4
Cheese & Chive, 50% Less Fat, Asda*	1 Pot/125g	261	21.5	209	4.5	9.0	17.2	0.0
Cheese & Chive, 50% Less Fat, Morrisons*	1 Serving/50g	86	6.4	172	8.8	5.2	12.7	0.2
Cheese & Chive, Asda*	1 Serving/43g	190	19.6	447	4.9	3.4	46.0	0.0
Cheese & Chive, Tesco*	¼ Pack/50g	268	27.6	535	4.3	4.3	55.1	0.1
Chilli Cheese, Asda*	1 Serving/50g	131	11.0	262	8.0	8.0	22.0	1.1
Chilli, M&S*	1 Pot/35g	103	0.1	295	0.4	73.2	0.2	0.4
Endamame & Pea, Waitrose*	¼ Pot/51g	85	5.9	166	6.3	8.0	11.6	2.0
Frijolemole, Cannellini Bean & Chick Pea, Waitrose*	¼ Pot/50g	104	7.6	208	4.3	12.2	15.2	2.6
Garlic & Herb	1 Serving/100g	584	62.4	584	1.4	4.1	62.4	0.2
Garlic & Herb, Big Dipper, Morrisons*	¼ Pot/75g	278	28.1	370	1.3	6.9	37.5	0.4
Garlic & Herb, Tesco*	¼ Pack/43g	257	27.8	604	0.9	3.2	65.4	0.3
Garlic Butter, for Dough Balls, Supermarket, Pizza Express*	½ Pot/8g	54	5.8	673	1.3	5.2	71.9	0.6
Garlic, Olive Oil & Butter, Pizza Express*	½ Pot/17g	106	11.5	621	1.5	2.8	67.4	0.5
Hot Salsa, Doritos, Walkers*	1 Jar/300g	99	0.3	33	1.1	6.4	0.1	0.9
Houmous, Black Olive, Wild Garden*	2 Tbsp/30g	35	2.0	117	6.7	13.3	6.7	3.3
Houmous, Red Pepper, Wild Garden*	2 Tbsp/30g	35	2.0	117	6.7	13.3	6.7	3.3
Houmous, Roasted Garlic, Wild Garden*	2 Tbsp/30g	35	2.0	117	6.7	13.3	6.7	3.3
Jalapeno, Greek Yoghurt, Skotidakis*	1 Tbsp/15g	25	1.8	167	6.7	13.3	11.7	0.0
Mature Cheddar Cheese & Chive, Fresh, Waitrose*	½ Pot/85g	393	40.5	462	5.8	2.4	47.7	1.7
Mild Salsa, Doritos, Walkers*	1 Tbsp/30g	9	0.1	30	0.8	6.0	0.3	1.5
Nacho Cheese, Average	*1 Serving/50g*	*175*	*17.2*	*350*	*6.3*	*3.4*	*34.4*	*0.9*
Nacho Cheese, Doritos, Walkers*	1 Serving/40g	92	8.1	231	3.4	8.5	20.2	0.6
Nacho Cheese, Primula*	1 Serving/57g	144	14.2	253	2.7	3.6	24.9	2.1
Nacho Cheese, Sainsbury's*	1 Serving/50g	244	25.1	487	4.8	3.9	50.2	0.0
Onion & Garlic, Average	*1 Tbsp/15g*	*62*	*6.4*	*410*	*1.7*	*4.8*	*42.7*	*0.4*
Onion & Garlic, Classic, Tesco*	1 Serving/30g	133	13.9	442	1.7	4.6	46.3	0.2
Onion & Garlic, GFY, Asda*	1/5 Pot/34g	56	4.8	166	2.1	8.0	14.0	0.2
Onion & Garlic, HE, Tesco*	1 Pot/170g	345	29.9	203	3.3	7.9	17.6	0.1
Onion & Garlic, HL, Tesco*	1 Serving/43g	80	7.2	188	2.5	6.3	17.0	0.1
Pea, Yogurt & Mint, Sainsbury's*	¼ Pack/50g	119	10.8	238	3.4	7.5	21.6	2.1
Peanut, Satay Selection, Occasions, Sainsbury's*	1 Serving/2g	4	0.2	186	7.1	13.8	11.4	1.1
Pecorino, Basil & Pine Nut, Fresh, Waitrose*	½ Pot/85g	338	33.7	398	5.1	5.1	39.7	0.0
Red Pepper, Nando's*	1 Serving/260g	490	7.2	188	5.2	35.2	2.8	1.6
Red Pepper, Sainsbury's*	1 Pot/100g	103	4.0	103	2.3	14.6	4.0	0.0
Salsa Mild, Asda*	1 Portion/100g	47	0.3	47	1.4	8.7	0.3	1.8
Salsa, Chunky Tomato, Tesco*	1 Pot/170g	68	2.2	40	1.1	5.9	1.3	1.1
Salsa, Chunky, Fresh, Sainsbury's*	1 Serving/100g	51	1.7	51	1.1	7.8	1.7	1.2
Smoked Salmon & Dill, Fresh, Waitrose*	½ Pot/85g	373	38.0	439	5.1	4.1	44.7	0.1
Smoky Red Pepper, Gazpacho, Graze*	1 Punnet/23g	54	1.3	242	5.7	40.1	5.9	3.7
Sour Cream & Chive, Average	*1 Tbsp/15g*	*48*	*4.8*	*317*	*3.2*	*4.0*	*32.0*	*0.3*
Sour Cream & Chive, Doritos, Walkers*	1 Tbsp/20g	52	4.9	258	1.9	6.9	24.7	1.9
Sour Cream & Chive, Fresh, Tesco*	½ Pot/75g	305	31.8	407	2.1	4.1	42.4	0.0
Sour Cream & Chive, Half Fat, Waitrose*	½ Pot/85g	133	9.9	157	5.5	7.6	11.6	0.1
Sour Cream & Chive, Primula*	1 Serving/57g	169	17.4	297	4.3	1.3	30.5	1.0
Sour Cream & Chive, Sainsbury's*	1 Serving/50g	141	13.8	282	3.1	5.4	27.5	0.1
Sour Cream & Chives, Mexican Style, Morrisons*	¼ Pack/25g	68	7.0	274	2.2	3.4	27.9	0.4
Sour Cream, Tesco*	1 Serving/38g	111	11.2	297	3.4	3.9	29.8	0.2

D

	Measure INFO/WEIGHT	per Measure KCAL	FAT	Nutrition Values per 100g / 100ml KCAL	PROT	CARB	FAT	FIBRE
DIP								
Soured Cream & Chive, BGTY, Sainsbury's*	1 Serving/170g	253	17.5	149	4.2	9.9	10.3	0.1
Soured Cream & Chive, Classic, Tesco*	1 Serving/25g	81	8.4	323	1.7	3.2	33.7	0.2
Soured Cream & Chive, HL, Tesco*	1 Serving/31g	45	3.3	145	3.8	7.5	10.6	0.2
Soured Cream & Chive, Morrisons*	1 Serving/100g	317	32.6	317	2.6	3.3	32.6	0.0
Sweet Chilli Mango, Encona*	1 Tbsp/15ml	22	0.1	148	0.4	35.4	0.6	0.0
Tortilla Chips, Cool Flavour, Big, Morrisons*	½ Pack/100g	453	22.0	453	6.4	57.4	22.0	8.1
DOLLY MIXTURES								
M&S*	1 Pack/115g	431	1.6	375	1.8	89.2	1.4	0.0
Sainsbury's*	1 Serving/10g	40	0.2	401	1.4	94.4	1.9	0.1
Smart Price, Asda*	1 Sweet/3g	11	0.0	380	0.5	91.0	1.6	0.0
Tesco*	1 Pack/100g	376	1.5	376	1.6	88.9	1.5	0.0
DOLMADES								
Stuffed with Rice, M&S*	1 Leaf/38g	40	1.6	105	2.6	14.2	4.1	1.2
DOPIAZA								
Mushroom, Retail	1oz/28g	19	1.6	69	1.3	3.7	5.7	1.1
DORITOS								
Chargrilled BBQ, Walkers*	1 Bag/35g	170	8.8	485	5.5	59.0	25.0	3.5
Chilli Heatwave, Walkers*	1 Bag/30g	150	7.8	500	7.0	60.0	26.0	3.0
Cool Original, Walkers*	1 Bag/40g	200	10.8	500	7.5	58.0	27.0	3.0
Cool, Ranch Chips, Walkers*	1 Pack/50g	250	13.0	504	8.1	64.5	26.2	4.0
Dippas, Hint of Chilli, Dipping Chips, Walkers*	1 Bag/35g	173	8.8	495	7.0	61.0	25.0	3.5
Dippas, Hint of Lime, Walkers*	1 Bag/35g	173	8.8	495	7.0	60.0	25.0	3.5
Dippas, Lightly Salted, Dipping Chips, Walkers*	1 Serving/35g	178	9.4	510	6.5	60.0	27.0	3.0
Lighly Salted, Corn Chips, Doritos*	1 Bag/30g	149	7.1	497	6.9	62.9	23.6	3.3
Mexican Hot, Walkers*	1 Bag/40g	202	10.8	505	8.0	57.0	27.0	3.5
Tangy Cheese, Walkers*	1 Bag/40g	200	10.8	500	7.0	57.0	27.0	3.0
DOUBLE DECKER								
Cadbury*	1 Bar/55g	251	10.3	460	4.4	68.4	18.9	0.6
Snack Size, Cadbury*	1 Bar/36g	165	7.4	465	4.8	64.5	20.9	0.0
DOUGH BALLS								
Cheese & Garlic, Occasions, Sainsbury's*	1 Ball/12g	41	2.2	341	10.3	33.4	18.5	2.1
Garlic & Herb, Asda*	4 Balls/48g	173	8.5	361	9.2	40.9	17.8	3.6
Garlic, Tesco*	1 Serving/10g	40	2.3	400	7.0	40.0	23.0	1.0
Garlic, Waitrose*	1 Ball/11g	38	1.8	347	8.5	41.4	16.4	3.3
Supermarket, Pizza Express*	8 Balls/100g	363	1.7	363	14.3	72.9	1.7	3.3
with Garlic & Herb Butter, Aldi*	1 Ball/12g	45	2.2	365	7.7	46.7	18.2	1.8
DOUGHNUTS								
Apple & Custard, Finger, Sainsbury's*	1 Doughnut/65g	136	6.0	210	4.4	27.5	9.2	1.9
Baked, HL, Tesco*	1 Doughnut/67g	166	3.9	248	6.4	42.2	5.9	1.4
Cream & Jam, Assorted Box, Sainsbury's*	1 Doughnut/71g	229	12.7	322	6.2	34.2	17.9	2.2
Cream & Jam, Tesco*	1 Doughnut/90g	288	14.1	320	5.4	39.4	15.7	2.0
Custard Filled, Average	***1 Doughnut/75g***	***268***	***14.2***	***358***	***6.2***	***43.3***	***19.0***	***0.0***
Custard, Sainsbury's*	1 Doughnut/70g	172	7.5	246	5.1	32.3	10.7	2.3
Custard, Tesco*	1 Doughnut/91g	266	14.4	292	4.1	33.4	15.8	1.1
Jam Filled, Average	***1 Doughnut/75g***	***252***	***10.9***	***336***	***5.7***	***48.8***	***14.5***	***0.0***
Jam, Fresh Cream, Sweet Fresh, Tesco*	1 Doughnut/74g	248	12.1	335	5.5	40.7	16.4	1.9
Jam, M&S*	1 Doughnut/49g	141	2.0	287	5.0	57.6	4.0	1.3
Jam, Mini, Frozen, Party, Tesco*	2 Doughnuts/25g	101	5.5	405	5.3	45.0	22.1	2.0
Mini, Sainsbury's*	1 Doughnut/14g	53	2.7	379	5.2	47.9	18.9	2.1
Plain, Ring, Average	***1 Doughnut/60g***	***238***	***13.0***	***397***	***6.1***	***47.2***	***21.7***	***0.0***
Raspberry Jam, Sainsbury's*	1 Doughnut/70g	241	10.4	344	5.3	47.4	14.8	2.5
Ring, Iced, Average	***1 Doughnut/70g***	***268***	***12.2***	***383***	***4.8***	***55.1***	***17.5***	***0.0***
Ring, Waitrose*	1 Doughnut/107g	396	21.3	370	4.2	43.5	19.9	0.7

	Measure			Nutrition Values per 100g / 100ml				
	INFO/WEIGHT	KCAL	FAT	KCAL	PROT	CARB	FAT	FIBRE
DOUGHNUTS								
Salted Caramel, Cake Shop, Morrisons*	1 Doughnut/75g	301	14.4	402	4.4	52.3	19.2	1.1
Strawberry Jam & Cream, Sainsbury's*	1 Doughnut/80g	299	18.5	374	5.3	36.2	23.2	1.3
Toffee, Tesco*	1 Doughnut/75g	235	8.7	313	8.0	44.2	11.6	1.6
Yum Yums, Glazed, Sweet, Waitrose*	1 Doughnut/45g	172	10.0	382	4.0	41.6	22.2	2.0
Yum Yums, M&S*	1 Doughnut/37g	155	8.9	420	4.9	45.7	23.9	1.6
Yum Yums, Tesco*	1 Doughnut/50g	220	13.2	440	4.7	43.7	26.4	3.1
DOVER SOLE								
Fillet, Raw, Average	*1oz/28g*	*25*	*0.5*	*89*	*18.1*	*0.0*	*1.8*	*0.0*
DR PEPPER*								
Coca-Cola*	1 Bottle/500ml	210	0.0	42	0.0	10.9	0.0	0.0
Zero, Coca-Cola*	1 Can/330ml	2	0.0	0	0.0	0.0	0.0	0.0
DRAGON FRUIT								
Raw, Edible Portion, Average	*1 Serving/100g*	*41*	*0.5*	*41*	*0.7*	*9.6*	*0.5*	*3.6*
DRAMBUIE								
39% Volume	*1 Pub Shot/35ml*	*125*	*0.0*	*358*	*0.0*	*23.0*	*0.0*	*0.0*
DREAM TOPPING								
Dry, Bird's*	1oz/28g	193	16.4	690	6.7	32.5	58.5	0.5
DRESSING								
Balsamic Vinegar, Asda*	1 Pack/44ml	121	11.9	275	0.9	7.0	27.0	0.0
Balsamic Vinegar, Light, Kraft*	1 Serving/15ml	15	0.9	100	0.3	9.6	6.3	0.5
Balsamic Vinegar, Morrisons*	1 Serving/15ml	17	0.2	111	0.1	22.9	1.6	0.1
Balsamic Vinegar, Olives & Herb, COU, M&S*	1 Serving/30g	22	0.6	75	0.5	14.3	2.0	0.5
Balsamic with Olive Oil, Pizza Express*	1 Serving/10g	42	4.1	421	0.3	10.3	41.2	0.0
Balsamic, Fig Glaze, Tesco*	1 Tbsp/15ml	31	0.0	208	1.4	47.9	0.0	0.0
Balsamic, Light Choices, Tesco*	1 Tbsp/14g	12	0.2	85	0.3	16.7	1.5	0.2
Balsamic, M&S*	1 Tbsp/15g	74	7.2	490	0.3	9.7	48.0	0.5
Balsamic, New, Sainsbury's*	1 Tbsp/15g	58	5.2	389	0.6	18.3	34.8	0.8
Balsamic, Oak Aged, TTD, Sainsbury's*	1 Tbsp/15ml	54	4.8	338	0.5	16.3	30.0	0.5
Balsamic, Sainsbury's*	1 Tbsp/15ml	47	4.3	316	0.4	13.8	28.8	0.4
Balsamic, Sweet, BGTY, Sainsbury's*	1 Tsp/5g	3	0.0	61	0.5	13.6	0.5	0.5
Balsamic, Sweet, Finest, Tesco*	1 Serving/10ml	16	0.0	155	0.4	36.9	0.1	0.4
Balsamic, Vinaigrette, Newman's Own*	1 Tbsp/15ml	56	5.7	372	0.1	7.2	38.2	0.5
Balsamic, Weight Watchers*	1 Serving/15ml	12	0.3	81	0.1	16.0	1.8	0.5
Blue Cheese, 60% Less Fat, BGTY, Sainsbury's*	1 Tbsp/15ml	26	2.3	172	1.9	7.3	15.1	0.2
Blue Cheese, Chunky, Lite, Marie's*	2 Tbsp/31g	72	7.2	233	3.3	3.3	23.3	0.0
Blue Cheese, HE, Tesco*	1 Tsp/5g	4	0.2	82	4.4	9.0	3.1	0.1
Blue Cheese, Hellmann's*	1 Tbsp/15g	69	7.1	459	0.7	6.3	47.2	1.1
Blue Cheese, Sainsbury's*	1 Serving/20g	64	6.0	321	2.3	10.6	29.9	0.4
Blue Cheese, Salad, Waitrose*	1 Serving/50g	265	25.2	530	2.1	17.3	50.3	4.1
Caesar Style, GFY, Asda*	1 Sachet/44ml	34	1.0	77	5.0	9.0	2.3	0.0
Caesar, 95% Fat Free, Tesco*	1 Tsp/6g	5	0.2	88	4.1	8.9	3.7	0.3
Caesar, Asiago, Briannas*	1 Tbsp/15ml	70	7.5	467	3.3	3.3	50.0	0.0
Caesar, Chilled, Reduced Fat, Tesco*	1 Tsp/5ml	13	1.2	252	6.5	3.1	23.7	0.1
Caesar, Classic, Sainsbury's*	1 Tsp/5ml	22	2.3	442	2.7	4.6	45.9	0.5
Caesar, Fat Free, Average	*1 Tsp/5g*	*4*	*0.2*	*84*	*4.6*	*11.0*	*4.1*	*0.2*
Caesar, Finest, Tesco*	1 Tbsp/15ml	72	7.6	477	1.9	2.8	50.9	0.2
Caesar, Fresh, Asda*	1 Dtsp/10ml	45	4.8	454	2.4	3.2	48.0	0.0
Caesar, Fresh, M&S*	1 Tsp/6g	32	3.4	525	2.0	1.8	56.4	0.2
Caesar, Fresh, Sainsbury's*	1 Tbsp/15ml	72	7.5	477	3.7	3.7	49.7	1.9
Caesar, Hellmann's*	1 Tsp/6g	30	3.1	499	2.5	4.5	51.7	0.3
Caesar, Less Than 3% Fat, BGTY, Sainsbury's*	1 Serving/20g	10	0.4	48	0.8	7.0	1.9	0.3
Caesar, Light Choices, Tesco*	1 Serving/15g	9	0.2	60	1.5	9.5	1.5	0.5
Caesar, Light, Kraft*	1 Serving/15g	22	1.6	148	0.5	11.5	11.0	0.2

DRESSING	Measure INFO/WEIGHT	per Measure KCAL	per Measure FAT	Nutrition Values per 100g / 100ml KCAL	PROT	CARB	FAT	FIBRE
Caesar, Low Fat, Average	*1 Tsp/5g*	*4*	*0.1*	*77*	*2.3*	*11.1*	*2.6*	*0.2*
Caesar, Loyd Grossman*	1 Dtsp/10g	34	3.4	342	2.1	7.0	33.9	0.0
Caesar, Luxury, Hellmann's*	1 Tsp/4g	20	2.1	498	2.5	4.4	51.7	0.3
Caesar, Original, Cardini's*	1 Serving/10g	56	6.0	555	2.3	1.5	60.0	0.2
Caesar, Tesco*	1 Tbsp/15ml	65	6.8	435	0.9	5.4	45.1	0.3
Caesar, Waitrose*	1 Serving/15ml	72	7.6	479	4.5	0.9	50.8	0.2
Citrus Salad, BGTY, Sainsbury's*	1 Tbsp/15ml	14	0.5	90	0.3	14.4	3.1	0.3
Classic French, Fresh, M&S*	1 Serving/10ml	52	5.3	515	0.6	8.2	53.1	0.2
Classic Italian, Get Dressed, Kraft*	1 Serving/25ml	30	2.6	120	0.1	5.6	10.3	0.5
Cream Cheese & Chive, Creamy Ranch, Kraft*	1 Serving/15ml	31	2.6	205	1.2	11.0	17.0	0.0
Creamy Caesar, Get Dressed, Kraft*	1 Serving/67g	68	2.3	102	2.1	15.0	3.5	0.1
Creamy Caesar, Waistline, Crosse & Blackwell*	1 Dtsp/11g	15	1.0	135	1.5	11.1	9.2	0.3
Creamy Ranch, 95% Fat Free, Kraft*	1 Tsp/6ml	7	0.3	111	1.4	14.5	5.0	0.3
Creamy Roasted Garlic, GFY, Asda*	1 Tbsp/15g	10	0.6	70	0.8	8.0	3.9	0.6
Creme Fraiche, Salad, Kraft*	1 Tbsp/15ml	12	0.4	78	0.8	12.5	2.5	0.0
Dijon Honey Mustard, Briannas*	1 Tbsp/15ml	65	6.0	433	0.0	20.0	40.0	0.0
Fat Free, Vinegar & Oil Based, Average	*1 Tsp/5g*	*2*	*0.0*	*37*	*0.4*	*7.9*	*0.2*	*0.4*
French Salad, M&S*	1 Serving/25ml	156	16.8	625	0.5	3.8	67.3	0.1
French Style Calorie-Wise Salad, Kraft*	1 Tbsp/15ml	24	1.6	160	0.0	18.7	10.7	0.0
French Style, BGTY, Sainsbury's*	1 Tbsp/15ml	11	0.4	76	0.7	12.6	2.5	0.5
French Style, Oil Free, HE, Tesco*	1 Tbsp/15g	4	0.0	30	0.3	6.0	0.2	1.4
French Vinaigrette, TTD, Sainsbury's*	1 Tbsp/15ml	69	6.7	460	0.6	13.9	44.5	0.5
French, Batts, Lidl*	2 Tbsp/30ml	95	8.7	317	1.7	12.0	29.0	0.0
French, BGTY, Organic, Sainsbury's*	1 Tbsp/15ml	11	0.6	71	0.2	8.3	4.1	0.5
French, Chilled, Tesco*	1 Tbsp/15ml	63	5.9	421	1.1	15.1	39.6	0.0
French, Cider Vinegar & Mustard, Tesco*	1 Tbsp/15ml	45	4.2	300	0.7	9.9	28.1	0.3
French, Classic, Fat Free, Kraft*	1 Tsp/5ml	2	0.0	39	0.1	8.7	0.0	0.5
French, Classic, Sachet, The English Provender Co.*	1 Sachet/25g	21	0.6	84	0.8	14.7	2.4	0.0
French, Classic, Sainsbury's*	1 Tbsp/15ml	71	7.4	473	1.0	5.7	49.6	0.5
French, Classics, M&S*	1 Tbsp/15ml	77	8.0	516	0.6	8.2	53.1	0.2
French, Essential, Waitrose*	1 Serving/15ml	34	2.3	228	0.1	22.9	15.1	0.5
French, Finest, Tesco*	1 Tbsp/15g	56	5.8	370	0.4	5.1	38.7	1.0
French, Fresh, Florette*	1 Bottle/175ml	763	73.2	436	0.8	14.1	41.8	0.0
French, Fresh, HE, Tesco*	1 Tbsp/15ml	8	0.4	56	1.1	6.7	2.8	0.0
French, Fresh, Morrisons*	1 Tbsp/15ml	75	7.3	499	1.5	13.6	48.7	0.0
French, Fresh, Organic, Sainsbury's*	1 Tbsp/15ml	45	4.6	301	0.4	5.5	31.0	0.4
French, Fresh, Sainsbury's*	1 Tbsp/15ml	64	6.7	429	0.6	6.6	44.6	0.6
French, GFY, Asda*	1 Tbsp/15g	8	0.3	50	0.7	7.0	2.1	0.1
French, Light Choices, Tesco*	1 Tbsp/16g	8	0.3	50	0.8	7.6	1.6	1.1
French, Luxury, Hellmann's*	1 Tbsp/15g	45	3.9	297	0.4	14.9	25.9	0.3
French, Oil Free, French, Waitrose*	1 Tsp/5ml	4	0.1	76	1.5	13.1	2.0	0.6
French, Organic, M&S*	1 Tbsp/15g	98	10.4	655	0.2	7.5	69.4	0.3
French, Reduced Fat, M&S*	1 Tbsp/15g	10	0.4	70	0.7	11.5	2.8	0.7
French, Sainsbury's*	1 Tbsp/15ml	33	2.9	219	0.6	9.8	19.1	0.5
French, Tesco*	1 Serving/25ml	110	11.2	441	0.7	7.2	44.9	0.2
French, Virtually Fat Free, Aldi*	1 Serving/10g	3	0.0	33	0.9	6.7	0.3	1.1
Garlic & Herb, Reduced Calorie, Hellmann's*	1 Tbsp/15ml	35	2.9	232	0.6	12.8	19.3	0.4
Garlic & Herb, Tesco*	1 Tbsp/15g	32	3.0	210	0.9	5.8	20.2	0.8
Ginger & Toasted Sesame, Naturally Righteous *	1 Serving/15ml	66	6.3	440	2.7	16.0	42.0	0.0
Herb & Garlic, Light, 5% Fat, Get Dressed, Kraft*	1 Serving/25ml	29	1.3	116	1.3	15.5	5.1	0.2
Honey & Mustard, BGTY, Sainsbury's*	1 Tbsp/20g	14	0.1	71	0.4	16.1	0.5	0.2
Honey & Mustard, Finest, Tesco*	1 Serving/25ml	72	5.6	288	1.7	19.6	22.5	0.7
Honey & Mustard, Fresh, M&S*	1 Serving/10ml	43	4.2	430	1.7	9.7	42.4	0.5

DRESSING

INFO/WEIGHT	Measure	per Measure KCAL	FAT	Nutrition Values per 100g / 100ml KCAL	PROT	CARB	FAT	FIBRE
Honey & Mustard, GFY, Asda*	1 Tbsp/15g	13	0.5	89	1.5	13.0	3.4	0.8
Honey & Mustard, Hellmann's*	1 Serving/15ml	27	0.2	182	0.7	13.7	1.6	0.3
Honey & Mustard, Light Choices, Tesco*	1 Tbsp/14g	9	0.2	65	1.3	11.6	1.1	0.6
Honey & Mustard, M&S*	1 Tbsp/15ml	64	6.4	427	1.7	9.7	42.4	0.6
Honey & Mustard, Sainsbury's*	1 Serving/10ml	37	3.3	366	1.0	15.4	33.0	0.1
Honey & Mustard, Tesco*	1 Serving/10ml	38	3.6	378	0.8	13.1	35.8	0.6
Honey & Mustard, The English Provender Co.*	1 Tbsp/15ml	17	0.2	111	2.5	21.8	1.5	1.0
Honey, Orange & Mustard, BGTY, Sainsbury's*	1 Tbsp/15ml	16	0.4	105	1.8	18.6	2.5	1.8
Italian Balsamic, Loyd Grossman*	1 Serving/10g	36	3.4	357	0.9	13.1	33.5	0.1
Italian Balsamic, The English Provender Co.*	1 Serving/30ml	20	0.8	67	0.8	9.9	2.7	0.2
Italian Salad, Hellmann's*	1 Serving/50g	103	8.4	206	0.7	12.8	16.7	0.0
Italian, M&S*	1 Tbsp/15ml	62	6.2	415	0.9	8.9	41.5	1.0
Italian, Waistline, 99% Fat Free, Crosse & Blackwell*	1 Tsp/6g	2	0.1	39	0.7	7.0	0.9	0.3
Lemon & Cracked Black Pepper, GFY, Asda*	1 Tbsp/15g	9	0.0	57	0.2	14.0	0.0	0.3
Lemon & Tarragon, HE, Tesco*	1 Serving/10ml	11	0.2	113	1.1	21.6	2.4	0.0
Lime & Coriander, Oil Free, Waitrose*	1 Tsp/5ml	3	0.1	65	1.5	11.9	1.3	0.4
Lime & Coriander, Sainsbury's*	1 Tbsp/15ml	61	6.1	409	0.4	10.0	40.8	0.5
Mayonnaise Style, 90% Fat Free, Weight Watchers*	1 Tsp/11g	14	1.0	125	1.7	8.9	9.2	0.0
Mild Mustard, Low Fat, Weight Watchers*	1 Tbsp/10g	6	0.4	63	2.0	5.7	3.6	0.0
Oil & Lemon	1 Tbsp/15g	97	10.6	647	0.3	2.8	70.6	0.0
Olive Oil & Balsamic Vinegar, Sainsbury's*	1 Serving/25ml	104	10.4	415	0.9	9.4	41.8	0.2
Orange Rosemary, Oil & Vinegar*	1 Tbsp/15ml	50	3.2	331	2.7	30.7	21.2	4.0
Passion Fruit & Mango, HE, Tesco*	1 Tbsp/15ml	25	0.3	169	0.6	36.7	2.2	0.4
Ranch Style, Asda*	1 Serving/44ml	37	1.7	85	3.5	9.0	3.9	0.0
Red Pepper, M&S*	1 Tbsp/15ml	58	5.9	385	0.6	7.6	39.2	0.5
Rich Poppy Seed, Briannas*	1 Tbsp/15ml	65	6.5	433	0.0	20.0	43.3	0.0
Salad, Blue Cheese, Heinz*	1 Serving/15g	55	5.5	369	1.2	7.8	36.9	0.2
Salad, Catalina, Kraft*	1 Serving/34g	100	6.0	294	0.0	29.4	17.6	0.0
Salad, Honey & Mustard, Light, Kraft*	1 Tbsp/15ml	19	0.7	126	1.2	19.0	4.6	1.1
Salad, Italian, Light, Kraft*	1 Tbsp/15ml	5	0.0	31	0.1	6.8	0.0	0.6
Salad, Italian, Newman's Own*	1 Tbsp/15g	82	9.0	545	0.2	1.0	59.8	0.0
Salad, Low Fat, Weight Watchers*	1 Tbsp/10g	10	0.4	106	1.5	15.4	4.3	0.0
Salad, Mary Berry*	1 Serving/15g	77	6.6	513	0.8	28.5	44.0	0.1
Salad, Pizza Express*	1 Serving/5g	29	3.2	573	1.4	3.4	63.0	0.0
Salad, Raspberry Balsamic, GFY, Asda*	1 Tbsp/15ml	6	0.1	40	0.7	9.3	0.7	1.3
Salad, Sun Dried Tomato & Chilli, Loyd Grossman*	1 Tsp/5g	18	1.9	361	0.9	5.3	37.3	0.9
Salad, Thousand Island, 95% Fat Free, Asda*	1 Tsp/6g	6	0.3	99	1.6	12.6	4.7	0.5
Seafood, M&S*	1 Tsp/7g	39	4.2	555	0.9	4.9	59.3	0.9
Sicilian Lemon, M&S*	1 Tbsp/15ml	73	7.4	485	0.1	10.5	49.1	0.0
Sweet Balsamic & Smoked Garlic, BGTY, Sainsbury's*	1 Serving/20g	10	0.1	51	0.2	11.9	0.3	0.2
Sweet Chilli & Mango, LL, Waitrose*	1 Serving/16ml	10	0.0	64	1.6	14.0	0.1	0.6
Sweet Chilli, COU, M&S*	1 Tbsp/15ml	9	0.1	60	0.5	14.5	0.5	0.4
Thousand Island	1 Tsp/6g	19	1.8	323	1.1	12.5	30.2	0.4
Thousand Island, BGTY, Sainsbury's*	1 Serving/20g	19	1.4	95	0.4	7.3	7.2	0.5
Thousand Island, COU, M&S*	1 Serving/30g	26	0.8	85	1.4	14.2	2.6	1.1
Thousand Island, Eat Smart, Morrisons*	1 Tbsp/15ml	38	3.2	253	0.0	0.0	21.3	0.0
Thousand Island, HE, Tesco*	1 Serving/25ml	47	3.8	189	2.9	10.0	15.1	0.0
Thousand Island, Light, Kraft*	1 Tbsp/15ml	16	0.0	105	0.6	23.0	0.2	3.0
Thousand Island, Reduced Calorie	1 Tsp/6g	12	0.9	195	0.7	14.7	15.2	0.0
Thousand Island, Tesco*	1 Tbsp/15g	55	4.7	360	1.1	19.5	30.5	0.3
True Blue Cheese, Briannas*	2 Tbsp/30ml	120	11.0	400	3.3	16.7	36.7	0.0
Yoghurt & Mint, HE, Tesco*	1 Tbsp/15g	20	0.4	135	1.5	26.2	2.7	0.0
Yoghurt Mint Cucumber, M&S*	1 Tsp/5ml	6	0.4	115	1.0	8.7	8.0	0.0

D

	Measure INFO/WEIGHT	per Measure KCAL	FAT	Nutrition Values per 100g / 100ml KCAL	PROT	CARB	FAT	FIBRE
DRIED FRUIT								
Banana, Bites, Kiddylicious, Babylicious*	1 Serving/15g	74	4.0	493	1.7	65.1	26.8	6.6
Beach Bum, Graze*	1 Pack/28g	93	4.2	332	4.0	46.0	15.0	9.0
Goji Berry, Graze*	1 Pack/45g	234	17.3	521	17.1	28.4	38.4	0.0
Honey Coated Banana Chips, Whitworths*	1 Serving/25g	132	7.8	526	1.0	59.9	31.4	1.7
Mixed, Value, Tesco*	1 Serving/25g	71	0.2	285	2.1	67.5	0.7	2.3
Pineapple, Sweetened, Whitworths*	1 Bag/35g	122	0.1	350	0.4	86.3	0.2	0.5
Prunes, Juicy, Whitworths*	1 Pack/500g	740	2.0	148	2.5	34.0	0.4	5.7
Strawberry, Banana & Cherry, Sunshine Mix, Graze*	1 Pack/50g	78	0.2	157	9.7	37.2	0.4	0.0
Trail Mix, Kick Start, Wholefoods, Asda*	1 Serving/50g	194	10.2	387	10.9	40.0	20.4	10.7
DRIED FRUIT & SEED MIX								
Sainsbury's*	1 Pack/50g	204	10.7	408	11.6	42.0	21.4	5.1
DRIED FRUIT MIX								
Agadoo, Pineapple, Jumbo & Green Raisins, Graze*	1 Pack/40g	110	0.4	275	2.1	69.0	0.9	0.0
Apple Strudel, Graze*	1 Pack/40g	99	0.3	247	2.2	58.7	0.7	5.9
Average	***1 Tbsp/25g***	***67***	***0.1***	***268***	***2.3***	***68.1***	***0.4***	***2.2***
Berry, LL, Waitrose*	1 Serving/30g	89	0.3	296	1.9	70.0	0.9	3.0
Dates, Raisins & Apricots, Wholefoods, Tesco*	1 Serving/20g	52	0.1	260	3.1	59.0	0.4	4.0
Eden, Graze*	1 Punnet/25g	69	0.2	275	2.0	63.7	1.0	8.1
Fruit & Oat Bites, Mixed Berry, Planet Lunch*	1 Bar/20g	53	0.6	265	3.9	56.0	2.8	8.0
Garden of England, Graze*	1 Punnet/25g	70	0.2	280	1.0	71.2	0.7	5.6
Little Figgy Went to Market, Graze*	1 Punnet/36g	97	0.3	272	2.0	66.0	0.9	7.0
Luxury, Co-Op*	1 Serving/40g	114	0.2	285	2.0	68.0	0.6	4.0
Pear Tatin, Graze*	1 Punnet/35g	143	6.3	408	7.0	57.2	18.1	5.9
Raisins & Berries, Tesco*	1 Pot/60g	200	0.3	334	2.2	78.2	0.5	3.8
Scandinavian Forest, Graze*	1 Punnet/28g	79	0.2	282	2.0	71.0	0.6	3.0
Scrumptious Blueberry Swirl, Graze*	1 Punnet/40g	155	3.2	392	1.2	76.0	8.0	3.0
Sultanas Raisins & Cranberries, Dunnes*	1 Sm Handful/15g	47	0.1	315	2.0	80.2	0.9	4.7
Sultanas, Currants, Raisins & Citrus Peel, Asda*	1 Serving/100g	283	0.5	283	2.6	67.0	0.5	1.7
Tesco*	1 Tbsp/25g	71	0.1	284	2.3	67.9	0.4	2.2
Tropical Sundae, Graze*	1 Punnet/29g	86	0.3	299	2.7	72.7	1.0	8.5
Tropical, Morrisons*	1 Pack/200g	368	1.0	184	1.7	50.6	0.5	6.3
Vine Fruit, Wholesome, Waitrose*	1 Serving/30g	87	0.1	289	2.1	69.3	0.4	5.3
DRIED MIXED FRUIT								
Rhubarb & Custard, Graze*	1 Punnet/43g	160	3.0	373	2.0	74.0	7.0	8.0
DRIFTER								
Nestle*	1 Finger/20g	99	4.3	484	4.1	68.9	20.9	1.2
DRINKING CHOCOLATE								
Cadbury*	1 Heap Tbsp/16g	64	0.9	400	6.2	76.0	5.8	9.1
Dry, Asda*	1 Serving/30g	111	1.8	370	6.0	73.0	6.0	0.0
Dry, M&S*	3 Heaped Tsp/20g	73	0.9	365	8.4	66.0	4.4	13.0
Dry, Tesco*	3 Tsp/25g	92	1.4	368	6.4	72.6	5.8	4.2
Dry, Waitrose*	3 Tsp/12g	48	0.7	403	7.2	79.9	6.1	2.9
Hot Chocolate, Light Choices, Tesco*	1 Cup/11g	38	0.8	345	13.8	54.9	7.7	13.1
Made Up with Semi-Skimmed Milk, Average	***1 Mug/227ml***	***129***	***4.3***	***57***	***3.5***	***7.0***	***1.9***	***0.2***
Made Up with Skimmed Milk, Average	***1 Mug/227ml***	***100***	***1.1***	***44***	***3.5***	***7.0***	***0.5***	***0.0***
Made Up with Whole Milk, Average	***1 Mug/227ml***	***173***	***9.5***	***76***	***3.4***	***6.8***	***4.2***	***0.2***
Made Up, BGTY, Sainsbury's*	1 Serving/178g	114	0.4	64	3.9	11.4	0.2	0.7
Maxpax, Light, Suchard*	1 Serving/11g	37	0.6	355	20.0	56.0	5.5	9.3
Milk, Instant Break, Cadbury*	4 Tsp/28g	119	3.9	425	10.9	64.2	14.0	0.0
Mix, Flavia*	1 Serving/18g	64	0.7	368	15.6	67.2	4.0	0.0
DRIPPING								
Beef	***1oz/28g***	***249***	***27.7***	***891***	***0.0***	***0.0***	***99.0***	***0.0***

	Measure INFO/WEIGHT	per Measure KCAL	FAT	Nutrition Values per 100g / 100ml KCAL	PROT	CARB	FAT	FIBRE
DUCK								
Breast, Cantonese Style Plum Sauce, Gressingham Foods*	1 Portion/200g	423	18.0	211	14.2	18.5	9.0	0.5
Breast, Meat Only, Cooked, Average	*1oz/28g*	*48*	*2.0*	*172*	*25.3*	*1.8*	*7.0*	*0.0*
Breast, Meat Only, Raw, Average	*1 Serving/160g*	*206*	*6.8*	*128*	*22.6*	*0.0*	*4.2*	*0.2*
Fillets, Gressingham, Mini, TTD, Sainsbury's*	½ Pack/90g	127	2.4	141	29.0	0.0	2.7	0.6
Leg, Meat & Skin, Average	*1oz/28g*	*80*	*5.6*	*286*	*17.2*	*0.5*	*20.0*	*0.4*
Legs, with Plum & Hoisin Sauce, Just Cook, Sainsbury's*	½ Pack/140g	344	17.1	246	21.4	12.3	12.2	0.5
Raw, Meat, Fat & Skin	*1oz/28g*	*109*	*10.4*	*388*	*13.1*	*0.0*	*37.3*	*0.0*
Roast, Duckling, Half, Irish, Crispy, Deluxe, Lidl*	1 Serving/50g	172	12.4	343	13.1	17.4	24.7	0.0
Roasted, Meat Only, Weighed with Fat, Skin & Bone	1 Serving/100g	41	2.2	41	5.3	0.0	2.2	0.0
Roasted, Meat, Fat & Skin	*1oz/28g*	*118*	*10.7*	*423*	*20.0*	*0.0*	*38.1*	*0.0*
DUCK &								
Plum Sauce, Roasted, Sainsbury's*	½ Pack/150g	174	3.8	116	6.9	16.0	2.5	1.8
DUCK AROMATIC								
Crispy, Asda*	1/3 Pack/166g	469	24.9	283	19.0	18.0	15.0	0.8
Crispy, Half Duck & Pancakes, M&S*	½ Pack/311g	590	26.7	190	13.9	14.0	8.6	2.1
Crispy, Half with Hoisin Sauce & 12 Pancakes, Tesco*	1/6 Pack/70g	162	7.4	232	18.3	15.9	10.6	1.1
with Plum Sauce, Tesco*	½ Pack/250g	350	11.5	140	9.3	15.2	4.6	0.3
DUCK CANTONESE								
Style, Roast, Tesco*	1 Pack/300g	375	6.9	125	8.2	17.9	2.3	0.5
DUCK IN								
Chinese Barbecue, Wings, Sainsbury's*	1 Serving/175g	430	25.0	246	19.4	9.7	14.3	0.0
Orange Sauce, Breast, Simply, Gressingham Foods*	½ Pack/175g	254	11.9	145	15.9	5.1	6.8	0.4
Orange Sauce, Iceland*	1 Serving/200g	336	20.8	168	11.3	7.4	10.4	1.2
Orange Sauce, Roast, a L'Orange, M&S*	½ Pack/270g	554	42.1	205	12.5	4.1	15.6	0.6
Red Wine Sauce, Free Range Fillets, Waitrose*	½ Pack/250g	378	19.2	151	16.4	4.1	7.7	2.2
DUCK PEKING								
Crispy, Aromatic, Sainsbury's*	½ Pack/300g	1236	110.7	412	19.5	0.6	36.9	0.1
Crispy, Cherry Valley*	1 Serving/270g	702	35.9	260	17.5	17.8	13.3	0.7
DUCK WITH								
Noodles, Shanghai Roast, Sainsbury's*	1 Pack/450g	580	17.1	129	5.6	18.0	3.8	1.2
Pancakes & Hoisin Sauce, M&S*	1 Pack/80g	136	3.2	170	13.0	19.9	4.0	0.9
Pancakes, Shredded, Iceland*	1 Pack/220g	471	5.9	214	20.4	27.0	2.7	1.5
DUMPLINGS								
Average	*1oz/28g*	*58*	*3.3*	*208*	*2.8*	*24.5*	*11.7*	*0.9*
Dim Sum, Chicken, Asian Fusion, Waitrose*	1 Dumpling/20g	30	0.4	152	9.5	22.8	2.2	1.4
Dim Sum, From Restaurant, Average	*1 Piece/12g*	*50*	*2.4*	*433*	*28.9*	*31.3*	*20.4*	*0.0*
Dim Sum, Steamed, Prawn, M&S*	6 Dim Sum/120g	222	3.2	185	1.1	39.0	2.7	1.5
Dim Sum, 177Chicken, Spicy, Zao, Taiko Foods*	1 Dumpling/18g	31	0.4	166	14.1	21.4	2.1	1.5
Dried Mix, Tesco*	1 Pack/137g	404	16.7	295	5.4	39.9	12.2	2.8
Farmhouse, Mix, Goldenfry Foods Ltd*	1 Serving/35g	148	5.3	422	9.1	62.0	15.1	1.0
Homestyle, Baked Weight, Frozen, Aunt Bessie's*	1 Dumpling/49g	188	8.6	384	9.7	44.4	17.6	2.8
Pork & Garlic Chive, Waitrose*	1 Pack/115g	215	8.1	187	9.4	20.4	7.0	1.1
Prawn, Siu Mai, Chinese, M&S*	8 Dumplings/170g	170	2.9	100	7.8	13.1	1.7	1.3

D

	Measure INFO/WEIGHT	per Measure KCAL	FAT	Nutrition Values per 100g / 100ml KCAL	PROT	CARB	FAT	FIBRE
EASTER EGG								
After Eight Giant Chocolate Egg, Nestle*	¼ Egg/50g	274	16.9	547	5.5	51.8	33.8	7.1
Buttons, Chocolate Egg Shell Only, Cadbury*	1 Med Egg/162g	859	48.6	530	7.5	56.8	30.0	0.7
Caramel, Chocolate Egg Shell Only, Cadbury*	1 Lge Egg/343g	1801	102.9	525	7.5	56.8	30.0	0.7
Chick, Dairy Milk, Chocolate Egg Shell Only, Cadbury*	1 Chick Egg/167g	877	50.1	525	7.5	56.8	30.0	0.7
Chocolate Egg Shell Only, Dairy Milk, Cadbury*	1 Med Egg/178g	943	53.4	530	7.5	56.8	30.0	0.7
Creme Egg, Chocolate Egg Shell Only, Cadbury*	1 Egg/178g	943	53.4	530	7.5	56.8	30.0	0.7
Dark Chocolate, 70%, Green & Black's*	1 Med Egg/165g	960	69.5	580	9.1	36.5	42.0	10.0
Dark Chocolate, Dairy, Gluten, Egg, & Nut Free, Kinnerton*	¼ Egg28g	149	9.6	543	5.5	47.6	35.0	7.5
Flake, Chocolate Egg Shell Only, Cadbury*	1 Med Shell/153g	811	46.7	530	7.6	56.5	30.5	0.7
Galaxy Ripple Indulgence, with Chocolate Egg, Mars*	1 Egg Shell/198g	1047	57.2	529	7.0	59.2	28.9	1.6
Kit Kat, Chunky, Nestle*	1 Med Egg/235g	1248	67.2	531	5.3	62.3	28.6	1.7
Mars*	1 Serving/63g	281	10.9	449	4.2	69.0	17.4	0.0
Milk Chocolate, Nestle*	½ Egg/42g	205	9.7	489	5.0	65.2	23.1	0.5
Milk Chocolate, Swiss, Hollow, M&S*	1 Egg/18g	100	6.3	555	6.7	53.2	34.8	2.5
Milky Bar, Nestle*	1 Egg/40g	182	6.9	454	4.2	70.8	17.2	0.0
Smarties, Nestle*	1 Med Egg/258g	1367	74.0	530	5.3	62.2	28.7	1.7
White Chocolate, Thorntons*	1 Egg/360g	1958	109.1	544	5.5	62.2	30.3	2.1
ECLAIR								
Chocolate & Fresh Cream, Tempting, Tesco*	1 Eclair/39g	158	11.2	405	6.5	29.1	28.8	1.1
Chocolate, Asda*	1 Eclair/33g	144	11.0	436	6.7	27.3	33.3	4.8
Chocolate, Cream, Fresh, Tesco*	1 Eclair/66g	285	20.5	430	6.0	31.1	30.9	1.8
Chocolate, Fresh Cream, M&S*	1 Eclair/44g	170	12.2	390	6.3	28.4	27.9	2.0
Chocolate, Fresh Cream, Sainsbury's*	1 Eclair/59g	212	13.9	360	4.2	32.7	23.6	0.5
Chocolate, Frozen, Morrisons*	1 Eclair/31g	116	9.6	374	5.0	18.8	31.0	1.3
Chocolate, HL, Tesco*	1 Eclair/77g	192	9.7	249	6.8	27.1	12.6	0.9
Chocolate, Mini, Iceland*	1 Eclair/13g	55	4.6	426	4.9	21.5	35.6	0.4
Chocolate, Cream filled, VLH Kitchens	1 Serving/66g	286	44.2	434	7.0	36.4	29.2	1.8
EEL								
Cooked or Smoked, Dry Heat, Average	**1 Serving/100g**	**236**	**15.0**	**236**	**23.6**	**0.0**	**15.0**	**0.0**
Jellied, Average	**1oz/28g**	**26**	**1.9**	**93**	**8.0**	**0.0**	**6.7**	**0.0**
Raw, Average	**1oz/28g**	**32**	**2.1**	**113**	**11.1**	**0.0**	**7.6**	**0.0**
EGGS								
Barn, Basics, Sainsbury's*	1 Egg/50g	72	4.8	143	4.1	0.5	9.6	0.5
Dried, White, Average	**1 Tbsp/14g**	**41**	**0.0**	**295**	**73.8**	**0.0**	**0.0**	**0.0**
Dried, Whole, Average	**1oz/28g**	**159**	**11.6**	**568**	**48.4**	**0.0**	**41.6**	**0.0**
Duck, Boiled & Salted, Average, Weight with Shell	**1 Egg/75g**	**148**	**11.6**	**198**	**14.6**	**0.0**	**15.5**	**0.0**
Duck, Whole, Raw, Average, Weight with Shell	**1 Egg/75g**	**122**	**8.8**	**163**	**14.3**	**0.0**	**11.8**	**0.0**
Free Range, Golden, TTD, Sainsbury's*	1 Egg/49g	72	5.3	147	12.5	0.0	10.8	0.0
Free Range, Large, Average, Weight with Shell	**1 Egg/68g**	**97**	**6.8**	**143**	**12.6**	**0.8**	**9.9**	**0.0**
Fried in Veg Oil, Average	**1 Med/60g**	**107**	**8.3**	**179**	**13.6**	**0.0**	**13.9**	**0.0**
Fried without Fat, Average	**1 Med/60g**	**104**	**7.6**	**174**	**15.0**	**0.0**	**12.7**	**0.0**
Goose, Whole, Raw, Average, Weight with Shell	**1 Egg/144g**	**232**	**16.6**	**161**	**12.1**	**1.2**	**11.5**	**0.0**
Large, Average, Weight with Shell	**1 Egg/68g**	**101**	**7.5**	**149**	**12.3**	**0.0**	**11.0**	**0.0**
Medium, Average, Weight with Shell	**1 Egg/58g**	**86**	**6.4**	**148**	**12.2**	**0.1**	**11.0**	**0.0**
Medium, Boiled, Average, Weight with Shell	**1 Egg/58g**	**85**	**6.3**	**147**	**12.5**	**0.5**	**10.8**	**0.1**
Poached, Weight with Shell	1 Med/50g	73	5.4	147	12.5	0.5	10.8	0.5
Quail, Whole, Raw, Weight with Shell	**1 Egg/13g**	**20**	**1.4**	**151**	**12.9**	**0.4**	**11.1**	**0.0**
Savoury, Bites, Mini, Sainsbury's*	1 Egg/12g	35	2.2	288	9.4	21.7	17.8	1.6
Savoury, Mini, Tesco*	1 Egg/20g	55	3.5	274	9.2	20.2	17.4	2.3
Scotch, All Day Breakfast, Tesco*	1 Egg/114g	279	18.4	245	13.3	11.1	16.1	1.1
Scotch, Asda*	1 Egg/114g	286	19.2	251	11.2	13.7	16.8	1.4
Scotch, Budgens*	1 Egg/113g	294	19.9	260	11.4	13.8	17.6	0.0
Scotch, Cumberland, Waitrose*	1 Egg/114g	243	14.3	214	13.0	12.1	12.6	1.6

	Measure	per Measure		Nutrition Values per 100g / 100ml				
	INFO/WEIGHT	KCAL	FAT	KCAL	PROT	CARB	FAT	FIBRE
EGGS								
Scotch, Finest, Tesco*	1 Egg/114g	280	20.1	247	11.6	10.4	17.7	1.1
Scotch, Free Range, Sainsbury's*	1 Egg/113g	284	19.0	252	12.4	12.5	16.9	2.5
Scotch, Ginsters*	1 Egg/95g	228	15.1	240	15.3	9.7	15.9	0.6
Scotch, Morrisons*	1 Egg/114g	286	19.1	251	11.2	13.7	16.8	1.4
Scotch, Retail	1 Egg/120g	301	20.5	251	12.0	13.1	17.1	0.0
Scotch, Sainsbury's*	1 Egg/113g	311	21.8	275	11.1	14.2	19.3	0.9
Scotch, Savoury, M&S*	1 Egg/21g	63	4.5	305	11.0	15.7	21.8	1.3
Scotch, Super Mini, Asda*	1 Egg/13g	38	2.6	305	10.0	19.0	21.0	2.1
Scotch, Value, Tesco*	1 Egg/114g	277	18.9	243	9.6	13.8	16.6	2.6
Scotch, Vegetarian, Holland & Barrett*	1 Egg/100g	209	8.0	209	13.0	19.9	8.0	2.9
Scrambled & Bacon, in Store Cafe, Sainsbury's*	1 Serving/403g	533	46.4	132	9.6	11.5	11.5	2.7
Scrambled with Milk, Average	*1 Serving/100g*	*257*	*23.4*	*257*	*10.9*	*0.7*	*23.4*	*0.0*
Scrambled, Average	*1 Serving/100g*	*160*	*11.6*	*160*	*13.8*	*0.0*	*11.6*	*0.0*
Turkey, Whole, Raw, Weight with Shell	*1 Egg/79g*	*135*	*9.6*	*171*	*13.7*	*1.2*	*12.2*	*0.0*
Very Large, Average, Weight with Shell	*1 Egg/78g*	*112*	*7.8*	*143*	*12.6*	*0.8*	*9.9*	*0.0*
White, Free Range, Liquid, Two Chicks*	3 Tbsp/45g	23	0.0	50	10.5	1.0	0.0	0.0
Whites Only, Raw, Average	*1 Lg Egg/33g*	*12*	*0.0*	*36*	*9.0*	*0.0*	*0.0*	*0.0*
Yolks, Raw	*1 Yolk/14g*	*47*	*4.3*	*339*	*16.1*	*0.0*	*30.5*	*0.0*
ELK								
Raw, Meat only	*1 Serving/100g*	*111*	*1.4*	*111*	*23.0*	*0.0*	*1.4*	*0.0*
Roasted, Meat only	1 Serving/100g	146	1.9	146	30.2	0.0	1.9	0.0
ENCHILADAS								
Chicken, Asda*	1 Serving/500g	690	30.0	138	10.0	17.0	6.0	1.0
Chicken, Average	*1 Serving/295g*	*483*	*18.8*	*164*	*11.6*	*16.0*	*6.4*	*1.7*
Spicy, Three Bean, Cooked, CBY, Asda*	1 Pack/400g	466	15.9	117	4.4	13.7	4.0	4.1
ENDIVE								
Raw	*1oz/28g*	*2*	*0.0*	*8*	*1.1*	*0.6*	*0.1*	*1.3*
ENERGY DRINK								
Average	*1 Can/250ml*	*118*	*0.0*	*47*	*0.0*	*11.4*	*0.0*	*0.0*
Isostar Sport, Isostar*	1 Glass/250ml	74	0.0	30	0.0	7.0	0.0	0.0
KX, Sugar Free, Diet, Tesco*	1 Can/250ml	5	0.0	2	0.0	0.0	0.0	0.0
KX, Sugar Free, Tesco*	1 Can/250ml	8	0.0	3	0.0	0.0	0.0	0.0
Lemon, Active Sport, Tesco*	1 Bottle/500ml	135	0.0	27	0.0	6.5	0.0	0.0
Monster*	1 Can/500ml	240	0.0	48	0.0	12.0	0.0	0.0
Powerade, Aqua+*	1 Bottle/500ml	80	0.0	16	0.0	3.7	0.0	0.0
Red Thunder, Diet, Low Calorie, Aldi*	1 Can/250ml	5	0.0	2	0.1	0.0	0.0	0.0
Relentless, Original, Relentless*	1 Can/500ml	230	0.0	46	0.0	10.4	0.0	0.0
Sugar Free, Boost Drinks Ltd*	1 Can/250ml	5	0.0	2	0.0	0.0	0.0	0.0

E

	Measure INFO/WEIGHT	per Measure KCAL	FAT	Nutrition Values per 100g / 100ml KCAL	PROT	CARB	FAT	FIBRE
FAGGOTS								
British Pork with Streaky Bacon, Essential, Waitrose*	2 Faggots/128g	255	14.5	199	16.7	7.5	11.3	0.9
Pork, in a West Country Sauce, Mr Brains*	2 Faggots/242g	307	15.9	127	5.5	10.9	6.6	1.0
FAJITA								
Chicken, Average	**1 Serving/275g**	**409**	**14.7**	**149**	**10.2**	**15.0**	**5.4**	**2.3**
Chicken, M&S*	1 Pack/230g	345	12.2	150	8.6	17.7	5.3	1.0
Crispy Chicken, Old El Paso*	1 Fajita/70g	183	5.4	263	7.6	41.0	7.8	1.8
Vegetable	1 Serving/275g	472	14.9	172	4.9	25.6	5.4	1.9
Vegetable, Tesco*	1 Fajita/112g	133	5.6	119	4.2	14.3	5.0	1.1
FALAFEL								
12 pack, Sainsbury's*	1 Falafel/17g	44	2.5	259	7.3	20.6	14.8	7.2
Asda*	½ Pack/50g	140	9.6	281	8.3	18.9	19.1	8.2
Balls, Meat Free, Meat Free, Tesco*	3 Balls/67g	135	5.3	205	7.1	21.7	8.1	6.3
Fried in Vegetable Oil, Average	**1 Falafel/25g**	**45**	**2.8**	**179**	**6.4**	**15.6**	**11.2**	**3.4**
Mini, M&S*	1 Falafel/14g	43	2.5	310	7.9	28.1	18.4	2.6
Mini, Sainsbury's*	1 Serving/168g	499	29.6	297	8.0	26.8	17.6	3.2
Organic, Cauldron Foods*	1 Falafel/25g	51	2.4	203	8.4	20.3	9.8	7.2
Original, Mediterranean, Great Food*	1 Falafel/22g	69	4.0	316	9.2	32.0	18.3	6.6
FANTA								
Fruit Twist, Coca-Cola*	1 Serving/250ml	132	0.0	53	0.0	13.0	0.0	0.0
Icy Lemon, Coca-Cola*	1 Can/330mls	112	0.0	34	0.0	8.3	0.0	0.0
Icy Lemon, Zero, Coca-Cola*	1 Can/330mls	7	0.0	2	0.0	0.2	0.0	0.0
Lemon, Coca-Cola*	1 Can/330ml	165	0.0	50	0.0	12.0	0.0	0.0
Orange, Coca-Cola*	1 Glass/250ml	75	0.0	30	0.0	7.1	0.0	0.0
Orange, Zero, Coca-Cola*	1 Can/330ml	11	0.0	3	0.0	0.5	0.0	0.0
FARFALLE								
Bows, Dry, Average	**1 Serving/75g**	**265**	**1.4**	**353**	**11.4**	**72.6**	**1.9**	**1.9**
Salmon, Hot Smoked, Slimming World*	1 Pack/550g	605	12.1	110	6.0	15.3	2.2	2.4
FENNEL								
Florence, Boiled in Salted Water	**1oz/28g**	**3**	**0.1**	**11**	**0.9**	**1.5**	**0.2**	**2.3**
Florence, Raw, Unprepared, Average	**1 Bulb/250g**	**24**	**0.4**	**10**	**0.7**	**1.4**	**0.2**	**1.9**
Florence, Steamed	**1 Serving/80g**	**9**	**0.2**	**11**	**9.0**	**1.5**	**0.2**	**2.3**
FENUGREEK								
Leaves, Raw, Fresh, Average	**1 Serving/80g**	**28**	**0.2**	**35**	**4.6**	**4.8**	**0.2**	**1.1**
FETTUCCINI								
Chicken, Cajun Spiced, COU, M&S*	1 Pack/400g	400	8.0	100	8.0	12.3	2.0	1.3
Dry Weight, Buitoni*	1 Serving/90g	326	1.5	362	12.2	74.4	1.7	0.0
FIG ROLLS								
Asda*	1 Biscuit/19g	71	1.7	372	4.8	68.0	9.0	0.0
Bolands*	1 Biscuit/17g	63	1.4	372	4.1	68.3	8.0	5.0
Go Ahead, McVitie's*	1 Biscuit/15g	55	0.7	365	4.2	76.8	4.6	2.9
Jacob's*	1 Biscuit/17g	66	1.5	386	3.4	72.2	8.6	3.0
Sainsbury's*	1 Biscuit/19g	67	1.6	360	4.3	64.5	8.7	3.4
Vitalinea, Jacob's*	1 Biscuit/18g	61	1.0	339	3.7	68.2	5.8	3.8
FIGS								
Dried, Average	**1 Fig/14g**	**32**	**0.1**	**232**	**3.6**	**53.2**	**1.1**	**8.6**
Dried, Organic, LL, Waitrose*	1 Fig/30g	66	0.4	221	3.3	48.6	1.5	9.8
Dried, Ready to Eat, CBY, Asda*	1 Serving/30g	70	0.4	234	3.3	48.4	1.5	6.9
Fresh, Black Bursa, Morrisons*	1 Fig/54g	119	0.8	221	3.3	48.6	1.5	6.9
in Light Syrup, Asda*	1 Serving/100g	75	0.1	75	0.4	18.0	0.1	0.7
Raw, Fresh, Average	**1 Fig/35g**	**16**	**0.1**	**45**	**1.3**	**9.8**	**0.2**	**1.5**
Rich & Jammy, Speciality, Fresh, Waitrose*	**1 Fig/50g**	**26**	**0.2**	**52**	**1.3**	**9.5**	**0.3**	**2.9**
FISH								
Balls, Gefilte, M&S*	1 Pack/200g	280	7.8	140	14.1	11.9	3.9	1.0

F

	Measure INFO/WEIGHT	per Measure KCAL	FAT	Nutrition Values per 100g / 100ml KCAL	PROT	CARB	FAT	FIBRE
FISH								
Battered, Portion, Ross*	1 Serving/110g	223	11.9	203	10.4	16.1	10.8	0.8
Chargrills, Jalepeno, Red Pepper & Honey, Birds Eye*	1 Chargrill/164g	125	2.3	76	14.0	1.9	1.4	0.3
Chargrills, Thai Coconut Lemongrass & Chilli, Birds Eye*	1 Chargrill/160g	125	2.6	78	14.4	1.3	1.6	0.4
Chargrills, Tomato, Basil & Oregano, Birds Eye*	1 Chargrill/158g	120	2.3	76	14.2	1.1	1.5	0.3
Crumbed, Pak-N-Save*	2 Pieces/140g	298	17.8	213	10.8	13.9	12.7	0.0
Fillets, Lemon & Pepper, Youngs*	1 Fillet/130g	283	16.7	218	10.3	15.3	12.9	4.3
Fillets, Lime & Chilli, Fish Fusions, Birds Eye*	1 Portion/160g	270	10.1	169	15.0	12.9	6.3	0.5
Fillets, White, Breaded, Tesco*	1 Piece/95g	198	10.4	208	10.6	16.9	10.9	1.0
Fillets, White, Breaded, Value, Tesco*	1 Serving/100g	192	9.7	192	10.6	15.6	9.7	2.2
Fillets, White, Natural, Tesco*	1 Fillet/100g	72	0.6	72	16.6	0.0	0.6	0.0
Goujons, Asda*	1 Serving/125g	240	8.0	192	12.8	20.8	6.4	0.2
Grouper	1 Serving/100g	92	1.0	92	19.4	0.0	1.0	0.0
Haddock, Fillets, Lightly Dusted, Seeded, M&S*	1 Fillet/144g	266	12.5	185	14.3	12.2	8.7	1.0
Hake Fillets in Tomato & Basil Marinage, Donegal Catch*	1 Fillet/135g	201	8.9	149	15.6	6.7	6.6	1.0
Pie Mix, Seasonal, Sainsbury's*	1 Pack/320g	480	28.2	150	17.7	0.0	8.8	0.0
Portions in Oven Crisp Batter, Value, Tesco*	1 Serving/100g	209	11.0	209	11.0	16.4	11.0	2.6
River Cobbler, Smoked, Tesco*	1 Fillet/165g	124	3.5	75	13.9	0.0	2.1	1.5
River Cobbler, Value, Tesco*	½ Pack/133g	133	5.3	100	15.1	0.1	4.0	0.1
Steaks, Chip Shop, Youngs*	1 Serving/100g	198	10.4	198	11.0	14.9	10.4	0.9
Sushi, Medium Pack, Tesco*	1 Pack/224g	336	3.8	150	4.0	29.4	1.7	1.0
White, Breaded, Fillets, Ocean Pure*	1 Fillet/113g	276	11.5	245	20.8	16.9	10.2	1.2
White, Smoked, Average	**1 Serving/100g**	**108**	**0.9**	**108**	**23.4**	**0.0**	**0.9**	**0.0**
White, Tesco*	1 Med Fillet/100g	78	0.6	78	16.6	0.0	0.6	0.0
FISH & CHIPS								
Mini Meal, 093, Wiltshire Farm Foods*	1 Serving/185g	255	8.3	138	6.9	17.7	4.5	2.8
with Mushy Peas, Kershaws*	1 Pack/315g	450	18.3	143	6.4	16.4	5.8	1.6
FISH CAKES								
Breaded, Sainsbury's*	1 Cake/42g	75	3.4	179	10.0	16.2	8.1	0.7
Bubbly Batter, Youngs*	1 Cake/44g	109	6.7	247	7.1	20.5	15.1	1.4
Cod & Pancetta, Cafe Culture, M&S*	1 Cake/85g	166	13.2	195	9.2	7.2	15.5	2.0
Cod Fillets, Melting Middle, M&S*	½ Pack/145g	228	9.6	157	8.0	15.9	6.6	0.9
Cod in Crunch Crumb, Birds Eye*	1 Cake/50g	93	4.3	187	11.4	16.0	8.6	1.0
Cod Mornay, Easy to Cook, Waitrose*	1 Cake/149g	234	9.1	157	10.5	15.0	6.1	1.4
Cod, Baked, Tesco*	1 Cake/135g	255	9.9	189	9.1	21.1	7.3	3.2
Cod, Birds Eye*	1 Cake/51g	93	4.4	182	10.0	16.0	8.7	1.1
Cod, Chunky, Breaded, Chilled, Youngs*	1 Cake/90g	192	11.5	213	9.5	14.9	12.8	1.2
Cod, Homemade, Average	**1 Cake/50g**	**120**	**8.3**	**241**	**9.3**	**14.4**	**16.6**	**0.7**
Cod, M&S*	1 Cake/85g	153	7.8	180	8.9	15.4	9.2	1.3
Crab & Prawn, Thai, Tesco*	1 Cake/115g	269	16.6	234	8.8	17.4	14.4	1.2
Fried in Blended Oil	1 Cake/50g	109	6.7	218	8.6	16.8	13.4	0.0
Frozen, Average	**1 Cake/85g**	**112**	**3.3**	**132**	**8.6**	**16.7**	**3.9**	**0.0**
Great Value, Iceland*	1 Cake/42g	74	2.7	175	9.1	20.3	6.4	1.6
Grilled, Average	**1 Cake/50g**	**77**	**2.2**	**154**	**9.9**	**19.7**	**4.5**	**0.0**
Haddock in Breadcrumbs, Sainsbury's*	1 Cake/88g	158	6.2	179	10.8	18.2	7.0	1.4
Haddock, & Cheese, Smoked, Harbour Fresh, Lidl*	1 Cake/145g	268	9.6	185	9.6	21.0	6.6	2.5
Haddock, Breaded, Asda*	1 Cake/90g	187	7.6	208	10.0	22.8	8.5	1.2
Haddock, Fresh Tastes, Asda*	1 Cake/75g	141	5.0	188	9.6	22.2	6.7	1.8
Haddock, Sainsbury's*	1 Cake/135g	253	10.0	188	10.8	18.7	7.4	1.5
Haddock, Smoked, ES, Asda*	1 Cake/115g	218	10.9	190	12.8	13.2	9.5	1.3
Haddock, Smoked, Frozen, Waitrose*	1 Cake/85g	186	10.3	219	9.6	17.8	12.1	0.8
Haddock, Smoked, M&S*	1 Cake/85g	153	8.0	180	10.6	13.4	9.4	2.6
Haddock, Smoked, Sainsbury's*	1 Cake/63g	127	6.0	201	11.0	17.8	9.5	2.1
Haddock, Smoked, Tesco*	1 Cake/135g	236	9.3	175	7.7	19.9	6.9	2.8

F

FISH CAKES

	Measure INFO/WEIGHT	per Measure KCAL	FAT	Nutrition Values per 100g / 100ml KCAL	PROT	CARB	FAT	FIBRE
FISH CAKES								
M&S*	1 Cake/80g	180	10.6	225	8.0	18.0	13.2	0.0
Prawn, Sainsbury's*	1 Cake/90g	184	7.8	204	9.6	21.7	8.7	1.2
Prawn, Thai Style, Finest, Tesco*	1 Cake/145g	305	13.5	210	6.7	24.2	9.3	1.0
Ross*	1 Cake/52g	83	3.8	160	7.4	15.9	7.4	1.2
Salmon & Dill, Cook*	1 Cake/95g	144	5.3	152	11.3	14.2	5.6	1.5
Salmon & Dill, Waitrose*	1 Cake/85g	206	11.9	242	11.5	17.5	14.0	1.8
Salmon & Haddock with Lemon & Dill Sauce, Waitrose*	1 Cake/187g	304	18.1	163	9.2	9.7	9.7	1.5
Salmon & Leek, Northern Catch, Aldi*	1 Cake/114g	212	9.0	186	9.5	19.3	7.9	0.9
Salmon & Tarragon, Waitrose*	1 Cake/85g	179	10.0	211	11.9	14.3	11.8	2.2
Salmon with Parsley Sauce, Finest, Tesco*	½ Pack/170g	350	23.6	206	8.6	11.7	13.9	1.0
Salmon, & Broccoli, Morrisons*	1 Cake/110g	211	10.3	191	9.0	16.7	9.3	2.2
Salmon, & Hollandaise Sauce, Saucy Fish Co*	1 Fishcake/135g	270	13.0	200	9.2	19.2	9.6	1.4
Salmon, Asda*	1 Cake/86g	215	12.0	250	8.0	23.0	14.0	1.4
Salmon, Ginger & Chilli, Sainsbury's*	1 Cake/150g	332	17.0	221	11.1	17.7	11.3	2.3
Salmon, Homemade, Average	***1 Cake/50g***	***136***	***9.8***	***273***	***10.4***	***14.4***	***19.7***	***0.7***
Salmon, in Light & Crispy Breadcrumbs, Tesco*	1 Cake/90g	212	10.8	235	9.7	21.0	12.0	1.2
Salmon, M&S*	1 Cake/86g	180	10.9	210	9.1	15.1	12.7	1.7
Salmon, Melting Middle, Lochmuir, M&S*	1 Pack/290g	551	30.4	190	9.1	14.3	10.5	1.5
Salmon, Morrisons*	1 Cake/90g	241	11.8	268	10.1	27.6	13.1	1.5
Salmon, Sainsbury's*	1 Cake/88g	171	7.6	194	12.6	16.5	8.6	1.6
Salmon, Spinach & Sicilian Lemon, Finest, Tesco*	1 Cake/145g	290	16.2	200	9.9	14.3	11.2	1.4
Salmon, Tesco*	1 Cake/90g	239	13.5	266	11.4	21.3	15.0	0.0
Salmon, VLH Kitchens	1 Cake/56g	156	35.7	278	10.5	14.4	20.0	0.6
Smart Price, Asda*	1 Cake/42g	78	3.3	188	7.0	22.0	8.0	0.9
Thai Style, Sainsbury's*	1 Cake/49g	69	2.1	141	12.0	13.8	4.2	1.7
Thai, Frozen, Sainsbury's*	1 Cake/15g	28	1.1	187	21.3	9.3	7.3	0.7
Thai, Oriental Selection, Waitrose*	1 Cake/11g	18	0.3	161	17.8	15.8	3.0	1.5
Thai, Tesco*	1 Cake/22g	37	1.1	166	17.4	12.8	5.0	1.1
Tuna, Lime & Coriander, BGTY, Sainsbury's*	1 Cake/91g	200	10.7	220	10.7	17.7	11.8	2.6
FISH FINGERS								
Atlantis*	1 Finger/30g	52	2.2	172	12.0	14.0	7.5	0.4
Brilliant, 10 Pack, Jamie Oliver, Youngs*	3 Fingers/86g	177	7.9	205	11.7	18.4	9.1	1.2
Chip Shop, Youngs*	1 Finger/30g	75	4.9	251	9.3	16.6	16.4	1.2
Chunky, Cooked, Tesco*	2 Fingers/98g	230	10.0	235	13.2	21.6	10.2	1.3
Cod, 100% Cod Fillet, Tesco*	1 Finger/30g	53	2.2	177	12.4	14.9	7.5	1.4
Cod, Chunky, Tesco*	1 Finger/40g	70	3.0	175	12.3	14.3	7.6	1.6
Cod, Fillets, Asda*	1 Finger/31g	66	3.1	214	13.0	18.0	10.0	0.0
Cod, Fillets, Chunky, M&S*	1 Finger/40g	70	2.4	175	12.0	17.2	6.0	1.0
Cod, Fillets, Chunky, TTD, Sainsbury's*	2 Fingers/120g	274	13.2	228	13.4	18.3	11.0	1.2
Cod, Fillets, Essential, Waitrose*	1 Finger/28g	57	2.2	205	13.6	19.1	8.0	1.1
Cod, Fillets, Waitrose*	1 Finger/30g	55	2.2	183	11.9	16.9	7.5	0.7
Cod, Fried in Blended Oil, Average	***1 Finger/28g***	***67***	***3.9***	***238***	***13.2***	***15.5***	***14.1***	***0.6***
Cod, Frozen, Average	***1 Finger/28g***	***48***	***2.2***	***170***	***11.6***	***14.2***	***7.8***	***0.6***
Cod, Grilled, Average	***1 Finger/28g***	***56***	***2.5***	***200***	***14.3***	***16.6***	***8.9***	***0.7***
Cod, Morrisons*	1 Finger/30g	54	2.2	180	11.7	16.4	7.5	1.1
Cod, Sainsbury's*	1 Finger/28g	53	2.1	190	12.5	17.7	7.7	1.0
Free From, Sainsbury's*	1 Finger/30g	56	2.3	188	11.4	18.0	7.8	0.7
Haddock in Crispy Batter, Birds Eye*	1 Finger/30g	56	2.3	188	14.3	15.1	7.8	0.7
Haddock in Crunchy Crumb, Morrisons*	1 Finger/30g	57	2.4	190	13.1	16.3	8.0	1.1
Haddock, Fillets, Asda*	1 Finger/30g	62	2.7	205	14.0	17.0	9.0	0.0
Iceland*	1 Finger/23g	44	2.0	192	11.5	17.3	8.5	1.3
Omega 3, Grilled, Tesco*	3 Fingers/71g	150	6.8	210	12.4	17.8	9.5	1.3
Plaice, Cider Battered, M&S*	½ Pack/140g	372	24.6	266	12.3	14.1	17.6	1.2

	Measure INFO/WEIGHT	per Measure KCAL	FAT	Nutrition Values per 100g / 100ml KCAL	PROT	CARB	FAT	FIBRE
Ross*	1 Finger/26g	50	2.3	193	10.7	17.7	8.8	0.8
FISH FINGERS								
Sainsbury's*	1 Finger/27g	52	2.3	194	13.4	16.0	8.5	0.7
Salmon, Birds Eye*	1 Finger/28g	63	2.7	225	13.2	21.7	9.5	0.9
Value, Tesco*	1 Finger/25g	42	2.0	170	11.5	11.9	8.1	1.7
FISH IN								
Batter, Light, Iceland*	1 Fillet/120g	230	12.1	192	13.6	11.6	10.1	0.7
Batter, Morrisons*	1 Fish/140g	235	8.1	168	14.0	15.0	5.8	0.2
Batter, Youngs*	1 Serving/100g	315	19.7	315	14.9	20.4	19.7	0.8
Butter Sauce, Steaks, Ross*	1 Serving/140g	111	4.0	84	10.6	3.6	3.0	0.3
Butter Sauce, Steaks, Youngs*	1 Steak/140g	102	2.9	73	9.6	3.7	2.1	0.5
Parsley Sauce, Steaks, Ross*	1 Serving/150g	123	5.6	82	9.1	3.1	3.7	0.1
FIVE SPICE								
Powder, Sharwood's*	1 Tsp/2g	3	0.2	172	12.2	11.6	8.6	23.4
FLAKE								
Luxury, Cadbury*	1 Bar/45g	240	13.6	533	7.3	57.8	30.2	0.0
FLAN								
Cheese & Potato, Hot, Tesco*	¼ Flan/100g	282	19.7	282	6.0	20.0	19.7	2.3
Pastry with Fruit	1oz/28g	33	1.2	118	1.4	19.3	4.4	0.7
Sponge with Fruit	1oz/28g	31	0.4	112	2.8	23.3	1.5	0.6
FLAN CASE								
Sponge, Average	***1oz/28g***	***90***	***1.5***	***320***	***7.0***	***62.5***	***5.4***	***0.7***
FLAPJACK								
Lemon Curd, Graze*	1 Punnet/53g	248	12.7	468	6.0	60.0	24.0	6.0
7 Fruits, Graze*	1 Punnet/55g	223	10.5	406	5.1	54.9	19.1	4.3
All Butter, Organic, Sainsbury's*	1 Serving/35g	156	8.0	446	5.3	54.5	23.0	2.7
All Butter, Sainsbury's*	1 Flapjack/35g	156	8.0	446	5.7	54.5	22.8	2.7
All Butter, Squares, M&S*	1 Flapjack/34g	150	7.2	441	6.2	56.2	21.2	4.4
All Butter, Waitrose*	1 Flapjack/34g	126	9.0	376	3.8	52.4	26.8	1.2
Almond, Hazelnut & Almond, Seriously Nutty, Waitrose*	1 Square/26g	133	8.4	517	9.2	46.7	32.6	3.1
Apple & Cinnamon, Graze*	1 Punnet/52g	236	12.0	453	5.0	54.0	23.0	5.0
Apple & Raspberry, Fox's*	1 Flapjack/26g	105	5.0	403	4.8	52.5	19.4	3.7
Apricot & Raisin, Waitrose*	1 Flapjack/38g	143	4.2	376	4.7	64.3	11.1	5.8
Average	***1 Flapjack/50g***	***242***	***13.3***	***484***	***4.5***	***60.4***	***26.6***	***2.7***
Banana, The Handmade Flapjack Company*	1 Flapjack/90g	379	13.1	421	5.3	67.2	14.6	0.0
Belgian Chocolate Dipped, Asda*	1 Flapjack/67g	321	16.8	477	6.0	57.0	25.0	3.2
Cherry Bakewell, Iced, Devondale*	1 Flapjack/95g	432	21.9	455	3.7	54.0	23.1	2.6
Cherry Sultana, Devondale*	1 Flapjack/95g	412	21.8	434	4.0	51.0	23.0	3.0
Chocolate Chip, Boots*	1 Flapjack/75g	313	11.2	417	5.6	65.0	15.0	3.5
Chocolate Chip, Happy Shopper*	1 Flapjack/35g	163	8.2	467	5.7	58.7	23.3	0.0
Chocolate Dipped, M&S*	1 Flapjack/96g	442	21.5	460	6.1	61.3	22.4	3.0
Chocolate, The Handmade Flapjack Company*	1 Flapjack/90g	392	17.6	435	6.0	58.6	19.6	0.0
Chunky Chocolate, M&S*	1 Flapjack/80g	348	15.1	435	5.8	59.9	18.9	2.2
Co-Op*	1 Flapjack/38g	175	9.4	465	5.0	54.0	25.0	4.0
Cranberry, Apple & Raisin, Light Choices, Tesco*	1 Flapjack/30g	98	1.7	325	5.7	63.1	5.6	5.7
Date & Walnut, The Handmade Flapjack Company*	1 Flapjack/90g	360	13.5	400	6.1	60.2	15.0	0.0
Fruit, Tesco*	1 Flapjack/33g	136	5.2	412	5.7	62.0	15.7	4.0
Fruit, Weight Watchers*	1 Flapjack/30g	106	1.9	353	6.0	68.3	6.3	4.7
Fruity, Waitrose*	1 Flapjack/50g	199	6.8	398	6.1	62.9	13.5	3.9
Golden Oaty, Fingers, Fabulous Bakin' Boys*	1 Flapjack/28g	130	6.8	464	4.5	60.2	24.3	3.1
Hobnobs, Milk Chocolate, McVitie's*	1 Flapjack/35g	155	6.0	443	5.8	64.2	17.2	4.2
Honey Almond, Multigrain, Devondale*	1 Flapjack/80g	352	20.5	440	4.7	49.0	25.6	3.2
Jaffa Cake, Graze*	1 Punnet/53g	242	12.7	457	6.0	53.0	24.0	5.0

F

	Measure INFO/WEIGHT	per Measure KCAL	FAT	Nutrition Values per 100g / 100ml KCAL	PROT	CARB	FAT	FIBRE
FLAPJACK								
M&S*	1 Flapjack/53g	228	10.1	430	6.0	59.1	19.0	3.5
Mighty Oat, Fabulous Bakin' Boys*	1 Flapjack/75g	349	16.5	466	5.7	58.8	22.0	4.9
Milk Chocolate Digestive, McVitie's*	1 Flapjack/65g	293	13.8	451	5.4	59.7	21.2	3.4
Mini, Sainsbury's*	1 Flapjack/15g	65	2.9	431	5.6	59.3	19.0	2.7
Mixed Fruit, Fabulous Bakin' Boys*	1 Flapjack/90g	350	9.4	389	5.5	71.0	10.5	4.0
Oat & Syrup, Oatjacks, McVitie's*	1 Flapjack/34g	153	7.5	450	5.3	57.6	22.0	5.0
Oats, Butter & Syrup, McVitie's*	1 Flapjack/79g	356	17.7	454	4.9	57.9	22.5	3.7
Orange & Ginger, Graze*	1 Punnet/54g	241	12.9	446	5.1	53.0	23.8	4.2
Organic, Wholebake*	1 Flapjack/90g	388	18.7	431	6.0	59.4	20.8	0.0
Red Berry, Finger, Fabulous Bakin' Boys*	1 Flapjack/27g	129	6.2	477	5.5	60.6	22.9	2.9
Snickers, McVitie's*	1 Flapjack/65g	315	18.5	484	7.9	49.0	28.5	6.0
Sultana, Tesco*	1 Flapjack/50g	173	10.0	346	5.0	36.2	20.1	3.7
Summer Berry, Graze*	1 Punnet/52g	230	10.9	442	5.0	56.0	21.0	5.0
Walnut & Maple, Devondale*	1 Flapjack/95g	445	27.6	468	4.0	45.2	29.0	3.2
Weight Watchers*	1 Flapjack/30g	109	1.8	363	6.7	71.0	6.0	4.0
FLATBREAD								
Caramelised Onion & Cheddar, Specially Selected, Aldi*	¼ Flatbread/65g	201	6.0	310	10.0	45.0	9.3	2.5
Chargrilled Chicken, COU, M&S*	1 Pack/163g	245	3.1	150	10.8	23.0	1.9	5.2
Cheddar & Black Pepper, Thins, Ryvita*	1 Thin/7g	30	0.7	422	17.5	63.8	10.0	3.3
Cheddar & Caramelised Red Onion, TTD, Sainsbury's*	1 Flatbread/140g	412	13.9	294	9.9	41.0	9.9	2.5
Cheddar & Garlic, Finest, Tesco*	¼ Flatbread/66g	188	6.3	285	7.2	41.8	9.6	2.6
Cheese & Tomato, Tesco*	¼ Pack/54g	160	3.5	295	11.6	45.7	6.4	1.9
Chicken & Mango Salad, Sainsbury's*	1 Pack/100g	251	2.5	251	16.9	40.4	2.5	2.5
Chicken Tikka, BGTY, Sainsbury's*	1 Flatbread/186g	292	4.5	157	11.6	20.5	2.4	3.5
Chicken Tikka, Shapers, Boots*	1 Flatbread/164g	269	4.1	164	11.0	24.0	2.5	1.5
Harissa Chicken & Roasted Vegetable, M&S*	1 Pack/186g	342	4.8	184	10.7	19.7	2.6	0.0
Multi Seed, Thins, Ryvita*	1 Thin/9g	39	1.3	434	16.4	56.2	14.1	8.1
Multiseed, Spelt, Suzie's*	1 Portion/100g	364	6.0	364	10.6	66.9	6.0	3.3
Red Pepper & Mozzarella, Morrisons*	¼ Pack/65g	148	2.6	226	10.1	36.4	3.9	2.7
Spicy Chicken, Shapers, Boots*	1 Pack/181g	292	4.5	161	11.0	23.0	2.5	0.0
Spicy Mexican, Shapers, Boots*	1 Pack/190g	296	7.6	156	7.0	23.0	4.0	3.7
Sweet Chilli, Thins, Ryvita*	1 Thin/8g	31	0.1	382	12.0	77.5	1.5	5.2
FLAXSEED								
Milled, Organic, Linwoods*	2 Dtsp/30g	152	12.0	508	22.1	3.0	40.0	23.7
Organic, Premium Ground, Prewett's*	1 Tbsp/15g	73	6.0	489	24.0	2.0	40.0	23.0
FLOUR								
00 Grade, Pasta, TTD, Sainsbury's*	1 Bag/1000g	3390	13.0	339	11.5	70.3	1.3	3.0
Arrowroot, Average	*1oz/28g*	*100*	*0.0*	*357*	*0.3*	*88.2*	*0.1*	*3.4*
Bread, White, Strong, Average	*1oz/28g*	*94*	*0.4*	*336*	*11.8*	*68.4*	*1.5*	*3.4*
Brown, Chapati, Average	*1 Tbsp/20g*	*67*	*0.2*	*333*	*11.5*	*73.7*	*1.2*	*0.0*
Brown, Wheat	*1oz/28g*	*90*	*0.5*	*323*	*12.6*	*68.5*	*1.8*	*6.4*
Chick Pea	*1oz/28g*	*88*	*1.5*	*313*	*19.7*	*49.6*	*5.4*	*10.7*
Coconut, Average	*1 Serving/100g*	*344*	*13.6*	*344*	*18.2*	*15.4*	*13.6*	*43.8*
Coconut, Organic, Sukrin*	1 Serving/100g	320	12.0	320	19.0	9.0	12.0	50.0
Millet	*1oz/28g*	*99*	*0.5*	*354*	*5.8*	*75.4*	*1.7*	*0.0*
Peanut, Protein Plus*	¼ Cup/30g	110	4.0	367	53.3	26.7	13.3	13.3
Plain, Average	*1oz/28g*	*98*	*0.4*	*349*	*10.3*	*73.8*	*1.5*	*2.2*
Potato	*1oz/28g*	*92*	*0.3*	*328*	*9.1*	*75.6*	*0.9*	*5.7*
Rice	*1 Tsp/5g*	*18*	*0.0*	*366*	*6.4*	*80.1*	*0.8*	*2.0*
Soya, Low Fat, Average	*1oz/28g*	*99*	*2.0*	*352*	*45.3*	*28.2*	*7.2*	*13.5*
Speciality Gluten Free, Dove's Farm*	1 Serving/100g	353	1.8	353	4.7	85.2	1.8	2.7
Spelt, Average	*1 Serving/57g*	*216*	*1.7*	*381*	*14.3*	*74.5*	*3.0*	*6.4*
Strong, Wholemeal, Average	*1 Serving/100g*	*315*	*2.2*	*315*	*13.2*	*60.6*	*2.2*	*9.0*

F

	Measure		per Measure		Nutrition Values per 100g / 100ml				
	INFO/WEIGHT		KCAL	FAT	KCAL	PROT	CARB	FAT	FIBRE
FLOUR									
White, Average	*1oz/28g*		*89*	*0.3*	*319*	*9.8*	*66.8*	*1.0*	*2.9*
White, Chapati, Average	*1 Tbsp/20g*		*67*	*0.1*	*335*	*9.8*	*77.6*	*0.5*	*0.0*
White, Self Raising, Average	*1oz/28g*		*94*	*0.4*	*336*	*9.9*	*71.8*	*1.3*	*2.9*
Wholemeal, Average	*1oz/28g*		*87*	*0.6*	*312*	*12.6*	*61.9*	*2.2*	*9.0*
FOOL									
Fruit, Average	*1 Pot/120g*		*196*	*11.2*	*163*	*1.0*	*20.2*	*9.3*	*1.2*
Gooseberry, Sainsbury's*	1 Pot/113g		214	12.9	189	2.6	19.1	11.4	1.1
Gooseberry, Tesco*	1 Pot/112g		225	14.1	200	3.0	17.8	12.5	0.7
Lemon, Fruit, BGTY, Sainsbury's*	1 Pot/113g		94	3.8	83	3.4	9.7	3.4	0.3
Lemon, Signature, Morrisons*	1 Pot/114g		213	11.8	187	3.0	20.0	10.4	0.5
Raspberry, Fruit, Tesco*	1 Pot/113g		234	12.8	207	2.6	23.6	11.3	0.3
Rhubarb, Fruit, Waitrose*	1 Pot/114g		182	12.9	160	2.7	11.9	11.3	0.3
Rhubarb, Sainsbury's*	1 Pot/113g		180	12.9	159	2.6	11.5	11.4	0.4
FRANKFURTERS									
Average	*1 Frankfurter/42g*	*123*		*11.2*	*292*	*12.0*	*1.3*	*26.6*	*0.0*
FRANKFURTERS VEGETARIAN									
Tivall*	1 Sausage/30g		73	4.8	244	18.0	7.0	16.0	3.0
FRAZZLES									
Bacon, Smith's, Walkers*	1 Bag/23g		113	5.3	488	7.5	62.0	23.0	1.3
FRENCH FRIES									
Cheese & Onion, Walkers*	1 Pack/22g		95	3.5	430	5.0	66.0	16.0	5.0
Ready Salted, Walkers*	1 Bag/22g		83	3.0	377	4.5	56.4	13.6	4.5
Salt & Vinegar, Walkers*	1 Bag/22g		95	3.5	430	5.0	66.0	16.0	5.0
Worcester Sauce, Walkers*	1 Bag/22g		96	3.5	435	5.0	65.0	16.0	5.0
FRENCH TOAST									
Co-Op*	1 Toast/8g		31	0.5	385	10.0	72.0	6.0	5.0
Sainsbury's*	1 Toast/8g		31	0.5	382	10.0	72.0	6.6	5.0
FRIES									
American Style, Frozen, Thin, Tesco*	1 Serving/125g		208	10.1	166	2.2	21.1	8.1	1.9
Crispy French, Weighed Deep Fried, McCain*	1 Serving/100g		193	8.5	193	1.9	27.4	8.5	0.9
Curly, Cajun, Weighed Frozen, McCain*	1 Serving/100g		156	8.7	156	1.6	17.7	8.7	1.8
Curly, Ovenbaked, Iceland*	1 Serving/100g		253	12.1	253	3.5	30.8	12.1	3.5
Curly, Southern Style, Tesco*	1 Serving/50g		124	3.6	248	3.8	41.7	7.3	3.8
Curly, Twisters, Frozen, Conagra Foods*	1 Serving/150g		273	14.0	182	2.5	22.0	9.3	2.2
Extra Chunky, Oven Baked, Homefries, McCain*	1 Serving/200g		306	6.2	153	3.2	28.0	3.1	2.3
Oven, American Style, Frozen, Asda*	1 Serving/180g		407	14.4	226	3.9	34.6	8.0	4.0
Seasoned, Conagra Foods*	1 Serving/150g		248	12.0	165	2.4	20.8	8.0	1.9
Southern, Oven Cook, Baked, Potato Winners, McCain*	1 Serving/100g		232	8.3	232	3.6	35.7	8.3	2.4
Southern, Oven Cook, Frozen, Potato Winners, McCain*	1 Serving/100g		176	6.7	176	2.4	26.5	6.7	1.6
Sweet Potato, Alexia*	12 Fries/84g		140	5.0	167	1.2	28.6	6.0	3.6
Sweet Potato, Crispy, McCain*	1 Serving/125g		170	5.7	136	1.6	20.4	4.6	3.5
Sweet Potato, Iceland*	1 Serving/125g		252	9.9	202	1.9	28.4	7.9	4.7
Sweet Potato, Oven Baked, CBY, Asda*	1 Serving/125g		188	6.5	150	5.6	19.0	5.2	2.4
Sweet Potato, Slims Kitchen *	1 Bowl/340g		578	25.5	170	1.5	22.0	7.5	0.0
FRISPS									
Tangy Salt & Vinegar, KP Snacks*	1 Bag/30g		160	10.0	532	5.0	52.6	33.5	2.9
Tasty Cheese & Onion, KP Snacks*	1 Bag/28g		150	9.4	537	5.5	53.2	33.6	3.2
FRITTATA									
Spinach & Courgette, Meat Free, Tesco*	1 Frittata/120g		199	12.8	166	5.8	10.2	10.7	2.9
Vegetable, CBY, Asda*	1 Frittatas/150g		183	7.8	122	6.2	12.1	5.2	1.0
FROG									
Legs, Raw, Meat Only	*1oz/28g*		*20*	*0.1*	*73*	*16.4*	*0.0*	*0.3*	*0.0*

F

	Measure INFO/WEIGHT	per Measure KCAL	per Measure FAT	Nutrition Values per 100g / 100ml KCAL	PROT	CARB	FAT	FIBRE
FROMAGE FRAIS								
0% Fat, Vitalinea, Danone*	1 Tbsp/28g	14	0.0	50	7.4	4.7	0.1	0.0
Apricot, Summer Fruit, Layered, Weight Watchers*	1 Pot/100g	46	0.1	46	5.4	5.8	0.1	0.2
Blackberry, Berry Fruits, Layered, Weight Watchers*	1 Pot/100g	49	0.2	49	5.5	5.7	0.2	0.4
Cherry, 0% Fat, Vitalinea, Danone*	1 Serving/150g	88	0.2	59	6.1	8.0	0.2	1.6
Fabby, Loved By Kids, M&S*	1 Pot/43g	45	1.6	105	6.2	12.3	3.7	0.0
Fat Free, Average	*1 Pot/60g*	*35*	*0.1*	*58*	*7.7*	*6.8*	*0.2*	*0.0*
Forest Fruit, Layered, Weight Watchers*	1 Pot/100g	47	0.2	47	5.5	5.7	0.2	0.4
Kids, Yeo Valley*	1 Serving/90g	111	4.8	123	6.6	12.6	5.3	0.0
Low Fat, Aldi*	1 Pot/100g	52	0.3	52	5.4	7.1	0.3	0.7
Natural, Creamy, Co-Op*	1 Pot/200g	204	14.6	102	6.1	2.9	7.3	0.0
Natural, GFY, Asda*	½ Pot/100g	52	0.3	52	7.3	5.0	0.3	0.0
Natural, HL, Tesco*	1 Serving/65g	30	0.1	46	7.8	3.3	0.2	0.0
Natural, Plain, Fat Free, Normandy, BGTY, Sainsbury's*	1 Serving/30g	15	0.0	49	8.0	4.2	0.1	0.0
Natural, Virtually Fat Free, French, Waitrose*	1 Tub/500g	260	1.5	52	7.3	5.0	0.3	0.0
Normandy, Light Choices, Tesco*	1 Serving/100g	46	0.2	46	7.8	3.3	0.2	0.0
Organic, Vrai*	1 Serving/100g	83	3.6	83	8.1	4.5	3.6	0.0
Peach, BGTY, Sainsbury's*	1 Pot/100g	53	0.2	53	7.2	5.5	0.2	0.5
Peach, Summer Fruit, Layered, Weight Watchers*	1 Pot/100g	46	0.1	46	5.0	8.0	0.1	0.0
Plain, Average	*1oz/28g*	*32*	*2.0*	*113*	*6.8*	*5.7*	*7.1*	*0.0*
Raspberry, Berry Fruits, Layered, Weight Watchers*	1 Pot/100g	47	0.2	47	5.5	5.7	0.2	0.4
Raspberry, Organic, Yeo Valley*	1 Pot/100g	127	6.5	127	6.1	11.1	6.5	0.4
Raspberry, Value, Tesco*	1 Serving/60g	56	0.8	93	7.2	13.5	1.3	0.0
Strawberry, HE, Tesco*	1 Pot/100g	54	0.2	54	6.2	6.8	0.2	0.1
Strawberry, Petits Filous, Yoplait*	1 Pot/50g	52	1.4	104	6.7	12.6	2.9	0.2
Strawberry, Thomas the Tank Engine, Yoplait*	1 Pot/50g	50	0.6	101	6.8	15.4	1.3	0.0
Strawberry, Value, Tesco*	1 Pot/60g	55	0.8	92	7.2	13.0	1.3	0.0
Virtually Fat Free, Tesco*	1 Pot/100g	56	0.1	56	5.6	8.2	0.1	0.0
Wildlife, Strawberry, Raspberry Or Peach, Yoplait*	1 Pot/50g	46	0.6	93	7.1	13.2	1.3	0.2
with Fruit, Average	*1 Pot/90g*	*74*	*2.2*	*83*	*6.1*	*9.0*	*2.5*	*0.8*
FROZEN YOGHURT								
Belgian Chocolate, Calorie Controlled, LL, Waitrose*	1/5 Pot/65g	90	1.7	139	6.6	21.6	2.6	1.3
Black Cherry, M&S*	1 Pot/125g	164	1.4	131	3.1	27.1	1.1	0.5
Cherry Garcia, Low Fat, Ben & Jerry's*	1 Serving/100g	143	2.4	143	3.0	26.0	2.4	1.0
Chocolate, Snog*	1 Serving/100g	109	1.6	109	4.5	19.9	1.6	1.7
Green Tea, Pinkberry*	1 Sm Pot/100g	110	0.0	110	4.0	25.0	0.0	0.0
Mango, Pinkberry*	1 Sm Pot/140g	140	0.0	100	3.0	23.0	0.0	0.0
Nakedmoo, Yoomoo*	1 Serving/125g	168	2.0	134	3.3	24.5	1.6	4.1
Natural, Average	*1 Portion/100g*	*101*	*0.8*	*101*	*3.8*	*19.9*	*0.8*	*0.9*
Natural, Snog*	1 Serving/100g	89	0.2	89	3.3	18.4	0.2	0.5
Original, Pinkberry*	1 Sm Pot/140g	140	0.0	100	3.0	21.0	0.0	0.0
Peanut Butter, Pinkberry*	1 Sm Pot/140g	238	9.8	170	7.0	23.0	7.0	1.0
Raspberry, Handmade Farmhouse, Sainsbury's*	1 Serving/100g	132	3.8	132	2.7	21.8	3.8	2.2
Strawberry Cheesecake, Low Fat, Ben & Jerry's*	1 Serving/100g	170	3.0	170	4.0	31.0	3.0	1.0
Strawberry, Average	*1 Portion/100g*	*114*	*2.2*	*114*	*2.6*	*21.2*	*2.2*	*0.5*
Strawberry, Tesco*	1 Pot/60g	82	1.3	136	2.6	26.5	2.2	0.8
Strawbmoo, Yoomoo*	1 Serving/100g	133	1.5	133	3.2	24.7	1.5	4.1
Tropicoolmoo, Yoomoo*	1 Pot/92g	134	1.2	146	2.9	28.9	1.3	3.6
FRUIT								
Apple & Pear, Snack Pack, Great Stuff, Asda*	1 Pack/80g	42	0.1	52	0.4	11.0	0.1	2.6
Apple, Pineapple & Grape, Ready to Eat, Sainsbury's*	1 Pack/180g	94	0.2	52	0.5	8.3	0.1	1.3
Baked, Nibbles, Cherry Berry, We Are Bear*	1 Pack/30g	87	0.0	290	1.2	76.0	0.2	10.3
Baked, Nibbles, Mango Pineapple, We Are Bear*	1 Bag/30g	85	0.0	285	1.4	73.0	0.2	11.0
Berry Medley, Freshly Prepared, M&S*	1 Pack/180g	90	0.4	50	0.7	10.9	0.2	2.9

F

	Measure			Nutrition Values per 100g / 100ml				
	INFO/WEIGHT	KCAL	FAT	KCAL	PROT	CARB	FAT	FIBRE

FRUIT

	Measure	KCAL	FAT	KCAL	PROT	CARB	FAT	FIBRE
Black Forest, Frozen, Tesco*	1 Serving/80g	37	0.0	46	0.8	10.5	0.0	1.8
Fabulous Fruity Fingers, Melon & Mango, M&S*	1 Pack/240g	96	0.5	40	0.6	8.2	0.2	1.0
Fingers, Melon & Pineapple, Sainsbury's*	1 Pack/240g	74	0.2	31	0.5	6.5	0.1	0.8
Grapefruit & Orange Segments, Breakfast, Del Monte*	1 Can/411g	193	0.4	47	1.0	10.2	0.1	1.0
Melon & Grape Munchies, Eat Well, M&S*	½ Pack/200g	70	0.2	35	0.5	8.3	0.1	0.7
Melon & Grape Pot, Co-Op*	1 Pot/125g	44	0.1	35	0.6	7.0	0.1	0.9
Melon & Grape, Sainsbury's*	½ Pack/200g	66	0.2	33	0.5	7.1	0.1	0.7
Melon & Grapes, Morrisons*	1 Pack/360g	112	0.4	31	0.6	6.4	0.1	0.8
Melon, Kiwi Fruit & Strawberries, Fresh Tastes, Asda*	1 Pack/240g	96	0.5	40	0.8	7.7	0.2	2.1
Mixed, Fresh, 5 a Day, Tesco*	1 Pack/400g	136	0.8	34	0.8	7.4	0.2	1.4
Mixed, Pieces, in Orange Jelly, Fruitini, Del Monte*	1 Can/140g	94	0.1	67	0.3	15.8	0.1	0.0
Outrageously Orange Melon, M&S*	1 Pack/180g	36	0.2	20	0.6	4.2	0.1	0.8
Peach, Slices, Frozen, Sainsbury's*	1 Serving/80g	30	0.0	37	1.0	7.6	0.0	1.5
Pieces, Mixed in Fruit Juice, Fruitini, Del Monte*	1 Serving/120g	61	0.1	51	0.4	12.0	0.1	0.5
Pineapple & Mango Tango, Eat Well, M&S*	1 Pack/200g	100	0.8	50	1.0	22.2	0.4	2.6
Pineapple, Grape & Kiwi, Fresh Tastes, Asda*	1 Pack/200g	106	0.6	53	0.6	11.0	0.3	1.8
Pineapple, Mango & Nectarine, Fresh Tastes, Asda*	1 Pack/240g	127	0.5	53	0.8	11.0	0.2	2.1
Summer Berries, M&S*	1 Pack/160g	80	0.3	50	0.7	10.0	0.2	3.0
Tropical in Juice, Dole*	1 Pot/113g	59	0.0	52	0.3	14.2	0.0	1.8

FRUIT & NUT

	Measure	KCAL	FAT	KCAL	PROT	CARB	FAT	FIBRE
Salted Caramel, Nibbles, N'akd*	1 Bag/40g	138	4.7	345	6.6	56.1	11.8	3.3

FRUIT & NUT MIX

	Measure	KCAL	FAT	KCAL	PROT	CARB	FAT	FIBRE
After Dinner Mint, Graze*	1 Pack/42g	203	12.2	483	10.0	42.0	29.0	7.0
Almonds & Raisins, LL, Waitrose*	1 Pack/150g	681	42.6	454	11.6	38.1	28.4	4.7
Bakewell Tart, Graze*	1 Pack/37g	154	8.1	416	8.9	48.3	21.8	4.7
Banoffee Pie, Graze*	1 Punnet/34g	149	9.2	438	7.0	42.0	27.0	5.0
Billionaire's Shortbread, Graze*	1 Punnet/41g	192	10.2	469	8.0	53.0	25.0	5.0
Bounty Hunter, Graze*	1 Punnet/31g	147	8.3	474	4.0	54.4	26.8	5.6
Cherry Fudge Sundae, Graze*	1 Punnet/45g	186	8.1	414	7.2	56.0	18.0	4.9
Date & Banana Loaf, Graze*	1 Punnet/41g	132	1.8	327	3.3	68.3	4.4	6.3
Dried, Selection, Wholesome, LL, Waitrose*	1 Serving/30g	144	9.6	479	9.8	38.0	32.0	4.4
Eleanor's Apple Crumble, Graze*	1 Pack/32g	115	4.0	356	6.4	62.0	12.5	8.0
Flapjack, Fruit & Seed, Graze*	1 Punnet/53g	226	11.1	426	6.0	54.0	21.0	5.0
Grandma's Apple Crumble, Graze*	1 Punnet/40g	154	7.8	385	0.0	48.9	19.6	4.0
Honeycomb Crunch, Graze*	1 Punnet/40g	181	9.7	446	9.0	50.0	24.0	4.0
Jaffa Cake, Graze*	1 Punnet/44g	208	13.7	472	7.0	43.0	31.0	6.0
Jam Doughnut, Graze*	1 Punnet/31g	131	4.7	422	7.0	65.0	15.0	6.0
Luxury, Asda*	1 Serving/50g	226	15.2	451	9.0	33.5	30.5	7.4
M&S*	1 Sm Pack/75g	338	19.0	450	12.4	44.3	25.3	6.0
Macadamias & Dried Cranberries, LL, Waitrose*	1 Serving/30g	143	9.2	477	3.3	47.1	30.8	6.2
Marvellous Macaroon, Graze*	1 Punnet/28g	157	10.9	562	11.0	41.0	39.0	6.0
Nuts & Raisins, Mixed, Natural, LL, Waitrose*	1 Serving/50g	258	16.4	515	16.5	38.4	32.8	7.2
Organic, Waitrose*	1 Pack/100g	489	32.6	489	15.0	33.8	32.6	5.4
Peanuts & Flame Raisins, Wholefoods, Tesco*	1 Serving/30g	142	8.3	475	18.6	34.7	27.8	4.5
Pure Vitality, Graze*	1 Punnet/45g	151	6.4	337	11.2	46.0	14.3	9.5
Seed, Nut & Sultana Sprinkle, LL, Waitrose*	1 Serving/30g	177	15.4	591	17.2	15.4	51.2	4.3
Selection, Starbucks*	1 Pack/40g	187	9.5	466	10.8	49.7	23.6	6.0
Strawberry Milkshake, Graze*	1 Pack/39g	148	3.9	380	2.0	72.0	10.0	2.0
The Foodie Market, Aldi*	1 Serving/25g	119	7.0	477	10.0	42.0	28.0	7.9
The Mix, Whitworths*	1 Pot/90g	341	13.1	379	4.1	63.1	14.6	7.3
The Waldorf, Graze*	1 Punnet/28g	109	6.2	389	6.0	43.5	22.1	5.7
Trail Mix, Average	*1oz/28g*	*121*	*8.0*	*432*	*9.1*	*37.2*	*28.5*	*4.3*
Trail Mix, LL, Waitrose*	1 Portion/30g	126	9.3	506	14.2	28.5	37.2	6.3

	Measure INFO/WEIGHT	per Measure KCAL	FAT	Nutrition Values per 100g / 100ml KCAL	PROT	CARB	FAT	FIBRE
FRUIT & NUT MIX								
Tropical Praline, Graze*	1 Punnet/35g	121	4.2	347	4.2	59.2	12.1	2.0
Unsalted, Tesco*	1 Serving/25g	112	4.6	449	12.6	58.1	18.5	12.2
Vanilla, Cherry, Frangipane, Graze*	1 Punnet/39g	201	13.2	516	15.0	38.0	34.0	6.0
Walnut & Vanilla Truffle, Graze*	1 Punnet/38g	187	12.1	496	10.0	43.9	32.2	6.0
White Chocolate & Raspberry Cheesecake, Graze*	1 Punnet/39g	204	13.7	524	7.5	44.7	35.1	4.5
FRUIT COCKTAIL								
Fresh & Ready, Sainsbury's*	1 Pack/300g	117	0.3	39	0.6	9.0	0.1	1.2
in Fruit Juice, Sainsbury's*	1 Serving/198g	97	0.2	49	0.3	11.9	0.1	1.3
in Juice, Del Monte*	1 Can/415g	203	0.4	49	0.4	11.2	0.1	0.0
in Light Syrup, Princes*	1 Serving/206g	64	0.0	31	0.4	7.3	0.0	1.0
in Light Syrup, Valfrutta*	1 Serving/206g	95	0.0	46	0.2	11.4	0.0	1.5
in Syrup, Morrisons*	½ Can/205g	129	0.2	63	0.3	14.9	0.1	0.0
Tropical, Canned, Asda*	½ Can/200g	120	0.0	60	0.0	15.0	0.0	1.6
Tropical, in Juice, Morrisons*	1 Serving/100g	56	0.0	56	0.0	14.0	0.0	0.0
FRUIT COMPOTE								
Apple, Strawberry & Blackberry, Organic, Yeo Valley*	½ Pot/112g	73	0.1	65	0.5	15.5	0.1	1.9
Apricot & Prune, Yeo Valley*	1 Pot/225g	207	0.2	92	0.6	22.3	0.1	1.6
HE, Tesco*	1 Pot/140g	113	0.3	81	0.9	19.1	0.2	1.6
Strawberry & Raspberry, M&S*	1 Serving/80g	72	0.1	90	0.7	23.5	0.1	2.3
Summerfruit, M&S*	¼ Pot/125g	119	0.8	95	0.9	22.7	0.6	0.8
FRUIT DRINK								
Multivitamin, Rejuvenation, Active Life, Purdy's*	1 Bottle/330ml	125	0.0	38	0.0	9.5	0.0	0.0
Sparkling Pink Grapefruit, Shapers, Boots*	1 Serving/200ml	6	0.0	3	0.0	0.3	0.0	0.0
FRUIT FLAKES								
Blackcurrant with Yoghurt Coating, Fruit Bowl*	1 Bag/25g	112	5.1	449	1.7	64.2	20.6	0.0
Raisins with Yoghurt Coating, Fruit Bowl*	1 Pack/30g	133	5.6	440	2.9	66.6	18.4	2.0
Raspberry with Yoghurt Coating, Fruit Bowl*	1 Serving/25g	112	5.2	449	1.7	64.2	20.6	0.0
Strawberry with Yoghurt Coating, Fruit Bowl*	1 Serving/25g	112	5.2	449	1.7	64.2	20.6	0.0
Strawberry, Fruit Bowl*	1 Pack/20g	66	0.4	330	1.0	78.0	2.0	2.0
FRUIT GUMS								
Rowntree's*	1 Tube/49g	170	0.1	344	4.8	81.3	0.2	0.0
FRUIT MEDLEY								
Dried, Tropical, Soft, LL, Waitrose*	1 Serving/30g	86	0.0	288	0.2	70.6	0.0	2.5
Exotic, Co-Op*	1 Serving/120g	54	0.2	45	0.6	10.0	0.2	0.0
Fresh, Tesco*	1 Pack/200g	86	0.2	43	0.4	10.0	0.1	1.1
Mango, Melon, Kiwi & Blueberry, Fresh, M&S*	1 Pack/260g	104	0.8	40	0.7	9.1	0.3	1.6
Nectarine, Mango & Blueberry, Fresh, M&S*	1 Pack/245g	122	0.5	50	1.0	11.1	0.2	2.1
Pineapple, Papaya & Mango, Waitrose*	1 Pack/550g	297	0.6	54	0.6	12.8	0.1	1.1
Shapers, Boots*	1 Pack/140g	55	0.3	39	0.7	8.6	0.2	1.0
FRUIT MIX								
Apple Cosmo, Graze*	1 Punnet/34g	100	0.2	292	1.5	69.8	0.7	4.6
Apricot, Torte, Graze*	1 Pack/45g	151	3.6	335	3.3	63.0	8.0	4.0
Banana, Coconut & Mango, Dried, Graze*	1 Punnet/45g	144	3.7	320	18.7	57.1	8.2	0.0
Forest Fruit, Dried, Graze*	1 Pack/50g	160	0.4	319	1.8	76.0	0.8	0.0
Frozen, Blueberries & Strawberries, Sainsbury's*	1 Portion/75g	26	0.2	34	0.7	6.5	0.2	1.5
Love Mix, Graze*	1 Pack/40g	99	0.4	245	4.0	58.0	0.9	5.9
Luxury, Sainsbury's*	1 Serving/30g	78	0.2	261	1.8	62.3	0.5	2.7
Melon, Strawberry & Grape, Sainsbury's*	1 Pack/180g	58	0.4	32	0.5	7.0	0.2	0.4
Nectarine, Raspberry & Blueberry, Seasonal, M&S*	1 Pack/160g	72	0.3	45	1.3	8.3	0.2	2.7
Pineapple, Kiwi, Mango & Blueberry, Waitrose*	1 Pack/330g	208	1.0	63	0.7	14.5	0.3	1.9
Pineapple, Melon, Mango, Tesco*	1 Pack/440g	242	0.9	55	1.1	11.4	0.2	1.3
Pumpkin Pie, Graze*	1 Pack/65g	274	11.2	422	11.4	48.2	17.2	0.0
Sour Mango Tangtastic, Graze*	1 Pack/34g	110	0.2	323	1.3	79.8	0.6	2.0

F

	Measure INFO/WEIGHT	per Measure KCAL	per Measure FAT	Nutrition Values per 100g / 100ml KCAL	PROT	CARB	FAT	FIBRE
FRUIT MIX								
Summer Fruits, British, Frozen, Waitrose*	1 Pack/380g	99	0.8	26	1.0	5.2	0.2	5.5
Summer Fruits, Frozen, Asda*	1 Serving/100g	28	0.0	28	0.9	6.0	0.0	2.5
Summer Fruits, Frozen, Sainsbury's*	1 Serving/80g	43	0.1	54	0.9	6.9	0.1	2.0
Summer Fruits, in Syrup, Sainsbury's*	1 Pudding/289g	188	0.3	65	0.5	15.6	0.1	1.2
Summer Pudding, Graze*	1 Punnet/32g	109	0.4	342	1.6	81.2	1.2	4.2
Super Wholefood with Blueberries & Mango, M&S*	1 Pack/215g	260	7.7	121	4.4	17.0	3.6	8.7
Tropical, Dried, Costa*	1 Pack/40g	135	0.7	338	3.4	72.1	1.8	0.0
Tropical, Fresh, Waitrose*	1 Pack/240g	122	0.5	51	0.6	11.6	0.2	1.9
Tutti Frutti, Graze*	1 Punnet/41g	120	0.4	292	1.9	72.3	0.9	4.0
FRUIT PUREE								
Apple & Blueberry, Organic, Clearspring*	1 Tub/100g	76	0.3	76	0.4	17.8	0.3	0.0
Apple & Peach, Organix*	1 Pot/100g	49	0.3	49	0.6	11.0	0.3	2.1
FRUIT SALAD								
Apple, Orange, Pineapple & Grape, Morrisons*	1 Serving/64g	40	0.1	62	0.8	13.1	0.1	2.6
Autumn, Fresh, M&S*	½ Pack/160g	64	0.2	40	0.7	9.4	0.1	2.9
Berry, Asda*	1 Pack/250g	122	0.2	49	0.6	10.9	0.1	0.0
Berry, Seasonal, Asda*	1 Pack/300g	93	0.3	31	0.6	7.0	0.1	2.1
Chunky in Fruit Juice, Canned, John West*	1 Can/411g	193	0.8	47	0.4	11.0	0.2	0.8
Citrus, Fresh, M&S*	½ Pack/225g	79	0.2	35	0.9	7.7	0.1	1.5
Classic, Co-Op*	1 Box/285g	142	0.3	50	0.6	11.0	0.1	2.3
Classic, Fresh, Prepared, Sainsbury's*	1 Pack/320g	157	0.3	49	0.6	10.3	0.1	2.0
Classic, Ocado*	1 Pack/265g	130	0.3	49	0.7	12.1	0.1	1.2
Exotic with Melon, Mango, Kiwi Fruit & Grapes, Asda*	1 Pot/300g	141	0.9	47	0.6	10.5	0.3	1.4
Exotic, Fresh, Tesco*	1 Serving/225g	86	0.4	38	0.7	8.4	0.2	1.5
Exotic, Fully Prepared, Sainsbury's*	1 Serving/200g	74	0.4	37	0.6	8.3	0.2	1.3
Exotic, Morrisons*	1 Serving/150g	78	0.3	52	0.6	12.2	0.2	0.0
Exotic, Waitrose*	1 Pack/300g	126	0.6	42	0.6	9.5	0.2	1.1
Fresh for You, Tesco*	1 Pack/160g	59	0.3	37	0.6	8.2	0.2	1.1
Fresh, Morrisons*	1 Tub/350g	150	0.4	43	0.7	9.9	0.1	0.0
Fresh, Sweet, Ripe & Moist, Tesco*	1 Serving/750g	345	0.8	46	0.7	10.6	0.1	1.6
Fresh, Tesco*	1 Pack/200g	84	0.4	42	0.7	9.3	0.2	1.5
Fresh, Washed, Ready to Eat, Tesco*	1 Pack/200g	92	0.2	46	0.7	10.6	0.1	1.6
Freshly Prepared, M&S*	1 Pack/350g	140	0.7	40	0.5	9.3	0.2	1.0
Green, M&S*	1 Pack/400g	200	0.8	50	0.6	10.9	0.2	1.2
Homemade, Unsweetened, Average	***1 Serving/140g***	***77***	***0.1***	***55***	***0.7***	***13.8***	***0.1***	***1.5***
Kiwi, Pineapple & Grape, Fresh Tastes, Asda*	1 Pack/200g	106	0.6	53	0.6	11.0	0.3	1.8
Layered, Tropical Rainbow, Freshly Prepared, M&S*	1 Pack/375g	206	1.1	55	0.7	12.6	0.3	1.7
Luxury, Frozen, Boylans*	1 Serving/100g	54	0.2	54	0.8	12.7	0.2	0.0
Melon & Mango, Shapers, Boots*	1 Pack/80g	29	0.1	36	0.6	7.8	0.1	1.2
Melon & Red Grape, Freshly Prepared, M&S*	1 Pack/450g	158	0.4	35	0.5	8.4	0.1	0.7
Melon, Kiwi, Grapes & Pomegranate Seeds, Morrisons*	1 Pack/400g	152	1.2	38	0.7	8.2	0.3	1.2
Melon, Kiwi, Strawberry, Way to Five, Sainsbury's*	1 Pack/245g	74	0.5	30	0.8	6.3	0.2	1.3
Melon, Pineapple & Grapes, Fresh, Tesco*	1 Pack/300g	120	0.3	40	0.5	9.2	0.1	1.0
Mixed, Average	***1 Bowl/100g***	***42***	***0.2***	***42***	***0.6***	***9.4***	***0.2***	***1.5***
Mixed, Food to Go, M&S*	1 Pack/400g	400	1.2	100	0.9	23.3	0.3	2.8
Mixed, Fresh, Sainsbury's*	1 Pack/200g	84	0.4	42	0.7	9.4	0.2	1.9
Mixed, Tesco*	1 Pack/225g	86	0.4	38	0.7	8.3	0.2	1.3
Oranges, Apple, Pineapple & Grapes, Fresh, Asda*	1 Pack/260g	120	0.3	46	0.6	10.5	0.1	2.1
Pineapple, Apple & Strawberries, Tesco*	1 Pack/190g	80	0.2	42	0.4	9.8	0.1	1.4
Pineapple, Apple, Melon & Grape, Shapers, Boots*	1 Serving/100g	49	0.1	49	0.4	10.5	0.1	1.2
Pineapple, Mango & Passion Fruit, Prepared, M&S*	1 Pack/400g	200	0.8	50	0.7	10.8	0.2	1.8
Pineapple, Mango, Apple & Grape, Waitrose*	1 Pack/300g	186	0.6	62	0.5	14.7	0.2	1.7
Plum, Blackberries, & Fig, Tesco*	1 Pot/260g	109	0.5	42	0.8	8.2	0.2	2.5

F

	INFO/WEIGHT	KCAL	FAT	KCAL	PROT	CARB	FAT	FIBRE
FRUIT SALAD								
Rainbow, Asda*	1 Pack/350g	140	1.0	40	0.6	8.8	0.3	1.4
Sharing, Fresh Tastes, Asda*	1 Pack/450g	220	0.9	49	0.4	10.4	0.2	0.0
Strawberry & Blueberry, Asda*	1 Pack/240g	86	0.2	36	0.9	7.0	0.1	1.5
Summer, Red, Fresh, M&S*	1 Pack/400g	160	0.8	40	0.0	10.0	0.2	1.2
Sunshine, Fresh, M&S*	1 Serving/200g	70	0.2	35	0.0	8.3	0.1	1.3
Tropical in Light Syrup, Passion Fruit Juice, Tesco*	½ Can/216g	130	0.2	60	0.3	14.1	0.1	1.1
Tropical Medley, Costa*	1 Pack/200g	84	0.4	42	0.5	8.9	0.2	2.9
Tropical Mix, Tesco*	½ Pack/140g	71	0.3	51	0.5	11.0	0.2	1.5
Tropical, Fresh, Asda*	1 Pack/400g	164	0.8	41	0.7	9.0	0.2	1.8
Tropical, Fruit Snacks, Frozen, Sainsbury's*	1 Serving/175g	79	0.2	45	0.7	10.4	0.1	1.6
FRUIT SHOOT								
Apple & Blackcurrant, Robinson's*	1 Bottle/200ml	10	0.0	5	0.1	0.8	0.0	0.0
Apple, Low Sugar, Robinson's*	1 Bottle/200ml	14	0.0	7	0.0	1.2	0.0	0.0
FRUIT SPREAD								
Cherries & Berries, Organic, Meridian Foods*	1 Tbsp/15g	16	0.0	109	0.5	26.0	0.3	1.1
Cherry & Berry, Meridian Foods*	1 Serving/10g	14	0.1	138	0.7	33.7	0.6	3.2
Raspberry & Cranberry, No Added Sugar, Superjam*	1 Spread/10g	22	0.0	216	2.1	47.0	0.3	0.0
FU YUNG								
Chicken, Chinese Takeaway, Tesco*	1 Pack/350g	315	3.5	90	5.6	14.5	1.0	0.8
Egg, Average	**1oz/28g**	**67**	**5.8**	**239**	**9.9**	**2.2**	**20.6**	**1.3**
FUDGE								
All Butter, Finest, Tesco*	1 Sweet/10g	43	1.4	429	1.3	73.4	14.5	0.0
Butter, Milk, Thorntons*	1 Sweet/13g	60	2.5	462	3.7	68.5	19.2	0.0
Cadbury*	1 Bar/25g	115	4.0	440	2.4	73.7	15.3	0.4
Cherry & Almond, Thorntons*	1 Bag/100g	464	19.1	464	3.2	70.5	19.1	0.4
Chocolate, Average	**1 Sweet/30g**	**132**	**4.1**	**441**	**3.3**	**81.1**	**13.7**	**0.0**
Chocolate, Thorntons*	1 Bag/100g	459	19.1	459	3.1	69.0	19.1	0.6
Chunks for Baking	1 Serving/100g	428	12.2	428	1.7	77.2	12.2	0.6
Chunks, Home Cooking, Asda*	1 Portion/10g	45	1.3	446	1.5	79.7	13.2	1.1
Clotted Cream, Sainsbury's*	1 Sweet/8g	35	0.9	430	1.9	81.5	10.7	0.7
Dairy, Co-Op*	1 Sweet/9g	39	1.2	430	2.0	76.0	13.0	0.0
Double Chocolate Bar, M&S*	1 Bar/43g	202	9.0	470	4.2	66.9	21.0	0.7
Pure Indulgence, Thorntons*	1 Bar/45g	210	9.9	466	1.8	65.9	21.9	0.0
Vanilla, Bar, Diabetic, Thorntons*	1 Bar/34g	121	6.7	356	3.2	69.7	19.7	0.6
Vanilla, Bar, M&S*	1 Bar/43g	205	10.0	476	3.7	63.0	23.3	0.4
Vanilla, Julian Graves*	1 Serving/10g	41	1.0	407	1.0	78.9	9.7	0.0
Vanilla, Thorntons*	1 Bag/100g	465	21.9	465	1.8	65.9	21.9	0.0
Vanilla, Whipped, M&S*	1 Serving/43g	210	10.3	490	3.8	65.4	23.9	0.3
FUSILLI								
Cooked, Average	**1 Serving/210g**	**248**	**1.4**	**118**	**4.2**	**23.8**	**0.6**	**1.2**
Dry, Average	**1 Serving/90g**	**316**	**1.4**	**352**	**12.3**	**72.0**	**1.6**	**2.2**
Fresh, Cooked, Average	**1 Serving/200g**	**329**	**3.6**	**164**	**6.4**	**30.6**	**1.8**	**1.8**
Fresh, Dry, Average	**1 Serving/75g**	**208**	**2.0**	**277**	**10.9**	**53.4**	**2.7**	**2.1**
Fusilloni, TTD, Sainsbury's*	1 Serving/90g	321	1.5	357	12.3	73.1	1.7	2.5
Tricolore, Dry, Average	**1 Serving/75g**	**264**	**1.3**	**351**	**12.2**	**71.8**	**1.7**	**2.7**
Twists, Quick Cook, Morrisons*	1 Serving/75g	265	1.5	353	12.0	72.0	2.0	3.1
Whole Wheat, Dry Weight, Average	**1 Serving/90g**	**290**	**2.1**	**322**	**13.1**	**62.3**	**2.3**	**9.0**
Wholewheat, Dry, Tesco*	1 Portion/75g	245	1.9	327	12.5	62.5	2.5	9.1
FYBOGEL								
Lemon, Reckitt Benckiser*	1 Serving/4g	4	0.0	95	2.4	11.3	1.1	64.8
Orange, Reckitt Benckiser*	1 Serving/4g	5	0.0	106	2.4	12.7	1.1	64.4

F

INFO/WEIGHT	Measure	per Measure KCAL	FAT	Nutrition Values per 100g / 100ml KCAL	PROT	CARB	FAT	FIBRE
GALANGAL								
Raw, Root, Average	*100g*	*71*	*0.6*	*71*	*1.2*	*15.3*	*0.6*	*2.4*
GALAXY								
Amicelli, Mars*	1 Serving/13g	66	3.5	507	6.2	59.7	27.1	0.0
Bubbles Filled, Chocolate Egg, Galaxy, Mars*	1 Egg/28g	155	9.5	555	6.5	54.7	34.1	1.5
Caramel Crunch, Promises, Mars*	1 Bar/100g	540	31.8	540	6.1	57.5	31.8	0.0
Caramel, Mars*	1 Bar/49g	254	13.0	518	5.8	64.2	26.4	0.0
Cookie Crumble, Mars*	1 Bar/114g	627	37.6	550	6.2	56.0	33.0	1.9
Fruit & Hazelnut, Milk, Mars*	1 Bar/47g	235	13.2	501	7.1	55.2	28.0	0.0
Hazelnut, Mars*	1 Piece/6g	37	2.5	582	7.8	49.4	39.2	0.0
Hazelnut, Roast, Promises, Mars*	1 Bar/100g	544	32.9	544	6.4	55.6	32.9	0.0
GAMMON								
Breaded, Average	*1oz/28g*	*34*	*0.9*	*120*	*22.5*	*1.0*	*3.0*	*0.0*
Dry Cured, Ready to Roast, M&S*	½ Joint/255g	255	3.8	100	20.5	0.5	1.5	0.5
Grills, Grilled, Savers, Morrisons*	1 Grill/97g	135	4.5	139	24.2	0.0	4.6	0.0
Honey & Mustard, Average	*½ Pack/190g*	*294*	*13.5*	*155*	*19.1*	*3.6*	*7.1*	*0.1*
Joint, Applewood Smoked, Tesco*	1 Serving/100g	152	9.0	152	17.5	0.2	9.0	0.0
Joint, Boiled, Average	*1 Serving/60g*	*122*	*7.4*	*204*	*23.3*	*0.0*	*12.3*	*0.0*
Joint, Raw, Average	*1 Serving/100g*	*138*	*7.5*	*138*	*17.5*	*0.0*	*7.5*	*0.0*
Joint, Unsmoked, Tesco*	2 Slices/150g	248	15.6	165	16.8	0.2	10.4	0.0
Steak with Egg & Fries	1 Serving/540g	684	26.9	127	10.3	10.1	5.0	0.0
Steaks, Cooked, Average	*1 Steak/97g*	*157*	*7.1*	*161*	*23.3*	*0.4*	*7.4*	*0.0*
Steaks, Healthy Range, Average	*1 Serving/110g*	*107*	*3.5*	*97*	*18.0*	*0.4*	*3.2*	*0.2*
Steaks, Honey Roast, Average	*1 Steak/100g*	*142*	*5.3*	*142*	*21.5*	*2.3*	*5.3*	*0.0*
Steaks, Smoked, Average	*1 Steak/110g*	*150*	*5.5*	*137*	*22.7*	*0.1*	*5.0*	*0.1*
Unsmoked, Dry Cured, TTD, Sainsbury's*	1 Serving/100g	214	11.2	214	27.7	0.5	11.2	0.8
GAMMON &								
Cheese, Ovenbaked, CBY, Asda*	½ Pack/182g	253	9.8	139	17.8	4.5	5.4	0.5
Parsley Sauce, Steak, Tesco*	½ Pack/140g	217	7.3	155	23.7	2.9	5.2	0.5
GAMMON WITH								
Pineapple, Steaks, Asda*	½ Pack/195g	254	2.7	130	17.8	11.5	1.4	0.7
GARAM MASALA								
Dry, Ground, Average	*1 Tbsp/15g*	*57*	*2.3*	*379*	*15.6*	*45.2*	*15.1*	*0.0*
GARLIC								
Crushed, Frozen, Taj*	1 Block/18g	18	0.1	102	7.5	14.0	0.6	4.0
Minced, Nishaan*	1 Tsp/5g	5	0.0	97	6.0	16.2	0.9	0.0
Pickled, Bevellini*	1 Serving/12g	5	0.0	42	2.5	0.8	0.1	0.0
Powder, Average	*1 Tsp/3g*	*7*	*0.0*	*246*	*18.7*	*42.7*	*1.2*	*9.9*
Raw, Asda*	1 Clove/3g	3	0.0	98	5.0	10.0	0.6	2.0
Raw, Average	*1 Clove/3g*	*3*	*0.0*	*98*	*7.9*	*16.3*	*0.6*	*2.1*
Spice Blend, Gourmet Garden*	1 Squeeze/10mls	32	2.4	210	4.5	10.8	16.2	10.3
Very Lazy, The English Provender Co.*	1 Tsp/3g	3	0.0	111	6.0	20.9	0.4	3.0
Wild	1 Clove/3g	1	0.0	23	2.8	1.7	0.6	1.9
GARLIC PUREE								
Average	*1 Tbsp/18g*	*68*	*6.0*	*380*	*3.5*	*16.9*	*33.6*	*0.0*
in Vegetable Oil, GIA*	1 Tsp/5g	12	0.9	248	3.6	18.8	17.7	0.0
GATEAU								
Black Forest, 500g Size, Tesco*	1 Cake/500g	1125	55.0	225	4.0	27.1	11.0	1.8
Black Forest, Family Size, 860g, Tesco*	1 Cake/860g	1978	113.5	230	3.4	24.8	13.2	0.9
Black Forest, Mini, Tesco*	1 Serving/55g	136	5.1	247	5.7	35.3	9.2	1.0
Black Forest, Sara Lee*	1 Serving/80g	221	9.8	276	3.6	37.9	12.3	1.2
Chocolate Layer, M&S*	1 Serving/86g	278	15.7	323	4.2	35.9	18.3	0.9
Chocolate, Asda*	1 Serving/100g	176	10.0	176	2.4	19.0	10.0	0.4
Chocolate, Swirl, Tesco*	1 Serving/83g	230	13.3	277	3.8	29.3	16.0	0.2

G

	Measure INFO/WEIGHT	per Measure KCAL	FAT	Nutrition Values per 100g / 100ml KCAL	PROT	CARB	FAT	FIBRE
GATEAU								
Double Chocolate, Frozen, Tesco*	1/5 Gateau/70g	119	4.7	265	5.0	35.8	10.4	4.0
Ice Cream, Chocolate & Vanilla, Iceland*	1 Serving/130g	252	12.2	194	3.3	24.1	9.4	0.6
Lemon & Lime, M&S*	1 Serving/100g	295	15.6	295	3.2	35.0	15.6	0.3
Orange & Lemon, Iceland*	1 Serving/90g	220	9.9	245	2.6	33.8	11.0	0.3
Strawberry, Co-Op*	1 Serving/77g	222	12.9	288	5.1	29.2	16.7	1.0
Strawberry, Frozen, Tesco*	1/5 Gateau/75g	155	6.3	205	2.8	28.8	8.3	0.9
Swiss, Cadbury*	1/6 Cake/60g	228	10.1	380	5.2	52.0	16.8	0.9
Triple Chocolate, Heinz*	¼ Cake/85g	209	9.5	245	5.1	31.2	11.1	2.4
GELATINE								
Average	*1 Tsp/3g*	*10*	*0.0*	*338*	*84.4*	*0.0*	*0.0*	*0.0*
GHEE								
Butter	*1oz/28g*	*251*	*27.9*	*898*	*0.0*	*0.0*	*99.8*	*0.0*
Vegetable	*1oz/28g*	*251*	*27.8*	*895*	*0.0*	*0.0*	*99.4*	*0.0*
GHERKINS								
Pickled, Average	*1 Gherkin/36g*	*4*	*0.0*	*12*	*0.8*	*2.1*	*0.1*	*1.0*
Pickled, Crunchy, with Dill Flower, Drained, Waitrose*	1 Serving/25g	10	0.1	41	1.7	6.0	0.5	1.1
GIN								
& Diet Tonic, Can, Greenalls*	1 Can/250ml	95	0.0	38	0.0	0.0	0.0	0.0
37.5% Volume	*1 Pub Shot/35ml*	*72*	*0.0*	*207*	*0.0*	*0.0*	*0.0*	*0.0*
40% Volume	*1 Pub Shot/35ml*	*78*	*0.0*	*224*	*0.0*	*0.0*	*0.0*	*0.0*
Gordons & Bitter Lemon, Premixed, Canned, Gordons*	1 Can/250ml	170	0.0	68	0.0	7.1	0.0	0.0
London Dry, Bombay Sapphire*	1 Serving/25ml	59	0.0	236	0.0	0.0	0.0	0.0
GINGER								
Chunks, Crystallised, Julian Graves*	1 Serving/10g	28	0.0	283	0.2	70.1	0.2	1.5
Crystalised, Graze*	1 Pack/25g	61	0.1	243	2.9	58.0	0.3	0.0
Ground, Average	*1 Tsp/2g*	*5*	*0.1*	*258*	*7.4*	*60.0*	*3.3*	*0.0*
Root, Raw, Pared, Average	*1 Tsp/2g*	*2*	*0.0*	*81*	*1.8*	*18.0*	*0.8*	*2.0*
Root, Raw, Unprepared, Average	*1 Tsp Chopped/2g*	*1*	*0.0*	*74*	*1.7*	*16.3*	*0.7*	*1.8*
Stem in Sugar Syrup, Sainsbury's*	1oz/28g	76	0.0	271	0.2	67.3	0.1	1.4
Stem in Syrup, Waitrose*	1 Jar/350g	1071	7.7	306	0.1	70.4	2.2	0.7
Very Lazy, The English Provender Co.*	1 Tsp/5g	3	0.0	52	0.7	10.9	0.8	0.8
GINGER ALE								
American, Finest, Tesco*	1 Serving/150ml	68	0.0	45	0.0	11.0	0.0	0.0
American, Low Calorie, Tesco*	1 fl oz/30ml	0	0.0	1	0.0	0.0	0.0	0.0
Dry	1 Glass/250ml	38	0.0	15	0.0	3.9	0.0	0.0
Dry, Sainsbury's*	1 Glass/250ml	95	0.2	38	0.1	9.1	0.1	0.1
GINGER BEER								
Alcoholic, Crabbies*	1 Bottle/500ml	254	0.0	51	0.0	7.1	0.0	0.0
Asda*	1 Can/330ml	144	0.0	44	0.0	10.9	0.0	0.0
Classic, Schweppes*	1 Can/330ml	115	0.0	35	0.0	8.4	0.0	0.0
D & G Old Jamaican*	1 Can/330ml	211	0.0	64	0.0	16.0	0.0	0.0
Fiery, Canned, Waitrose*	1 Can/330ml	178	0.0	54	0.0	13.3	0.0	0.0
Fiery, Low Calorie, Waitrose*	1 Can/330ml	3	0.0	1	0.1	0.0	0.0	0.0
Light, Waitrose*	1 Glass/250ml	2	0.2	1	0.0	0.0	0.1	0.1
No Added Sugar, Canned, Tesco*	1 Can/330ml	3	0.3	1	0.0	0.1	0.1	0.1
Sparkling, Organic, Whole Earth*	1 Can/330ml	116	0.0	35	0.0	8.2	0.0	0.0
Tesco*	1 Serving/200ml	70	0.2	35	0.1	8.2	0.1	0.0
Traditional, Fentiman's*	1 Bottle/275ml	130	0.0	47	0.0	11.3	0.0	0.0
GINGER WINE								
Green Ginger Wine & Scots Whisky, Crabbies*	1 Glass/125ml	192	0.0	153	14.3	14.3	0.0	0.0
GINGERBREAD								
Average	*1oz/28g*	*106*	*3.5*	*379*	*5.7*	*64.7*	*12.6*	*1.2*
Men, Mini, Asda*	1 Biscuit/11g	46	1.4	433	5.0	74.0	13.0	1.8

G

	Measure INFO/WEIGHT	per Measure KCAL	FAT	Nutrition Values per 100g / 100ml KCAL	PROT	CARB	FAT	FIBRE
GINGERBREAD								
Men, Mini, M&S*	1 Biscuit/17g	78	3.1	470	6.2	63.9	18.6	1.7
Men, Mini, Sainsbury's*	1 Biscuit/12g	56	1.4	463	5.7	83.4	11.8	1.5
GNOCCHI								
Aldi*	1 Serving/100g	160	0.3	160	3.8	35.6	0.3	0.0
Di Patate, Italfresco*	½ Pack/200g	296	0.4	148	3.3	33.2	0.2	0.0
Fresh, Italian, Chilled, Sainsbury's*	¼ Pack/125g	190	0.4	152	3.8	33.6	0.3	1.4
Potato, Cooked, Average	*1 Serving/150g*	*200*	*0.0*	*133*	*0.0*	*33.2*	*0.0*	*0.0*
GNOCCHI								
Potato, Fresh, Dell'ugo*	¼ Pack/87g	124	0.3	142	4.0	30.2	0.4	1.0
GOAT								
Meat, Uncooked	1 Portion/100g	109	2.3	109	20.0	0.0	2.3	0.0
GOJI BERRIES								
Average	*1 Serving/100g*	*287*	*0.7*	*287*	*6.6*	*65.1*	*0.7*	*6.8*
Dried, LL, Waitrose*	1 Sm Handful/30g	91	0.5	302	13.6	57.8	1.8	12.2
Whole, Sun-Dried, Linwoods*	30g Serving/30g	80	0.7	268	13.0	48.8	2.3	14.9
GOOSE								
Leg with Skin, Fire Roasted	*1 Leg/174g*	*482*	*29.8*	*277*	*28.8*	*0.0*	*17.1*	*0.0*
Meat & Skin, Roasted	*½ Goose/774g*	*2361*	*169.5*	*305*	*25.2*	*0.0*	*21.9*	*0.0*
Meat, Fat & Skin, Raw	*1oz/28g*	*101*	*9.2*	*361*	*16.5*	*0.0*	*32.8*	*0.0*
Meat, Raw	*1 Portion/185g*	*298*	*13.0*	*161*	*23.0*	*0.0*	*7.0*	*0.0*
Meat, Roasted	*1 Portion/143g*	*340*	*18.6*	*238*	*29.0*	*0.0*	*13.0*	*0.0*
GOOSEBERRIES								
Dessert, Raw, Tops & Tails Removed	*1oz/28g*	*11*	*0.1*	*40*	*0.7*	*9.2*	*0.3*	*2.4*
Stewed with Sugar	*25g*	*14*	*0.1*	*54*	*0.7*	*12.9*	*0.3*	*4.2*
Stewed without Sugar	*25g*	*4*	*0.1*	*16*	*0.9*	*2.5*	*0.3*	*4.4*
GOULASH								
Beef with Tagliatelle, COU, M&S*	1 Pack/360g	414	8.3	115	8.5	14.5	2.3	1.0
Beef, Average	*1 Serving/300g*	*310*	*9.5*	*103*	*8.1*	*10.4*	*3.2*	*0.9*
Beef, Weight Watchers*	1 Pack/330g	241	5.6	73	4.8	9.5	1.7	0.6
GRAPEFRUIT								
in Juice, Average	*1oz/28g*	*13*	*0.0*	*46*	*0.5*	*10.6*	*0.0*	*0.4*
in Syrup, Average	*1oz/28g*	*19*	*0.0*	*69*	*0.5*	*16.8*	*0.1*	*0.5*
Raw, Flesh Only, Average	*½ Fruit/160g*	*48*	*0.2*	*30*	*0.8*	*6.8*	*0.1*	*1.3*
Raw, Weighed with Skin & Seeds, Average	*1 Large/340g*	*54*	*0.2*	*16*	*0.3*	*4.0*	*0.0*	*0.6*
Ruby Red in Juice, Average	*1 Serving/135g*	*54*	*0.1*	*40*	*0.6*	*9.4*	*0.0*	*0.5*
GRAPES								
Cotton Candy, Black, Seedless, Finest, Tesco*	1 Portion/80g	53	0.1	66	0.4	15.4	0.1	0.7
Green, Average	*1 Grape/5g*	*3*	*0.0*	*62*	*0.4*	*15.2*	*0.1*	*0.7*
Red & Green Selection, Average	*1 Grape/5g*	*3*	*0.0*	*62*	*0.4*	*15.2*	*0.1*	*0.8*
Red, Average	*1 Grape/5g*	*3*	*0.0*	*65*	*0.4*	*15.8*	*0.1*	*0.6*
Seedless, Black, Asda*	1 Serving/80g	51	0.1	64	0.4	15.4	0.1	0.7
GRAPPA								
	1 Serving/30ml	85	0.0	283	0.0	6.7	0.0	0.0
GRATIN								
Cauliflower, Findus*	1 Pack/400g	340	20.0	85	3.5	7.0	5.0	0.0
Dauphinoise, Budgens*	½ Pack/218g	277	15.7	127	3.0	12.5	7.2	2.5
Leek & Carrot, Findus*	1 Pack/400g	440	26.0	110	3.5	9.5	6.5	0.0
Potato, Creamy, M&S*	½ Pack/225g	360	25.0	160	2.2	11.9	11.1	0.9
Potato, HL, Tesco*	1 Serving/225g	169	5.0	75	2.3	11.4	2.2	0.6
Potato, Sainsbury's*	½ Pack/225g	448	34.0	199	4.4	11.4	15.1	1.0
GRAVY								
Beef, Aunt Bessie's*	1 Serving/100g	73	5.3	73	1.0	5.3	5.3	0.5
Beef, Favourite, Granules, Made Up, Bisto*	1 Serving/50ml	13	0.5	26	0.0	4.2	1.0	0.0

G

GRAVY

	Measure INFO/WEIGHT	per Measure KCAL	FAT	Nutrition Values per 100g / 100ml KCAL	PROT	CARB	FAT	FIBRE
Beef, Free From, Sainsbury's*	½ Pack/151g	47	1.5	31	1.5	4.1	1.0	0.2
Beef, Fresh, Sainsbury's*	1 Serving/83ml	47	2.7	56	2.4	4.5	3.2	0.6
Beef, Fresh, Signature, TTD, Sainsbury's*	¼ Pot/123g	38	1.1	31	1.9	3.7	0.9	0.6
Beef, Heat & Serve, Morrisons*	1 Serving/150g	27	0.4	18	0.3	3.9	0.3	0.5
Beef, Home Style, Savoury, Heinz*	¼ Cup/60g	30	1.0	50	1.7	6.7	1.7	0.0
Beef, Rich, Ready to Heat, Schwartz*	½ Pack/100g	31	1.6	31	0.8	3.4	1.6	0.5
Caramelised Onion, Made Up, Bisto*	1 Serving/70ml	20	0.3	29	0.1	6.1	0.4	0.1
Chicken, Granules For, Dry Weight, Bisto*	1 Serving/20g	80	3.2	400	1.9	62.5	15.8	0.2
Chicken, Rich, Ready to Heat, Schwartz*	½ Pack/100g	27	1.2	27	0.8	3.3	1.2	0.5
Chicken, with White Wine & Tarragon, Atkins & Potts*	1 Pack/350g	136	3.2	39	0.7	6.2	0.9	0.0
Favourite, Granules, Made Up, Bisto*	1 Serving/50ml	15	0.6	30	0.2	4.4	1.2	0.0
Granules for Chicken, Made Up, Smart Price, Asda*	1 Serving/100ml	34	2.3	34	0.2	3.0	2.3	0.1
Granules for Meat, Made Up, Asda*	1 Serving/100ml	38	2.4	38	0.6	4.0	2.4	0.1
Granules for Meat, Made Up, Sainsbury's*	1 Serving/100ml	37	2.4	37	0.4	3.5	2.4	0.1
Granules for Vegetarian Dishes, Dry Weight, Bisto*	1 Serving/28g	100	3.7	356	2.7	56.0	13.3	4.5
Granules, Beef, Dry, Tesco*	1 Serving/6g	29	2.1	480	5.5	36.4	34.7	1.5
Granules, Beef, Made Up, Tesco*	1 Serving/140ml	48	3.6	35	0.3	2.6	2.5	0.1
Granules, Chicken & Hint of Sage & Onion, Oxo*	1 Serving/30g	95	1.8	316	11.1	54.2	6.1	0.7
Granules, Chicken, Dry, Average	*1 Tsp/4g*	*17*	*0.9*	*428*	*4.5*	*49.4*	*23.6*	*1.2*
Granules, Chicken, Made Up, Oxo*	1 fl oz/30ml	5	0.1	18	0.7	3.3	0.3	0.0
Granules, Chicken, Morrisons*	1 Serving/100ml	34	2.3	34	0.2	3.2	2.3	0.0
Granules, Dry, Bisto*	1 Serving/10g	38	1.6	384	3.1	56.4	16.2	1.5
Granules, Instant, Dry	*1oz/28g*	*129*	*9.1*	*462*	*4.4*	*40.6*	*32.5*	*0.0*
Granules, Instant, Made Up	*1oz/28g*	*10*	*0.7*	*34*	*0.3*	*3.0*	*2.4*	*0.0*
Granules, Lamb, Dry, Average	*1 Tsp/4g*	*14*	*0.3*	*344*	*10.8*	*56.2*	*8.4*	*2.8*
Granules, Lamb, Hint of Mint, Made Up, Oxo*	1 Serving/100ml	25	0.5	25	0.7	4.3	0.5	0.0
Granules, Made Up, Oxo*	1 Serving/150ml	28	0.4	19	0.6	3.4	0.3	0.0
Granules, Onion, Dry, Morrisons*	1 Serving/25g	124	8.7	495	3.4	44.0	34.7	0.0
Granules, Onion, Made Up, Oxo*	1 fl oz/30ml	6	0.1	20	0.5	3.7	0.3	0.0
Granules, Vegetable, Dry, Tesco*	½ Pint/20g	94	6.7	470	3.8	38.5	33.4	3.7
Instant, Dry Weight, Morrisons*	1 Serving/25g	80	0.1	320	3.5	77.0	0.3	1.2
Instant, Made Up, BGTY, Sainsbury's*	1 fl oz/30ml	10	0.0	32	0.3	7.4	0.1	0.1
Meat, Granules, As Consumed, Quixo, Aldi*	1 Serving/71ml	24	1.6	34	0.5	3.0	2.3	0.5
Onion, Fresh, Asda*	1/6 Pot/77g	30	1.6	39	1.7	3.3	2.1	0.4
Onion, Granules For, Dry Weight, Bisto*	4 Tsp/20g	78	2.9	391	2.4	62.3	14.7	2.3
Onion, Granules, Made Up, Bisto*	1 Serving/50ml	14	0.3	28	0.2	5.6	0.6	0.0
Onion, Rich, M&S*	½ Pack/150g	60	1.8	40	2.0	5.9	1.2	0.3
Onion, Rich, Ready to Heat, Schwartz*	½ Sachet/100g	24	0.6	24	0.4	4.3	0.6	0.5
Pork, Best, Made Up, Bisto*	1 Serving/50ml	14	0.2	28	0.6	5.8	0.4	0.0
Poultry, Fresh, Sainsbury's*	1 Serving/100g	46	1.2	46	3.5	4.9	1.2	0.5
Poultry, Fresh, Signature, TTD, Sainsbury's*	¼ Pot/126g	58	2.0	46	3.1	4.9	1.6	0.6
Poultry, TTD, Sainsbury's*	1 Portion/125g	76	5.6	61	1.8	3.5	4.5	0.8
Powder, Made Up, Sainsbury's*	1 Serving/100ml	15	0.1	15	0.4	3.2	0.1	0.1
Powder, Vegetarian, Organic, Marigold*	1 Serving/22g	79	1.7	361	10.6	61.5	7.7	1.3
Roast Beef, Best in Glass Jar, Made Up, Bisto*	1 Serving/70ml	21	0.3	30	0.3	6.1	0.4	0.0
Roast Beef, Classic, Dry, Schwartz*	1 Pack/27g	83	0.8	306	11.2	58.8	2.9	3.8
Roast Chicken, Classic, Dry, Schwartz*	1 Pack/26g	49	1.5	189	10.3	23.6	5.9	2.5
Roast Lamb, Bisto*	1 Serving/20g	60	0.9	302	3.4	62.3	4.3	0.0
Roast Lamb, Classic, Dry, Schwartz*	1 Pack/26g	87	1.2	336	10.4	63.6	4.5	0.0
Roast Onion, Classic, Dry, Schwartz*	1 Pack/27g	85	1.1	315	8.8	61.0	4.0	4.6
Roast Pork & Sage, Classic, Dry, Schwartz*	1 Pack/25g	88	1.4	354	11.8	63.8	5.8	0.0
Roast Pork, Best, in Glass Jar, Dry Weight, Bisto*	4 Tsp/20g	63	0.9	314	4.3	64.1	4.5	0.0
Roast Turkey, Dry, Schwartz*	1 Pack/25g	91	1.6	365	10.8	64.7	6.5	2.4

	Measure INFO/WEIGHT	per Measure KCAL	FAT	Nutrition Values per 100g / 100ml KCAL	PROT	CARB	FAT	FIBRE
GRAVY								
Turkey, Granules For, Dry Weight, Bisto*	4 Tsp/20g	75	3.1	377	2.4	57.2	15.5	1.0
Turkey, Granules, Made Up, Bisto*	1 Serving/50ml	14	0.6	28	0.2	4.0	1.2	0.2
Turkey, Rich, Ready to Heat, Schwartz*	1 Pack/200g	62	2.4	31	1.9	3.1	1.2	0.5
Vegetable, Granules For, Dry Weight, Bisto*	1 Tsp/4g	15	0.5	380	2.1	63.0	13.3	4.5
Vegetable, Granules For, Made Up, Bisto*	1 Serving/50ml	14	0.2	28	0.2	5.6	0.4	0.2
GREENGAGES								
Raw, Average	*1 Fruit/23g*	*9*	*0.0*	*37*	*0.7*	*9.2*	*0.1*	*2.0*
GRILLS								
Cheese & Bacon, Danepak*	1 Grill/85g	241	16.0	284	15.0	13.4	18.9	1.2
Vegetable, Dalepak*	1 Grill/83g	125	4.1	151	4.0	22.5	5.0	1.6
Vegetable, Tesco*	1 Grill/72g	129	7.2	179	4.2	18.0	10.0	2.2
GROUSE								
Meat Only, Roasted	*1oz/28g*	*36*	*0.6*	*128*	*27.6*	*0.0*	*2.0*	*0.0*
GUACAMOLE								
Average	*1 Tbsp/17g*	*33*	*3.3*	*194*	*1.6*	*3.4*	*19.2*	*2.4*
Chunky, M&S*	1 Pot/170g	221	19.2	130	1.5	5.1	11.3	1.7
Chunky, Sainsbury's*	½ Pot/65g	120	11.9	185	1.6	3.2	18.4	3.8
Fresh, VLH Kitchens	1 Serving/17g	26.9	85.9	158	1.5	3.0	14.6	2.5
Mexican Style, Dip Selection, Morrisons*	½ Pack/50g	102	10.2	204	1.5	3.7	20.4	0.9
Reduced Fat, Dip, BGTY, Sainsbury's*	¼ Pot/43g	62	5.7	146	1.3	2.9	13.5	4.0
Style, Topping, Dip, Discovery*	1 Seving/37g	29	2.1	79	1.2	6.0	5.6	1.2
GUAVA								
Canned in Syrup	*1oz/28g*	*17*	*0.0*	*60*	*0.4*	*15.7*	*0.0*	*3.0*
Raw, Flesh Only, Average	*1 Fruit/55g*	*37*	*0.6*	*68*	*3.0*	*14.0*	*1.0*	*5.0*
GUINEA FOWL								
Boned & Stuffed, Fresh, Fayrefield Foods*	1 Serving/325g	650	39.3	200	19.1	3.3	12.1	0.5
Fresh, Free Range, Waitrose*	1 Portion/193g	258	11.9	134	19.5	0.0	6.2	0.3
GUMS								
American Hard, Sainsbury's*	1 Sweet/6g	22	0.0	360	0.1	90.0	0.1	0.0
American Hard, Tesco*	1 Serving/200g	646	0.0	323	0.0	80.8	0.0	0.0
Milk Bottles, Bassett's*	1 Pack/25g	88	0.4	353	6.2	78.3	1.6	0.0

G

INFO/WEIGHT	Measure	per Measure KCAL	FAT	Nutrition Values per 100g / 100ml KCAL	PROT	CARB	FAT	FIBRE
HADDOCK								
Fillets, Battered, Average	*1oz/28g*	*64*	*3.4*	*228*	*13.4*	*16.3*	*12.2*	*1.1*
Fillets, in Breadcrumbs, Average	*1 Fillet/125g*	*253*	*12.4*	*203*	*13.5*	*14.9*	*9.9*	*1.2*
Fillets, Raw, Average	*1 Fillet/140g*	*111*	*1.2*	*79*	*17.7*	*0.2*	*0.8*	*0.0*
Fillets, Smoked, Cooked, Average	*1 Pack/300g*	*337*	*7.7*	*112*	*21.9*	*0.4*	*2.6*	*0.1*
Fillets, Smoked, Harbour Fresh, Lidl*	1 Fillet/107g	109	0.5	102	23.0	1.0	0.5	0.6
Fillets, Smoked, in Mustard & Dill, The Saucy Fish Co.*	2 Fillets/270g	262	9.7	97	15.5	0.1	3.6	0.0
Fillets, Smoked, Raw, Average	*1 Pack/227g*	*190*	*1.0*	*84*	*19.9*	*0.1*	*0.4*	*0.2*
Flour, Fried in Blended Oil	1oz/28g	39	1.1	138	21.1	4.5	4.1	0.2
Goujons, Batter, Crispy, M&S*	1 Serving/100g	250	14.1	250	11.7	18.5	14.1	0.8
Mornay, COU, M&S*	½ Pack/194g	165	3.9	85	14.5	2.6	2.0	0.6
HADDOCK IN								
Butter Sauce, Steaks, Youngs*	1 Serving/150g	134	5.6	89	9.9	4.0	3.7	0.5
Lemon & Chive Sauce, Inspirations, Birds Eye*	1 Fillet/148g	200	11.8	135	15.4	0.3	8.0	0.1
White Wine, Mustard & Spring Onion Sauce, Birds Eye*	1 Fillet/148g	175	7.9	118	16.0	1.6	5.3	0.1
HADDOCK WITH								
a Rich Cheese Crust, Smoked, Sainsbury's*	1 Serving/199g	295	18.9	148	13.0	2.5	9.5	0.9
Cheddar & Chive Sauce, Smoked, The Saucy Fish Co.*	1 Pack/240g	307	9.8	128	21.5	1.0	4.1	0.6
Creme Fraiche & Chive Sauce, Smoked, Tesco*	1 Serving/150g	154	4.6	103	16.8	2.1	3.1	0.3
HAGGIS								
Hall's*	1 Whole/454g	1053	64.5	232	9.7	15.1	14.2	2.5
Neeps & Tatties, M&S*	1 Pack/300g	330	14.4	110	3.8	12.3	4.8	0.8
Traditional, Average	*1 Serving/454g*	*1119*	*66.5*	*246*	*12.4*	*17.2*	*14.6*	*1.0*
Traditional, Macsween*	1 Haggis/454g	1149	70.8	253	11.1	19.1	15.6	2.1
Vegetarian, Macsween*	1 Serving/100g	208	11.5	208	5.9	25.9	11.5	2.4
HAKE								
Fillets, in Breadcrumbs, Average	*1oz/28g*	*66*	*3.7*	*234*	*12.9*	*16.0*	*13.4*	*1.0*
Fillets, with Roast Garlic & Herb Butter, Lidl*	1 Fillet/125g	152	7.6	122	16.0	0.5	6.1	0.5
Goujons, Average	*1 Serving/150g*	*345*	*17.8*	*230*	*12.4*	*18.6*	*11.9*	*1.3*
Raw, Average	*1oz/28g*	*28*	*0.6*	*100*	*20.1*	*0.0*	*2.2*	*0.0*
with Tomato & Basil Sauce, Vegetable Selection, Tesco*	1 Pack/450g	248	5.8	55	4.3	6.7	1.3	1.5
HALIBUT								
Cooked, Dry Heat, Average	*1oz/28g*	*38*	*1.1*	*135*	*24.6*	*0.4*	*4.0*	*0.0*
Raw	*1oz/28g*	*28*	*0.5*	*101*	*21.1*	*0.0*	*1.9*	*0.0*
with Roasted Pepper Sauce, Fillets, M&S*	1 Serving/145g	218	14.4	150	12.7	2.4	9.9	0.6
HALVA								
Average	*1oz/28g*	*107*	*3.7*	*381*	*1.8*	*68.0*	*13.2*	*0.0*
HAM								
Applewood Smoked, Average	*1 Slice/28g*	*31*	*0.8*	*112*	*21.2*	*0.6*	*2.8*	*0.2*
Baked, Average	*1 Slice/74g*	*98*	*3.7*	*133*	*21.0*	*1.0*	*5.0*	*0.0*
Beechwood Smoked, Morrisons*	1 Slice/20g	32	1.8	160	19.5	0.5	9.0	0.0
Boiled, Average	*1 Pack/113g*	*154*	*6.5*	*136*	*20.6*	*0.6*	*5.8*	*0.0*
Breaded, Average	*1 Slice/37g*	*57*	*2.3*	*155*	*23.1*	*1.8*	*6.3*	*1.6*
Breaded, British, TTD, Sainsbury's*	1 Slice/28g	34	0.8	121	22.1	1.4	3.0	0.0
Breaded, Dry Cured, Average	*1 Slice/33g*	*47*	*1.8*	*142*	*22.2*	*1.4*	*5.4*	*0.0*
Breaded, Dry Cured, Sliced, Morrisons*	1 Slice/24g	28	0.5	118	21.9	2.6	2.1	0.5
Breaded, M&S*	1 Slice/20g	23	0.6	115	22.2	0.7	2.8	0.1
Breaded, Thick Cut, TTD, Sainsbury's*	1 Slice/42g	63	2.6	150	22.7	0.6	6.3	0.0
Breaded, Wiltshire, TTD, Sainsbury's*	1 Slice/30g	44	1.8	147	22.5	0.6	6.1	0.2
British, Honey Roast, M&S*	1 Slice/20g	21	0.4	105	20.2	1.7	2.0	0.1
British, Oak Smoked & Flame Grilled, M&S*	½ Pack/50g	62	2.0	123	21.3	0.5	3.9	0.0
Brunswick, Average	*1 Slice/20g*	*32*	*1.8*	*160*	*19.5*	*0.6*	*8.8*	*0.0*
Carvery, Thinly Sliced, Dry-Cured, Morrisons*	1 Slice/15g	21	0.7	140	23.0	1.1	4.8	0.5
Cooked, Sliced, Average	*1 Slice/17g*	*18*	*0.5*	*109*	*19.0*	*1.0*	*3.2*	*0.1*

H

HAM

INFO/WEIGHT	Measure	per Measure KCAL	FAT	Nutrition Values per 100g / 100ml KCAL	PROT	CARB	FAT	FIBRE
Cooked, Slices, Value, Tesco*	1 Slice/13g	14	0.5	113	16.0	3.2	4.0	0.0
Crumbed, Sliced, Average	*1 Slice/28g*	*33*	*0.9*	*117*	*21.5*	*0.9*	*3.1*	*0.0*
Crumbed, Wafer Thin, Denny*	8 Slices/100g	112	2.3	112	21.8	2.4	2.3	0.0
Danish, Average	*1 Slice/11g*	*14*	*0.6*	*125*	*18.4*	*1.0*	*5.4*	*0.0*
Danish, Lean, Average	*1 Slice/15g*	*14*	*0.3*	*92*	*17.8*	*1.0*	*1.8*	*0.0*
Deli Hand Carved, Asda*	1 Slice/43g	62	2.4	145	26.9	1.0	5.5	0.5
Dry Cured, Average	*1 Slice/18g*	*26*	*1.0*	*144*	*22.4*	*1.0*	*5.6*	*0.2*
Dry Cured, British, TTD, Sainsbury's*	1 Slice/28g	34	0.8	120	21.3	1.9	3.0	0.0
Extra Lean, Average	*1 Slice/11g*	*10*	*0.2*	*90*	*18.0*	*1.4*	*1.4*	*0.0*
Gammon, Applewood Smoked, Dry Cured, Waitrose*	1 Slice/20g	29	1.3	145	21.4	0.0	6.6	0.0
Gammon, Breaded, Average	*1 Serving/25g*	*31*	*0.8*	*122*	*22.0*	*1.5*	*3.1*	*0.0*
Gammon, Dry Cured, Sliced, Average	*1 Slice/33g*	*43*	*1.4*	*131*	*22.9*	*0.4*	*4.2*	*0.0*
Gammon, Honey Roast, Average	*1 Serving/60g*	*81*	*2.8*	*134*	*22.4*	*0.4*	*4.8*	*0.0*
Gammon, Smoked, Average	*1 Slice/43g*	*59*	*2.1*	*137*	*22.3*	*0.7*	*4.9*	*0.2*
German Black Forest, Average	*½ Pack/35g*	*93*	*6.0*	*267*	*27.2*	*1.3*	*17.0*	*0.5*
Hock, Caramelised Apple, M&S*	½ Pack/60g	104	2.0	173	19.2	16.4	3.4	0.0
Hock, Cooked, Shredded, Sainsbury's*	½ Pack50g	69	1.6	138	26.3	0.7	3.3	0.0
Honey & Mustard, Average	*1oz/28g*	*39*	*1.2*	*140*	*20.8*	*4.6*	*4.3*	*0.0*
Honey Roast, Average	*1 Slice/20g*	*25*	*0.8*	*123*	*20.3*	*1.6*	*3.8*	*0.1*
Honey Roast, British, TTD, Sainsbury's*	1 Slice/28g	34	0.8	121	21.0	2.5	3.0	0.0
Honey Roast, Dry Cured, Average	*1 Slice/33g*	*46*	*1.5*	*140*	*22.7*	*2.3*	*4.4*	*0.2*
Honey Roast, Lean, Average	*1 Serving/25g*	*28*	*0.8*	*111*	*18.2*	*2.7*	*3.1*	*0.0*
Honey Roast, Wafer Thin, Average	*1 Slice/10g*	*11*	*0.3*	*113*	*17.4*	*3.7*	*3.2*	*0.3*
Honey Roast, Wafer Thin, Premium, Average	*1 Slice/10g*	*15*	*0.6*	*149*	*22.0*	*1.6*	*6.0*	*0.0*
Honey Roast, Wafer Thin, Tesco*	1 Slice/15g	18	0.4	118	21.6	1.8	2.6	0.6
Jamon de Trevelez, Antonio Alvarez Jamones*	1 Slice/10g	19	0.9	192	35.6	0.0	8.6	0.0
Joint, Cured, Roasted, Average	1 Serving/100g	138	5.2	138	21.7	1.0	5.2	0.1
Joint, Roast, Christmas, Tesco*	1/6 Joint/167g	225	10.8	135	17.9	1.1	6.5	0.0
Lean, Average	*1 Slice/18g*	*19*	*0.4*	*104*	*19.5*	*1.1*	*2.4*	*0.3*
Oak Smoked, Average	*1 Slice/20g*	*26*	*0.9*	*130*	*21.0*	*1.0*	*4.7*	*0.3*
Parma, Average	*1 Slice/10g*	*21*	*1.1*	*213*	*29.3*	*0.0*	*10.6*	*0.0*
Parma, Premium, Average	*1 Slice/14g*	*36*	*2.3*	*258*	*27.9*	*0.3*	*16.1*	*0.0*
Parma, TTD, Sainsbury's*	1 Slice/12g	31	1.9	258	27.8	0.8	15.9	0.5
Peppered, Average	*1 Slice/12g*	*13*	*0.3*	*110*	*18.5*	*2.0*	*2.7*	*0.0*
Peppered, Dry Cured, Average	*1 Slice/31g*	*43*	*1.5*	*140*	*23.1*	*1.3*	*4.7*	*0.2*
Prosciutto Cotto, TTD, Sainsbury's*	1 Slice/25g	40	2.3	162	18.6	0.4	9.5	0.1
Prosciutto Di Speck, TTD, Sainsbury's*	2 Slices/20g	59	4.0	293	26.0	1.5	20.0	0.5
Prosciutto, Average	*1 Slice/12g*	*27*	*1.5*	*226*	*28.7*	*0.0*	*12.4*	*0.4*
Prosciutto, Crudo, Cremona, Casa Emilia, Deluxe, Lidl*	1 Slice/13g	33	2.1	256	28.0	0.0	16.0	0.0
San Daniele, Finest, Tesco*	1 Slice/10g	24	1.3	242	30.5	0.5	13.1	0.0
Serrano, Average	*1 Slice/20g*	*46*	*2.4*	*230*	*30.5*	*0.4*	*11.8*	*0.0*
Serrano, Jamon, Deluxe, Lidl*	1 Slice/13g	30	1.6	232	30.0	1.0	12.0	0.0
Smoked, Average	*1Slice/18g*	*21*	*0.7*	*117*	*19.7*	*0.9*	*3.7*	*0.0*
Smoked, Dry Cured, Average	1 Slice/28g	38	1.2	137	23.0	1.4	4.4	0.2
Smoked, Wafer Thin, Average	*1 Serving/40g*	*41*	*1.2*	*102*	*17.7*	*1.2*	*2.9*	*0.2*
Thick Cut, Average	*1 Slice/74g*	*94*	*2.9*	*127*	*22.4*	*0.6*	*3.9*	*0.1*
Tinned, Average	*½ Can/100g*	*136*	*8.8*	*136*	*12.2*	*2.0*	*8.8*	*0.0*
Tinned, Lean, Average	*½ Can/100g*	*94*	*2.3*	*94*	*18.1*	*0.2*	*2.3*	*0.4*
Wafer Thin Cooked, CBY, Asda*	1 Serving/100g	92	2.5	92	16.5	0.8	2.5	0.0
Wafer Thin, Average	*1 Slice/10g*	*10*	*0.3*	*101*	*17.9*	*1.4*	*2.6*	*0.1*
Wafer Thin, Organic, Tesco*	1 Slice/14g	15	0.3	108	21.1	0.6	2.4	0.5
Wholemeal Crumbed, Slices, Light Choices, Tesco*	1 Slice/21g	23	0.4	110	21.5	0.2	2.1	0.0
Wiltshire, Average	*1oz/28g*	*41*	*1.7*	*148*	*23.1*	*0.0*	*6.0*	*0.0*

H

	Measure INFO/WEIGHT	per Measure KCAL	FAT	Nutrition Values per 100g / 100ml KCAL	PROT	CARB	FAT	FIBRE
HAM								
Wiltshire, Breaded, Average	*1oz/28g*	*41*	*1.4*	*145*	*23.9*	*1.0*	*5.0*	*0.0*
Wiltshire, Dry Cured, TTD, Sainsbury's*	1 Slice/30g	41	1.4	137	23.6	0.0	4.7	0.0
Wiltshire, Orange Marmalade Roasted, Finest, Tesco*	1 Slice/40g	67	2.4	167	23.6	0.0	4.7	0.0
Wiltshire, Smoked, Finely Sliced, TTD, Sainsbury's*	1 Serving/34g	44	1.3	129	23.8	0.0	3.7	0.0
HARE								
Raw, Lean Only, Average	*1oz/28g*	*35*	*1.0*	*125*	*23.5*	*0.2*	*3.5*	*0.0*
Stewed, Lean Only, Average	*1oz/28g*	*48*	*1.5*	*170*	*29.5*	*0.2*	*5.5*	*0.0*
HARIBO*								
Cola Bottles, Fizzy, Haribo*	1 Med Pack/175g	595	0.4	340	6.3	78.3	0.2	0.3
Cola Bottles, Haribo*	1 Sm Pack/16g	56	0.0	348	7.7	78.9	0.2	0.3
Dolly Mixtures, Haribo*	1 Pack/175g	719	8.4	411	1.8	90.2	4.8	0.2
Fantasy Mix, Haribo*	1 Sm Pack/100g	344	0.2	344	6.6	79.0	0.2	0.3
Gold Bears, Haribo*	1 Pack/100g	348	0.2	348	7.7	78.9	0.2	0.3
Happy Cherries, Haribo*	1 Serving/40g	139	0.1	348	7.7	78.9	0.2	0.3
Horror Mix, Haribo*	1 Sm Pack/100g	344	0.2	344	6.6	79.0	0.2	0.3
Jelly Beans, Haribo*	1 Pack/100g	379	0.2	379	0.6	93.8	0.2	0.1
Kiddies Super Mix, Haribo*	1 Pack/100g	344	0.2	344	6.6	79.0	0.2	0.3
Liquorice Favourites, Haribo*	1 Serving/40g	143	1.2	357	2.8	78.8	3.0	2.3
Liquorice with Stevia, Stevi-Lakritz, Haribo*	¼ Bag/25g	46	0.0	185	8.1	16.0	0.1	48.6
Magic Mix, Haribo*	1oz/28g	102	0.5	366	5.4	82.0	1.9	0.3
Maoam Stripes, Haribo*	1 Chew/7g	27	0.4	384	1.2	81.7	6.1	0.3
Milky Mix, Haribo*	1 Pack/175g	607	0.4	347	7.1	79.6	0.2	0.4
Mint Imperials, Haribo*	1 Pack/175g	695	0.9	397	0.4	98.8	0.5	0.1
Peaches, Haribo*	1oz/28g	98	0.4	350	4.3	82.1	0.0	0.0
Pontefract Cakes, Haribo*	1 Serving/40g	118	0.1	296	5.3	68.2	0.2	0.5
Shrimps, Haribo*	1oz/28g	99	0.1	352	6.1	81.5	0.2	0.1
Snakes, Haribo*	1 Snake/8g	28	0.0	348	7.7	78.9	0.2	0.3
Starmix, Haribo*	1 Pack/100g	344	0.2	344	6.6	79.0	0.2	0.3
Tangfastics, Haribo*	1 Pack/100g	359	2.3	359	6.3	78.3	2.3	0.5
Tropifruit, Haribo*	1oz/28g	97	0.1	348	4.5	82.1	0.2	0.5
HARISSA PASTE								
Average	*1 Tsp/5g*	*6*	*0.3*	*123*	*2.9*	*12.9*	*6.7*	*2.8*
Barts*	1 Tbsp/15g	11	0.3	76	4.0	10.7	1.9	0.0
CBY, Asda*	¼ Jar/24g	22	1.0	91	2.1	9.3	4.0	4.8
Easy, M&S*	1 Tbsp/15g	16	0.8	105	2.5	11.2	5.5	4.4
Moroccan Style, Al'fez*	1 Tsp/10g	19	1.1	190	4.0	18.2	11.2	3.4
Sainsbury's*	¼ Jar/23g	60	4.5	266	2.1	6.6	20.1	5.1
HASH								
Corned Beef, Asda*	1 Pack/400g	416	14.4	104	6.0	12.0	3.6	1.1
Corned Beef, Canned, Princes*	1 Can/410g	726	45.1	177	11.5	7.1	11.0	1.9
Corned Beef, M&S*	½ Pack/321g	385	20.2	120	8.1	7.4	6.3	1.3
Corned Beef, Meal for One, M&S*	1 Pack/400g	420	18.0	105	7.7	7.7	4.5	1.5
Corned Beef, Tesco*	1 Serving/400g	416	10.4	104	5.3	14.8	2.6	1.7
HASH BROWNS								
Homestyle, Aunt Bessie's*	2 Pieces/98g	182	9.2	186	1.6	23.0	9.4	1.9
Oven Baked, Weighed Cooked, McCain*	1 Piece/38g	80	4.3	214	2.1	25.7	11.4	2.2
Oven Baked, Weighed Frozen, McCain*	1 Piece/40g	75	4.1	187	1.7	21.8	10.3	2.1
Uncooked, Average	*1 Piece/45g*	*78*	*3.7*	*173*	*2.0*	*22.5*	*8.3*	*1.9*
HAZELNUTS								
Blanched, Average	*1 Serving/25g*	*164*	*15.9*	*656*	*15.4*	*5.8*	*63.5*	*6.5*
Chopped, Average	*1 Serving/10g*	*67*	*6.4*	*666*	*16.8*	*5.6*	*64.0*	*6.6*
Roasted, Graze*	1 Pack/26g	173	16.9	665	14.0	6.1	65.0	0.0
Whole, Average	*10 Whole/10g*	*66*	*6.4*	*655*	*15.4*	*5.8*	*63.5*	*6.5*

	Measure INFO/WEIGHT	per Measure		Nutrition Values per 100g / 100ml				
		KCAL	FAT	KCAL	PROT	CARB	FAT	FIBRE
HEART								
Lambs, Average	**1 Heart/75g**	**92**	**4.5**	**122**	**16.0**	**1.0**	**6.0**	**0.0**
Ox, Raw	**1oz/28g**	**23**	**0.8**	**82**	**14.4**	**0.0**	**2.8**	**0.0**
Ox, Stewed	**1oz/28g**	**44**	**1.4**	**157**	**27.8**	**0.0**	**5.1**	**0.0**
HERMESETAS								
Powdered, Hermes*	1 Tsp/0.78g	3	0.0	387	1.0	96.8	0.0	0.0
The Classic Sweetener, Hermes*	1 Tablet/0.5g	0	0.0	294	14.2	59.3	0.0	0.0
HEROES								
Dairy Milk, Whole Nut, Cadbury*	1 Chocolate/11g	60	3.9	545	9.1	48.2	35.2	0.0
Fudge, Cadbury*	1 Sweet/10g	44	1.5	435	2.5	72.7	14.9	0.0
HERRING								
Bismark, Drained, Ocean Sea, Lidl*	1 Can/85g	119	7.7	140	14.1	0.1	9.1	0.0
Canned in Tomato Sauce, Average	**1oz/28g**	**57**	**4.3**	**204**	**11.9**	**4.1**	**15.5**	**0.1**
Dried, Salted, Average	**1oz/28g**	**47**	**2.1**	**168**	**25.3**	**0.0**	**7.4**	**0.0**
Fillets in Mustard & Dill Sauce, John West*	1 Can/190g	332	26.6	175	9.4	2.9	14.0	0.1
Fillets in Olive Oil, Succulent, Princes*	1 Serving/50g	108	7.5	215	20.0	0.0	15.0	0.0
Fillets, Raw, Average	**1 Herring/100g**	**139**	**9.4**	**139**	**13.8**	**0.0**	**9.4**	**0.0**
Fillets, Smoked, & Peppered, Sainsbury's*	½ Pack/80g	163	8.7	204	22.8	3.5	10.9	0.0
Grilled, Average	**1oz/28g**	**51**	**3.1**	**181**	**20.1**	**0.0**	**11.2**	**0.0**
in Cream Sauce, with Cucumber & Dill, Vitakrone, Lidl*	1 Pack/360g	1296	121.7	360	7.2	6.6	33.8	0.0
Pickled in Mustard Sauce, Abba*	1 Serving/58g	150	10.9	260	7.0	16.0	19.0	0.0
Pickled, Average	**1oz/28g**	**42**	**2.9**	**149**	**8.1**	**5.5**	**10.3**	**0.0**
Rollmops, Tesco*	1 Rollmop/65g	110	5.5	170	12.0	10.4	8.4	0.4
Rollmops, with Onion, Asda*	1 Rollmop/65g	89	3.1	137	13.2	10.3	4.8	0.8
Whole, Raw, Average	**1 Serving/100g**	**95**	**6.6**	**95**	**8.9**	**0.0**	**6.6**	**0.0**
HIGHLIGHTS								
Caffe Latte, Made Up, Cadbury*	1 Serving/200g	40	1.4	20	1.0	2.5	0.7	0.0
Choc Mint, Made Up, Cadbury*	1 Serving/200ml	40	1.4	20	1.0	2.5	0.7	0.3
Chocolate Orange, Made Up, Cadbury*	1 Serving/200ml	40	1.4	20	1.0	2.3	0.7	0.3
Chocolate, Dairy Fudge, Dry Weight, Cadbury*	1 Serving/11g	40	1.1	363	17.0	50.0	10.0	0.0
Dairy Fudge, Hot Chocolate, Made Up, Cadbury*	1 Serving/200ml	40	1.0	20	1.0	2.7	0.5	0.2
Dark Chocolate, Cadbury*	1 Sachet/11g	35	0.9	315	23.1	37.3	8.1	0.0
Dark, Hot Chocolate, Bournville, Made Up, Cadbury*	1 Serving/200ml	35	0.9	18	1.2	2.0	0.4	0.0
Hot Chocolate Drink, Instant, Dry Weight, Cadbury*	1 Sachet/11g	42	1.4	380	16.8	46.9	13.1	3.4
Hot Chocolate Drink, Instant, Made Up, Cadbury*	1 Cup/200ml	40	1.4	20	1.0	2.5	0.7	0.3
Instant Hot Chocolate, Cadbury*	1 Sachet/22g	80	2.8	364	17.3	44.6	12.7	0.0
Mint, Cadbury*	1 Serving/200ml	40	1.4	20	1.0	2.5	0.7	0.0
Toffee Flavour, Made Up, Cadbury*	1 Serving/200ml	40	1.4	20	1.0	2.6	0.7	0.0
HOKI								
Grilled	**1oz/28g**	**34**	**0.8**	**121**	**24.1**	**0.0**	**2.7**	**0.0**
Raw	**1oz/28g**	**24**	**0.5**	**85**	**16.9**	**0.0**	**1.9**	**0.0**
HONEY								
Acacia Blossom, Sainsbury's*	1 Serving/24g	81	0.0	339	0.1	84.7	0.1	0.3
Acacia, Tesco*	1 Tsp/4g	12	0.0	307	0.4	76.4	0.0	0.0
Australian Eucalyptus, Finest, Tesco*	1 Tsp/4g	12	0.0	307	0.4	76.4	0.0	0.0
Clear, Basics, Sainsbury's*	1 Tsp/15g	46	0.0	307	0.4	76.4	0.1	0.0
Clear, Runny, Sainsbury's*	1 Serving/15g	51	0.0	339	0.1	84.7	0.1	0.3
Clear, Value, Tesco*	1 Serving/27g	86	0.0	320	1.0	78.0	0.0	0.0
Clover, Canadian, TTD, Sainsbury's*	1 Tbsp/15g	50	0.0	336	0.2	83.6	0.1	0.1
Costa*	1 Portion/28g	64	0.0	228	0.4	76.4	0.0	0.0
Florida Orange, ES, Asda*	1 Tbsp/15g	50	0.0	334	0.5	83.0	0.0	0.0
Greek, Waitrose*	1 Tsp/6g	18	0.0	307	0.4	76.4	0.0	0.0
Pure, Clear, Average	**1 Tbsp/20g**	**63**	**0.0**	**315**	**0.5**	**78.5**	**0.0**	**0.0**
Pure, Clear, Squeezy, Oak Lane*	1 Tsp/5ml	16	0.0	330	0.5	81.0	0.0	0.0

	Measure INFO/WEIGHT	per Measure		Nutrition Values per 100g / 100ml				
		KCAL	FAT	KCAL	PROT	CARB	FAT	FIBRE
HONEY								
Pure, Set, Average	*1 Tbsp/20g*	*62*	*0.0*	*312*	*0.4*	*77.6*	*0.0*	*0.0*
Raw, British Wildflower, Hilltop*	1 Tsp/5g	17	0.0	333	0.2	83.1	0.2	0.0
Runny, Organic, Ocado *	1 Tsp/15g	49	0.0	324	0.0	81.0	0.0	0.0
Scottish Heather, Waitrose*	1 Serving/20g	61	0.0	307	0.4	76.4	0.0	0.0
Spanish Orange Blossom, Sainsbury's*	1 Tbsp/15g	51	0.0	339	0.1	84.7	0.0	0.3
HONEYCOMB								
Natural, Epicure*	1 Serving/100g	290	4.6	290	0.4	74.4	4.6	0.0
HOOCH*								
Vodka, Calculated Estimate, Hooch*	1 Bottle/330ml	145	0.0	44	0.3	5.1	0.0	0.0
HORLICKS								
Malted Drink, Extra Light, Instant, Dry Weight, Horlicks*	1 Serving/11g	35	0.7	319	8.4	57.4	6.2	10.5
Malted Drink, Light, Dry Weight, Horlicks*	1 Serving/32g	116	1.2	364	14.8	72.2	3.8	1.9
Malted Drink, Light, Made Up, Horlicks*	1 Mug/200ml	116	1.2	58	2.4	11.6	0.6	0.3
Powder, Made Up with Semi-Skimmed Milk	1 Mug/227ml	184	4.3	81	4.3	12.9	1.9	0.0
HORSERADISH								
Prepared, Average	*1 Tsp/5g*	*1*	*0.0*	*28*	*2.0*	*5.0*	*0.1*	*2.8*
HOT CHOCOLATE								
Balanced Lifestyle, Camelot*	1 Sachet/11g	40	1.6	363	18.5	40.6	14.1	0.5
Cadbury*	1 Serving/12g	44	0.7	370	6.3	73.3	5.9	0.0
Caramel, Whittards of Chelsea*	1 Serving/20g	71	1.5	355	7.5	64.5	7.5	13.0
Chococino, Dulce Gusto, Nescafe*	1 Serving/34g	149	5.5	437	14.6	58.6	16.1	4.6
Chocolate Break, Dry, Tesco*	1 Serving/21g	110	6.0	524	7.9	58.9	28.5	1.7
Cocoa, Lidl*	1 Serving/20g	77	1.2	386	6.1	74.1	6.2	0.0
Drink, Organic, Green & Black's*	1 Tsp/4g	13	0.3	374	9.1	63.5	9.3	0.1
Drink, Twinings*	1 Serving/21g	81	0.7	387	5.0	82.0	3.3	6.0
Dry Weight, Tassimo, Suchard*	1 Cup/27g	88	2.4	325	3.2	58.0	8.9	2.6
Fairtrade, Whittards of Chelsea*	4 Tsp/20g	68	0.8	342	7.8	69.0	3.9	10.9
From Coffee Shop, Waitrose*	1 Serving/298ml	217	5.9	73	3.6	10.9	2.0	0.0
Galaxy, Mars*	1 Sachet/25g	97	1.9	386	4.8	71.9	7.7	4.7
Instant Break, Cadbury*	1 Sachet/28g	119	3.9	425	10.9	64.2	14.0	0.0
Instant, BGTY, Made Up, Sainsbury's*	1 Sachet/28g	16	0.2	56	2.1	10.6	0.6	0.3
Instant, Tesco*	1 Serving/32g	155	10.3	485	10.5	38.1	32.3	5.0
Luxury, Skinny, Whittards of Chelsea*	1 Serving/28g	92	0.8	328	12.9	67.1	2.8	13.5
Made Up, Tassimo, Suchard*	1 Serving/280ml	88	2.4	31	0.3	5.5	0.9	0.2
Maltesers, Malt Drink, Instant, Made Up, Mars*	1 Serving/220ml	104	3.0	47	0.9	7.7	1.4	0.0
Velvet, Cadbury*	1 Serving/28g	136	6.9	487	8.6	57.8	24.6	2.0
Wispa, Hot Frothy, Cadbury*	1 Sachet/27g	107	1.4	395	11.0	74.0	5.3	2.9
HOT DOG								
Feasters, Eat Well, M&S*	1 Sausage/140g	326	11.3	233	11.0	29.1	8.1	1.6
in Brine, McEnnedy American Way, Lidl*	1 Sausage/23g	47	3.7	204	10.0	3.5	16.1	0.0
Sausage, American Style, Average	*1 Sausage/75g*	*180*	*14.3*	*241*	*11.6*	*6.2*	*19.0*	*0.0*
Sausage, Average	*1 Sausage/23g*	*40*	*3.0*	*175*	*10.8*	*4.3*	*12.8*	*0.3*
HOT DOG VEGETARIAN								
Meat Free, Sainsbury's*	1 Sausage/30g	71	4.5	237	18.0	7.6	15.0	1.0
Tesco*	1 Sausage/30g	66	4.5	220	18.0	2.7	15.0	2.0
HOT POT								
Beef, Classic, 800g, Asda*	1 Serving/400g	400	20.8	100	5.7	7.1	5.2	1.2
Beef, Minced, Sainsbury's*	1 Pack/450g	464	22.1	103	5.3	9.5	4.9	2.2
Beef, Ross*	1 Pack/310g	255	11.2	82	2.2	9.4	3.6	1.5
Beef, Weight Watchers*	1 Pack/320g	231	7.7	72	3.6	8.4	2.4	1.6
Chicken, & Mushroom, HL, Tesco*	1 Serving/450g	369	6.8	82	6.3	11.8	1.5	0.5
Chicken, Chunky, Weight Watchers*	1 Pack/320g	275	9.0	86	4.7	10.4	2.8	0.6
Chicken, GFY, Asda*	1 Serving/400g	256	5.2	64	4.8	8.2	1.3	1.4

	Measure INFO/WEIGHT	per Measure KCAL	FAT	Nutrition Values per 100g / 100ml KCAL	PROT	CARB	FAT	FIBRE
HOT POT								
Chicken, Good Choice, Iceland*	1 Pack/400g	276	5.2	69	5.0	9.3	1.3	1.0
Chicken, Light Choices, Tesco*	1 Pack/347g	260	5.2	75	4.9	8.7	1.5	1.4
Chicken, Sainsbury's*	1 Pack/400g	340	11.0	85	5.2	9.8	2.8	1.3
Chicken, Weight Watchers*	1 Pack/320g	226	4.5	71	6.4	7.3	1.4	1.8
Lamb Shank, ES, Asda*	1 Pack/450g	508	20.2	113	10.2	7.8	4.5	1.3
Lamb, Classic, CBY, Asda*	1 Pack/399g	323	13.6	81	3.9	8.1	3.4	1.2
Lamb, Classic, Tesco*	1 Pack/335g	429	18.1	128	5.1	13.7	5.4	1.9
Lamb, Cumbrian, Look What We Found*	1 Pack/300g	276	5.4	92	8.9	10.1	1.8	3.0
Lamb, Diet Chef Ltd*	1 Pack/300g	276	5.4	92	8.9	10.1	1.8	3.0
Lamb, Minced, Classic Kitchen, Tesco*	1 Pack/450g	374	11.2	83	4.6	10.0	2.5	0.9
Lamb, Minced, Morrison*	1 Pack/400g	376	11.6	94	4.1	11.7	2.9	2.2
Lamb, Minced, New Zealand, Sainsbury's*	1 Pack/450g	580	30.2	129	7.3	8.2	6.7	3.6
Lancashire, Asda*	1 Pack/401g	269	5.2	67	3.8	10.0	1.3	0.9
Lancashire, M&S*	1 Pack/454g	431	15.0	95	10.1	6.7	3.3	1.0
Lancashire, Tesco*	½ Pack/225g	205	7.0	91	6.0	9.7	3.1	0.5
Liver & Bacon, Tesco*	1 Pack/550g	693	31.4	126	6.4	12.3	5.7	1.5
Minced Beef & Vegetable, COU, M&S*	1 Pack/400g	380	6.8	95	10.3	9.0	1.7	2.4
Minced Beef, Bisto*	1 Pack/375g	363	13.5	97	4.1	11.3	3.6	1.4
Minced Beef, Classic, Asda*	1 Pack/375g	398	17.2	106	6.8	8.7	4.6	1.1
Minced Beef, Iceland*	1 Pack/500g	505	15.5	101	5.5	12.7	3.1	1.3
Minced Lamb & Vegetable, COU, M&S*	1 Pack/400g	340	10.8	85	5.7	12.5	2.7	1.8
Roast, Vegetable with Gravy, Hometown Buffet*	1 Serving/113g	50	0.5	44	0.9	11.5	0.4	1.8
Sausage, Smart Price, Asda*	1 Pack/300g	239	7.0	80	3.7	11.0	2.3	0.4
Vegetable, Gluten, Yeast & Dairy Free, GranoVita*	1 Can/420g	290	8.4	69	3.2	9.5	2.0	1.6
Vegetable, Ready Meal, Average	**1 Serving/400g**	**261**	**7.4**	**65**	**1.9**	**10.7**	**1.9**	**1.9**
Vegetable, Weight Watchers*	1 Pack/335g	228	6.4	68	2.6	9.9	1.9	1.5
Vegetarian Sausage & Vegetable, Linda McCartney*	1 Pot/400g	516	20.4	129	6.4	15.7	5.1	2.3
HOUMOUS								
40% Less fat, Eat Smart, Morrisons*	½ Pack/85g	209	15.0	246	7.9	13.8	17.7	2.7
Avocado, Fresh, San Amvrosia*	1 Serving/50g	172	16.0	344	5.4	8.5	32.1	2.5
Broad Bean, Asparagus & Mint, Tesco*	¼ Pot/42g	120	9.7	285	7.1	9.7	23.0	3.7
Caramelised Onion, Tesco*	¼ Pack/50g	125	9.7	250	5.5	13.0	19.4	4.2
Caramelised Onion, The Deli, Aldi*	½ Pack/42g	94	5.9	224	7.4	15.0	14.0	4.1
Chargrilled Red Pepper & Chilli, 30% Less Fat, Asda*	1 Serving/50g	116	8.2	233	7.5	11.5	16.4	4.9
Chilli & Red Pepper, Topped, Tesco*	½ Pack/100g	281	25.1	281	7.1	6.6	25.1	8.1
Classic, The Deli, Aldi*	1 Serving/30g	104	8.7	346	7.7	12.0	29.0	3.3
Feta, Fresh, Sainsbury's*	1 Serving/100g	292	27.4	292	8.0	3.5	27.4	6.7
Fresh, Sainsbury's*	1 Serving/50g	156	13.8	312	7.3	8.9	27.5	2.2
Fresh, Waitrose*	1 Serving/75g	219	19.8	292	7.2	6.3	26.4	7.6
Garlic & Pesto, Asda*	1 Serving/34g	107	8.8	314	8.0	12.0	26.0	0.0
GFY, Asda*	1 Serving/50g	136	10.0	272	9.0	14.0	20.0	3.8
Jalapeno, Asda*	1 Serving/50g	166	14.5	331	7.0	10.6	29.0	4.5
Jalapeno, Tesco*	½ Pot/100g	360	31.1	360	7.5	11.4	31.1	3.9
Lemon & Coriander, BGTY, Sainsbury's*	½ Tub/100g	145	9.0	145	6.3	9.7	9.0	5.9
Lemon & Coriander, GFY, Asda*	1 Serving/50g	130	9.9	259	8.3	12.0	19.8	5.1
Lemon & Coriander, Reduced Fat, Tesco*	1 Pot/60g	135	9.2	225	7.4	13.8	15.3	4.7
Lemon & Coriander, Sainsbury's*	¼ Tub/50g	146	12.6	291	7.0	9.1	25.1	6.0
Lemon & Coriander, Tesco*	1 Serving/50g	170	14.5	340	7.0	12.7	29.0	2.1
Light, Morrisons*	½ Pack/85g	200	15.3	235	7.4	10.9	18.0	0.0
Mediterranean Deli, M&S*	¼ Pack/70g	203	17.7	290	7.8	8.0	25.3	6.5
Moroccan Style Topped, M&S*	1 Serving/100g	220	15.3	220	6.5	13.2	15.3	9.2
Moroccan Style, Sainsbury's*	¼ Pot/50g	114	9.8	227	5.5	7.3	19.5	6.6
Moroccan, Tesco*	¼ Pot/50g	144	12.8	289	6.8	8.1	25.5	7.3

	INFO/WEIGHT	KCAL	FAT	KCAL	PROT	CARB	FAT	FIBRE
HOUMOUS								
Organic, M&S*	¼ Pack/25g	82	7.4	330	6.9	9.1	29.7	3.3
Organic, Sainsbury's*	¼ Pot/43g	139	12.1	326	6.8	10.7	28.4	3.5
Organic, Tesco*	¼ Tub/42g	134	11.4	320	6.5	12.3	27.2	2.4
Pesto Style Houmous, Sainsbury's*	1 Spread/25g	85	7.4	339	7.9	10.8	29.4	5.7
Red Pepper Pesto, Tesco*	¼ Pot/50g	138	11.3	275	7.4	9.7	22.6	5.7
Red Pepper, Reduced Fat, Tesco*	¼ Pot/57g	120	7.4	205	7.7	12.5	12.6	5.3
Reduced Fat, Average	***1 Tbsp/30g***	***72***	***5.0***	***241***	***9.2***	***13.3***	***16.8***	***3.6***
Reduced Fat, BGTY, Sainsbury's*	1 Serving/60g	108	6.3	180	6.4	11.0	10.5	8.4
Reduced Fat, Classic, The Deli, Aldi*	1 Serving/50g	108	7.0	217	8.1	13.0	14.0	5.2
Reduced Fat, Co-Op*	¼ Pack/50g	72	4.3	145	6.5	10.7	8.6	7.3
Reduced Fat, LBU, Co-Op*	1 Serving/50g	82	4.5	165	6.8	9.6	9.0	9.0
Reduced Fat, Mediterranean Deli, M&S*	1 Mini Pot/60g	126	9.7	210	7.5	8.3	16.2	9.3
Reduced Fat, Moroccan Style, Topped, M&S*	1 Tub/170g	374	26.0	220	6.6	13.2	15.3	9.2
Reduced Fat, Selection, The Deli, Aldi*	1 Pot/60g	148	9.6	246	8.0	16.0	16.0	4.7
Reduced Fat, Snack Pots, Mini, BGTY, Sainsbury's*	1 Mini Pot/60g	100	7.3	167	7.0	13.8	12.1	5.5
Roasted Red Pepper VLH Kitchens	1 Serving/17g	31	49.4	183.4	6.5	15.6	8.4	6.2
Roasted Red Pepper, 50% Less Fat, Tesco*	½ Pot/85g	156	10.5	184	7.3	10.9	12.4	9.5
Roasted Red Pepper, Sainsbury's*	½ Pot/100g	317	27.2	317	6.2	9.0	27.2	5.7
Roasted Red Pepper, Tesco*	1 Serving/75g	255	22.3	340	7.1	11.1	29.7	2.4
So Organic, Sainsbury's*	¼ Pack/50g	157	13.5	314	6.7	8.5	27.0	5.0
Spicy Red Pepper with Crudite Dippers, M&S*	1 Pack/130g	124	7.9	95	3.3	7.1	6.1	3.4
Sun Dried Tomato, Chunky, Tesco*	½ Pot/95g	322	27.0	339	6.7	14.0	28.4	3.3
Sweet Chilli, Tesco*	¼ Pot/50g	120	8.4	240	6.9	15.2	16.7	5.4
Tesco*	¼ Pot/51g	160	13.6	315	7.4	9.8	26.8	3.4
with Extra Virgin Olive Oil, Tesco*	1 Pack/190g	564	46.2	297	7.9	11.7	24.3	5.1
Zorba Delicacies Ltd*	1 Serving/50g	156	13.3	313	7.6	10.7	26.6	3.0
HULA HOOPS								
BBQ Beef, 55% Less Saturated Fat, KP Snacks*	1 Pack/34g	172	9.0	505	3.7	61.8	26.4	2.2
Cheese & Onion 55% Less Saturated Fat, KP Snacks*	1 Bag/34g	175	9.7	515	3.6	61.0	28.5	1.9
Cheese, Puft, KP Snacks*	1 Pack/28g	132	5.6	471	8.8	61.0	20.0	4.1
Minis, Original, KP Snacks*	1 Tub/140g	752	48.7	537	3.0	52.9	34.8	1.7
Multigrain, KP Snacks*	1 Pack/23g	113	5.9	491	5.6	60.0	25.6	4.4
Original, 55% Less Saturated Fat, KP Snacks*	1 Bag/34g	175	9.7	515	3.2	61.6	28.4	1.8
Ready Salted, Puft, KP Snacks*	1 Pack/15g	72	3.2	482	8.3	64.0	21.0	4.0
Salt & Vinegar, 50% Less Saturated Fat, KP Snacks*	1 Multi Pack/25g	128	7.0	510	3.1	60.9	28.2	1.8
Salt & Vinegar, Puft, KP Snacks*	1 Pack/15g	72	3.0	478	8.1	63.0	20.0	3.9

H

ICE CREAM

	Measure INFO/WEIGHT	per Measure KCAL	FAT	Nutrition Values per 100g / 100ml KCAL	PROT	CARB	FAT	FIBRE
After Eight, Nestle*	1 Serving/55g	114	5.2	207	3.6	27.1	9.4	0.3
Almond Indulgence, Sainsbury's*	1 Serving/120g	286	18.8	238	2.8	21.4	15.7	0.6
Baked Alaska, Ben & Jerry's*	1 Serving/100g	260	15.0	260	4.0	29.0	15.0	0.1
Banana Split, Tesco*	1 Scoop/53g	115	4.5	215	2.8	30.9	8.4	0.8
Belgian Milk Chocolate, Tesco*	1 Lolly/85g	255	15.5	300	3.9	29.8	18.2	0.7
Bounty, Mini Bar, Mars*	1 Bar/25ml	72	4.8	288	4.5	24.8	19.0	1.0
Caramel Craze, Organic, Tesco*	1 Serving/100g	253	15.3	253	3.3	25.5	15.3	0.0
Caramel, Carte d'Or*	2 Boules/50g	106	4.4	212	2.6	30.8	8.7	0.0
Caramella, Tesco*	1 Serving/51g	120	5.5	235	2.6	32.0	10.7	1.1
Cheesecake Brownie, Ben & Jerry's*	1 Serving 100g	260	16.0	260	4.0	26.0	16.0	0.0
Cherry Garcia, Ben & Jerry's*	1 Serving/100g	250	15.0	250	3.0	26.0	15.0	0.0
Chocolate & Orange, Organic, Green & Black's*	1 Serving/100g	248	14.1	248	5.0	25.3	14.1	0.1
Chocolate Brownie with Walnuts, Haagen-Dazs*	1 Cup/101g	223	16.4	221	4.4	21.0	16.2	0.0
Chocolate Chip, Baskin Robbins*	1 Serving/75g	170	10.0	227	4.0	24.0	13.3	0.0
Chocolate Flavour, Average	*1 Serving/70g*	*149*	*7.9*	*212*	*4.1*	*23.7*	*11.3*	*0.6*
Chocolate Flavour, Soft Scoop, Sainsbury's*	1 Serving/70g	122	5.2	174	3.1	23.6	7.5	0.3
Chocolate Honeycomb, Co-Op*	¼ Pot/81g	186	10.5	230	4.0	26.0	13.0	0.3
Chocolate Macadamia, Ben & Jerry's*	1 Serving/100g	260	18.0	260	4.0	22.0	18.0	0.8
Chocolate, Gelatelli, Lidl*	1 Portion/50g	126	6.8	251	3.8	27.3	13.6	2.1
Chocolate, Haagen-Dazs*	1 Serving/120ml	269	18.0	224	4.0	19.0	15.0	0.0
Chocolate, Organic, Green & Black's*	1 Serving/125g	310	17.6	248	5.0	25.3	14.1	1.1
Chocolate, Soft Scoop, Asda*	1 Scoop/47g	84	3.8	179	3.7	23.0	8.0	0.0
Chocolate, Soft Scoop, Tesco*	1 Serving/50g	93	4.0	186	3.2	25.1	8.1	0.3
Chocolatino, Sundae, Tesco*	1 Tub/80g	160	5.9	200	4.4	29.0	7.4	2.4
Chocolatino, Tesco*	1 Serving/56g	115	3.8	205	3.4	31.4	6.8	1.8
Chunky Monkey, Ben & Jerry's*	1 Serving/100g	290	17.0	290	4.0	27.0	17.0	1.0
Chunky Monkey, Fairtrade, Ben & Jerry's*	1 Serving/100g	290	17.0	290	4.0	27.0	17.0	1.0
Clotted Cream, Cornish, Kelly's of Cornwall*	1 Serving/125g	282	18.6	226	2.9	20.1	14.9	0.1
Coconut, Carte d'Or*	1 Serving/100ml	125	7.1	125	1.8	14.0	7.1	0.5
Coffee, Haagen-Dazs*	1 Serving/120ml	271	18.4	226	4.1	17.9	15.3	0.0
Coffee, Waitrose*	¼ Tub/125ml	292	16.4	234	3.6	25.4	13.1	0.0
Cookie Dough, Ben & Jerry's*	1 Serving/100g	270	14.0	270	4.0	31.0	14.0	0.0
Cookie Dough, Tesco*	1 Serving/125g	301	14.2	241	3.3	31.0	11.4	0.6
Cookies & Cream, Haagen-Dazs*	1 Sm Tub/100ml	226	14.7	226	4.0	19.5	14.7	0.0
Cornish Clotted, M&S*	1 Pot/90g	207	13.0	230	2.8	21.8	14.5	0.1
Cornish Dairy, Waitrose*	1 Serving/125ml	121	6.6	97	1.7	10.7	5.3	0.1
Crema Di Mascarpone, Carte d'Or*	1 Serving/100g	207	8.9	207	2.8	29.0	8.9	0.0
Crunchie, Blast, Cadbury*	1 Lolly/100ml	230	13.9	230	2.8	23.1	13.9	0.1
Dairy Cornish, Tesco*	1 Serving/49g	112	6.0	228	3.2	24.7	12.3	0.1
Dairy Milk, Orange, Cadbury*	1 Serving/120ml	259	13.9	216	3.5	26.0	11.6	0.0
Dairy, Flavoured	1oz/28g	50	2.2	179	3.5	24.7	8.0	0.0
Dulce De Leche, Bar, Haagen-Dazs*	1 Bar/105g	370	24.0	352	3.8	32.3	22.9	0.0
Farmhouse Toffee, TTD, Sainsbury's*	¼ Pot/100g	293	18.6	293	3.2	28.3	18.6	0.6
Fig & Orange Blossom Honey, Waitrose*	1 Serving/100g	219	11.8	219	3.9	24.3	11.8	0.4
Gelato, Vanilla	1 Serving/100g	162	7.2	162	2.4	22.6	7.2	0.3
Greek Yoghurt & Honey, Carte d'Or*	1 Serving/55g	114	4.8	207	2.7	29.0	8.8	0.0
Half Baked, Ben & Jerry's*	1 Serving/100g	270	13.0	270	5.0	32.0	13.0	1.0
Honeycomb Harvest, Mackies*	1 Serving/100g	209	10.0	209	4.0	25.0	10.0	0.0
Hunky Punky Chocolate, Booja-Booja*	1 Tub/500ml	685	33.0	137	3.3	17.5	6.6	0.0
Lavazza, Carte d'Or*	1 Serving/55g	120	5.4	218	3.5	29.0	9.9	0.0
Lemon Cream, Dairy, Sainsbury's*	1 Serving/100g	199	9.3	199	3.0	25.9	9.3	0.1
Lemon Curd Swirl, Duchy Originals*	¼ Pot/101g	247	14.2	245	3.7	25.8	14.1	0.0
Light Chocolate Ices, Co-Op*	1 Ice/62g	121	8.1	195	2.0	18.0	13.0	0.5

ICE CREAM

	Measure INFO/WEIGHT	KCAL	FAT	KCAL	PROT	CARB	FAT	FIBRE
Log, Mint Chocolate, Sainsbury's*	1 Serving/51g	100	5.1	197	3.0	23.8	10.0	0.2
Luscious Mint Choc Chip, Morrisons*	1 Serving/50g	99	5.2	198	2.9	23.1	10.5	0.7
Lychee Cream & Ginger, Haagen-Dazs*	1 Serving/120ml	258	12.7	215	3.6	26.1	10.6	0.0
Mango, 98% Fat Free, Bulla*	1 Serving/70g	94	1.1	134	4.2	25.4	1.6	0.0
Mini Mix, Chocolate Coated, Gelatelli, Lidl*	1 Lolly/36g	123	7.8	342	3.9	32.0	21.8	1.2
Mini Sticks, Milk Chocolate, Weight Watchers*	1 Mini Stick/45ml	96	5.0	213	2.7	25.8	11.1	0.7
Mint & Chocolate Flavour, Average	***1 Serving/70g***	***129***	***6.3***	***184***	***3.0***	***22.6***	***9.0***	***1.2***
Mint & Chocolate, Sainsbury's*	1 Serving/71g	137	6.7	192	3.4	23.5	9.4	0.4
Mint Choc Chip Soft Scoop, Asda*	1 Serving/46g	86	4.1	189	2.9	24.0	9.0	0.3
Mint Chocolate Chip, Baskin Robbins*	1 Scoop/113g	270	16.0	239	4.4	24.8	14.2	0.9
Mint Crunch, Dairy Milk, Cadbury*	1 Serving/60ml	162	13.3	270	3.0	29.0	22.2	0.0
Mint, Majestic Luxury, Iceland*	1 Serving/80g	269	14.6	337	3.8	39.3	18.3	1.3
Mocha Coffee Indulgence, Sainsbury's*	¼ Pot/82g	178	10.6	217	3.2	22.1	12.9	0.1
My Carte D'or, Caramel, Carte d'Or*	1 Tub/200ml	210	8.0	105	1.5	16.0	4.0	0.2
My Carte D'or, Chocolate, Carte d'Or*	1 Tub/200ml	220	11.0	110	1.8	12.5	5.5	0.4
Neapolitan, Average	***1 Serving/70g***	***111***	***4.6***	***158***	***3.1***	***21.9***	***6.5***	***0.6***
Neapolitan, Brick, Tesco*	1 Serving/50g	82	3.4	163	3.3	21.9	6.9	0.4
Neapolitan, Lidl*	1 Serving/48g	108	4.8	226	4.3	29.5	10.0	0.0
Neapolitan, Soft Scoop, Asda*	1 Scoop/47g	82	3.8	175	2.8	23.0	8.0	0.2
Neapolitan, Soft Scoop, Sainsbury's*	1 Serving/75g	124	5.2	165	2.8	22.8	6.9	0.2
Neapolitan, Soft Scoop, Tesco*	1 Serving/43g	70	3.0	163	3.3	21.9	6.9	0.4
Non-Dairy, Reduced Calorie	1oz/28g	33	1.7	119	3.4	13.7	6.0	0.0
Nuts About Caramel, Cadbury*	1 Serving/100ml	290	17.1	290	4.3	28.1	17.1	2.6
Organic, Madagascan Vanilla, Yeo Valley*	1 Serving/40ml	45	2.5	112	2.4	11.4	6.3	0.1
Panna Cotta, & Raspberry Swirl, Haagen-Dazs*	1 Serving/120ml	250	14.9	208	3.2	21.0	12.4	0.0
Pistachio, Haagen-Dazs*	1 Serving/120ml	276	18.8	230	4.4	17.7	15.7	0.0
Pistachio, Seriously Nutty, Waitrose*	1 fl oz/30ml	48	3.2	161	3.2	12.6	10.8	0.3
Praline, Green & Black's*	1 Sm Pot/100g	191	10.8	191	3.5	20.0	10.8	0.9
Pralines & Cream, Baskin Robbins*	1 Serving/100g	252	13.6	252	4.5	27.7	13.6	0.3
Raspberries, Clotted Cream, Waitrose*	1 Tub/500ml	790	39.5	158	2.9	18.9	7.9	0.1
Raspberry Ripple, Average	***1 Serving/70g***	***93***	***3.3***	***134***	***1.9***	***20.8***	***4.7***	***0.1***
Raspberry Ripple, Dairy, Waitrose*	1 Serving/186ml	195	10.0	105	1.9	12.3	5.4	0.0
Raspberry Ripple, Soft Scoop, Asda*	1 Scoop/46g	78	3.2	170	2.5	24.0	7.0	0.3
Raspberry Ripple, Soft Scoop, Tesco*	1 Scoop/25g	39	1.5	157	2.5	23.0	6.1	0.2
Really Creamy Toffee, Asda*	1 Serving/120ml	146	6.0	122	1.8	17.5	5.0	0.1
Rum & Raisin, Carte d'Or*	2 Scoops/50g	100	4.0	200	2.5	24.0	8.0	1.0
Rum & Raisin, Haagen-Dazs*	1 Serving/120ml	264	17.6	220	3.4	18.6	14.7	0.0
Rum & Raisin, TTD, Sainsbury's*	¼ Pot/100g	220	10.4	220	3.8	27.7	10.4	1.0
Screwball, Asda*	1 Screwball/60g	122	6.0	203	3.3	25.0	10.0	1.5
Screwball, Raspberry Ripple, Asda*	1 Screwball/100ml	100	3.7	100	1.3	15.4	3.7	0.1
Soft Scoop, Neapolitan, Value, Tesco*	1 Serving/100g	125	5.1	125	2.7	16.2	5.1	1.4
Soft Scoop, Vanilla, Light, Weighed in Grams, Wall's*	1 Serving/100g	140	6.0	140	3.0	19.0	6.0	2.0
Stem Ginger with Belgian Chocolate, Waitrose*	1 Lolly/110g	255	14.4	232	2.9	25.5	13.1	1.7
Sticky Toffee, Cream O' Galloway*	1 Serving/30g	80	4.4	266	4.7	28.7	14.7	0.0
Strawberry & Cream, Mivvi, Nestle*	1 Serving/60g	118	4.6	196	2.6	29.4	7.6	0.2
Strawberry & Cream, Organic, Sainsbury's*	1 Serving/100g	193	9.8	193	3.6	22.6	9.8	0.4
Strawberry & Yoghurt Delice, Carte d'Or*	1 Portion/54g	95	2.0	175	1.5	34.0	3.6	0.0
Strawberry Cheesecake, Ben & Jerry's*	1 Serving 100g	240	14.0	240	3.0	27.0	14.0	0.0
Strawberry Cheesecake, Co-Op*	1/6 Pot/86g	163	6.0	190	3.0	29.0	7.0	0.2
Strawberry Cheesecake, Haagen-Dazs*	¼ Tub/125ml	295	17.0	236	3.3	25.1	13.6	0.3
Strawberry, Majestic, Luxury, Iceland*	1 Lolly/100g	281	18.6	281	2.7	25.8	18.6	0.1
Strawberry, Soft Scoop, Tesco*	1 Serving/46g	78	3.4	170	2.8	23.1	7.4	0.1
Strawberry, Weight Watchers*	1 Pot/57g	81	2.2	142	2.5	23.4	3.9	0.2

ICE CREAM

	Measure INFO/WEIGHT	KCAL	FAT	KCAL	PROT	CARB	FAT	FIBRE
Taste of Carrot Cake, Iced Dessert, Perfect World*	1 Tub/120ml	170	12.0	142	3.1	14.0	10.0	2.6
Tiramisu, Haagen-Dazs*	1 Serving/120ml	303	19.6	253	3.8	22.7	16.3	0.0
Toblerone, Carte d'Or*	1 Serving/100g	211	9.1	211	3.7	29.0	9.1	0.0
Toffee & Honeycomb Sundaes, Weight Watchers*	1 Pot/98g	119	1.8	122	1.7	18.1	1.8	5.9
Toffee & Vanilla, Sainsbury's*	1 Serving/71g	146	6.8	205	3.1	26.7	9.5	0.1
Toffee Fudge, Soft Scoop, Asda*	1 Serving/50g	92	3.5	185	2.6	28.0	7.0	0.0
Triple Chocolate Centenary, Cadbury*	1 Serving/100ml	255	15.6	255	2.5	27.1	15.6	0.0
Triple Chocolate, Carte d'Or*	1 Serving/58g	122	5.7	210	3.7	27.0	9.8	0.0
Triple Chocolate, Dairy, Sainsbury's*	1/8 Litre/67g	123	4.4	184	3.5	27.6	6.6	1.0
Vanilla & Cinnamon, Finest, Tesco*	1 Serving/50g	114	7.4	229	3.9	20.2	14.7	0.4
Vanilla Bean, Light, Deluxe, Lidl*	1 Serving/64g	110	2.5	172	4.7	26.6	3.9	0.0
Vanilla Bean, Purbeck*	1 Serving/100g	198	11.5	198	4.8	18.7	11.5	0.0
Vanilla Caramel Brownie, Haagen-Dazs*	1 Serving/150g	410	24.8	273	4.5	26.8	16.5	0.0
Vanilla Chocolate, Taste Sensation, Frosty's, Aldi*	1 Pot/73g	164	7.0	224	2.1	32.4	9.6	0.7
Vanilla Flavour, Soft Scoop, Measured in Ml, Wall's*	1 Scoop/45ml	27	1.1	60	1.5	8.0	2.5	0.9
Vanilla Flavour, Soft Scoop, Sainsbury's*	1 Serving/71g	96	3.9	136	2.9	18.8	5.5	0.2
Vanilla Flavour, Soft VLH Kitchens	1 Serving/100g	235	15.0	235	4.0	22.1	15.0	0.2
Vanilla with Strawberry Swirl, Mini Tub, Weight Watchers*	1 Mini Tub/57g	81	2.2	142	2.5	23.4	3.9	0.2
Vanilla with Vanilla Pods, Sainsbury's*	1 Serving/100g	195	10.1	195	3.5	22.5	10.1	0.1
Vanilla, Carte d'Or*	1 Serving/50g	105	4.8	210	3.0	26.0	9.5	0.0
Vanilla, COU, M&S*	¼ Pot/79g	111	2.2	140	1.7	25.9	2.8	0.8
Vanilla, Dairy, Average	*1 Scoop/40g*	*80*	*4.4*	*201*	*3.5*	*23.6*	*11.0*	*0.7*
Vanilla, Dairy, Finest, Tesco*	1 Serving/92g	227	16.0	247	4.5	18.0	17.4	0.3
Vanilla, Dairy, Organic, Yeo Valley*	1 Serving/100g	206	11.2	206	4.9	21.3	11.2	0.0
Vanilla, Light, Carte d'Or*	1 Serving/100g	136	4.4	136	2.4	22.0	4.4	4.0
Vanilla, Low Fat, Average	*1 Scoop/50g*	*59*	*1.7*	*118*	*2.3*	*19.4*	*3.4*	*0.6*
Vanilla, Low Fat, Weight Watchers*	1 Scoop/125ml	75	2.1	60	1.1	9.7	1.7	0.1
Vanilla, Mackies*	1 Serving/100g	193	11.0	193	4.0	18.0	11.0	0.0
Vanilla, Non-Dairy, Average	*1 Serving/60g*	*107*	*5.2*	*178*	*3.2*	*23.1*	*8.7*	*0.0*
Vanilla, Organic, Tesco*	1 Serving/100g	237	17.2	237	3.7	16.8	17.2	0.0
Vanilla, Organic, Waitrose*	1 Serving/125g	178	11.2	142	2.7	12.4	9.0	0.0
Vanilla, Pecan, Haagen-Dazs*	1 Serving/120ml	316	23.5	263	4.3	17.1	19.6	0.0
Vanilla, Pizza Express*	1 Serving/100g	119	6.8	119	0.9	13.8	6.8	0.0
Vanilla, Really Creamy, Asda*	1 Serving/50g	98	5.0	196	3.5	23.0	10.0	0.1
Vanilla, Smart Price, Asda*	1 Scoop/40g	55	2.4	137	2.8	19.0	6.0	0.2
Vanilla, Soft Scoop, BGTY, Sainsbury's*	1 Serving/75g	88	1.3	117	3.1	22.2	1.7	0.2
Vanilla, Soft Scoop, Light, Wall's*, Wall's Ice Cream*	1 Scoop/50ml	31	1.3	62	1.3	7.0	2.6	0.9
Vanilla, Soft Scoop, Value, Tesco*	1 Scoop/42g	57	2.4	137	2.8	18.7	5.7	0.2
Vanilla, Soft Slice, Wall's Ice Cream*	1 Serving/100ml	90	4.4	90	1.4	11.2	4.4	0.1
Vanilla, Toffe Crunch, Fairtrade, Ben & Jerry's*	1 Serving/100g	280	16.0	280	4.0	29.0	16.0	0.5
Vanilla, Toffee Crunch, Ben & Jerry's*	1 Tub/407g	1099	65.1	270	4.0	29.0	16.0	0.5
Vanilla, TTD, Sainsbury's*	¼ Pot/100g	246	16.9	246	5.2	18.2	16.9	0.0
Vanilla, Waitrose*	1 Serving/100ml	156	10.8	156	2.6	12.0	10.8	0.0
Viennetta, Chocolate, Wall's Ice Cream*	¼ Pot/80g	200	12.2	250	4.1	24.0	15.2	0.0
Viennetta, Mint, Wall's Ice Cream*	1 Serving/80g	204	13.3	255	3.4	23.0	16.6	0.0
Viennetta, Strawberry, Wall's Ice Cream*	1 Serving/80g	204	13.4	255	3.4	22.1	16.8	0.0
Viennetta, Vanilla, Wall's Ice Cream*	¼ Bar/80g	204	13.4	255	3.3	23.0	16.7	0.0
with Cherry Sauce, Tesco*	1 Serving/58g	121	3.2	210	2.8	37.0	5.6	0.2
Zesty Lemon Meringue, COU, M&S*	¼ Pot/73g	120	1.8	165	2.6	33.0	2.5	0.5

ICE CREAM BAR

	Measure INFO/WEIGHT	KCAL	FAT	KCAL	PROT	CARB	FAT	FIBRE
Chocolate Covered	1 Bar/40g	128	9.3	320	5.0	24.0	23.3	0.0
Chunky Chocolate, Co-Op*	1 Bar/60g	204	12.0	340	5.0	35.0	20.0	1.0
Dairy Milk, Caramel, Cadbury*	1 Bar/60ml	175	10.3	290	3.6	30.2	17.1	0.0

	Measure INFO/WEIGHT	per Measure KCAL	FAT	Nutrition Values per 100g / 100ml KCAL	PROT	CARB	FAT	FIBRE
ICE CREAM BAR								
Dairy Milk, Fruit & Nut, Cadbury*	1 Bar/90ml	243	15.3	270	3.5	26.1	17.0	0.0
Dairy Milk, Lolly, Cadbury*	1 Lolly/100g	235	15.0	235	3.0	25.1	15.0	0.0
Dream, Cadbury*	1 Serving/118g	260	14.0	220	3.6	26.0	11.9	0.0
Galaxy, Mars*	1 Bar/54g	184	12.2	341	3.8	30.7	22.5	0.6
Lion, Nestle*	1 Bar/45g	166	9.9	370	4.2	39.1	21.9	1.0
Maltesers, Mars*	1 Bar/45ml	113	7.0	252	2.9	25.0	15.6	0.7
Mars, Mars*	1 Bar/65g	182	10.5	280	3.4	29.7	16.2	0.8
Peanut, Farmfoods*	1 Bar/60ml	216	12.8	360	5.3	36.6	21.4	1.2
Racer, Aldi*	1 Bar/59g	194	11.0	328	6.0	34.2	18.6	0.0
Snickers, Mars*	1 Bar/53ml	179	10.4	337	6.5	33.2	19.6	0.0
Twix, Mars*	1 Serving/43ml	128	7.3	301	4.0	32.0	17.1	1.2
Vanilla & Raspberry, Weight Watchers*	1 Serving/100g	81	0.3	81	2.0	23.0	0.3	0.0
ICE CREAM CONE								
After Eight, Nestle*	1 Cone/100ml	174	8.0	174	2.4	23.0	8.0	0.9
Average	**1 Cone/75g**	**140**	**6.4**	**186**	**3.5**	**25.5**	**8.5**	**0.0**
Chocolate & Nut, Co-Op*	1 Cone/110g	307	17.0	279	3.9	31.0	15.5	0.6
Chocolate & Vanilla, Good Choice, Iceland*	1 Cone/110ml	161	7.2	146	2.7	22.9	6.5	0.8
Chocolate Chip, Soft, Cornetto, Wall's Ice Cream*	1 Cone/80g	256	13.6	320	3.5	37.0	17.0	1.5
Chocolate, Mini, Cornetto, Wall's Ice Cream*	1 Cone/36g	110	5.9	300	3.5	34.0	16.0	2.0
Chocolate, Vanilla & Hazelnut, Sainsbury's*	1 Cone/62g	190	10.5	306	4.5	33.9	16.9	0.6
Classico, Cornetto, Wall's Ice Cream*	1 Cone/98g	200	12.6	205	2.7	19.7	12.9	0.0
Classico, Mini, Cornetto, Wall's Ice Cream*	1 Cone/36g	120	6.8	320	3.5	35.0	18.0	1.0
Cornet, Wafer Cone, Askeys*	1 Cone/4g	13	0.1	376	10.7	77.6	2.5	0.0
Cornetto, GFY, Asda*	1 Cone/67g	162	6.0	241	3.0	37.0	9.0	0.1
Cornetto, Wall's Ice Cream*	1 Cone/75g	195	9.7	260	3.7	34.5	12.9	0.0
Creme Egg, Cadbury*	1 Cone/115ml	270	13.3	235	2.9	29.3	11.6	0.0
Cup Cornet, Wafer Cone, Askeys*	1 Cone/4g	13	0.1	376	10.7	77.6	2.5	0.0
Dairy Milk Buttons, Cadbury*	1 Cone/100ml	204	10.4	204	0.0	24.6	10.4	0.6
Dairy Milk, Mint, Cadbury*	1 Cone/115ml	190	8.9	165	2.4	21.5	7.7	0.0
Flake 99, Cadbury*	1 Cone/125ml	244	12.5	195	2.6	23.2	10.0	0.0
Flake 99, Strawberry, Cadbury*	1 Cone/125g	250	10.9	200	2.6	27.3	8.7	0.0
Kit Kat, Nestle*	1 Cone/87g	201	8.9	230	2.8	31.4	10.2	0.7
Mini, Sainsbury's*	1 Cone/18g	66	3.8	366	4.4	39.8	21.0	3.4
Mini, Tesco*	1 Cone/48g	152	9.3	316	4.1	31.5	19.3	0.8
Mint Chocolate Chip, Soft, Cornetto, Wall's Ice Cream*	1 Cone/80g	240	13.6	300	4.0	33.0	17.0	1.0
Mint, Cornetto, Wall's Ice Cream*	1 Cone/75g	190	9.9	250	4.0	31.0	13.0	0.8
Smarties, Nestle*	1 Cone/100g	177	8.1	177	2.4	23.6	8.1	0.7
Sticky Toffee, Farmfoods*	1 Cone/120ml	326	15.4	272	3.2	36.0	12.8	2.0
Strawberry & Vanilla, Asda*	1 Cone/115ml	193	9.0	168	1.8	22.6	7.8	0.1
Strawberry & Vanilla, Iceland*	1 Cone/70g	182	7.6	260	3.3	37.5	10.8	0.7
Strawberry & Vanilla, Sainsbury's*	1 Cone/70g	171	6.8	243	3.4	35.6	9.7	1.0
Strawberry & Vanilla, Tesco*	1 Cone/70g	194	9.4	277	3.0	35.9	13.5	0.3
Strawberry, BGTY, Sainsbury's*	1 Cone/69g	151	4.5	219	2.6	37.5	6.5	1.3
Strawberry, Soft, Cornetto, Wall's Ice Cream*	1 Cone/80g	208	8.0	260	2.5	38.0	10.0	1.0
Tropical, GFY, Asda*	1 Cone/100g	135	5.0	135	2.6	20.0	5.0	0.3
Vanilla & Chocolate, Everyday Value, Tesco*	1 Cone/58g	170	7.4	285	3.8	38.9	12.4	1.3
Vanilla, Soft, Cornetto, Wall's Ice Cream*	1 Cone/80g	264	16.0	330	4.5	33.0	20.0	0.0
ICE CREAM ROLL								
Arctic, Average	**1 Serving/70g**	**140**	**4.6**	**200**	**4.1**	**33.3**	**6.6**	**0.0**
Tesco*	¼ Roll/57g	131	4.9	230	3.7	34.5	8.6	0.4
ICE CREAM SANDWICH								
Chocolate, Skinny Cow*	1 Portion/36g	101	2.8	280	6.0	46.0	7.9	2.9
Neapolitan, Gelatelli, Lidl*	1 Sandwich/106g	233	9.5	220	4.9	29.0	9.0	1.9

ICE CREAM SANDWICH	Measure INFO/WEIGHT	per Measure KCAL	FAT	Nutrition Values per 100g / 100ml KCAL	PROT	CARB	FAT	FIBRE
ICE CREAM SANDWICH								
Vanilla, Chocolate Coated, Lidl*	1 Serving/51g	145	9.5	284	1.8	21.6	18.6	0.0
Vanilla, Skinny Cow*	1 Portion/36g	100	3.0	277	5.4	45.1	8.2	2.1
Wich, Ben & Jerry's*	1 Pack/117g	398	19.9	340	4.0	44.0	17.0	1.0
ICE CREAM STICK								
Chocolate Cookies, Haagen-Dazs*	1 Stick/43g	162	10.9	376	4.9	31.8	25.4	0.0
Mint Double Chocolate, Skinny Cow*	1 Stick/110ml	94	1.8	85	2.7	15.1	1.6	2.4
Toffee, Skinny Cow*	1 Stick/72g	87	0.4	121	3.9	25.2	0.5	4.2
Tropical Moment, Asda*	1 Lolly/75g	112	3.1	150	1.7	26.1	4.2	0.4
ICE LOLLY								
Assorted, Iceland*	1 Lolly/51g	33	0.0	65	0.0	16.2	0.0	0.0
Baby, Tesco*	1 Lolly/32g	26	0.0	80	0.1	20.0	0.0	0.1
Berry Burst, Sainsbury's*	1 Lolly/90ml	93	1.6	103	1.1	20.8	1.8	0.7
Blackcurrant Split, Iceland*	1 Lolly/75g	61	2.4	81	1.1	12.0	3.2	0.1
Blackcurrant, Ribena*	1 Lolly/35ml	25	0.0	68	0.0	16.4	0.0	0.0
Calippo, Lemon Lime, Mini, Wall's Ice Cream*	1 Lolly/80g	68	0.0	85	0.0	21.0	0.0	0.2
Calippo, Orange, Mini, Wall's Ice Cream*	1 Lolly/78g	70	0.0	90	0.0	21.9	0.0	0.2
Calippo, Strawberry Tropical, Wall's Ice Cream*	1 Lolly/105g	89	0.1	85	0.1	21.0	0.1	0.0
Choc & Almond, Mini, Tesco*	1 Lolly/31g	103	7.4	331	4.4	24.8	23.8	0.9
Chocolate, Mini Milk, Milk Time, Wall's Ice Cream*	1 Lolly/23g	31	0.7	135	4.3	22.0	3.1	1.0
Chocolate, Plain, Mini, Tesco*	1 Lolly/31g	94	6.6	304	3.1	24.8	21.4	1.2
Cider Refresher, Treats*	1 Lolly/70ml	54	0.0	77	0.0	19.2	0.0	0.0
Exotic Fruit, Ice Cream, Gelatelli, Lidl*	1 Lolly/110g	148	2.8	135	1.8	25.6	2.5	0.0
Exotic Fruit, Mini, HL, Tesco*	1 Lolly/31g	41	0.6	131	1.0	26.4	2.0	1.0
Fab, Nestle*	1 Lolly/64g	90	3.2	141	0.5	23.4	5.0	0.4
Fab, Orange, Nestle*	1 Lolly/58g	81	2.7	140	0.6	24.0	4.7	0.0
Feast, Chocolate, Mini, Wall's Ice Cream*	1 Lolly/52g	165	11.9	318	3.3	24.0	23.0	0.0
Feast, Ice Cream, Original, Wall's Ice Cream*	1 Lolly/90ml	252	18.0	280	2.5	20.0	20.0	0.0
Fruit Flavour, Assorted, Basics, Sainsbury's*	1 Lolly/50g	33	0.0	66	0.0	16.5	0.0	0.0
Fruit Ices, Made with Orange Juice, Del Monte*	1 Lolly/75ml	79	0.0	105	0.5	25.7	0.0	0.0
Fruit Luxury, Mini, Co-Op*	1 Lolly/45g	58	2.7	130	2.0	18.0	6.0	0.2
Fruit Pastilles, Rowntree's*	1 Lolly/65ml	61	0.0	94	0.2	23.2	0.0	0.0
Fruit Split, Asda*	1 Lolly/74g	85	2.7	115	1.7	19.0	3.6	0.0
Fruit Split, Assorted, Co-Op*	1 Lolly/73g	80	2.2	110	1.0	20.0	3.0	0.1
Fruit Split, BFY, Morrisons*	1 Lolly/73g	50	0.5	69	1.6	13.9	0.7	0.1
Fruit Split, Waitrose*	1 Lolly/73g	91	2.6	124	2.5	21.7	3.6	0.4
Fruit, Assorted, Waitrose*	1 Lolly/73g	59	0.0	81	0.0	20.0	0.0	0.1
Fruits of the Forest, Ice Cream, Gelatelli, Lidl*	1 Lolly/110g	145	2.8	132	1.9	24.5	2.5	0.0
Funny Foot, Wall's Ice Cream*	1 Lolly/81ml	83	4.9	102	2.0	12.5	6.0	0.0
Ice Burst, Aldi*	1 Lolly/60g	67	1.1	112	0.5	24.0	1.8	0.5
Icicles, All Flavours, Freezepops, Calypso*	1 Lolly/50ml	1	0.0	1	0.0	0.3	0.0	0.0
Kiwi Burst, Pineapple Sorbet in Kiwi Ice, Sainsbury's*	1 Lolly/90ml	76	0.1	84	0.1	20.7	0.1	0.4
Lemon & Lime, Mini Bar, M&S*	1 Lolly/50g	48	0.0	95	0.1	23.6	0.1	0.2
Lemon & Lime, Rocket Split, De Roma*	1 Lolly/60ml	65	2.6	108	1.0	16.0	4.3	0.2
Lemonade & Cola, Morrisons*	1 Lolly/55ml	36	0.0	65	0.0	16.2	0.0	0.0
Lemonade Flavour, R White*	1 Lolly/75ml	56	1.1	75	0.5	15.1	1.5	0.1
Lemonade Sparkle, Wall's Ice Cream*	1 Lolly/55g	40	0.0	73	0.0	18.2	0.0	0.0
Mango & Passion Fruit Smoothie, Waitrose*	1 Lolly/73g	60	0.3	82	0.7	18.9	0.4	0.7
Milk, Blue Parrot Cafe, Sainsbury's*	1 Lolly/30ml	34	1.0	113	2.7	18.0	3.3	0.3
Minis, Caramel & Chocolate, Skinny Cow*	1 Lolly/38ml	62	1.9	162	3.4	24.3	5.0	3.3
Mint Chocolate, Tesco*	1 Lolly/70g	234	13.9	334	3.6	35.4	19.8	1.2
Nobbly Bobbly, Nestle*	1 Lolly/70ml	219	11.6	312	2.9	38.1	16.5	0.6
Orange Juice, Asda*	1 Lolly/70g	58	0.0	83	0.7	20.0	0.0	0.0
Orange Juice, Bar, M&S*	1 Lolly/75g	64	0.0	86	0.5	21.0	0.0	0.1

	Measure INFO/WEIGHT	per Measure KCAL	FAT	Nutrition Values per 100g / 100ml KCAL	PROT	CARB	FAT	FIBRE
ICE LOLLY								
Orange Juice, Freshly Squeezed, Finest, Tesco*	1 Lolly/80ml	89	0.0	111	0.7	27.0	0.0	0.0
Orange Juice, Freshly Squeezed, Waitrose*	1 Lolly/73g	88	0.1	120	0.6	29.7	0.1	0.0
Orange, Average	*1 Lolly/72g*	*66*	*0.0*	*92*	*0.4*	*22.4*	*0.0*	*0.1*
Orange, Real Fruit Juice, Sainsbury's*	1 Lolly/73ml	49	0.1	67	0.2	16.5	0.1	0.1
Orange, Real Juice, Sainsbury's*	1 Lolly/72ml	63	0.1	88	0.7	21.0	0.1	0.1
Orange, Real Juice, Tesco*	1 Lolly/32g	25	0.0	78	0.6	18.7	0.0	0.3
Orange, Tesco*	1 Lolly/77g	53	0.0	68	0.2	16.8	0.0	0.3
Pineapple & Coconut Colada, Waitrose*	1 Lolly/73ml	79	1.5	108	1.0	21.0	2.1	0.6
Pineapple, Dairy Split, Sainsbury's*	1 Lolly/72ml	84	2.6	116	1.8	19.0	3.6	0.1
Pineapple, Real Fruit Juice, Sainsbury's*	1 Lolly/73ml	55	0.1	76	0.1	19.0	0.1	0.1
Pop Up, CBY, Asda*	1 Lolly/80ml	65	0.0	81	0.0	20.1	0.0	0.3
Raspberry, Real Fruit Juice, Sainsbury's*	1 Lolly/72g	62	0.1	86	0.3	21.0	0.1	0.1
Raspberry, Smoothie, Iced, Del Monte*	1 Lolly/90ml	84	0.0	94	0.3	22.8	0.0	0.8
Real Fruit, Dairy Split, Sainsbury's*	1 Lolly/73ml	100	3.1	137	2.1	22.8	4.2	0.1
Refresher, Fruit Flavour, Bassett's*	1 Lolly/45g	56	0.7	125	1.6	26.0	1.6	0.3
Rocket, Co-Op*	1 Lolly/60g	42	0.0	70	0.0	17.0	0.0	0.0
Rocket, Sainsbury's*	1 Lolly/60g	50	0.3	83	0.5	19.9	0.5	0.5
Rolo, Nestle*	1 Lolly/75ml	243	14.1	324	3.8	36.5	18.8	0.0
Salted Caramel, Tesco*	1 Lolly/70g	227	12.5	324	3.6	36.7	17.9	1.1
Scooby Doo, Freezepops, Calypso*	1 Lolly/45ml	13	0.0	28	0.0	7.0	0.0	0.0
Seriously Fruity, Mango Sorbet, Waitrose*	1 Lolly/100ml	79	0.3	79	0.8	18.4	0.3	0.5
Solero, Exotic, Wall's Ice Cream*	1 Lolly/70g	94	1.1	134	1.5	28.0	1.5	0.5
Solero, Orange Fresh, Wall's Ice Cream*	1 Lolly/96g	78	0.0	81	0.2	20.0	0.0	0.0
Solero, Red Fruits, Wall's Ice Cream*	1 Lolly/95g	99	2.1	104	1.3	21.0	2.2	0.0
Spotty Dotty, Sainsbury's*	1 Lolly/47g	111	6.5	236	1.8	25.5	13.8	1.3
Sprinkle Tops, Sainsbury's*	1 Lolly/40g	51	1.2	126	0.2	24.8	2.9	0.1
Strawberry & Banana, Smoothies, Sainsbury's*	1 Lolly/60g	100	3.2	166	1.5	28.0	5.3	0.2
Strawberry Split, Average	*1 Lolly/72g*	*78*	*2.3*	*108*	*1.5*	*18.5*	*3.2*	*0.2*
Strawberry, Dairy Split, Sainsbury's*	1 Lolly/73ml	86	2.6	118	1.7	19.8	3.6	0.1
Strawberry, Fruit Split, Iceland*	1 Lolly/73g	77	2.4	105	0.9	17.8	3.3	0.5
Strawberry, Mini Milk, Milk Time, Wall's Ice Cream*	1 Lolly/23g	30	0.7	131	4.0	22.0	2.9	0.5
Tropical Fruit Sorbet, Waitrose*	1 Lolly/110g	90	2.2	82	1.5	14.5	2.0	0.2
Twister, Choc, Mini, Wall's Ice Cream*	1 Lolly/27g	40	1.6	150	3.5	22.0	6.0	0.9
Twister, Wall's Ice Cream*	1 Lolly/80ml	76	1.5	95	0.6	18.4	1.9	0.0
Vanilla, Mini Milk, Milk Time, Wall's Ice Cream*	1 Lolly/23g	29	0.7	127	3.8	21.0	2.9	0.3
Zoom, Nestle*	1 Lolly/58ml	54	0.4	93	0.9	20.6	0.7	0.0
INDIAN MEAL								
Banquet for One, COU, M&S*	1 Pack/500g	400	6.0	80	6.7	10.2	1.2	3.1
for Two, Hot, Takeaway, Tesco*	1 Pack/825g	1215	60.6	147	6.6	13.6	7.4	1.9
for Two, Menu, Tesco*	1 Serving/537g	811	34.4	151	6.3	17.0	6.4	0.8
INSTANT WHIP								
Strawberry Flavour, Dry, Bird's*	1oz/28g	112	1.5	400	2.5	85.0	5.4	0.4
IRN BRU								
Diet, Barr's*	1 Can/330ml	2	0.0	1	0.1	0.1	0.0	0.0
Original, Barr's*	1 Bottle/500ml	214	0.0	43	0.0	10.5	0.0	0.0

I

	Measure INFO/WEIGHT	per Measure KCAL	FAT	Nutrition Values per 100g / 100ml KCAL	PROT	CARB	FAT	FIBRE
JACKFRUIT								
Raw, Average, Flesh Only	**1 Portion/162g**	**155**	**0.5**	**95**	**1.5**	**24.4**	**0.3**	**1.6**
JALFREZI								
Chicken with Basmati Rice, Weight Watchers*	1 Pack/330g	238	1.6	72	5.0	11.8	0.5	0.5
Chicken with Lemon Pilau Rice, Finest, Tesco*	1 Pack/493g	665	21.7	135	6.9	16.4	4.4	1.8
Chicken with Pilau Basmati Rice, Frozen, Patak's*	1 Pack/400g	556	18.4	139	9.8	14.7	4.6	0.9
Chicken with Pilau Rice, Tesco*	1 Pack/460g	506	17.5	110	5.3	13.6	3.8	0.9
Chicken with Rice, Morrisons*	1 Pack/400g	564	20.8	141	7.7	15.9	5.2	1.4
Chicken with Rice, Tesco*	1 Pack/550g	732	26.4	133	5.5	17.0	4.8	1.0
Chicken, & Coriander Rice, TTD, Sainsbury's*	1 Pack/473g	501	15.1	106	6.2	13.2	3.2	3.1
Chicken, & Pilau Rice, Sainsbury's*	1 Pack/500g	600	20.5	120	6.9	13.9	4.1	1.5
Chicken, & Pilau Rice, Takeaway, Asda*	1 Pack/558g	792	23.4	142	7.0	19.0	4.2	1.3
Chicken, & Rice, Serves 1, Tesco*	1 Serving/475g	589	38.0	124	7.4	5.7	8.0	1.6
Chicken, Asda*	1 Pack/340g	415	20.4	122	10.0	7.0	6.0	1.6
Chicken, Canned, Tesco*	½ Can/200g	190	6.8	95	10.8	4.1	3.4	1.4
Chicken, Diet Chef Ltd*	1 Pack/300g	285	5.7	95	10.5	9.0	1.9	2.2
Chicken, Finest, Tesco*	1 Pack/350g	402	16.4	115	10.4	6.9	4.7	1.2
Chicken, Hot & Spicy, Sainsbury's*	½ Pack/200g	228	11.4	114	12.8	2.9	5.7	1.0
Chicken, Indian Takeaway, Tesco*	1 Serving/350g	245	8.7	70	7.4	4.3	2.5	1.8
Chicken, Thali, Meal for One, M&S*	1 Pack/500g	680	28.5	136	7.0	12.7	5.7	3.1
Chicken, with Rice, Ready Meal, Average	**1 Serving/450g**	**557**	**18.9**	**124**	**6.9**	**14.5**	**4.2**	**1.5**
Meal for One, M&S*	1 Serving/500g	700	35.0	140	6.1	13.4	7.0	3.0
Vegetable, Indian, Sainsbury's*	½ Pack/200g	156	9.0	78	2.0	5.3	4.5	4.2
JAM								
Apricot, Average	**1 Tbsp/15g**	**37**	**0.0**	**248**	**0.2**	**61.6**	**0.0**	**1.5**
Apricot, Reduced Sugar, Average	**1 Serving/20g**	**37**	**0.1**	**186**	**0.4**	**46.0**	**0.3**	**0.4**
Black Cherry, Average	**1 Tsp/5g**	**12**	**0.0**	**247**	**0.4**	**61.2**	**0.3**	**0.4**
Blackberry, ES, Asda*	1 Tbsp/15g	29	0.1	190	0.9	45.0	0.7	0.0
Blackcurrant, Average	**1 Tbsp/15g**	**38**	**0.0**	**250**	**0.2**	**62.3**	**0.0**	**1.0**
Blackcurrant, Reduced Sugar, Average	**1 Tsp/6g**	**10**	**0.0**	**178**	**0.4**	**44.4**	**0.2**	**1.0**
Blueberry & Blackberry, Baxters*	1 Tsp/15g	38	0.0	252	0.0	63.0	0.0	1.2
Blueberry, Best, Hartley's*	1 Tsp/20g	49	0.0	244	0.3	60.6	0.1	0.0
Blueberry, St Dalfour*	1 Serving/20g	46	0.0	228	0.5	56.0	0.2	2.2
Country Berries, Luxury, Baxters*	1 Tsp/15g	37	0.0	247	0.5	60.0	0.1	2.0
Damson, Extra Fruit, Best, Hartley's*	1 Tsp/5g	12	0.0	244	0.2	60.8	0.0	0.0
Fig	1 Tsp/15g	36	0.0	242	0.5	60.0	0.0	0.0
Golden Peach, Rhapsodie De Fruit, St Dalfour*	1 Tsp/10g	23	0.0	227	0.5	56.0	0.1	1.3
Kiwi & Gooseberry, 66% Fruit, Asda*	1 Serving/30g	56	0.2	187	0.5	45.0	0.5	0.0
Mixed Fruit, Average	**1 Tbsp/15g**	**38**	**0.0**	**252**	**0.3**	**63.5**	**0.0**	**0.5**
Mixed Fruit, Value, Tesco*	1 Tsp/5g	12	0.0	250	0.1	62.1	0.0	0.8
Plum, Tesco*	1 Serving/50g	130	0.0	261	0.2	64.4	0.0	0.6
Raspberry, Average	**1 Tbsp/15g**	**36**	**0.0**	**239**	**0.6**	**58.6**	**0.1**	**0.9**
Raspberry, GFY, Asda*	1 Tbsp/19g	24	0.1	124	0.6	29.0	0.6	1.5
Raspberry, Grandessa, Aldi*	1 Serving/25g	45	0.1	179	1.0	41.0	0.2	1.8
Raspberry, Reduced Sugar, Average	**1 Tsp/6g**	**10**	**0.0**	**160**	**0.5**	**39.3**	**0.2**	**0.6**
Raspberry, Reduced Sugar, Tesco*	1 Tsp/8g	14	0.0	170	1.2	39.6	0.2	1.9
Raspberry, Seedless, Average	**1 Tsp/10g**	**26**	**0.0**	**257**	**0.4**	**63.6**	**0.0**	**0.3**
Rhubarb & Ginger, Baxters*	1 Tsp/15g	40	0.0	264	0.4	65.0	0.1	0.8
Strawberry, Average	**1 Tsp/10g**	**24**	**0.0**	**243**	**0.3**	**60.2**	**0.1**	**0.7**
Strawberry, Less Sugar, Hartley's*	1 Tsp/15g	28	0.0	184	0.4	44.4	0.2	0.8
Strawberry, Reduced Sugar, Average	**1 Tbsp/15g**	**28**	**0.0**	**187**	**0.4**	**45.8**	**0.3**	**0.2**
Strawberry, Smooth, Squeezy, Hartley's*	1 Tsp/5g	10	0.0	196	0.4	48.6	0.0	0.0
Strawberry, Value, Tesco*	1 Tbsp/15g	37	0.0	246	0.3	61.2	0.0	0.5
Wild Blackberry Jelly, Baxters*	1 Tsp/15g	32	0.0	210	0.0	53.0	0.0	1.2

J

	Measure INFO/WEIGHT	per Measure KCAL	FAT	Nutrition Values per 100g / 100ml KCAL	PROT	CARB	FAT	FIBRE
JAMBALAYA								
American Style, Tesco*	1 Serving/275g	432	19.2	157	7.7	16.0	7.0	0.5
Cajun Chicken, Cooked, BGTY, Sainsbury's*	1 Pack/400g	392	6.5	103	6.6	14.6	1.7	1.6
Chicken & Prawn, LL, Waitrose*	1 Pack/390g	417	10.9	107	5.2	14.3	2.8	1.9
Chicken, Smoky Cajun, COU, M&S*	1 Pack/400g	360	4.0	90	5.9	13.9	1.0	1.5
COU, M&S*	1 Pack/400g	340	8.0	85	6.5	10.8	2.0	0.9
Ready Meal, Average	**1 Pack/450g**	**569**	**18.2**	**126**	**6.4**	**15.7**	**4.0**	**1.3**
JELLY								
Apple & Watermelon, Low Calorie, Hartley's*	1 Serving/175g	5	0.0	3	0.0	0.3	0.0	0.3
Blackberry, Unprepared, Morrisons*	1 Serving/20g	52	0.0	261	0.3	65.0	0.0	0.0
Blackcurrant & Tahitian Vanilla, M&S*	¼ Pack/143g	77	0.4	54	0.3	12.1	0.3	0.6
Blackcurrant, Made Up, Rowntree's*	¼ Jelly/140ml	100	0.1	71	1.4	16.4	0.1	0.0
Blackcurrant, Tesco*	1 Serving/100g	84	0.1	84	0.2	20.5	0.1	0.4
Bramble, Tesco*	1 Serving/100g	257	0.1	257	0.3	63.7	0.1	1.3
Crystals, Orange, Sugar Free, Bird's*	1 Sachet/12g	39	0.1	335	62.5	6.4	0.9	0.0
Crystals, Strawberry, Made Up, Tesco*	1 Serving/145g	9	0.0	6	1.3	0.3	0.0	0.0
Exotic Fruit, M&S*	1 Pot/175g	140	0.4	80	0.1	18.9	0.2	0.9
Fresh Fruit, M&S*	1 Pot/175g	131	0.2	75	0.2	18.4	0.1	0.3
Lime Flavour, Cubes, Hartley's*	1 Cube/12g	36	0.0	296	5.1	68.9	0.0	0.0
Lime, Made Up, Rowntree's*	¼ Jelly/140ml	100	0.1	71	1.4	16.4	0.1	0.0
Made Up with Water, Average	**1oz/28g**	**17**	**0.0**	**61**	**1.2**	**15.1**	**0.0**	**0.0**
Mandarin & Pineapple, Sainsbury's*	1 Pot/125g	95	0.1	76	0.2	18.9	0.1	1.2
Orange, Sugar Free, Made Up, Hartley's*	1 Serving/140ml	9	0.0	6	1.3	0.3	0.0	0.0
Orange, Sugar Free, Rowntree's*	1 Serving/140ml	8	0.0	6	1.4	0.1	0.0	0.0
Raspberry Flavour, Sugar Free, Made Up, Rowntree's*	1 Serving/140ml	9	0.0	6	1.4	0.1	0.0	0.0
Raspberry Flavour, Tesco*	1 Serving/34g	22	0.0	64	1.0	15.0	0.0	0.1
Raspberry, Unprepared, Rowntree's*	1 Serving/135g	405	0.5	300	5.6	67.3	0.4	0.0
Redcurrant, Average	**1oz/28g**	**70**	**0.0**	**250**	**0.2**	**64.4**	**0.0**	**0.0**
Strawberry & Raspberry, Sainsbury's*	½ Pot/280g	230	0.0	82	0.2	20.2	0.0	1.2
Strawberry, No Added Sugar, Hartley's*	1 Pot/115g	4	0.0	4	0.0	0.4	0.0	0.3
Sugar Free, Dry, Tesco*	1 Pack/13g	36	0.0	285	55.4	15.6	0.0	0.2
JELLY BABIES								
Bassett's*	1 Sweet/6g	20	0.0	335	3.5	79.7	0.0	0.0
M&S*	1 Pack/125g	418	0.0	334	5.2	78.0	0.0	0.0
Mini, Rowntree's*	1 Sm Bag/35g	128	0.0	366	4.6	86.9	0.0	0.0
Sainsbury's*	1 Serving/70g	247	0.5	353	4.1	82.5	0.7	0.3
JELLY BEANS								
Asda*	1 Bag/100g	364	0.4	364	0.1	90.0	0.4	0.2
Jelly Belly*	35 Beans/40g	140	0.0	350	0.0	90.0	0.0	0.0
M&S*	1 Bag/113g	407	0.0	360	0.1	89.6	0.0	0.0
	1 Serving/100g	365	0.1	365	0.1	91.2	0.1	0.1
JELLY BEARS								
Co-Op*	1 Sweet/3g	10	0.0	325	6.0	76.0	0.1	0.0
JELLY TOTS								
Rowntree's*	1 Pack/42g	145	0.0	346	0.1	86.5	0.0	0.0
JERKY								
Beef, BBQ Flavour, Texas Joe's*	1 Pack/50g	180	2.7	359	41.9	35.7	5.4	0.5
Beef, Honey BBQ, Wild West*	1 Pack/50g	150	2.4	300	34.2	29.9	4.8	0.5
Beef, Peppered, Jack Link's*	1 Serving/28g	80	0.5	286	53.6	14.3	1.8	0.0
Beef, with Tomato Relish, Graze*	1 Pack/36g	91	1.0	253	22.2	30.6	2.8	2.5
Soy, Cajun Chick'n, Vegan, Tasty Eats*	1 Pack/28g	90	3.0	321	42.9	14.3	10.7	7.1
JUICE								
Aloe Vera, Organic, Pukka Herbs*	1 Glass/50ml	1	0.1	2	0.1	0.4	0.2	100.0
Apple & Cranberry, Average	**1 Glass/250ml**	**114**	**0.0**	**46**	**0.1**	**10.2**	**0.0**	**0.0**

J

	Measure INFO/WEIGHT	per Measure		Nutrition Values per 100g / 100ml				
		KCAL	FAT	KCAL	PROT	CARB	FAT	FIBRE
JUICE								
Apple & Elderflower, Copella*	1 Glass/250ml	108	0.2	43	0.4	10.2	0.1	0.0
Apple & Mango, Average	*1 Glass/200ml*	*108*	*0.1*	*54*	*0.3*	*12.6*	*0.0*	*0.1*
Apple & Orange, Fresh Up*	1 Serving/250ml	105	0.0	42	0.0	10.3	0.0	0.0
Apple & Raspberry, Average	*1 Serving/200ml*	*89*	*0.1*	*44*	*0.4*	*10.2*	*0.0*	*0.2*
Apple & Rhubarb, Pressed, Cawston Vale*	1 Glass/200ml	92	0.8	46	0.2	9.7	0.4	0.0
Apple with Ginger, Waitrose*	1 Glass/150ml	72	0.0	48	0.3	11.0	0.0	0.5
Apple, Cloudy, Pressed, Copella*	1 Glass/100ml	46	0.0	46	0.2	10.7	0.0	0.7
Apple, Concentrate, Average	*1 Tbsp/15ml*	*45*	*0.0*	*302*	*0.0*	*73.6*	*0.2*	*0.0*
Apple, Peach & Pear, Innocent*	1 Serving/100ml	45	0.1	45	0.4	10.0	0.1	1.4
Apple, Pressed, Not from Concentrate, Co-Op*	1 Glass/100ml	45	0.1	45	0.1	10.4	0.1	0.0
Apple, Pure, Average	*1 Glass/100ml*	*47*	*0.0*	*47*	*0.1*	*11.2*	*0.0*	*0.0*
Apple, Pure, Organic, Average	*1 Serving/200ml*	*92*	*0.1*	*46*	*0.0*	*11.2*	*0.0*	*0.0*
Apple, Pure, Value, Tesco*	1 Glass/200ml	94	0.0	47	0.1	11.4	0.0	0.0
Apple, Raspberry & Grape, Pressed, Sainsbury's*	1 Serving/200ml	92	0.2	46	0.3	11.2	0.1	0.5
Beetroot, Organic, James White*	1 Glass/250ml	105	0.2	42	0.9	9.3	0.1	0.0
Breakfast, Ruby, Tropicana*	1 Glass/200ml	90	0.0	45	0.8	9.7	0.0	0.7
Breakfast, Sainsbury's*	1 Serving/200ml	94	0.2	47	0.7	11.3	0.1	0.3
Carrot, & Wild Strawberry, Kubus*	1 Glass/200ml	93	0.3	47	0.0	11.3	0.2	1.0
Carrot, Average	*1 Glass/200ml*	*48*	*0.2*	*24*	*0.5*	*5.7*	*0.1*	*0.0*
Clementine, Morrisons*	1 Serving/100ml	48	0.1	48	0.5	10.9	0.1	0.1
Cranberry, Average	*1 Bottle/250ml*	*139*	*0.2*	*56*	*0.1*	*13.4*	*0.1*	*0.3*
Cranberry, No Added Sugar, Average	*1 Glass/200ml*	*11*	*0.1*	*6*	*0.1*	*0.8*	*0.0*	*0.0*
Froot Refresh, Orange & Passion Fruit, Minute Maid*	1 Bottle/330ml	79	0.0	24	0.0	6.0	0.0	0.0
Fruit, Tropical in Sparkling Spring Water, Light, Rio*	1 Can/330ml	17	0.0	5	0.1	1.1	0.0	0.0
Fruit, Tropical, Pure Premium, Tropicana*	1 Glass/200ml	98	0.0	49	0.5	11.0	0.0	0.8
Grape, Purple, Light, Welch's*	1 Serving/100ml	27	0.3	27	0.2	6.1	0.3	0.3
Grape, Purple, Welch's*	1 Serving/200ml	136	0.0	68	0.1	16.5	0.0	0.0
Grape, Red, Average	*1 Serving/100ml*	*62*	*0.0*	*62*	*0.2*	*15.2*	*0.0*	*0.0*
Grape, White, Average	*1 Can/160ml*	*95*	*0.1*	*60*	*0.2*	*14.3*	*0.1*	*0.1*
Grapefruit, Pink, Average	*1 Glass/200ml*	*81*	*0.1*	*40*	*0.6*	*9.0*	*0.0*	*0.2*
Grapefruit, Pure, Average	*1 Glass/200ml*	*77*	*0.2*	*38*	*0.5*	*8.5*	*0.1*	*0.1*
Lemon, Fresh, Average	*1 Lemon/36ml*	*2*	*0.0*	*7*	*0.3*	*1.6*	*0.0*	*0.1*
Lime, Fresh, Average	*1 Tsp/5ml*	*0*	*0.0*	*9*	*0.4*	*1.6*	*0.1*	*0.1*
Mandarin Orange, Tropicana*	1 Serving/200ml	94	0.0	47	0.6	10.0	0.0	0.8
Mango Veggie, Naked Juice Co*	1 Serving/240ml	150	1.0	62	1.2	15.8	0.4	2.1
Mango, Peach, Papaya, Pure, Premium, Tropicana*	1 Glass/200ml	88	0.0	44	0.5	9.8	0.0	0.1
Mango, Pure, Canned	*1 Glass/250ml*	*98*	*0.5*	*39*	*0.1*	*9.8*	*0.2*	*0.0*
Multivitamin, Fruit, Vitafit, Lidl*	1 Carton/250ml	135	0.2	54	0.3	12.5	0.1	0.5
Orange & Banana, Pure, Average	*1 Glass/150ml*	*79*	*0.1*	*53*	*0.7*	*12.1*	*0.1*	*0.2*
Orange & Grapefruit, Average	*1 Glass/200ml*	*84*	*0.2*	*42*	*0.8*	*9.2*	*0.1*	*0.4*
Orange & Kiwi Fruit, Tropicana*	1 Serving/175ml	90	0.0	51	0.5	12.0	0.0	0.0
Orange & Lime, Tropicana*	1 Serving/250ml	115	0.0	46	1.1	9.4	0.0	0.6
Orange & Mango, Average	*1 Bottle/375ml*	*176*	*0.4*	*47*	*0.5*	*10.7*	*0.1*	*0.2*
Orange & Passionfruit, Tropicana*	1 Serving/200ml	94	0.0	47	0.8	10.0	0.0	0.7
Orange & Pineapple, Average	*1 Glass/120ml*	*56*	*0.6*	*46*	*0.4*	*10.5*	*0.5*	*0.5*
Orange & Raspberry, Average	*1 fl oz/30ml*	*15*	*0.0*	*50*	*0.6*	*11.4*	*0.1*	*0.2*
Orange & Raspberry, Tropicana*	1 Bottle/330ml	139	0.0	42	0.4	9.0	0.0	0.8
Orange 100% from Concentrate, Farmfoods*	1 Serving/200ml	84	0.2	42	0.6	9.1	0.1	0.1
Orange with Bits, Innocent*	1 Glass/250ml	120	0.0	48	0.8	10.9	0.0	0.3
Orange with Bits, Not From Concentrate, Tesco*	1 Glass/250ml	110	0.0	44	0.4	10.6	0.0	0.0
Orange, Freshly Squeezed, Average	*1 Serving/200ml*	*66*	*0.0*	*33*	*0.6*	*8.1*	*0.0*	*1.0*
Orange, No Bits, Innocent*	1 Glass/250ml	120	0.0	48	0.8	10.9	0.0	0.2
Orange, Pure from Concentrate, Carton, Value, Tesco*	1 Serving/250ml	115	0.0	46	0.5	10.4	0.0	0.0

J

	Measure INFO/WEIGHT	per Measure KCAL	FAT	Nutrition Values per 100g / 100ml KCAL	PROT	CARB	FAT	FIBRE
JUICE								
Orange, Pure Premium, Smooth, No Bits, Tropicana*	1 Glass/200ml	96	0.0	48	0.8	10.0	0.0	0.4
Orange, Pure with Bits, Average	*1 Glass/200ml*	*90*	*0.1*	*45*	*0.6*	*10.2*	*0.1*	*0.1*
Orange, Pure, Smooth, Average	*1 Glass/200ml*	*88*	*0.1*	*44*	*0.7*	*9.8*	*0.0*	*0.2*
Orange, Pure, Smooth, from Concentrate, Sainsbury's*	1 Serving/200ml	84	0.2	42	0.5	9.1	0.1	0.1
Orange, Pure, Tesco*	1 Glass/200ml	94	0.0	47	0.5	10.5	0.0	0.0
Orange, Red, Average	*1 Glass/250ml*	*115*	*0.1*	*46*	*0.4*	*10.7*	*0.0*	*0.2*
Orange, Smooth, Freshly Squeezed, TTD, Sainsbury's*	1 Serving/249g	132	0.0	53	0.7	11.4	0.0	0.2
Orange, Sparkling, 55, Britvic*	1 Bottle/275ml	135	0.3	49	0.3	11.3	0.1	0.1
Passion Fruit, Average	*1 Glass/200ml*	*94*	*0.2*	*47*	*0.8*	*10.7*	*0.1*	*0.0*
Peach, Mango & Passion Fruit, Sainsbury's*	1 Glass/200ml	92	0.2	46	0.3	10.3	0.1	0.5
Pear with a Hint of Ginger, Pressed, M&S*	1 Glass/250ml	125	0.2	50	0.3	11.7	0.1	0.0
Pear, Concentrate, Meridian Foods*	1 Serving/45ml	134	0.0	298	0.0	74.6	0.0	0.0
Pear, Pure, Heinz*	1 Serving/100ml	41	0.1	41	0.1	9.8	0.1	0.0
Pineapple & Coconut, Sainsbury's*	1 Glass/250ml	152	3.5	61	0.5	11.6	1.4	0.1
Pineapple & Coconut, Tesco*	1 Serving/250ml	138	1.0	55	0.4	11.3	0.4	0.0
Pineapple, Average	*1 Glass/200ml*	*100*	*0.1*	*50*	*0.3*	*11.7*	*0.1*	*0.2*
Pomegranate, Grape & Apple, Tropicana*	1 Bottle/330ml	211	0.0	64	0.2	15.5	0.0	0.6
Pomegranate, Pomegreat*	1 Glass/200ml	88	0.0	44	0.1	11.1	0.0	0.0
Prune, Average	*1 Serving/200ml*	*123*	*0.1*	*61*	*0.6*	*15.3*	*0.1*	*1.8*
Prune, Pure Squeezed, Sunraysia*	1 Glass/250ml	182	0.2	73	0.6	18.4	0.1	0.6
Simpleberry 100 Purple, Pressed, The Berry Company*	1 Glass/200ml	122	0.2	61	0.6	14.0	0.1	0.1
Sweet Carrot & Orange, Shapers, Boots*	1 Serving/250ml	100	0.4	40	0.9	8.8	0.2	0.4
Tomato from Concentrate, Sainsbury's*	1 Glass/250ml	40	0.2	16	0.7	2.7	0.1	0.7
Tomato, Average	*1 Glass/200ml*	*40*	*0.1*	*20*	*0.8*	*4.0*	*0.0*	*0.4*
Tomato, Tangy, Princes*	1 Serving/200ml	34	0.0	17	0.8	3.1	0.0	0.6
Tropical, Pure, Sainsbury's*	1 Glass/200ml	104	0.2	52	0.5	12.0	0.1	0.1
V Fusion, Passion Fruit, Mango & Carrot, V8*	1 Serving/150ml	72	0.0	48	0.3	11.8	0.0	0.4
Vegetable, Organic, James White*	1 Glass/100g	22	0.2	22	0.6	4.4	0.2	0.0
Vegetable, Original, V8*	1 Glass/150ml	26	0.2	17	0.9	2.8	0.1	0.9
JUICE DRINK								
Apple & Elderflower, Tesco*	1 Serving/200ml	76	0.0	38	0.0	9.4	0.0	0.0
Apple & Mango, CBY, Asda*	1 Carton/250ml	115	0.0	46	0.0	11.0	0.0	0.0
Apple & Pomegranate, Sparkling Water, Sainsbury's*	1 Serving/200ml	4	0.0	2	0.0	0.3	0.0	0.0
Apple & Raspberry, Sainsbury's*	1 Serving/200ml	112	0.2	56	0.1	13.8	0.1	0.1
Apple & Raspberry, Tesco*	1 Serving/300ml	138	0.0	46	0.1	11.2	0.0	0.0
Apple, No Added Sugar, Asda*	1 Glass/200ml	10	0.0	5	0.0	1.0	0.0	0.0
Apple, No Added Sugar, Light Choices, Tesco*	1 Glass/250ml	12	0.0	5	0.0	0.9	0.0	0.0
Apple, Plum & Pear, Pure Pressed, CBY, Asda*	1 Glass/200ml	92	0.0	46	0.4	10.5	0.0	0.2
Apple, Sparkling, Zing*	1 Can/250ml	92	0.0	37	0.1	8.5	0.0	0.0
Berry & Elderberry, Fusion, Oasis*	1 Bottle/375ml	11	0.0	3	0.0	0.4	0.0	0.0
Blackcurrant & Apple, Oasis*	1 Serving/500ml	90	0.0	18	0.0	4.1	0.0	0.0
Blackcurrant, Extra Light, Ribena*	1 Serving/200ml	8	0.0	4	0.0	0.5	0.0	0.0
Cherry & Cinnamon Presse, CBY, Asda*	1 Can/250ml	95	1.3	37	0.5	9.2	0.5	0.5
Cherry, No Added Sugar, Sainsbury's*	1 Carton/250ml	25	0.1	10	0.2	1.9	0.0	0.0
Cranberry & Blackberry, Ocean Spray*	1 Glass/250ml	120	0.2	48	0.1	11.3	0.1	0.2
Cranberry & Blackcurrant, Ocean Spray*	1 Bottle/500ml	265	0.0	53	0.2	12.7	0.0	0.0
Cranberry & Mango, Light, Ocean Spray*	1 Glass/250ml	22	0.0	9	0.0	2.0	0.0	0.1
Cranberry & Orange, HE, Tesco*	1 Glass/200ml	10	0.0	5	0.0	0.8	0.0	0.0
Cranberry & Pomegranate, Ocean Spray*	1 Glass/250ml	120	0.0	48	0.0	11.5	0.0	0.0
Cranberry & Raspberry, BGTY, Sainsbury's*	1 Glass/250ml	10	0.2	4	0.1	0.7	0.1	0.1
Cranberry & Raspberry, Ocean Spray*	1 Glass/200ml	96	0.0	48	0.0	11.6	0.0	0.0
Cranberry & Raspberry, Tesco*	1 Serving/200ml	96	0.0	48	0.0	11.6	0.0	0.0
Cranberry, Classic, Ocean Spray*	1 Bottle/500ml	245	0.5	49	0.1	11.7	0.1	0.1

J

JUICE DRINK

	Measure INFO/WEIGHT	per Measure KCAL	FAT	Nutrition Values per 100g / 100ml KCAL	PROT	CARB	FAT	FIBRE
Cranberry, Grape & Apple, Ocean Spray*	1 Glass/200ml	108	0.0	54	0.1	12.9	0.0	0.0
Cranberry, Juice Burst, Purity*	1 Bottle/500ml	245	0.0	49	0.0	12.0	0.0	0.0
Cranberry, Light, Classic, Ocean Spray*	1 Glass/200ml	16	0.0	8	0.0	1.4	0.0	0.0
Cranberry, M&S*	1 Serving/100ml	60	0.0	60	0.1	14.3	0.0	0.0
Cranberry, No Added Sugar, BGTY, Sainsbury's*	1 Glass/200ml	4	0.0	2	0.0	0.3	0.0	0.0
Cranberry, No Added Sugar, HL, Tesco*	1 Glass/200ml	8	0.0	4	0.0	1.1	0.0	0.0
Cranberry, Organic, Sainsbury's*	1 Serving/200ml	100	0.0	50	0.0	11.9	0.0	0.0
Cranberry, Solevita*	1 Serving/200ml	98	0.0	49	0.5	11.7	0.0	0.0
Cranberry, Tesco*	1 Serving/250ml	127	0.0	51	0.1	12.2	0.0	0.0
Cranberry, Waitrose*	1 Serving/250ml	145	0.0	58	0.1	13.9	0.0	0.1
Fruit Cocktail, Sainsbury's*	1 Glass/200ml	90	0.0	45	0.2	10.6	0.0	0.1
Fruit Shoot, My-5, Apple & Pear, Robinson's*	1 Bottle/200ml	78	0.2	39	0.2	8.9	0.1	0.0
Grape & Elderflower, White, Sparkling, Shloer*	1 Glass/200ml	74	0.0	37	0.0	9.2	0.0	0.0
Grape, Apple & Raspberry, Asda*	1 Glass/200ml	90	0.0	45	0.2	11.0	0.0	0.0
Grape, Red, Sparkling, Shloer*	1 Glass/200ml	84	0.0	42	0.0	10.4	0.0	0.0
Grape, White, Sparkling, Shloer*	1 Serving/120ml	59	0.0	49	0.0	11.6	0.0	0.0
Guava Exotic, Rubicon*	1 Carton/288ml	150	0.3	52	0.2	12.9	0.1	0.0
J2O, Apple & Mango, Britvic*	1 Bottle/275ml	83	0.0	30	0.1	6.8	0.0	0.2
J2O, Apple & Raspberry, Britvic*	1 Bottle/275ml	88	0.0	32	0.1	7.3	0.0	0.3
J2O, Apple & Watermelon, Sparkling Spritz, Britvic*	1 Serving/250ml	58	0.0	23	0.0	5.4	0.0	0.0
J2O, Glitterberry, Britvic*	1 Bottle/275ml	110	0.0	40	0.2	9.4	0.0	0.0
J2O, Midnight Forest, Orange, Cherry & Chocolate, Britvic*	1 Bottle/275ml	77	0.0	28	0.0	6.3	0.0	0.0
J2O, Orange & Passion Fruit, Britvic*	1 Bottle/275ml	88	0.0	32	0.3	7.2	0.0	0.2
J2O, Peach & Apricot, Sparkling Spritz, Britvic*	1 Serving/250ml	52	0.0	21	0.0	4.9	0.0	0.0
J2O, Pear & Raspberry, Sparkling, Spritz, Britvic*	1 Serving/250ml	55	0.0	22	0.0	5.2	0.0	0.0
Lemon & Lime, Light, Oasis*	1 Bottle/250ml	6	0.0	3	0.0	0.2	0.0	0.0
Lemon, The Feel Good Drinks Co*	1 Bottle/171ml	78	0.2	46	0.1	10.8	0.1	0.0
Lychee, Sparkling, Rubicon*	1 Can/330g	182	0.0	55	0.0	13.6	0.0	0.0
Mango & Passionfruit, Shot, Big Shotz*	1 Shot/120ml	67	0.5	56	0.0	12.1	0.4	3.4
Mango, Rubicon*	1 Serving/100ml	54	0.1	54	0.1	13.1	0.1	0.0
Mango, Sparkling, Rubicon*	1 Can/330ml	172	0.0	52	0.0	12.8	0.0	0.0
Orange, Caprisun*	1 Pouch/200ml	89	0.0	45	0.0	10.8	0.0	0.0
Orange, Carrot & Lemon, Pago*	1 Serving/200g	90	0.2	45	0.2	10.5	0.1	0.0
Orange, Juice Burst, Purity*	1 Bottle/500ml	220	0.0	44	1.0	10.2	0.0	0.0
Orange, No Added Sugar, Tesco*	1 fl oz/30ml	1	0.0	4	0.0	0.7	0.0	0.0
Orange, Value, Tesco*	1 Glass/250ml	32	0.0	13	0.0	3.3	0.0	0.0
Orange, Zero, Vive, Aldi*	1 Serving/200g	2	1.0	1	0.5	0.5	0.5	0.5
Passion Fruit, Exotic, Rubicon*	1 Serving/200ml	110	0.0	55	0.1	13.6	0.0	0.0
Peach & Passionfruit Fruit, Sunmagic*	1 Serving/330ml	172	0.0	52	0.3	13.0	0.0	0.1
Peach, Passion Fruit, Extra Light, Oasis*	1 Bottle/500ml	18	0.0	4	0.0	0.6	0.0	0.0
Pineapple & Grapefruit, Shapers, Boots*	1 Bottle/500ml	10	0.5	2	0.1	0.2	0.1	0.0
Pink Grapefruit, Juice Burst, Purity*	1 Bottle/500ml	210	0.0	42	0.4	10.0	0.0	0.0
Raspberry & Pear, Tesco*	1 Serving/250ml	118	0.0	47	0.0	11.3	0.0	0.0
Spirit, Lemon & Grapefruit, Tropicana*	1 Bottle/400ml	184	0.0	46	0.3	10.4	0.0	0.6
Summer Fruits, Fresh, Tesco*	1 Glass/250ml	112	0.2	45	0.1	10.8	0.1	0.3
Summer Fruits, Oasis*	1 Bottle/500ml	90	0.0	18	0.0	4.2	0.0	0.0
Tropical Fruit, Tesco*	1 Glass/250ml	118	0.0	47	0.0	11.4	0.0	0.0
Tropical, Be Light, Aldi*	1 Glass/250mls	62	0.2	25	0.2	5.4	0.1	0.2
Tropical, No Added Sugar, Tesco*	1 Carton/250ml	12	0.0	5	0.0	1.1	0.0	0.0
White Cranberry & Lychee, Ocean Spray*	1 Glass/200ml	86	0.0	43	0.0	11.5	0.0	0.0
White Grape & Peach, Sainsbury's*	1 Glass/250ml	95	0.2	38	0.2	9.0	0.1	0.1

J

INFO/WEIGHT	Measure	per Measure		Nutrition Values per 100g / 100ml				
		KCAL	FAT	KCAL	PROT	CARB	FAT	FIBRE

KALE

	INFO/WEIGHT	KCAL	FAT	KCAL	PROT	CARB	FAT	FIBRE
Curly, Boiled in Salted Water, Average	1 Sm Serving/60g	14	0.7	24	2.4	1.0	1.1	2.8
Curly, Raw, Average	1 Serving/90g	25	1.2	28	2.9	1.2	1.4	2.6

KANGAROO

	INFO/WEIGHT	KCAL	FAT	KCAL	PROT	CARB	FAT	FIBRE
Raw, Average	1 Serving/200g	196	2.0	98	22.0	1.0	1.0	0.0
Steak, Grilled, Average	1 Fillet/150g	198	1.8	132	30.0	0.0	1.2	0.0

KANGAROO

	INFO/WEIGHT	KCAL	FAT	KCAL	PROT	CARB	FAT	FIBRE
Leg, Steaks, Kraken Meat Gmbh*	1 Steak/150g	137	1.7	91	20.2	0.0	1.1	0.0

KEBAB

	INFO/WEIGHT	KCAL	FAT	KCAL	PROT	CARB	FAT	FIBRE
BBQ Pork, Sainsbury's*	1 Serving/90g	65	2.2	72	11.0	1.4	2.4	0.9
Beef & Pepper, Kofta, Waitrose*	1 Kebab/138g	223	13.9	162	14.8	2.9	10.1	0.6
Beef with Onion, Dulano, Lidl*	1 Serving/100g	224	16.0	224	18.0	2.0	16.0	0.0
Beef, Hot & Spicy, Tesco*	1 Kebab/41g	111	8.4	270	15.7	4.4	20.6	1.6
Beef, Kofta, Uncooked, Tesco*	1 Kebab/73g	163	12.5	225	14.0	3.2	17.3	1.2
Cajun Salmon, Tesco*	1 Kebab/75g	100	3.2	133	19.8	3.9	4.2	1.3
Chicken Tikka, Oakhurst, Aldi*	1 Kebab/59g	52	0.7	88	14.0	5.1	1.2	0.5
Chicken, & Chorizo, Waitrose*	1 Kebab/70g	135	8.2	195	20.4	1.3	11.8	1.1
Chicken, & Pineapple, Aldi*	1 Kebab/85g	89	2.6	105	13.9	5.3	3.1	0.0
Chicken, & Pineapple, Caribbean Style, Iceland*	1 Kebab/44g	41	0.6	93	11.6	8.7	1.4	1.4
Chicken, & Sausage with Teriyaki Sauce, Asda*	1 Serving/110g	257	15.4	234	17.0	10.0	14.0	1.0
Chicken, Barbecue, Sainsbury's*	1 Pack/200g	238	3.4	119	24.4	1.5	1.7	1.8
Chicken, Breast, Mediterranean, Sainsbury's*	1 Kebab/65g	73	2.1	113	16.5	4.6	3.2	0.6
Chicken, Chilli & Lime, Breast Fillets, Sainsbury's*	1 Kebab/77g	120	0.7	156	29.9	6.2	0.9	0.3
Chicken, Citrus Tikka, Mini, Sainsbury's*	1 Serving/48g	72	1.1	151	30.3	2.7	2.3	0.2
Chicken, Fillets, Mini with a Tikka Marinade, Sainsbury's*	1 Kebab/25g	41	0.8	164	33.4	0.6	3.1	0.1
Chicken, Shish in Pitta Bread with Salad	1 Kebab/250g	388	10.2	155	13.5	17.2	4.1	1.0
Chicken, Shish, Meat Only, Average	1 Kebab/250g	312	5.2	125	25.7	0.9	2.1	0.1
Chicken, Thigh, Sticky Barbecue, M&S*	1 Kebab/100g	160	7.5	160	15.6	7.4	7.5	0.8
Chicken, Thin Sliced, Heat 'n' Eat, Asda*	½ Pack/50g	92	6.0	184	15.0	3.9	12.0	1.1
Chicken, with Sweet Chilli Sauce, Finest, Tesco*	½ Pack/175g	242	1.4	138	17.9	14.7	0.8	1.2
Chicken, with Sweet Chilli Sauce, M&S*	1 Serving/165g	228	1.3	138	17.9	14.7	0.8	1.2
Chinese Chicken, Tesco*	1 Kebab/21g	37	1.6	175	19.5	5.8	7.8	0.5
Citrus Tikka Chicken Breast, Sainsbury's*	1 Kebab/61g	79	0.3	129	25.6	5.4	0.5	0.9
Doner, Iceland*	1 Serving/152g	268	7.1	176	9.2	24.4	4.6	2.4
Green Thai Chicken, Waitrose*	1 Serving/180g	223	7.2	124	20.5	1.4	4.0	1.4
Halloumi & Vegetable, Waitrose*	1 Kebab/127g	235	21.6	185	5.6	2.2	17.0	2.4
Lamb Shami with a Mint Raita Dip, M&S*	½ Pack/90g	189	12.1	210	12.8	9.7	13.4	3.5
Lamb with Halloumi Cheese & Olives, Waitrose*	1 Kebab/75g	123	6.2	164	20.0	2.4	8.3	0.2
Lamb with Mint, Tesco*	1 Serving/80g	192	13.4	240	16.0	5.5	16.7	0.4
Lamb, Greek Style, Lakeland*	1 Serving/100g	196	15.6	196	11.8	1.9	15.6	0.0
Lamb, Greek Style, Sainsbury's*	1 Serving/70g	196	15.3	282	16.1	4.9	22.0	1.8
Lamb, Kofta, Citrus Tikka, Sainsbury's*	1 Kebab/84g	199	11.6	235	18.1	9.8	13.7	2.6
Lamb, Kofta, Indian Style, Waitrose*	1 Kebab/125g	266	19.8	213	12.3	5.5	15.8	1.6
Lamb, Minted, Ashfield Farm, Aldi*	1 Kebab/54g	137	9.2	254	18.5	5.7	17.0	0.0
Lamb, Shish, Sainsbury's*	1 Kebab/85g	178	11.3	210	19.7	2.8	13.3	0.7
Lamb, Shish, Waitrose*	1 Kebab/56g	114	7.1	203	15.3	6.8	12.7	1.1
Lamb, Shoulder, M&S*	½ Pack/250g	312	10.8	125	20.4	0.9	4.3	1.7
Lemon & Ginger Chicken, Delicatezze, Waitrose*	1 Kebab/25g	50	2.8	201	24.5	0.3	11.3	2.7
Pork & Pepper, BBQ, Sainsbury's*	1 Kebab/41g	65	2.2	158	24.1	3.1	5.4	1.9
Salmon, Hot & Spicy, Tesco*	1 Kebab/75g	88	2.2	118	22.0	1.1	2.9	0.0
Spicy Tomato Creole King Prawn, M&S*	1 Pack/240g	240	7.9	100	14.3	2.9	3.3	0.7
Sweetcorn, Tesco*	1 Kebab/130g	74	1.3	57	2.0	9.9	1.0	0.9
Turkey with Chinese Style Dressing, Sainsbury's*	1 Kebab/54g	84	2.7	157	21.4	6.4	5.1	1.7
Vegetable, Asda*	1 Kebab/40g	25	1.7	63	1.8	4.5	4.3	2.4

K

	Measure INFO/WEIGHT	per Measure KCAL	FAT	Nutrition Values per 100g / 100ml KCAL	PROT	CARB	FAT	FIBRE
KEBAB								
Vegetable, Sainsbury's*	1 Kebab/100g	36	0.5	36	1.5	6.4	0.5	1.2
KEDGEREE								
356, Oakhouse Foods Ltd.*	1 Meal/400g	432	15.6	108	8.2	9.8	3.9	0.6
Average	*1oz/28g*	*48*	*2.4*	*171*	*15.9*	*7.8*	*8.7*	*0.1*
COU, M&S*	1 Pack/370g	388	8.1	105	7.6	13.7	2.2	2.1
Smoked Haddock, Big Dish, M&S*	1 Pack/450g	585	22.5	130	8.5	13.0	5.0	1.9
KETCHUP								
Barbeque, Asda*	1 Tbsp/15g	20	0.0	136	0.9	33.0	0.0	0.0
BBQ, Heinz*	1 Serving/10g	14	0.0	137	1.3	31.3	0.3	0.3
Mild Chilli, Twisted, Heinz*	1 Tbsp/15g	16	0.0	108	1.0	24.9	0.2	0.7
Tomato with Indian Spices, Heinz*	1 Tbsp/15g	17	0.1	114	1.1	24.8	0.4	0.8
Tomato, Average	*1 Tsp/5g*	*6*	*0.0*	*120*	*1.5*	*28.1*	*0.2*	*0.8*
Tomato, Branston, Crosse & Blackwell*	1 Serving/15g	18	0.0	119	1.4	28.1	0.0	0.6
Tomato, Everyday Value, Tesco*	1 Tbsp/15ml	21	0.0	140	0.9	32.6	0.2	0.5
Tomato, Morrisons*	1 Serving/15g	16	0.0	110	1.6	24.0	0.2	1.6
Tomato, Reduced Sugar, Average	*1 Tbsp/10g*	*9*	*0.1*	*87*	*2.0*	*16.9*	*1.2*	*0.9*
KIDNEY								
Lamb, Fried, Average	*1oz/28g*	*53*	*2.9*	*188*	*23.7*	*0.0*	*10.3*	*0.0*
Lamb, Raw, Average	*1oz/28g*	*25*	*0.7*	*91*	*17.0*	*0.0*	*2.6*	*0.0*
Ox, Raw	*1oz/28g*	*22*	*0.5*	*77*	*15.1*	*0.0*	*1.8*	*0.0*
Ox, Stewed	*1oz/28g*	*39*	*1.2*	*138*	*24.5*	*0.0*	*4.4*	*0.0*
Pig, Fried	*1oz/28g*	*57*	*2.7*	*202*	*29.2*	*0.0*	*9.5*	*0.0*
Pig, Raw	*1oz/28g*	*22*	*0.7*	*77*	*14.0*	*0.0*	*2.4*	*0.0*
Pig, Stewed	*1oz/28g*	*43*	*1.7*	*153*	*24.4*	*0.0*	*6.1*	*0.0*
Veal, Raw, Average	*1 Serving/100g*	*99*	*3.1*	*99*	*15.8*	*0.8*	*3.1*	*0.0*
KIPPER								
Baked, Average	*1oz/28g*	*57*	*3.2*	*205*	*25.5*	*0.0*	*11.4*	*0.0*
Fillets in Brine, John West*	1 Can/140g	269	16.8	192	21.0	0.0	12.0	0.0
Fillets in Sunflower Oil, John West*	1 Can/140g	321	23.8	229	19.0	0.0	17.0	0.0
Fillets, Raw, Average	*1 Serving/200g*	*384*	*29.1*	*192*	*14.5*	*0.0*	*14.6*	*0.0*
Fillets, Smoked, TTD, Sainsbury's*	1 Serving/100g	255	19.4	255	20.1	0.1	19.4	0.0
Grilled, Average	*1oz/28g*	*71*	*5.4*	*255*	*20.1*	*0.0*	*19.4*	*0.0*
Smoked, Average	*1 Serving/150g*	*322*	*23.0*	*214*	*18.9*	*0.0*	*15.4*	*0.0*
Whole, with Bone, Grilled, Average	*1 Serving/100g*	*161*	*12.2*	*161*	*12.7*	*0.0*	*12.2*	*0.0*
KIT KAT								
2 Finger, Nestle*	2 Fingers/21g	107	5.3	512	6.0	63.5	25.5	2.1
4 Finger, Nestle*	4 Fingers/45g	233	11.7	513	5.9	63.3	25.7	2.1
Caramac, 4 Finger, Nestle*	4 Fingers/49g	259	14.1	532	5.9	61.9	29.0	0.6
Chunky, Caramel, Nestle*	1 Bar/48g	259	15.3	539	5.2	58.6	31.8	0.0
Chunky, Double Caramel, Nestle*	½ Bar/21g	109	5.8	520	6.5	61.0	27.6	1.0
Chunky, Nestle*	1 Bar/48g	248	12.6	516	5.9	62.5	26.3	2.1
Chunky, Orange, Nestle*	1 Bar/48g	247	12.5	515	5.8	62.0	26.1	0.0
Chunky, Peanut, Nestle*	1 Bar/50g	268	15.8	537	8.4	54.9	31.5	0.0
Chunky, Snack Size, Nestle*	1 Bar/26g	133	7.1	513	6.6	60.4	27.2	1.1
Cookies & Cream, Nestle*	2 Finger Bar/21g	107	5.2	510	6.3	64.0	25.0	1.4
Cookies & Cream, Snap & Share, Nestle*	1 Row/16g	81	4.2	522	7.2	61.5	26.9	1.5
Editions, Seville Orange, Nestle*	1 Bar/45g	223	10.4	496	4.6	69.3	23.0	0.8
Kubes, Nestle*	1 Pack/50g	258	13.8	515	5.9	60.9	27.5	1.0
Low Carb, 2 Finger, Nestle*	2 Fingers/21g	92	6.6	438	9.2	28.3	31.3	1.3
Mini, Nestle*	1 Bar/15g	75	3.9	502	7.5	59.4	26.0	0.0
Mint, 4 Finger, Nestle*	4 Fingers/48g	244	12.7	508	6.0	61.5	26.4	1.1
Orange, 2 Finger, Nestle*	2 Fingers/21g	107	5.6	507	5.5	61.7	26.5	0.0
White, Chunky, Nestle*	1 Bar/53g	276	14.6	521	8.3	60.3	27.5	0.7

K

	Measure	per Measure		Nutrition Values per 100g / 100ml				
	INFO/WEIGHT	KCAL	FAT	KCAL	PROT	CARB	FAT	FIBRE
KIWI BERRY								
Tesco*	1 Serving/80g	70	0.5	87	1.2	17.6	0.6	3.2
KIWI FRUIT								
Fresh, Raw, Flesh & Seeds, Average	*1 Kiwi/60g*	*29*	*0.3*	*49*	*1.1*	*10.6*	*0.5*	*1.9*
Hayward, Perfectly Ripe, Waitrose*	1 Fruit/85g	45	0.4	53	1.1	10.6	0.5	3.0
Weighed with Skin, Average	*1 Kiwi/60g*	*25*	*0.3*	*42*	*0.9*	*9.1*	*0.4*	*1.6*
KOHLRABI								
Boiled in Salted Water	*1oz/28g*	*5*	*0.1*	*18*	*1.2*	*3.1*	*0.2*	*1.9*
Raw	*1oz/28g*	*5*	*0.0*	*16*	*1.1*	*2.6*	*0.1*	*1.5*
KORMA								
Chicken with Pilau Rice, Asda*	1 Serving/350g	735	49.0	210	12.0	9.0	14.0	2.0
Chicken with Pilau Rice, Co-Op*	1 Pack/400g	520	20.4	130	10.3	10.7	5.1	2.6
Chicken with Pilau Rice, Sharwood's*	1 Pack/375g	489	16.2	130	5.2	17.1	4.3	1.2
Chicken, & Basmati Rice, Tesco*	1 Pot/350g	588	32.6	168	4.3	16.9	9.3	2.3
Chicken, & Pilau Rice, Morrisons*	1 Pack/450g	889	48.2	198	9.4	15.9	10.7	1.4
Chicken, & Pilau Rice, Tesco*	1 Serving/460g	722	45.1	157	5.6	11.5	9.8	1.3
Chicken, & White Rice, BGTY, Frozen, Sainsbury's*	1 Pack/375g	341	3.8	91	5.6	14.9	1.0	0.5
Chicken, Fresh, Chilled, Tesco*	1 Pack/350g	819	60.9	234	13.1	6.3	17.4	2.3
Chicken, Indian Meal for 2, Finest, Tesco*	½ Pack/200g	348	24.0	174	10.3	6.2	12.0	2.5
Chicken, Indian Takeaway for One, Sainsbury's*	1 Serving/300g	498	30.9	166	13.0	5.3	10.3	1.6
Chicken, Indian Takeaway, Iceland*	1 Pack/400g	656	44.0	164	11.8	4.5	11.0	1.4
Chicken, Indian Takeaway, Tesco*	½ Pack/175g	222	13.5	127	9.0	5.5	7.7	1.8
Chicken, Morrisons*	1 Pack/350g	707	46.6	202	13.6	7.0	13.3	0.7
Chicken, Tesco*	1 Pack/350g	620	41.3	177	10.8	6.8	11.8	0.6
Chicken, Waitrose*	1 Pack/400g	680	46.8	170	13.7	2.4	11.7	1.9
Chicken, with Rice, Ready Meal, Average	*1 Sm Pack/350g*	*648*	*30.4*	*185*	*8.4*	*18.1*	*8.7*	*1.7*
Chicken, with Rice, Ready Meal, Healthy Range	*1 Serving/400g*	*450*	*8.2*	*112*	*7.3*	*16.1*	*2.1*	*1.2*
Vegetable & Rice, Tesco*	1 Pack/450g	621	26.6	138	2.9	18.3	5.9	1.6
KRISPROLLS								
Cracked Wheat, Original, Pagen*	1 Krisproll/13g	48	0.9	380	12.0	67.0	7.0	9.0
Golden, Swedish Toasts, Pagen*	1 Krisproll/12g	48	1.0	400	11.0	69.0	8.5	5.0
Swedish Toasts, Wholegrain, Pagen*	1 Toast/13g	51	0.8	390	11.0	67.0	6.5	8.5
KULFI								
Average	*1oz/28g*	*119*	*11.2*	*424*	*5.4*	*11.8*	*39.9*	*0.6*
KUMQUATS								
Raw	*1oz/28g*	*12*	*0.1*	*43*	*0.9*	*9.3*	*0.5*	*3.8*
KUNG PO								
Chicken, Sainsbury's*	½ Pack/175g	131	4.4	75	9.2	4.0	2.5	1.0
Chicken, Waitrose*	1 Pack/350g	318	3.9	91	8.2	12.1	1.1	1.2
Chicken, with Egg Fried Rice, Asda*	1 Pack/450g	688	22.5	153	6.0	21.0	5.0	1.0

	Measure INFO/WEIGHT	per Measure		Nutrition Values per 100g / 100ml				
		KCAL	FAT	KCAL	PROT	CARB	FAT	FIBRE
LAGER								
Alcohol Free, Becks*	1 Serving/275ml	55	0.0	20	0.7	5.0	0.0	0.0
Amstel, Heineken*	1 Pint/568ml	227	0.0	40	0.5	3.0	0.0	0.0
Average	*½ Pint/284ml*	*117*	*0.0*	*41*	*0.3*	*3.1*	*0.0*	*0.0*
Basics, Sainsbury's*	1 Can/440g	71	0.0	16	0.0	1.0	0.0	0.0
Becks*	1 Can/275ml	113	0.0	41	0.0	3.0	0.0	0.0
Boston, Samuel Adams*	1 Bottle/355ml	160	0.0	45	0.0	0.0	0.0	0.0
Bottled, Brahma*	1 Bottle/330ml	125	0.0	38	0.0	0.0	0.0	0.0
Budweiser, 66, Anheuser-Busch*	1 Bottle/330ml	102	0.0	31	0.0	0.0	0.0	0.0
C2, Carling*	½ Pint/284ml	80	0.0	28	0.0	3.5	0.0	0.0
Can, Carlsberg*	1 Can/440ml	141	0.0	32	0.0	2.0	0.0	0.0
Draught, Carling*	1 Pint/568ml	189	0.0	33	0.0	1.4	0.0	0.0
Export, Carlsberg*	1 Can/440ml	185	0.0	42	0.4	2.8	0.0	0.4
Foster's*	1 Pint/568ml	193	0.0	34	0.0	3.1	0.0	0.0
German, Low Alcohol, Sainsbury's*	1 Bottle/330ml	92	0.3	28	0.4	5.9	0.1	0.1
Gold, Foster's, Heineken*	1 Can/440ml	145	0.0	33	0.3	1.2	0.0	0.0
Grolsch*	1 Sm Can/330ml	145	0.0	44	0.0	2.2	0.0	0.0
Heineken v 5, Heineken*	1 Pint/568ml	256	0.0	45	0.5	3.0	0.0	0.0
Heineken*, 5%, Heineken*	1 Bottle/250ml	110	0.0	44	0.4	3.4	0.0	0.0
Kaliber, Guinness*	1 Can/440ml	110	0.0	25	0.2	6.0	0.0	0.0
Light, Coors*	1 Pint/500ml	150	0.0	30	0.3	1.5	0.0	0.0
Light, Corona*	1 Bottle/330ml	105	0.0	32	1.5	0.0	0.0	0.0
Low Alcohol	1 Can/440ml	44	0.0	10	0.2	1.5	0.0	0.0
Pils, Holsten*	1 Can/440ml	167	0.0	38	0.3	2.4	0.0	0.0
Pilsner, Efes*	1 Can/500ml	226	0.0	45	0.0	7.6	0.0	0.0
Premier, Kronenbourg*	½ Pint/284ml	136	0.0	48	0.0	0.0	0.0	0.0
Premium	1 Can/440ml	260	0.0	59	0.3	2.4	0.0	0.0
Premium, French, Biere Speciale, Tesco*	1 Serving/250ml	105	0.0	42	0.3	3.3	0.0	0.0
Premium, Light, Amstel*	1 Can/355ml	95	0.0	27	0.0	1.4	0.0	0.0
Premium, San Miguel*	1 Bottle/330ml	148	0.0	45	0.3	3.7	0.0	0.0
Shandy, Traditional Style, Asda*	1 Serving/200ml	44	0.0	22	0.0	4.6	0.0	0.0
Tuborg Green, Carlsberg*	1 Serving/200ml	78	0.0	39	0.5	2.5	0.0	0.0
Vier, Becks*	1 Bottle/275ml	110	0.0	40	0.0	3.0	0.0	0.0
LAMB								
Breast, Lean, Roasted, Average	*1 Serving/100g*	*273*	*18.5*	*273*	*26.7*	*0.0*	*18.5*	*0.0*
Chops, Average	*1 Chop/82g*	*190*	*13.4*	*231*	*20.6*	*0.4*	*16.4*	*0.0*
Chops, Leg, De-boned, Grilled, Simply Cook, Tesco*	1 Chop/105g	330	17.7	314	39.2	0.0	16.9	0.0
Chops, Minted, Average	*1 Chop/100g*	*260*	*15.1*	*260*	*25.9*	*5.1*	*15.1*	*0.3*
Cutlets, Neck, Raw, Lean & Fat, Weighed with Bone	*1 Pack 210g*	*359*	*31.7*	*171*	*8.8*	*0.0*	*15.1*	*0.0*
Cutlets, TTD, Sainsbury's*	1 Serving/100g	238	13.8	238	28.5	0.0	13.8	0.0
Diced, From Supermarket, Healthy Range, Average	*½ Pack/200g*	*277*	*8.9*	*138*	*24.6*	*0.1*	*4.5*	*0.0*
Escalope, Asda*	1 Serving/100g	173	5.0	173	32.0	0.0	5.0	0.0
Escalope, British, HL, Tesco*	1 Piece/95g	104	3.1	110	20.1	0.0	3.3	0.0
Grill Steak, Average	*1oz/28g*	*70*	*4.7*	*250*	*20.2*	*4.4*	*16.9*	*0.4*
Grill Steak, Prime, Average	*1 Steak/63g*	*197*	*16.1*	*312*	*18.5*	*2.0*	*25.5*	*0.1*
Grill Steak, Rosemary & Mint, Tesco*	1 Steak/62g	172	10.9	277	24.4	5.6	17.6	1.8
Leg, Joint, Raw, Average	*1 Joint/510g*	*858*	*45.5*	*168*	*20.9*	*1.4*	*8.9*	*0.2*
Leg, Roasted, Lean & Fat, Average	*1oz/28g*	*66*	*3.8*	*237*	*28.6*	*0.0*	*13.6*	*0.0*
Leg, Roasted, Lean, Average	*1oz/28g*	*58*	*2.7*	*206*	*29.9*	*0.0*	*9.6*	*0.0*
Leg, Welsh Hill Carvery, TTD, Sainsbury's*	1 Serving/100g	187	12.3	187	19.0	0.0	12.3	0.0
Loin, Chop, Grilled, Lean & Fat, Weighed with Bone	1 Serving/100g	193	14.0	193	16.8	0.0	14.0	0.0
Loin, Chops, Raw, Lean & Fat, Weighed with Bone	*1 Serving/100g*	*216*	*17.9*	*216*	*13.7*	*0.0*	*17.9*	*0.0*
Mince, Average	*1oz/28g*	*58*	*4.2*	*207*	*17.6*	*0.5*	*14.8*	*0.0*
Mince, Extra Lean, Sainsbury's*	1 Serving/225g	324	11.9	144	24.1	0.0	5.3	0.1

L

	Measure INFO/WEIGHT	per Measure KCAL	FAT	Nutrition Values per 100g / 100ml KCAL	PROT	CARB	FAT	FIBRE

LAMB

	Measure INFO/WEIGHT	KCAL	FAT	KCAL	PROT	CARB	FAT	FIBRE
Mince, Lean, Raw, Tesco*	1 Pack/400g	860	63.6	215	17.6	0.0	15.9	0.0
Neck Fillet, Lean, Raw	*1 Serving/100g*	*232*	*17.6*	*232*	*18.4*	*0.0*	*17.6*	*0.0*
Pulled, Spiced, with Garlic Mayo & Chilli Sauce, Tesco*	½ Pack/117g	300	20.2	256	21.1	3.8	17.3	0.5
Rack, Raw, Lean & Fat	*1oz/28g*	*79*	*6.7*	*283*	*17.3*	*0.0*	*23.8*	*0.0*
Rack, Raw, Lean Only, Weighed with Bone	*1oz/28g*	*21*	*1.1*	*73*	*8.6*	*0.0*	*4.0*	*0.0*
Rack, Roasted, Lean	*1oz/28g*	*63*	*3.6*	*225*	*27.1*	*0.0*	*13.0*	*0.0*
Rack, Roasted, Lean & Fat	*1oz/28g*	*102*	*8.4*	*363*	*23.0*	*0.0*	*30.1*	*0.0*
Shoulder, Cooked, Lean & Fat	*1oz/28g*	*84*	*6.3*	*301*	*24.4*	*0.0*	*22.5*	*0.0*
Shoulder, Fillet, Average	*1oz/28g*	*66*	*5.1*	*235*	*17.6*	*0.0*	*18.3*	*0.0*
Shoulder, Raw, Average	*1oz/28g*	*70*	*5.7*	*248*	*16.8*	*0.0*	*20.2*	*0.0*
Shoulder, Roasted, Whole, Lean	*1oz/28g*	*61*	*3.4*	*218*	*27.2*	*0.0*	*12.1*	*0.0*
Steak, Leg, Raw, Average	*1 Steak/150g*	*169*	*5.5*	*112*	*20.0*	*0.0*	*3.6*	*0.0*
Steak, Minted, Average	*1 Steak/125g*	*212*	*9.0*	*170*	*22.7*	*3.4*	*7.2*	*0.9*
Steak, Raw, Average	*1 Steak/140g*	*190*	*7.6*	*136*	*21.7*	*0.2*	*5.4*	*0.0*
Stewing, Raw, Lean & Fat	*1oz/28g*	*57*	*3.5*	*203*	*22.5*	*0.0*	*12.6*	*0.0*
Stewing, Stewed, Lean	*1oz/28g*	*67*	*4.1*	*240*	*26.6*	*0.0*	*14.8*	*0.0*
Stewing, Stewed, Lean & Fat	*1oz/28g*	*78*	*5.6*	*279*	*24.4*	*0.0*	*20.1*	*0.0*

LAMB IN

Garlic & Rosemary Gravy, Shank, Asda*	1 Shank/280g	451	23.2	161	19.8	1.7	8.3	0.5
Minted Gravy, Shank, Iceland*	1 Shank/350g	651	45.2	186	15.0	2.4	12.9	0.5
Rich Minted Gravy, Shank, Morrisons*	1 Pack/400g	612	26.4	153	18.8	5.2	6.6	0.0

LAMB WITH

Chunky Vegetables, Shanks, Braised, M&S*	½ Pack/425g	808	38.2	190	24.7	2.0	9.0	0.7
Mint Glaze & Redcurrant Sauce, Steaks, Leg, Asda*	½ Pack/145g	247	8.7	170	18.0	11.0	6.0	0.5
Roasted Vegetables, Shank, M&S*	½ Pack/420g	660	30.6	157	14.9	8.3	7.3	0.7
Rosemary Gravy, Shank, Sainsbury's*	1 Serving/200g	204	8.2	102	13.2	3.1	4.1	0.3

LARD

Average	*1oz/28g*	*249*	*27.7*	*891*	*0.0*	*0.0*	*99.0*	*0.0*

LASAGNE

Al Forno, Beef, with a Chianti Classico Ragu, M&S*	1 Pack/400g	640	38.0	160	8.2	10.7	9.5	2.8
Al Forno, Finest, Tesco*	1 Pack/400g	700	38.4	175	8.4	13.3	9.6	1.0
Al Forno, TTD, Sainsbury's*	1 Pack/383g	571	30.3	149	8.6	10.9	7.9	2.1
Alla Bolognese, Weight Watchers*	1 Pack/350g	416	8.8	119	8.0	16.0	2.5	0.0
Asda*	1 Pack/398g	502	23.9	126	7.3	10.6	6.0	1.1
Beef & Chunky Vegetable, HL, Tesco*	1 Pack/340g	354	9.5	104	5.9	13.8	2.8	1.2
Beef & Red Wine, & Seasoned Wedges, Weight Watchers*	1 Pack/400g	400	13.2	100	5.1	12.5	3.3	0.2
Beef, BGTY, Sainsbury's*	1 Pack/390g	376	8.5	102	6.2	13.2	2.3	1.7
Beef, Cooked, Italian, Sainsbury's*	1 Serving/375g	555	32.2	148	7.8	6.8	8.6	6.7
Beef, Frozen, Co-Op*	1 Pack/340g	388	15.6	114	7.5	10.7	4.6	1.4
Beef, Frozen, Tesco*	1 Pack/450g	608	25.2	135	7.5	12.6	5.6	0.8
Beef, Great Stuff, Asda*	1 Pack/300g	327	12.0	109	6.7	11.0	4.0	1.1
Beef, Italian, Classic, Tesco*	1 Pack/600g	948	51.0	158	7.5	12.7	8.5	0.5
Beef, Italian, M Kitchen, Morrisons*	1 Pack/400g	551	24.5	137	7.8	11.8	6.1	2.0
Beef, Ready Meal, Average	*1 Serving/400g*	*553*	*24.0*	*138*	*8.2*	*12.7*	*6.0*	*1.4*
Beef, Ready Meals, Waitrose*	1 Pack/400g	444	20.5	111	5.8	10.4	5.1	0.8
Bolognese, & Vegetable, Weight Watchers*	1 Pack/300g	279	7.8	93	5.0	12.4	2.6	0.0
Bolognese, Co-Op*	1 Pack/500g	758	35.5	152	8.1	13.8	7.1	0.0
Bolognese, Lidl*	1 Serving/200g	336	18.0	168	8.0	13.7	9.0	0.0
Bolognese, Trattorie Alfredo*	1 Serving/125g	204	11.2	163	9.0	13.0	9.0	0.0
Charlie Bigham's*	½ Pack/344g	557	29.2	162	8.5	11.3	8.5	0.7
Chicken, Italian, Sainsbury's*	1 Pack/450g	549	18.9	122	8.4	12.6	4.2	0.5
Chicken, Italiano, Tesco*	1 Serving/450g	490	13.5	109	8.6	12.0	3.0	0.6
Chicken, Mushroom & Asparagus, Finest, Tesco*	½ Pack/300g	360	16.2	120	7.6	10.2	5.4	0.8

L

LASAGNE	Measure INFO/WEIGHT	per Measure KCAL	FAT	Nutrition Values per 100g / 100ml KCAL	PROT	CARB	FAT	FIBRE
Chicken, Ready Meals, Waitrose*	1 Pack/300g	411	19.8	137	6.3	13.0	6.6	0.9
Classic, Deep Filled, M&S*	1 Pack/400g	760	47.6	190	10.0	11.2	11.9	0.6
ES, Asda*	½ Pack/291g	416	20.4	143	7.0	13.0	7.0	0.3
Frozen, You Count, LL, Waitrose*	1 Pack/380g	359	10.3	94	5.0	12.2	2.7	0.6
GFY, Asda*	1 Pack/410g	344	8.2	84	5.5	11.0	2.0	0.3
Italian, Fresh, Chilled, Sainsbury's*	1 Pack/400g	480	22.0	120	10.1	7.5	5.5	1.4
Italian, Tesco*	1 Sm Pack/400g	540	28.8	135	6.3	11.1	7.2	1.5
Kit, Original, No Meat, Dolmio*	1 Serving/213g	279	7.5	131	3.3	20.6	3.5	0.0
Low Fat, Co-Op*	1 Pack/300g	255	9.0	85	6.0	10.0	3.0	1.0
Low Saturated Fat, Waitrose*	1 Pack/400g	312	6.0	78	4.7	11.4	1.5	0.4
M&S*	1/3 Pack/333g	466	24.6	140	8.5	10.4	7.4	0.9
Minced Beef, Great Stuff, Asda*	1 Pack/300g	333	13.2	111	6.2	11.7	4.4	1.3
Mushroom & Spinach, Waitrose*	1 Pack/400g	373	14.0	93	3.1	12.3	3.5	1.3
Ovenbaked, Smart Price, Asda*	1 Pack/300g	279	12.3	93	5.5	7.8	4.1	1.5
Primana, Aldi*	1 Serving/250g	422	22.5	169	8.0	14.0	9.0	0.0
Reduced Calorie, CBY, Asda*	1 Pack/400g	332	10.0	83	6.0	8.4	2.5	1.3
Roasted Vegetable, M&S*	1 Pack/400g	440	20.4	110	3.4	12.8	5.1	1.7
Salmon, King Prawn & Spinach, Finest, Tesco*	1 Pack/400g	600	29.6	150	10.6	9.6	7.4	0.8
Sheets, Boiled, Average	*1 Sheet/20g*	*20*	*0.1*	*100*	*3.0*	*22.0*	*0.6*	*0.9*
Sheets, Dry, Average	*1 Sheet/20g*	*70*	*0.3*	*349*	*11.9*	*72.1*	*1.5*	*2.9*
Sheets, Verdi, Dry, Average	*1 Sheet/20g*	*71*	*0.4*	*356*	*12.6*	*71.1*	*2.2*	*2.8*
Smoked Salmon & Asparagus, Sainsbury's*	1 Pack/350g	665	37.4	190	7.9	15.6	10.7	0.7
Spinach & Cheese, Italian, Sainsbury's*	1 Pack/450g	666	30.6	148	6.0	15.5	6.8	0.5
Spinach & Ricotta, Asda*	1 Pack/400g	488	24.0	122	4.9	12.0	6.0	1.5
Spinach & Ricotta, Finest, Tesco*	1 Pack/350g	584	37.1	167	6.1	11.7	10.6	1.2
Spinach & Ricotta, Giovanni Rana*	1 Pack/350g	728	39.6	208	7.4	19.2	11.3	0.0
Vegetable, BGTY, Sainsbury's*	1 Pack/385g	339	7.7	88	3.5	13.9	2.0	2.3
Vegetable, Healthy Range, Average	*1 Serving/400g*	*318*	*8.2*	*80*	*3.5*	*11.8*	*2.1*	*1.5*
Vegetable, Italian Roasted, Asda*	1 Serving/200g	234	14.0	117	2.6	11.0	7.0	0.7
Vegetable, Italian Three Layer, Sainsbury's*	1 Pack/450g	554	23.4	123	4.8	14.3	5.2	0.5
Vegetable, Italiano, Tesco*	1 Pack/425g	382	14.0	90	2.7	11.7	3.3	1.2
Vegetable, Morrisons*	1 Pack/400g	464	22.8	116	3.8	12.3	5.7	0.7
Vegetable, Ready Meal, Average	*1 Serving/400g*	*408*	*17.6*	*102*	*4.1*	*12.4*	*4.4*	*1.0*
Vegetable, Waitrose*	1 Pack/400g	440	23.2	110	3.2	11.3	5.8	1.2
Vegetable, You Count, LL, Waitrose*	1 Pack/400g	319	28.3	80	3.2	11.9	7.1	1.5
Vegetarian, Meat Substitute, Ready Meal, Average	*1 Serving/400g*	*468*	*20.8*	*117*	*5.3*	*12.2*	*5.2*	*1.6*
You Count, LL, Waitrose*	1 Pack/385g	343	8.1	89	6.8	9.9	2.1	1.5
LASAGNE VEGETARIAN								
Linda McCartney*	1 Pack/360g	451	20.2	125	6.3	12.4	5.6	1.4
Tesco*	1 Pack/450g	630	34.6	140	6.0	11.6	7.7	1.6
LAVERBREAD								
Average	*1oz/28g*	*15*	*1.0*	*52*	*3.2*	*1.6*	*3.7*	*0.0*
LEEKS								
Boiled, Average	*1oz/28g*	*6*	*0.2*	*21*	*1.2*	*2.6*	*0.7*	*1.7*
Creamed, Frozen, Waitrose*	1 Serving/225g	115	5.4	51	1.8	5.5	2.4	0.0
Frozen, Sliced, Asda*	1 Serving/100g	27	0.5	27	1.6	2.9	0.5	2.2
Raw, Unprepared, Average	*1 Leek/166g*	*37*	*0.8*	*22*	*1.6*	*2.9*	*0.5*	*2.2*
LEMON								
Fresh, Raw, Average	*1 Slice/5g*	*1*	*0.0*	*18*	*0.9*	*2.9*	*0.3*	*2.1*
Fresh, Raw, Unwaxed, Sainsbury's*	½ Lemon/60g	12	0.2	20	1.0	3.2	0.3	0.0
Peel, Raw, Average	*1 Tbsp/6g*	*3*	*0.0*	*47*	*1.5*	*16.0*	*0.3*	*10.6*
LEMON CURD								
Average	*1 Tbsp/15g*	*44*	*0.7*	*294*	*0.7*	*62.9*	*4.7*	*0.1*

L

	Measure INFO/WEIGHT	per Measure KCAL	per Measure FAT	Nutrition Values per 100g / 100ml KCAL	PROT	CARB	FAT	FIBRE
LEMON CURD								
Luxury, Average	*1 Tsp/7g*	*23*	*0.6*	*326*	*2.8*	*59.7*	*8.4*	*0.1*
Sainsbury's*	1 Portion/20g	51	1.0	254	0.7	51.3	4.8	1.3
Value, Tesco*	1 Serving/15g	44	0.7	290	0.7	61.1	4.8	0.4
LEMON GRASS								
Stalks, Tesco*	1 Stalk/13g	12	0.1	99	1.8	25.3	0.5	0.0
LEMON SOLE								
Fillets, Raw, Average	*1 Serving/220g*	*177*	*2.8*	*81*	*17.0*	*0.2*	*1.3*	*0.3*
Goujons, Average	*1 Serving/150g*	*359*	*18.3*	*239*	*13.9*	*18.5*	*12.2*	*1.0*
Grilled, Average	*1oz/28g*	*27*	*0.5*	*97*	*20.2*	*0.0*	*1.7*	*0.0*
in Breadcrumbs, Average	*1 Fillet/142g*	*322*	*17.4*	*228*	*13.7*	*15.7*	*12.3*	*1.0*
in White Wine & Herb Butter, Fillets, M&S*	1 Pack/220g	385	27.7	175	15.1	0.1	12.6	0.0
Steamed, Average	*1oz/28g*	*25*	*0.3*	*91*	*20.6*	*0.0*	*0.9*	*0.0*
LEMONADE								
7 Up, Zero, Britvic*	1 Can/330ml	6	0.0	2	0.1	0.1	0.0	0.0
7-Up, Light, Britvic*	1 Can/330ml	4	0.0	1	0.1	0.2	0.0	0.0
Average	*1 Glass/250ml*	*52*	*0.2*	*21*	*0.1*	*5.0*	*0.1*	*0.1*
Cloudy, Diet, Sainsbury's*	1 Can/330ml	7	0.3	2	0.1	0.2	0.1	0.3
Cloudy, Diet, Tesco*	1 Serving/200ml	6	0.0	3	0.0	0.8	0.0	0.0
Cloudy, Gastropub, M&S*	1 Bottle/500ml	25	0.0	5	0.0	0.0	0.0	0.0
Cloudy, Sainsbury's*	1 Glass/250ml	118	0.2	47	0.1	12.0	0.1	0.1
Cloudy, Shapers, Boots*	1 Bottle/500ml	15	0.0	3	0.0	0.3	0.0	0.0
Cloudy, Waitrose*	1 Glass/250ml	125	0.0	50	0.0	12.2	0.0	0.0
Diet, Average	*1 Glass/250ml*	*4*	*0.1*	*2*	*0.1*	*0.2*	*0.0*	*0.0*
Diet, Premium, Tesco*	1 Glass/250ml	8	0.0	3	0.0	0.4	0.0	0.0
Low Calorie, Smart Price, Asda*	1 Glass/250ml	1	0.0	0	0.0	0.1	0.0	0.0
Pink, Pret a Manger*	1 Serving/250ml	75	0.0	30	0.1	7.1	0.0	0.0
R White*	1 Glass/250ml	65	0.0	26	0.1	6.2	0.0	0.0
Schweppes*	1 Glass/250ml	45	0.0	18	0.0	4.2	0.0	0.0
Sicilian, Sainsbury's*	1 Glass/200ml	98	0.2	49	0.1	11.5	0.1	0.1
Sparkling with Spanish Lemon Juice, Waitrose*	1 Glass/250ml	85	0.0	34	0.0	8.3	0.0	0.0
Still, Freshly Squeezed, M&S*	½ Bottle/250ml	100	0.5	40	0.1	9.0	0.2	0.5
Sugar Free, Everyday Value, Tesco*	1 Glass/250ml	1	0.0	0	0.0	0.0	0.0	0.0
Traditional Style, Tesco*	1 Glass/200ml	100	0.0	50	0.0	12.3	0.0	0.0
Victorian, Fentiman's*	1 Bottle/275ml	130	0.0	47	0.0	11.3	0.0	0.0
LEMSIP								
Beechams*	1 Sachet/3g	11	0.0	387	0.0	100.0	0.0	0.0
LENTILS								
Black Beluga, Ready to Eat, Merchant Gourmet*	1 Serving/63g	92	0.8	147	10.9	20.5	1.2	5.2
Green & Brown, Dried, Boiled in Salted Water, Average	*1 Tbsp/30g*	*32*	*0.2*	*105*	*8.8*	*16.9*	*0.7*	*3.8*
Green or Brown in Water, Tinned, Average	*½ Can/132g*	*131*	*0.8*	*99*	*8.1*	*15.4*	*0.6*	*3.8*
Green or Brown, Dried, Average	*1 Serving/50g*	*150*	*0.8*	*301*	*22.8*	*49.8*	*1.5*	*9.6*
Organic, Mr Organic*	1 Can/400g	216	1.2	54	4.0	6.8	0.3	4.0
Puy, Green, Dry, Average	*1 Serving/100g*	*306*	*1.4*	*306*	*24.7*	*49.5*	*1.4*	*10.3*
Red, Boiled in Unsalted Water, Average	*1oz/28g*	*28*	*0.1*	*102*	*7.6*	*17.5*	*0.4*	*2.6*
Red, Dried, Average	*1oz/28g*	*88*	*0.4*	*315*	*23.8*	*53.8*	*1.3*	*4.9*
Red, Split, Wholefoods, Tesco*	1 Serving/100g	335	1.3	335	23.8	56.3	1.3	4.9
LETTUCE								
Average, Raw	*½ Cup/28g*	*4*	*0.1*	*13*	*1.0*	*1.7*	*0.3*	*1.1*
Crest, Sainsbury's*	1 Serving/80g	11	0.4	14	0.8	1.7	0.5	0.0
Curly Leaf, Sainsbury's*	1 Serving/80g	11	0.4	14	0.8	1.7	0.5	0.0
Iceberg, Average	*1 Serving/80g*	*10*	*0.2*	*13*	*0.8*	*1.8*	*0.3*	*0.4*
Lamb's, Average	*1 Serving/80g*	*12*	*0.2*	*14*	*1.4*	*1.6*	*0.2*	*1.0*
Leafy, Tesco*	1 Serving/80g	11	0.3	14	1.2	1.5	0.4	1.9

L

	Measure INFO/WEIGHT	per Measure KCAL	FAT	Nutrition Values per 100g / 100ml KCAL	PROT	CARB	FAT	FIBRE
LETTUCE								
Little Gem, Average	*1 Lettuce/90g*	*14*	*0.4*	*15*	*0.8*	*1.8*	*0.5*	*0.7*
Radicchio, Red, Raw, Average	*1 Med Head/220g*	*29*	*0.2*	*13*	*1.4*	*1.6*	*0.1*	*3.0*
Red Gem, Tesco*	½ Lettuce/45g	7	0.2	15	0.8	1.7	0.5	0.9
Romaine, Average	*1 Serving/80g*	*12*	*0.4*	*15*	*0.9*	*1.7*	*0.5*	*0.7*
Romaine, Hearts, Average	*1 Serving/80g*	*12*	*0.4*	*16*	*0.9*	*1.7*	*0.6*	*1.0*
Romaine, Sweet, Average	*1 Serving/80g*	*12*	*0.4*	*16*	*0.9*	*1.6*	*0.6*	*0.8*
Round, Average	*1 Serving/80g*	*10*	*0.2*	*13*	*1.4*	*2.2*	*0.2*	*1.1*
Sweet Gem, TTD, Sainsbury's*	1 Serving/100g	15	0.5	15	0.8	1.7	0.5	0.9
LILT								
Fruit Crush, Coca-Cola*	1 Can/330ml	66	0.0	20	0.0	4.6	0.0	0.0
Fruit Crush, Zero, Coca-Cola*	1 Can/330ml	12	0.0	4	0.0	0.3	0.0	0.0
LIME								
Peel, Raw	*1 Tbsp/6g*	*3*	*0.0*	*47*	*1.5*	*16.0*	*0.3*	*10.6*
Raw, Flesh Only, Average	*1 Lime/71g*	*18*	*0.1*	*25*	*0.6*	*8.8*	*0.2*	*2.4*
Raw, Weighed with Peel & Seeds, Average	*1 Lime/85g*	*21*	*0.1*	*25*	*0.6*	*8.9*	*0.2*	*2.4*
LINGUINE								
Cooked	1 Serving/100g	133	0.7	133	5.1	26.3	0.7	1.1
Crab & Chilli, Waitrose*	1 Pack/350g	770	45.0	220	7.7	18.0	12.9	1.8
Crab, Rocket & Chilli, Italian, Finest, Tesco*	1 Pack/350g	718	36.4	205	6.5	20.7	10.4	1.7
Dry Weight, De Cecco*	1 Serving/100g	350	1.5	350	13.0	71.0	1.5	2.9
Dry, Average	*1 Serving/100g*	*352*	*2.2*	*352*	*13.1*	*70.0*	*2.2*	*2.8*
Fresh, Dry, Average	*1 Pack/250g*	*681*	*6.5*	*272*	*12.3*	*51.7*	*2.6*	*4.0*
King Prawn, Asda*	1 Pack/400g	380	10.4	95	6.4	11.5	2.6	1.5
King Prawn, FreshTastes, Asda*	1 Serving/356g	338	9.3	95	6.4	11.5	2.6	1.5
King Prawn, Meal For One, CBY, Asda*	1 Pack/380g	338	9.1	89	5.1	10.5	2.4	2.3
King Prawn, Meal for One, M&S*	1 Pack/400g	380	6.8	95	6.6	13.1	1.7	2.2
Salmon & Prawn, Iceland*	1 Meal/450g	540	19.8	120	4.5	15.8	4.4	1.5
with Chicken & Basil Dressing, HL, Tesco*	1 Pack/359g	503	15.4	140	8.6	16.6	4.3	2.2
with Mushrooms, Vegelicious, Tesco*	1 Bowl/380g	399	12.5	105	4.3	13.7	3.3	2.0
with Prawns & Scallops, BGTY, Sainsbury's*	1 Pack/400g	320	2.0	80	6.2	12.7	0.5	0.8
LINSEEDS								
Average	*1 Tsp/5g*	*23*	*1.7*	*464*	*21.7*	*18.5*	*33.5*	*26.3*
Brown, Wholefoods, Tesco*	1 Portion/10g	52	4.2	515	18.3	1.6	42.2	27.3
LION BAR								
Mini, Nestle*	1 Bar/16g	80	3.6	486	4.6	67.7	21.7	0.0
Nestle*	1 Bar/52g	248	11.2	478	6.5	64.6	21.6	0.0
Peanut, Nestle*	1 Bar/40g	195	10.0	488	8.1	57.1	25.0	2.3
LIQUEURS								
Amaretto, Average	*1 Pub Shot/25ml*	*97*	*0.0*	*388*	*0.0*	*60.0*	*0.0*	*0.0*
Cointreau, Specialite De France	1 Serving/37ml	80	0.0	215	0.0	8.5	0.0	0.0
Cream, Average	*1 Shot/25ml*	*81*	*4.0*	*325*	*0.0*	*22.8*	*16.1*	*0.0*
*Gr& Marnier**	*1 Pub Shot/35ml*	*94*	*0.0*	*268*	*0.0*	*22.9*	*0.0*	*0.0*
High Strength, Average	*1 Shot/25ml*	*78*	*0.0*	*314*	*0.0*	*24.4*	*0.0*	*0.0*
Kirsch, Average	*1 Shot/25ml*	*67*	*0.0*	*267*	*0.0*	*20.0*	*0.0*	*0.0*
Marula Fruit & Cream Cocktail, Amarula*	1 fl oz/30ml	103	0.0	343	0.0	36.7	0.0	0.0
LIQUORICE								
Allsorts, Average	*1 Sm Bag/56g*	*195*	*2.9*	*349*	*3.7*	*76.7*	*5.2*	*2.0*
Allsorts, Bassett's*	1 Pack/225g	855	11.0	380	5.6	77.8	4.9	1.6
Allsorts, Fruit, Bassett's*	1 Serving/50g	160	0.2	320	1.8	76.9	0.4	0.0
Allsorts, Julian Graves*	1 Serving/30g	113	2.2	376	3.4	78.7	7.2	1.2
Allsorts, Spar*	1 Serving/100g	325	3.6	325	2.2	71.0	3.6	1.6
Assorted, Filled, Panda*	1 Sweet/4g	15	0.4	385	3.7	68.0	11.0	0.0
Bars, Panda*	1 Bar/32g	99	0.1	308	3.7	72.0	0.4	0.9

L

	INFO/WEIGHT	KCAL	FAT	KCAL	PROT	CARB	FAT	FIBRE
LIQUORICE								
Catherine Wheels, Barratt*	1 Wheel/22g	65	0.1	290	3.8	67.2	0.3	0.7
Catherine Wheels, Sainsbury's*	1 Wheel/17g	49	0.1	286	3.8	67.2	0.3	0.7
Organic, Laidback Liquorice*	1 Bar/28g	90	0.3	320	4.7	75.0	1.0	3.0
Panda*	1 Bar/32g	109	0.2	340	3.8	78.0	0.5	0.0
Piglets, Black, Old Fashioned, Route 29 Napa Inc*	1 Sweet/2g	5	0.0	325	2.5	70.0	2.5	0.0
Red, Fresh, 98% Fat Free, RJ's Licorice Ltd*	1oz/28g	96	0.5	342	3.0	75.0	1.7	0.0
Shapes, Average	**1oz/28g**	**78**	**0.4**	**278**	**5.5**	**65.0**	**1.4**	**1.9**
Soft Eating, Australia, Darrell Lea*	1 Piece/20g	68	0.4	338	2.8	76.1	1.9	0.0
Sweets, Blackcurrant, Tesco*	1 Sweet/8g	32	0.3	410	0.0	92.3	3.8	0.0
Torpedos, Panda*	1 Serving/25g	92	0.0	366	1.9	88.0	0.2	1.4
Twists, Tesco*	1 Serving/63g	186	0.2	297	2.7	71.0	0.3	0.7
LIVER								
Calves with Fresh Sage Butter, M&S*	1 Serving/117g	210	12.5	180	12.8	10.1	10.7	1.5
Calves, Fried	**1oz/28g**	**49**	**2.7**	**176**	**22.3**	**0.0**	**9.6**	**0.0**
Calves, Raw	**1oz/28g**	**29**	**1.0**	**104**	**18.3**	**0.0**	**3.4**	**0.0**
Chicken, Cooked, Simmered, Average	**1 Serving/100g**	**167**	**6.5**	**167**	**24.5**	**0.9**	**6.5**	**0.0**
Chicken, Fried, Average	**1oz/28g**	**47**	**2.5**	**169**	**22.1**	**0.0**	**8.9**	**0.0**
Chicken, Raw, Average	**1oz/28g**	**26**	**0.6**	**92**	**17.7**	**0.0**	**2.3**	**0.0**
Lamb's, Braised, Average	**1 Serving/100g**	**220**	**8.8**	**220**	**30.6**	**2.5**	**8.8**	**0.0**
Lamb's, Fried, Average	**1oz/28g**	**66**	**3.6**	**237**	**30.1**	**0.0**	**12.9**	**0.0**
Lamb's, Raw, Average	**1 Serving/125g**	**171**	**7.8**	**137**	**20.3**	**0.0**	**6.2**	**0.0**
Ox, Raw	**1oz/28g**	**43**	**2.2**	**155**	**21.1**	**0.0**	**7.8**	**0.0**
Ox, Stewed	**1oz/28g**	**55**	**2.7**	**198**	**24.8**	**3.6**	**9.5**	**0.0**
Pig's, Raw	**1oz/28g**	**32**	**0.9**	**113**	**21.3**	**0.0**	**3.1**	**0.0**
Pig's, Stewed	**1 Serving/70g**	**132**	**5.7**	**189**	**25.6**	**3.6**	**8.1**	**0.0**
LIVER & BACON								
Meal for One, M&S*	1 Pack/452g	430	16.7	95	7.0	8.0	3.7	1.2
with Fresh Mashed Potato, Waitrose*	1 Pack/400g	416	17.2	104	7.3	9.0	4.3	1.3
with Mash, Cooked, British Classics, Tesco*	1 Pack/450g	562	20.2	125	11.9	7.6	4.5	1.0
with Mash, M Kitchen, Morrisons*	1 Pack/450g	463	16.6	103	7.4	9.3	3.7	1.4
LIVER & ONIONS								
British Classics, Tesco*	1 Pack/250g	265	12.0	106	9.7	5.9	4.8	0.5
Finest, Tesco*	½ Pack/225g	349	18.7	155	15.6	3.7	8.3	1.6
LIVER SAUSAGE								
Average	**1 Slice/10g**	**22**	**1.5**	**216**	**15.3**	**4.4**	**15.2**	**0.2**
LOBSTER								
Boiled, Average	**1oz/28g**	**29**	**0.4**	**103**	**22.1**	**0.0**	**1.6**	**0.0**
Canadian, Whole, Cooked, Meat Only, Frozen, Iceland*	1 Pack/140g	122	1.0	87	18.9	1.0	0.7	0.6
Dressed, John West*	1 Can/43g	45	2.2	105	13.0	2.0	5.0	0.0
Raw, Average	**1 Serving/100g**	**92**	**1.4**	**92**	**18.7**	**0.3**	**1.4**	**0.0**
Thermidor, Finest, Tesco*	½ Pack/140g	381	25.2	272	15.3	12.1	18.0	1.0
Thermidor, M&S*	1 Serving/140g	287	19.2	205	10.7	9.7	13.7	0.0
LOGANBERRIES								
Raw	**1oz/28g**	**5**	**0.0**	**17**	**1.1**	**3.4**	**0.0**	**2.5**
LOLLIPOPS								
Assorted Flavours, Asda*	1 Lolly/7g	27	0.0	380	0.0	95.0	0.0	0.0
Assorted, Co-Op*	1 Lolly/10g	40	0.0	400	0.0	97.0	0.0	0.0
Chocolate Lolly, M&S*	1 Lolly/45g	248	15.8	550	6.8	54.0	35.1	2.7
Chupa Chups*	1 Lolly/18g	44	0.2	247	0.0	96.5	1.3	0.0
Refreshers, Bassett's*	1 Lolly/6g	25	0.0	417	0.0	108.3	0.0	0.0
LOQUATS								
Raw	**1oz/28g**	**5**	**0.0**	**18**	**0.4**	**4.0**	**0.1**	**0.0**

L

	Measure INFO/WEIGHT	per Measure		Nutrition Values per 100g / 100ml				
		KCAL	FAT	KCAL	PROT	CARB	FAT	FIBRE
LOZENGES								
Blackcurrant Flavour, Fishermans Friend*	1 Lozenge/1g	3	0.0	251	0.1	97.2	1.3	0.0
Original Extra Strong Lozenge, Fisherman's Friend*	1 Lozenge/1g	4	0.0	382	0.3	94.9	0.0	0.5
LUCOZADE								
Caribbean Crush, Energy, Lucozade*	1 Bottle/380ml	217	0.0	57	0.0	13.9	0.0	0.0
Energy, Original, GlaxoSmithKline UK Limited*	1 Bottle/380ml	266	0.0	70	0.0	17.2	0.0	0.0
Orange Energy Drink, GlaxoSmithKline UK Limited*	1 Bottle/500ml	350	0.0	70	0.0	17.2	0.0	0.0
Orange, Sport Lite, GlaxoSmithKline UK Limited*	1 Serving/500g	50	0.0	10	0.0	2.0	0.0	0.0
LUNCHEON MEAT								
Pork, Average	*1oz/28g*	*81*	*6.8*	*288*	*13.3*	*4.0*	*24.3*	*0.0*
Pork, Value, Tesco*	1 Slice/14g	33	2.7	240	13.5	3.3	19.2	0.0
LYCHEES								
Fresh, Raw, Flesh Only	*1oz/28g*	*16*	*0.0*	*58*	*0.9*	*14.3*	*0.1*	*0.7*
in Syrup, Average	*1oz/28g*	*19*	*0.0*	*69*	*0.4*	*17.7*	*0.0*	*0.4*
Raw, Weighed with Skin & Stone	*1oz/28g*	*6*	*0.0*	*22*	*0.3*	*5.5*	*0.1*	*0.2*

L

M

	Measure INFO/WEIGHT	per Measure KCAL	FAT	Nutrition Values per 100g / 100ml KCAL	PROT	CARB	FAT	FIBRE
M&M'S								
Crispy, Mars*	1 Serving/36g	179	8.8	498	4.1	63.9	24.4	2.7
Mars*	1 Pack/45g	218	9.7	485	5.0	68.0	21.5	0.0
Mini, Mars*	1 Sm Pack/36g	176	8.4	489	6.3	63.6	23.2	0.0
Peanut Butter, Mars*	1 Pack/46g	240	14.0	520	8.7	56.3	30.3	2.2
Peanut, Mars*	1 Pack/45g	228	11.4	506	9.4	60.1	25.4	2.7
MACADAMIA NUTS								
LL, Waitrose*	1 Serving/15g	113	11.4	754	7.8	5.4	76.1	8.0
Plain, Average	*1 Pack/100g*	*750*	*77.6*	*750*	*7.9*	*4.8*	*77.6*	*5.3*
Roasted, Salted, Average	*6 Nuts/10g*	*75*	*7.8*	*748*	*7.9*	*4.8*	*77.6*	*5.3*
MACARONI								
Dry, Average	*1oz/28g*	*99*	*0.5*	*354*	*11.9*	*73.5*	*1.7*	*2.6*
MACARONI CHEESE								
Birds Eye*	1 Pack/300g	470	15.0	157	5.7	22.3	5.0	0.8
Canned	1oz/28g	39	1.8	138	4.5	16.4	6.5	0.4
Canned, Sainsbury's*	1 Can/400g	480	24.0	120	4.4	12.0	6.0	0.3
Charlie Bigham's*	½ Pack/335g	771	36.9	230	10.5	21.8	11.0	0.2
Combino, Lidl*	1 Can/410g	472	25.8	115	4.5	10.1	6.3	0.3
COU, M&S*	1 Pack/360g	360	8.6	100	5.8	13.9	2.4	1.2
Finest, Tesco*	1 Serving/450g	735	30.3	165	7.6	17.8	6.8	1.8
Italian, Sainsbury's*	½ Pack/225g	360	15.8	160	6.9	17.3	7.0	1.5
Italian, Tesco*	1 Pack/420g	830	40.7	198	9.2	18.2	9.7	1.2
Light Choices, Tesco*	1 Pack/385g	465	7.3	121	7.0	18.7	1.9	1.5
M&S*	1 Pack/400g	700	28.4	175	7.0	20.9	7.1	0.9
Made with Fresh Pasta, Findus*	1 Pack/360g	360	7.2	100	5.0	16.0	2.0	0.5
Pasta, Italian Kitchen, Tesco*	1 Pack/450g	801	36.0	178	7.1	18.3	8.0	2.3
Ready Meal, Average	*1 Serving/300g*	*435*	*19.1*	*145*	*6.0*	*15.8*	*6.4*	*1.0*
Smart Price, Asda*	1 Can/410g	291	6.2	71	2.6	11.8	1.5	0.4
Value, Tesco*	1 Pack/300g	375	14.7	125	4.4	15.0	4.9	1.2
Waitrose*	1 Pack/350g	466	32.9	133	6.8	5.2	9.4	0.0
MACAROONS								
Butterscotch, Picard*	1 Macaroon/20g	85	3.6	424	9.7	55.1	18.2	0.0
Coconut, Sainsbury's*	1 Macaroon/33g	146	6.1	441	4.7	63.7	18.6	0.8
Coconut, Tesco*	1 Macaroon/33g	140	6.1	425	4.4	59.0	18.6	5.7
French, Average	*1 Serving/60g*	*225*	*11.0*	*375*	*6.7*	*46.7*	*18.3*	*3.3*
MACKEREL								
Atlantic, Raw, Average	*1 Fillet/75g*	*154*	*10.4*	*205*	*18.6*	*0.0*	*13.9*	*0.0*
Fillets in a Hot Chilli Dressing, Princes*	1 Pack/125g	370	33.8	296	13.3	0.0	27.0	0.0
Fillets in Brine, Average	*1 Can/88g*	*206*	*15.3*	*234*	*19.4*	*0.0*	*17.4*	*0.0*
Fillets in Curry Sauce, John West*	1 Can/125g	275	20.8	220	14.2	3.5	16.6	0.2
Fillets in Green Peppercorn Sauce, John West*	1 Can/125g	329	26.2	263	14.0	4.5	21.0	0.1
Fillets in Mustard Sauce, Average	*1 Can/125g*	*274*	*19.4*	*219*	*14.1*	*5.4*	*15.5*	*0.0*
Fillets in Olive Oil, Average	*1 Serving/50g*	*149*	*12.2*	*298*	*18.5*	*1.0*	*24.4*	*0.0*
Fillets in Olive Oil, Sainsbury's*	1 Can/125g	325	25.0	260	20.0	0.0	20.0	0.0
Fillets in Spicy Tomato Sauce, Average	*1oz/28g*	*56*	*3.9*	*199*	*14.3*	*3.8*	*14.0*	*0.0*
Fillets in Sunflower Oil, Average	*1 Can/94g*	*262*	*20.6*	*279*	*20.2*	*0.2*	*21.9*	*0.2*
Fillets in Teriyaki Sauce, Boneless & Skinless, Tesco*	1 Can/125g	320	20.3	255	12.6	13.4	16.2	2.0
Fillets in Tomato Sauce, Average	1 Can/125g	251	18.3	200	14.3	2.7	14.7	0.0
Fillets with Red Pepper & Onion, Smoked, Asda*	1 Serving/90g	319	27.9	354	18.0	0.8	31.0	1.2
Fillets, Honey Roast Smoked, Sainsbury's*	1 Serving/100g	349	27.3	349	21.5	4.5	27.3	12.4
Fillets, in Hot Smoked Peppered, Asda*	1 Fillet/100g	341	28.0	341	19.0	3.3	28.0	0.6
Fillets, Lemon & Parsley, Smoked, Fishmonger, Aldi*	1 Pack/200g	658	53.0	329	19.6	2.9	26.5	0.0
Fillets, Mexican, Canned, Princes*	1 Can/125g	241	13.8	193	11.4	11.8	11.0	0.5
Fillets, Peppered with Red & Green Peppers, LL, Waitrose*	½ Pack/120g	282	20.9	235	17.4	2.1	17.4	1.3

	Measure	per Measure		Nutrition Values per 100g / 100ml				
	INFO/WEIGHT	KCAL	FAT	KCAL	PROT	CARB	FAT	FIBRE
MACKEREL								
Fillets, Smoked, Average	*1 Fillet/75g*	*251*	*21.1*	*334*	*19.7*	*0.5*	*28.2*	*0.3*
Fried in Blended Oil	*1oz/28g*	*76*	*5.5*	*272*	*24.0*	*0.0*	*19.5*	*0.0*
Grilled	*1oz/28g*	*67*	*4.8*	*239*	*20.8*	*0.0*	*17.3*	*0.0*
Raw with Skin, Weighed with Bone, Average	*1oz/28g*	*64*	*4.7*	*227*	*18.9*	*0.0*	*16.8*	*0.0*
Roasted with Piri-piri, Tesco*	1 Fillet/80g	240	19.0	300	20.7	0.0	23.8	1.0
Smoked, Peppered, Average	*1oz/28g*	*87*	*7.0*	*310*	*20.4*	*0.3*	*25.2*	*0.2*
Whole, Raw, Average	*1 Serving/100g*	*156*	*11.4*	*156*	*13.3*	*0.0*	*11.4*	*0.0*
MADRAS								
Beef, Canned, BGTY, Sainsbury's*	1 Can/400g	344	14.4	86	9.5	4.0	3.6	0.9
Beef, Indian, Takeaway, CBY, Asda*	½ Pack/200g	246	14.2	123	8.9	4.7	7.1	2.5
Beef, Tesco*	1 Pack/460g	616	37.7	134	10.6	4.5	8.2	1.2
Beef, Weight Watchers*	1 Pack/320g	317	4.8	99	5.6	15.8	1.5	0.3
Chicken & Pilau Rice, Asda*	1 Pack/400g	588	28.0	147	8.0	13.0	7.0	1.7
Chicken & Rice, Hot & Spicy, Sainsbury's*	1 Pack/500g	670	25.5	134	7.1	14.9	5.1	2.2
Chicken, Asda*	1 Serving/350g	430	31.5	123	7.0	3.6	9.0	2.3
Chicken, Iceland*	1 Pack/400g	376	19.2	94	7.7	4.9	4.8	1.1
Chicken, Indian Take Away, Tesco*	1 Serving/175g	254	17.7	145	8.2	4.8	10.1	1.7
Chicken, Indian, Tesco*	1 Pack/350g	518	31.2	148	11.3	5.6	8.9	1.9
Chicken, Morrisons*	1 Pack/350g	448	30.4	128	9.6	2.8	8.7	2.4
Chicken, Sainsbury's*	1 Pack/400g	468	27.2	117	11.7	2.2	6.8	2.8
Chicken, Waitrose*	1 Pack/400g	672	42.0	168	14.6	3.7	10.5	1.8
MAGNUM								
After Dinner Bites, Vanilla, Magnum, Wall's Ice Cream*	1 Serving/29g	100	6.7	344	3.4	31.0	23.0	1.4
Almond, Wall's Ice Cream*	1 Bar/82g	270	17.2	330	5.0	30.0	21.0	1.5
Caramel & Almond, Temptation, Wall's Ice Cream*	1 Lolly/68g	239	15.0	351	5.4	34.0	22.0	0.0
Chocolate Desire, Wall's Ice Cream*	1 Dessert/85g	374	24.0	440	5.3	40.0	28.2	0.0
Classic, Mini, Wall's Ice Cream*	1 Lolly/50g	170	11.0	340	4.0	30.0	22.0	0.0
Classic, Wall's Ice Cream*	1 Lolly/86g	239	15.0	278	3.5	26.7	17.4	1.2
Double Chocolate, Wall's Ice Cream*	1 Bar/92g	346	22.0	378	4.5	36.0	24.0	0.0
Infinity, Chocolate & Caramel, Wall's Ice Cream*	1 Lolly/82g	260	18.0	317	4.9	29.3	22.0	4.9
Moments, Wall's Ice Cream*	1 Serving/18ml	58	3.7	323	4.0	30.0	20.8	0.0
Pistachio, Wall's Ice Cream*	1 Bar/86g	275	18.9	320	4.0	30.0	22.0	0.0
White, Wall's Ice Cream*	1 Lolly/77g	250	16.0	325	3.9	29.9	20.8	0.0
MAKHANI								
Chicken Tikka, Waitrose*	1 Pack/400g	560	30.4	140	14.0	3.8	7.6	2.1
Chicken, Sainsbury's*	½ Pack/199g	313	21.3	157	12.2	2.9	10.7	2.5
King Prawns, Finest, Tesco*	1 Pack/350g	514	38.8	147	6.0	6.0	11.1	1.3
MALTESERS								
MaltEaster, Chocolate Bunny, Mars*	1 Bunny/29g	156	9.0	539	6.9	57.6	31.0	1.2
Mars*	1 Reg Bag/37g	187	9.3	505	8.0	61.8	25.0	0.9
Mini Bunnies, Mars*	1 Bunny/12g	64	3.6	534	8.0	53.5	30.2	0.0
MANDARIN ORANGES								
Broken, Segments in Fruit Juice, Basics, Sainsbury's*	½ Can/149g	51	0.0	34	0.7	7.7	0.0	0.3
in Juice, Average	*1oz/28g*	*11*	*0.0*	*39*	*0.7*	*9.0*	*0.0*	*0.5*
in Light Syrup, Average	*1 Can/298g*	*201*	*0.1*	*68*	*0.6*	*16.0*	*0.0*	*0.1*
Weighed with Peel, Average	*1 Sm Fruit/50g*	*14*	*0.0*	*27*	*0.7*	*6.2*	*0.1*	*0.9*
MANGE TOUT								
& Sugar Snap Peas, Tesco*	1 Pack/150g	102	0.6	68	7.0	9.2	0.4	3.8
Boiled in Salted Water	*1oz/28g*	*7*	*0.0*	*26*	*3.2*	*3.3*	*0.1*	*2.2*
Raw, Average	*1 Serving/80g*	*25*	*0.2*	*31*	*3.5*	*4.0*	*0.2*	*1.1*
Stir-Fried in Blended Oil	*1oz/28g*	*20*	*1.3*	*71*	*3.8*	*3.5*	*4.8*	*2.4*
MANGO								
Chunks, Fresh, Morrisons*	1 Serving/80g	50	0.2	63	0.7	13.6	0.2	1.8

	Measure INFO/WEIGHT	per Measure		Nutrition Values per 100g / 100ml				
		KCAL	FAT	KCAL	PROT	CARB	FAT	FIBRE
MANGO								
Dried, Average	**1 Serving/50g**	**174**	**0.5**	**347**	**1.4**	**83.1**	**1.0**	**4.9**
Dried, Pieces, Jus Fruit, Yu!*	1 Pack/24g	87	0.1	364	1.0	84.7	0.4	0.0
Dried, Sweetened, Whitworths*	1 Pack/30g	80	0.4	260	0.3	61.3	1.3	0.5
in Syrup, Average	**1oz/28g**	**22**	**0.0**	**80**	**0.3**	**20.5**	**0.0**	**0.9**
Organic, Dried, LL, Waitrose*	1 Serving/50g	148	0.4	297	3.4	68.7	0.9	12.0
Pieces in Juice, Natures Finest*	1 Pot/220g	123	0.4	56	0.5	12.3	0.2	1.5
Pineapple & Passionfruit, M&S*	1 Pack/400g	200	0.8	50	0.6	10.9	0.2	1.7
Ripe, Raw, Weighed with Skin & Stone, Average	**1 Mango/225g**	**60**	**0.2**	**27**	**0.3**	**6.5**	**0.1**	**1.2**
Ripe, Raw, without Peel & Stone, Flesh Only, Average	**1 Mango/207g**	**81**	**1.0**	**39**	**0.5**	**9.6**	**0.5**	**1.8**
Slices, in Juice, SPC Nature's Finest*	1 Pot/400g	224	0.8	56	5.0	12.3	0.2	1.5
MANGOSTEEN								
Raw, Fresh, Average	**1 Serving/80g**	**50**	**0.5**	**63**	**0.6**	**15.6**	**0.6**	**5.1**
MARGARINE								
Average	**1 Thin Spread/7g**	**51**	**5.7**	**726**	**0.1**	**0.5**	**81.0**	**0.0**
Butter Style, Average	**1 Thin Spread/7g**	**44**	**4.8**	**627**	**0.7**	**1.1**	**68.9**	**0.0**
Buttery, Pro Activ, Flora*	1 Serving/10g	55	6.0	550	0.0	0.0	60.0	0.0
for Baking, Average	**1 Thin Spread/7g**	**42**	**4.7**	**607**	**0.2**	**0.4**	**67.2**	**0.0**
No Salt, Flora*	1 Thin Spread/7g	37	4.1	531	0.0	0.0	59.0	0.0
Pro Activ with Olive Oil, Flora*	1 Thin Spread/7g	23	2.4	331	0.1	4.0	35.0	0.0
Pro Activ, Extra Light, Flora*	1 Thin Spread/7g	15	1.6	218	0.1	2.9	23.0	0.2
Pro Activ, Light, Flora*	1 Thin Spread/7g	23	2.4	331	0.1	4.0	35.0	0.0
Pro Active, Becel*	1 Serving/7g	22	1.8	320	0.0	0.0	25.0	0.0
Reduced Fat, Average	**1 Thin Spread/7g**	**25**	**2.7**	**356**	**0.6**	**3.0**	**38.0**	**0.0**
Utterly Butterly*	1 Thin Spread/7g	32	3.4	452	0.3	2.5	49.0	0.0
White, Flora*	1 Thin Spread/7g	60	6.6	855	0.0	0.0	95.0	0.0
MARINADE								
Barbeque, Sticky, Sainsbury's*	¼ Jar/77g	112	2.8	145	0.8	26.7	3.6	1.0
BBQ, Sticky, Newman's Own*	1/3 Jar/83ml	139	0.7	167	0.9	39.0	0.8	2.5
Cajun Spice, The English Provender Co.*	1 Serving/50g	94	6.7	187	1.3	15.3	13.4	1.6
Coat 'n Cook, Medium, Nando's*	1 Sachet/120g	94	5.4	78	1.1	9.6	4.5	2.8
Hot & Spicy Barbecue, M&S*	1 Serving/18g	23	0.1	130	1.0	31.1	0.3	0.8
Lemon & Rosemary, Nando's*	1fl oz/30ml	44	3.9	147	1.0	11.8	13.0	0.2
Lime & Coriander with Peri Peri, Nando's*	1 Tsp/5g	9	0.8	182	0.0	13.1	16.6	0.2
Peri Peri, Hot, Nando's*	1 Serving/40g	46	2.2	115	1.4	15.2	5.4	0.9
Peri Peri, Portuguese BBQ, Nando's*	1 Serving/40g	36	0.6	90	1.1	17.7	1.6	1.0
Sticky Barbecue, Tesco*	¼ Jar/70g	80	0.1	115	0.7	26.7	0.2	0.6
Sun Dried Tomato & Basil with Peri-Peri, Nando's*	1 Bottle/270g	319	25.6	118	0.1	15.3	9.5	0.8
MARJORAM								
Dried	**1 Tsp/1g**	**2**	**0.0**	**271**	**12.7**	**42.5**	**7.0**	**0.0**
MARMALADE								
3 Fruit, Thick Cut, Waitrose*	1 Tsp/15g	39	0.0	262	0.4	64.8	0.1	0.7
Blood Orange, TTD, Sainsbury's*	1 Tbsp/15g	40	0.0	264	0.3	65.7	0.0	0.8
Citrus Shred, Robertson*	1 Tsp/5g	13	0.0	253	0.2	63.0	0.0	0.0
Five Fruit, Tesco*	1 Serving/10g	28	0.0	278	0.2	68.2	0.1	0.9
Fresh Fruit, Three Fruits, TTD, Sainsbury's*	1 Tbsp/15g	40	0.0	268	0.3	66.7	0.0	0.8
Grapefruit, Fine Cut, Duerr's*	1 Tsp/15g	39	0.0	261	0.2	65.0	0.0	0.0
Lemon & Lime, Average	**1 Tbsp/20g**	**53**	**0.0**	**267**	**0.2**	**66.4**	**0.1**	**0.4**
Lemon Jelly, No Peel, Tesco*	1 Tsp/15g	39	0.0	263	0.1	65.0	0.0	0.4
Lemon with Shred, Average	**1 Serving/20g**	**50**	**0.0**	**248**	**0.2**	**61.6**	**0.0**	**0.6**
Lemon, Fine Cut, Tesco*	1 Serving/15g	39	0.0	257	0.2	64.0	0.0	0.5
Lime with Shred, Average	**1 Tbsp/15g**	**39**	**0.0**	**261**	**0.2**	**65.0**	**0.1**	**0.4**
Onion, Organic, Antony Worrall Thompson's*	1 Serving/11g	20	0.1	191	1.1	44.9	0.8	1.8
Onion, Organic, Duchy Originals*	1 Serving/40g	103	1.0	257	1.0	57.8	2.4	2.6

	Measure INFO/WEIGHT	per Measure KCAL	FAT	Nutrition Values per 100g / 100ml KCAL	PROT	CARB	FAT	FIBRE
MARMALADE								
Orange & Ginger, Average	*1 Tbsp/15g*	*40*	*0.0*	*264*	*0.2*	*65.7*	*0.1*	*0.3*
Orange & Tangerine, Tiptree, Wilkin & Sons*	1 Tsp/15g	40	0.0	268	0.0	67.0	0.0	0.0
Orange Shred, Medium Cut, Tesco*	1 Serving/15g	39	0.0	260	0.3	64.7	0.0	0.5
Orange with Shred, Average	*1 Tsp/5g*	*13*	*0.0*	*263*	*0.2*	*65.2*	*0.0*	*0.3*
Orange, Fine Shred, Bonne Maman*	1 Tsp/5g	12	0.0	238	0.3	59.0	0.1	0.6
Orange, Lemon & Grapefruit, Baxters*	1 Tsp/15g	38	0.0	252	0.0	63.0	0.0	0.1
Orange, Reduced Sugar, Average	*1 Tbsp/15g*	*26*	*0.0*	*170*	*0.4*	*42.0*	*0.1*	*0.6*
Orange, Reduced Sugar, Thin Cut, Streamline*	1 Serving/10g	18	0.0	178	0.5	43.0	0.3	0.0
Orange, Shredless, Average	*1 Tsp/10g*	*26*	*0.0*	*261*	*0.2*	*65.0*	*0.0*	*0.1*
Pink Grapefruit, Thin Cut, Waitrose*	1 Serving/10g	26	0.0	261	0.2	65.0	0.0	0.4
Seville Orange, with Scotch Whisky, Deluxe, Lidl*	1 Tsp/5g	13	0.0	262	0.5	63.0	0.5	1.8
Seville, Thick Cut, Organic, Fair Trade, Tesco*	1 Tbsp/15g	37	0.0	245	0.3	60.3	0.1	0.7
Three Fruits, Fresh Fruit, Sainsbury's*	1 Tsp/15g	38	0.0	250	0.0	61.3	0.0	0.0
MARMITE*								
XO, Marmite*	1 Serving/4g	10	0.0	250	37.5	25.0	0.2	0.2
Yeast Extract with Gold Coloured Flecks, Marmite*	1 Serving/4g	10	0.0	250	39.0	24.0	0.1	3.5
Yeast Extract, Marmite*	1 Tsp/9g	22	0.0	250	39.0	24.0	0.1	3.5
MARROW								
Boiled, Average	*1oz/28g*	*3*	*0.1*	*9*	*0.4*	*1.6*	*0.2*	*0.6*
Raw	*1oz/28g*	*2*	*0.0*	*6*	*0.3*	*1.2*	*0.1*	*0.3*
MARS								
Bar, 5 Little Ones, Mars*	1 Piece/8g	38	1.5	477	4.5	73.6	18.3	0.0
Bar, Duo, Mars*	1 Bar/42g	191	7.6	450	4.4	67.5	18.0	1.2
Bar, Funsize, Mars*	1 Bar/18g	80	3.0	446	3.5	70.1	16.8	1.1
Bar, Mars*	1 Bar/51g	229	8.7	449	4.0	69.0	17.0	1.0
Bar, Medium, 58g, Mars*	1 Bar/58g	263	10.5	453	4.6	67.9	18.1	0.0
Bar, Minis, Mars*	1 Bar/18g	80	11.6	444	3.3	0.0	64.4	1.1
Triple Choc, Limited Edition, Mars*	1 Bar/52g	233	9.0	448	4.5	67.7	17.3	2.0
MARSHMALLOWS								
Average	*1 Mallow/5g*	*16*	*0.0*	*327*	*3.9*	*83.1*	*0.0*	*0.0*
Chocolate Mallows, Cadbury*	1 Mallow/13g	56	2.2	435	4.7	64.7	17.4	0.8
Fat Free, Tesco*	1 Mallow/7g	24	0.0	339	3.4	80.8	0.2	0.5
Haribo*	1 Mallow/5g	16	0.0	330	3.0	80.0	0.0	0.0
No Added Sugar, Sainsbury's*	1 Mallow/2g	5	0.0	206	3.3	77.0	0.1	0.0
Pascall*	1 Mallow/5g	15	0.0	335	2.6	80.0	0.0	0.0
Pink & White, Co-Op*	1 Mallow/7g	24	0.0	340	3.0	82.0	0.0	0.0
Princess*	1 Mallow/5g	16	0.0	314	3.4	80.0	0.0	0.0
Raspberry & Cream, Sainsbury's*	1 Mallow/7g	23	0.0	330	4.1	78.5	0.0	0.5
Sainsbury's*	1 Mallow/7g	23	0.0	330	4.1	78.5	0.0	0.5
MARZIPAN								
Bar, Chocolate, Plain, Thorntons*	1 Bar/46g	206	8.0	448	5.2	69.1	17.4	2.0
Dark Chocolate, Thorntons*	1 Serving/46g	207	8.0	451	5.2	69.4	17.4	2.1
Plain, Average	*1oz/28g*	*115*	*4.0*	*412*	*5.8*	*67.5*	*14.2*	*1.7*
MASALA								
Dal with Channa & Toor Lentils, Waitrose*	½ Pack/150g	166	6.1	111	6.6	12.0	4.1	5.0
Prawn Mango, Waitrose*	½ Pack/175g	175	11.2	100	5.8	4.3	6.4	1.3
Prawn, King, Waitrose*	1 Pack/350g	385	25.9	110	7.1	3.8	7.4	1.8
Vegetable, Waitrose*	1 Serving/400g	288	19.2	72	2.2	4.9	4.8	2.5
MASH								
Carrot & Swede, M Kitchen, Morrisons*	½ Pack/250g	155	4.8	62	0.9	9.0	1.9	2.6
Carrot, Parsnip & Turnip, Mash Direct*	1 Serving/100g	63	2.0	63	1.0	10.2	2.0	2.8
Potato, Carrot, Swede, Parsnip, Cream & Butter, Asda*	½ Pack/200g	94	3.0	47	1.0	7.2	1.5	3.3
Root Vegetable, Finest, Tesco*	½ Pack/250g	225	12.5	90	1.1	9.1	5.0	3.4

M

	Measure INFO/WEIGHT	per Measure KCAL	FAT	Nutrition Values per 100g / 100ml KCAL	PROT	CARB	FAT	FIBRE
MASH								
Root, Asda*	½ Pack/200g	142	8.0	71	0.7	8.0	4.0	3.1
Vegetables, Mousline, Maggi*	1 Bag/39g	127	1.2	328	8.2	67.0	3.0	10.4
Winter Root, Sainsbury's*	1 Serving/140g	157	2.1	112	2.7	22.0	1.5	0.9
MAYONNAISE								
50% Less Fat, GFY, Asda*	1 Tbsp/10g	32	3.1	322	0.8	10.0	31.0	0.0
60% Less Fat, BGTY, Sainsbury's*	1 Tbsp/15ml	42	4.1	277	0.4	7.3	27.3	0.0
Aioli, Finest, Tesco*	1 Tsp/5g	20	2.1	408	0.8	8.5	41.2	0.0
Average	*1 Tsp/5g*	*35*	*3.8*	*690*	*0.9*	*1.6*	*75.5*	*0.0*
Bramwells, Extra Light, Specially Selected, Aldi*	1 Tbsp/33g	40	3.2	121	1.1	7.2	9.7	2.4
Branston, with a Twist of Pesto, Crosse & Blackwell*	1 Tbsp/30ml	124	11.6	412	1.2	14.1	38.6	0.2
Branston, with a Twist, Petri Peri, Crosse & Blackwell*	1 Serving/15g	64	5.6	430	0.9	21.4	37.5	0.2
Deli, Moroccan, Heinz*	1 Tbsp/15g	80	8.5	532	0.9	4.6	56.5	0.1
Deli, Roasted Garlic, Heinz*	1 Tbsp/15g	81	8.5	537	1.1	5.5	56.6	0.0
Egg, Dairy & Gluten Free, Solesse*	1 Serving/100g	319	29.7	319	0.4	11.7	29.7	0.0
Extra Light, Asda*	1 Tbsp/10ml	12	0.7	119	0.7	13.1	7.1	0.2
Extra Light, Average	*1 Tbsp/33g*	*34*	*2.0*	*102*	*0.7*	*10.5*	*6.2*	*0.8*
Extra Light, Heinz*	1 Tbsp/12ml	9	0.4	75	0.6	11.4	3.0	0.6
Extra Light, Now Only 3% Fat, Hellmann's*	1 Serving/16g	12	0.5	73	0.6	11.0	3.0	0.6
Extra Light, Sainsbury's*	1 Tbsp/15ml	17	1.0	115	0.7	11.9	7.0	0.0
Extra Light, Tesco*	1 Serving/45ml	40	2.1	90	0.6	10.2	4.7	0.0
Extra Light, Top Down, Tesco*	1 Tbsp/15g	14	0.8	95	0.6	10.4	5.5	0.0
Extra Light, Weight Watchers*	1 Serving/15g	15	0.9	97	1.1	9.6	5.9	3.2
Finest, Tesco*	1 Dtsp/22g	155	16.9	703	1.1	1.5	77.0	0.0
French Style, BGTY, Sainsbury's*	1 Tbsp/15ml	55	5.5	366	0.6	7.5	36.9	0.0
French, Light, Sainsbury's*	1 Serving/15ml	46	4.7	307	0.4	6.1	31.1	0.2
Garlic & Herb, M&S*	1 Tsp/6g	43	4.6	712	3.4	2.4	76.9	0.9
Garlic & Herb, Reduced Calorie, Hellmann's*	1 Serving/25ml	58	4.8	233	0.7	13.1	19.3	0.4
Garlic Flavoured, Frank Cooper*	1 Tsp/6g	28	2.8	460	2.2	8.8	46.2	0.1
Garlic, Morrisons*	1 Tbsp/15ml	55	5.4	365	0.7	8.8	36.0	0.0
Garlic, Retail, Average	*1 Tsp/11g*	*44*	*4.4*	*403*	*1.2*	*8.6*	*40.3*	*0.0*
Garlic, Waitrose*	1 Tsp/6g	21	2.1	346	0.6	8.6	34.3	0.0
Heinz*	1 Tbsp/15g	99	10.8	663	0.9	3.0	71.8	0.0
Lemon, Waitrose*	1 Tsp/8ml	56	6.1	694	1.2	1.3	76.0	5.4
Lett Majones, Mills*	1 Serving/10g	44	4.7	436	0.4	3.5	46.7	0.0
Light & Squeezy, Co-Op*	1 Tbsp/15ml	45	4.2	315	1.0	11.4	29.6	0.0
Light Dijon, Benedicta*	1 Tbsp/15g	44	4.4	292	0.7	6.7	29.2	0.0
Light, Asda*	2 Tsp/10g	36	3.3	364	1.0	16.1	32.8	0.0
Light, BGTY, Sainsbury's*	1 Tbsp/15g	44	4.4	296	0.5	7.2	29.3	0.0
Light, Hellmann's*	1 Serving/10g	30	3.0	298	0.7	6.5	29.8	0.1
Light, Knorr*	1 Tbsp/15g	50	5.0	333	0.0	6.7	33.3	0.0
Light, Kraft*	1 Serving/25g	61	5.0	245	0.6	15.0	20.0	0.0
Light, Morrisons*	1 Tsp/11g	32	3.0	287	1.4	8.5	27.5	0.0
Light, Reduced Calorie, Hellmann's*	1 Tsp/10g	30	3.0	297	0.7	6.5	29.8	0.0
Light, Reduced Fat, Heinz*	1 Tbsp/15g	42	4.0	279	1.1	7.7	26.8	0.5
Light, Squeezable, Hellmann's*	1 Tbsp/15g	44	4.4	293	0.7	6.4	29.4	0.0
Light, Tesco*	1 Tbsp/15ml	41	4.0	275	0.8	7.1	26.7	0.0
Lighter than Light, Bramwells, Aldi*	1 Tbsp/15ml	10	0.4	67	0.4	10.4	2.6	0.0
Made with Free Range Eggs, M&S*	1 Tbsp/15g	108	11.8	720	1.1	1.2	78.5	0.0
Organic, Evernat*	1 Tsp/11g	83	8.9	752	1.3	2.8	81.0	0.0
Organic, Whole Foods*	1 Tbsp/14g	100	11.0	714	0.0	7.1	78.6	0.0
Original, Egg, Dairy & Gluten Free, Tiger Tiger*	1 Tbsp/15g	66	6.8	440	1.4	5.8	45.6	0.3
Real, Asda*	1 Serving/10g	72	7.9	721	1.3	1.2	79.0	0.1
Real, Hellmann's*	1 Tsp/5g	36	4.0	720	1.1	1.5	79.1	0.0

	Measure INFO/WEIGHT	per Measure KCAL	per Measure FAT	Nutrition Values per 100g / 100ml KCAL	PROT	CARB	FAT	FIBRE
MAYONNAISE								
Real, The Big Squeeze, Hellmann's*	1 Tbsp/15ml	101	11.1	676	1.0	1.2	74.0	0.0
Reduced Calorie, Average	*1 HeapTsp/11g*	*33*	*3.2*	*301*	*0.7*	*8.9*	*29.0*	*0.1*
Reduced Calorie, Tesco*	1 Tbsp/15g	49	4.7	326	0.8	9.8	31.5	0.0
Reduced Calorie, Waitrose*	1 Tsp/11g	32	3.0	287	1.4	8.5	27.5	0.0
Reduced Fat, Tesco*	1 Tbsp/15ml	44	4.3	292	0.8	7.9	28.6	0.0
Sainsbury's*	1 Tsp/11g	75	8.3	686	0.4	1.2	75.4	0.0
Value, Tesco*	1 Tbsp/15g	73	7.7	488	0.8	5.4	51.4	0.0
Waitrose*	1 Tbsp/15ml	106	11.7	709	1.3	0.8	77.8	0.0
with a Spark of Chilli, Hellmann's*	1 Tbsp/15ml	41	4.0	276	0.8	7.5	27.0	0.3
with Dijon Mustard, Hellmann's*	1 Tbsp/15ml	32	3.0	210	2.9	5.1	19.7	0.0
MEAL REPLACEMENT								
Caramel Flavour Shake, Celebrity Slim*	1 Pack/55g	212	2.4	385	34.2	50.9	4.4	0.6
Chocolate Flavour Shake, Celebrity Slim*	1 Sachet/55g	211	2.5	383	34.0	49.1	4.6	2.2
Chocolate, Slender Shake, Boots*	1 Serving/30g	116	2.1	385	15.0	60.0	7.0	11.0
Shake, Chocolate, Advantage, Atkins*	1 Serving/34g	121	4.2	361	49.0	8.1	12.5	15.5
Shake, Chocolate, Ready to Drink, Advantage, Atkins*	1 Carton/330ml	172	9.2	52	6.0	0.6	2.8	1.2
Shake, Herbalife*	1 Serving/250ml	245	6.4	98	10.0	8.8	2.6	1.0
Shake, Vanilla, Ready to Drink, Advantage, Atkins*	1 Carton/330ml	175	8.9	53	6.2	0.6	2.7	0.9
Strawberry Flavour Shake, Celebrity Slim*	1 Sachet/55g	214	2.4	389	34.4	51.6	4.4	0.6
Strawberry, High Protein, Energy Meal, Spiru-tein*	1 Serving/34g	99	0.0	291	41.2	32.4	0.0	2.9
Ultra Slim, Ready to Drink, Strawberry, Tesco*	1 Carton/330ml	231	3.0	70	4.2	10.5	0.9	1.5
Ultra-Slim, Ready to Drink, Chocolate, Tesco*	1 Carton/330ml	214	3.6	65	4.0	9.8	1.1	1.3
MEAT LOAF								
Beef & Pork, Co-Op*	¼ Loaf/114g	314	25.1	275	13.0	7.0	22.0	1.0
Beef, Wrapped in Prosciutto Crudo, Waitrose*	1/3 Pack/196g	378	27.4	193	14.2	2.6	14.0	0.7
Iceland*	1 Serving/150g	332	23.6	221	10.8	9.3	15.7	0.9
Turkey & Bacon, Tesco*	1 Serving/225g	400	22.3	178	14.7	7.4	9.9	1.1
MEATBALLS								
& Mashed Potato, Tesco*	1 Pack/450g	526	29.7	117	4.0	10.4	6.6	1.0
& Pasta in Tomato Sauce, Wayfayrer*	1 Pack/300g	375	17.4	125	9.0	9.2	5.8	1.0
& Pasta, Sainsbury's*	1 Serving/300g	333	9.3	111	5.3	15.5	3.1	1.9
& Pasta, Spicy Tomato Sauce, Slimming World, Iceland*	1 Pack/550g	605	9.9	110	8.3	14.0	1.8	2.5
Aberdeen Angus, Fresh, Chilled, Waitrose*	1 Meatball/36g	92	7.1	256	18.0	1.5	19.8	0.0
Al Forno, Charlie Bigham's*	½ Pack/324g	532	32.4	164	7.0	11.5	10.0	1.1
Beef & Pork, with Spaghetti, in Chilli Sauce, LL, Waitrose*	1 Pack/363g	388	11.6	107	7.7	10.3	3.2	2.9
Beef in Tomato Sauce, Diet Chef Ltd*	1 Pack/300g	408	18.6	136	11.3	8.7	6.2	2.7
Beef, Aberdeen Angus, with Tomato Sauce, Tesco*	½ Pack/250g	362	19.5	145	10.7	7.1	7.8	1.2
Beef, Ashfield Farm, Aldi*	1 Meatball/20g	45	2.7	232	23.0	3.9	14.0	0.5
Beef, British, Duchy Originals, As Prepared, Waitrose*	¼ Pack56g	124	6.6	221	28.6	0.2	11.7	0.1
Beef, Italian Style, As Consumed, Morrisons*	3 Meatballs/104g	235	14.7	226	19.7	4.5	14.1	0.9
Beef, Italian Style, Ocado*	1 Meatball/24g	56	4.0	235	17.0	3.2	17.0	1.4
Beef, Sainsbury's*	1 Meatball/24g	59	4.0	251	19.6	4.8	16.9	0.5
Beef, Scotch, Strathvale, Lidl*	1 Meatball/30g	73	5.6	243	17.4	0.2	18.8	1.7
Beef, Tesco*	3 Meatballs/53g	140	11.4	265	15.0	2.9	21.5	0.9
Beef, TTD, Sainsbury's*	1 Meatball/35g	73	5.2	208	16.7	1.5	15.0	0.1
Chicken in Tomato Sauce, Average	*1 Can/392g*	*580*	*32.9*	*148*	*7.7*	*10.4*	*8.4*	*0.0*
Chicken, Basil & Garlic, in a Tomato Sauce, Ilumi*	½ Pack/125g	116	3.9	93	7.8	7.8	3.1	0.0
in Bolognese Sauce, Fray Bentos*	½ Can/204g	188	5.9	92	4.8	11.6	2.9	0.7
in Gravy, Campbell's*	½ Can/205g	164	5.3	80	5.6	8.6	2.6	0.0
in Gravy, Fray Bentos*	1 Meatball/21g	17	0.6	79	4.6	8.7	2.9	0.6
in Sherry Sauce, Tapas, Waitrose*	1 Serving/185g	272	7.4	147	18.8	5.9	4.0	1.2
in Tomato & Basil Sauce, Go Cook, Asda*	½ Pack/270g	526	38.3	195	12.4	4.4	14.2	2.4
in Tomato Sauce, Canned, Average	*1 Can/410g*	*387*	*15.1*	*94*	*5.6*	*9.8*	*3.7*	*0.0*

MEATBALLS

	Measure INFO/WEIGHT	per Measure KCAL	FAT	Nutrition Values per 100g / 100ml KCAL	PROT	CARB	FAT	FIBRE
in Tomato Sauce, Tapas, Waitrose*	1 Pack/185g	285	16.8	154	10.8	7.2	9.1	1.3
Italian Pork, Al Forno, Sainsbury's*	1 Pack/450g	644	23.8	143	6.1	17.6	5.3	1.4
Lamb, Asda*	1 Pack/340g	928	71.4	273	16.0	5.1	21.0	0.6
Pork & Beef, Swedish Style, Tesco*	1 Meatball/14g	34	2.5	245	14.3	6.5	17.7	2.0
Pork & Chorizo with Paprika Potatoes, Finest, Tesco*	½ Pack/425g	527	25.9	124	7.5	9.8	6.1	2.8
Pork, & Chorizo, Sweet Tomato Sauce, Finest, Tesco*	½ Pack/245g	380	22.5	155	6.7	10.1	9.2	0.9
Pork, British, Simply, M&S*	½ Pack/180g	396	27.2	220	17.0	4.3	15.1	0.5
Pork, Duchy Originals, Waitrose*	5 Meatballs/68g	184	12.6	270	21.7	4.0	18.6	0.0
Pork, Menu, Waitrose*	½ Pack/240g	458	34.1	191	10.9	4.2	14.2	1.7
Spicy, Deli Melt, Sainsbury's*	1 Pack/200g	338	21.4	169	12.7	5.5	10.7	2.9
Swedish, Average	*¼ Pack/88g*	*198*	*13.8*	*224*	*14.0*	*7.4*	*15.7*	*1.3*
Turkey, GFY, Asda*	½ Pack/330g	333	12.2	101	10.0	7.0	3.7	0.0
Venison, Uncooked, Tesco*	1 Ball/30g	62	3.7	205	17.8	5.4	12.3	0.5
with Spicy Potato Wedges, Bistro, TTD, Sainsbury's*	½ Pack/500g	678	8.5	136	9.4	17.3	1.7	7.1

MEATBALLS VEGETARIAN

Swedish Style, Sainsbury's*	1 Ball/27g	53	2.6	194	21.5	5.5	9.5	4.0

MEDLAR

Raw, Flesh Only	*1 Fruit/28g*	*11*	*0.1*	*40*	*0.5*	*10.6*	*0.4*	*10.0*

MELBA TOAST

Asda*	1 Slice/3g	13	0.2	395	12.0	76.0	4.8	4.6
Average	*1 Serving/3g*	*13*	*0.2*	*396*	*12.0*	*76.0*	*4.9*	*4.6*
Dutch, Light Choices, Tesco*	1 Pack/20g	75	0.5	375	13.1	75.0	2.4	4.6
NUME, Morrisons*	6 Slices/20g	77	0.5	384	11.8	76.9	2.4	3.9
Original, Van Der Meulen*	1 Slice/3g	12	0.1	399	12.8	80.5	2.9	3.9
Thinly Sliced Toasted Wheat Bread, Sainsbury's*	1 Slice/3g	12	0.1	374	13.1	75.1	2.4	4.6
Wholegrain, HL, Tesco*	1 Pack/20g	74	1.0	370	16.8	63.8	4.9	8.9
Wholegrain, Morrisons*	6 Toasts/20g	73	1.0	367	16.8	63.8	4.9	8.9

MELON

Cantaloupe, Flesh Only, Average	*½ Melon/255g*	*87*	*0.5*	*34*	*0.8*	*8.2*	*0.2*	*0.9*
Cantaloupe, Weighed with Rind, Average	*1 Wedge/100g*	*18*	*0.2*	*18*	*0.4*	*4.2*	*0.2*	*0.4*
Galia	1 Serving/240g	60	0.1	25	0.8	5.8	0.0	0.2
Honeydew, Raw, Flesh Only, Average	*1oz/28g*	*8*	*0.0*	*30*	*0.7*	*7.0*	*0.1*	*0.5*
Medley, Pre Packed, Average	*1 Pack/240g*	*66*	*0.3*	*27*	*0.6*	*6.0*	*0.1*	*0.5*
Piel de Sapo, Waitrose*	1 Pack/200g	80	0.4	40	0.8	8.2	0.2	0.9
Pineapple & Strawberry, Fully Prepared, Sainsbury's*	1 Serving/245g	86	0.2	35	0.6	7.8	0.1	0.9

MELON & GRAPES

Ocado*	½ Pack/170g	65	0.2	38	0.6	8.4	0.1	0.0

MERINGUE

Average	*1 Meringue/8g*	*30*	*0.0*	*379*	*5.3*	*95.4*	*0.0*	*0.0*
Belgian Chocolate, Mini, ES, Asda*	1 Meringue/6g	28	0.9	459	6.0	75.0	15.0	0.7
Bombe, Raspberry & Vanilla, M&S*	1 Bombe/100g	155	1.8	155	3.4	33.3	1.8	2.6
Coffee Fresh Cream, Asda*	1 Meringue/28g	109	4.7	396	3.8	57.0	17.0	0.3
Cream, Fresh, Sainsbury's*	1 Meringue/35g	142	5.1	407	3.5	65.4	14.6	0.5
Cream, M&S*	1 Meringue/34g	145	7.6	425	4.1	52.6	22.2	1.4
Lemon, Morrisons*	1 Serving/120g	295	14.4	246	2.5	32.0	12.0	0.5
Mini, ES, Asda*	1 Meringue/4g	14	0.0	394	5.0	93.0	0.2	0.5
Mini, M&S*	1 Meringue/4g	15	0.0	395	6.1	91.6	0.0	0.2
Nests, Asda*	1 Nest/15g	59	0.0	394	5.0	93.0	0.2	0.5
Nests, Average	*1 Nest/16g*	*63*	*0.0*	*397*	*4.8*	*93.3*	*0.1*	*0.1*
Nests, M&S*	1 Nest/12g	47	0.0	390	6.1	91.6	0.0	0.0
Nests, Mini, Tesco*	1 Nest/5g	19	0.0	386	4.8	91.2	0.2	0.0
Nests, Morrisons*	1 Nest/15g	62	0.0	414	4.5	94.7	0.0	0.0

	Measure INFO/WEIGHT	per Measure KCAL	FAT	Nutrition Values per 100g / 100ml KCAL	PROT	CARB	FAT	FIBRE
MERINGUE								
Nests, Sainsbury's*	1 Nest/13g	52	0.0	392	4.2	93.6	0.1	0.1
Nests, Tropical Fruit, Sainsbury's*	1 Nest/95g	234	7.4	246	2.0	42.0	7.8	2.4
Raspberry, M&S*	1 Serving/105g	215	13.8	205	1.8	20.6	13.1	3.1
Shells, Sainsbury's*	2 Shells/24g	93	0.0	387	3.9	92.8	0.0	0.0
Strawberry, Mini, ES, Asda*	1 Meringue/4g	15	0.0	387	5.0	91.0	0.3	0.5
Toffee Cream, British, CBY, Asda*	1 Meringue/77g	320	14.4	416	3.7	58.1	18.7	0.1
Toffee Cream, Tesco*	1 Meringue/30g	114	5.0	380	4.2	52.9	16.5	0.0
Toffee, M&S*	1 Meringue/30g	124	6.3	415	4.1	52.2	20.9	0.8
MIDGET GEMS								
M&S*	1 Bag/113g	367	0.1	325	6.3	75.1	0.1	0.0
Smart Price, Asda*	1 Pack/178g	586	0.2	329	6.0	76.0	0.1	0.0
MILK								
1% Fat, Fresh, Arla*	1 Glass/202ml	83	2.0	41	3.3	4.8	1.0	0.0
2% Low Fat, Dunkley's*	1 Cup/240ml	130	5.0	54	3.3	5.4	2.1	0.0
Alternative, Original, Good Hemp*	1 Glass/250ml	90	6.0	36	1.3	2.2	2.4	0.2
Cashew Nut, Provamel*	1 Serving/100ml	47	2.8	47	0.9	4.4	2.8	0.3
Condensed, Caramel, Carnation, Nestle*	1 Serving/50g	148	3.0	296	5.5	55.1	6.0	0.0
Condensed, Semi Skimmed, Sweetened	*1oz/28g*	*75*	*0.1*	*267*	*10.0*	*60.0*	*0.2*	*0.0*
Condensed, Skimmed, Unsweetened, Average	*1oz/28g*	*30*	*1.1*	*108*	*7.5*	*10.5*	*4.0*	*0.0*
Condensed, Whole, Sweetened, Average	*1oz/28g*	*93*	*2.8*	*333*	*8.5*	*55.5*	*10.1*	*0.0*
Dried, Skimmed, Average	*1oz/28g*	*99*	*0.3*	*355*	*35.4*	*52.3*	*0.9*	*0.0*
Dried, Skimmed, Powder, Value, Tesco*	1 Serving/50g	180	0.3	361	36.1	52.9	0.6	0.0
Dried, Whole, Average	*1oz/28g*	*137*	*7.4*	*490*	*26.3*	*39.4*	*26.3*	*0.0*
Evaporated, Average	*1 Serving/85g*	*136*	*7.6*	*160*	*8.2*	*11.6*	*9.0*	*0.0*
Evaporated, Reduced Fat, Average	*1oz/28g*	*33*	*1.5*	*118*	*7.4*	*10.5*	*5.2*	*0.0*
Evaporated, Sainsbury's*	1 Serving/50g	80	4.5	161	8.4	11.7	9.0	0.0
Goats Semi Skimmed, Waitrose*	1 Serving/250ml	98	4.0	39	3.0	4.5	1.6	0.0
Goats, Pasteurised	*1 fl oz/30ml*	*18*	*1.0*	*60*	*3.1*	*4.4*	*3.5*	*0.0*
Goats, Semi Skimmed, St Helen's Farm*	1 Serving/250ml	109	4.0	44	3.0	4.3	1.6	0.0
Goats, Skimmed, St Helen's Farm*	1 Serving/125ml	38	0.1	30	3.0	4.3	0.1	0.0
Gold Top, Original, Graham's*	1 Tbsp/15ml	12	0.8	80	3.7	4.7	5.0	0.0
Powder, Instant, Skimmed, Basics, Sainsbury's*	1 Serving/60g	209	0.4	349	35.6	50.4	0.6	0.0
Rice, Organic, Provamel*	1 Serving/250ml	122	3.8	49	0.1	9.5	1.5	0.0
Rice, Original, Rice Dream*	1 Serving/150ml	70	1.5	47	0.1	9.4	1.0	0.1
Semi Skimmed, Advance with Omega 3, St Ivel*	1 Glass/250ml	122	4.2	49	3.4	5.0	1.7	0.0
Semi Skimmed, Asda*	1 Serving/100ml	50	1.8	50	3.6	4.8	1.8	0.0
Semi Skimmed, Average	*1 fl oz/30ml*	*15*	*0.5*	*49*	*3.4*	*5.0*	*1.7*	*0.0*
Semi Skimmed, Long Life, Average	*1 fl oz/30ml*	*15*	*0.5*	*49*	*3.4*	*5.0*	*1.7*	*0.0*
Semi Skimmed, Low Lactose, Lactofree, Arla*	1 Glass/125ml	50	1.9	40	3.6	3.0	1.5	0.0
Semi Skimmed, Low Lactose, UHT, Lactofree, Arla*	1 Serving/100ml	38	1.5	38	3.5	3.7	1.5	0.0
Semi Skimmed, Organic, Country Life*	1 fl oz/30ml	15	0.5	49	3.4	5.0	1.7	0.0
Skimmed 1% Fat, Waitrose*	1 Serving/200ml	70	0.2	35	3.4	5.0	0.1	0.0
Skimmed, Average	*1 Pint/568ml*	*194*	*0.5*	*34*	*3.3*	*5.0*	*0.1*	*0.0*
Skimmed, Lactofree, Arla*	1 Serving/200ml	66	0.8	33	3.8	3.6	0.4	0.0
Skimmed, Uht, Average	*1 fl oz/30ml*	*10*	*0.0*	*34*	*3.4*	*5.0*	*0.1*	*0.0*
Soya, Banana Flavour, Provamel*	1 Serving/250ml	195	5.5	78	3.8	10.4	2.2	0.6
Soya, Chocolate, So Good Beverages*	1 Serving/250ml	160	2.5	64	3.6	10.8	1.0	0.0
Soya, Flavoured, Average	*1floz/30mls*	*12*	*0.5*	*40*	*2.8*	*3.6*	*1.7*	*0.0*
Soya, No Added Sugar, Unsweetened, Average	*1 Serving/250ml*	*85*	*4.8*	*34*	*3.3*	*0.9*	*1.9*	*0.4*
Soya, Plain, Organic, Kirkland*	1 Glass/250ml	118	5.5	47	4.0	3.7	2.2	0.5
Soya, Strawberry Flavour, Provamel*	1 Serving/250ml	160	5.2	64	3.6	7.7	2.1	1.2
Soya, Sweetened, Average	*1 Glass/200ml*	*94*	*4.2*	*47*	*3.4*	*3.7*	*2.1*	*0.4*
Soya, Sweetened, Calcium Enriched, Average	*1 Glass/200ml*	*91*	*3.9*	*46*	*3.4*	*3.7*	*2.0*	*0.3*

M

MILK

INFO/WEIGHT	Measure	per Measure KCAL	FAT	Nutrition Values per 100g / 100ml KCAL	PROT	CARB	FAT	FIBRE
Soya, Unsweetened, Organic, Waitrose*	1 Serving/60ml	19	1.1	31	3.3	0.2	1.9	0.0
Soya, Unsweetened, Uht, Organic, Tesco*	1 Serving/150ml	50	2.8	33	3.4	0.4	1.9	0.6
Soya, Vanilla Flavour, Organic, Provamel*	1 Serving/250ml	150	5.5	60	3.8	6.2	2.2	0.6
Soya, Vanilla, Organic, Heinz*	1 Serving/200ml	106	3.2	53	2.6	6.9	1.6	0.2
Soya, Vanilla, So Good Beverages*	1 Serving/250ml	180	5.0	72	3.6	10.4	2.0	0.0
Soya, Vitasoy*	1 Serving/250ml	130	3.8	52	3.0	5.5	1.5	2.0
Super Milk Low Fat 1%, Avonmore*	1 Litre/1000ml	420	10.0	42	3.4	5.0	1.0	0.0
Whole, Average	*1 Serving/200ml*	*134*	*7.8*	*67*	*3.3*	*4.7*	*3.9*	*0.0*
Whole, Lactose Free, Lactofree, Arla*	1 Serving/200ml	114	7.0	57	3.4	2.8	3.5	0.0

MILK DRINK

INFO/WEIGHT	Measure	per Measure KCAL	FAT	KCAL	PROT	CARB	FAT	FIBRE
Banana Flavour, Sterilised, Low Fat, Gulp*	1 Bottle/500ml	425	9.0	85	5.2	11.9	1.8	0.0
Chocolate Flavoured, Goodness for Kids, Tesco*	1 Bottlel/330ml	248	5.9	75	3.8	10.3	1.8	0.7
Chocolate Sterilised Skimmed, Happy Shopper*	1 Bottle/500ml	295	1.5	59	3.6	10.4	0.3	0.0
Chocolate, Spar*	1 Serving/500ml	290	1.5	58	3.6	10.2	0.3	0.0
Chocolatte, Cafe Met*	1 Bottle/290ml	174	4.1	60	3.7	9.1	1.4	0.3
Original, Mars*	1 Serving/330g	284	6.9	86	3.1	13.7	2.1	0.0
Refuel, Mars*	1 Bottle/388ml	299	5.8	77	3.1	13.5	1.5	0.0
Semi Skimmed, Cholesterol Lowering, Pro Activ, Flora*	1 Serving/250ml	125	4.5	50	3.6	4.8	1.8	0.0

MILK SHAKE

INFO/WEIGHT	Measure	per Measure KCAL	FAT	KCAL	PROT	CARB	FAT	FIBRE
Banana & Cashew, Almond, Dairy Free, Pret a Manger*	1 Pack/264g	232	13.4	88	2.6	8.4	5.1	0.0
Banana Flavour, Frijj*	1 Bottle/500ml	325	4.5	65	3.7	10.5	0.9	0.0
Banana, Shudda, Aldi*	½ Bottle/236g	163	2.1	69	3.4	12.0	0.9	0.5
Banana, Yazoo, Campina*	1 Bottle/200ml	120	2.4	60	3.1	9.6	1.2	0.0
Chocolate Flavoured, Fresh, Thick, Frijj*	1 Bottle/500ml	350	5.0	70	3.5	11.7	1.0	0.0
Chocolate, Asda*	1 Serving/250ml	198	9.2	79	4.4	7.0	3.7	0.4
Honeycomb Choc Swirl Flavour, The Incredible, Frijj*	1 Bottle/500ml	450	12.5	90	4.0	13.0	2.5	0.2
Strawberry Flavour, Thick, Low Fat, Frijj*	1 Bottle/250ml	155	2.0	62	3.4	10.1	0.8	0.0
Strawberry, Yazoo, Campina*	1 Bottle/475ml	300	6.0	60	3.1	9.5	1.2	0.0

MILKY BAR

INFO/WEIGHT	Measure	per Measure KCAL	FAT	KCAL	PROT	CARB	FAT	FIBRE
Buttons, Nestle*	1 Pack/30g	164	9.5	547	7.3	58.4	31.7	0.0
Eggs, Mini, Nestle*	1 Pack/100g	503	22.0	503	5.4	70.5	22.0	0.5
Funsize (17g), Mars*	1 Funsize Bar/17g	75	2.7	449	3.8	71.8	16.3	0.6
Nestle*	1 Sm Bar/13g	68	4.0	547	7.3	58.4	31.7	0.0

MILKY WAY

INFO/WEIGHT	Measure	per Measure KCAL	FAT	KCAL	PROT	CARB	FAT	FIBRE
Fun Size, Mars*	1 Bar/17g	75	2.7	447	3.8	71.6	16.2	0.0
Mars*	1 Bar/22g	96	3.3	446	3.9	72.4	15.5	0.6

MINCEMEAT

INFO/WEIGHT	Measure	per Measure KCAL	FAT	KCAL	PROT	CARB	FAT	FIBRE
Average	*1oz/28g*	*77*	*1.2*	*274*	*0.6*	*62.1*	*4.3*	*1.3*
Traditional, Sainsbury's*	1 Tbsp/23g	65	0.7	282	0.9	62.4	3.2	1.4

MINI BITES

INFO/WEIGHT	Measure	per Measure KCAL	FAT	KCAL	PROT	CARB	FAT	FIBRE
Blueberry & Yoghurt Clusters, M&S*	1 Mini Bite/13g	60	2.7	465	5.0	64.4	20.7	4.7
Chocolate Caramel, M&S*	1 Bite/21g	95	5.1	460	5.6	53.5	24.6	1.6
Chocolate Cornflake, M&S*	1 Bite/12g	55	2.4	470	6.2	66.3	20.1	3.6
Chocolate Orange, M&S*	1 Bite/22g	95	4.8	430	5.5	54.6	21.6	1.8
Extremely Chocolatey Caramel Crispy, M&S*	1 Bite/11g	50	2.0	455	4.7	68.2	17.9	2.8
Extremely Chocolatey, M&S*	1 Bite/20g	90	4.9	450	5.7	52.4	24.6	1.6
Flapjack, M&S*	1 Bite/14g	70	3.5	500	6.4	62.1	25.0	3.6
Rocky Road, M&S*	1 Bite/12g	50	1.6	410	5.2	66.9	13.3	2.5

MINSTRELS

INFO/WEIGHT	Measure	per Measure KCAL	FAT	KCAL	PROT	CARB	FAT	FIBRE
Galaxy, Mars*	1 Serving/100g	503	22.3	503	5.2	70.3	22.3	1.1

MINT

INFO/WEIGHT	Measure	per Measure KCAL	FAT	KCAL	PROT	CARB	FAT	FIBRE
Dried, Average	*1 Tsp/5g*	*14*	*0.2*	*279*	*24.8*	*34.6*	*4.6*	*0.0*
Fresh, Average	*2 Tbsp/3g*	*1*	*0.0*	*43*	*3.8*	*5.3*	*0.7*	*0.0*

	Measure INFO/WEIGHT	per Measure KCAL	FAT	Nutrition Values per 100g / 100ml KCAL	PROT	CARB	FAT	FIBRE
MINTS								
After Dinner, Dark, Elizabeth Shaw*	1 Sweet/9g	42	2.1	469	2.8	62.5	23.1	0.0
After Dinner, Sainsbury's*	1 Mint/7g	32	1.5	456	4.1	62.1	21.2	4.1
Butter Mintoes, M&S*	1 Sweet/9g	35	0.6	391	0.0	84.0	6.8	0.0
Butter Mintoes, Tesco*	1 Sweet/7g	24	0.5	349	0.0	71.3	7.1	0.0
Clear, Co-Op*	1 Sweet/6g	24	0.0	395	0.0	98.0	0.0	0.0
Cream, Luxury, Thorntons*	1 Sweet/13g	62	3.1	477	4.2	62.3	23.8	2.3
Creams, Bassett's*	1 Sweet/11g	40	0.0	365	0.0	91.8	0.0	0.0
Curiously Strong, M&S*	1 Sweet/1g	4	0.0	390	0.4	97.5	0.0	0.0
Everton, Co-Op*	1 Sweet/6g	25	0.2	410	0.6	92.0	4.0	0.0
Extra Strong, Peppermint, Trebor*	1 Mint/2g	10	0.0	395	0.3	98.5	0.0	0.0
Extra Strong, Spearmint, Trebor*	1 Pack/44g	174	0.0	395	0.4	98.7	0.0	0.0
Extra, Peppermint Coolburst, Wrigleys*	1 Pack/22g	53	0.2	240	0.0	98.0	1.0	0.0
Extra, Spearmint, Sugar Free, Wrigleys*	1 Sweet/1g	3	0.0	244	0.0	98.5	0.8	0.0
Glacier, Fox's*	1 Sweet/5g	19	0.0	386	0.0	96.4	0.0	0.0
Humbugs, Co-Op*	1 Sweet/8g	34	0.6	425	0.6	89.9	7.0	0.0
Humbugs, M&S*	1 Sweet/9g	37	0.4	407	0.6	91.1	4.4	0.0
Humbugs, Thorntons*	1 Sweet/9g	31	0.4	340	1.0	87.8	4.4	0.0
Imperials, Co-Op*	1 Sweet/3g	12	0.0	395	0.3	98.0	0.2	0.0
Imperials, M&S*	1 Sweet/3g	12	0.0	391	0.0	97.8	0.0	0.0
Imperials, Sainsbury's*	1 Sweet/3g	10	0.0	374	0.0	92.1	0.0	0.0
Imperials, Tesco*	1 Sweet/3g	12	0.0	397	0.6	98.7	0.0	0.0
Mento, Sugar Free, Mentos*	1 Sweet/2g	5	0.1	260	1.0	87.0	5.5	0.0
Mint Assortment, M&S*	1 Sweet/7g	26	0.5	375	0.4	78.2	6.9	0.0
Mint Favourites, Bassett's*	1 Sweet/6g	22	0.4	367	0.9	77.4	5.9	0.0
Soft, Trebor*	1 Pack/48g	182	0.0	380	0.0	94.9	0.0	0.0
Softmints, Peppermint, Trebor*	1 Pack/48g	170	0.0	355	0.0	88.9	0.0	0.0
Softmints, Spearmint, Trebor*	1 Pack/45g	170	0.0	375	0.0	94.3	0.0	0.0
MIRIN								
Rice Wine, Sweetened, Average	1 Tbsp/15ml	35	0.0	231	0.2	41.6	0.0	0.0
MISO								
Average	1oz/28g	57	1.7	203	13.3	23.5	6.2	0.0
MIXED HERBS								
Average	1 Tsp/5g	13	0.4	260	13.0	37.5	8.5	6.7
Herbes De Provence, Dried, Schwartz*	1 Tsp/2g	7	0.1	364	12.9	65.0	5.8	0.0
MIXED SPICE								
Schwartz*	1 Tsp/2g	8	0.2	390	10.4	65.8	9.5	2.0
MOLASSES								
Average	1 Tsp/5g	13	0.0	266	0.0	68.8	0.1	0.0
MONKEY NUTS								
without Shell, Average	1oz/28g	158	13.4	565	25.6	8.2	48.0	6.3
MONKFISH								
Grilled	1oz/28g	27	0.2	96	22.7	0.0	0.6	0.0
Raw	1oz/28g	18	0.1	66	15.7	0.0	0.4	0.0
MONSTER MUNCH								
Pickled Onion, Walkers*	1 Bag/22g	108	5.5	490	6.0	60.0	25.0	1.7
Roast Beef, Walkers*	1 Bag/22g	108	5.5	490	7.0	59.0	25.0	1.7
Spicy, Walkers*	1 Bag/25g	125	7.2	500	5.0	55.0	29.0	1.3
MOUSSAKA								
Beef, HL, Tesco*	1 Pack/450g	396	12.2	88	5.0	10.9	2.7	0.8
Cafe Culture, M&S*	1 Serving/375g	619	39.4	165	9.2	7.8	10.5	0.8
Charlie Bigham's*	½ Pack/328g	396	24.2	121	7.0	7.0	7.4	0.9
COU, M&S*	1 Pack/340g	272	9.9	80	5.3	8.5	2.9	1.4
Lamb, Finest, Tesco*	1 Pack/335g	543	37.5	162	6.7	7.9	11.2	1.5

	Measure INFO/WEIGHT	per Measure KCAL	per Measure FAT	Nutrition Values per 100g / 100ml KCAL	PROT	CARB	FAT	FIBRE
MOUSSAKA								
Low Saturated Fat, Waitrose*	1 Pack/350g	304	10.8	87	6.3	8.4	3.1	3.1
Vegetable, COU, M&S*	1 Pack/400g	280	10.8	70	2.7	9.1	2.7	2.4
MOUSSE								
Aero Chocolate, Nestle*	1 Pot/58g	101	3.0	174	4.8	27.3	5.1	1.1
Apricot, Lite, Onken*	1 Pot/150g	156	2.2	104	4.6	18.0	1.5	0.3
Belgian Chocolate & Vanilla, Weight Watchers*	1 Pot/80g	106	2.2	132	4.4	22.2	2.8	0.9
Belgian Chocolate, Finest, Tesco*	1 Pot/120g	360	22.7	300	5.1	26.6	18.9	1.1
Blackcurrant, Onken*	1 Pot/150g	210	10.2	140	5.2	14.6	6.8	0.0
Cappuccino, Essential, Waitrose*	1 Pot/100g	279	16.7	279	4.2	27.7	16.7	0.5
Chocolate	1 Pot/60g	83	3.2	139	4.0	19.9	5.4	0.0
Chocolate & Mint, COU, M&S*	1 Pot/70g	84	1.8	120	6.2	18.7	2.5	1.0
Chocolate & Orange, COU, M&S*	1 Pot/70g	77	1.8	110	5.9	16.0	2.6	0.9
Chocolate Orange, Low Fat, Cadbury*	1 Pot/100g	110	3.0	110	5.6	15.1	3.0	0.0
Chocolate, Asda*	1 Pot/61g	134	6.1	219	3.7	26.0	10.0	1.0
Chocolate, Basics, Sainsbury's*	1 Pot/63g	94	3.8	150	5.1	18.9	6.0	0.0
Chocolate, BGTY, Sainsbury's*	1 Pot/63g	83	1.8	133	4.9	21.8	2.9	0.5
Chocolate, Cadbury*	1 Pot/55g	107	4.5	195	6.1	24.6	8.2	0.0
Chocolate, COU, M&S*	1 Pot/70g	84	1.9	120	5.2	20.3	2.7	1.0
Chocolate, Light Choices, Light Choices, Tesco*	1 Pot/63g	80	1.3	125	5.0	20.8	2.1	1.5
Chocolate, Light, Cadbury*	1 Pot/55g	60	1.9	110	4.6	14.2	3.4	0.0
Chocolate, Low Fat, Danette, Danone*	1 Pot/60g	73	1.1	121	5.1	20.8	1.9	1.5
Chocolate, Minty, Bubbly, Dessert, Aero, Nestle*	1 Pot/58g	108	5.9	186	4.6	18.9	10.2	0.3
Chocolate, Sainsbury's*	1 Pot/63g	119	5.3	190	4.7	23.8	8.5	1.0
Chocolate, Tesco*	1 Pot/60g	120	5.0	200	3.6	27.6	8.4	0.9
Chocolate, Value, Tesco*	1 Pot/63g	101	3.3	161	4.9	23.3	5.2	1.3
Chocolate, White, Bubbly, Dessert, Aero, Nestle*	1 Pot/58g	99	4.4	170	4.3	21.0	7.5	0.2
Layered Strawberry, Co-Op*	1 Pot/100g	120	3.0	120	3.0	19.0	3.0	0.2
Lemon with Meringue Style Sauce, Ski, Nestle*	1 Pot/60g	81	2.8	137	3.1	19.8	4.8	0.0
Lemon, COU, M&S*	1 Pot/70g	91	1.8	130	3.1	23.7	2.5	0.6
Lemon, Dessert, Sainsbury's*	1 Pot/63g	114	5.9	182	3.6	20.7	9.4	0.6
Lemon, Low Fat, Morrisons*	1 Pot/63g	99	5.8	158	3.7	15.4	9.3	0.3
Lemon, Tesco*	1 Pot/60g	67	1.6	111	3.4	18.2	2.7	0.0
Milk Chocolate, M&S*	1 Pot/90g	180	7.8	200	5.3	24.8	8.7	1.5
Mint Chocolate, Cadbury*	1 Pot/45g	90	3.6	200	6.0	25.6	8.1	0.0
Raspberry Ripple, Value, Tesco*	1 Pot/47g	70	2.9	149	2.1	21.3	6.1	0.1
Rhubarb, COU, M&S*	1 Pot/70g	88	1.5	125	2.9	25.7	2.1	4.2
Strawberry with Strawberry Sauce, Ski, Nestle*	1 Pot/60g	79	3.1	131	3.1	18.1	5.2	0.0
Strawberry, Light, Muller*	1 Pot/150g	147	0.6	98	4.3	19.4	0.4	0.0
Strawberry, Sainsbury's*	1 Pot/63g	106	5.9	168	3.4	17.5	9.4	0.1
Strawberry, Tesco*	1 Pot/63g	106	5.8	169	3.5	17.9	9.3	0.2
Summer Fruits, Light, Muller*	1 Pot/149g	143	0.6	96	4.3	18.7	0.4	0.0
Toffee, M&S*	1 Pot/90g	180	7.2	200	4.5	27.6	8.0	0.6
White Chocolate, Finest, Tesco*	1 Pot/92g	436	34.5	474	3.9	30.2	37.5	0.0
MUFFIN								
All Butter, M&S*	1 Muffin/65g	175	4.7	270	10.3	40.8	7.3	2.1
Apple, Sultana & Cinnamon, GFY, Asda*	1 Muffin/50g	134	1.8	268	6.0	53.0	3.5	3.9
Banana & Walnut, The Handmade Flapjack Company*	1 Muffin/135g	520	30.6	385	5.3	40.5	22.7	0.0
Banana Pecan, Organic, Honeyrose Bakery*	1 Muffin/110g	300	12.6	273	4.1	38.3	11.5	4.3
Berry Burst, Asda*	1 Muffin/60g	139	1.4	232	6.2	46.7	2.3	1.7
Blueberry, American Style, Aldi*	1 Muffin/85g	344	17.3	405	4.3	51.2	20.3	0.0
Blueberry, American Style, Sainsbury's*	1 Muffin/72g	256	13.1	355	5.1	42.7	18.2	1.9
Blueberry, Asda*	1 Muffin/77g	273	13.1	353	5.0	45.0	17.0	1.3
Blueberry, M&S*	1 Muffin/75g	255	12.6	340	4.9	41.9	16.8	1.3

MUFFIN

INFO/WEIGHT	Measure	per Measure		Nutrition Values per 100g / 100ml				
		KCAL	FAT	KCAL	PROT	CARB	FAT	FIBRE
Blueberry, Mini, Sainsbury's*	1 Muffin/28g	82	2.3	293	6.3	48.9	8.1	1.9
Blueberry, Mini, Tesco*	1 Muffin/28g	104	5.4	370	5.6	43.5	19.3	1.2
Blueberry, Tesco*	1 Muffin/73g	248	12.5	340	4.7	41.0	17.1	1.9
Blueberry, Waitrose*	1 Muffin/65g	239	9.2	367	4.7	55.2	14.2	1.7
Bran & Sultana, Weight Watchers*	1 Muffin/60g	144	1.3	240	4.5	50.7	2.1	2.3
Bran, Average	*1 Muffin/57g*	*155*	*4.4*	*272*	*7.8*	*45.6*	*7.7*	*7.7*
Caramel, Salted, TTD, Sainsbury's*	1 Muffin/113g	447	22.0	396	4.8	49.6	19.5	1.5
Carrot Cake, Entenmann's*	1 Muffin/105g	344	15.9	328	5.1	45.8	15.1	3.0
Carrot, Asda*	1 Muffin/59g	138	1.4	233	6.0	47.0	2.3	1.6
Cheese, Tesco*	1 Muffin/67g	150	1.9	224	13.0	36.4	2.9	3.0
Chocolate Chip, American Style, Sainsbury's*	1 Muffin/72g	284	14.4	395	5.0	48.8	20.0	2.1
Chocolate Chip, BGTY, Sainsbury's*	1 Muffin/75g	282	12.3	376	5.2	51.8	16.4	1.6
Chocolate Chip, Gluten Free, Antoinette Savill*	1 Muffin/100g	472	31.9	472	5.3	44.9	31.9	3.3
Chocolate Chip, Mini, Asda*	1 Muffin/22g	77	2.9	349	7.0	51.0	13.0	2.1
Chocolate Chip, Mini, BGTY, Sainsbury's*	1 Muffin/28g	91	2.4	324	6.5	55.1	8.7	1.6
Chocolate Chip, Mini, Essential, Waitrose*	1 Muffin/27g	108	5.1	399	5.9	49.8	19.0	2.5
Chocolate Chip, Plain, Tesco*	1 Muffin/72g	270	12.7	375	5.0	48.1	17.6	1.4
Chocolate Indulgence, McVitie's*	1 Muffin/75g	254	6.9	338	5.8	57.9	9.2	1.3
Chocolate, Galaxy, McVitie's*	1 Muffin/88g	319	17.1	364	5.0	44.5	19.5	0.0
Cinnamon & Sultana, Baked by Us, Morrisons*	1 Muffin/68g	166	1.0	244	8.3	48.2	1.4	2.9
Cranberry & White Chocolate, Sainsbury's*	1 Muffin/72g	253	13.3	352	5.7	40.7	18.5	1.5
Double Berry Burst, Entenmann's*	1 Muffin/59g	140	1.2	238	4.6	50.1	2.1	1.6
Double Chocolate Chip, American Style, Sainsbury's*	1 Muffin/72g	276	14.6	384	5.2	45.0	20.3	2.9
Double Chocolate Chip, Co-Op*	1 Muffin/70g	308	16.8	440	6.6	49.4	24.0	2.5
Double Chocolate Chip, Co-Op*	1 Muffin/60g	246	12.6	410	6.0	49.0	21.0	3.0
Double Chocolate Chip, Mini, Asda*	1 Muffin/19g	76	3.7	400	7.4	48.5	19.6	2.7
Double Chocolate Chip, Tesco*	1 Muffin/100g	360	17.9	360	6.1	44.9	17.9	5.4
Double Chocolate, CBY, Asda*	1 Muffin/100g	398	19.8	398	6.0	47.9	19.8	0.0
Double Chocolate, Chocolate Chip, Mini, Tesco*	1 Muffin/28g	116	6.4	414	6.3	45.7	23.0	1.4
Double Chocolate, Free From, Tesco*	1 Muffin/70g	281	12.7	402	4.7	54.8	18.2	1.7
Double Chocolate, Mini, M&S*	1 Muffin/32g	133	6.9	416	5.4	49.8	21.7	1.1
English	1 Muffin/57g	120	1.0	211	7.0	43.9	1.8	1.8
English, Butter, Tesco*	1 Muffin/67g	170	3.6	253	11.2	39.8	5.4	2.0
English, Gluten, Wheat & Milk Free, Free From, Livwell*	1 Muffin/50g	160	4.9	320	4.6	52.8	9.8	3.2
English, Kingsmill*	1 Muffin/75g	167	1.4	222	9.7	40.4	1.8	2.6
English, M&S*	1 Muffin/60g	135	1.1	225	11.2	43.7	1.9	2.9
English, Tesco*	1 Muffin/72g	171	2.3	238	11.2	41.7	3.2	2.8
Fruit, Spiced, TTD, Sainsbury's*	1 Muffin/70g	181	3.6	259	10.1	43.1	5.1	2.1
Jammy, Kate's Cakes Ltd*	1 Muffin/100g	393	20.7	393	4.0	47.8	20.7	1.1
Lemon & Poppy Seed, M&S*	1 Muffin/72g	281	14.3	390	6.3	46.1	19.8	1.5
Lemon & Poppy Seed, Waitrose*	1 Muffin/121g	460	23.1	380	4.3	46.8	19.1	1.8
Lemon Curd, Patisserie, TTD, Sainsbury's*	1 Muffin/108g	418	20.9	386	5.4	47.1	19.3	1.4
Lemon, Boots*	1 Muffin/110g	424	20.9	385	3.6	50.0	19.0	1.3
Mini, Chocolate Chip, CBY, Asda*	1 Muffin/100g	425	22.5	425	5.0	50.0	22.5	0.0
Mini, Tesco*	1 Muffin/28g	120	6.3	428	6.4	50.0	22.6	1.2
Muesli, Breakfast, LL, Waitrose*	1 Muffin/68g	216	6.2	318	9.1	50.0	9.1	3.4
Orange, Apricot & Almond, Organic, Honeyrose Bakery*	1 Muffin/110g	312	11.4	284	3.5	44.2	10.4	1.9
Organic Wholemeal, LL, Waitrose*	1 Muffin/100g	245	3.6	245	11.7	40.8	3.6	6.3
Oven Bottom, Aldi*	1 Muffin/68g	173	1.0	255	10.0	50.4	1.5	2.2
Oven Bottom, Asda*	1 Muffin/68g	173	1.0	255	10.0	50.4	1.5	2.2
Oven Bottom, Tesco*	1 Muffin/68g	173	1.0	255	10.0	50.4	1.5	2.2
Oven Bottom, Warburton's*	1 Muffin/69g	175	2.0	253	10.9	45.8	2.9	0.0
Plain, Co-Op*	1 Muffin/60g	135	1.1	225	11.2	41.3	1.9	2.4

MUFFIN

INFO/WEIGHT	per Measure KCAL	FAT	Nutrition Values per 100g / 100ml KCAL	PROT	CARB	FAT	FIBRE
Plain, Morrisons*	1 Muffin/70g	140	0.8	200	8.0	41.4	1.1	0.0
Plain, Prepared From Recipe, Average	*1 Sm Muffin/57g*	*169*	*6.5*	*296*	*6.9*	*41.4*	*11.4*	*2.7*
Raspberry Cream, Sainsbury's*	1 Muffin/90g	314	19.8	349	3.9	33.8	22.0	1.3
Sausage, Egg & Cheese, American Style, Tesco*	1 Muffin/155g	383	20.5	247	12.2	19.9	13.2	1.0
Spiced Fruit, Toasting, Finest, Tesco*	1 Muffin/77g	215	5.2	279	9.2	43.2	6.8	3.9
Spicy Fruit, Quality Bakers*	1 Muffin/65g	146	1.0	225	9.4	38.0	1.5	3.3
Strawberry Cakelet, The Handmade Flapjack Company*	1 Muffin/135g	526	29.6	390	4.5	43.6	21.9	0.0
Sunblest*	1 Muffin/72g	166	1.3	230	9.6	43.9	1.8	2.2
Toasting, Warburton's*	1 Muffin/64g	138	1.0	216	8.9	41.4	1.6	2.9
Toffee & Pecan, Finest, Tesco*	1 Muffin/127g	551	29.0	434	5.4	51.8	22.8	0.9
Toffee, The Handmade Flapjack Company*	1 Muffin/135g	533	31.6	395	4.4	41.2	23.4	0.0
White Chocolate & Strawberry Filled, Tesco*	1 Muffin/103g	415	20.3	405	5.2	51.3	19.8	1.3
White Chocolate Chunk Lemon, Mini, M&S*	1 Muffin/28g	130	6.7	464	6.4	55.4	23.9	2.1
White, All Butter, Sainsbury's*	1 Muffin/67g	173	4.2	258	10.6	39.6	6.3	3.6
White, Asda*	1 Muffin/67g	148	1.3	222	11.0	40.0	2.0	2.5
White, Finest, Tesco*	1 Muffin/70g	159	0.8	227	8.4	45.7	1.2	2.1
White, Tesco*	1 Muffin/72g	173	2.3	240	11.3	41.6	3.2	2.8
Wholemeal, Tesco*	1 Muffin/65g	130	1.3	200	12.6	32.9	2.0	5.7

MULBERRIES

Raw	*1oz/28g*	*10*	*0.0*	*36*	*1.3*	*8.1*	*0.0*	*0.0*

MULLET

Grey, Grilled	*1oz/28g*	*42*	*1.5*	*150*	*25.7*	*0.0*	*5.2*	*0.0*
Grey, Raw	*1oz/28g*	*16*	*0.6*	*58*	*9.9*	*0.0*	*2.0*	*0.0*
Red, Grilled	*1oz/28g*	*34*	*1.2*	*121*	*20.4*	*0.0*	*4.4*	*0.0*
Red, Raw, Weighed Whole, Flesh Only	*1 Portion/100g*	*25*	*0.9*	*25*	*4.3*	*0.0*	*0.9*	*0.0*

MUNCHIES

Original, Tube, Nestle*	1 Pack/55g	266	12.3	487	5.4	64.6	22.5	1.4

MUSHROOMS

Breaded, Average	*3 Mushrooms/51g*	*77*	*2.9*	*152*	*4.3*	*20.8*	*5.7*	*0.6*
Breaded, Garlic, Average	*3 Mushrooms/50g*	*92*	*4.9*	*183*	*5.2*	*18.7*	*9.7*	*1.7*
Buna Shimeji, Livesey Brothers*	½ Pack/75g	29	0.3	39	2.7	5.9	0.4	1.2
Button, Raw, Average	*1 Serving/50g*	*7*	*0.2*	*15*	*2.3*	*0.5*	*0.4*	*1.2*
Chestnut, Average	*1 Med/5g*	*1*	*0.0*	*13*	*1.8*	*0.4*	*0.5*	*0.6*
Chinese, Dried, Raw	*1oz/28g*	*80*	*0.5*	*284*	*10.0*	*59.9*	*1.8*	*0.0*
Closed Cup, Average	*1 Handfull/30g*	*4*	*0.2*	*14*	*1.8*	*0.4*	*0.5*	*1.1*
Closed Cup, Co-Op*	1 Portion/85g	13	0.4	15	1.8	0.4	0.5	1.0
Common, Boiled in Salted Water, Average	*1oz/28g*	*3*	*0.1*	*11*	*1.8*	*0.4*	*0.3*	*1.1*
Common, Fried, Average	*1oz/28g*	*44*	*4.5*	*157*	*2.4*	*0.3*	*16.2*	*1.5*
Common, Raw, Average	*1 Serving/80g*	*10*	*0.4*	*12*	*1.8*	*0.3*	*0.5*	*1.1*
Creamed, Average	*1oz/28g*	*23*	*1.5*	*82*	*1.3*	*6.8*	*5.5*	*0.5*
Dried	*1oz/28g*	*45*	*1.7*	*159*	*21.8*	*4.8*	*6.0*	*13.3*
Enoki, Average	*1 Serving/80g*	*34*	*0.0*	*42*	*3.0*	*7.0*	*0.0*	*3.0*
Family Pack, Tesco*	1 Serving/100g	16	0.5	16	1.8	0.4	0.5	1.1
Flat, Large, Average	*1 Mushroom/52g*	*10*	*0.3*	*20*	*3.3*	*0.5*	*0.5*	*0.7*
Frozen, Cooks' Ingredients, Waitrose*	1 Portion/75g	14	0.2	18	2.1	1.8	0.3	2.5
Garlic, Average	*½ Pack/150g*	*159*	*14.0*	*106*	*2.1*	*3.7*	*9.3*	*1.7*
Garlic, Cooked, World Cafe, Waitrose*	½ Pack/51g	177	16.7	350	4.0	8.2	33.0	2.3
Giant with Tomatoes & Mozzarella, M&S*	1 Serving/145g	218	15.8	150	6.3	7.1	10.9	5.5
Hon Shimeji, Sainsbury's*	1 Serving/80g	18	0.4	22	4.0	3.9	0.5	1.1
Oyster, Average	*1 Serving/80g*	*10*	*0.2*	*13*	*1.4*	*1.4*	*0.2*	*1.1*
Porcini, Dried, Asda*	1 Bag/25g	65	1.2	260	30.4	24.1	4.7	17.5
Porcini, Wild, Dried, Merchant Gourmet*	1 Pack/25g	66	0.8	265	27.9	30.6	3.4	18.7
Portobello, Mini, Sainsbury's*	1 Serving/100g	16	0.5	16	1.8	0.4	0.5	1.1

	Measure INFO/WEIGHT	per Measure KCAL	per Measure FAT	Nutrition Values per 100g / 100ml KCAL	PROT	CARB	FAT	FIBRE
MUSHROOMS								
Shiitake, Cooked	**1oz/28g**	**15**	**0.1**	**55**	**1.6**	**12.3**	**0.2**	**0.0**
Shiitake, Dried, Raw	**1oz/28g**	**83**	**0.3**	**296**	**9.6**	**63.9**	**1.0**	**0.0**
Shiitake, Raw, Waitrose*	1 Serving/100g	32	0.5	32	2.2	48.0	0.5	25.0
Shiitake, TTD, Sainsbury's*	1 Serving/100g	40	0.5	40	5.5	3.4	0.5	4.9
Sliced, Average	**1oz/28g**	**3**	**0.1**	**12**	**1.8**	**0.4**	**0.3**	**1.1**
Sliced, Canned in Water, Everyday Value, Tesco*	½ Can/78g	14	0.3	18	2.1	0.2	0.4	2.8
Straw, Canned, Drained	**1oz/28g**	**4**	**0.1**	**15**	**2.1**	**1.2**	**0.2**	**0.0**
Stuffed, & Mediterranean Vegetables, Sainsbury's*	1 Pack/270g	219	11.1	81	2.6	7.4	4.1	2.2
Stuffed, Cheesy, Asda*	1 Serving/290g	322	17.4	111	4.3	10.0	6.0	0.0
Stuffed, Garlic & Cream Cheese, Aldi*	1 Serving/100g	130	7.5	130	5.3	9.7	7.5	1.4
Stuffed, Ready to Roast, Waitrose*	1 Serving/125g	94	4.6	75	3.9	6.5	3.7	1.5
Stuffed, Stilton & Leek, Portobello, Asda*	1 Mushroom/200g	292	19.0	146	9.2	5.5	9.5	1.0
MUSSELS								
Boiled, Weighed in Shell, Average	**1 Mussel/7g**	**2**	**0.1**	**28**	**4.5**	**0.9**	**0.7**	**0.0**
Cooked & Shelled, Meat, Tesco*	1 Pack/240g	216	5.0	90	13.9	3.8	2.1	0.0
Pickled, Drained, Average	**1oz/28g**	**32**	**0.6**	**112**	**20.0**	**1.5**	**2.2**	**0.0**
Raw, Weighed in Shell, Average	**1oz/28g**	**7**	**0.2**	**23**	**3.4**	**1.0**	**0.7**	**0.0**
MUSSELS IN								
Seasoned White Wine Sauce, Bantry Bay*	1 Serving/450g	270	9.0	60	6.3	4.1	2.0	0.1
Thai Sauce, Scottish, Waitrose*	1 Serving/250g	135	6.2	54	5.4	2.6	2.5	0.6
White Wine & Garlic Sauce,,Scottish, Tesco*	1 Pouch/155g	130	6.2	84	9.8	1.9	4.0	0.6
White Wine Sauce, Sainsbury's*	½ Pack/250g	221	9.2	88	8.0	5.8	3.7	0.0
MUSTARD								
American, Average	**1 Tsp/5g**	**5**	**0.2**	**102**	**4.4**	**10.5**	**5.0**	**2.5**
Cajun, Colman's*	1 Tsp/6g	11	0.4	187	7.0	23.0	6.5	2.7
Coarse Grain, Average	**1 Tsp/5g**	**7**	**0.4**	**141**	**7.7**	**8.4**	**8.3**	**5.9**
Dijon, Average	**1 Tsp/5g**	**8**	**0.6**	**163**	**7.4**	**7.7**	**11.3**	**1.1**
English, Average	**1 Tsp/5g**	**9**	**0.4**	**173**	**6.8**	**19.2**	**7.6**	**1.2**
English, Original,,Colman's*	1 Tsp/5g	8	0.3	160	8.2	8.7	5.6	2.1
French, Average	**1 Tsp/5g**	**5**	**0.3**	**106**	**5.4**	**8.1**	**5.6**	**1.8**
French, Tesco*	1 Tsp/5g	7	0.3	140	6.4	11.9	6.3	3.0
German Style, Sainsbury's*	1 Serving/10g	9	0.6	92	5.5	2.8	6.5	0.0
Honey, Colman's*	1 Tsp/6g	12	0.5	208	7.4	24.0	8.2	0.0
Powder, Average	**1 Tsp/3g**	**15**	**0.9**	**452**	**28.9**	**20.7**	**28.7**	**0.0**
Smooth, Average	**1 Tsp/8g**	**11**	**0.7**	**139**	**7.1**	**9.7**	**8.2**	**0.0**
Whole Grain, Average	**1 Tsp/8g**	**11**	**0.8**	**140**	**8.2**	**4.2**	**10.2**	**4.9**
Wholegrain, Essential, Waitrose*	1 Serving/10g	16	1.0	161	7.4	10.6	9.9	2.5
Yellow, Prepared	**1 Tbsp/15ml**	**11**	**0.6**	**73**	**4.0**	**6.0**	**4.0**	**0.0**
MUSTARD CRESS								
Raw	**1oz/28g**	**4**	**0.2**	**13**	**1.6**	**0.4**	**0.6**	**1.1**

M

	Measure INFO/WEIGHT	per Measure KCAL	FAT	Nutrition Values per 100g / 100ml KCAL	PROT	CARB	FAT	FIBRE
NACHOS								
American Chilli Beef, Asda*	1 Serving/200g	208	10.0	104	10.0	4.7	5.0	0.8
Cheesy with Salsa & Soured Cream, Sainsbury's*	½ Pack/170g	449	26.9	264	8.8	21.5	15.8	1.4
Chilli, Sainsbury's*	½ Pack/250g	695	32.2	278	10.9	29.5	12.9	1.3
Kit, Old El Paso*	½ Pack/260g	598	26.0	230	4.0	31.0	10.0	0.0
NASI GORENG								
Indonesian, Asda*	1 Pack/360g	778	22.7	216	7.4	32.3	6.3	1.3
Vitasia, Lidl*	1 Bowl/250g	438	11.0	175	7.3	25.8	4.4	1.1
NECTARINES								
Fresh, Raw, Weighed with Stone, Average	*1 Med/140g*	*50*	*0.1*	*36*	*1.2*	*8.0*	*0.1*	*1.1*
White Flesh, LL, Waitrose*	1 Fruit/130g	60	0.1	46	1.4	9.0	0.1	1.6
NESQUIK								
Chocolate, Powder, Dry Weight, Nesquik, Nestle*	1 Serving/15g	56	0.5	372	3.0	82.9	3.1	6.5
Strawberry, Powder, Dry Weight, Nesquik, Nestle*	1 Serving/15g	59	0.0	393	0.0	98.1	0.0	0.0
NIK NAKS								
Cream 'n' Cheesy, KP Snacks*	1 Bag/34g	196	13.0	575	5.2	52.7	38.1	0.2
Nice 'n' Spicy, KP Snacks*	1 Bag/30g	171	11.5	571	4.6	51.6	38.4	1.6
Rib 'n' Saucy, Golden Wonder*	1 Sm Bag/25g	143	9.4	571	4.5	53.7	37.6	0.5
Scampi 'n' Lemon, KP Snacks*	1 Bag/25g	143	9.4	573	4.9	53.1	37.5	0.1
NOODLES								
Barbecue Beef, Instant, Asda*	1 Pack/333g	420	16.0	126	2.6	18.0	4.8	0.0
BBQ Beef, Instant, Cooked, Aldi*	1 Serving/324g	515	19.4	159	3.7	21.9	6.0	1.1
Cellophane, Glass, Dry Weight	1 Serving/100g	351	0.1	351	0.1	86.1	0.1	0.5
Chicken & Mushroom, Mugfull, Batchelors*	1 Portion245g	198	1.2	81	2.5	16.0	0.5	0.7
Chicken & Mushroom, Speedy, Newgate, Lidl*	1 Pot/302g	438	14.8	145	3.6	21.0	4.9	1.1
Chicken Curry, Instant, Sainsbury's*	1 Pack/85g	167	6.2	196	4.6	27.9	7.3	0.8
Chicken Teriyaki, Pot, Tesco*	1 Pot/300g	315	4.8	105	5.8	15.9	1.6	1.8
Chicken Teriyaki, Skinny, City Kitchen, Tesco*	1 Pack/385g	366	5.0	95	7.2	13.0	1.3	1.4
Chicken, 3 Minute, Dry, Blue Dragon*	1 Pack/85g	403	18.2	475	9.3	61.2	21.4	0.0
Chicken, Dry, Eldorado*	1 Pack/85g	360	12.8	423	14.0	61.0	15.0	0.0
Chicken, Instant, Basics, Sainsbury's*	½ Pack/132g	209	7.0	158	4.0	23.5	5.3	0.6
Chicken, Instant, Cooked, Aldi*	½ Pack/204g	318	12.6	156	3.4	21.1	6.2	1.1
Chicken, Instant, Cooked, Smart Price, Asda*	1 Serving/246g	293	11.1	111	2.8	14.9	4.2	1.0
Chicken, Instant, Made Up, Tesco*	½ Pack/168g	285	10.6	170	4.1	23.7	6.3	1.5
Chicken, Instant, Sainsbury's*	1 Pack/335g	549	21.4	164	4.4	22.3	6.4	1.3
Chicken, Snack, Made Up, Mug Shot, Symingtons*	1 Mug/243g	246	1.5	101	2.7	21.0	0.6	1.0
Chilli Infused, Blue Dragon*	1 Serving/150g	286	1.0	191	6.1	33.6	0.7	0.3
Chinese Pork, CBY, Asda*	1 Pack/400g	380	6.4	95	6.7	12.6	1.6	1.8
Chinese, Stir Fry, Sainsbury's*	1 Serving/100g	185	4.8	185	6.0	29.5	4.8	1.5
Chow Mein, Snack in a Pot, Light Choices, Tesco*	1 Pot/235g	235	1.2	100	3.7	19.4	0.5	1.8
Crispy, Dry, Blue Dragon*	1 Box/125g	438	0.6	350	2.4	84.0	0.5	0.0
Curry Flavour, Instant, Dry, Asda*	1 Serving/65g	415	11.0	638	20.0	101.5	16.9	0.9
Curry Flavour, Instant, Sainsbury's*	1 Pack/335g	412	15.4	123	2.6	17.8	4.6	0.1
Curry Flavour, Instant, Value, Made Up, Tesco*	1 Pack/65g	83	2.4	127	3.1	20.3	3.7	0.8
Curry, Instant, Dry, Heinz*	1 Serving/85g	261	0.3	307	9.5	66.4	0.4	2.7
Curry, Spicy, Speedy, Newgate, Lidl*	1 Pot/312g	443	13.7	142	3.6	21.0	4.4	2.1
Egg & Bean Sprouts, Cooked, Tesco*	1 Pack/250g	238	5.2	95	4.4	14.6	2.1	1.5
Egg, Asda*	1 Pack/184g	213	12.9	116	2.3	11.0	7.0	0.6
Egg, Boiled	*1oz/28g*	*17*	*0.1*	*62*	*2.2*	*13.0*	*0.5*	*0.6*
Egg, Chilli & Ginger, Asian Fusion, Waitrose*	½ Pack/137g	188	3.3	137	4.4	24.0	2.4	0.8
Egg, Dry, Average	*1 Block/63g*	*218*	*1.2*	*348*	*12.1*	*70.1*	*1.9*	*2.6*
Egg, Fine Thread, Dry, M&S*	1 Serving/63g	220	0.6	350	14.3	71.6	0.9	5.1
Egg, Fine, Blue Dragon*	1 Serving/100g	356	1.7	356	13.8	70.0	1.7	3.4
Egg, Fine, Dry Weight, Sharwood's*	1 Block/63g	216	1.3	346	12.0	70.0	2.1	2.5

NOODLES

	Measure INFO/WEIGHT	per Measure KCAL	FAT	Nutrition Values per 100g / 100ml KCAL	PROT	CARB	FAT	FIBRE
Egg, Fine, Fresh, M&S*	1 Pack/275g	330	6.1	120	4.4	20.7	2.2	1.5
Egg, Fine, Waitrose*	¼ Pack/63g	221	1.6	353	15.0	67.3	2.6	3.8
Egg, Free Range, Asda*	1 Serving/125g	205	4.9	164	5.1	27.0	3.9	1.8
Egg, Free Range, Fresh, Sainsbury's*	½ Pack/205g	340	7.0	166	5.0	28.0	3.4	1.8
Egg, Free Range, Morrisons*	1 Pack/300g	372	8.7	124	4.9	19.7	2.9	1.3
Egg, Fresh, Just Stir Fry, Sainsbury's*	½ Pack/192g	314	6.5	163	5.0	28.1	3.4	1.8
Egg, Fresh, Tesco*	½ Pack/205g	287	3.9	140	4.9	25.3	1.9	2.0
Egg, Medium, Asda*	1 Serving/83g	125	0.7	150	4.8	31.0	0.8	1.3
Egg, Medium, Dry, Blue Dragon*	1 Serving/50g	158	1.2	317	10.1	62.3	2.4	3.1
Egg, Medium, Dry, Sharwood's*	1 Serving/63g	216	1.3	346	12.0	70.0	2.1	2.5
Egg, Medium, Sainsbury's*	1 Serving/122g	168	1.0	138	5.7	26.9	0.8	1.0
Egg, Raw, Medium, Waitrose*	¼ Pack/63g	221	1.6	353	15.0	67.3	2.6	3.8
Egg, Tossed in Sesame Oil, Asda*	½ Pack/150g	174	10.5	116	2.3	11.0	7.0	0.6
Fried, Average	*1oz/28g*	*43*	*3.2*	*153*	*1.9*	*11.3*	*11.5*	*0.5*
Instant, Express, Dry, Blue Dragon*	1 Serving/75g	338	12.8	450	10.0	65.0	17.0	2.0
Instant, Fat Free, Koka*	1 Piece/80g	143	0.0	179	6.2	38.5	0.0	1.0
Instant, Vegetable Flavour, Made Up, Indo Mie*	1 Pack/349g	373	15.7	107	2.6	14.0	4.5	0.8
Japanese Udon, Sainsbury's*	1 Serving/150g	210	2.7	140	3.9	27.1	1.8	1.2
Medium, Egg, Dry Nests, Cooks' Ingredients, Waitrose*	1 Nest/54g	189	0.9	350	13.2	70.4	1.7	2.4
Medium, Soft, Ready to Wok, Asia Specialities, Aldi*	1 Serving/150g	232	0.9	155	6.6	30.0	0.6	1.6
Oriental, Chinese, Tesco*	1 Pack/200g	184	5.0	92	2.8	14.7	2.5	1.0
Pad Thai, Ribbon, Ready to Wok, Sharwood's*	1 Serving/150g	206	1.7	137	5.0	26.3	1.1	1.0
Plain, Boiled	*1oz/28g*	*17*	*0.1*	*62*	*2.4*	*13.0*	*0.4*	*0.7*
Plain, Dry	*1oz/28g*	*109*	*1.7*	*388*	*11.7*	*76.1*	*6.2*	*2.9*
Ramen with Chilli Beef, M&S*	1 Pack/484g	532	17.4	110	8.1	11.9	3.6	0.8
Ribbon, Thai Style, Ready to Wok, Sharwood's*	1 Pack/150g	206	1.7	137	5.0	26.3	1.1	1.0
Rice with Spring Onions, Fresh Tastes, Asda*	½ Pack/188g	248	4.1	132	2.2	25.9	2.2	1.4
Rice, Brown, 100%, Organic, King Soba*	1 Pack/83g	252	2.0	303	6.0	64.4	2.4	0.0
Rice, Cooked	1 Cup/176g	192	0.4	109	0.9	24.9	0.2	1.0
Rice, Cooked, Sharwood's*	1 Serving/200g	239	0.6	120	2.0	27.2	0.3	0.8
Rice, Fresh, Sainsbury's*	½ Pack/150g	202	3.3	135	2.2	25.9	2.2	1.4
Rice, Oriental, Thai, Stir Fry, Dry Weight, Sharwood's*	1 Serving/63g	226	0.6	361	6.5	86.8	1.0	2.4
Rice, Stir Fry, Tesco*	½ Pack/190g	304	10.8	160	2.0	24.8	5.7	1.0
Rice, Thick, Thai, Dry, M&S*	1 Serving/100g	355	0.7	355	6.5	80.6	0.7	1.4
Savoury Vegetable, COU, M&S*	1 Pack/450g	270	2.7	60	2.9	11.5	0.6	1.2
Shanghai Beef, COU, M&S*	1 Pack/400g	380	6.4	95	6.8	13.1	1.6	1.5
Singapore Style, Asda*	1 Pack/400g	688	32.0	172	7.0	18.0	8.0	1.0
Singapore, BGTY, Sainsbury's*	1 Pack/369g	317	10.0	86	7.2	8.2	2.7	2.1
Singapore, Morrisons*	1 Serving/400g	480	26.8	120	4.8	11.6	6.7	1.6
Singapore, Sainsbury's*	1 Pack/400g	432	15.6	108	6.5	11.7	3.9	2.8
Singapore, Waitrose*	1 Pack/400g	476	17.6	119	7.3	12.6	4.4	2.1
Special, Chinese Takeaway, Iceland*	1 Pack/340g	422	10.9	124	6.5	17.2	3.2	0.6
Stir Fry, Tesco*	1 Serving/150g	202	3.6	135	5.3	23.0	2.4	1.5
Straight to Wok, Medium, Amoy*	1 Pack/150g	240	2.2	160	5.8	31.7	1.5	0.0
Straight to Wok, Rice, Amoy*	1 Pack/150g	174	0.2	116	1.6	27.4	0.1	0.0
Straight to Wok, Singapore, Amoy*	1 Serving/150g	232	4.2	155	4.8	28.4	2.8	0.0
Straight to Wok, Udon, Amoy*	1 Pack/150g	212	2.0	141	4.4	28.8	1.3	0.0
Super, Barbecue Beef, Made Up, Batchelors*	1 Serving/100g	156	6.7	156	3.2	20.9	6.7	1.1
Super, Chicken & Herb, Low Fat, Made Up, Batchelors*	1 Pack/170g	322	1.6	189	6.1	39.2	0.9	1.2
Super, Chicken Flavour, Dry Weight, Batchelors*	1 Serving/100g	449	19.2	449	8.7	60.3	19.2	2.5
Super, Chicken Flavour, Made Up, Batchelors*	1 Serving/150g	264	11.8	176	3.1	23.0	7.9	0.4
Super, Chow Mein Flavour, Made Up, Batchelors*	½ Pack/150g	262	11.8	175	3.0	23.0	7.9	0.4
Super, Mild Curry Flavour, Made Up, Batchelors*	1 Serving/100g	157	6.7	157	3.2	20.9	6.7	1.0

	Measure INFO/WEIGHT	per Measure		Nutrition Values per 100g / 100ml				
		KCAL	FAT	KCAL	PROT	CARB	FAT	FIBRE
NOODLES								
Super, Mild Curry, Dry Weight, Batchelors*	½ Pack/50g	260	11.7	520	9.4	67.8	23.4	1.4
Super, Southern Fried Chicken, Made Up, Batchelors*	1 Serving/100g	171	7.2	171	3.3	23.2	7.2	0.5
Sweet Chilli, Wok, Findus*	1 Pack/300g	300	1.5	100	3.0	20.0	0.5	0.0
Tiger Prawn, Stir Fry, Tesco*	1 Pack/400g	596	14.8	149	6.0	23.0	3.7	2.7
Udon Style, Thick, Ready to Wok, Sharwood's*	1 Pack/150g	233	0.6	155	5.4	32.5	0.4	2.1
Vermicelli Rice, Mama*	1 Serving/45g	166	0.4	370	7.0	81.0	1.0	0.0
Whole Wheat, Dry, Blue Dragon*	1 Serving/65g	208	1.3	320	12.5	63.0	2.0	8.0
Zero, Glow Nutrition Ltd*	1 Serving/100g	5	0.0	5	0.0	4.0	0.0	4.0
NOUGAT								
Almond & Cherry, M&S*	1 Sweet/7g	28	0.6	405	4.5	76.0	9.1	1.1
Average	*1 Sm Bar/28g*	*108*	*2.4*	*384*	*4.4*	*77.3*	*8.5*	*0.9*
Soft, Bar, Bassett's*	1 Bar/25g	94	1.0	375	4.0	82.0	4.0	0.0
NUT ROAST								
Average	*1 Serving/200g*	*704*	*51.4*	*352*	*13.3*	*18.3*	*25.7*	*4.2*
Lentil, Average	*1oz/28g*	*62*	*3.4*	*222*	*10.6*	*18.8*	*12.1*	*3.8*
Roasted Butternut, Almond & Pecan, M&S*	1 Pack/245g	551	35.0	225	7.3	14.6	14.3	4.3
NUTMEG								
Ground, Average	*1 Tsp/3g*	*16*	*1.1*	*525*	*5.8*	*45.3*	*36.3*	*0.0*
NUTS								
Assortment, Eat Well, M&S*	1 Pack/70g	441	41.2	630	16.7	8.5	58.9	5.3
Brazil, Chocolate, Dark, Bolivian, Hotel Chocolat*	½ Pack/50g	303	24.0	606	10.0	34.0	48.0	4.0
Brazil, Chocolate, Natural Ketosis Company*	1 Pack/15g	87	7.2	580	7.9	38.9	48.1	0.0
Cashews & Peanuts, Honey Roasted, Average	*1 Serving/50g*	*290*	*21.4*	*579*	*21.6*	*26.6*	*42.9*	*4.2*
Luxury Assortment, Tesco*	1 Serving/10g	68	6.5	676	17.5	6.1	64.6	5.0
Mixed	1 Pack/40g	243	21.6	607	22.9	7.9	54.1	6.0
Mixed, Almonds, Brazil, Hazel & Walnuts, M&S*	1 Serving/25g	168	16.0	670	16.0	4.8	64.0	5.4
Mixed, Chopped, Sainsbury's*	1 Serving/100g	605	50.9	605	27.1	9.6	50.9	6.0
Mixed, Chopped, Tesco*	1 Serving/25g	149	12.6	595	23.5	10.5	50.6	6.0
Mixed, Cookies & Cream, Graze*	1 Punnet/38g	214	16.0	562	12.0	36.0	42.0	5.0
Mixed, Honey Roasted, Waitrose*	1 Serving/50g	292	22.5	583	17.1	27.5	45.0	5.3
Mixed, Natural Energy, Graze*	1 Punnet/36g	227	21.3	629	19.0	8.0	59.0	8.0
Mixed, Natural, Asda*	1 Snack/30g	197	18.8	656	18.0	4.3	62.7	7.4
Mixed, Roasted, Salted, Waitrose*	1 Pack/200g	1252	116.8	626	13.7	11.3	58.4	4.4
Mixed, Roasted, Waitrose*	1 Serving/25g	166	16.0	662	15.2	6.2	64.0	8.2
Mixed, Unsalted, Sainsbury's*	1 Serving/50g	311	28.8	622	18.5	7.2	57.7	8.7
Mixed, Wholesome, LL, Waitrose*	1 Serving/30g	206	19.6	685	14.6	5.0	65.2	5.4
Natural Roasted Peanuts, LL, Waitrose*	1 Pack/250g	1595	131.5	638	27.1	15.6	52.6	5.1
Natural, Mixed, LL, Waitrose*	1 Serving/50g	314	25.8	628	17.4	24.9	51.6	12.1
Omega Booster Seeds, Graze*	1 Punnet/34g	189	16.5	553	22.1	16.4	48.3	11.1
Peanuts & Cashews, Honey Roast, Tesco*	1 Serving/25g	145	10.7	579	21.6	26.6	42.9	4.2
Peanuts, Roasted, Salted, Value, Tesco*	1/8 Pack/25g	151	12.4	604	25.5	13.8	49.6	6.8
Pecan, Wholesome, LL, Waitrose*	1 Serving/30g	207	21.0	691	9.2	5.8	70.1	9.6
Pine, Tesco*	1 Pack/100g	699	68.6	699	16.5	4.0	68.6	1.9
Pine, Wholefoods, Tesco*	1 Serving/10g	69	6.9	690	14.0	4.0	68.6	1.9
Soya Beans, Roasted & Salted, Chinese Style, Tesco*	1 Serving/26g	100	5.0	385	46.1	6.9	19.2	21.8
Soya, Dry Roasted, The Food Doctor*	1 Serving/50g	203	10.7	406	37.5	15.9	21.4	16.1
Unsalted, Selection, Sainsbury's*	1 Serving/75g	491	48.0	655	14.7	5.0	64.0	6.7
Walnut Pieces, Morrisons*	7 Peices/6g	41	4.1	689	14.7	3.3	68.5	3.5
NUTS & RAISINS								
Mixed, Average	*1 Serving/30g*	*144*	*10.2*	*481*	*14.1*	*31.5*	*34.1*	*4.5*
Mixed, Tesco*	1 Serving/25g	115	6.9	450	18.6	32.6	26.8	12.5
Peanuts, Mixed, Average	*1 Pack/40g*	*174*	*10.4*	*435*	*15.3*	*37.5*	*26.0*	*4.4*
Yoghurt Coated, Waitrose*	1 Serving/50g	264	18.4	527	10.9	38.2	36.7	3.0

	Measure INFO/WEIGHT	per Measure KCAL	FAT	Nutrition Values per 100g / 100ml KCAL	PROT	CARB	FAT	FIBRE

OAT CAKES

	Measure INFO/WEIGHT	KCAL	FAT	KCAL	PROT	CARB	FAT	FIBRE
Bran, Paterson's*	1 Cake/13g	52	2.0	416	10.0	58.5	15.8	9.5
Cheese, Nairn's*	1 Cake/8g	39	2.3	471	13.2	43.3	27.2	6.8
Fine Milled, Nairn's*	1 Cake/8g	35	1.7	449	10.5	52.6	21.8	8.6
Herb & Pumpkin Seed, Nairn's*	1 Cake/10g	43	2.1	426	12.2	46.8	21.1	13.0
Highland, Organic, Sainsbury's*	1 Cake/13g	57	2.4	456	10.2	59.8	19.5	5.5
Highland, Walkers*	1 Cake/12g	54	2.5	451	10.3	56.0	20.6	6.7
Oatmeal, Rough, Nairn's*	1 Cake/11g	45	2.0	421	10.6	52.8	18.6	10.5
Oatmeal, Rough, Organic, Nairn's*	1 Cake/10g	43	1.7	418	10.2	57.7	16.3	7.5
Organic, The Village Bakery*	1 Cake/13g	56	2.7	452	10.9	54.5	21.3	5.6
Retail, Average	*1 Cake/13g*	*57*	*2.4*	*441*	*10.0*	*63.0*	*18.3*	*2.0*
Rough Scottish, Sainsbury's*	1 Cake/11g	51	2.1	462	12.3	59.9	19.3	6.5
Rough with Olive Oil, Paterson's*	1 Cake/13g	54	2.2	431	10.6	58.4	17.2	8.1
Rough, Sainsbury's*	1 Cake/11g	45	1.8	426	11.7	65.2	16.9	8.6
Rough, Scottish, Tesco*	1 Cake/10g	45	1.9	435	11.4	55.3	18.4	8.0
Traditional, M&S*	1 Cake/11g	49	2.0	445	11.0	59.3	18.3	6.6
with Cracked Black Pepper, Walkers*	1 Cake/10g	41	1.8	433	10.4	55.0	19.0	8.5

OAT DRINK

Healthy, Enriched, Oatly*	1 Serving/250ml	112	3.8	45	1.0	6.5	1.5	0.8
Oat Milk, Organic, Healthy, Oatly*	1 Serving/250ml	88	1.8	35	1.0	6.5	0.7	0.8

OCTOPUS

Chunks in Olive Oil, Palacio De Oriente*	1 Tin/111g	148	4.0	133	21.6	4.5	3.6	0.0
Raw	*1oz/28g*	*18*	*0.3*	*66*	*14.1*	*0.0*	*1.0*	*0.0*

OIL

Avocado, Olivado*	1 Tsp/5ml	40	4.4	802	0.0	0.0	88.0	0.0
Black Truffle, Grapeseed, Cuisine Perel*	1 Tsp/5ml	43	5.0	857	0.0	7.1	100.0	0.0
Butter, Cooking Mist, Spray, Cook's Range, Lurpak*	1 Spray/0.2ml	2	0.2	792	0.3	0.2	87.9	0.0
Chilli, Average	*1 Tsp/5ml*	*41*	*4.6*	*824*	*0.0*	*0.0*	*91.5*	*0.0*
Chinese Stir Fry, Asda*	1 Tbsp/15ml	123	13.7	823	0.0	0.0	91.4	0.0
Coconut Oil, Virgin Oil, Raw, Biona Organic*	1 Serving/5g	43	5.0	857	0.0	0.0	100.0	0.0
Coconut, Average	*1 Tsp/5ml*	*45*	*5.0*	*899*	*0.0*	*0.0*	*99.9*	*0.0*
Coconut, Extra Virgin, Organic, Fair Trade, Tiana*	1 Tbsp/15g	135	15.0	900	0.0	0.0	100.0	0.0
Coconut, Virgin, Organic, Groovy Food Company*	1 Tsp/5ml	38	4.6	767	0.0	0.0	92.5	0.0
Cod Liver, Average	*1 Capsule/1g*	*9*	*1.0*	*900*	*0.0*	*0.0*	*100.0*	*0.0*
Corn, Average	*1 Tsp/5ml*	*43*	*4.8*	*864*	*0.0*	*0.0*	*96.0*	*0.0*
Cuisine, Flora*	1 Tsp/5ml	32	3.5	630	0.1	1.0	70.3	0.0
Dipping, Herb, Italian Style, Finest, Tesco*	1 Serving/5g	44	4.8	877	0.4	0.9	96.9	0.4
Evening Primrose, Average	*1 Serving/1g*	*9*	*1.0*	*900*	*0.0*	*0.0*	*100.0*	*0.0*
Fish, Average	*1 Serving/1g*	*9*	*1.0*	*900*	*0.0*	*0.0*	*100.0*	*0.0*
Fish, Omega 3, Capsule, Holland & Barrett*	1 Capsule/1g	10	1.0	1000	0.1	0.1	100.0	0.1
Flax Seed, Average	*1 Tbsp/15ml*	*124*	*13.9*	*829*	*0.0*	*0.0*	*92.6*	*0.0*
Fry Light, Bodyline*	1 Spray/0.25ml	1	0.1	522	0.0	0.0	55.2	0.0
Grapeseed, Average	*1 Tsp/5ml*	*43*	*4.8*	*866*	*0.0*	*0.0*	*96.2*	*0.0*
Groundnut, Average	*1 Tsp/5ml*	*41*	*4.6*	*824*	*0.0*	*0.0*	*91.8*	*0.0*
Hazelnut, Average	*1 Tsp/5ml*	*45*	*5.0*	*899*	*0.0*	*0.0*	*99.9*	*0.0*
Macadamia Nut, Oz Tukka*	1 Tsp/5ml	40	4.6	805	0.0	0.0	91.0	0.0
Olive, Average	*1 Tsp/5ml*	*43*	*4.7*	*855*	*0.0*	*0.0*	*94.9*	*0.0*
Olive, Basil Infused, Tesco*	1 Serving/20ml	180	20.0	900	0.0	0.0	100.0	0.0
Olive, Extra Virgin, Average	*1 Tsp/5ml*	*42*	*4.7*	*848*	*0.0*	*0.0*	*94.5*	*0.0*
Olive, Extra Virgin, Only 1 Cal, Spray, Fry Light*	1 Spray/0.2ml	1	0.1	498	0.0	0.0	55.2	0.0
Olive, Garlic, Average	*1 Tbsp/15ml*	*127*	*14.1*	*848*	*0.0*	*0.0*	*94.3*	*0.0*
Olive, Lemon Flavoured, Sainsbury's*	1 Tbsp/15ml	123	13.7	823	0.1	0.0	91.4	0.1
Olive, Mild, Average	*1 Tbsp/15ml*	*129*	*14.4*	*862*	*0.0*	*0.0*	*95.7*	*0.0*
Olive, Spray, Fry Light*	5 Sprays/1ml	5	0.5	520	0.0	0.0	54.2	0.0

O

	Measure INFO/WEIGHT	per Measure KCAL	FAT	Nutrition Values per 100g / 100ml KCAL	PROT	CARB	FAT	FIBRE
OIL								
Palm, Average	*1 Tsp/5ml*	*45*	*5.0*	*899*	*0.0*	*0.0*	*99.9*	*0.0*
Peanut, Average	*1 Tsp/5ml*	*45*	*5.0*	*899*	*0.0*	*0.0*	*99.9*	*0.0*
Rapeseed, Average	*1 Tbsp/15ml*	*130*	*14.4*	*864*	*0.0*	*0.0*	*96.0*	*0.0*
Red Palm & Canola, Carotino*	1 Tsp/5ml	41	4.6	812	0.0	0.0	92.0	0.0
Rice Bran, Alpha One, Hansells Foods*	1 Serving/4ml	32	3.7	812	0.0	0.0	92.0	0.0
Rice Bran, Alphaone*	1 Tbsp/14g	120	13.6	880	0.0	0.0	100.0	0.0
Rice Bran, Average	*1 Tbsp/14g*	*120*	*13.6*	*884*	*0.0*	*0.0*	*100.0*	*0.0*
Safflower, Average	*1 Tsp/5ml*	*45*	*5.0*	*899*	*0.0*	*0.0*	*99.9*	*0.0*
Sesame, Average	*1 Tsp/5ml*	*45*	*5.0*	*892*	*0.1*	*0.0*	*99.9*	*0.0*
Soya, Average	*1 Tsp/5ml*	*45*	*5.0*	*899*	*0.0*	*0.0*	*99.9*	*0.0*
Sunflower, Average	*1 Tsp/5ml*	*43*	*4.8*	*869*	*0.0*	*0.0*	*96.6*	*0.0*
Sunflower, Spray, Fry Light*	1 Spray/0.2ml	1	0.1	522	0.0	0.0	55.2	0.0
Ultimate Blend, Udo's Choice*	1 Capsule/1ml	9	1.0	900	1.3	0.0	96.8	0.0
Vegetable, Average	*1 Tbsp/15ml*	*129*	*14.3*	*858*	*0.0*	*0.0*	*95.3*	*0.0*
Virgin Coconut, Spray, Groovy Food Company*	1 Spray/0.2ml	1	0.1	475	0.0	0.0	53.3	0.0
Walnut, Average	*1 Tsp/5ml*	*45*	*5.0*	*899*	*0.0*	*0.0*	*99.9*	*0.0*
OKRA								
Boiled in Unsalted Water, Average	*1 Serving/80g*	*22*	*0.7*	*28*	*2.5*	*2.7*	*0.9*	*3.6*
Raw, Average	*1 Serving/80g*	*18*	*0.6*	*23*	*2.1*	*2.2*	*0.7*	*3.0*
Stir-Fried in Corn Oil, Average	*1 Serving/80g*	*215*	*20.9*	*269*	*4.3*	*4.4*	*26.1*	*6.3*
OLIVES								
Black & Green with Greek Feta Cheese, Tesco*	1 Pot/100g	200	20.1	200	3.4	0.3	20.1	4.6
Black, Pitted, Average	*½ Jar/82g*	*135*	*13.3*	*164*	*1.0*	*3.5*	*16.2*	*3.1*
Green & Harissa, Graze*	1 Punnet/44g	110	11.6	255	0.8	2.0	27.0	3.0
Green with Chilli & Garlic, Delicious, Boots*	1 Pack/70g	113	10.5	161	1.3	4.4	15.0	2.0
Green with Chilli & Garlic, Graze*	1 Punnet/44g	133	13.6	301	0.6	1.4	30.9	2.9
Green, Garlic Stuffed, Asda*	1 Olive/3g	6	0.6	174	1.8	3.5	17.0	0.0
Green, Lightly Flavoured with Lemon & Garlic, Attis*	1 Serving/50g	82	8.2	164	1.7	2.2	16.5	0.0
Green, Pitted, Average	*1 Olive/3g*	*4*	*0.4*	*130*	*1.1*	*0.9*	*13.3*	*2.5*
Green, Queen, & Garlic, Herb Dressing, LBU, Co-Op*	1/3 Pot/50g	56	5.5	113	1.8	1.0	11.0	3.0
Green, Stuffed with Almonds, Pitted, Waitrose*	1 Serving/50g	90	8.4	180	3.8	3.2	16.9	2.5
Green, Stuffed with Anchovy, Waitrose*	½ Can/40g	38	3.1	94	1.5	4.7	7.7	2.3
Kalamata & Halkidiki with Chilli & Garlic, Graze*	1 Punnet/51g	144	14.8	281	0.7	1.5	28.8	3.0
Manzanilla, Marinated with Chilli, Lidl*	1 Pot/140g	230	23.1	164	1.4	0.3	16.5	0.0
Marinated, Mixed, M&S*	1 Serving/20g	33	3.0	165	1.6	6.5	14.9	3.0
Marinated, Selection, M&S*	4 Olives/20g	44	4.4	225	1.4	3.9	22.6	2.1
Mixed, Chilli & Garlic, Asda*	1 Serving/30g	43	4.7	144	0.9	0.0	15.6	6.1
Mixed, Marinated with Feta & Red Peppers, Asda*	1 Pot/120g	233	21.6	194	5.8	2.2	18.0	1.7
Mixed, Marinated, Anti Pasti, Asda*	1 Serving/100g	215	22.0	215	1.8	0.7	22.0	3.1
Pimento Stuffed in Brine, Drained, Tesco*	1 Serving/25g	35	3.2	140	0.7	4.0	12.8	2.9
OMELETTE								
Cheese & Mushroom, Apetito*	1 Serving/320g	486	25.0	152	6.2	14.4	7.8	1.9
Cheese, 2 Egg, Average	*1 Omelette/180g*	*479*	*40.7*	*266*	*15.9*	*0.0*	*22.6*	*0.0*
Cheese, Asda*	1 Omelette/119g	268	22.6	225	12.0	1.5	19.0	0.0
Ham & Mushroom, Farmfoods*	1 Omelette/120g	200	16.7	167	8.7	1.8	13.9	0.1
Mushroom & Cheese, Tesco*	1 Omelette/120g	248	21.5	207	9.8	1.6	17.9	0.0
Plain, 2 Egg	1 Omelette/120g	229	19.7	191	10.9	0.0	16.4	0.0
Spanish	1oz/28g	34	2.3	120	5.7	6.2	8.3	1.4
Spanish, Potato, Rapido, Unearthed*	1 Pack/300g	492	32.7	164	5.2	10.5	10.9	2.2
ONION POWDER								
Average	1 Tsp/2g	7	0.0	341	10.4	79.1	1.0	15.2
ONION RINGS								
Battered, Asda*	1 Serving/100g	343	22.7	343	3.8	31.0	22.7	1.7

	Measure	per Measure		Nutrition Values per 100g / 100ml				
	INFO/WEIGHT	KCAL	FAT	KCAL	PROT	CARB	FAT	FIBRE
ONION RINGS								
Battered, Oven Baked, Tesco*	1 Serving/50g	110	5.0	219	3.9	28.4	10.0	3.5
Battered, Sainsbury's*	1 Ring/12g	26	1.2	219	3.9	28.4	10.0	3.5
Breadcrumbs, Tesco*	1 Serving/100g	294	15.6	294	4.3	34.1	15.6	2.3
Breaded, Asda*	1 Serving/10g	29	1.5	289	4.4	34.0	15.0	2.7
Breaded, Iceland*	1 Ring/11g	33	1.7	293	4.4	34.2	15.4	2.7
Breaded, Sainsbury's*	4 Rings/48g	128	5.8	266	3.8	33.7	12.1	3.6
Oven Crisp Batter, Tesco*	1 Ring/17g	40	2.3	236	4.2	24.8	13.3	2.5
Value, Tesco*	1 Bag/14g	73	3.8	520	7.0	61.4	27.0	1.2
ONIONS								
Baked	*1oz/28g*	*29*	*0.2*	*103*	*3.5*	*22.3*	*0.6*	*3.9*
Boiled in Unsalted Water	*1oz/28g*	*5*	*0.0*	*17*	*0.6*	*3.7*	*0.1*	*0.7*
Brown, Value, Tesco*	1 Onion/100g	36	0.2	36	1.3	7.8	0.2	1.8
Dried, Raw, Average	*1oz/28g*	*88*	*0.5*	*313*	*10.2*	*68.6*	*1.7*	*12.1*
Fried, Average	*1oz/28g*	*46*	*3.1*	*164*	*2.3*	*14.1*	*11.2*	*3.1*
Pickled, Average	*1 Onion/15g*	*3*	*0.0*	*19*	*0.7*	*4.1*	*0.1*	*0.6*
Pickled, Strong, Drained, Haywards*	1 Onion/42g	10	0.0	23	0.7	4.8	0.1	0.0
Raw, Average	*1 Med/180g*	*69*	*0.4*	*38*	*1.2*	*7.9*	*0.2*	*1.3*
Red, Raw, Average	*1 Med/180g*	*66*	*0.4*	*37*	*1.2*	*7.9*	*0.2*	*1.5*
Sliced, Frozen, Farmfoods*	1 Serving/80g	29	0.2	36	1.2	7.9	0.2	1.4
Spring, Raw, Average	*1 Med/15g*	*4*	*0.1*	*24*	*1.9*	*2.9*	*0.5*	*1.4*
Sweet, TTD, Sainsbury's*	1 Serving/100g	39	0.2	39	1.3	7.9	0.2	1.4
OPTIONS								
Choca Mocha Drink, Ovaltine*	1 Sachet/11g	39	1.3	359	14.1	50.1	11.4	7.0
Chocolate Au Lait, Ovaltine*	1 Sachet/10g	36	1.0	355	11.8	54.5	10.0	7.3
Dreamy Caramel, Hot Chocolate, Ovaltine*	1 Sachet/11g	39	0.9	354	12.3	48.5	7.8	0.0
Mint Madness, Belgian, Ovaltine*	1 Serving/11g	38	0.8	348	12.3	49.2	6.9	20.0
Outrageous Orange, Hot Chocolate, Ovaltine*	1 Serving/11g	38	0.8	348	12.3	49.3	6.9	20.0
Tempting Toffee, Ovaltine*	1 Sachet/11g	43	1.0	391	13.6	66.4	9.1	0.0
Wicked White, Hot Chocolate, Ovaltine*	1 Sachet/11g	44	1.1	398	10.5	64.6	10.0	3.7
ORANGE CURD								
Sainsbury's*	2 Tsps/12g	34	0.5	282	1.1	59.2	4.4	0.4
ORANGES								
Blood, Average	*1 Orange/140g*	*82*	*0.0*	*58*	*0.8*	*13.3*	*0.0*	*2.5*
Fresh, Weighed with Peel, Average	*1oz/28g*	*7*	*0.0*	*26*	*0.8*	*6.0*	*0.0*	*1.2*
Fresh, without Peel, Average	*1 Med/145g*	*54*	*0.1*	*37*	*1.1*	*8.5*	*0.1*	*1.7*
Market, Value, Tesco*	1 Orange/150g	56	0.2	37	1.1	8.5	0.1	1.7
Peel Only, Raw, Average	*1 Tbsp/6g*	*6*	*0.0*	*97*	*1.5*	*25.0*	*0.2*	*10.6*
Ruby Red, Tesco*	1 Med/130g	51	0.1	39	1.1	8.5	0.1	1.7
TTD, Sainsbury's*	1 Serving/100g	37	0.1	37	1.1	8.5	0.1	1.7
OREGANO								
Dried,	*1 Tsp/1g*	*3*	*0.1*	*306*	*11.0*	*49.5*	*10.3*	*0.0*
Fresh	*1 Tsp/1g*	*1*	*0.0*	*66*	*2.2*	*9.7*	*2.0*	*0.0*
OVALTINE*								
Chocolate, Light, Ovaltine*	4 Tsp/20g	76	1.2	380	8.5	70.5	6.0	4.5
Hi Malt, Light, Instant Drink, Ovaltine*	1 Sachet/20g	72	1.2	358	9.1	67.1	5.9	2.8
OXTAIL								
Raw	*1oz/28g*	*18*	*1.1*	*65*	*7.6*	*0.0*	*3.8*	*0.0*
Stewed, Bone Removed	*1oz/28g*	*68*	*3.8*	*243*	*30.5*	*0.0*	*13.4*	*0.0*
OYSTERS								
in Vegetable Oil, Smoked, John West*	1oz/28g	64	3.9	230	16.0	10.0	14.0	0.0
Raw, Shelled, Shucked	*1 Oyster/14g*	*9*	*0.2*	*65*	*10.8*	*2.7*	*1.3*	*0.0*

O

	Measure INFO/WEIGHT	per Measure KCAL	FAT	Nutrition Values per 100g / 100ml KCAL	PROT	CARB	FAT	FIBRE
PAELLA								
Chicken & Chorizo, Asda*	1 Pack/390g	484	8.6	124	10.0	16.0	2.2	2.6
Chicken & Chorizo, LowLow*	1 Pack/320g	333	3.8	104	5.6	17.1	1.2	1.2
Chicken & Chorizo, M Kitchen, Morrisons*	1 Pack/402g	482	14.1	120	4.4	18.3	3.5	1.3
Chicken & Prawn, HL, Tesco*	1 Pack/380g	370	6.9	97	6.5	13.0	1.8	1.8
Chicken, Chorizo & King Prawn, Finest, Tesco*	½ Pack/400g	520	19.6	130	7.0	14.2	4.9	1.2
Chicken, HL, Tesco*	1 Pack/400g	432	2.0	108	6.7	19.2	0.5	1.7
Chicken, King Prawns & Chorizo, Fuller Longer, M&S*	1 Pack/390g	410	11.3	105	9.8	10.1	2.9	1.6
Diet Chef Ltd*	1 Pack/250g	355	3.0	142	11.2	21.7	1.2	0.4
King Prawn & Chargrilled Chicken, Valencia, COU, M&S*	1 Pack/400g	552	11.2	138	7.5	20.4	2.8	0.8
King Prawn, Chicken & Chorizo, City Kitchen, Tesco*	1 Pack/400g	540	20.0	135	4.7	17.0	5.0	1.4
Seafood, Espana, M&S*	1 Bowl/380g	565	12.1	150	5.5	25.2	3.2	0.5
Seafood, Finest, Tesco*	1 Pack/400g	756	23.6	189	6.8	27.2	5.9	1.0
Seafood, M&S*	1 Pack/450g	518	17.1	115	6.4	13.7	3.8	3.2
Seafood, Sainsbury's*	1 Pack/400g	504	5.2	126	8.3	20.3	1.3	0.6
Vegetable, Espana, M&S*	1 Pack/375g	505	13.5	135	2.8	22.4	3.6	1.3
with Prawns & Cajun Chicken, COU, M&S*	1 Pack/400g	360	4.4	90	7.0	13.2	1.1	1.6
PAIN AU CHOCOLAT								
All Butter, Tesco*	1 Serving/59g	242	11.6	410	8.2	49.4	19.7	2.3
Asda*	1 Serving/58g	244	13.9	420	8.0	43.0	24.0	3.3
Average	*1 Serving/60g*	*253*	*13.7*	*422*	*8.0*	*45.8*	*22.8*	*3.1*
Chocolate Filled, CBY, Asda*	1 Pain/45g	198	11.3	441	7.1	44.9	25.2	2.9
M&S*	1 Pastry/60g	210	11.5	350	5.9	38.0	19.2	1.6
Mini, Asda*	1 Pastry/23g	96	5.5	420	8.0	43.0	24.0	3.3
Sainsbury's*	1 Serving/58g	241	13.8	415	7.9	42.5	23.7	3.3
Small, Asda*	1 Serving/23g	106	6.0	462	8.0	49.0	26.0	0.0
Waitrose*	1 Pastry/53g	230	12.6	435	8.8	45.5	23.9	3.7
PAIN AU RAISIN								
Takeaway, Average	*1 Pastry/100g*	*313*	*13.2*	*313*	*5.2*	*43.0*	*13.2*	*1.3*
PAK CHOI								
Raw, Average	*1 Leaf/14g*	*2*	*0.0*	*11*	*1.3*	*1.9*	*0.2*	*0.9*
PAKORA								
Bhaji, Onion, Fried in Vegetable Oil	1oz/28g	76	4.1	271	9.8	26.2	14.7	5.5
Bhajia, Potato Carrot & Pea, Fried in Vegetable Oil	1oz/28g	100	6.3	357	10.9	28.8	22.6	6.1
Bhajia, Vegetable, Retail	1oz/28g	66	4.1	235	6.4	21.4	14.7	3.6
Chicken, Tikka, Asda*	1 Pack/350g	696	38.5	199	16.0	9.0	11.0	1.1
Potato & Spinach, Waitrose*	1 Pakora/50g	120	8.2	240	5.5	17.3	16.5	4.7
Prawn, Indian Appetisers, Waitrose*	1 Pakora/21g	35	1.7	165	16.8	5.9	8.2	1.5
Sainsbury's*	1 Pakora/55g	166	10.1	302	7.3	26.8	18.3	1.1
Spinach, Sainsbury's*	1 Pakora/18g	35	1.9	195	5.1	19.4	10.8	3.8
Vegetable, Indian Selection, Party, Co-Op*	1 Pakora/23g	47	1.6	205	6.0	28.0	7.0	4.0
Vegetable, Indian Starter Selection, M&S*	1 Pakora/23g	61	4.2	265	6.3	19.6	18.1	2.9
Vegetable, Mini, Indian Snack Collection, Tesco*	1 Pakora/21g	36	1.9	173	6.0	16.8	9.1	4.9
PANCAKE								
& Maple Syrup, Mini, Burger King*	6 Pancakes/78g	268	10.1	346	3.7	53.0	13.1	1.3
Apple, GFY, Asda*	1 Pancake/74g	100	1.8	135	4.2	24.0	2.5	1.0
Asda*	1 Pancake/23g	59	1.6	254	4.8	43.0	7.0	4.0
Big, Crafty, Genesis*	1 Pancake/70g	149	3.6	213	5.6	38.4	5.2	4.1
Blueberry, Tesco*	1 Pancake/75g	195	3.1	260	4.8	49.5	4.1	2.0
Chinese Roll, Farmfoods*	1 Pancake/88g	125	3.8	142	4.3	21.6	4.3	1.0
Chocolate, M&S*	1 Pancake/80g	125	4.9	156	3.1	22.1	6.1	0.2
for Duck, Sainsbury's*	1 Pancake/10g	33	0.9	333	10.9	51.7	9.3	2.4
HL, Tesco*	1 Pancake/25g	60	0.5	240	5.8	48.8	2.0	1.9
Lemon & Raisin, Morrisons*	1 Pancake/36g	55	0.4	153	5.3	30.4	1.2	0.9

	Measure INFO/WEIGHT	per Measure KCAL	FAT	Nutrition Values per 100g / 100ml KCAL	PROT	CARB	FAT	FIBRE
PANCAKE								
M&S*	1 Pancake/62g	170	7.7	275	5.7	33.9	12.5	1.5
Maple & Raisin, M&S*	1 Pancake/35g	102	2.4	290	5.6	50.4	6.9	2.2
Mini for Kids, Tesco*	1 Pancake/16g	45	0.9	283	6.6	51.7	5.5	1.3
Mini, Scotch, Tesco*	1 Pancake/16g	44	0.9	277	6.7	50.0	5.6	1.4
Morrisons*	1 Pancake/60g	133	3.0	221	8.4	37.3	5.0	1.5
North Staffordshire Oatcakes Ltd*	1 Pancake/71g	166	4.3	234	5.0	40.9	6.1	1.0
Perfect, Kingsmill*	1 Pancake/27g	71	1.2	264	6.2	49.7	4.5	1.2
Plain, Sainsbury's*	1 Pancake/46g	102	2.4	221	6.9	36.1	5.3	1.2
Pockets, Strawberry, Kingsmill*	1 Pancake/44g	112	1.6	254	4.3	50.5	3.6	1.3
Raisin & Lemon, Asda*	1 Pancake/30g	92	2.4	304	6.0	52.0	8.0	1.4
Raisin & Lemon, Sainsbury's*	1 Pancake/35g	95	1.5	272	6.3	51.8	4.4	2.2
Ready Made, Average	*1 Sm Pancake/30g*	*77*	*1.9*	*258*	*6.1*	*44.2*	*6.4*	*1.7*
Savoury, Made with Whole Milk, Average	*6" Pancake/77g*	*210*	*13.5*	*273*	*6.3*	*24.0*	*17.5*	*0.8*
Scotch	1 Pancake/50g	146	5.8	292	5.8	43.6	11.7	1.4
Scotch, Essential, Waitrose*	1 Pancake/31g	82	2.6	265	6.4	40.9	8.4	2.4
Scotch, Hovis*	1 Pancake/30g	88	2.5	295	5.5	48.1	8.4	2.3
Scotch, M&S*	1 Pancake/34g	95	1.4	280	6.5	54.5	4.0	1.6
Scotch, Sainsbury's*	1 Pancake/30g	78	1.3	260	5.9	48.8	4.4	1.0
Sultana & Syrup, Asda*	1 Pancake/34g	89	2.4	263	5.9	43.7	7.2	1.5
Syrup, Gluten, Wheat & Dairy Free, Free From, Livwell*	1 Pancake/40g	108	2.9	270	2.5	49.0	7.2	0.8
Traditional, Aunt Bessie's*	1 Pancake/60g	90	1.9	150	6.1	24.6	3.1	1.1
Traditional, Tesco*	1 Pancake/62g	137	3.1	221	8.4	35.6	5.0	1.5
with Syrup, American Style, Large, Tesco*	1 Pancake/38g	102	1.3	268	5.1	54.2	3.4	0.9
PANCAKE MIX								
4 Grain, Wheat & Gluten Free, Organic, Hale & Hearty*	½ Pack/180g	562	2.9	312	7.8	66.6	1.6	5.7
Batter, Shake to Make, Made Up, Betty Crocker*	1 Serving/74g	114	4.0	154	3.5	22.7	5.4	1.0
PANCETTA								
Average	*½ Pack/65g*	*212*	*18.7*	*326*	*17.0*	*0.1*	*28.7*	*0.0*
Cubes, Tesco*	1 Serving/38g	135	12.2	355	17.5	0.5	32.2	0.0
PANINI								
Chargrilled Chicken, Mozzarella & Pesto, Udo's Choice*	1 Panini/170g	389	14.6	229	16.4	21.6	8.6	2.0
Cheese, Tesco*	1 Panini/100g	249	9.1	249	10.5	31.3	9.1	3.1
Mozzarella & Tomato, M&S*	1 Serving/176g	484	28.5	275	11.3	21.3	16.2	2.1
Tuna & Sweetcorn, Tesco*	1 Serving/250g	559	16.4	224	12.0	29.3	6.6	1.4
PANNA COTTA								
Caramel, Sainsbury's*	1 Pot/120g	335	15.7	279	2.5	34.6	13.1	3.3
Sainsbury's*	1 Pot/100g	304	15.7	304	3.0	41.5	15.7	4.0
Strawberry, COU, M&S*	1 Pot/145g	145	3.8	100	2.6	15.7	2.6	0.8
PAPAYA								
Dried, Strips, Tropical Wholefoods*	1 Strip/10g	31	0.1	310	3.9	71.4	0.9	1.5
Raw, Flesh Only, Average	*1 Serving/140g*	*37*	*0.1*	*26*	*0.4*	*6.6*	*0.1*	*1.2*
Raw, Weighed with Seeds & Skin	*1 Cup/140g*	*37*	*0.1*	*26*	*0.4*	*6.6*	*0.1*	*1.2*
PAPPARDELLE								
Buitoni*	1 Serving/65g	242	3.1	373	15.0	67.5	4.8	0.0
Egg, Dry, Average	*1 Serving/100g*	*364*	*3.7*	*364*	*14.1*	*68.5*	*3.7*	*2.1*
Egg, Fresh, Waitrose*	¼ Pack/125g	350	3.4	280	12.9	51.0	2.7	1.9
with Salmon, COU, M&S*	1 Pack/358g	340	6.8	95	6.3	13.0	1.9	0.8
PAPRIKA								
Average	*1 Tsp/2g*	*6*	*0.3*	*289*	*14.8*	*34.9*	*13.0*	*0.0*
PARATHA								
Average	*1 Paratha/80g*	*258*	*11.4*	*322*	*8.0*	*43.2*	*14.3*	*4.0*
Lachha, Waitrose*	1 Paratha/75g	322	17.8	429	7.8	46.0	23.8	1.8
Roti, Plain, Crown Farms*	1 Slice/80g	250	10.0	312	5.0	46.2	12.5	1.2

P

	Measure INFO/WEIGHT	per Measure KCAL	FAT	Nutrition Values per 100g / 100ml KCAL	PROT	CARB	FAT	FIBRE
PARCELS								
Beef Steak, Sainsbury's*	½ Pack/226g	488	35.3	216	12.2	6.6	15.6	1.0
Cheese & Ham, Sainsbury's*	1 Pack/250g	445	19.0	178	7.4	19.9	7.6	1.5
Filo, Brie & Cranberry, Finest, Tesco*	1 Parcel/22g	73	3.7	330	9.8	33.2	17.0	1.4
Filo, Feta & Spinach, Sainsbury's*	1 Parcel/27g	83	5.6	307	5.8	23.8	20.7	1.8
Filo, Mushroom Leek & Gruyere, Finest, Tesco*	1 Serving/160g	440	33.6	275	6.9	20.5	21.0	1.5
Smoked Salmon with Soft Cheese & Herb, Waitrose*	1 Pack/100g	246	20.2	246	14.6	1.2	20.2	0.0
Smoked Salmon, Sainsbury's*	1 Pack/115g	269	20.2	234	15.8	3.5	17.6	0.2
PARSLEY								
Dried	*1 Tsp/1g*	*2*	*0.1*	*181*	*15.8*	*14.5*	*7.0*	*26.9*
Fresh, Average	*1 Tbsp/4g*	*1*	*0.0*	*27*	*2.4*	*2.2*	*1.0*	*4.0*
PARSNIP								
Boiled, Average	*1 Serving/80g*	*53*	*1.0*	*66*	*1.6*	*12.9*	*1.2*	*4.7*
Honey Roasted, Tesco*	½ Pack/125g	165	6.6	130	1.3	16.7	5.2	5.2
Raw, Savers, Morrisons*	1 Serving/80g	61	0.9	76	1.8	12.5	1.1	4.6
Raw, Unprepared, Average	*1oz/28g*	*17*	*0.3*	*62*	*1.7*	*11.6*	*1.0*	*4.3*
Roast, Honey Glazed, Baked, Aunt Bessie's*	1 Serving/80g	177	11.9	221	1.4	18.7	14.9	3.4
Roasting, Freshly Frozen, CBY, Asda*	1 Serving/110g	221	8.5	201	2.5	30.4	7.7	7.8
PARTRIDGE								
Breast, Fillets, Raw, Skinned, Abel & Cole*	1 Serving/100g	145	4.7	145	25.8	0.0	4.7	0.0
Meat Only, Roasted	*1oz/28g*	*59*	*2.0*	*212*	*36.7*	*0.0*	*7.2*	*0.0*
PASSATA								
Napolina*	1 Bottle/690g	172	0.7	25	1.4	4.5	0.1	0.0
Sieved Tomato, Valfrutta*	1 Pack/500g	110	0.5	22	1.2	4.0	0.1	0.0
Smart Price, Asda*	1 Serving/100g	30	0.1	30	1.1	5.6	0.1	0.9
So Organic, Sainsbury's*	¼ Jar/175g	38	0.7	22	0.9	3.8	0.4	0.9
with Fresh Leaf Basil, Waitrose*	¼ Jar/170g	44	0.2	26	1.0	5.2	0.1	0.8
with Garlic & Italian Herbs, Tesco*	1 Serving/165g	53	0.3	32	1.2	6.4	0.2	1.1
PASSION FRUIT								
Raw, Fresh, Average	*1 Fruit/30g*	*11*	*0.1*	*36*	*2.6*	*5.8*	*0.4*	*3.3*
Weighed with Skin, Average	*1 Fruit/30g*	*7*	*0.1*	*22*	*1.6*	*3.5*	*0.2*	*2.0*
PASTA								
& Chargrilled Mushrooms, Finest, Tesco*	1 Pack/200g	410	22.4	205	6.1	19.6	11.2	1.4
Arrabbiata Nodini, Asda*	1 Serving/150g	302	8.7	201	7.8	29.3	5.8	2.7
Boccoletti, Dried, Sainsbury's*	1 Serving/90g	321	1.5	357	12.3	73.1	1.7	2.5
Bolognese Flavour, Mugfull, As Consumed, Batchelors*	1 Portion/245g	197	1.2	80	2.7	15.9	0.5	0.8
Bolognese, Diet Chef Ltd*	1 Pack/300g	255	10.2	85	7.9	5.8	3.4	4.4
Bolognese, Diet Chef Ltd*	1 Serving/300g	288	10.2	96	7.9	5.8	3.4	4.4
Brown Rice, Fusilli, Gluten Free, Dove's Farm*	1 Serving/30g	101	0.4	338	7.9	70.3	1.5	4.1
Cappelletti, Meat, Sainsbury's*	1 Pack/420g	816	23.9	195	10.0	25.8	5.7	2.3
Carbonara, Pasta Vita, Dolmio*	1 Pack/270g	335	12.4	124	4.5	15.8	4.6	0.0
Carbonara, Pasta Vita, Dolmio*	1 Pot/300g	372	13.8	124	4.5	15.8	4.6	0.0
Chargrilled Chicken & Bacon, Tesco*	1 Pack/200g	420	23.6	210	6.7	18.8	11.8	1.3
Cheese & Broccoli, Made Up, Smart Price, Asda*	1 Serving/120g	198	8.4	165	4.6	21.0	7.0	2.1
Cheese & Broccoli, Sauce Mix, Made Up, Sainsbury's*	1 Pack/120g	164	6.8	137	4.2	17.2	5.7	1.1
Cheese & Broccoli, Tubes, Tesco*	1 Serving/202g	319	13.9	158	5.0	19.1	6.9	2.3
Cheese, Leek & Ham, Pasta n Sauce, Batchelors*	1 Pack/120g	454	6.1	378	16.1	67.0	5.1	2.0
Cheese, Tomato & Pesto, Boots*	1 Pack/250g	355	11.0	142	5.9	20.0	4.4	2.0
Cheesy Spirals, Curly Whirly, Asda*	1/3 Pack/200g	214	5.2	107	6.0	15.0	2.6	0.5
Chicken & Chorizo, Quadrotti, TTD, Sainsbury's*	1 Pack/320g	675	28.8	211	11.8	20.6	9.0	2.7
Chicken & Mushroom, Made Up, Smart Price, Asda*	1 Pack/110g	183	6.6	166	5.0	23.0	6.0	2.2
Chicken & Mushroom, Pasta n Sauce, Batchelors*	½ Pack/63g	227	1.1	361	14.1	72.3	1.7	2.8
Chicken & Mushroom, Snack Pot, Asda*	1 Pot/228g	269	6.4	118	3.4	19.8	2.8	2.3
Chicken & Mushroom, Snack Stop, Crosse & Blackwell*	1 Pot/60g	251	5.3	418	10.3	74.3	8.8	0.0

	Measure INFO/WEIGHT	per Measure KCAL	per Measure FAT	Nutrition Values per 100g / 100ml KCAL	PROT	CARB	FAT	FIBRE
PASTA								
Chicken & Vegetable, Mediterranean, Waitrose*	1 Serving/400g	375	9.2	94	7.5	10.5	2.3	2.2
Chicken Penne, Weight Watchers*	1 Pot/261g	248	3.7	95	5.0	14.6	1.4	2.1
Courgette, Green Bean & Basil Pappardelle, M&S*	1 Pack/270g	324	15.9	120	4.7	11.8	5.9	1.6
Creamy Mushroom, Light Choices, Tesco*	1 Pack/350g	455	4.9	130	4.3	25.0	1.4	1.3
Creamy Mushroom, Sainsbury's*	1 Serving/63g	148	9.1	237	4.5	21.7	14.6	1.2
Fagottini, Wild Mushroom, Sainsbury's*	½ Pack/125g	274	9.4	219	10.2	27.7	7.5	2.7
Feta & Slow Roasted Tomato, Tesco*	1 Pack/290g	365	11.6	126	5.2	16.7	4.0	1.2
Filled, Tomato & Mozzarella Caramella, Jamie Oliver*	½ Pack/165g	294	9.2	178	8.9	24.9	5.6	2.0
Fiorelli, Goats Cheese & Caramelised Red Onion, Waitrose*	½ Pack/155g	226	8.8	146	6.3	17.3	5.7	2.2
Fiorelli, Mozzarella, Tomato & Basil, Waitrose*	1 Serving/125g	352	11.6	282	10.8	38.9	9.3	1.7
Fresh, Pumpkin & Sage Quadrotti, TTD, Sainsbury's*	½ Pack/160g	261	8.0	163	6.6	21.3	5.0	3.4
Garlic & Tomato, Pasta Vita, Dolmio*	1 Pot/300g	336	5.7	112	4.4	18.4	1.9	1.4
Garlic Mushroom Filled, ES, Asda*	1 Serving/125g	224	8.8	179	8.0	21.0	7.0	2.5
Girasole, Filled with Red Pepper & Goats Cheese, Asda*	½ Pack/150g	261	9.9	174	7.2	21.4	6.6	1.8
High Fibre, Uncooked, Fiber Gourmet*	1 Serving/56g	130	1.0	232	12.5	75.0	1.8	32.1
in Rich Tomato & Mushroom Sauce, Spirals, Tesco*	1 Serving/217g	326	13.7	150	4.6	18.8	6.3	2.5
Lumaconi, TTD, Sainsbury's*	1 Serving/90g	321	1.5	357	12.3	73.1	1.7	2.5
Macaroni Cheese, Dry, Pasta n Sauce, Batchelors*	1 Pack/108g	402	5.1	372	17.2	65.2	4.7	2.7
Margherite, Basil & Pinenut, TTD, Sainsbury's*	½ Pack/150g	275	11.1	184	8.7	19.4	7.4	2.3
Medaglioni, Bolognese, Rich Red Wine, Waitrose*	½ Pack/125g	266	7.0	213	12.5	28.1	5.6	2.6
Mediterranean Vegetable, Low Fat, LBU, Co-Op*	1 Pack/399g	395	10.0	99	4.6	14.0	2.5	1.4
Mild Cheese & Broccoli, Pasta n Sauce, Batchelors*	½ Pack/61g	221	2.4	363	15.0	67.0	3.9	4.0
Mushroom & Emmental Stuffed, Sainsbury's*	1 Pack/250g	650	23.0	260	11.3	33.5	9.2	3.7
Orecchiette, Tesco*	1 Serving75g	270	1.1	360	13.5	72.5	1.5	1.6
Organic, Gluten Free, Dove's Farm*	1 Serving/100g	338	1.5	338	7.9	70.3	1.5	4.1
Orzo, Dry, Average	*1 Serving/100g*	*348*	*1.5*	*348*	*12.4*	*71.9*	*1.5*	*3.0*
Penne Arrabiata, with Chicken, Birds Eye*	1 Bag/350g	360	10.0	103	6.0	12.6	2.8	1.3
Penne, Cajun Steak, Balanced for You, M&S*	1 Serving/360g	392	7.6	109	7.1	14.8	2.1	1.2
Penne, Creamy Mushroom, Prepared, Tesco*	½ Pack/200g	288	12.8	144	4.5	17.4	6.4	3.3
Peperonata, Pasta King*	1 Serving/100g	104	1.4	104	3.5	19.4	1.4	1.8
Pomodoro, Pasta King*	1 Serving/100g	109	1.8	109	3.6	19.6	1.8	1.8
Pumpkin & Pine Nut Stuffed, Fiorelli, Fresh, Waitrose*	½ Pack/125g	225	7.5	180	8.0	22.3	6.0	2.3
Pumpkin & Sage, Mezze Lune, Whole Foods, Co-Op*	½ Pack/146g	256	6.3	175	6.8	26.0	4.3	2.6
Seafood, Retail	1oz/28g	31	1.3	110	8.9	7.6	4.8	0.4
Sweet Pepper, Pasta Vita, Dolmio*	1 Pot/300g	327	5.7	109	4.4	17.9	1.9	1.4
Sweet Pepper, Pasta Vita, Dolmio*	1 Pot/300g	327	5.7	109	4.4	17.9	1.9	1.4
Tagliatelle, Mushroom & Creamy Cheese Sauce, Birds Eye*	1 Serving/350g	620	29.0	177	4.9	19.7	8.3	2.5
Tomato & Chilli, Pasta Vita, Dolmio*	1 Pot/300g	330	5.4	110	4.4	18.4	1.8	1.5
Tomato & Herb, Snackpot, Made Up, CBY, Asda*	1 Pot/225g	259	1.6	115	3.8	23.4	0.7	2.0
Tomato & Vegetable, Diet Chef Ltd*	1 Pack/300g	216	6.0	72	2.6	10.9	2.0	1.8
Tomato, Onion & Herb, Made Up, Morrisons*	1 Serving/110g	141	5.0	128	3.2	18.7	4.5	2.3
Tortelloni, Spinach & Ricotta, Giovanni Rana*	½ Pack/125g	319	10.0	255	9.0	35.5	8.0	3.1
Tuna Rigatoni, Diet Chef Ltd*	1 Pack/300g	336	13.2	112	5.9	12.2	4.4	1.0
Wholewheat, Cooked, Tesco*	1 Serving/200g	284	1.8	142	5.7	27.9	0.9	4.5
PASTA BAKE								
Aberdeen Angus Meatball, Waitrose*	½ Pack/350g	501	28.0	143	5.2	12.5	8.0	0.9
Bacon & Leek, Average	*1 Serving/400g*	*633*	*32.3*	*158*	*6.7*	*14.8*	*8.1*	*1.3*
Bolognese, Finest, Tesco*	1 Serving/250g	375	15.8	150	7.3	16.1	6.3	1.1
Bolognese, Weight Watchers*	1 Pack/400g	324	8.0	81	6.1	9.6	2.0	1.3
Cheese & Bacon, Fresh Italian, Asda*	1 Serving/250g	265	20.0	106	6.0	2.6	8.0	0.5
Cheese & Tomato, Italiano, Tesco*	1 Bake/300g	354	12.6	118	3.9	16.1	4.2	1.0
Cheese & Tomato, Tesco*	1 Pack/400g	388	5.6	97	3.4	17.8	1.4	1.2
Chicken & Bacon, Asda*	¼ Pack/374g	610	26.2	163	9.0	16.0	7.0	4.1

	Measure	per Measure		Nutrition Values per 100g / 100ml				
	INFO/WEIGHT	KCAL	FAT	KCAL	PROT	CARB	FAT	FIBRE
PASTA BAKE								
Chicken & Bacon, Average	**1 Serving/400g**	**627**	**28.7**	**157**	**9.0**	**13.7**	**7.2**	**1.6**
Chicken & Broccoli, Morrisons*	1 Pack/400g	452	16.0	113	6.1	13.3	4.0	0.6
Chicken & Broccoli, Pasta Presto, Findus*	1 Pack/321g	449	22.5	140	7.5	12.0	7.0	0.0
Chicken & Leek, HL, Tesco*	1 Pack/400g	460	7.6	115	10.8	13.1	1.9	1.6
Chicken & Mushroom, Waitrose*	1 Pack/400g	532	30.8	133	6.7	9.1	7.7	0.8
Chicken, Bacon & Mushroom, Average	**1 Serving/400g**	**632**	**29.2**	**158**	**7.8**	**15.1**	**7.3**	**2.3**
Chicken, Bacon & Mushroom, Sainsbury's*	1 Serving/400g	548	20.0	137	7.0	15.3	5.0	1.3
Chicken, Morrisons*	1 Pack/402g	442	14.5	110	4.6	14.8	3.6	0.9
Chicken, Weight Watchers*	1 Pack/300g	249	2.7	83	6.0	12.1	0.9	1.1
Chilli Beef, Asda*	1 Pack/1500g	2010	90.0	134	7.0	13.0	6.0	1.2
Creamy Mushroom, Dolmio*	½ Jar/245g	267	22.5	109	1.1	5.5	9.2	0.0
Creamy Tomato, Dolmio*	1 Serving/125g	141	9.0	113	2.3	8.4	7.2	0.0
Ham & Broccoli, Asda*	1 Pack/340g	309	13.9	91	3.4	10.0	4.1	0.5
Meat Feast, Average	**1 Serving/400g**	**601**	**21.4**	**150**	**5.8**	**19.2**	**5.4**	**1.4**
Meat Feast, Italian, Sainsbury's*	½ Pack/400g	562	19.1	141	5.4	18.1	4.8	1.5
Mix, Tuna & Pasta, Colman's*	1 Pack/45g	149	2.4	331	10.4	60.5	5.3	4.4
Mix, Tuna, Colman's*	1 Sachet/45g	145	2.3	323	9.2	60.0	5.2	4.7
Mozzarella & Tomato, Asda*	1 Pack/400g	532	19.2	133	4.4	18.1	4.8	1.8
Penne Mozzarella, Tesco*	1 Pack/340g	408	8.5	120	4.7	19.7	2.5	0.6
Roasted Mediterranean Vegetables, Dolmio*	1 Portion/125g	66	2.1	53	1.3	8.1	1.7	1.2
Sausage, Average	**1 Serving/400g**	**591**	**24.0**	**148**	**5.5**	**17.7**	**6.0**	**1.9**
Spicy Tomato & Pepperoni, Asda*	1 Pack/440g	431	26.4	98	1.1	10.0	6.0	1.2
Tomato & Mozzarella, Average	**1 Serving/400g**	**500**	**12.4**	**125**	**5.3**	**17.3**	**3.1**	**1.5**
Tomato & Mozzarella, Italiano, Tesco*	1 Pack/340g	398	8.5	117	4.8	18.9	2.5	1.7
Tuna & Sweetcorn, Average	**1 Pack/400g**	**423**	**22.4**	**106**	**5.0**	**8.6**	**5.6**	**1.9**
Tuna, Co-Op*	1 Serving/340g	306	6.8	90	7.0	12.0	2.0	1.0
Vegetable, M&S*	½ Pack/175g	201	8.8	115	4.1	12.6	5.0	2.2
Vegetable, Mediterranean, HL, Tesco*	1 Serving/450g	374	3.6	83	2.9	16.0	0.8	1.5
Vegetable, Mediterranean, Tesco*	1 Serving/450g	495	20.7	110	4.3	12.9	4.6	1.3
with Tomato & Mozzarella, Sainsbury's*	1 Pack/400g	480	12.8	120	5.0	17.9	3.2	2.1
PASTA QUILLS								
Dry, Average	**1 Serving/75g**	**256**	**0.9**	**342**	**12.0**	**72.3**	**1.2**	**2.0**
Dry, Value, Tesco*	1 Serving/75g	261	1.1	348	12.0	71.7	1.5	3.0
Gluten Free, Salute*	1 Serving/75g	269	1.4	359	7.5	78.0	1.9	0.0
PASTA SALAD								
& Mixed Leaf with Basil Pesto Dressing, Tesco*	1 Pack/220g	528	37.6	240	4.7	16.9	17.1	0.7
Bacon, Budgens*	1 Salad/200g	570	47.8	285	5.1	12.6	23.9	0.7
Basil & Parmesan, Tesco*	1 Serving/50g	65	1.8	130	4.3	20.2	3.6	0.6
BBQ Bean, Tesco*	1 Pack/850g	1139	43.3	134	3.6	18.5	5.1	1.8
Caesar & Santa Tomatoes, M&S*	1 Serving/220g	495	33.7	225	5.2	15.9	15.3	0.8
Chargrilled Chicken & Pesto Pasta, Sainsbury's*	1 Pack/240g	454	22.1	189	7.2	19.4	9.2	0.0
Chargrilled Chicken, Italian Style, Fresh, Asda*	1 Pack/200g	318	14.0	159	7.0	17.0	7.0	0.4
Cheese Layered, Asda*	1 Pack/440g	471	21.6	107	5.2	10.4	4.9	2.0
Cheese, Asda*	1 Serving/40g	118	9.0	296	6.5	16.6	22.6	0.5
Cheese, Layered, Asda*	1 Pack/440g	647	40.9	147	4.5	11.4	9.3	0.0
Cheese, Morrisons*	½ Pot/125g	341	26.6	273	5.7	14.7	21.3	1.0
Cherry Tomato & Rocket, HE, Tesco*	1 Pack/225g	223	5.6	99	3.2	15.8	2.5	1.0
Chicken & Bacon Caesar, Tesco*	1 Pack/265g	442	23.6	167	10.2	10.8	8.9	1.3
Chicken & Bacon Layered, Fresh Tastes, Asda*	1 Pack/375g	266	30.0	71	5.9	11.5	8.0	0.0
Chicken & Bacon Layered, Fresh Tastes, Asda*	1 Pack/197g	290	16.9	147	6.5	10.3	8.6	0.0
Chicken & Smoked Bacon, M&S*	1 Pack/380g	817	46.7	215	7.5	19.0	12.3	1.9
Chicken, Tomato & Basil, Sainsbury's*	1 Pack/350g	626	27.6	179	7.4	19.0	7.9	1.1
Chicken, Tomato & Basil, Tesco *	1 Pack/300g	414	9.3	138	6.2	20.6	3.1	1.6

	Measure INFO/WEIGHT	per Measure KCAL	FAT	Nutrition Values per 100g / 100ml KCAL	PROT	CARB	FAT	FIBRE
PASTA SALAD								
Chicken, with Basil & Tomato, Creamy, COU, M&S*	1 Pack/327g	360	6.9	110	7.8	13.8	2.1	1.6
Crayfish, Rocket & Lemon, Finest, Tesco*	1 Serving/250g	728	39.8	291	8.9	28.0	15.9	4.2
Farfalle, Prawns Tomatoes & Cucumber, Sainsbury's*	1 Serving/260g	270	12.2	104	4.5	10.9	4.7	0.7
Goats Cheese & Mixed Pepper, Sainsbury's*	1 Pack/200g	366	18.8	183	6.4	18.2	9.4	1.5
Ham, Sainsbury's*	1 Pot/250g	610	48.2	244	4.1	13.4	19.3	0.8
Honey & Mustard Chicken, M&S*	1 Serving/190g	304	4.8	160	8.7	26.7	2.5	1.5
Honey & Mustard Chicken, Sainsbury's*	1 Pack/190g	344	16.9	181	7.1	18.0	8.9	0.0
Italian, Tesco*	½ Pack/225g	315	8.3	140	3.5	22.6	3.7	2.3
Mixed Bean, Diet Chef Ltd*	1 Pack/300g	300	3.6	100	4.7	17.5	1.2	2.8
Mozzarella & Sun Dried Tomato, Waitrose*	1 Serving/150g	312	18.3	208	5.8	18.8	12.2	1.3
Pepper & Tomato, Fire Roasted, Finest, Tesco*	1 Pack/200g	260	8.2	130	3.7	19.4	4.1	2.5
Pepper, HE, Tesco*	1 Salad/210g	139	0.8	66	2.4	13.3	0.4	1.0
Pesto, Creamy, Pot, Diet Chef*	1 Pot/248g	236	3.7	95	3.6	16.2	1.5	1.0
Poached Salmon, M&S*	1 Serving/200g	340	16.8	170	7.8	16.2	8.4	1.4
Prawn Cocktail, Layered, Shapers, Boots*	1 Pot/210g	181	5.2	86	3.6	13.0	2.5	1.3
Prawn, Layered, Asda*	½ Pack/220g	279	11.4	127	5.2	14.2	5.2	2.0
Prawn, Tesco*	½ Pack/250g	488	27.8	195	4.9	18.9	11.1	2.0
Prawns, King & Juicy Fresh Tomatoes, COU, M&S*	1 Serving/270g	256	4.0	95	5.1	16.4	1.5	0.9
Roasted Mushroom, Spinach & Tarragon, Tesco*	1 Pot/200g	216	4.8	108	4.3	17.2	2.4	0.8
Sainsbury's*	½ Pack/160g	235	9.6	147	3.2	20.0	6.0	1.5
Spicy Chilli Pesto, Sainsbury's*	¼ Pot/63g	170	12.3	272	3.8	20.1	19.6	1.6
Sun Dried Tomato Dressing, Sainsbury's*	1 Pack/320g	442	14.1	138	3.7	20.8	4.4	3.6
Tomato & Basil Chicken, M&S*	1 Serving/279g	446	22.0	160	7.0	14.8	7.9	1.8
Tomato & Basil with Red & Green Pepper, Sainsbury's*	¼ Pot/63g	89	4.3	141	3.2	16.4	6.9	3.8
Tomato & Basil, Chicken, Waitrose*	1 Pack/205g	434	24.6	212	8.3	17.7	12.0	1.1
Tomato & Basil, M&S*	1 Pot/225g	484	35.8	215	2.9	15.0	15.9	1.2
Tomato & Basil, Pot, HL, Tesco*	1 Pot/200g	242	5.4	121	2.0	22.1	2.7	2.2
Tomato & Basil, Sainsbury's*	1 Serving/62g	87	4.3	141	3.2	16.4	6.9	3.8
Tomato & Chargrilled Vegetable, Tesco*	1 Serving/200g	248	7.8	124	3.7	18.6	3.9	1.4
Tomato & Mozzarella, Sainsbury's*	1 Pack/200g	440	22.6	220	7.5	22.2	11.3	1.3
Tomato & Mozzarella, Waitrose*	1 Pack/225g	380	27.9	169	4.3	10.0	12.4	0.6
Tomato, Aldi*	1 Serving/50g	58	1.8	117	3.9	18.6	3.6	0.0
Tuna & Sweetcorn, COU, M&S*	1 Pack/200g	210	1.8	105	7.1	18.3	0.9	1.2
Tuna & Sweetcorn, HE, Tesco*	1 Pot/200g	230	5.4	115	5.7	17.0	2.7	1.3
Tuna & Sweetcorn, Sainsbury's*	1 Serving/100g	111	1.2	111	7.1	18.3	1.2	1.2
Tuna Nicoise, Waitrose*	1 Pot/190g	306	17.1	161	5.1	14.9	9.0	1.1
PASTA SAUCE								
Amatriciana, Tesco*	1 Serving/175g	108	7.2	62	2.3	4.0	4.1	0.7
Arrabbiata, Barilla*	1 Serving/100g	47	3.0	47	1.5	3.5	3.0	0.0
Arrabbiata, Fresh, Co-Op*	½ Pot/150g	82	4.5	55	1.0	5.0	3.0	1.0
Arrabbiata, Fresh, Morrisons*	1 Pot/350g	139	5.2	40	1.9	5.4	1.5	0.0
Arrabbiata, GFY, Asda*	1 Serving/350g	133	3.9	38	1.1	6.0	1.1	0.0
Arrabbiata, Italian, Waitrose*	1 Jar/320g	115	3.2	36	1.5	6.7	1.0	1.4
Arrabbiata, M&S*	1 Jar/320g	240	17.0	75	1.2	6.2	5.3	0.8
Arrabbiata, Red Pepper, Sainsbury's*	½ Pot/175g	79	5.1	45	1.4	3.3	2.9	1.6
Arrabbiata, Romano*	1 Serving/100g	69	3.4	69	2.5	7.0	3.4	0.6
Bolognese with Beef, Tesco*	½ Can/213g	179	10.0	84	4.9	5.5	4.7	0.0
Bolognese, Finest, Tesco*	1 Serving/175g	170	10.7	97	7.0	3.8	6.1	0.5
Bolognese, Fresh, Sainsbury's*	½ Pot/150g	120	6.1	80	6.0	4.7	4.1	1.2
Bolognese, GFY, Asda*	1 Jar/500g	210	1.5	42	0.7	7.9	0.3	2.4
Bolognese, Italiano, Tesco*	1 Serving/175g	194	13.1	111	5.9	4.8	7.5	0.8
Bolognese, Mediterranean Vegetable, Chunky, Dolmio*	½ Jar/250g	138	4.0	55	1.3	8.8	1.6	1.1
Bolognese, Organic, Seeds of Change*	1 Jar/500g	290	6.0	58	1.3	10.4	1.2	0.8

P

PASTA SAUCE

	Measure INFO/WEIGHT	per Measure		Nutrition Values per 100g / 100ml				
		KCAL	FAT	KCAL	PROT	CARB	FAT	FIBRE
Bolognese, Original, Asda*	1 Serving/158g	73	2.2	46	1.4	7.0	1.4	0.8
Bolognese, Original, Light, Low Fat, Dolmio*	1 Serving/125g	41	0.1	33	1.2	5.9	0.1	0.9
Bolognese, Original, Sainsbury's*	¼ Jar/136g	90	2.9	66	1.9	9.9	2.1	1.3
Bolognese, Tesco*	¼ Jar/125g	51	1.8	41	1.0	6.1	1.4	2.3
Bolognese, Tomato, Beef & Red Wine, Fresh, Waitrose*	1 Pot/350g	301	17.2	86	5.4	5.3	4.9	2.0
Bolognese, Traditional, Ragu, Knorr*	1 Jar/320g	157	5.4	49	1.3	7.1	1.7	1.2
Bolognese, VLH Kitchens	1 Serving/380g	316	1.1	83	6.0	4.7	4.1	1.2
Bolognese, with Red Wine, Weight Watchers*	1 Jar/350g	98	0.4	28	1.4	5.3	0.1	1.3
Cacciatore, Fresh, Sainsbury's*	½ Pot/150g	152	8.8	101	5.4	8.1	5.9	1.5
Carbonara, Asda*	½ Pot/175g	359	29.8	205	7.0	6.0	17.0	0.1
Carbonara, Co-Op*	½ Pot/150g	270	25.5	180	3.0	4.0	17.0	0.1
Carbonara, Creamy, Dolmio Express, Dolmio*	1 Pack/150g	171	13.8	114	3.1	4.7	9.2	0.1
Carbonara, Creamy, Stir in Sauce, Dolmio*	1 Serving/75g	98	8.0	130	3.3	5.2	10.6	0.2
Carbonara, Fresh, Chilled, Finest, Tesco*	½ Tub/175g	298	24.8	170	5.5	4.2	14.2	0.0
Carbonara, Fresh, Chilled, Italiano, Tesco*	½ Tub/175g	201	11.4	115	6.1	7.2	6.5	0.1
Carbonara, Italian, Fresh, Sainsbury's*	½ Pot/176g	209	16.3	119	5.4	3.4	9.3	0.9
Cherry Tomato & Basil, Sacla*	1 Serving/96g	90	7.1	94	1.2	5.3	7.4	0.0
Cherry Tomato & Roasted Pepper, Asda*	1 Jar/172g	91	5.2	53	1.5	5.0	3.0	2.4
Creamy Tomato & Basil, BGTY, Sainsbury's*	½ Jar/250g	172	9.0	69	1.7	7.6	3.6	1.0
Five Cheese, Italiano, Tesco*	½ Tub/175g	271	20.1	155	6.8	6.0	11.5	0.0
for Bolognese, Extra Mushrooms, Dolmio*	1 Jar/500g	240	6.5	48	1.6	7.6	1.3	1.1
for Bolognese, Extra Onion & Garlic, Dolmio*	1 Serving/125g	51	0.8	41	1.4	6.6	0.6	1.0
for Bolognese, Extra Spicy, Dolmio*	1 Jar/500g	260	5.5	52	1.7	8.8	1.1	0.8
for Lasagne, White, Ragu, Knorr*	1 Jar/475g	755	72.2	159	0.5	5.1	15.2	0.3
Four Cheese, BGTY, Sainsbury's*	1 Serving/150g	104	6.0	69	2.9	5.5	4.0	0.1
Four Cheese, Fresh, Asda*	½ Pot/162g	309	28.8	191	5.4	2.2	17.8	0.5
Four Cheese, Sainsbury's*	1 Serving/150g	296	25.5	197	6.6	4.5	17.0	0.8
Hot & Spicy, Morrisons*	1 Serving/130g	81	3.1	62	1.4	8.5	2.4	1.1
Hot Pepper & Mozzarella, Stir Through, Sacla*	½ Jar/95g	229	20.4	241	4.7	7.2	21.5	0.0
Italian Cheese, Finest, Tesco*	½ Pot/175g	172	8.9	98	4.8	8.4	5.1	0.0
Italian Tomato & Herb, for Pasta, Sainsbury's*	½ Jar/146g	102	2.9	70	2.0	11.1	2.0	1.4
Italian, Amatriciana, Sainsbury's*	½ Pot/175g	136	3.0	78	2.6	5.7	1.7	0.5
Italian, Vongole, Waitrose*	1 Serving/175g	116	5.6	66	4.2	5.2	3.2	0.7
Mediterranean Tomato, Asda*	1 Jar/500g	285	6.0	57	1.5	10.0	1.2	0.0
Mediterranean Vegetable Pasta, Tesco*	1 Serving/166g	95	2.8	57	1.4	9.0	1.7	1.2
Mediterranean Vegetable, Organic, Seeds of Change*	1 Jar/350g	210	10.2	60	1.2	6.6	2.9	1.4
Mediterranean Vegetable, Rustico, Bertolli*	½ Jar/160g	141	11.5	88	1.7	4.1	7.2	0.7
Mediterranean, Fresh, Waitrose*	1 Pot/350g	214	13.6	61	1.4	5.0	3.9	2.4
Mushroom & Marsala Wine, Sacla*	½ Pot/85g	165	16.0	194	2.2	3.9	18.8	0.0
Mushroom, Fresh, Waitrose*	1 Serving/175g	142	10.0	81	1.6	5.7	5.7	0.5
Mushroom, GFY, Asda*	1 Serving/175g	112	4.9	64	2.7	7.0	2.8	0.0
Mushroom, Morrisons*	1 Serving/128g	76	2.9	59	1.6	7.9	2.3	1.1
Mushroom, Sainsbury's*	1 Serving/100g	66	2.1	66	2.0	9.8	2.1	1.7
Mushroom, Tesco*	1 Jar/500g	225	5.5	45	1.0	7.7	1.1	1.8
Napoletana, Fresh, Asda*	1 Pot/330g	148	7.3	45	1.4	5.0	2.2	2.8
Napoletana, Fresh, Waitrose*	1 Serving/175g	82	3.0	47	1.3	6.6	1.7	1.0
Napoletana, Morrisons*	1 Serving/175g	82	2.6	47	2.6	6.7	1.5	0.0
Olive & Tomato, Sacla*	1 Serving/95g	87	7.6	92	1.3	3.6	8.0	0.0
Olive, Barilla*	1 Serving/100g	92	5.0	92	1.5	10.3	5.0	0.0
Original with Tomato & Onions, Morrisons*	1 Serving/125g	51	1.4	41	1.4	6.3	1.1	1.2
Original with Tomatoes & Onions, Morrisons*	1 Serving/100g	64	2.5	64	1.2	9.3	2.5	1.0
Original, BFY, Morrisons*	1/3 Jar/200g	100	0.2	50	1.6	10.6	0.1	1.2
Original, Tesco*	1 Jar/300g	123	4.2	41	1.0	6.1	1.4	2.3

PASTA SAUCE

	Measure INFO/WEIGHT	per Measure KCAL	FAT	Nutrition Values per 100g / 100ml KCAL	PROT	CARB	FAT	FIBRE
Parmesan & Pesto, Weight Watchers*	½ Jar/175g	86	2.8	49	1.8	6.7	1.6	1.0
Pepper & Tomato, M&S*	1 Jar/320g	224	13.4	70	1.6	6.1	4.2	0.9
Pomodoro, Cirio*	1 Serving/200g	116	4.6	58	1.4	8.4	2.3	0.0
Puttanesca, Italian, Waitrose*	1 Jar/350g	195	9.8	56	1.5	6.1	2.8	1.3
Puttanesca, Loyd Grossman*	1 Jar/350g	315	21.7	90	1.7	6.8	6.2	0.9
Puttanesca, M&S*	1 Jar/320g	256	17.6	80	1.5	6.2	5.5	1.9
Red Pepper & Italian Cheese, Stir Through, Asda*	½ Jar/95g	86	4.7	90	2.9	8.5	4.9	0.9
Rich Tomato with Basil Pesto, Express, Dolmio*	1 Pack/170g	146	10.0	86	2.0	6.2	5.9	0.0
Roasted Aubergine & Mascarpone, Stir Through, M&S*	½ Jar/95g	111	8.9	117	1.0	6.3	9.4	1.7
Roasted Garlic & Onion, Weight Watchers*	1 Jar/175g	65	0.7	37	1.3	6.4	0.4	1.2
Roasted Red Pepper & Tomato, Finest, Tesco*	1 Serving/145g	117	7.8	81	1.2	6.8	5.4	2.2
Roasted Vegetable, Sainsbury's*	½ Pot/151g	103	5.9	68	1.6	6.7	3.9	0.4
Roasted Vegetable, Tesco*	1 Pack/175g	114	5.2	65	1.5	8.0	3.0	0.8
Salsina with Onions & Garlic, Valfrutta*	1 Serving/150g	36	0.0	24	1.6	4.5	0.0	1.4
Seasonal, Bolognese, Dolmio*	1 Jar/500g	205	1.0	41	1.5	7.4	0.2	1.4
Siciliana, Sainsbury's*	1/3 Jar/113g	168	14.7	149	1.8	6.2	13.0	0.0
Smoky Bacon, Loyd Grossman*	½ Jar/175g	142	8.4	81	3.0	6.1	4.8	0.8
Spicy Italian Chilli, Express, Dolmio*	1 Serving/170g	87	2.7	51	1.5	7.5	1.6	0.0
Spicy Pepper & Tomato, Sacla*	½ Jar/95g	132	11.2	139	1.4	6.8	11.8	0.0
Spicy Red Pepper & Roasted Vegetable, Asda*	1 Serving/175g	140	7.7	80	1.2	9.0	4.4	1.0
Spicy Roasted Garlic, Seeds of Change*	1 Serving/195g	123	3.9	63	1.5	9.7	2.0	1.2
Spicy Tomato, Asda*	1 Serving/155g	76	1.9	49	1.5	8.0	1.2	1.0
Spicy Tomato, with Mixed Peppers, Combino, Lidl*	1 Jar/500g	270	5.0	54	2.3	8.4	1.0	1.2
Spicy with Peppers, Tesco*	1 Jar/500g	240	4.5	48	2.2	7.8	0.9	1.8
Sun Dried Tomato & Basil, Organic, Seeds of Change*	½ Jar/100g	155	13.1	155	1.6	7.7	13.1	0.0
Sun Dried Tomato & Garlic, M&S*	½ Jar/95g	147	13.0	155	2.9	4.4	13.7	0.8
Sun Dried Tomato, Asda*	½ Jar/159g	165	12.7	104	1.9	6.0	8.0	1.5
Sun Dried Tomato, Garlic & Basil, Finest, Tesco*	1 Jar/340g	493	39.1	145	1.8	7.7	11.5	2.3
Sun Dried Tomato, Stir In, Light, Dolmio*	1 Serving/75g	62	3.5	83	1.7	9.8	4.7	0.0
Sun Ripened Tomato & Basil, Dolmio*	1 Serving/150g	117	6.9	78	1.3	7.9	4.6	0.0
Sun Ripened Tomato & Basil, Express, Dolmio*	1 Pouch/170g	88	2.7	52	1.5	7.9	1.6	0.0
Sun Ripened Tomato & Basil, Microwaveable, Dolmio*	½ Pack/190g	106	4.0	56	1.4	7.9	2.1	0.0
Sweet Pepper, Dolmio*	1 Serving/150g	238	20.1	159	1.6	8.8	13.4	0.0
Sweet Red Pepper, Loyd Grossman*	1 Jar/350g	304	19.6	87	1.7	7.3	5.6	1.2
Tomato & Basil, Bertolli*	1 Jar/500g	215	5.0	43	1.2	7.3	1.0	0.4
Tomato & Basil, Dolmio*	1 Serving/170g	95	3.6	56	1.4	7.9	2.1	0.0
Tomato & Basil, LBU, Co-Op*	½ Pot/150g	90	4.4	60	1.6	6.1	2.9	1.0
Tomato & Basil, Loyd Grossman*	½ Jar/175g	107	6.0	61	1.5	5.8	3.4	0.8
Tomato & Basil, M&S*	1 Jar/340g	119	7.1	35	2.0	2.1	2.1	0.9
Tomato & Basil, Morrisons*	½ Jar/140g	76	0.7	54	1.7	10.1	0.5	1.3
Tomato & Basil, Organic, Pasta Reale*	1 Pack/300g	216	15.9	72	1.0	5.1	5.3	0.4
Tomato & Basil, Organic, Simply Organic*	1 Pot/300g	183	12.9	61	1.5	4.2	4.3	0.6
Tomato & Chilli, Pour Over, M&S*	1 Jar/330g	231	12.5	70	1.3	7.6	3.8	1.8
Tomato & Garlic, CBY, Asda*	½ Jar/160g	74	0.8	46	1.6	7.9	0.5	1.7
Tomato & Herb with Extra Garlic, Sainsbury's*	½ Pot/150g	62	1.7	41	1.4	6.3	1.1	1.6
Tomato & Herb, Co-Op*	1 Serving/125g	75	2.5	60	1.0	9.0	2.0	1.0
Tomato & Herb, for Bolognese, Lighter, Sainsbury's*	¼ Jar/125g	35	0.4	28	1.1	4.4	0.3	1.5
Tomato & Herb, M&S*	1 Jar/500g	400	15.5	80	2.6	10.1	3.1	1.7
Tomato & Herb, Organic, M&S*	1 Jar/550g	302	19.8	55	1.4	4.2	3.6	2.6
Tomato & Mascarpone, BGTY, Sainsbury's*	1 Pot/300g	150	9.0	50	2.0	3.6	3.0	3.6
Tomato & Mascarpone, Finest, Tesco*	1 Serving/175g	135	8.8	77	2.7	5.4	5.0	0.8
Tomato & Mascarpone, Italiano, Tesco*	½ Pot/175g	168	12.2	96	2.8	5.5	7.0	0.7
Tomato & Mascarpone, Morrisons*	½ Pot/175g	217	16.8	124	2.9	6.5	9.6	1.1

	Measure INFO/WEIGHT	per Measure		Nutrition Values per 100g / 100ml				
		KCAL	FAT	KCAL	PROT	CARB	FAT	FIBRE
PASTA SAUCE								
Tomato & Mascarpone, Sainsbury's*	½ Pot/150g	137	9.9	91	2.1	5.9	6.6	1.2
Tomato & Mascarpone, So Organic, Sainsbury's*	1/3 Jar/146g	180	13.2	123	1.9	8.7	9.0	2.8
Tomato & Mascarpone, Tesco*	1 Serving/175g	194	15.2	111	2.8	5.4	8.7	0.6
Tomato & Mascarpone, Waitrose*	½ Pot/175g	184	14.7	105	1.9	5.5	8.4	1.1
Tomato & Olives, La Doria*	1 Jar/90g	76	5.9	84	1.2	5.0	6.6	0.0
Tomato & Parmesan, Seeds of Change*	1 Serving/150g	100	4.4	67	2.5	7.8	2.9	1.1
Tomato & Ricotta, Italian, Sainsbury's*	1 Pack/390g	238	11.7	61	2.5	6.1	3.0	1.2
Tomato & Roasted Garlic, CBY, Asda*	1 Pot/350g	122	2.1	35	1.5	5.0	0.6	1.7
Tomato & Roasted Garlic, Loyd Grossman*	½ Jar/175g	107	5.4	61	1.5	6.3	3.1	0.8
Tomato & Tuna, Loyd Grossman*	½ Jar/175g	154	7.7	88	4.4	7.5	4.4	0.8
Tomato & Wild Mushroom, Loyd Grossman*	½ Jar/175g	154	9.8	88	2.1	7.4	5.6	1.5
Tomato & Wild Mushroom, Waitrose*	1 Serving/175g	65	1.2	37	1.7	6.0	0.7	0.9
Tomato with Red Wine & Herbs, Ragu, Knorr*	1 Jar/500g	215	0.5	43	1.3	9.3	0.1	1.1
Tomato, Low Price, Sainsbury's*	1 Jar/440g	220	3.1	50	0.6	10.1	0.7	0.4
Tomato, Pecorino Romano Cheese & Garlic, Bertolli*	1 Serving/125g	76	3.5	61	2.3	6.5	2.8	0.9
Vegetable, Chunky, Tesco*	1 Jar/500g	235	5.0	47	1.8	6.8	1.0	1.8
Vine Ripened Tomato & Black Olive, Bertolli*	½ Jar/93g	145	12.3	157	2.3	7.3	13.3	0.0
Whole Cherry Tomato & Roasted Pepper, Sacla*	½ Jar/145g	93	5.9	64	1.5	5.2	4.1	0.0
PASTA SHAPES								
Alphabetti, in Tomato Sauce, Heinz*	1 Can/200g	118	1.0	59	1.8	11.7	0.5	1.5
Cooked, Tesco*	1 Serving/260g	356	2.1	137	5.1	26.3	0.8	1.1
Disney Princess in Tomato Sauce, Heinz*	1 Can/200g	114	0.6	57	1.8	11.9	0.3	1.5
Dried, Tesco*	1 Serving/100g	345	2.0	345	13.2	68.5	2.0	2.9
Durum Wheat, Dry, Basics, Sainsbury's*	1 Serving/75g	260	1.5	346	12.0	70.0	2.0	4.0
Spiderman, & Mini Sausages in Tomato Sauce, Heinz*	1 Can/200g	178	6.2	89	3.6	11.6	3.1	0.5
PASTA SHELLS								
Conchiglie, Dry Weight, Parioli, Cucina*	1 Serving/75g	266	1.0	355	12.5	73.0	1.4	2.6
Dry, Average	*1 Serving/75g*	*265*	*1.5*	*353*	*11.1*	*71.8*	*2.0*	*2.0*
Egg, Fresh, Average	*1 Serving/125g*	*344*	*3.6*	*275*	*11.5*	*49.8*	*2.8*	*3.4*
PASTA SNACK								
Mug Shot, Creamy Cheese, Symingtons*	1 Sachet/271g	301	6.0	111	3.7	19.1	2.2	1.0
Mug Shot, Roast Chicken, Symingtons*	1 Sachet/258g	204	2.6	79	1.4	16.2	1.0	0.8
Tomato & Herb in a Pot, Dry, Tesco*	1 Pot/59g	207	1.4	352	11.8	70.7	2.4	2.6
Tomato 'n' Herb, Mug Shot*	1 Sachet/257g	265	2.1	103	2.3	21.6	0.8	1.2
PASTA SPIRALS								
Co-Op*	1 Serving/100g	350	1.0	350	12.0	73.0	1.0	3.0
PASTA TWIRLS								
Dry, Asda*	1 Serving/50g	173	0.8	346	12.0	71.0	1.5	3.0
Tri-Colour, Sainsbury's*	1 Serving/75g	268	1.3	357	12.3	73.1	1.7	2.5
PASTA TWISTS								
Dry, Average	*1oz/28g*	*99*	*0.4*	*354*	*12.2*	*71.8*	*1.5*	*2.2*
Wheat & Gluten Free, Glutafin*	1 Serving/75g	262	1.5	350	8.0	75.0	2.0	0.1
PASTA WITH								
Feta Cheese & Slow Roasted Tomatoes, M&S*	1 Pack/190g	332	13.3	175	6.0	22.3	7.0	2.5
Pesto, Spinach & Pine Nuts, Tesco*	1 Pack/300g	480	22.2	160	5.2	17.1	7.4	1.5
Spicy Chicken, Sainsbury's*	1 Pot/300g	489	18.3	163	7.1	20.1	6.1	2.3
Spicy Sausage, Pasta King*	1 Serving/100g	117	2.2	117	4.8	19.7	2.2	1.7
Tomato & Basil Chicken, BGTY, Sainsbury's*	1 Pack/189g	250	2.1	132	9.2	21.2	1.1	2.7
PASTE								
Beef, Princes*	1 Serving/18g	40	2.8	220	14.4	5.2	15.8	0.0
Beef, Sainsbury's*	1 Jar/75g	142	9.9	189	16.0	1.5	13.2	1.4
Chicken & Ham, Princes*	1 Jar/100g	233	18.6	233	13.6	2.8	18.6	0.0
Chicken & Stuffing, Princes*	1 Jar/100g	229	17.0	229	15.7	3.3	17.0	0.0

P

	Measure INFO/WEIGHT	per Measure KCAL	FAT	Nutrition Values per 100g / 100ml KCAL	PROT	CARB	FAT	FIBRE
PASTE								
Chicken, Princes*	1 Thin Spread/9g	22	1.7	240	12.6	5.6	18.5	0.0
Crab, Princes*	1 Pot/35g	36	1.2	104	13.4	4.8	3.5	0.0
Crab, Sainsbury's*	1 Thick Spread/5g	6	0.2	115	16.5	1.7	4.7	0.5
Crab, Tesco*	1 Jar/75g	116	6.3	155	14.4	4.6	8.4	0.1
Fruit, Golden Quince, Lowry Peaks*	1 Tsp/5g	16	0.0	321	0.8	83.6	0.2	0.0
Salmon, Asda*	1 Serving/53g	76	3.7	143	15.0	5.0	7.0	0.0
Salmon, Value, Tesco*	1 Serving/10g	16	1.0	165	14.0	4.6	10.1	0.8
Sardine & Tomato, Asda*	1 Thin Spread/9g	11	0.5	123	14.0	3.3	6.0	0.0
Sardine & Tomato, Princes*	1 Jar/75g	130	8.1	173	13.9	3.4	10.8	3.2
Sardine & Tomato, Sainsbury's*	1 Mini Pot/35g	60	3.8	170	16.9	1.2	10.8	1.3
Sardine & Tomato, Tesco*	1 Jar/75g	98	4.4	130	14.6	4.8	5.8	0.1
Tuna & Mayonnaise, Princes*	1 Pot/75g	86	12.3	115	16.8	3.8	16.4	0.0
Tuna & Mayonnaise, Tesco*	1 Serving/15g	32	2.3	215	15.8	0.7	15.6	2.2
PASTILLES								
Blackcurrant, Rowntree's*	1 Tube/53g	188	0.0	353	4.4	84.0	0.0	0.0
Fruit, Average	*1 Tube/33g*	*108*	*0.0*	*327*	*2.8*	*84.2*	*0.0*	*0.0*
Fruit, Co-Op*	1 Sweet/6g	20	0.0	337	2.8	81.5	0.0	0.0
Fruit, Rowntree's*	1 Tube/53g	186	0.0	351	4.4	83.7	0.0	0.0
Fruit, Sainsbury's*	1 Sweet/7g	23	0.0	332	3.4	78.7	0.1	0.1
Wine, Maynards*	1 Sweet/5g	15	0.0	325	6.1	75.0	0.0	0.0
PASTRAMI								
Beef, Average	*1 Serving/40g*	*51*	*1.4*	*128*	*23.1*	*1.1*	*3.6*	*0.2*
TTD, Sainsbury's*	1 Slice/10g	12	0.3	121	21.6	1.0	3.4	0.4
Turkey, Average	*½ Pack/35g*	*38*	*0.5*	*107*	*21.8*	*1.7*	*1.5*	*0.5*
with a Spicy Coating, Hazelmeade Farm, Lidl*	1 Slice/10g	14	0.4	136	24.0	1.3	3.7	0.5
PASTRY								
Case, From Supermarket, Average	*1 Case/230g*	*1081*	*58.9*	*470*	*5.8*	*55.9*	*25.6*	*1.2*
Choux, Cooked, Average	*1oz/28g*	*91*	*5.5*	*325*	*8.5*	*29.8*	*19.8*	*1.2*
Choux, Raw, Average	*1oz/28g*	*59*	*3.6*	*211*	*5.5*	*19.4*	*12.9*	*0.8*
Cinnamon Swirls, Bake it Fresh, Jus-Rol*	1 Swirl/45g	162	7.1	360	6.2	47.7	15.7	1.6
Cream Horn, Fresh, Tesco*	1 Horn/57g	244	15.8	428	4.1	40.3	27.8	0.3
Filo, Average	*1 Sheet/45g*	*137*	*1.2*	*304*	*9.0*	*61.4*	*2.7*	*0.9*
Filo, Cooked, Ready Roll Sheets, Jus-Rol*	½ Sheet/8g	26	0.2	335	9.1	66.3	3.0	2.8
Filo, Frozen, Ready Roll Sheets, Jus-Rol*	1 Sheet/45g	123	1.2	273	8.1	52.1	2.7	2.1
Flaky, Cooked, Average	*1oz/28g*	*157*	*11.4*	*560*	*5.6*	*45.9*	*40.6*	*1.8*
Flaky, Raw, Average	*1oz/28g*	*119*	*8.6*	*424*	*4.2*	*34.8*	*30.7*	*1.4*
Pain Au Chocolat, Bake it Fresh, Jus-Rol*	1 Pain/46g	170	8.7	369	7.4	41.0	19.0	2.2
Puff, Fresh, Sainsbury's*	½ Pack/250g	1112	85.7	445	5.4	28.8	34.3	1.3
Puff, Frozen, Average	*1 Serving/47g*	*188*	*12.0*	*400*	*5.0*	*29.2*	*25.6*	*0.0*
Puff, Light, Frozen, Ready Roll Sheets, Jus-Rol*	1/6 Sheet/53g	176	8.7	332	6.4	38.3	16.5	2.3
Puff, Light, Sheet, Jus-Rol*	1 Serving/50g	166	8.2	332	6.4	38.3	16.5	2.3
Puff, Ready Rolled, As Sold, Greenvale, Aldi*	1 Pack/375g	1320	72.4	352	5.4	36.5	19.3	5.5
Shortcrust, Chilled, Ready to Roll Blocks, Jus-Rol*	1 Block/500g	2295	155.0	459	7.0	39.0	31.0	2.0
Shortcrust, Cooked, Average	*1oz/28g*	*146*	*9.0*	*521*	*6.6*	*54.2*	*32.3*	*2.2*
Shortcrust, Raw, Average	*1oz/28g*	*127*	*8.1*	*453*	*5.6*	*44.0*	*29.1*	*1.3*
Wholemeal, Cooked, Average	*1oz/28g*	*140*	*9.2*	*499*	*8.9*	*44.6*	*32.9*	*6.3*
PASTY								
Beef, Port Royal*	1 Pattie/130g	299	13.3	230	10.2	24.4	10.2	0.0
Cheese & Onion, Average	*1 Pasty/150g*	*435*	*27.6*	*290*	*7.3*	*24.5*	*18.4*	*1.4*
Cheese & Onion, Co-Op*	1 Pasty/75g	235	14.8	313	9.2	24.5	19.8	1.7
Cheese & Onion, Farmfoods*	1 Pasty/191g	485	26.7	254	6.6	25.5	14.0	2.0
Cheese & Onion, Tesco*	1 Pasty/150g	416	26.4	277	5.9	23.7	17.6	2.2
Chicken & Vegetable, Proper Cornish Ltd*	1 Pasty/255g	671	34.7	263	7.4	30.2	13.6	2.4

P

	Measure INFO/WEIGHT	per Measure KCAL	FAT	Nutrition Values per 100g / 100ml KCAL	PROT	CARB	FAT	FIBRE
PASTY								
Chicken, Port Royal*	1 Pattie/130g	289	10.9	222	5.5	31.2	8.4	0.0
Cornish, Asda*	1 Pasty/100g	287	19.0	287	7.0	22.0	19.0	1.2
Cornish, Average	**1 Pasty/160g**	**450**	**27.7**	**281**	**7.0**	**24.2**	**17.3**	**1.6**
Cornish, BGTY, Sainsbury's*	1 Pasty/135g	308	12.7	228	7.7	28.2	9.4	1.6
Cornish, Cheese & Onion, Ginsters*	1 Pasty/130g	511	33.0	393	10.4	30.7	25.4	2.3
Cornish, Mini, M&S*	1 Pasty/75g	244	17.6	325	7.3	21.9	23.4	1.8
Cornish, Mini, Sainsbury's*	1 Pasty/70g	280	20.1	400	7.3	28.1	28.7	1.5
Cornish, Mini, Tesco*	1 Pasty/24g	66	4.2	274	5.6	23.2	17.7	0.5
Cornish, Morrisons*	1 Pasty/200g	626	37.0	313	7.5	29.1	18.5	0.0
Cornish, Multi Pack, Ginsters*	1 Pasty/130g	358	24.3	275	6.0	20.6	18.7	2.6
Cornish, Original, Ginsters*	1 Pasty/227g	549	32.2	242	5.3	23.2	14.2	3.1
Cornish, Pork Farms*	1 Pasty/250g	672	40.8	269	7.7	22.8	16.3	0.0
Cornish, Sainsbury's*	1 Pasty/150g	489	32.1	326	6.7	26.6	21.4	2.0
Cornish, Tesco*	1 Pasty/150g	466	32.7	311	6.8	21.9	21.8	1.6
Cornish, Traditional Style, Geo Adams*	1 Pasty/165g	488	30.4	296	7.1	25.4	18.4	1.3
Lamb, Port Royal*	1 Pattie/130g	352	17.4	271	7.2	30.5	13.4	0.0
Salt Fish, Port Royal*	1 Pattie/130g	300	13.4	231	6.8	27.8	10.3	0.0
Tandoori & Vegetable, Holland & Barrett*	1 Pack/110g	232	9.4	211	4.3	29.4	8.5	1.8
Vegetable, Average	**1oz/28g**	**77**	**4.2**	**274**	**4.1**	**33.3**	**14.9**	**1.9**
Vegetable, Hand Crimped, Waitrose*	1 Pasty/200g	454	22.6	227	4.5	26.8	11.3	2.2
Vegetarian, Country Slice, Linda McCartney*	1 Pasty/150g	373	20.2	249	5.6	26.5	13.5	2.9
PATE								
Ardennes with Bacon, Tesco*	½ Pack/85g	241	20.6	284	11.4	5.1	24.2	1.1
Ardennes, Asda*	1 Serving/50g	143	12.0	286	13.9	3.6	24.0	1.3
Ardennes, BGTY, Sainsbury's*	¼ Pack/50g	90	5.7	180	16.6	2.9	11.4	0.0
Ardennes, Course, Deli Continental, Aldi*	1 Serving/35g	124	12.0	362	10.0	2.5	35.0	0.5
Ardennes, HL, Tesco*	½ Pack/88g	154	11.0	176	12.1	3.6	12.6	1.8
Ardennes, Reduced Fat, Waitrose*	¼ Pack/42g	94	7.1	224	15.4	2.6	16.9	0.5
Ardennes, Tesco*	1 Tbsp/15g	53	5.0	354	13.3	0.5	33.2	1.2
Bean Feast, The Redwood Co*	1 Serving/60g	161	10.2	268	7.3	21.1	17.0	3.8
Breton, Country with Apricots, Coarse, Sainsbury's*	1 Serving/21g	60	4.7	285	13.5	7.0	22.5	0.5
Brussels & Garlic, Reduced Fat, Tesco*	1 Serving/65g	135	8.0	208	16.2	8.1	12.3	0.6
Brussels & Garlic, Tesco*	1 Serving/40g	145	13.5	363	8.7	6.0	33.8	0.0
Brussels Style, Organic, The Redwood Co*	¼ Pack/30g	82	6.1	273	15.2	8.0	20.4	1.3
Brussels with Garlic, Asda*	1 Serving/50g	170	15.6	340	10.7	4.0	31.3	2.5
Brussels, 25% Less Fat, Morrisons*	¼ Pack/43g	106	8.8	249	14.2	0.7	20.6	0.0
Brussels, BGTY, 50% Less Fat, Sainsbury's*	1 Serving/100g	223	16.0	223	14.6	5.1	16.0	0.1
Brussels, Co-Op*	1 Serving/15g	51	4.6	340	11.0	4.0	31.0	2.0
Brussels, HL, Tesco*	1 Serving/29g	66	4.4	229	14.4	8.4	15.3	1.8
Brussels, M&S*	1 Pot/170g	518	45.2	305	13.3	2.8	26.6	1.0
Brussels, Reduced Fat, Tesco*	1 Pack/175g	420	33.2	240	11.1	5.8	19.0	1.4
Brussels, Sainsbury's*	1 Pack/170g	663	64.9	390	10.6	1.1	38.2	0.1
Brussels, Smooth, 50% Less Fat, Tesco*	1 Pack/175g	350	26.8	200	14.1	1.2	15.3	1.8
Brussels, Smooth, Reduced Fat, Tesco*	1 Serving/40g	98	7.5	245	12.0	6.4	18.7	0.5
Brussels, Smooth, Reduced, Tesco*	1 Serving/40g	82	6.4	205	10.7	4.5	16.0	0.6
Brussels, Smooth, Spreadable, Sainsbury's*	1 Serving/30g	97	8.7	323	10.7	4.7	29.0	0.0
Brussels, Tesco*	1 Serving/28g	92	8.5	330	11.0	3.0	30.5	1.1
Chick Pea & Black Olive, Cauldron Foods*	1 Pot/113g	193	11.9	171	7.6	11.4	10.5	6.6
Chicken & Brandy, Morrisons*	1 Serving/44g	133	11.8	303	10.8	4.3	26.9	0.8
Chicken Liver & Brandy, Asda*	1 Serving/50g	176	16.4	353	9.0	5.5	32.8	3.2
Chicken Liver & Garlic, Smooth, Asda*	1 Serving/31g	119	11.1	388	9.0	7.0	36.0	3.2
Chicken Liver with Madeira, Sainsbury's*	1 Serving/30g	84	7.3	279	13.1	1.9	24.3	0.0
Chicken Liver, Asda*	1 Serving/65g	131	10.4	202	13.0	4.0	16.0	0.8

	Measure	per Measure		Nutrition Values per 100g / 100ml				
	INFO/WEIGHT	KCAL	FAT	KCAL	PROT	CARB	FAT	FIBRE

PATE

Chicken Liver, Madeira, Garlic, Thyme & Bay Leaves, M&S*	1/6 Tub/87g	271	25.2	312	10.4	2.0	29.0	0.5
Chicken Liver, Organic, Waitrose*	½ Tub/88g	204	16.1	233	12.6	1.8	18.4	1.4
Chicken Liver, Parfait, Waitrose*	1 Pack/100g	258	22.9	258	7.5	4.8	22.9	1.1
Coarse Farmhouse, Organic, Sainsbury's*	1 Serving/56g	138	11.0	246	13.3	3.7	19.7	0.8
Coarse Pork &d Onion, Christmas, Belgian, Waitrose*	¼ Pack/40g	122	9.4	306	14.1	8.9	23.6	0.8
Coarse Pork Liver with Garlic, Asda*	1 Pack/40g	130	12.0	326	13.0	1.0	30.0	0.0
Crab, Ready to Eat, Asda*	1 Pot/115g	210	13.2	183	12.7	6.9	11.5	0.5
Crab, Terrine, Orkney, Luxury, Castle MacLellan*	1 Tub/113g	250	21.4	221	7.3	5.5	18.9	0.9
Crab, Waitrose*	1 Pot/113g	218	16.7	193	12.4	2.5	14.8	0.9
De Campagne, Sainsbury's*	1 Serving/55g	129	10.0	235	16.3	1.4	18.2	0.0
Duck & Orange, Asda*	1 Serving/40g	94	7.2	235	16.0	2.2	18.0	0.0
Duck & Orange, Smooth, Tesco*	1 Serving/50g	188	17.7	377	10.5	4.0	35.4	0.5
Duck Liver, Gr& Marnier & Orange Jelly, M&S*	½ Pot/75g	218	18.5	291	8.7	8.2	24.7	0.6
Farmhouse Mushroom, Asda*	1 Serving/50g	126	10.0	252	13.0	5.0	20.0	0.7
Farmhouse Style, Finest, Tesco*	1 Serving/28g	83	7.3	295	11.9	3.6	25.9	1.0
Farmhouse with Herbes De Provence, Tesco*	1 Serving/50g	136	10.8	273	13.9	5.4	21.6	1.0
Farmhouse with Mushrooms & Garlic, Tesco*	1 Serving/90g	256	22.8	285	13.8	0.6	25.3	1.3
Farmhouse, Simply, M&S*	¼ Pack/42g	113	9.7	265	11.4	3.4	22.8	0.4
Liver & Pork, HE, Tesco*	1 Serving/28g	64	4.3	229	14.4	8.4	15.3	1.3
Mackerel, Smoked	1oz/28g	103	9.6	368	13.4	1.3	34.4	0.0
Mackerel, Tesco*	1 Serving/29g	102	9.5	353	14.3	0.5	32.6	0.0
Mousse De Canard, French, Weight Watchers*	1 Portion/50g	122	9.5	245	14.0	4.4	19.0	0.0
Mushroom & Tarragon, Waitrose*	1 Serving/30g	46	4.0	155	2.8	5.5	13.5	1.4
Mushroom, BGTY, Sainsbury's*	½ Pot/58g	29	0.3	50	4.6	6.7	0.5	3.0
Mushroom, M&S*	1 Pot/115g	224	20.1	195	4.2	4.8	17.5	1.5
Mushroom, Roast, Tesco*	1 Serving/25g	36	3.2	145	3.6	3.6	12.9	4.5
Mushroom, Sainsbury's*	½ Pot/58g	89	7.0	153	3.3	7.8	12.1	2.1
Pork & Mushroom, Morrisons*	1 Serving/30g	108	10.0	360	12.8	2.5	33.2	0.0
Pork with Apple & Cider, Sainsbury's*	1 Serving/50g	152	12.6	303	12.5	6.3	25.3	1.1
Pork with Peppercorns, Tesco*	1 Serving/28g	84	7.5	300	12.9	1.4	26.8	0.7
Salmon Sensation, Deluxe, Lidl*	1 Portion/50g	191	17.8	382	6.3	1.4	35.7	0.5
Salmon, Smoked, Isle of Skye, TTD, Sainsbury's*	½ Pot/58g	133	9.8	231	17.5	1.8	17.1	0.2
Scottish Smoked Salmon, Castle MacLellan*	¼ Tub/28g	76	6.4	271	9.0	7.0	22.9	0.0
Smoked Mackerel, Sainsbury's*	½ Pot/57g	215	20.1	378	14.2	0.8	35.3	0.0
Smoked Mackerel, Scottish, M&S*	½ Pot/58g	158	13.3	275	15.9	0.6	23.2	0.1
Smoked Salmon, Luxury, Morrisons*	½ Pot/57g	150	12.4	266	16.0	0.9	22.0	0.5
Smoked Salmon, Tesco*	1 Pack/115g	282	22.0	245	15.0	3.0	19.1	1.0
Smoked Trout, Waitrose*	½ Pot/56g	130	10.3	232	15.8	0.9	18.4	0.6
Spicy Mexican, Organic, Waitrose*	1 Serving/50g	58	3.1	115	6.2	8.6	6.2	3.5
Tofu, Spicy Mexican, Organic, GranoVita*	1 Serving/50g	108	10.0	216	6.0	3.0	20.0	0.0
Tomato, Lentil & Basil, Cauldron Foods*	1 Pot/115g	161	7.8	140	6.8	14.0	6.8	3.2
Tuna with Butter & Lemon Juice, Sainsbury's*	½ Pot/58g	209	18.3	360	19.0	0.1	31.6	0.3
Tuna, Tesco*	1 Pack/115g	332	26.7	289	19.8	0.3	23.2	0.2
Turkey, Pork & Duck Liver, Deluxe, Lidl*	1 Pack/125g	366	30.6	293	13.1	4.5	24.5	1.0
Vegetable	1oz/28g	48	3.8	173	7.5	5.9	13.4	0.0
Vegetarian with Mushrooms, Organic, Tartex*	¼ Tube/50g	102	8.0	203	7.7	7.0	16.0	0.0
Yeast, Garlic & Herb, Tartex*	1 Serving/30g	69	5.4	230	7.0	10.0	18.0	0.0
Yeast, Pateole, GranoVita*	1 Portion/30g	66	5.3	219	10.2	4.5	17.8	0.0

PAVLOVA

Raspberry, Individual, M&S*	1 Pavlova/65g	133	1.6	205	4.0	41.8	2.4	0.2
Raspberry, M&S*	1 Serving/84g	193	8.1	230	2.3	33.3	9.6	0.3
Raspberry, Mini, Co-Op*	1 Pavlova/19g	61	1.7	320	3.0	56.0	9.0	0.6
Raspberry, Sara Lee*	1/6 Pavlova/55g	168	8.5	303	2.7	38.5	15.3	1.1

	Measure INFO/WEIGHT	per Measure KCAL	FAT	KCAL	PROT	CARB	FAT	FIBRE
PAVLOVA								
Raspberry, Tesco*	1 Serving/65g	191	8.4	294	2.7	41.8	12.9	1.1
PAW-PAW								
Raw, Fresh	*1oz/28g*	*10*	*0.0*	*36*	*0.5*	*8.8*	*0.1*	*2.2*
Raw, Weighed with Skin & Pips	*1oz/28g*	*6*	*0.0*	*20*	*0.3*	*5.0*	*0.1*	*1.3*
PEACH								
Dried, Average	*1 Pack/250g*	*472*	*1.6*	*189*	*2.6*	*45.0*	*0.6*	*6.9*
in Fruit Juice, Average	*1oz/28g*	*13*	*0.0*	*47*	*0.5*	*11.2*	*0.0*	*0.7*
in Light Syrup, Canned, As Sold	1 Serving/100g	66	0.0	66	0.4	15.9	0.0	1.0
in Syrup, Average	*1oz/28g*	*19*	*0.0*	*67*	*0.4*	*16.3*	*0.1*	*0.4*
Raw, Stoned, Average	*1oz/28g*	*9*	*0.0*	*33*	*1.0*	*7.6*	*0.1*	*1.5*
Raw, Weighed with Stone, Average	*1 Peach/125g*	*39*	*0.1*	*31*	*1.0*	*7.2*	*0.1*	*1.3*
Slices in Fruit Juice, Average	*1 Serving/100g*	*49*	*0.0*	*49*	*0.6*	*11.6*	*0.0*	*0.5*
Slices in Fruit Juice, Tesco*	½ Can/125g	51	0.0	41	0.6	9.7	0.0	0.8
Slices in Light Syrup, Value, Tesco*	4 Serving/238g	159	0.2	67	0.4	16.0	0.1	0.8
PEANUT BRITTLE								
Thorntons*	2 Pieces/32g	163	8.6	509	12.4	54.3	26.9	2.6
PEANUT BUTTER								
& Grape Jelly Stripes in Jar, Goober*	1 Tsp/15g	68	3.4	450	13.2	65.0	22.6	3.8
30% Less Fat, Tesco*	1 Tbsp/15g	86	5.7	570	18.4	37.1	37.9	3.6
Chocolate Flavour, Nuts 'n More*	1 Serving/10g	59	3.8	588	43.8	18.8	37.5	15.6
Creamy, Smooth, Sun Pat*	1 Serving/15g	93	7.5	620	24.0	17.5	50.2	6.1
Crunchy, Basics, Sainsbury's*	1 Serving/20g	134	11.7	672	26.4	6.8	58.8	4.9
Crunchy, Bettabuy, Morrisons*	1 Serving/10g	61	5.2	606	22.5	17.3	52.2	5.7
Crunchy, CBY, Asda*	1 Serving/10g	60	4.9	603	24.5	15.5	49.2	6.6
Crunchy, Harvest Spread*	1 Serving/25g	148	12.4	592	23.6	12.5	49.7	6.9
Crunchy, Natural, No Added Sugar or Salt, Average	*1 Tsp/5g*	*30*	*2.4*	*606*	*27.6*	*12.2*	*48.4*	*7.0*
Crunchy, No Added Sugar, Organic, Whole Earth*	1 Serving/25g	148	12.6	592	24.9	10.1	50.2	7.3
Crunchy, Organic, No Added Sugar, Waitrose*	1 Serving/12g	71	6.0	592	24.9	10.1	50.2	7.3
Crunchy, Organic, Tesco*	1 Serving/25g	149	12.4	595	23.6	12.5	49.7	6.9
Crunchy, Original Style, No Added Sugar, Whole Earth*	1 Serving/20g	129	10.9	643	27.7	7.4	54.3	6.7
Crunchy, Sainsbury's*	1 Serving/10g	62	5.0	620	28.6	12.6	49.6	4.3
Crunchy, Smart Price, Asda*	1 Thin Spread/12g	73	6.0	610	23.2	16.0	50.4	6.2
Crunchy, Sun Pat*	1 Serving/50g	308	24.4	615	25.3	15.1	48.9	6.8
Crunchy, Tesco*	1 Serving/20g	123	10.2	615	23.8	14.6	50.8	6.4
Crunchy, Value, Tesco*	1 Serving/10g	62	5.4	615	21.5	11.7	53.6	5.4
Crunchy, Whole Nut, Organic, Meridian Foods*	1 Serving/28g	171	13.6	612	31.2	12.2	48.7	6.5
Extra Crunch, Skippy*	2 Tbsps/40g	252	20.0	630	22.7	22.9	50.0	7.7
Extra Crunchy, Sun Pat*	1 Serving/20g	119	10.2	597	21.9	12.6	51.0	7.3
Powdered, PB2, Bell Plantation*	2 Tbsp/12g	45	1.5	375	41.7	41.7	12.5	16.7
Smart Price, Asda*	1 Serving/15g	87	7.5	582	23.0	10.0	50.0	6.0
Smooth, 33% Less Fat, BGTY, Sainsbury's*	1 Serving/10g	53	3.5	533	22.6	31.7	35.1	6.7
Smooth, Average	*1 Serving/20g*	*125*	*10.7*	*623*	*22.6*	*13.1*	*53.7*	*5.4*
Smooth, CBY, Asda*	1 Serving/15g	91	7.4	604	24.1	15.7	49.4	6.0
Smooth, Light, Kraft*	1 Serving/20g	114	7.7	571	16.3	40.1	38.6	0.0
Smooth, Morrisons*	1 Serving/15g	92	7.8	616	23.1	14.5	51.8	6.2
Smooth, No Added Sugar, Organic, Whole Earth*	1 Serving/20g	126	10.2	628	25.6	13.7	51.2	4.9
Smooth, No Added Sugar, Sun Pat*	1 Tsp/5g	31	2.5	614	25.3	13.7	49.4	0.0
Smooth, Organic, Meridian Foods*	1 Serving/10g	61	4.9	612	31.2	12.2	48.7	6.5
Smooth, Organic, Tesco*	1 Serving/15g	90	7.5	600	23.3	12.4	50.3	6.5
Smooth, Organic, Waitrose*	1 Serving/12g	71	6.1	595	24.6	9.9	50.8	7.1
Smooth, Original, No Added Sugar, Whole Earth*	1 Serving/10g	64	5.4	645	26.3	9.2	54.5	6.5
Smooth, Sun Pat*	1 Serving/20g	123	9.8	614	25.0	15.2	48.9	6.7
Smooth, Tesco*	1 Serving/20g	123	10.1	614	27.8	12.0	50.5	6.5

P

	Measure INFO/WEIGHT	per Measure KCAL	FAT	Nutrition Values per 100g / 100ml KCAL	PROT	CARB	FAT	FIBRE
PEANUT BUTTER								
Whole Nut, Crunchy, Average	**1 Tsp/10g**	**61**	**5.3**	**606**	**24.9**	**7.7**	**53.1**	**6.0**
Wholenut, Sainsbury's*	1 Serving/15g	90	7.7	598	24.2	9.8	51.3	7.0
Wholenut, Tesco*	1 Tbsp/15g	90	7.6	590	24.9	10.1	50.0	6.3
Wholenut, Waitrose*	1 Serving/12g	70	6.0	587	24.9	9.3	50.0	6.3
PEANUTS								
Chilli, Average	**½ Pack/50g**	**303**	**25.3**	**605**	**28.2**	**9.3**	**50.6**	**6.8**
Dry Roasted, Average	**1 Serving/20g**	**117**	**9.8**	**587**	**25.7**	**11.5**	**48.8**	**6.5**
Dry Roasted, Classic, Nobbys*	1 Bag/50g	302	24.0	603	25.0	12.0	48.0	9.0
Honey Roasted, Average	**1oz/28g**	**169**	**13.2**	**605**	**26.8**	**23.6**	**47.0**	**5.5**
Hot Chilli, Holland & Barrett*	1 Pack/100g	523	31.0	523	14.0	47.0	31.0	5.5
Milk Chocolate Coated, Graze*	1 Pack/35g	187	13.1	533	14.6	34.9	37.3	0.0
Original, Salted, KP Snacks*	1 Pack/50g	308	25.5	615	30.0	5.6	51.0	8.5
Plain, Average	**10 Whole/10g**	**59**	**5.0**	**592**	**24.7**	**11.0**	**50.0**	**6.3**
Roast, Salted, Average	**10 Whole/12g**	**74**	**6.3**	**614**	**27.8**	**7.9**	**52.4**	**4.9**
Roasted, Californian Honey & Salt, Sensations, Walkers*	1 Serving/30g	173	12.3	575	21.0	27.0	41.0	5.0
Roasted, LL, Waitrose*	1 Serving/30g	170	13.8	567	25.6	12.5	46.1	8.0
Salted, Average	**10 Whole/6g**	**37**	**3.1**	**609**	**27.0**	**8.3**	**52.0**	**5.4**
Salted, Classic, Nobbys*	1 Bag/50g	315	26.0	630	27.0	11.0	52.0	7.0
Sweet Chilli, Nobby's*	1 Bag/40g	214	13.6	535	15.0	42.0	34.0	3.0
Yoghurt Coated, Graze*	1 Pack/35g	189	12.3	540	9.9	48.1	35.1	0.0
PEARL BARLEY								
Boiled	**1oz/28g**	**34**	**0.1**	**123**	**2.3**	**28.2**	**0.4**	**3.8**
Dried, Cooked, LL, Waitrose*	1 Serving/80g	101	0.4	126	2.2	28.2	0.5	3.8
Raw, Average	**1oz/28g**	**99**	**0.3**	**352**	**9.9**	**77.7**	**1.2**	**15.6**
PEARS								
Abate Fetel, Average	**1 Med/133g**	**48**	**0.1**	**36**	**0.4**	**8.3**	**0.1**	**2.2**
Asian, Nashi, Raw, Average	**1 Lge Pear/209g**	**80**	**0.4**	**38**	**0.5**	**9.7**	**0.2**	**3.3**
Blush, Morrisons*	1 Sm Pear/148g	86	0.2	58	0.4	15.5	0.1	3.1
Cape, Quartered, Tesco*	1 Serving/100g	35	0.0	35	0.3	8.5	0.0	1.4
Comice, Raw, Weighed with Core	**1 Med/170g**	**56**	**0.0**	**33**	**0.3**	**8.5**	**0.0**	**2.0**
Conference, Average	**1 Lge Pear/209g**	**88**	**0.2**	**42**	**0.3**	**10.1**	**0.1**	**2.0**
Dessert, Green, Sainsbury's*	1 Sm/135g	53	0.1	39	0.3	9.2	0.1	2.0
Dried, Average	**1 Pear Half/16g**	**33**	**0.1**	**204**	**1.9**	**48.4**	**0.5**	**9.7**
in Fruit Juice, Average	**1 Serving/225g**	**102**	**0.1**	**45**	**0.3**	**10.9**	**0.0**	**1.2**
in Syrup, Average	**1oz/28g**	**16**	**0.0**	**58**	**0.2**	**14.4**	**0.1**	**1.4**
Prickly, Raw, Fresh	**1oz/28g**	**8**	**0.1**	**30**	**0.4**	**7.0**	**0.2**	**0.0**
Raw, Weighed with Core, Average	**1 Med/166g**	**58**	**0.2**	**35**	**0.3**	**8.4**	**0.1**	**1.3**
Red, Tesco*	1 Med/180g	65	0.2	36	0.4	8.3	0.1	2.2
TTD, Sainsbury's*	1 Serving/100g	40	0.1	40	0.3	10.0	0.1	2.2
William, Raw, Average	**1 Med/170g**	**58**	**0.2**	**34**	**0.4**	**8.3**	**0.1**	**2.2**
PEAS								
Dried, Boiled in Unsalted Water, Average	**1oz/28g**	**31**	**0.2**	**109**	**6.9**	**19.9**	**0.8**	**5.5**
Dried, Raw, Average	**1oz/28g**	**85**	**0.7**	**303**	**21.6**	**52.0**	**2.4**	**13.0**
Edible Podded, Raw	**1 Cup/63g**	**25**	**0.1**	**39**	**2.6**	**7.1**	**0.2**	**2.4**
Frozen, Average	**1 Serving/85g**	**62**	**0.8**	**73**	**6.0**	**9.7**	**1.0**	**4.5**
Frozen, Boiled, Average	**1 Serving/75g**	**51**	**0.7**	**68**	**6.0**	**9.4**	**0.9**	**5.1**
Frozen, Value, Tesco*	1 Serving/75g	60	0.7	80	5.9	9.0	0.9	5.5
Garden, Canned with Sugar & Salt, Average	**1 Serving/90g**	**59**	**0.6**	**66**	**5.3**	**9.3**	**0.7**	**5.1**
Garden, Canned, Asda*	1 Sm Tin/90g	66	0.7	73	5.7	7.6	0.8	6.4
Garden, Canned, No Sugar Or Salt, Average	**1 Can/80g**	**36**	**0.3**	**45**	**4.4**	**6.0**	**0.4**	**2.8**
Garden, Frozen for Freshness, CBY, Asda*	1 Serving/80g	72	1.3	90	6.7	10.0	1.6	4.5
Garden, Frozen, Average	**1 Serving/90g**	**66**	**1.0**	**74**	**6.3**	**9.8**	**1.1**	**3.3**
Garden, Frozen, Essential, Waitrose*	1 Portion/80g	52	0.7	65	5.7	8.6	0.9	4.7

P

	Measure INFO/WEIGHT	per Measure KCAL	FAT	Nutrition Values per 100g / 100ml KCAL	PROT	CARB	FAT	FIBRE
PEAS								
Garden, Minted, Average	*1 Serving/80g*	*59*	*0.9*	*74*	*6.3*	*9.7*	*1.1*	*5.9*
Garden, Value, Tesco*	3 Tbsp/80g	54	0.7	67	5.3	9.4	0.9	5.1
Giant, Marrowfat, Processed, Canned, Farrows*	1 Serving/80g	70	0.6	88	6.7	13.8	0.7	5.9
Marrowfat, Average	*1 Sm Can/160g*	*134*	*0.9*	*84*	*6.1*	*13.7*	*0.6*	*3.7*
Marrowfat, Processed, Canned, Drained, Value, Tesco*	1 Can/180g	162	1.3	90	6.5	14.5	0.7	3.9
Mushy, Average	*1 Can/200g*	*173*	*1.0*	*86*	*6.2*	*14.4*	*0.5*	*2.2*
Mushy, Frozen, Cooked, CBY, Asda*	1 Serving/80g	75	0.6	94	6.5	11.8	0.8	7.2
Processed, Canned, Average	*1 Sm Can/220g*	*162*	*1.6*	*74*	*5.6*	*11.3*	*0.7*	*3.4*
Snow	*1 Serving/80g*	*24*	*0.2*	*29*	*3.3*	*3.9*	*0.2*	*2.1*
Sugar Snap, Average	*1 Serving/80g*	*27*	*0.2*	*33*	*3.2*	*4.8*	*0.2*	*1.4*
Wasabi, Average	*1 Serving/28g*	*114*	*3.8*	*406*	*15.2*	*54.0*	*13.7*	*8.6*
Wasabi, Delicious, Boots*	½ Bag/25g	98	2.4	393	19.0	51.0	9.6	15.0
PEASE PUDDING								
Canned, Re-Heated, Drained	1oz/28g	26	0.2	93	6.8	16.1	0.6	1.8
PECAN NUTS								
Average	*3 Nuts/6g*	*42*	*4.2*	*692*	*10.0*	*5.6*	*70.1*	*4.7*
Honey, Golden, Graze*	1 Pack/26g	168	15.4	647	7.6	23.4	59.4	0.0
PENNE								
Arrabbiata, BGTY, Sainsbury's*	1 Pack/450g	414	7.2	92	2.9	16.5	1.6	1.9
Brown Rice, Gluten Free, Organic, Dove's Farm*	1 Serving/100g	338	1.5	338	7.9	70.3	1.5	4.1
Chicken & Tomato, Italian, Sainsbury's*	½ Pack/350g	472	11.2	135	7.6	19.0	3.2	1.6
Chilli, Asda*	1 Serving/100g	148	0.7	148	5.1	30.2	0.7	2.4
Cooked, Average	*1 Serving/185g*	*244*	*1.3*	*132*	*4.7*	*26.7*	*0.7*	*1.1*
Dry Weight, Parioli, Cucina*	1 Serving/76g	270	1.1	355	12.5	73.0	1.4	2.6
Dry, Average	*1 Serving/100g*	*352*	*1.9*	*352*	*12.4*	*71.3*	*1.9*	*2.7*
Egg, Fresh, Average	*1 Serving/125g*	*352*	*4.0*	*282*	*11.1*	*52.2*	*3.2*	*2.0*
Free From, Tesco*	1 Serving/100g	340	2.0	340	8.0	72.5	2.0	2.5
Fresh, Dry, Average	*1 Serving/125g*	*222*	*2.4*	*178*	*7.3*	*32.2*	*1.9*	*1.6*
in Tomato & Basil Sauce, Sainsbury's*	½ Pack/110g	118	0.7	107	3.6	21.8	0.6	1.1
Organic, Dry, Average	*1 Serving/100g*	*352*	*1.8*	*352*	*12.4*	*71.6*	*1.8*	*1.9*
Rigate, Dry Weight, Average	*1 Serving/90g*	*318*	*1.6*	*353*	*12.3*	*72.1*	*1.8*	*1.8*
Roasted Red Pepper, GFY, Asda*	1 Pack/400g	212	2.4	53	1.9	10.0	0.6	0.8
Smoked Salmon, Bistro, Morrisons*	½ Pack/350g	612	23.8	175	9.7	18.0	6.8	1.4
Tomato & Basil Sauce, Asda*	½ Pack/314g	185	11.0	59	0.8	6.0	3.5	2.0
Tomato & Roasted Vegetable, Big Eat, Heinz*	1 Pot/351g	281	10.5	80	2.5	10.7	3.0	4.6
Whole Wheat, Asda*	1 Serving/100g	333	2.1	333	12.1	66.3	2.1	6.9
Wholewheat, Cooked, Authentic, Italiano, Tesco*	1 Portion/75g	244	1.9	325	12.5	62.5	2.5	9.0
with Chicken & Vegetables, Eat Positive, Birds Eye*	1 Meal/396g	325	5.2	82	7.7	9.8	1.3	1.2
with Roasted Vegetables, Waitrose*	1 Pack/400g	424	15.6	106	2.8	15.0	3.9	0.8
PEPERAMI*								
Firestick, Peperami*	1 Stick/25g	127	11.0	508	24.5	3.5	44.0	1.2
Hot, Peperami*	1 Stick/25g	126	11.0	504	24.5	2.5	44.0	1.2
Lunchbox Minis, 30% Less Fat, Peperami*	1 Stick/10g	38	3.0	379	25.0	1.5	30.0	3.0
Original, Peperami*	1 Stick/25g	126	11.0	504	24.0	2.5	44.0	0.1
Wideboy, Peperami*	1 Stick/40g	202	17.6	504	24.0	2.5	44.0	0.1
PEPPER								
Black, Freshly Ground, Average	*1 Tsp/2g*	*5*	*0.1*	*255*	*11.0*	*64.8*	*3.3*	*26.5*
Cayenne, Ground	*1 Tsp/2g*	*6*	*0.3*	*318*	*12.0*	*31.7*	*17.3*	*0.0*
White	*½ Tsp/1g*	*3*	*0.0*	*296*	*10.4*	*68.6*	*2.1*	*26.2*
PEPPERCORNS								
Black, Schwartz*	1 Tsp/2g	11	0.4	529	13.0	68.7	22.5	27.0
Green, Average	*1 Tsp/10g*	*4*	*0.1*	*44*	*1.6*	*5.3*	*0.8*	*4.7*

P

Measure INFO/WEIGHT		per Measure KCAL	FAT	Nutrition Values per 100g / 100ml KCAL	PROT	CARB	FAT	FIBRE
PEPPERS								
Cheesy Rice, Stuffed, Growers Selection, Asda*	1 Pack/252g	244	9.6	97	3.0	12.0	3.8	1.4
Cherrybell, with Goats Cheese, Deli, M&S*	1 Pot/140g	433	35.6	309	5.2	14.4	25.4	1.1
Chilli, Crushed, Schwartz*	1 Tsp/0.5g	2	0.1	321	12.0	29.0	17.0	27.0
Chilli, Dried, Flakes, Average	*1 Tsp/3g*	*13*	*0.4*	*425*	*16.0*	*56.0*	*15.0*	*44.0*
Chilli, Dried, Whole, Red, Schwartz*	1 Tsp/0.5g	2	0.1	425	15.9	56.4	15.1	0.0
Chilli, Green, Raw, Unprepared, Average	*1 Med/13g*	*4*	*0.0*	*29*	*1.5*	*6.9*	*0.1*	*1.1*
Chilli, Green, Very Lazy, The English Provender Co.*	1 Serving/10g	11	0.4	114	4.2	15.3	4.0	0.5
Chilli, Red, Raw, Unprepared, Average	*1 Sm Pepper/13g*	*4*	*0.0*	*29*	*1.5*	*6.9*	*0.1*	*1.1*
Chilli, Red, Very Lazy, The English Provender Co.*	1 Serving/15g	17	0.6	114	4.2	15.3	4.0	0.5
Green, Boiled in Salted Water	*1oz/28g*	*5*	*0.1*	*18*	*1.0*	*2.6*	*0.5*	*1.8*
Green, Raw, Unprepared, Average	*1 Med/160g*	*20*	*0.4*	*13*	*0.7*	*2.2*	*0.3*	*1.3*
Italian Style, Sainsbury's*	1 Serving/150g	160	7.5	107	3.5	14.1	5.0	2.1
Jalapeno, Raw	*1 Cup, Sliced/90g*	*25*	*0.5*	*28*	*1.2*	*5.4*	*0.6*	*2.6*
Mixed Bag, From Supermarket, Average	*1oz/28g*	*7*	*0.1*	*25*	*1.0*	*4.4*	*0.4*	*1.7*
Mixed, Sliced, Morrisons*	1 Pack/120g	34	0.4	28	1.0	4.5	0.3	1.6
Orange, Sweet, Raw, Average	*1oz/28g*	*8*	*0.1*	*30*	*1.8*	*5.0*	*0.3*	*1.5*
Pickled, Hot, Turkish, Melis, Melis*	1 Serving/25g	9	0.0	35	1.0	7.9	0.0	1.0
Ramiro, Red, Sainsbury's*	1 Serving/100g	30	0.3	30	1.6	5.1	0.3	2.2
Red, Boiled in Salted Water	*1oz/28g*	*10*	*0.1*	*34*	*1.1*	*7.0*	*0.4*	*1.7*
Red, Filled, Halves, Vegetarian, M&S*	1 Pack/295g	239	9.7	81	2.4	9.7	3.3	1.6
Red, Raw, Unprepared, Average	*1oz/28g*	*7*	*0.1*	*27*	*0.8*	*5.3*	*0.3*	*1.3*
Red, Roasted, in Brine, Cooks & Co*	1 Serving/100g	23	0.3	23	1.6	4.5	0.3	0.0
Red, Roasted, Melis*	1 Serving/100g	90	1.0	90	1.1	18.8	1.0	0.2
Red, Sweet Pointed, Organic, Tesco*	1 Serving/100g	33	0.4	33	1.0	6.4	0.4	1.6
Red, Sweet, Pointed, TTD, Sainsbury's*	1 Serving/100g	32	0.4	32	1.0	6.4	0.4	0.0
Stuffed with Rice Based Filling, Average	*1oz/28g*	*24*	*0.7*	*85*	*1.5*	*15.4*	*2.4*	*1.3*
Stuffed with Vegetables, Cheese Topping, Average	*1oz/28g*	*31*	*1.9*	*111*	*3.4*	*9.8*	*6.7*	*1.5*
Stuffed, Fresh, Asda	*1 Pepper/150g*	*144*	*7.5*	*96*	*3.8*	*9.0*	*5.0*	*1.2*
Stuffed, Sainsbury's*	1 Serving/137g	169	9.5	123	3.3	11.8	6.9	1.0
Stuffed, Yellow, Italian, Ready to Roast, Sainsbury's*	1 Pack/136g	144	6.8	106	5.3	9.9	5.0	1.3
Sweet, Pointed, ES, Asda*	1 Serving/100g	36	0.4	36	1.0	6.4	0.4	1.6
Yellow, Raw, Unprepared, Average	*1 Med/160g*	*35*	*0.3*	*22*	*1.0*	*4.4*	*0.2*	*1.4*
PERCH								
Raw, Atlantic	*1oz/28g*	*26*	*0.5*	*94*	*18.6*	*0.0*	*1.6*	*0.0*
PERNOD*								
19% Volume, Pernod	*1 Pub Shot/35ml*	*46*	*0.0*	*130*	*0.0*	*0.0*	*0.0*	*0.0*
PESTO								
Chargrilled Aubergine, Sacla*	1 Serving/30g	102	10.5	339	2.4	3.8	34.9	0.0
Green, Asda*	1 Tsp/5g	21	2.2	429	4.7	3.5	44.0	1.4
Red, Alla Siciliana, Finest, Tesco*	¼ Jar/48g	110	10.0	230	4.9	4.4	20.9	3.0
Sauce, Basil, M&S*	1 Serving/65g	348	30.5	535	7.5	20.7	46.9	1.4
Sauce, Fiery Chilli, Sacla*	½ Jar/95g	342	29.3	360	4.8	16.0	30.8	3.4
Sauce, Green, Alla Genovese, Finest, Tesco*	1 Serving/65g	188	25.7	290	5.7	1.5	39.6	2.8
Sauce, Green, Alla Genovese, TTD, Sainsbury's*	1 Serving/30g	192	19.8	640	6.2	5.4	65.9	3.1
Sauce, Green, Asda*	2 Dtsp/25g	92	7.4	368	7.6	16.6	29.7	2.0
Sauce, Green, Average	*1 Tbsp/20g*	*103*	*9.5*	*517*	*20.4*	*2.0*	*47.5*	*0.0*
Sauce, Green, Classic, Sacla*	1 Serving/40g	185	18.6	462	5.2	7.6	46.5	0.0
Sauce, Green, Fresh, Sainsbury's*	1 Serving/60g	328	31.7	546	9.4	8.3	52.8	0.1
Sauce, Green, Morrisons*	1 Serving/50g	255	24.9	510	10.7	4.7	49.8	0.0
Sauce, Green, Reduced Fat, Tesco*	¼ Jar/49g	96	9.5	195	2.6	0.7	19.4	3.4
Sauce, Green, Sainsbury's*	1 Tsp/5g	23	2.2	451	5.9	10.1	43.0	2.0
Sauce, Green, Tesco*	¼ Jar/48g	192	20.0	405	5.6	0.6	42.2	4.4
Sauce, Red, Garlic & Chilli, Jamie Oliver*	1 Jar/190g	494	48.8	260	1.1	5.6	25.7	1.1

P

	Measure INFO/WEIGHT	per Measure KCAL	FAT	Nutrition Values per 100g / 100ml KCAL	PROT	CARB	FAT	FIBRE
PESTO								
Sauce, Red, Italian, Tesco*	1 Serving/38g	128	11.5	340	8.2	8.2	30.6	1.2
Sauce, Red, Morrisons*	1 Tbsp/15g	47	4.4	311	5.7	6.6	29.0	5.9
Sauce, Red, Rosso, Bertolli*	1 Jar/185g	703	64.8	380	6.8	9.5	35.0	2.0
Sauce, Red, Tesco*	¼ Jar/50g	162	15.2	325	5.6	6.3	30.3	6.0
Sauce, Ricotta & Red Pepper, CBY, Asda*	1 Jar/190g	486	37.2	256	4.2	14.4	19.6	2.4
Sauce, Spinach & Parmesan, Sainsbury's*	¼ Jar/46g	162	16.0	349	4.6	5.3	34.4	2.5
Sauce, Sun Dried Tomato, Sacla*	1 Serving/30g	87	8.4	289	4.2	5.2	27.9	0.0
Sauce, Verde, Traditional Italian, Sacla*	1 Serving/100g	454	45.4	454	5.3	6.0	45.4	0.0
Wild Rocket, Sacla*	1 Serving/30g	128	13.0	425	5.2	3.2	43.5	4.5
PETIT POIS								
& Baby Carrots, Canned, Drained, Average	**½ Can/122g**	**58**	**0.8**	**47**	**2.9**	**7.0**	**0.7**	**3.2**
Canned, Drained, Average	**1 Sm Can/200g**	**125**	**1.0**	**63**	**4.8**	**8.9**	**0.5**	**2.6**
Fresh, Frozen, Average	**1 Serving/80g**	**51**	**0.8**	**63**	**5.4**	**7.1**	**1.0**	**4.8**
PHEASANT								
Breast, Fillets, Skinless, Cooked, Gressingham Foods*	1 Serving/100g	127	2.4	127	32.7	0.0	2.4	0.0
Meat Only, Roasted	**1oz/28g**	**62**	**3.4**	**220**	**27.9**	**0.0**	**12.0**	**0.0**
Meat Only, Roasted, Weighed with Bone	**1oz/28g**	**32**	**1.7**	**114**	**14.5**	**0.0**	**6.2**	**0.0**
Stuffed, Easy Carve, Finest, Tesco*	1 Serving/200g	540	37.4	270	23.2	2.2	18.7	0.9
Whole with Bacon, Cooked, Gressingham Foods*	1 Serving/100g	220	14.5	220	21.9	0.0	14.5	0.0
PHYSALIS								
Goldenberries, Dried, Neal's Yard*	1 Serving/20g	60	1.6	302	6.0	42.8	8.0	17.4
Raw, without Husk, Average	**5 Fruits/30g**	**16**	**0.2**	**53**	**1.9**	**11.2**	**0.7**	**0.4**
PICCALILLI								
Haywards*	1 Serving/28g	18	0.1	66	1.4	13.9	0.5	0.0
Heinz*	1 Serving/10g	10	0.1	99	1.0	20.5	0.6	0.6
M&S*	1 Serving/20g	21	0.1	105	1.3	23.0	0.6	1.1
Morrisons*	1 Serving/50g	38	0.4	75	1.6	15.0	0.7	0.6
Sainsbury's*	1 Dtsp/15g	9	0.1	60	1.8	11.9	0.6	0.7
Sandwich, Tesco*	1 Serving/20g	16	0.0	80	0.4	18.5	0.0	1.6
Sweet, Asda*	1 Tbsp/15g	17	0.0	112	0.5	27.0	0.2	0.6
Tesco*	1 Serving/50g	51	1.8	102	0.5	17.8	3.6	2.0
Three Mustard, Finest, Tesco*	1 Serving/30g	40	0.2	134	1.3	30.7	0.7	1.0
TTD, Sainsbury's*	1 Serving/19g	13	0.2	67	0.7	13.9	0.9	1.8
PICKLE								
Branston, Beetroot, Crosse & Blackwell*	1 Tsp/20g	25	0.1	123	1.2	28.2	0.3	1.6
Branston, Original, Crosse & Blackwell*	1 Serving/12g	19	0.1	157	0.5	34.0	0.7	1.8
Branston, Red Onion & Cranberry, Crosse & Blackwell*	1 Tbsp/14g	13	0.1	92	0.6	21.4	0.4	0.8
Branston, Red Pepper & Tomato, Crosse & Blackwell*	1 Tbsp/14g	12	0.0	84	1.2	17.7	0.3	1.1
Branston, Small Chunk, Squeezy, Crosse & Blackwell*	1 Serving/15g	19	0.0	127	0.9	29.8	0.2	1.1
Branston, Smooth, Squeezy, Crosse & Blackwell*	1 Serving/15g	19	0.0	127	0.9	29.8	0.2	1.1
Branston, Sweet, Small Chunk, Crosse & Blackwell*	1 Serving/20g	22	0.0	109	0.8	26.1	0.2	1.1
Brinjal, Patak's*	1 Tsp/16g	59	3.9	367	2.2	34.6	24.4	0.9
Chilli, Patak's*	1 Tsp/16g	52	5.4	325	4.3	1.3	33.7	0.0
Cornichons, in Sweet & Sour Vinegar, Waitrose*	1 Serving/10g	3	0.0	28	0.6	6.1	0.1	0.6
Garlic, Patak's*	1 Tsp/16g	42	3.0	261	3.6	20.0	18.5	1.6
Hot Chilli Jam, What a Pickle*	1 Tsp/8g	14	0.0	178	0.6	44.0	0.1	1.2
Lime, Hot, Asda*	1 Dtsp/10g	12	1.0	123	2.2	6.0	10.0	1.0
Lime, Hot, Patak's*	1 Tsp/16g	31	3.0	194	2.2	4.0	18.7	0.4
Lime, M&S*	1 Tsp/16g	34	0.8	215	0.8	42.5	4.8	2.4
Lime, Sharwood's*	1 Tbsp/20g	28	2.0	142	1.7	11.5	9.9	1.3
Mango, Hot, Patak's*	1 Tsp/16g	43	4.1	270	2.3	7.4	25.7	1.9
Mild Mustard, Heinz*	1 Tbsp/10g	13	0.1	129	2.2	25.7	1.3	0.9
Mixed, Drained	1 Serving/100g	14	0.2	14	1.0	1.9	0.2	1.0

INFO/WEIGHT	Measure	per Measure		Nutrition Values per 100g / 100ml				
		KCAL	FAT	KCAL	PROT	CARB	FAT	FIBRE

PICKLE
Mixed, Drained, Haywards*	½ Jar/120g	22	0.4	18	1.4	2.4	0.3	0.0
Mixed, Patak's*	1 Serving/30g	78	7.7	259	2.3	4.7	25.7	0.8
Red Cabbage, Asda*	1 Serving/50g	16	0.0	32	1.6	6.0	0.1	0.0
Sweet	**1 Tsp/10g**	**14**	**0.0**	**141**	**0.6**	**36.0**	**0.1**	**1.2**
Sweet Harvest, Asda*	1 Serving/25g	38	0.1	154	0.8	37.0	0.3	0.8
Sweet, Country, Morrisons*	1 Tbsp/15g	20	0.0	130	0.9	31.1	0.2	0.0
Sweet, Low Price, Sainsbury's*	1 Serving/23g	23	0.1	98	0.7	23.2	0.3	0.7
Sweet, Original, Tesco*	1 Tbsp/15g	20	0.0	135	0.5	31.5	0.1	2.1
Sweet, Value, Tesco*	1 Serving/10g	10	0.0	96	0.6	23.0	0.2	0.7
Tomato, Tangy, Heinz*	1 Tsp/10g	10	0.0	102	2.0	22.0	0.3	1.5

PICNIC
Cadbury*	1 Bar/48g	230	10.9	475	7.3	60.9	22.6	2.1

PIE
2 Mini Pork, Ploughmans, Ginsters*	1 Pie/50g	190	12.6	380	8.9	29.2	25.3	2.0
Admiral's, Ross*	1 Pie/340g	357	15.6	105	4.8	10.9	4.6	0.7
All Steak, Pukka Pies Ltd*	1 Pie/233g	499	29.8	214	6.9	17.6	12.8	3.1
Apple & Blackberry, Co-Op*	1 Serving/138g	338	15.2	245	3.0	33.0	11.0	2.0
Apple & Blackberry, Fruit, Finest, Tesco*	1 Pie/95g	265	11.3	279	13.7	29.3	11.9	2.8
Apple & Blackberry, Shortcrust, M&S*	1 Serving/142g	469	17.8	330	4.3	50.2	12.5	1.1
Apple & Blackcurrant, Mr Kipling*	1 Pie/66g	211	8.4	320	3.3	47.9	12.8	1.2
Apple with Custard	1 Serving/217g	353	18.8	163	2.4	25.2	8.7	1.1
Apple, Asda*	¼ Pack/107g	287	11.7	269	3.6	39.0	11.0	1.7
Apple, Bramley, Aunt Bessie's*	¼ Pie/138g	386	15.1	281	2.4	42.0	11.0	1.1
Apple, Bramley, Free From, Tesco*	1 Pie/60g	225	7.5	375	1.7	63.8	12.5	0.8
Apple, Bramley, Individual, Mr Kipling*	1 Pie/66g	228	8.6	346	3.4	53.8	13.0	1.4
Apple, Bramley, Individual, Tesco*	1 Pie/61g	210	7.9	344	3.4	53.1	13.0	1.5
Apple, Bramley, Large, Tesco*	1/8 Pie/87g	311	13.0	358	3.9	51.9	15.0	1.9
Apple, Bramley, Tesco*	1 Serving/106g	284	11.6	268	3.6	38.8	10.9	1.7
Apple, Deep Filled, Iceland*	1 Serving/116g	332	15.3	286	2.5	39.2	13.2	1.1
Apple, Family, Asda*	1/6 Pie/119g	314	13.0	265	3.6	38.0	11.0	2.9
Apple, Family, Morrisons*	1/6 Pie/116g	326	14.0	281	3.1	39.9	12.1	3.1
Apple, Lattice, Tesco*	1 Serving/145g	325	13.3	224	2.2	33.2	9.2	1.4
Apple, Pastry Top & Bottom	1oz/28g	74	3.7	266	2.9	35.8	13.3	1.7
Apple, Puff Pastry, M&S*	1 Pie/135g	338	17.1	250	2.4	31.3	12.7	1.0
Apple, VLH Kitchens	1 Serving/50g	136	22.4	272	3.7	40.0	11.2	1.7
Banoffee, Mini, Waitrose*	1 Pie/26g	115	5.8	444	3.3	57.0	22.5	1.2
Banoffee, Tesco*	1/6 Pie/94g	365	19.7	390	3.9	45.8	21.1	1.5
Beef & Onion, Pukka Pies Ltd*	1 Serving/231g	529	32.6	229	7.6	17.9	14.1	3.0
Beef & Vegetable, Macdougalls, McDougalls*	¼ Pie/114g	292	19.3	256	5.3	20.6	16.9	0.3
Beef Steak, Aberdeen Angus, Top Crust, Waitrose*	½ Pie/280g	476	24.1	170	10.0	13.4	8.6	4.1
Beef, Sainsbury's*	1 Pie/210g	535	30.0	255	10.3	21.2	14.3	2.0
Blackcurrant, Deep Filled, Sainsbury's*	1 Slice/137g	440	19.3	321	5.8	42.6	14.1	2.2
Blackcurrant, Shortcrust, M&S*	1 Pie/142g	412	14.3	290	3.9	45.6	10.1	1.3
Bramley Apple & Blackberry, Aunt Bessie's*	¼ Pie/138g	344	12.5	250	2.1	40.1	9.1	2.6
Bramley Apple & Blackberry, M&S*	¼ Pie/146g	380	14.5	260	3.4	39.8	9.9	1.3
Bramley Apple, M&S*	1 Pie/55g	184	6.4	335	2.9	57.6	11.7	1.6
Butternut Squash & Feta, Little, Higgidy*	1 Pie/160g	437	29.1	273	7.2	21.4	18.2	1.2
Cheese & Onion, Hollands*	1 Pie/200g	516	24.4	258	6.3	30.9	12.2	0.0
Cheese & Onion, Oven Baked, Average	**1 Serving/200g**	**654**	**40.0**	**327**	**8.2**	**30.4**	**20.0**	**1.2**
Cheese & Potato	1oz/28g	39	2.3	139	4.8	12.6	8.1	0.7
Cheese & Potato, Aunt Bessie's*	¼ Serving/200g	288	18.8	144	4.6	11.7	9.4	1.5
Cherry, Asda*	1/6 Pie/117g	337	14.5	289	3.1	41.2	12.4	1.8
Cherry, Sainsbury's*	1 Serving/117g	325	13.6	278	3.9	39.6	11.6	1.7

PIE

	INFO/WEIGHT	KCAL	FAT	KCAL	PROT	CARB	FAT	FIBRE
Cherry, Tesco*	1 Serving/106g	294	12.7	277	4.0	38.3	12.0	1.8
Chicken & Asparagus, McDougalls*	1 Serving/170g	394	21.9	232	7.4	21.6	12.9	1.5
Chicken & Bacon with Cheese Sauce, Tesco*	1 Serving/200g	540	33.6	270	12.0	17.6	16.8	0.8
Chicken & Bacon, Filo Pastry, Finest, Tesco*	1 Serving/160g	362	18.7	226	11.3	18.9	11.7	1.7
Chicken & Bacon, Puff Pastry, Deep Fill, Sainsbury's*	1/3 Pie/200g	532	34.0	266	9.1	19.1	17.0	1.3
Chicken & Broccoli Potato, Top, Asda*	1 Pack/400g	319	7.0	80	5.2	10.8	1.8	0.6
Chicken & Broccoli, Lattice, Tesco*	½ Pie/200g	496	30.8	248	8.5	18.9	15.4	2.1
Chicken & Gravy, Deep Fill, Asda*	1 Serving/130g	370	22.1	285	10.0	23.0	17.0	0.8
Chicken & Gravy, Shortcrust Pastry, Large, Tesco*	1 Pie/600g	1578	91.2	263	8.2	23.4	15.2	1.0
Chicken & Gravy, Shortcrust Pastry, Sainsbury's*	1 Serving/235g	610	33.4	259	12.5	19.7	14.2	1.5
Chicken & Gravy, Shortcrust Pastry, Tesco*	1 Pie/250g	618	34.5	247	6.8	23.9	13.8	1.0
Chicken & Ham, Deep Filled, Sainsbury's*	1 Pie/210g	594	37.2	283	8.0	23.0	17.7	1.0
Chicken & Ham, Morrisons*	¼ Pie/115g	267	13.7	232	8.7	22.5	11.9	0.8
Chicken & Ham, Sainsbury's*	1 Pie/128g	461	28.7	360	11.0	28.5	22.4	2.0
Chicken & Ham, Tesco*	1 Serving/113g	293	17.6	259	9.4	20.2	15.6	1.2
Chicken & Leek, Deep Filled, Puff Pastry, Sainsbury's*	1/3 Pie/451g	1109	65.4	246	10.1	18.7	14.5	1.5
Chicken & Leek, Light Choices, Tesco*	1 Pie/350g	298	5.6	85	6.6	10.3	1.6	1.3
Chicken & Leek, Shortcrust, TTD, Sainsbury's*	½ Pie/300g	824	48.8	275	12.2	19.8	16.3	1.1
Chicken & Mushroom, Average	**1 Serving/200g**	**540**	**31.7**	**270**	**8.0**	**23.8**	**15.9**	**1.0**
Chicken & Mushroom, Chilled, Weight Watchers*	1 Pack/400g	304	4.8	76	5.7	9.8	1.2	1.5
Chicken & Mushroom, Deep Filled, Frozen, Tesco*	¼ Pie/198g	465	22.2	235	9.0	23.8	11.2	1.2
Chicken & Mushroom, Finest, Tesco*	1 Pie/250g	742	46.8	297	9.3	21.1	18.7	0.9
Chicken & Mushroom, Fray Bentos*	1 Pie/425g	684	40.4	161	6.7	11.5	9.5	0.0
Chicken & Mushroom, Individual, Frozen, Tesco*	1 Pie/142g	347	17.9	245	8.9	23.5	12.6	1.2
Chicken & Mushroom, Puff Pastry, Birds Eye*	1 Pie/152g	415	21.3	273	11.9	24.9	14.0	1.6
Chicken & Mushroom, Puff Pastry, Sainsbury's*	1 Pie/150g	417	25.0	278	9.0	22.1	16.7	1.5
Chicken & Mushroom, Pukka Pies Ltd*	1 Pie/226g	475	29.2	210	7.6	15.7	12.9	3.5
Chicken & Mushroom, Weight Watchers*	1 Pie/136g	317	15.1	233	8.0	25.1	11.1	1.5
Chicken & Potato, Cheeky, Eat Fussy, Annabel Karmel*	1 Pack/220g	202	7.0	92	5.6	10.0	3.2	1.3
Chicken & Vegetable, Freshbake*	1 Pie/125g	319	19.6	255	6.5	21.8	15.7	2.7
Chicken & Vegetable, Value, Tesco*	1 Pie/121g	321	16.9	265	6.6	26.9	14.0	1.1
Chicken & Wiltshire Ham, Finest, Tesco*	1 Pie/250g	688	37.2	275	11.6	22.7	14.9	1.1
Chicken Balti, Ginsters*	1 Pie/180g	416	25.0	231	7.3	19.2	13.9	1.9
Chicken Curry, Iceland*	1 Pie/156g	440	23.7	282	10.2	26.2	15.2	2.0
Chicken Leek & Sweetcorn, LL, Waitrose*	1 Pie/421g	358	14.3	85	5.2	8.6	3.4	1.7
Chicken Pot with Ham & Leek, Higgidy*	1 Pie/250g	710	33.5	284	13.1	19.1	13.4	1.1
Chicken, Cheese & Bacon, HL, Tesco*	1 Pack/450g	382	9.9	85	5.9	9.4	2.2	1.6
Chicken, Cheese & Leek Lattice, Sun Valley*	1 Lattice/125g	315	21.9	252	15.2	8.6	17.5	1.0
Chicken, Cottage, Frozen, Tesco*	1 Pack/450g	292	2.2	65	2.8	11.7	0.5	1.0
Chicken, Deep Filled, Puff Pastry, Sainsbury's*	1 Pie/210g	538	31.9	256	10.0	19.9	15.2	3.1
Chicken, Finest, Tesco*	1 Pie/250g	615	32.2	246	10.7	21.9	12.9	1.2
Chicken, Garlic, Lattice, Crumb Top, Gastropub, M&S*	½ Lattice/110g	299	18.2	272	11.1	19.1	16.5	1.1
Chicken, Individual, Made with 100% Breast, Birds Eye*	1 Pie/154g	455	28.1	296	7.9	25.0	18.3	1.0
Chicken, Leek & Bacon, Aldi*	1 Pie/210g	601	37.6	286	10.9	19.7	17.9	1.0
Chicken, Leek & Bacon, Deluxe, Lidl*	1/3 Pie/171g	511	30.8	299	11.0	22.0	18.0	2.7
Chicken, Leek & Ham, Morrisons*	1 Serving/113g	305	16.6	270	8.8	25.7	14.7	1.1
Chicken, Newgate, Lidl*	1 Pie/142g	358	23.6	252	6.1	23.1	16.6	1.0
Chicken, Puff Pastry, Tesco*	¼ Pie/114g	250	12.7	220	8.6	21.3	11.2	1.4
Chicken, Roast, in Gravy, Deep Fill, Tesco*	1 Pie/700g	1540	68.6	220	11.2	20.2	9.8	2.0
Chicken, Roast, Puff Pastry, Deep Fill, Asda*	½ Pie/259g	739	44.1	285	10.0	23.0	17.0	0.8
Chicken, Roast, Sainsbury's*	1/3 Pie/173g	538	30.8	311	10.5	27.2	17.8	0.9
Chicken, Short Crust, M&S*	1 Pie/170g	510	29.6	300	9.7	26.2	17.4	1.7
Chocolate, Mini, Waitrose*	1 Pie/24g	109	6.1	455	5.3	51.4	25.3	1.7

P

PIE

	Measure INFO/WEIGHT	per Measure KCAL	FAT	Nutrition Values per 100g / 100ml KCAL	PROT	CARB	FAT	FIBRE
Cod & Smoked Haddock, COU, M&S*	1 Pack/400g	320	9.6	80	6.1	9.0	2.4	1.2
Cottage with Cheddar Mash, TTD, Sainsbury's*	1 Pack/400g	601	27.6	150	9.2	11.6	6.9	2.4
Cottage, Aberdeen Angus, Waitrose*	1 Pie/350g	340	12.2	97	5.3	11.0	3.5	0.9
Cottage, Aldi*	1 Pack/440g	484	27.3	110	4.1	9.5	6.2	0.2
Cottage, Asda*	1 Pack/400g	360	9.6	90	6.5	10.6	2.4	1.0
Cottage, Aunt Bessie's*	1 Pack/350g	413	18.2	118	4.8	12.1	5.2	1.0
Cottage, Basics, Sainsbury's*	1 Pack/300g	228	9.0	76	4.4	7.9	3.0	1.5
Cottage, Beef, Delicious, Annabel Karmel*	1 Pack/200g	206	9.6	103	4.7	9.8	4.8	1.1
Cottage, British Pies, Chilled, Tesco*	1 Pack/500g	450	14.0	90	4.6	10.3	2.8	1.5
Cottage, Cheesy Mash, & Red Wine Gravy, Gastro, M&S*	1 Pack/400g	500	21.6	125	11.1	7.2	5.4	1.4
Cottage, Classic British, Sainsbury's*	1 Pack/450g	436	16.2	97	5.3	9.9	3.6	1.7
Cottage, Classics, Asda*	½ Pack/450g	531	27.0	118	7.0	9.0	6.0	1.0
Cottage, COU, M&S*	1 Pack/400g	340	8.0	85	6.0	11.0	2.0	1.5
Cottage, Diet Chef Ltd*	1 Pack/270g	235	9.7	87	3.7	9.8	3.6	1.7
Cottage, Fresh, M&S*	1 Pie/400g	460	22.4	115	6.8	9.9	5.6	0.6
Cottage, Healthy Living, Co-Op*	1 Pack/400g	320	6.4	80	5.0	11.0	1.6	2.0
Cottage, Iceland*	1 Pack/400g	468	18.8	117	5.1	13.6	4.7	0.7
Cottage, Individual, Smart Price, Asda*	1 Pie/159g	149	5.9	94	3.1	12.0	3.7	0.7
Cottage, Lentil & Vegetable, Linda McCartney*	1 Pot/398g	374	10.3	94	2.8	13.5	2.6	2.5
Cottage, Light Choices, Tesco*	1 Pack/500g	400	8.5	80	4.5	11.4	1.7	1.7
Cottage, Luxury, M&S*	½ Pack/310g	403	21.7	130	7.9	8.3	7.0	1.8
Cottage, Meal for One, M&S*	1 Pack/445g	356	16.0	80	5.4	6.2	3.6	1.7
Cottage, Mini, Waitrose*	1 Pack/250g	268	10.5	107	6.4	11.1	4.2	1.4
Cottage, Morrisons*	1 Pack/450g	450	18.4	100	5.2	10.7	4.1	1.2
Cottage, Ready Meals,,Tesco*	1 Pack/400g	380	12.0	95	6.1	10.8	3.0	1.6
Cottage, Retail, Average	*1 Pack/400g*	*399*	*15.7*	*100*	*5.5*	*10.5*	*3.9*	*1.3*
Cottage, Sainsbury's*	1 Pack/300g	297	10.2	99	6.4	10.7	3.4	1.1
Cottage, Salmon, Sainsbury's*	1 Serving/299g	218	4.2	73	4.6	10.4	1.4	1.3
Cottage, The Best, Morrisons*	½ Pack/400g	424	16.4	106	7.7	9.5	4.1	1.2
Cottage, Vegetarian, 694, Wiltshire Farm Foods*	1 Serving/415g	320	3.7	77	3.4	12.0	0.9	2.3
Cottage, Vegetarian, Sainsbury's*	1 Pack/450g	328	9.9	73	3.0	10.2	2.2	1.8
Cottage, Waitrose*	1 Pack/400g	424	19.6	106	3.4	12.1	4.9	1.2
Cottage, Weight Watchers*	1 Pack/300g	186	3.9	62	3.6	9.0	1.3	0.3
Cottage, You Count, LL, Waitrose*	1 Pack/402g	291	7.0	82	4.4	10.9	2.0	1.2
Cumberland, HL, Tesco*	1 Pie/500g	430	13.5	86	4.5	10.8	2.7	1.2
Cumberland, M&S*	1 Pie/195g	312	20.3	160	6.9	10.1	10.4	1.1
Farmhouse, Vegetable, Linda McCartney*	1 Pie/146g	380	23.2	260	5.8	23.4	15.9	1.6
Fish	1 Serving/250g	262	7.5	105	8.0	12.3	3.0	0.7
Fish with Cheese, Ross*	1 Pack/300g	321	13.5	107	4.7	12.0	4.5	0.8
Fish, Chilled, GFY, Asda*	1 Pie/450g	405	12.6	90	6.8	9.3	2.8	1.4
Fish, Co-Op*	1 Pack/400g	380	16.0	95	4.0	12.0	4.0	0.9
Fish, Creamy, Classics, Large, Finest, Tesco*	½ Pack/350g	402	19.6	115	6.4	8.6	5.6	0.9
Fish, Crunchy Topped, Menu, Waitrose*	1 Pack/400g	444	19.2	111	7.5	8.4	4.8	1.8
Fish, Cumberland, BGTY, Sainsbury's*	1 Serving/450g	342	8.6	76	7.3	7.3	1.9	1.8
Fish, Cumberland, Cod & Prawn, Tesco*	1 Pack/450g	428	11.2	95	7.9	9.5	2.5	1.3
Fish, ES, Asda*	1 Pack/400g	540	30.8	135	9.8	6.5	7.7	1.1
Fish, Frozen, GFY, Asda*	1 Pack/360g	342	8.6	95	5.8	12.5	2.4	0.9
Fish, HL, Tesco*	1 Pack/400g	316	8.8	79	4.0	10.8	2.2	1.7
Fish, Large, Oven Baked (700g), ES, Asda*	1 Pack/700g	714	29.4	102	8.0	7.4	4.2	1.1
Fish, Luxury, Cafe Culture, M&S*	1 Pack/660g	627	26.4	95	7.1	7.8	4.0	1.1
Fish, Luxury, M&S*	1 Pack/300g	330	16.8	110	7.3	7.6	5.6	1.5
Fish, Mariner's, Frozen, Oven Baked, Youngs*	1 Pack/340g	444	20.3	140	5.1	15.1	6.4	1.0
Fish, Potato Topped, Mini Meal, M&S*	1 Serving/220g	216	7.7	98	7.0	9.1	3.5	0.9

PIE

	Measure INFO/WEIGHT	per Measure KCAL	FAT	Nutrition Values per 100g / 100ml KCAL	PROT	CARB	FAT	FIBRE
Fish, The Best, Morrisons*	½ Pack/225g	250	11.9	111	6.6	9.3	5.3	0.8
Fishermans, British Recipe, Waitrose*	1 Pack/400g	408	16.4	102	7.7	8.5	4.1	1.2
Fisherman's, Chilled, Co-Op*	1 Pie/300g	345	18.0	115	4.0	11.0	6.0	0.7
Fisherman's, Famous, Chilled, Youngs*	1 Pack/400g	448	22.8	112	7.6	7.6	5.7	0.9
Fishermans, Smart Price, Asda*	1 Pack/300g	213	3.6	71	3.1	12.0	1.2	1.9
Fisherman's, Tesco*	1 Pie/400g	400	19.6	100	4.2	9.8	4.9	1.1
Fruit, Pastry Top & Bottom	1oz/28g	73	3.7	260	3.0	34.0	13.3	1.8
Fruit, Selection, Mr Kipling*	1 Pie/66g	232	9.0	350	3.5	53.5	13.6	1.3
Gala, Tesco*	1 Serving/70g	241	17.6	344	10.6	24.5	25.2	0.0
Just Chicken in Gravy, Fray Bentos*	½ Pie/215g	267	7.3	124	5.6	17.2	3.4	0.6
Key Lime, Sainsbury's*	¼ Pie/80g	280	11.2	350	4.2	51.8	14.0	0.7
Lamb & Mint, Shortcrust Pasty, Tesco*	¼ Pack/150g	412	26.1	275	5.9	23.6	17.4	1.6
Lemon Meringue	1 Portion/120g	383	17.3	319	4.5	45.9	14.4	0.7
Lemon Meringue, Mini, Asda*	1 Pie/26g	101	3.3	396	3.7	66.0	13.0	1.8
Lemon Meringue, Sainsbury's*	¼ Pie/110g	351	9.9	319	2.3	57.3	9.0	0.5
Lemon Meringue, Tesco*	1 Pie/385g	989	28.1	257	4.0	43.7	7.3	0.5
Macaroni Cheese, Countryside*	1 Serving/144g	282	10.1	196	4.9	28.3	7.0	1.2
Mariner's, Light & Easy, Youngs*	1 Pack/350g	368	14.3	105	5.0	12.0	4.1	1.1
Mashed Potato Topped Cumberland, M&S*	1/3 Pack/300g	360	17.7	120	5.8	9.6	5.9	1.0
Meat & Potato, Hollands*	1 Pie/175g	410	19.2	234	6.1	27.5	11.0	0.0
Meat & Potato, Shortcrust, Co-Op*	¼ Pie/137g	403	26.2	294	7.3	23.3	19.1	1.4
Meat & Potato, Tesco*	1 Serving/150g	414	26.8	276	5.1	23.6	17.9	1.6
Meat, Freshbake*	1 Pie/49g	152	10.5	313	6.6	23.2	21.6	1.0
Mince Puff, Tesco*	1 Pie/25g	105	4.4	420	3.3	62.0	17.6	2.0
Mince, Christmas, Classic, Asda*	1 Pie/54g	217	8.6	401	3.5	59.0	16.0	3.5
Mince, Christmas, Finest, Tesco*	1 Pie/64g	255	9.4	395	4.6	60.3	14.5	1.4
Mince, Christmas, Sainsbury's*	1 Pie/37g	147	6.0	397	4.5	58.0	16.3	2.6
Mince, Crumble, Handcrafted, Delicious, Boots*	1 Pie/72g	289	8.9	401	3.6	68.0	12.3	2.2
Mince, Deep Filled, Christmas, Tesco*	1 Pie/65g	255	9.3	395	4.0	60.0	14.4	2.8
Mince, Deep Filled, Morrisons*	1 Pie/66g	257	9.7	386	3.7	57.9	14.6	4.2
Mince, Deep Filled, Sainsbury's*	1 Pie/66g	262	10.2	394	4.2	58.8	15.4	1.8
Mince, Deep, Morrisons*	1 Pie/65g	243	9.1	371	3.7	57.8	13.9	1.5
Mince, Dusted, Mini, Finest, Tesco*	1 Pie/20g	76	2.4	379	7.3	62.9	12.2	5.0
Mince, ES, Asda*	1 Pie/60g	225	8.3	378	3.9	59.0	14.0	2.2
Mince, Iced Top, Asda*	1 Pie/57g	221	6.7	391	2.7	67.3	11.9	1.9
Mince, Iced Top, Tesco*	1 Pie/58g	223	7.1	381	3.8	62.8	12.2	2.5
Mince, Iceland*	1 Pie/39g	156	6.4	405	4.4	59.6	16.6	3.8
Mince, Individual, Average	**1 Pie/48g**	**203**	**9.8**	**423**	**4.3**	**59.0**	**20.4**	**2.1**
Mince, Individual, Mr Kipling*	1 Pie/66g	253	9.2	381	3.7	59.5	13.8	1.3
Mince, Lattice, Classics, M&S*	1 Pie/53g	210	8.0	400	4.0	61.7	15.2	2.4
Mince, Luxury, Deep Filled, M&S*	1 Pie/65g	234	9.0	360	4.3	55.0	13.8	3.8
Mince, Mini, Aldi*	1 Pie/31g	120	4.6	387	4.2	59.0	15.0	1.7
Mince, Mini, ES, Asda*	1 Pie/22g	86	2.8	390	4.1	63.7	12.7	2.1
Mince, Mini, M&S*	1 Pie/28g	105	4.0	380	4.3	57.8	14.6	4.0
Mince, Mini, Selection, Waitrose*	1 Pie/29g	118	4.8	408	4.0	59.1	16.5	3.3
Mince, Organic, Sainsbury's*	1 Pie/46g	177	7.5	384	5.0	54.5	16.2	5.6
Mince, Puff Pastry, Bakery, Tesco*	1 Pie/65g	246	10.3	379	4.7	53.1	15.9	2.2
Mince, Puff Pastry, Co-Op*	1 Pie/72g	245	11.9	340	5.0	43.1	16.5	2.6
Mince, Rowan Hill Bakery, Lidl*	1 Pie/55g	202	8.2	370	3.8	54.8	15.1	0.0
Mince, Shortcrust, Waitrose*	1 Pie/55g	210	8.0	385	3.6	60.0	14.6	20.9
Mince, Smart Price, Asda*	1 Pie/44g	178	7.6	409	4.6	55.6	17.4	3.2
Mince, Star Motif, Mini, Finest, Tesco*	1 Pie/17g	62	2.1	365	3.8	59.9	12.1	3.8
Mince, Trufree*	1 Pie/60g	238	9.8	397	2.1	58.5	16.4	3.6

PIE

	Measure INFO/WEIGHT	per Measure KCAL	FAT	Nutrition Values per 100g / 100ml KCAL	PROT	CARB	FAT	FIBRE
Mince, Value, Tesco*	1 Pie/41g	168	7.0	410	4.4	58.8	17.0	1.6
Minced Beef & Onion, Farmfoods*	1 Pie/128g	378	23.9	295	7.3	24.4	18.7	1.0
Minced Beef & Onion, Tesco*	1 Pie/150g	454	28.5	303	5.7	27.4	19.0	1.7
Minced Beef, & Onion, Frozen, Greggs, Iceland*	½ Pie/125g	390	25.8	310	0.0	25.0	20.5	0.0
Minced Beef, Aberdeen Angus, Shortcrust, M&S*	1 Pie/171g	435	26.6	255	9.3	19.3	15.6	3.0
Moroccan Vegetable & Feta, Little, Higgidy*	1 Pie/180g	418	22.5	232	5.1	24.7	12.5	0.6
Mushroom & Leaf Spinach, Little, Higgidy*	1 Pie/180g	441	25.9	245	6.6	22.3	14.4	0.7
Ocean, M&S*	1 Pie/650g	618	22.8	95	8.2	7.6	3.5	0.9
Ocean, Weight Watchers*	1 Pack/300g	196	3.3	65	4.2	9.2	1.1	0.8
Pork & Egg, M&S*	¼ Pie/108g	379	28.0	351	9.7	19.8	25.9	0.8
Pork, Buffet, Bowyers*	1 Pie/60g	217	14.7	362	10.4	24.9	24.5	0.0
Pork, Cheddar & Pickle, Mini, Finest, Tesco*	1 Pie/50g	185	10.8	365	10.0	31.3	21.4	1.9
Pork, Cheese & Pickle, Mini, Tesco*	1 Pie/49g	191	12.8	389	9.2	29.3	26.1	1.2
Pork, Crusty Bake, Mini, Sainsbury's*	1 Pie/43g	165	11.2	384	11.5	26.0	26.0	1.5
Pork, Crusty Bake, Sainsbury's*	1 Pie/75g	292	20.0	390	10.5	27.0	26.7	1.0
Pork, Geo Adams*	1 Pie/125g	488	34.8	390	11.8	23.1	27.8	0.9
Pork, Individual	1 Pie/75g	272	19.3	363	10.8	23.7	25.7	0.9
Pork, Melton Mowbray, Cured, M&S*	1 Pie/290g	1044	71.0	360	10.1	25.9	24.5	1.0
Pork, Melton Mowbray, Cured, Mini, M&S*	1 Pie/50g	192	12.2	385	9.8	32.6	24.4	1.0
Pork, Melton Mowbray, Individual, Sainsbury's*	1 Pie/75g	296	20.8	395	10.2	26.1	27.7	2.4
Pork, Melton Mowbray, Large, Co-Op*	¼ Pie/110g	418	35.2	380	11.0	12.0	32.0	5.0
Pork, Melton Mowbray, Lattice, Sainsbury's*	1 Serving/100g	342	23.6	342	10.8	21.7	23.6	1.2
Pork, Melton Mowbray, Mini, Co-Op*	1 Pie/49g	189	13.2	385	11.0	24.0	27.0	2.0
Pork, Melton Mowbray, Mini, Finest, Tesco*	1 Pie/50g	180	11.4	359	12.1	26.6	22.7	0.9
Pork, Melton Mowbray, Mini, M&S*	1 Pie/50g	185	12.1	370	11.6	26.1	24.2	1.6
Pork, Melton Mowbray, Mini, Morrisons*	1 Pie/50g	197	12.5	393	10.9	31.3	24.9	0.9
Pork, Melton Mowbray, Mini, Tesco*	1 Pie/50g	196	14.4	392	12.6	20.8	28.7	2.9
Pork, Melton Mowbray, Snack, Tesco*	1 Pie/75g	289	19.4	385	10.1	27.0	25.9	2.7
Pork, Melton, Mini, Pork Farms*	1 Pie/50g	200	14.6	399	8.9	26.2	29.2	0.0
Pork, Mini	1 Pie/50g	196	13.9	391	10.6	26.3	27.8	1.0
Pork, Mini, Tesco*	1 Pie/45g	162	10.7	359	10.2	25.9	23.8	1.0
Pork, Sliced	1 Slice/100g	380	29.9	380	10.2	18.7	29.9	0.0
Pork, VLH Kitchens	1 Serving/36g	168	100.0	466	11.0	26.0	36.0	2.5
Potato & Meat, Farmfoods*	1 Pie/158g	416	26.9	263	5.4	22.0	17.0	1.0
Rhubarb, Sara Lee*	1 Serving/90g	224	12.4	250	2.9	28.7	13.8	1.3
Roast Chicken, M&S*	1/3 Pie/182g	465	24.1	255	7.8	26.4	13.2	2.2
Salmon & Broccoli Lattice Bar, Asda*	1/3 Bar/133g	360	20.0	271	6.0	28.0	15.0	0.8
Salmon & Broccoli, Filo Pastry, Finest, Tesco*	1 Pie/170g	386	22.6	227	7.9	18.9	13.3	2.1
Salmon & Broccoli, Premium, Tesco*	1 Serving/170g	425	29.2	250	6.1	17.7	17.2	0.7
Sausage & Onion, Tesco*	1 Pack/300g	333	18.3	111	2.3	11.7	6.1	0.5
Scotch, Co-Op*	1 Pie/132g	408	24.9	309	7.3	27.3	18.9	1.5
Scotch, Farmfoods*	1 Pie/151g	430	24.6	285	7.8	26.8	16.3	1.2
Shepherd's, Average	**1oz/28g**	**31**	**1.7**	**112**	**6.0**	**9.3**	**5.9**	**0.7**
Shepherd's, British Classic, Serves 1, Sainsbury's*	1 Pack/450g	454	22.1	101	6.2	7.9	4.9	1.7
Shepherd's, Charlie Bigham's*	½ Pack/324g	496	28.8	153	8.1	9.6	8.9	0.9
Shepherd's, Chilled, Finest, Tesco*	½ Pack/400g	460	16.4	115	6.9	8.0	4.1	1.9
Shepherd's, COU, M&S*	1 Pack/300g	210	3.9	70	5.2	8.6	1.3	1.6
Shepherd's, Diet Chef Ltd*	1 Serving/270g	235	10.5	87	3.2	9.8	3.9	1.9
Shepherd's, Frozen, Tesco*	1 Pack/400g	270	9.1	68	4.1	7.6	2.3	1.2
Shepherd's, TTD, Sainsbury's*	1 Pack/397g	524	27.8	132	7.6	9.7	7.0	1.7
Shepherd's, Vegetarian, Average	**1 Serving/400g**	**371**	**14.6**	**93**	**4.0**	**10.4**	**3.6**	**2.5**
Shepherd's, Weight Watchers*	1 Pack/320g	211	5.8	66	3.2	8.8	1.8	1.1
Shepherd's, Welsh Hill Lamb, Gastropub, M&S*	½ Pack/330g	314	11.6	95	5.4	10.2	3.5	1.5

	Measure INFO/WEIGHT	per Measure KCAL	FAT	Nutrition Values per 100g / 100ml KCAL	PROT	CARB	FAT	FIBRE
PIE								
Steak & Ale with Chips & Gravy	1 Serving/400g	825	42.2	206	7.2	20.5	10.6	0.5
Steak & Ale, Average	***1 Pie/200g***	***507***	***28.7***	***253***	***9.8***	***21.1***	***14.4***	***1.3***
Steak & Ale, Charlie Bigham's*	1 Pie/300g	774	48.9	258	13.4	14.1	16.3	1.1
Steak & Ale, Deep Fill, Puff Pastry, Tesco*	¼ Pie/150g	324	19.6	216	8.0	16.6	13.1	2.3
Steak & Ale, Fray Bentos*	1 Pie/425g	697	38.7	164	7.6	13.0	9.1	0.0
Steak & Ale, Pub Style, Co-Op*	1 Pie/250g	538	30.0	215	9.0	17.0	12.0	2.0
Steak & Ale, Puff Pastry, Asda*	1/3 Pie/200g	520	30.2	260	10.6	20.4	15.1	1.6
Steak & Ale, Sainsbury's*	1 Serving/190g	445	23.4	234	8.3	22.6	12.3	0.9
Steak & Ale, TTD, Sainsbury's*	1 Pie/250g	681	35.6	272	11.6	24.4	14.2	1.4
Steak & Dorset Ale, Mini, Finest, Tesco*	1 Pie/30g	92	4.9	305	7.9	31.4	16.4	1.9
Steak & Guinness, Sainsbury's*	¼ Pie/137g	399	25.5	291	8.7	22.2	18.6	1.0
Steak & Kidney, Birds Eye*	1 Pie/146g	447	28.5	306	9.0	23.7	19.5	2.3
Steak & Kidney, Deep Fill, Sainsbury's*	½ Pie/125g	314	18.6	251	8.4	21.0	14.9	2.0
Steak & Kidney, Family, Co-Op*	1/6 Pie/87g	278	17.4	320	9.0	26.0	20.0	0.9
Steak & Kidney, Individual	1 Pie/200g	646	42.4	323	9.1	25.6	21.2	0.9
Steak & Kidney, Premium, Tesco*	1 Serving/170g	428	26.4	252	9.9	18.3	15.5	1.2
Steak & Kidney, Pukka Pies Ltd*	1 Pie/238g	488	25.9	205	9.1	17.7	10.9	3.6
Steak & Kidney, Tesco*	1 Pie/150g	420	27.3	280	7.3	21.9	18.2	3.7
Steak & Kidney, Tinned, Fray Bentos*	½ Pie/212g	346	18.7	163	8.2	12.9	8.8	0.0
Steak & Mushroom, Co-Op*	1 Pie/454g	1158	68.1	255	9.0	20.0	15.0	1.0
Steak & Mushroom, Finest, Tesco*	1 Pie/250g	640	36.5	256	9.2	21.9	14.6	1.1
Steak & Mushroom, Individual, Birds Eye*	1 Pie/142g	389	24.1	274	7.5	22.7	17.0	2.0
Steak & Peppered Sauce, Gastro Style, McDougalls*	1 Pie/192g	495	28.8	258	8.9	21.4	15.0	0.9
Steak & Potato, Asda*	1/3 Pie/173g	442	26.0	255	6.9	23.1	15.0	0.9
Steak in Rich Gravy, Aunt Bessie's*	¼ Pie/200g	440	20.6	220	9.6	22.0	10.3	1.5
Steak, Deep Fill, Tesco*	¼ Pie/195g	468	25.5	240	9.7	20.0	13.1	1.5
Steak, Individual, British Classics, Tesco*	1 Pie/150g	450	27.6	300	9.1	23.3	18.4	2.5
Steak, Mushroom & Ale, Topcrust, Waitrose*	1 Pie/250g	500	29.5	200	11.1	12.2	11.8	1.1
Steak, Puff Pastry, Deep Filled, Sainsbury's*	1 Pie/210g	536	30.0	255	10.3	21.2	14.3	2.0
Steak, Scotch, Bell's Bakery*	1 Serving/150g	378	20.2	252	13.6	18.6	13.5	0.7
Steak, Short Crust, Sainsbury's*	½ Pie/118g	314	24.1	267	10.9	22.2	20.5	1.7
Steak, Shortcrust Pastry, Finest, Tesco*	1 Pie/250g	660	37.8	264	10.9	21.2	15.1	0.8
Turkey & Ham, Farmfoods*	1 Pie/147g	404	21.9	275	8.6	26.5	14.9	1.4
Turkey & Ham, Shortcrust, M&S*	1/3 Pie/183g	494	29.1	270	11.9	19.5	15.9	1.0
Vegetable	1oz/28g	42	2.1	151	3.0	18.9	7.6	1.5
Vegetable & Cheddar Cheese, Waitrose*	1 Pie/210g	475	31.5	226	4.9	17.8	15.0	1.2
Vegetable & Cheese, Asda*	1 Pie/141g	330	16.2	234	5.8	26.9	11.5	1.0
Vegetable, Retail, Average	***1 Serving/200g***	***348***	***19.0***	***174***	***3.7***	***18.6***	***9.5***	***1.1***
Vegetarian, Deep Country, Linda McCartney*	1 Pie/166g	413	23.6	249	5.2	24.9	14.2	2.6
Vegetarian, Mushroom & Ale, Linda McCartney*	1 Pie/200g	439	23.5	219	4.1	25.0	11.7	1.2
Vegetarian, Vegetable Cumberland, M&S*	½ Pack/211g	190	5.5	90	2.8	13.4	2.6	1.6
Wild Shroom, Pieminister*	1 Pie/270g	513	26.2	190	5.2	19.5	9.7	2.7
PIE FILLING								
Apple, Sainsbury's*	1 Serving/75g	67	0.1	89	0.1	22.1	0.1	1.0
Black Cherry, Fruit, Sainsbury's*	1 Serving/100g	73	0.1	73	0.3	17.7	0.1	0.3
Fruit	1oz/28g	22	0.0	77	0.4	20.1	0.0	1.0
Summer Fruits, Fruit, Tesco*	1 Can/385g	377	0.0	98	0.4	24.1	0.0	0.9
PIGEON								
Meat Only, Roasted, Average	***1 Pigeon/115g***	***215***	***9.1***	***187***	***29.0***	***0.0***	***7.9***	***0.0***
Meat Only, Roasted, Weighed with Bone, Average	***1oz/28g***	***12***	***0.5***	***41***	***6.4***	***0.0***	***1.7***	***0.0***
PIKELETS								
Classics, M&S*	1 Pikelet/35g	70	0.5	200	7.3	39.1	1.3	1.6
Tesco*	1 Pikelet/35g	68	0.2	193	5.8	40.9	0.7	1.7

P

	Measure INFO/WEIGHT	per Measure KCAL	FAT	Nutrition Values per 100g / 100ml KCAL	PROT	CARB	FAT	FIBRE
PILCHARDS								
Fillets in Tomato Sauce, Average	*1 Can/120g*	*158*	*7.8*	*132*	*16.2*	*2.2*	*6.5*	*0.1*
in Brine, Average	*½ Can/77g*	*114*	*5.6*	*148*	*20.8*	*0.0*	*7.3*	*0.0*
PIMMS*								
& Lemonade, Premixed, Canned, Pimms*	1 Can/250ml	160	0.0	64	0.0	8.4	0.0	0.0
25% Volume, Pimms*	1 Serving/50ml	80	0.0	160	0.0	5.0	0.0	0.0
PINE NUTS								
Average	*1oz/28g*	*195*	*19.2*	*695*	*15.7*	*3.9*	*68.6*	*1.9*
Kernels, LL, Waitrose*	1 Serving/30g	204	20.6	680	14.0	4.0	68.6	41.4
PINEAPPLE								
& Papaya, Dried, Garden Gang, Asda*	1 Pack/50g	142	0.8	283	2.8	64.0	1.7	8.0
Chunks, Average	*1 Serving/100g*	*66*	*0.1*	*66*	*0.5*	*15.5*	*0.1*	*0.3*
Deliciously Refreshing & Sweet, LL, Waitrose*	8 Chunks/80g	47	0.1	59	0.5	13.1	0.1	1.4
Dried, Soft, LL, Waitrose*	1 Serving/30g	93	0.1	309	3.0	73.7	0.2	3.1
Dried, Unsweetened, Sainsbury's*	1 Bag/75g	255	1.5	340	1.7	84.7	2.0	6.0
Fingers, Good to Go, Waitrose*	1 Pack/160g	90	0.2	56	0.5	13.1	0.1	1.4
in Juice, Canned, Average	*1 Can/106g*	*57*	*0.0*	*53*	*0.3*	*12.9*	*0.0*	*0.6*
Lolly, Fresh, Great Stuff, Asda*	1 Pack/80g	36	0.2	45	0.4	9.8	0.2	1.2
Raw, Diced, Medley, Lozzas	1 Pack/400g	200	0.9	42	0.4	10.0	0.2	1.0
Raw, Flesh Only, Average	*1 Fruit/472g*	*200*	*0.9*	*42*	*0.4*	*10.0*	*0.2*	*1.0*
Sliced, Snack, Shapers, Boots*	1 Pack/80g	35	0.2	44	0.4	10.0	0.2	1.2
Tidbits, Dried, Graze*	1 Pack/30g	79	0.2	263	0.6	72.0	0.6	1.0
PISTACHIO NUTS								
As Consumed, Wholefoods, Morrisons*	1 Serving/25g	151	12.4	602	26.0	12.9	49.6	5.7
Black Pepper, Graze*	1 Punnet/31g	104	9.7	331	10.0	5.0	31.0	3.0
Lightly Toasted, Graze*	1 Punnet/31g	104	9.7	331	10.0	5.0	31.0	3.0
Raw, Average, without Shells	*1 Serving/20g*	*111*	*8.9*	*557*	*20.6*	*28.0*	*44.4*	*10.3*
Roasted & Salted, LL, Waitrose*	1 Serving/25g	144	13.0	576	18.5	8.2	52.1	6.1
Roasted & Salted, without Shells, Average	*1 Serving/25g*	*152*	*13.6*	*608*	*19.6*	*9.9*	*54.5*	*6.1*
Roasted, Graze*	1 Pack/50g	166	15.5	333	9.9	4.6	31.0	0.0
Salted, Roasted, Weighed with Shell	1 Serving/100g	331	30.5	331	9.8	4.5	30.5	3.4
Salted, Roasted, without Shells	1 Serving/100g	601	55.4	601	17.9	8.2	55.4	6.1
Shelled, Kernels, Wholesome, LL, Waitrose*	1 Serving/30g	181	16.6	603	17.9	8.2	55.4	10.3
PIZZA								
American Hot, 12 Inch, Supermarket, Pizza Express*	½ Pizza/264g	562	19.8	213	10.5	25.9	7.5	2.6
American Hot, 8 Inch, Supermarket, Pizza Express*	1 Pizza/295g	652	22.4	221	11.0	27.3	7.6	3.5
Bacon & Mushroom, Thin & Crispy, Sainsbury's*	½ Pizza/150g	396	15.9	264	12.9	29.2	10.6	1.7
Bacon & Mushroom, with Capers, Lozzas	1 Slice/157g	352	14.8	224	10.5	24.3	9.4	3.3
Bacon, Mushroom & Tomato, Stonebaked, Tesco*	1 Serving/173g	351	12.8	203	9.9	24.1	7.4	2.0
Baguette, Cheese & Tomato, Tesco*	1 Baguette/125g	275	8.5	220	11.0	28.0	6.8	2.8
Balsamic Roast Vegetable & Mozzarella, Sainsbury's*	½ Pizza/200g	444	15.6	222	8.5	29.4	7.8	2.4
BBQ Chicken, M&S*	½ Pizza/210g	430	11.8	205	11.6	27.5	5.6	1.8
BBQ Chicken, Stonebaked, Tesco*	½ Pizza/158g	285	9.5	180	10.5	20.9	6.0	3.9
BBQ Chicken, Thin & Crispy, Sainsbury's*	½ Pizza/167g	399	12.4	238	11.4	30.4	7.4	2.2
BBQ Pulled Pork, Deep Pan, Goodfellas*	¼ Pizza/102g	244	6.9	239	11.0	33.0	6.8	0.0
Bistro Caramelised Onion, Feta & Rosemary, Waitrose*	½ Pizza/230g	607	32.0	264	8.6	26.1	13.9	2.4
Bistro Salami & Pepperoni, Waitrose*	½ Pizza/190g	492	19.4	259	12.9	28.8	10.2	1.5
Cajun Style Chicken, Stonebaked, Tesco*	1 Pizza/561g	1318	55.0	235	11.9	24.8	9.8	1.4
Capricciosa, Pizza Express*	1 Serving/300g	753	29.3	251	13.6	29.0	9.8	0.0
Caprina, Pizza Express*	1 Pizza/300g	635	22.0	212	8.0	31.0	7.3	0.0
Charged Up Chilli Beef, Goodfella's*	½ Pizza/357g	857	32.8	240	12.8	26.4	9.2	1.6
Chargrilled Chicken, Thin & Crispy, Asda*	1 Pizza/373g	780	18.6	209	9.0	32.0	5.0	1.6
Chargrilled Vegetable, Frozen, BGTY, Sainsbury's*	1 Pizza/290g	548	13.3	189	10.2	26.7	4.6	3.0
Chargrilled Vegetable, HE, Tesco*	½ Pizza/143g	320	3.9	224	10.4	39.6	2.7	1.1

PIZZA

INFO/WEIGHT	Measure	per Measure KCAL	FAT	Nutrition Values per 100g / 100ml KCAL	PROT	CARB	FAT	FIBRE
Chargrilled Vegetable, Thin & Crispy, GFY, Asda*	1 Serving/188g	290	3.8	154	6.0	28.0	2.0	3.1
Cheese & Tomato French Bread, Findus*	1 Serving/143g	322	11.6	225	9.4	29.0	8.1	0.0
Cheese & Tomato Range, Italiano, Tesco*	1 Pizza/380g	969	35.0	255	11.4	31.7	9.2	3.3
Cheese & Tomato Slice, Ross*	1 Slice/77g	148	6.6	192	6.5	22.2	8.6	2.0
Cheese & Tomato Thin & Crispy, Stonebaked, Tesco*	1 Pizza/155g	355	12.1	229	11.6	28.1	7.8	1.3
Cheese & Tomato, 12 inch, Fresh, Tesco*	1/3 Pizza/160g	413	13.8	258	9.6	36.3	8.6	1.4
Cheese & Tomato, Average	***1 Serving/300g***	***711***	***35.4***	***237***	***9.1***	***25.2***	***11.8***	***1.4***
Cheese & Tomato, Bistro, Waitrose*	½ Pizza/205g	488	19.9	238	10.0	27.6	9.7	1.2
Cheese & Tomato, Deep & Crispy, Tesco*	1 Serving/197g	455	13.4	231	10.8	31.7	6.8	1.2
Cheese & Tomato, Deep Pan, Goodfella's*	¼ Pizza/102g	259	10.8	253	11.5	29.6	10.5	3.7
Cheese & Tomato, Deep Pan, Sainsbury's*	1 Pizza/182g	470	15.8	258	11.7	33.1	8.7	1.9
Cheese & Tomato, Everyday Value, Tesco*	1 Pizza/150g	423	9.2	282	9.6	46.0	6.1	2.2
Cheese & Tomato, French Bread, Co-Op*	1 Pizza/135g	270	8.1	200	9.0	27.0	6.0	2.0
Cheese & Tomato, Kids, Tesco*	1 Pizza/95g	219	5.2	231	11.5	33.9	5.5	1.9
Cheese & Tomato, Mini, Bruschetta, Iceland*	1 Pizza/34g	63	2.3	188	8.0	23.0	7.0	2.1
Cheese & Tomato, Slices, CBY, Asda*	1 Slice/14g	62	2.5	453	8.2	63.2	18.1	2.3
Cheese & Tomato, Smart Price, Asda*	1 Pizza/151g	393	7.6	260	4.7	27.0	5.0	1.6
Cheese & Tomato, Square, Sainsbury's*	1 Square/160g	435	11.7	272	14.0	37.6	7.3	2.1
Cheese & Tomato, Stonebaked, Co-Op*	1 Pizza/325g	699	26.0	215	10.0	26.0	8.0	3.0
Cheese & Tomato, Stonebaked, Thin & Crispy, Tesco*	½ Pizza/161g	388	13.8	241	11.6	29.4	8.6	2.1
Cheese & Tomato, Thin & Crispy, Asda*	1 Pizza/366g	827	36.6	226	11.0	23.0	10.0	2.0
Cheese & Tomato, Thin & Crispy, Carlos*	1 Pizza/155g	405	13.0	261	11.4	35.0	8.4	1.2
Cheese & Tomato, Thin & Crispy, Morrisons*	1 Pizza/335g	734	23.8	219	11.2	27.7	7.1	3.1
Cheese & Tomato, Thin & Crispy, Sainsbury's*	1 Serving/135g	344	10.0	255	14.9	32.2	7.4	5.0
Cheese & Tomato, Thin & Crispy, Stonebaked, Tesco*	1/3 Pizza/212g	509	19.5	240	10.1	29.2	9.2	1.4
Cheese & Tomato, Thin & Crispy, Waitrose*	1 Pizza/280g	658	28.3	235	12.3	23.6	10.1	2.3
Cheese Feast, Deep Crust, Carlos, Aldi*	1 Pizza/155g	432	14.9	279	9.7	37.3	9.6	2.1
Cheese Feast, Deep Pan, Asda*	½ Pizza/210g	422	18.9	201	13.0	17.0	9.0	2.3
Cheese Feast, Stuffed Crust, Take Away, Carlos, Aldi*	½ Pizza/238g	650	27.0	273	11.8	29.4	11.3	2.7
Cheese Feast, Thin Crust, Chilled, Tesco*	½ Pizza/175g	467	22.4	267	14.7	23.4	12.8	2.5
Cheese, Thin & Crispy, Goodfella's*	1 Serving/275g	729	27.8	265	15.7	27.6	10.1	1.8
Cheesefeast, Deep & Crispy 12", Takeaway, Iceland*	1 Slice/132g	342	11.1	259	13.1	32.8	8.4	1.5
Chicken & Bacon, Loaded, Tesco*	1 Serving/258g	622	25.3	241	12.8	25.4	9.8	1.9
Chicken & Bacon, Pizzeria, Italian, Sainsbury's*	½ Pizza/170g	508	24.1	300	13.6	29.4	14.2	2.7
Chicken & Chorizo, 12", TTD, Sainsbury's*	½ Pizza/290g	702	20.9	242	12.2	32.1	7.2	2.6
Chicken & Sweetcorn, Stonebaked, Tesco*	1 Serving/177g	354	9.6	200	11.9	26.0	5.4	2.0
Chicken Alfredo, Chicago Town*	1 Pizza/265g	583	24.9	220	11.9	21.9	9.4	1.8
Chicken Arrabiata, Italian Style, M&S*	½ Pizza/225g	495	15.8	220	12.3	26.3	7.0	2.0
Chicken Fajita, Stoneground, Carlos, Aldi*	½ Pizza/172g	382	11.2	222	11.0	29.0	6.5	2.5
Chicken Fajita, Thin & Crispy, Iceland*	1 Pizza/361g	729	21.3	202	9.6	26.5	5.9	1.8
Chicken Provencal, Goodfella's*	½ Pizza/143g	388	18.0	272	13.7	25.9	12.6	2.1
Chicken Tikka, Stonebaked, Tesco*	1 Serving/153g	326	10.4	213	10.7	27.3	6.8	1.3
Chicken, Thin & Crispy, Iceland*	½ Pizza/157g	469	19.9	299	13.0	33.2	12.7	3.1
Chilli Beef, Stone Bake, M&S*	1 Pizza/395g	790	22.9	200	9.6	26.7	5.8	1.9
Classic Italian, Stonebaked, Spinach & Ricotta, Tesco*	½ Pizza/190g	460	16.3	240	10.3	29.0	8.5	1.2
Diavolo Romano, Main, Supermarket, Pizza Express*	1 Pizza/477g	978	52.5	205	11.0	20.2	11.0	1.6
Diavolo, Pizza Express*	½ Pizza/164g	322	11.0	197	9.4	24.6	6.7	2.1
Double Pepperoni, Thin & Crispy, LBU, Co-Op*	½ Pizza/173g	389	18.9	225	10.5	27.3	10.9	3.4
Etruscan Pepperoni, TTD, Sainsbury's*	½ Pizza/252g	676	20.9	268	13.2	35.1	8.3	2.4
Fajita Chicken, 10 Inch, CBY, Asda*	½ Pizza/151g	319	9.8	211	10.7	26.3	6.5	2.4
Fajita Chicken, COU, M&S*	1 Pizza/255g	434	6.1	170	9.9	25.5	2.4	1.2
Fajita Chicken, Takeaway, Goodfella's*	¼ Pizza/150g	339	12.0	226	10.8	27.5	8.0	1.7
Fire Roasted Peppers & Vegetables, Waitrose*	½ Pizza/235g	442	16.7	188	9.8	21.3	7.1	2.7

P

PIZZA

	Measure INFO/WEIGHT	per Measure KCAL	FAT	Nutrition Values per 100g / 100ml KCAL	PROT	CARB	FAT	FIBRE
Flamed Chicken & Vegetables, BGTY, Sainsbury's*	1 Pizza/260g	660	11.4	254	14.2	39.3	4.4	2.3
Four Cheese, Deep Pan, Iceland*	1/3 Pizza/132g	337	12.1	255	11.3	30.6	9.2	2.6
Four Cheese, Finest, Tesco*	½ Pizza/230g	575	21.2	250	12.1	29.8	9.2	1.3
Four Cheese, Thin & Crispy, Iceland*	½ Pizza/148g	354	12.6	239	10.7	29.1	8.5	1.6
Four Cheese, Thin Crust, Tesco*	½ Pizza/142g	386	13.6	272	14.5	31.8	9.6	1.8
Four Cheese, Wood Fired, Iceland*	½ Pizza/129g	301	10.6	233	11.3	27.3	8.2	2.4
Four Seasons, Stonebaked, Truly Irresistible, Co-Op*	½ Pizza/245g	502	16.2	205	9.5	26.6	6.6	2.6
Four Seasons, Waitrose*	1/3 Pizza/174g	382	14.6	220	9.9	26.2	8.4	2.6
French Bread, Blue Parrot Cafe, Sainsbury's*	1 Pizza/132g	271	5.7	205	10.7	30.8	4.3	1.3
Frutti Di Mare, Express, Pizza Express*	1 Pizza/373g	500	9.5	134	9.1	20.1	2.6	0.0
Funghi, Ristorante, Dr Oetker*	1 Pizza/365g	847	43.4	232	7.6	22.5	11.9	1.8
Garlic & Mushroom, Asda*	½ Pizza/241g	696	41.0	289	10.0	24.0	17.0	1.6
Garlic Bread, Stonebaked, Italiano, Tesco*	1 Serving/117g	403	18.2	346	7.8	43.6	15.6	1.5
Garlic Chicken, Deep Pan, Sainsbury's*	½ Pizza/214g	464	13.9	217	11.2	28.3	6.5	3.3
Garlic Chicken, Thin & Crispy, Stonebake, Sainsbury's*	½ Pizza/160g	386	17.3	241	10.7	25.2	10.8	3.5
Garlic Mushroom, Classico, Tesco*	½ Pizza/208g	415	13.9	200	10.0	24.9	6.7	2.6
Giardiniera from Supermarket, Pizza Express*	½ Pizza/144g	291	10.5	202	8.6	25.5	7.3	2.1
Ham & Cheese, Ultra Thin, Sodebo*	1 Pizza/200g	400	8.6	200	11.3	29.1	4.3	0.0
Ham & Mushroom Slices, Farmfoods*	1 Slice/89g	170	2.3	191	8.0	34.0	2.6	0.9
Ham & Mushroom, Average	*1 Serving/250g*	*533*	*16.0*	*213*	*10.5*	*28.4*	*6.4*	*2.1*
Ham & Mushroom, Deep Pan, Waitrose*	½ Pizza/220g	453	13.6	206	10.9	26.6	6.2	1.0
Ham & Mushroom, Finest, Tesco*	½ Pizza/240g	576	26.4	240	9.5	25.9	11.0	2.2
Ham & Mushroom, Stone Baked, Goodfella's*	½ Pizza/175g	439	20.0	251	9.6	27.6	11.4	1.2
Ham & Mushroom, Thin & Crispy, Asda*	1 Pizza/360g	760	25.2	211	11.0	26.0	7.0	2.4
Ham & Pineapple Deep, Asda*	1 Pizza/486g	1055	22.4	217	11.3	32.5	4.6	3.0
Ham & Pineapple, Average	*1 Serving/250g*	*555*	*16.8*	*222*	*11.0*	*29.2*	*6.7*	*2.1*
Ham & Pineapple, Deep Dish, Individual, Chicago Town*	1 Pizza/170g	410	15.1	241	9.9	30.4	8.9	1.6
Ham & Pineapple, Deep Pan, Tesco*	1 Pizza/237g	437	6.9	184	9.8	29.8	2.9	1.9
Ham & Pineapple, Pizzerai, Simply Italian, Sainsbury's*	½ Pizza/178g	434	15.1	244	11.5	30.4	8.5	2.4
Ham & Pineapple, Stone Bake, M&S*	1 Pizza/345g	690	19.7	200	10.1	28.3	5.7	1.6
Ham & Pineapple, Stonebaked, Tesco*	1 Pizza/161g	293	9.2	182	9.2	23.5	5.7	3.5
Ham & Pineapple, Tesco*	1/6 Pizza/56g	134	4.6	240	10.4	30.9	8.3	2.1
Ham & Pineapple, Thin & Crispy Italian, Morrisons*	1 Pizza/375g	746	22.9	199	10.2	24.9	6.1	0.0
Ham & Pineapple, Thin & Crispy, 2 Pack, Sainsbury's*	1 Pizza/163g	417	13.2	256	13.8	32.0	8.1	1.7
Ham & Pineapple, Thin & Crispy, Goodfella's*	1 Serving/163g	333	12.7	204	10.6	22.8	7.8	2.4
Ham & Pineapple, Thin & Crispy, Iceland*	1 Serving/110g	301	13.1	274	9.9	31.9	11.9	3.0
Ham & Pineapple, Thin & Crispy, Iceland*	½ Pizza/172g	353	10.8	205	8.6	27.9	6.3	1.5
Ham & Pineapple, Thin & Crispy, Sainsbury's*	1 Pizza/330g	719	21.1	218	10.8	29.4	6.4	2.4
Ham & Pineapple, Thin Crust, Tesco*	½ Pizza/175g	385	10.0	220	12.3	29.6	5.7	2.5
Ham, Mushroom & Gruyere, Sainsbury's*	¼ Pizza/169g	404	13.7	239	10.2	31.3	8.1	3.7
Ham, Mushroom & Mascarpone, Italian Style, M&S*	1 Pizza/224g	515	21.7	230	10.0	25.5	9.7	2.9
Ham, Pepperoni & Milano, M&S*	1 Pizza/290g	696	28.4	240	14.0	23.3	9.8	1.1
Hawaiian, San Marco*	¼ Pizza/90g	208	8.3	231	8.9	29.7	9.2	1.5
Hawaiian, Thin Crust, Tesco*	½ Pizza/192g	365	9.4	190	10.3	25.6	4.9	1.8
Hickory Steak, M&S*	1 Pizza/400g	820	26.8	205	9.9	25.7	6.7	1.4
Honey Roast Salmon & Broccoli, BGTY, Sainsbury's*	1 Serving/280g	613	12.6	219	10.2	34.4	4.5	3.5
Hot & Spicy Chicken, Deep Pan, Morrisons*	½ Pizza/233g	521	13.0	224	10.5	32.9	5.6	1.0
Hot & Spicy Chicken, Deep Pan, Tesco*	½ Pizza/222g	423	7.3	191	10.5	30.0	3.3	2.1
Hot & Spicy, Pizzeria Style, Sainsbury's*	1 Pizza/376g	986	46.3	262	12.5	25.5	12.3	2.4
Hot & Spicy, Thin & Crispy, Morrisons*	½ Pizza/170g	393	15.8	231	10.5	26.5	9.3	3.2
Italian Meat Feast, Thin & Crispy, Waitrose*	1 Pizza/182g	477	22.9	262	10.7	26.5	12.6	1.8
Italian Meats, Finest, Tesco*	½ Pizza/217g	449	8.5	207	13.6	29.4	3.9	1.3
Italian Sausage & Roasted Peppers, Finest, Tesco*	1 Pizza/325g	650	13.6	200	7.8	31.7	4.2	1.9

PIZZA

INFO/WEIGHT	Measure	per Measure KCAL	FAT	Nutrition Values per 100g / 100ml KCAL	PROT	CARB	FAT	FIBRE
Le Reine, 8 Inch, Supermarket, Pizza Express*	1 Pizza/283g	546	16.4	193	10.2	25.0	5.8	2.7
Loaded Cheese, Goodfella's*	1 Pizza/410g	1115	49.6	272	11.4	29.4	12.1	1.7
Margherita, 12 Inch, Supermarket, Pizza Express*	½ Pizza/230g	494	13.8	215	10.1	28.3	6.0	3.6
Margherita, Average	**1 Slice/108g**	**239**	**8.6**	**239**	**11.0**	**30.5**	**8.6**	**1.2**
Margherita, Cheese & Tomato, San Marco*	½ Pizza/200g	454	14.4	227	10.7	29.8	7.2	1.2
Margherita, Classico, Tesco*	1 Serving/150g	342	11.4	228	11.3	28.5	7.6	1.8
Margherita, Finest, Tesco*	1 Serving/207g	441	10.8	213	11.0	30.5	5.2	1.2
Margherita, Italiano, Tesco*	1 Serving/173g	414	20.9	240	11.4	21.0	12.1	2.0
Margherita, Italiano, Tesco*	½ Pizza/168g	395	12.1	235	11.7	29.9	7.2	1.2
Margherita, Morrisons*	½ Pizza/163g	416	18.0	256	12.9	26.1	11.1	2.3
Margherita, Pizzeria, Italian, Sainsbury's*	½ Pizza/169g	426	17.4	253	12.2	27.9	10.3	2.5
Margherita, Stone Baked, Goodfella's*	1 Slice/36g	95	4.1	263	10.9	31.9	11.4	7.6
Margherita, Stonebaked, 10", Sainsbury's*	½ Pizza/139g	359	11.3	258	12.4	32.2	8.1	3.5
Margherita, Stonebaked, Co-Op*	1 Pizza/350g	840	29.1	240	13.2	27.6	8.3	3.0
Margherita, Thin & Crispy, Iceland*	½ Pizza/170g	391	14.4	230	12.7	25.9	8.5	2.8
Margherita, Thin Crust, Tesco*	1 Serving/170g	354	13.4	208	10.1	24.1	7.9	3.6
Margherita, Truly Irresistible, Co-Op*	1 Pizza/465g	1023	36.7	220	8.1	27.4	7.9	3.3
Meat Feast, Hot & Spicy, Thin & Crispy, Sainsbury's*	½ Pizza/170g	462	21.6	272	13.0	26.5	12.7	3.2
Meat Feast, Loaded, Deep Pan, Large, Tesco*	½ Pizza/282g	776	38.4	275	12.0	26.1	13.6	1.9
Meat Feast, Stuffed Crust, Asda*	½ Pizza/238g	597	24.0	251	14.6	25.5	10.1	3.1
Meat Feast, Thin & Crispy, Asda*	½ Pizza/183g	410	14.6	224	11.0	27.0	8.0	1.4
Meat Feast, Thin Crust, Tesco*	½ Pizza/178g	430	20.2	242	13.6	21.3	11.4	2.3
Mediterranean Vegetable, Pizzeria, Sainsbury's*	1 Serving/211g	397	13.5	188	8.0	24.7	6.4	3.2
Mediterranean Vegetable, Stonebaked, Sainsbury's*	½ Pizza/260g	622	16.4	239	9.8	35.7	6.3	3.1
Mini, Party, Tesco*	1 Pizza/11g	26	1.1	248	11.4	28.6	10.5	1.9
Mozzarella & Sunblush Tomato, 12", TTD, Sainsbury's*	½ Pizza/251g	638	17.8	254	12.4	35.0	7.1	2.6
Mozzarella, Ristorante, Dr Oetker*	1 Pizza/335g	874	44.6	261	10.4	23.9	13.3	1.7
Mushroom & Ham, COU, M&S*	1 Pizza/245g	355	4.4	145	8.8	24.0	1.8	2.2
Mushroom & Mascarpone, 12", TTD, Sainsbury's*	½ Pizza/255g	638	18.6	250	12.1	34.0	7.3	2.4
Mushroom & Roasted Onion, Waitrose*	½ Pizza/187g	403	12.6	215	9.8	28.9	6.7	1.3
Napoli Ham & Mushroom, San Marco*	½ Pizza/219g	449	13.4	205	10.0	27.5	6.1	2.8
Napoli, Tesco*	½ Pizza/184g	431	11.6	235	11.9	32.6	6.3	1.4
Pepperoni, Aldi*	1 Serving/55g	123	4.3	224	8.7	29.5	7.9	1.4
Pepperoni, Asda*	½ Pizza/150g	386	13.5	257	10.0	34.0	9.0	2.7
Pepperoni, Average	**1 Serving/250g**	**671**	**28.4**	**269**	**11.8**	**29.6**	**11.4**	**2.1**
Pepperoni, Deep Crust, Carlos, Aldi*	1 Pizza/162g	472	19.0	291	9.9	58.0	11.7	1.6
Pepperoni, Deep Pan, Frozen, Tesco*	½ Pizza/215g	527	17.4	245	11.9	31.1	8.1	2.6
Pepperoni, Deep Pan, Goodfella's*	¼ Pizza/109g	294	12.6	270	12.7	28.9	11.6	1.6
Pepperoni, Goodfella's*	1 Pizza/337g	900	43.5	267	13.2	26.3	12.9	1.7
Pepperoni, Hot & Spicy, Thin Crust, Chilled, Tesco*	½ Pizza/174g	486	25.5	280	12.4	24.0	14.7	2.2
Pepperoni, Italian, Tesco*	½ Pizza/186g	484	20.6	260	11.4	28.0	11.1	1.1
Pepperoni, Mini, Tesco*	1 Serving/22g	71	3.7	323	11.8	30.5	16.8	2.7
Pepperoni, Pizzeria Style, Sainsbury's*	½ Pizza/183g	515	23.3	281	13.5	28.0	12.7	2.2
Pepperoni, Stone Baked, Carlos*	1 Pizza/330g	832	39.6	252	13.0	23.0	12.0	0.0
Pepperoni, Stonebake, 10", Asda*	½ Pizza/170g	435	19.0	256	12.9	25.9	11.2	2.5
Pepperoni, Stonebaked, 12", Sainsbury's*	¼ Pizza/103g	301	13.3	292	13.2	29.2	12.9	3.1
Pepperoni, Stonebaked, American Hot, Sainsbury's*	½ Pizza/276g	674	30.9	244	11.6	24.1	11.2	2.9
Pepperoni, Thin & Crispy, Co-Op*	1 Pizza/270g	688	29.7	255	11.0	26.0	11.0	1.0
Pepperoni, Thin & Crispy, Essential, Waitrose*	½ Pizza/133g	380	18.0	286	12.3	28.8	13.5	1.0
Pepperoni, Thin & Crispy, Goodfella's*	1 Pizza/593g	1595	70.0	269	13.8	26.9	11.8	2.3
Pepperoni, Thin & Crispy, Sainsbury's*	½ Pizza/132g	405	18.9	307	13.9	30.7	14.3	2.6
Pepperoni, Thin Crust, Chilled, Tesco*	½ Pizza/163g	479	24.4	295	13.5	25.4	15.0	1.8
Pollo Ad Astra, Pizza Express*	1 Pizza/317g	602	14.9	190	11.6	25.2	4.7	2.7

	INFO/WEIGHT	KCAL	FAT	KCAL	PROT	CARB	FAT	FIBRE
PIZZA								
Pollo Pesto, Supermarket, Pizza Express*	1 Pizza/265g	500	10.1	189	9.2	25.0	3.8	2.0
Pollo, Ristorante, As Sold, Dr Oetker*	½ Pizza/183g	408	16.5	223	8.8	25.7	9.0	1.8
Prosciutto, Classico, Tesco*	½ Pizza/205g	461	10.0	225	11.7	33.6	4.9	2.5
Prosciutto, Italian Style, Co-Op*	½ Pizza/183g	421	12.8	230	13.0	29.0	7.0	3.0
Prosciutto, Ristorante, Dr Oetker*	1 Pizza/330g	752	32.3	228	10.3	24.6	9.8	0.0
Quattro Formaggi, 8 Inch, Supermarket, Pizza Express*	1 Pizza/266g	646	26.1	243	12.1	26.5	9.8	2.3
Quattro Formaggi, Ristorante, Dr Oetker*	½ Pizza/170g	457	23.8	269	10.8	24.1	14.0	1.6
Salame, Ristorante, Dr Oetker*	½ Pizza/160g	455	24.5	285	10.4	26.3	15.3	0.0
Salami & Ham, Pizzeria, Waitrose*	½ Pizza/205g	443	13.7	216	10.1	28.7	6.7	1.8
Salami, Lidl*	1 Pizza/350g	854	32.2	244	8.1	29.4	9.2	0.0
Salami, Ultra Thin Italian, Tesco*	1 Serving/263g	692	25.5	263	12.0	31.9	9.7	1.0
Slice Selection, M&S*	1 Serving/52g	120	4.1	230	9.4	30.3	7.8	1.9
Sloppy Joe, Take Away, Chicago Town*	¼ Pizza/158g	374	12.6	237	8.2	26.1	8.0	2.1
Smoked Ham & Mushroom, Thin & Crispy, Co-Op*	1 Pizza/400g	792	18.0	198	9.0	30.3	4.5	1.7
Smoked Ham & Pineapple, Deep Pan, Co-Op*	1 Pizza/395g	1142	41.9	289	11.6	36.7	10.6	1.7
Smoked Ham & Pineapple, Weight Watchers*	1 Pizza/241g	429	7.0	178	10.3	27.6	2.9	1.5
Spicy Beef, Goodfella's*	½ Pizza/148g	391	17.8	265	12.4	26.5	12.1	2.2
Spicy Chicken, BBQ, Deep Pan, Asda*	1 Pizza/476g	1033	25.2	217	10.9	31.4	5.3	0.0
Spicy Chicken, Foccacia, Sainsbury's*	½ Pizza/245g	581	18.6	237	12.0	30.3	7.6	2.5
Spicy Chicken, Iceland*	1 Pizza/345g	797	22.8	231	13.4	29.9	6.6	1.5
Spicy Chorizo, Red Pepper & Chilli, Classico, Tesco*	1 Serving/218g	474	17.4	218	10.3	26.4	8.0	2.5
Spinach & Ricotta, BGTY, Sainsbury's*	1 Pizza/265g	535	6.6	202	10.4	34.4	2.5	2.6
Spinach & Ricotta, ES, Asda*	1 Pizza/400g	940	28.0	235	9.0	34.0	7.0	1.9
Spinach & Ricotta, Italian, Chilled, Sainsbury's*	1 Pizza/361g	859	34.7	238	9.3	28.7	9.6	2.3
Spinach & Ricotta, Pizzaria, Waitrose*	½ Pizza/238g	501	21.1	211	10.7	21.9	8.9	2.6
Spinach & Ricotta, Thin Crust, Italian, Tesco*	½ Pizza/190g	365	16.7	192	9.6	18.7	8.8	1.9
Supreme, Deep Dish, Individual, Chicago Town*	1 Pizza/170g	456	20.4	268	9.2	30.8	12.0	1.0
Supreme, McCain*	1 Serving/125g	267	8.6	214	10.9	27.0	6.9	0.0
Three Cheese, Ultra Thin, Sodebo*	1 Pizza/180g	450	18.4	250	10.9	28.5	10.2	1.8
Three Cheeses & Tomato, Stonebaked, Co-Op*	1 Pizza/415g	888	33.6	214	10.0	25.2	8.1	1.5
Tomato	1oz/28g	54	3.0	193	3.3	22.6	10.6	1.4
Tomato & Cheese, Stone Bake, M&S*	1 Pizza/340g	782	28.6	230	10.8	30.1	8.4	1.6
Tomato & Cheese, Thin & Crispy, M&S*	1 Pizza/300g	705	28.2	235	11.0	27.7	9.4	1.2
Tomato & Pesto, Tesco*	1 Serving/176g	449	23.2	256	8.4	25.9	13.2	1.1
Tomato, Aubergine & Spinach, Pizzeria, Waitrose*	½ Pizza/193g	403	7.7	209	7.8	35.4	4.0	3.6
Tomato, Mushroom & Bacon, Deep Pan, Co-Op*	1 Pizza/420g	882	33.6	210	9.0	25.0	8.0	2.0
Triple Cheese, Deep Dish, Chicago Town*	1 Serving/170g	418	18.2	246	9.9	27.6	10.7	0.0
Triple Cheese, Deep Pan, Morrisons*	1/6 Pizza/75g	198	9.2	265	10.4	28.2	12.3	1.9
Tuna & Caramelised Red Onion, COU, M&S*	1 Pizza/245g	429	5.6	175	9.6	26.7	2.3	1.2
Tuna Sweetcorn, BGTY, Sainsbury's*	1 Pizza/304g	602	5.8	198	13.5	31.7	1.9	2.7
Vegetable Feast, Thin & Crispy, Iceland*	1 Slice/63g	148	6.9	237	7.8	26.5	11.1	1.8
Vegetable, Average	***1 Serving/250g***	***475***	***13.1***	***190***	***8.2***	***27.5***	***5.2***	***2.4***
Vegetable, COU, M&S*	1 Pizza/294g	397	7.1	135	6.4	23.2	2.4	1.9
Vegetable, Deep Pan, Co-Op*	1 Pizza/425g	829	29.8	195	8.0	25.0	7.0	2.0
Vegetable, Frozen, HL, Tesco*	1 Pizza/400g	604	10.8	151	8.1	23.5	2.7	4.4
Vegetable, GFY, Asda*	¼ Pizza/94g	141	2.7	150	7.0	24.0	2.9	3.7
Vegetable, Ristorante, Dr Oetker*	½ Pizza/185g	386	16.6	209	8.1	23.9	9.0	0.0
PIZZA BASE								
Deep Pan, Italian, Sainsbury's*	1 Base/220g	684	11.0	311	7.0	59.5	5.0	1.4
Everyday Value, Tesco*	½ Base/125g	401	2.8	320	9.6	65.2	2.2	0.7
Garlic Bread, Sainsbury's*	¼ Base/59g	109	4.2	186	5.1	25.4	7.1	1.8
Italian, Classic, Sainsbury's*	1 Base/150g	452	7.2	301	7.6	57.0	4.8	1.5
Light & Crispy, Napolina*	1 Base/150g	436	4.5	291	7.9	58.0	3.0	0.2

	Measure INFO/WEIGHT	per Measure KCAL	FAT	Nutrition Values per 100g / 100ml KCAL	PROT	CARB	FAT	FIBRE
PIZZA BASE								
Mini, Napolina*	1 Base/75g	218	2.2	291	7.9	58.0	3.0	0.2
Thin & Crispy, Sainsbury's*	1 Base/150g	504	7.8	336	9.9	62.3	5.2	4.3
Thin & Crispy, Tesco*	1 Serving/110g	348	8.2	316	9.2	52.9	7.5	1.5
PIZZA BASE MIX								
Sainsbury's*	1 Pack/145g	486	5.5	335	12.8	62.3	3.8	2.9
PLAICE								
Fillets in Breadcrumbs, Average	*1 Serving/150g*	*331*	*17.9*	*221*	*12.8*	*15.5*	*11.9*	*0.8*
Fillets, Garlic & Herb Dusted, Gastro, Youngs*	1 Fillet/106g	200	10.4	189	13.4	11.5	9.8	0.7
Fillets, Lightly Dusted, Average	*1 Fillet/113g*	*188*	*9.2*	*166*	*12.9*	*10.4*	*8.2*	*0.6*
Fillets, Raw, Average	*1oz/28g*	*24*	*0.4*	*87*	*18.2*	*0.0*	*1.5*	*0.0*
Fillets, with Spinach & Cheddar Cheese, Sainsbury's*	1 Serving/154g	222	13.3	144	13.6	3.1	8.6	0.8
Goujons, Baked	1oz/28g	85	5.1	304	8.8	27.7	18.3	0.0
Goujons, Fried in Blended Oil	1oz/28g	119	9.0	426	8.5	27.0	32.3	0.0
Goujons, Oven Baked, Gastro, Youngs*	½ Pack/119g	296	13.6	249	13.0	22.5	11.4	2.3
Grilled	*1oz/28g*	*27*	*0.5*	*96*	*20.1*	*0.0*	*1.7*	*0.0*
in Batter, Fried in Blended Oil	1oz/28g	72	4.7	257	15.2	12.0	16.8	0.5
Steamed	*1oz/28g*	*26*	*0.5*	*93*	*18.9*	*0.0*	*1.9*	*0.0*
Whole, with Spinach & Ricotta Cheese, Sainsbury's*	1 Serving/159g	334	16.7	210	11.6	17.2	10.5	0.8
with Mushrooms & Prawns, Sainsbury's*	1 Serving/170g	354	18.2	208	12.0	15.9	10.7	1.7
PLANTAIN								
Boiled in Unsalted Water	*1oz/28g*	*31*	*0.1*	*112*	*0.8*	*28.5*	*0.2*	*1.2*
Raw, Average	*1 Med/179g*	*218*	*0.7*	*122*	*1.3*	*31.9*	*0.4*	*2.3*
Ripe, Fried in Vegetable Oil	*1oz/28g*	*75*	*2.6*	*267*	*1.5*	*47.5*	*9.2*	*2.3*
PLUMS								
Average, Stewed without Sugar	*1oz/28g*	*8*	*0.0*	*30*	*0.5*	*7.3*	*0.1*	*1.3*
Fresh, Raw, Weighed without Stone, Average	*1 Plum/66g*	*24*	*0.1*	*36*	*0.6*	*8.6*	*0.1*	*1.9*
Fresh, Sweet & Juicy, Oaklands, Lidl*	1 Serving/80g	34	0.1	42	0.6	8.8	0.1	1.6
Soft Dried, Blue Parrot Cafe, Sainsbury's*	1 Pack/50g	118	0.2	237	2.6	55.6	0.5	7.1
Weighed with Stone, Average	*1 Plum/90g*	*31*	*0.1*	*34*	*0.5*	*8.1*	*0.1*	*1.8*
Yellow, Waitrose*	1 Plum/50g	20	0.0	39	0.6	8.8	0.1	1.5
POLENTA								
Dry, Merchant Gourmet*	1 Serving/65g	232	0.9	357	7.4	78.8	1.4	1.3
POLLOCK								
Alaskan, Value, Tesco*	1 Serving/200g	150	1.2	75	16.6	0.0	0.6	0.0
Breaded, Asda*	1 Serving/97g	200	9.7	206	12.0	17.0	10.0	1.0
Fillets, Breaded, Cooked, Tesco*	1 Fillet/125g	315	12.2	250	15.0	24.4	9.7	2.0
Fillets, British, Sainsbury's*	1 Pack/218g	157	1.3	72	16.6	0.0	0.6	0.0
POLO								
Fruits, Nestle*	1 Tube/37g	142	0.0	383	0.0	96.0	0.0	0.0
Mints, Original, Nestle*	1 Sweet/2g	8	0.0	402	0.0	98.2	1.0	0.0
Spearmint, Nestle*	1 Tube/35g	141	0.4	402	0.0	98.2	1.1	0.0
POMEGRANATE								
Fresh, Good to Go, Waitrose*	1 Pack/110g	101	1.3	92	1.7	18.7	1.2	4.0
Raw, Fresh, Flesh Only, Average	*1 Sm Fruit/86g*	*59*	*0.3*	*68*	*1.0*	*17.2*	*0.3*	*0.6*
Raw, Weighed with Rind & Skin, Average	*1 Sm Fruit/154g*	*59*	*0.3*	*38*	*0.5*	*9.6*	*0.2*	*0.0*
Snack Pot, Morrisons*	1 Pot/100g	38	0.1	38	0.9	7.3	0.1	2.2
POMELO								
Fresh, Raw, Weighed with Skin & Seeds	*100 Grams/100g*	*11*	*0.1*	*11*	*0.2*	*2.5*	*0.1*	*0.0*
Raw, Flesh Only, Average	*1 Fruit/340g*	*129*	*0.1*	*38*	*0.8*	*9.6*	*0.0*	*1.0*
POP TARTS								
Chocolate Chip Cookie Dough, Kellogg's*	1 Pastry/50g	190	5.0	380	4.0	70.0	10.0	2.0
Chocolate, Kellogg's*	1 Pastry/50g	198	8.5	396	5.0	136.0	17.0	2.0
Cinnamon Roll, Kelloggs*	1 Pastry/50g	210	7.0	420	4.0	68.0	14.0	2.0

	Measure INFO/WEIGHT	per Measure		Nutrition Values per 100g / 100ml				
		KCAL	FAT	KCAL	PROT	CARB	FAT	FIBRE
POP TARTS								
Frosted Cherry, Kellogg's*	1 Pastry/52g	200	5.0	385	3.8	73.1	9.6	2.3
Frosted Raspberry, Kellogg's*	1 Pastry/52g	200	5.0	385	3.8	73.1	9.6	1.9
Strawberry Sensation, Kellogg's*	1 Tart/50g	198	5.5	395	4.0	70.0	11.0	2.0
POPCORN								
Air Popped, Plain, Average	*1 Sm Bag/17g*	*66*	*0.8*	*387*	*12.9*	*77.9*	*4.5*	*14.5*
Butter Flavour, Microwave, Popz*	1 Serving/100g	480	27.5	480	7.5	51.1	27.5	9.2
Butter Toffee, Asda*	1 Serving/100g	364	8.0	364	2.1	71.0	8.0	4.1
Butter Toffee, Belgian Milk Chocolate Coated, M&S*	1 Pack/100g	505	25.0	505	6.5	60.4	25.0	4.1
Butter Toffee, Tesco*	1 Pack/175g	709	13.5	405	2.2	81.7	7.7	4.3
Butter, Microwave, 94% Fat Free, Act II*	½ Bag/41g	130	2.5	317	9.8	68.3	6.1	12.2
Butter, Microwave, Butterkist*	1 Bag/100g	395	18.5	395	8.3	49.5	18.5	8.5
Choc Full of, Cadbury*	¼ Bag/32g	160	7.6	495	4.5	64.5	23.5	2.9
Chocolate & Pecan, M&S*	1 Pack/27g	130	5.2	480	3.3	72.9	19.3	3.6
Chocolate Trickle, Skinny, Topcorn, Metcalfe's Food Co*	1 Pack/55g	221	8.4	401	5.2	59.6	15.2	7.1
Chocolate, Toffee, Snack-A-Jacks, Quaker Oats*	1 Bag/35g	126	3.4	359	2.2	65.0	9.8	3.0
Maple, Shapers, Boots*	1 Bag/20g	94	3.6	469	12.0	59.0	18.0	10.0
Organic Amaranth*	1 Serving/10g	36	0.9	365	14.6	26.8	8.8	0.0
Plain, Oil Popped, Average	*1 Bag/74g*	*439*	*31.7*	*593*	*6.2*	*48.7*	*42.8*	*0.0*
Popping Corn, Average	*1 Serving/30g*	*112*	*1.3*	*375*	*10.9*	*73.1*	*4.3*	*12.7*
Popping Corn, Lightly Salted, Graze*	1 Punnet/28g	127	7.0	454	8.0	44.0	25.0	13.0
Popping Corn, Slightly Sweet, Graze*	1 Punnet/23g	95	3.6	415	8.1	55.9	15.5	13.3
Ready Salted, Microwave, Popz*	1 Serving/20g	101	6.0	504	7.0	51.5	30.0	9.2
Salt & Sweet, Pure*	1 Serving/25g	119	5.5	476	6.0	61.1	22.1	7.8
Salt & Vinegar, Diet Chef Ltd*	1 Serving/23g	106	3.6	461	10.4	69.8	15.8	13.0
Salt & Vinegar, Snack-A-Jacks, Quaker Oats*	1 Sm Pack/13g	47	1.3	360	12.0	55.0	9.9	14.0
Salted, Blockbuster*	1 Bowl/25g	99	2.9	397	10.6	62.2	11.7	8.6
Salted, Diet Chef Ltd*	1 Pack/23g	107	3.8	465	10.5	68.6	16.6	14.0
Salted, Light, Microwave, Act II*	1 Pack/85g	336	6.5	395	10.6	71.0	7.6	15.8
Salted, M&S*	1 Pack/25g	132	7.8	530	9.4	50.4	31.1	6.4
Salted, Manhatten Peanuts Limited*	1 Bag/30g	135	4.3	450	10.0	70.0	14.3	13.7
Salted, Sold At Cinema, Playtime Popcorn*	1 Sm Serving/74g	384	24.9	519	8.3	45.9	33.6	0.0
Sea Salt Flavour, Skinny, Topcorn, Metcalfe's Food Co*	1 Pack/23g	108	5.6	471	6.6	63.7	24.4	15.2
Super, Perri*	1 Pack/30g	139	7.0	464	8.4	55.5	23.2	8.5
Sweet & Salted Microwave Popcorn, Butterkist*	½ Bag/30g	119	4.2	398	9.0	48.1	13.9	22.1
Sweet & Salty, Propercorn*	1 Pack/30g	128	4.2	428	5.9	63.5	13.9	12.7
Sweet & Salty, Shapers, Boots*	1 Bag/20g	89	3.2	443	5.8	65.0	16.0	10.0
Sweet Maple, Diet Chef Ltd*	1 Pack/23g	111	3.6	483	9.7	75.2	15.7	13.0
Sweet, Butterkist, Butterkist*	1 Pack/120g	612	29.8	510	2.8	68.5	24.8	5.6
Sweet, Cinema Style, Butterkist*	1 Bag/120g	612	29.8	510	2.8	68.5	24.8	5.6
Sweet, Microwave, Butterkist*	½ Pack/50g	235	10.0	470	9.8	60.5	20.1	4.4
Sweet, Microwave, Cinema, Popz*	1 Bag/85g	420	21.7	494	6.0	60.0	25.5	8.2
Toffee, Butterkist*	1 Bag/30g	124	3.0	415	2.3	79.3	10.0	4.4
Toffee, Milk Chocolate Coated, Sainsbury's*	¼ Bag/25g	130	6.6	520	6.5	64.1	26.4	1.3
Toffee, Snack Pack, Butterkist*	1 Bag/25g	105	2.2	420	2.1	81.3	9.0	3.5
Twist of Black Pepper, Graze*	1 Punnet/28g	127	7.0	452	8.0	44.0	25.0	13.0
Vanilla, Cinema Sweet Microwave, Act II*	½ Pack/50g	234	8.0	468	9.0	71.0	16.0	12.0
Wasabi Flavour, Skinny, Topcorn, Metcalfe's Food Co*	1 Bag/25g	121	6.6	484	8.4	54.1	26.2	9.7
Wasabi, Pret a Manger*	1 Pack/29g	137	6.4	472	7.2	55.2	22.1	10.7
White Cheddar Cheese, Manhatten Peanuts Limited*	1 Bag/30g	132	4.1	440	10.0	70.0	13.7	13.0
Yellow, Kernel, (Unpopped), Jolly Time*	2 Tbsp/33g	110	1.0	333	12.1	78.8	3.0	21.2
POPPADOMS								
Cracked Black Pepper, Ready to Eat, Sharwood's*	1 Poppadom/9g	41	2.4	461	16.7	37.2	27.3	7.3
Fried in Vegetable Oil, Takeaway, Average	*1 Poppadom/13g*	*65*	*5.0*	*501*	*11.5*	*28.3*	*38.8*	*5.8*

P

	Measure INFO/WEIGHT	per Measure KCAL	FAT	Nutrition Values per 100g / 100ml KCAL	PROT	CARB	FAT	FIBRE
POPPADOMS								
Garlic & Coriander, Ready to Eat, Sharwood's*	1 Popppadom/9g	39	1.9	438	18.4	43.0	21.4	6.5
Indian, Asda*	1 Pack/45g	232	15.7	516	14.5	36.2	34.8	7.8
Mini, Sainsbury's*	½ Pack/50g	249	16.2	498	14.9	36.9	32.3	7.6
Plain, Asda*	1 Poppadom/9g	44	2.5	484	18.0	40.0	28.0	0.0
Plain, Bilash, Aldi*	1 Poppadom/10g	46	2.2	463	15.2	48.7	22.3	0.0
Plain, Cook to Eat, Sharwood's*	1 Poppadom/12g	32	0.1	273	21.9	45.7	1.0	10.1
Plain, Indian to Go, Sainsbury's*	1 Poppadom/8g	34	1.5	405	18.4	43.4	17.5	9.0
Plain, Ready to Eat, Sharwood's*	1 Poppadom/8g	37	1.8	461	19.4	46.3	22.0	5.6
Plain, Tesco*	1 Poppadom/9g	41	2.0	439	17.8	44.4	21.1	4.6
Plain, Waitrose*	1 Poppadom/9g	37	1.7	408	21.0	39.3	18.6	9.1
Spicy, Cook to Eat, Sharwood's*	1 Popppadom/12g	30	0.1	257	20.2	43.0	0.5	13.0
Spicy, COU, M&S*	1 Pack/26g	84	0.6	325	23.5	51.9	2.4	8.1
Tesco*	1 Poppadom/9g	39	1.9	440	17.8	44.4	21.1	4.6
POPPETS*								
Chocolate Raisins, Poppets*	1 Pack/35g	140	4.7	401	4.9	65.4	13.3	0.0
Mint Cream, Poppets*	1oz/28g	119	3.6	424	2.0	75.0	13.0	0.0
Peanut, Poppets*	1 Box/100g	544	37.0	544	16.4	37.0	37.0	0.0
Toffee, Milk Chocolate, Poppets*	1 Box/100g	491	23.0	491	5.3	68.0	23.0	0.0
PORK								
& Apricots, Aromatic, Cafe Culture, M&S*	½ Pack/420g	672	31.1	160	10.3	12.5	7.4	2.1
Belly, Fresh, Raw, Weighed with Skin, Average	**1 Serving/100g**	**518**	**53.0**	**518**	**9.3**	**0.0**	**53.0**	**0.0**
Belly, Roasted, Lean & Fat	1oz/28g	82	6.0	293	25.1	0.0	21.4	0.0
Belly, Slow Cooked, Waitrose*	1 Serving/225g	590	45.9	262	17.3	2.2	20.4	0.0
Chop, Lean & Fat, Boneless, Raw, Average	**1oz/28g**	**67**	**3.8**	**240**	**29.2**	**0.0**	**13.7**	**0.0**
Chopped, Canned, Pek*	1 Can/240g	497	37.2	207	16.9	0.1	15.5	0.0
Diced, Lean, Average	**1oz/28g**	**31**	**0.5**	**109**	**22.0**	**0.0**	**1.8**	**0.0**
Escalope, Average	**1 Escalope/75g**	**108**	**1.7**	**144**	**31.0**	**0.0**	**2.2**	**0.0**
Escalope, Lean, Healthy Range, Average	**1 Escalope/75g**	**80**	**1.5**	**106**	**22.0**	**0.0**	**2.0**	**0.0**
Escalope, Tangy Gruyere & Mustard Crust, Waitrose*	1 Escalope/122g	239	10.7	196	19.8	9.3	8.8	0.8
Joint with Crackling, Ready to Roast, Average	**1 Joint/567g**	**1283**	**80.1**	**226**	**24.2**	**0.8**	**14.1**	**0.0**
Joint, Ready to Roast, Average	**½ Joint/254g**	**375**	**18.0**	**148**	**19.2**	**2.3**	**7.1**	**0.2**
Leg, Joint, Healthy Range, Average	**1 Serving/200g**	**206**	**4.4**	**103**	**20.0**	**0.6**	**2.2**	**0.0**
Loin, Applewood Smoked, Asda*	1 Slice/15g	18	0.5	122	21.8	0.5	3.6	0.0
Loin, Chops, Boneless, Grilled, Average	**1oz/28g**	**83**	**4.1**	**298**	**27.0**	**0.0**	**14.6**	**0.0**
Loin, Chops, Grilled, Lean	**1oz/28g**	**52**	**1.8**	**184**	**31.6**	**0.0**	**6.4**	**0.0**
Loin, Chops, Raw, Lean & Fat, Weighed with Bone	**1 Chop/130g**	**248**	**19.9**	**191**	**13.2**	**0.0**	**15.3**	**0.0**
Loin, Joint, Roast, Lean	**1oz/28g**	**51**	**1.9**	**182**	**30.1**	**0.0**	**6.8**	**0.0**
Loin, Joint, Roasted, Lean & Fat	**1oz/28g**	**71**	**4.3**	**253**	**26.3**	**0.0**	**15.3**	**0.0**
Loin, Joint, Salt & Pepper, Butchers Selection, Asda*	1 Serving/100g	333	24.2	333	27.4	1.1	24.2	0.5
Loin, Medallions, Extra Lean, Ashfield Farm*	1 Pack/400g	468	9.6	117	24.0	0.5	2.4	0.5
Loin, Roasted with Rosemary, Arista, Sainsbury's*	1 Slice/17g	24	1.2	144	20.8	0.1	6.8	0.7
Loin, Steak, Fried, Lean	**1oz/28g**	**53**	**2.0**	**191**	**31.5**	**0.0**	**7.2**	**0.0**
Loin, Steak, Fried, Lean & Fat	**1oz/28g**	**77**	**5.2**	**276**	**27.5**	**0.0**	**18.4**	**0.0**
Loin, Steak, Lean, Raw, Average	**1 Serving/175g**	**345**	**19.6**	**197**	**22.7**	**0.0**	**11.2**	**0.4**
Loin, Stuffed, Roast, M&S*	1 Slice/12g	22	0.9	180	24.4	2.4	7.9	0.0
Loin, Sweet Cured, Sliced, Tesco*	1 Slice/12g	17	0.5	141	23.0	2.1	4.4	0.5
Medallions, Average	**1 Medallion/125g**	**140**	**2.6**	**112**	**22.6**	**0.0**	**2.0**	**0.0**
Mince, Lean, Healthy Range, Average	**1 Pack/400g**	**504**	**20.2**	**126**	**19.8**	**0.4**	**5.0**	**0.3**
Mince, Raw	**1oz/28g**	**46**	**2.7**	**164**	**19.2**	**0.0**	**9.7**	**0.0**
Mince, Stewed	**1oz/28g**	**53**	**2.9**	**191**	**24.4**	**0.0**	**10.4**	**0.0**
Pulled, with BBQ Sauce, Shoulder, British, Sainsburys*	1 Serving/120g	290	18.1	242	24.6	1.6	15.1	0.5
Rashers, Streaky, British, Sainsbury's*	1 Serving/100g	320	23.4	320	27.4	0.0	23.4	0.0
Raw, Lean, Average	**1oz/28g**	**42**	**1.2**	**151**	**28.6**	**0.0**	**4.1**	**0.0**

	Measure INFO/WEIGHT	per Measure KCAL	FAT	Nutrition Values per 100g / 100ml KCAL	PROT	CARB	FAT	FIBRE
PORK								
Roast, Lean Only, Average	*1oz/28g*	*34*	*0.9*	*121*	*22.7*	*0.3*	*3.3*	*0.0*
Roast, Slices, Average	*1 Slice/30g*	*40*	*1.4*	*134*	*22.7*	*0.4*	*4.5*	*0.0*
Shoulder Steak, Boneless, Frozen, (Grilled), Tesco*	1 Steak/125g	156	4.9	125	0.0	0.0	3.9	0.0
Shoulder, Slices, Cured	*1oz/28g*	*29*	*1.0*	*103*	*16.9*	*0.9*	*3.6*	*0.0*
Shoulder, Whole, Lean & Fat, Raw, Average	*100g*	*236*	*18.0*	*236*	*17.2*	*0.0*	*18.0*	*0.0*
Shoulder, Whole, Lean Only, Roasted	1 Serving/150g	345	20.3	230	25.3	0.0	13.5	0.0
Slow Cooked with Smoked Chilli Beans, HL, Tesco*	1 Pack/365g	256	4.7	70	6.6	8.0	1.3	2.5
Steak, Lean & Fat, Average	*1oz/28g*	*61*	*3.8*	*219*	*23.8*	*0.0*	*13.7*	*0.1*
Steak, Lean, Stewed	*1oz/28g*	*49*	*1.3*	*176*	*33.6*	*0.0*	*4.6*	*0.0*
Stir Fry Strips, Lean, Healthy Range, Average	*¼ Pack/113g*	*118*	*2.3*	*104*	*21.3*	*0.0*	*2.0*	*0.0*
Tenderloin, Lean, Boneless, Raw, Average	*1 Serving/100g*	*109*	*2.2*	*109*	*21.0*	*0.0*	*2.2*	*0.0*
PORK CHAR SUI								
in Cantonese Sauce, Asda*	1 Pack/360g	623	7.9	173	9.8	28.4	2.2	0.5
Takeaway, Iceland*	1 Pack/400g	412	9.6	103	7.9	12.5	2.4	1.2
with Chicken & Egg Fried Rice, Tesco*	1 Serving/450g	602	16.2	134	7.1	18.3	3.6	0.9
PORK DINNER								
Roast, 103, Oakhouse Foods Ltd*	1 Dinner/400g	376	14.8	94	6.7	8.3	3.7	1.4
Roast, Birds Eye*	1 Pack/340g	410	12.0	121	7.6	14.7	3.5	1.6
PORK IN								
Light Mustard Sauce, Fillets, COU, M&S*	1 Pack/390g	312	9.4	80	10.9	3.5	2.4	0.7
Mustard & Cream, Chops	1oz/28g	73	6.0	261	14.5	2.4	21.6	0.3
PORK SCRATCHINGS								
Crunch, Mr Porky*	1 Pack/30g	159	9.6	531	60.4	0.5	31.9	4.6
Tavern Snacks*	1 Pack/30g	187	14.4	624	47.3	0.5	48.1	0.5
PORK WITH								
Crispy Garlic Infused Potatoes, Belly, Gastropub, M&S*	½ Pack/335g	616	38.2	184	13.8	5.8	11.4	1.7
Leek & Bacon Stuffing, Roast, Shoulder, Sainsbury's*	1 Serving/150g	237	12.5	158	18.8	2.4	8.3	0.5
Medallions with Bramley Apple, M&S*	1 Serving/380g	418	12.9	110	17.7	2.5	3.4	0.5
Noodles, Chinese, Tesco*	1 Serving/450g	464	13.5	103	5.3	13.7	3.0	1.4
Peppers, Marinated, Tapas, Waitrose*	1 Serving/105g	181	6.7	172	26.3	2.2	6.4	0.3
Rice & Beans, Jerk, LL, Waitrose*	1 Pack/380g	384	12.2	101	4.9	13.0	3.2	2.1
Sage & Onion Stuffing, Joint, Tesco*	1 Serving/200g	208	5.6	104	17.1	2.7	2.8	0.0
Spiced Apple Stuffing, Steaks, Easy Cook, Waitrose*	1 Serving/190g	237	7.8	124	19.3	2.4	4.1	0.5
Tomato & Apricot Sauce, Loin Steaks, Sainsbury's*	½ Pack/110g	216	10.6	196	24.4	3.1	9.6	0.6
PORT								
Average	*1 Serving/50ml*	*78*	*0.0*	*157*	*0.1*	*12.0*	*0.0*	*0.0*
POT NOODLE*								
Beef & Tomato, King, Made Up, Pot Noodle*	1 Pot/420g	543	19.8	129	3.3	18.5	4.7	1.1
Beef & Tomato, Made Up, Pot Noodle*	1 Pot/320g	426	14.7	133	3.4	19.4	4.6	1.3
Bombay Bad Boy, King, Made Up,,Pot Noodle*	1 Pot/420g	542	19.7	129	3.3	18.5	4.7	1.1
Bombay Bad Boy, Made Up, Pot Noodle*	1 Pot/320g	415	15.3	130	3.3	18.4	4.8	1.1
Chicken & Mushroom, Made Up, Pot Noodle*	1 Pot/305g	430	18.0	141	3.0	19.0	5.9	1.0
Chilli Beef, Made Up, Pot Noodle*	1 Pot/305g	384	14.6	126	3.0	17.7	4.8	0.8
Chow Mein Chinese, Made Up, Pot Noodle*	1 Pot/320g	416	14.7	130	3.2	19.0	4.6	1.3
Curry, Balti, Made Up, Pot Noodle*	1 Pot/301g	268	1.5	89	3.1	17.8	0.5	0.5
Curry, Original, King, Made Up, Pot Noodle*	1 Pot/420g	507	18.1	121	2.6	17.9	4.3	1.0
Curry, Original, Made Up, Pot Noodle*	1 Pot/320g	431	15.0	135	3.1	20.0	4.7	1.2
Curry, Spicy, Made Up, Pot Noodle*	1 Pot/300g	393	14.4	131	2.9	19.1	4.8	1.1
Jamaican Jerk, Made Up, Pot Noodle*	1 Pot/310g	430	15.4	140	3.0	21.0	5.0	1.5
Piri Piri Chicken, Made Up, Pot Noodle*	1 Pot/307g	430	15.4	140	3.0	20.0	5.0	0.0
Sweet & Sour, Oriental, Posh, Made Up, Pot Noodle*	1 Pot/300g	375	13.8	125	1.7	19.2	4.6	0.5
POTATO BOMBAY								
Average	*½ Pack/150g*	*176*	*10.2*	*117*	*2.0*	*13.7*	*6.8*	*1.2*

P

	Measure INFO/WEIGHT	per Measure		Nutrition Values per 100g / 100ml				
		KCAL	FAT	KCAL	PROT	CARB	FAT	FIBRE
POTATO BOMBAY								
Indian, Waitrose*	½ Pack/150g	125	5.4	83	1.6	9.7	3.6	3.0
Tesco*	1 Pack/300g	240	12.6	80	1.3	9.3	4.2	2.1
TTD, Sainsbury's*	½ Pack/113g	79	3.2	70	1.9	9.3	2.8	3.9
POTATO CAKES								
Average	*1 Cake/70g*	*127*	*1.2*	*180*	*3.8*	*37.5*	*1.7*	*2.4*
Fried, Average	*1oz/28g*	*66*	*2.5*	*237*	*4.9*	*35.0*	*9.0*	*0.8*
POTATO CREAMED								
with Cabbage, Asda*	1 Pack/350g	256	9.1	73	1.3	11.0	2.6	0.0
POTATO MASH								
Cheddar, Irish, Finest, Tesco*	½ Pack/250g	350	19.8	140	6.3	10.2	7.9	1.4
Cheese & Chive, Snack in a Pot, Tesco*	1 Pot/230g	304	21.6	132	2.2	9.6	9.4	0.9
Cheese & Onion, Eat Smart, Morrisons*	1 Pack/400g	340	6.4	85	4.4	13.2	1.6	1.3
Cheese & Onion, Tesco*	1 Serving/200g	210	9.4	105	3.2	12.6	4.7	1.0
Roast Onion, Snack in a Pot, Tesco*	1 Pot/218g	257	12.9	118	1.6	14.7	5.9	0.6
Sun Dried Tomato & Basil, COU, M&S*	1 Serving/170g	128	2.6	75	1.0	14.4	1.5	1.2
with Cracked Pepper & Sea Salt, Luxury, Sainsbury's*	½ Pack/225g	389	28.4	173	1.6	13.2	12.6	1.0
POTATO SALAD								
& Egg with Mayonnaise, Tesco*	½ Tub/150g	115	8.5	77	2.9	3.1	5.7	1.2
& Egg, M&S*	1 Serving/250g	150	7.2	60	3.0	4.6	2.9	0.9
& Yoghurt, Meadow Fresh, Lidl*	1 Portion/50g	72	4.0	144	1.8	15.4	8.0	1.8
30% Less Fat, BGTY, Sainsbury's*	1 Serving/60g	64	3.7	106	1.7	11.1	6.1	1.1
Asda*	¼ Pot/57g	67	4.0	117	0.9	12.5	7.0	1.1
Baby, & Coleslaw, TTD, Sainsbury's*	1 Serving/100g	300	30.4	300	1.2	5.4	30.4	1.6
Creamy, Asda*	½ Tub/150g	226	16.0	151	1.1	11.3	10.7	2.5
Creamy, Waitrose*	1 Serving/100g	163	11.9	163	1.3	12.7	11.9	1.1
Finest, Tesco*	1 Tub/250g	588	51.5	235	2.4	9.7	20.6	1.2
From Salad Selection, Sainsbury's*	1 Serving/50g	102	8.8	204	1.0	10.5	17.5	1.3
HL, Tesco*	1 Tub/250g	288	12.0	115	1.7	15.4	4.8	1.2
Iceland*	1 Serving/75g	162	14.7	216	1.1	8.9	19.6	0.6
Light Choices, Tesco*	1 Pack/100g	110	5.9	110	1.3	12.5	5.9	0.9
New, & Free Range Egg, Side, Sainsbury's*	1 Pack/290g	174	12.2	60	2.5	3.1	4.2	1.4
New, & King Prawn, COU, M&S*	1 Pack/300g	180	6.9	60	3.0	6.9	2.3	0.8
New, Co-Op*	1 Serving/50g	98	8.0	195	1.0	10.0	16.0	2.0
New, Less Than 5% Fat, M&S*	1 Serving/110g	88	3.4	80	1.3	12.1	3.1	1.5
New, M&S*	1 Serving/60g	114	9.8	190	0.9	9.9	16.3	1.3
Reduced Calorie, Pre Packed	1oz/28g	27	1.1	97	1.3	14.8	4.1	0.8
Seasonal, Salad Bar, Waitrose*	1 Serving/100g	109	3.4	109	0.0	0.0	3.4	0.0
Spar*	1 Serving/50g	180	18.2	360	1.8	10.2	36.3	1.2
Tesco*	1 Serving/100g	165	13.5	165	1.3	9.5	13.5	1.3
with Mayonnaise, Pre Packed	1oz/28g	67	5.8	239	1.6	12.2	20.8	0.9
with Mayonnaise, Retail	1oz/28g	80	7.4	287	1.5	11.4	26.5	0.8
with Onions & Chives, Co-Op*	1 Serving/50g	80	6.0	160	1.0	12.0	12.0	1.0
POTATO SKINS								
American Style, Loaded, Asda*	1 Serving/78g	294	18.0	375	15.0	27.0	23.0	2.4
American Style, Loaded, Tesco*	1 Serving/340g	388	8.2	114	6.8	16.3	2.4	3.3
Cheese & Bacon, Loaded, Asda*	½ Pack/125g	275	15.0	220	13.0	15.0	12.0	3.3
Cheese & Bacon, Loaded, Tesco*	1 Skin/59g	150	9.1	255	9.2	19.5	15.5	3.0
Cheese & Bacon, Sainsbury's*	1 Serving/140g	349	21.6	249	10.3	17.3	15.4	2.5
Cheese & Bacon, Waitrose*	1 Serving/75g	146	9.4	195	7.3	13.1	12.6	3.5
Cheese & Chive, Sainsbury's*	2 Skins/150g	286	17.8	191	7.7	13.3	11.9	2.8
Cheese & Ham, Iceland*	2 Skins/108g	155	4.9	143	6.3	19.3	4.5	2.0
Soured Cream, Loaded, M&S*	½ Pack/150g	308	17.8	205	9.1	15.8	11.9	0.9
with Sour Cream	1 Serving/275g	541	34.6	197	7.2	13.8	12.6	2.2

POTATO WAFFLES	Measure INFO/WEIGHT	per Measure KCAL	per Measure FAT	Nutrition Values per 100g / 100ml KCAL	PROT	CARB	FAT	FIBRE
Frozen, Cooked	1oz/28g	56	2.3	200	3.2	30.3	8.2	2.3
Frozen, Grilled, Asda*	1 Waffle/57g	104	5.8	183	2.0	21.0	10.1	1.7
Mini, Sainsbury's*	1 Waffle/11g	27	1.8	242	2.8	20.1	16.7	1.0
Oven Baked, Mini, McCain*	1oz/28g	62	2.4	221	3.9	32.0	8.6	0.0
Uncooked, Average	*1 Waffle/62g*	*113*	*5.1*	*182*	*2.4*	*24.4*	*8.3*	*1.8*
POTATO WEDGES								
& Dip, M&S*	1 Pack/450g	698	33.3	155	2.5	20.4	7.4	1.8
Aldi*	1 Serving/100g	150	6.8	150	2.1	20.2	6.8	0.0
Asda*	1 Wedge/40g	57	2.0	142	3.4	21.0	4.9	1.7
Baked, GFY, Asda*	1 Pack/450g	616	11.7	137	3.4	25.0	2.6	3.4
BBQ Flavour, Asda*	1 Serving/100g	185	9.0	185	2.9	23.0	9.0	1.7
BGTY, Sainsbury's*	½ Pack/190g	179	3.4	94	3.0	16.4	1.8	3.4
Crispy, M&S*	1 Serving/200g	340	14.2	170	1.3	25.3	7.1	1.7
Frozen, Average	*1 Serving/120g*	*145*	*4.1*	*121*	*2.0*	*20.5*	*3.4*	*2.2*
Garlic & Herb, COU, M&S*	1 Pack/300g	300	7.8	100	2.3	16.4	2.6	3.2
Harvest Basket, Lidl*	1 Serving/100g	147	5.7	147	2.2	20.5	5.7	0.0
Jacket, Spicy, American Style, Frozen, Sainsbury's*	1 Serving/125g	156	5.0	125	1.9	20.3	4.0	1.1
Jumbo, Finest, Tesco*	1 Serving/126g	145	2.6	115	1.4	22.7	2.1	1.7
Mexican, Inspire, Asda*	1 Pack/500g	525	17.0	105	2.2	16.5	3.4	1.8
New York Style, HL, Tesco*	1 Serving/125g	129	3.0	103	2.0	18.3	2.4	2.3
Onion & Garlic, Spicy, Cooked, Champion, Aldi*	1 Serving/100g	135	4.7	135	2.5	19.4	4.7	2.7
Only 5% Fat, Weighed Baked, McCain*	1 Serving/100g	173	4.3	173	3.3	30.2	4.3	2.8
Savoury, Waitrose*	1/3 Bag/250g	350	10.8	140	2.3	22.9	4.3	1.9
Sea Salt & Black Pepper, Finest, Tesco*	½ Pack/200g	200	3.2	100	1.8	18.0	1.6	3.4
Slightly Spiced, Weighed Baked, McCain*	1 Serving/100g	187	5.2	187	2.7	26.9	5.2	1.8
Slightly Spiced, Weighed Frozen, McCain*	1 Serving/100g	144	5.9	144	2.0	20.8	5.9	1.7
Southern Fried Style, Tesco*	1 Serving/155g	232	14.1	150	3.0	14.1	9.1	2.0
Southern Fried, Asda*	1 Serving/100g	157	4.5	157	3.0	26.0	4.5	3.5
Spicy, Asda*	1 Serving/100g	145	5.7	145	1.8	21.8	5.7	2.1
Spicy, M&S*	½ Pack/225g	349	14.6	155	2.4	21.8	6.5	1.3
Spicy, Occasions, Sainsbury's*	1 Serving/100g	144	4.3	144	2.5	23.7	4.3	0.4
with a Parsley & Oil Dressing, Tesco*	½ Pack/280g	168	2.8	60	1.0	11.5	1.0	1.8
POTATOES								
Alphabites, Captain Birds Eye, Birds Eye*	9 Bites/56g	75	3.0	134	2.0	19.5	5.3	1.4
Anya, Raw, TTD, Sainsbury's*	1 Serving/100g	75	0.3	75	1.5	17.8	0.3	1.1
Baby with Butter & Herbs, Sainsbury's*	¼ Pack/148g	103	0.9	70	1.9	14.2	0.6	2.0
Baby with Herbs & Butter, Morrisons*	1 Serving/100g	94	2.3	94	1.9	14.6	2.3	1.9
Baby with Paprika & Chilli Dressing, Morrisons*	1 Serving/120g	124	5.3	103	1.7	13.6	4.4	1.3
Baby, Dressed with Garlic & Rosemary, M&S*	1 Serving/185g	130	5.2	70	2.0	9.0	2.8	2.4
Baby, Garlic & Sea Salt Roasted, Finest, Tesco*	1 Serving/200g	192	6.6	96	3.1	13.5	3.3	1.0
Baby, New with Butter, Mint & Parsley, Organic, Asda*	1 Pack/360g	414	10.4	115	1.7	20.4	2.9	2.5
Baby, New, Ocado*	¼ Bag/188g	141	0.6	75	1.7	16.1	0.3	1.3
Baby, Oven Bake, Aunt Bessie's*	1 Serving/120g	103	1.7	86	2.2	16.3	1.4	3.0
Baked in Microwave, Flesh & Skin, Average	*1oz/28g*	*29*	*0.0*	*105*	*2.4*	*24.1*	*0.1*	*2.3*
Baked in Microwave, Flesh Only, Average	*1oz/28g*	*28*	*0.0*	*100*	*2.1*	*23.3*	*0.1*	*1.6*
Baked in Microwave, Skin Only, Average	*1oz/28g*	*37*	*0.0*	*132*	*4.4*	*29.6*	*0.1*	*5.5*
Baked with Cheddar Cheese, Farmfoods*	1 Potato/143g	196	5.4	137	4.7	21.0	3.8	1.9
Baked, Flesh & Skin, Average	*1 Med/200g*	*218*	*0.2*	*109*	*2.3*	*25.2*	*0.1*	*2.4*
Baked, Flesh Only, Weighed with Skin, Average	*1oz/28g*	*20*	*0.0*	*72*	*1.5*	*16.6*	*0.1*	*1.2*
Baked, Jacket with Beef Chilli, Asda*	1 Pack/300g	381	7.8	127	5.0	21.0	2.6	2.0
Baked, Jacket with Beef Chilli, M&S*	1 Pack/360g	288	7.2	80	5.9	9.6	2.0	0.9
Baked, Jacket with Cheese & Butter, Tesco*	1 Potato/225g	263	11.2	117	3.1	14.9	5.0	2.3
Baked, Jacket with Cheese, Freshly Prepared, Tesco*	½ Pack/215g	150	3.0	70	3.9	9.7	1.4	2.8

P

POTATOES

INFO/WEIGHT	Measure	per Measure KCAL	per Measure FAT	Nutrition Values per 100g / 100ml KCAL	PROT	CARB	FAT	FIBRE
Baked, Jacket, Cheddar Cheese, COU, M&S*	1 Potato/164g	164	3.1	100	2.9	17.3	1.9	2.0
Baked, Jacket, Chicken Tikka, Spar*	1 Serving/300g	309	3.1	103	5.5	19.2	1.0	5.0
Baked, Jacket, Chilli Con Carne, Pro Cuisine*	1 Pack/340g	347	3.4	102	4.6	18.7	1.0	0.0
Baked, Jacket, Garlic Butter Filling, Morrisons*	1 Potato/210g	239	12.4	114	1.7	13.6	5.9	0.9
Baked, Jacket, Garlic, Mini, Asda*	1 Serving/65g	59	2.1	91	2.2	13.0	3.3	0.0
Baked, Jacket, Ham & Cheddar Cheese, Asda*	1 Pack/300g	435	11.1	145	7.0	21.0	3.7	1.6
Baked, Jacket, Mature Cheddar Cheese, Finest, Tesco*	1 Potato/245g	360	18.4	147	5.4	14.6	7.5	2.3
Baked, Jacket, Mature Cheddar Cheese, M&S*	½ Pack/206g	225	6.6	109	3.6	16.9	3.2	1.0
Baked, Jacket, Mature Cheddar Cheese, Morrisons*	1 Serving/400g	520	20.4	130	4.4	16.6	5.1	1.5
Baked, Jacket, Spicy Chilli Con Carne, Spar*	1 Pack/340g	265	5.4	78	3.4	12.4	1.6	1.5
Baked, Jacket, Tuna & Sweetcorn, Average	*1 Serving/300g*	*273*	*6.8*	*91*	*5.0*	*12.6*	*2.2*	*0.9*
Baked, Jacket, Tuna & Sweetcorn, BGTY, Sainsbury's*	1 Pack/350g	360	9.4	103	6.5	13.2	2.7	1.3
Baked, Jacket, Tuna & Sweetcorn, COU, M&S*	1 Pack/300g	270	5.4	90	5.1	12.8	1.8	1.4
Baked, Jackets, Stuffed, Mini, Tesco*	1 Serving/108g	130	6.3	120	2.3	14.6	5.8	2.3
Baked, M&S*	1 Potato/205g	215	5.1	105	3.6	16.9	2.5	1.0
Baked, Skin Only, Average	*1oz/28g*	*55*	*0.0*	*198*	*4.3*	*46.1*	*0.1*	*7.9*
Baking, Raw, Average	*1 Med/250g*	*198*	*0.2*	*79*	*2.1*	*18.0*	*0.1*	*1.6*
Boiled with Skin	*1 Potato/125g*	*98*	*0.1*	*78*	*2.9*	*17.2*	*0.1*	*3.3*
Boiled, Average	*1 Serving/120g*	*86*	*0.1*	*72*	*1.8*	*17.0*	*0.1*	*1.2*
Boulangere, M&S*	½ Pack/225g	180	2.0	80	2.8	15.9	0.9	0.9
Charlotte, Average	*1 Serving/184g*	*139*	*0.5*	*76*	*1.6*	*17.4*	*0.2*	*3.3*
Crispy Bites, Weighed Frozen, McCain*	1 Serving/100g	141	4.4	141	2.5	20.4	4.4	1.5
Crispy Slices, M&S*	1/3 Pack/159g	231	8.3	145	2.9	22.2	5.2	1.9
Crispy Slices, Weighed Baked, McCain*	1 Serving/100g	240	11.0	240	3.2	32.1	11.0	2.1
Dauphinoise, Average	*1 Serving/200g*	*335*	*23.9*	*168*	*2.2*	*12.8*	*12.0*	*1.5*
Dauphinoise, Cook*	1 Pack/225g	320	18.7	142	5.3	11.0	8.3	1.8
Dauphinoise, TTD, Sainsbury's*	½ Pack/174g	240	16.2	138	2.9	10.8	9.3	2.7
Desiree, Average	*1 Serving/200g*	*152*	*0.4*	*76*	*2.2*	*16.4*	*0.2*	*0.6*
Exquisa, Finest, Tesco*	¼ Pack/247g	185	0.7	75	1.7	16.1	0.3	1.0
Frites, Fries, Golden, Crunchy, M&S*	½ Pack/100g	158	6.2	158	2.2	23.4	6.2	1.0
Fritters, Crispy, Oven Baked, Birds Eye*	1 Fritter/20g	29	1.6	145	2.0	16.3	8.0	1.2
Fritters, with Sweetcorn, M&S*	1 Pack/135g	304	17.0	225	4.4	24.1	12.6	2.3
Garlic, Tapas Selection, Sainsbury's*	1 Serving/22g	49	4.2	224	2.6	10.4	19.1	0.7
Hasselback, Average	*1 Serving/175g*	*182*	*1.6*	*104*	*1.9*	*22.0*	*0.9*	*2.9*
Hassleback, Dine in Side, Eat Well, M&S*	½ Pack/175g	195	6.0	110	2.1	18.3	3.4	1.9
Jacket, Ready Baked, Frozen, McCain*	1 Potato/200g	190	1.0	95	1.7	20.9	0.5	1.4
Jersey Royal, Canned, Average	*1 Can/186g*	*116*	*0.2*	*62*	*1.4*	*14.0*	*0.1*	*1.2*
Jersey Royal, New, Raw, Average	*1oz/28g*	*21*	*0.1*	*75*	*1.6*	*17.2*	*0.2*	*1.5*
King Edward, Tesco*	1 Serving/100g	77	0.2	77	2.1	16.8	0.2	1.3
Maris Piper, Mashed, Eat Fresh, Tesco*	½ Pack/213g	191	4.0	90	1.9	14.7	1.9	1.6
Maris Piper, Raw, Average	*1 Serving/200g*	*151*	*0.4*	*75*	*2.0*	*16.5*	*0.2*	*1.4*
Mashed with Cabbage & Spring Onion, COU, M&S*	½ Pack/225g	158	4.0	70	1.7	11.4	1.8	2.1
Mashed with Carrot & Swede, Morrisons*	1 Serving/100g	71	1.6	71	1.5	12.6	1.6	2.2
Mashed, Buttery, Sainsbury's*	1 Pack/450g	454	25.6	101	1.3	11.1	5.7	3.0
Mashed, CBY, Asda*	½ Pack/250g	177	5.5	71	1.0	10.3	2.2	2.8
Mashed, Colcannon, Co-Op*	1 Pack/500g	325	10.0	65	2.0	10.0	2.0	2.0
Mashed, Colcannon, Sainsbury's*	½ Pack/300g	192	12.0	64	0.4	6.7	4.0	1.4
Mashed, From Supermarket, Average	*½ Pack/200g*	*197*	*8.1*	*98*	*1.8*	*13.3*	*4.1*	*1.5*
Mashed, From Supermarket, Healthy Range, Average	*1 Serving/200g*	*160*	*3.1*	*80*	*1.8*	*14.6*	*1.6*	*1.3*
Mashed, From Supermarket, Premium, Average	*1 Serving/225g*	*305*	*17.8*	*136*	*1.7*	*14.4*	*7.9*	*1.1*
Mashed, Home Prepared with Whole Milk	1 Cup/210g	162	1.2	77	1.9	17.6	0.6	2.0
Mashed, Maris Piper with Cream & Butter, M&S*	½ Pack/200g	180	7.2	90	1.1	12.9	3.6	0.4
Mashed, Mash Direct*	½ Pack/200g	190	3.8	95	1.7	17.7	1.9	1.3

P

	Measure INFO/WEIGHT	per Measure KCAL	FAT	Nutrition Values per 100g / 100ml KCAL	PROT	CARB	FAT	FIBRE
POTATOES								
Mashed, Olive Oil, HE, Tesco*	1 Serving/100g	90	2.2	90	2.1	15.5	2.2	0.9
Mashed, Ready to Eat, Sainsbury's*	½ Pack/200g	142	3.8	71	1.4	12.1	1.9	2.0
Mashed, Vintage Cheddar Cheese, M&S*	½ Pack/225g	248	11.9	110	4.6	12.6	5.3	1.0
Mashed, with Cream & Butter, Ultimate, M&S*	½ Pack/225g	268	13.7	119	2.5	12.8	6.1	1.2
Mashed, with Milk Cream & Butter, Fresh, Ocado*	½ Pack/225g	207	7.2	92	1.7	13.3	3.2	1.6
New in a Herb Marinade, Tesco*	¼ Pack/150g	152	7.4	101	1.3	13.0	4.9	1.5
New with Butter, Chives & Mint, M&S*	¼ Pack/145g	116	2.0	80	1.1	16.2	1.4	2.3
New with English Churned Butter, M&S*	1 Pack/180g	261	4.0	145	1.3	29.5	2.2	2.1
New with Herbs & Butter, Asda*	½ Pack/170g	146	2.9	86	1.7	16.0	1.7	1.5
New with Herbs & Butter, Waitrose*	1 Serving/385g	443	22.7	115	1.7	13.8	5.9	1.2
New, Average	**1 Serving/100g**	**75**	**0.3**	**75**	**1.5**	**17.8**	**0.3**	**1.1**
New, Baby, Average	**1 Serving/180g**	**135**	**0.5**	**75**	**1.7**	**17.0**	**0.3**	**1.6**
New, Baby, Canned, Average	**1 Can/120g**	**69**	**0.2**	**58**	**1.4**	**12.9**	**0.2**	**1.4**
New, Easy Steam with Herbs & Butter, Tesco*	1 Serving/125g	94	3.5	75	1.8	9.6	2.8	1.7
New, Garlic, Herb & Parsley Butter, Co-Op*	1 Serving/100g	115	5.0	115	1.0	15.0	5.0	2.0
Pan Fried, Aldi*	1 Serving/250g	182	2.0	73	2.7	13.7	0.8	0.0
Raw, Peeled, Flesh Only	**1 Serving/100g**	**75**	**0.2**	**75**	**2.0**	**17.3**	**0.2**	**1.4**
Red, Flesh Only, Average	**1 Serving/300g**	**218**	**0.4**	**72**	**2.0**	**16.4**	**0.2**	**1.2**
Roast in Lard, Average	**1oz/28g**	**42**	**1.3**	**149**	**2.9**	**25.9**	**4.5**	**1.8**
Roast in Oil, Average	**1oz/28g**	**42**	**1.3**	**149**	**2.9**	**25.9**	**4.5**	**1.8**
Roast, Basted in Beef Dripping, Waitrose*	1 Serving/165g	213	8.9	129	2.2	18.0	5.4	1.9
Roast, Dry, No Oil, No fat	1 Serving/100g	79	0.1	79	2.7	18.0	0.1	1.6
Roast, Extra Crispy, Oven Baked, Aunt Bessie's*	1 Serving/100g	223	11.8	223	2.9	26.1	11.8	3.6
Roast, Frozen, Average	**1 Potato/70g**	**105**	**3.5**	**149**	**2.6**	**23.5**	**5.0**	**1.4**
Roast, Garlic & Rosemary, Miniature, Tesco*	¼ Pack/125g	85	0.9	68	1.8	12.5	0.7	2.3
Roast, New, Rosemary, Ainsley Harriott*	1 Serving/150g	133	4.0	89	2.0	16.0	2.7	1.3
Roast, Oven Baked, Aunt Bessie's*	1 Serving/165g	305	15.3	185	2.3	22.9	9.3	1.8
Roast, Roasties, Mini, Midweek, Aunt Bessie's*	1 Serving/100g	129	2.7	129	2.1	23.0	2.7	2.0
Roast, Seasoned, Butter Basted, Tesco*	½ Pack/225g	338	12.8	150	2.3	21.9	5.7	2.4
Roasting, Average	**1 Serving/150g**	**202**	**5.2**	**135**	**2.5**	**23.4**	**3.5**	**1.6**
Rooster, Boiled, Unsalted, Albert Bartlett & Sons Ltd*	1 Potato/175g	126	0.2	72	1.8	17.0	0.1	1.2
Salad, Value, Tesco*	1 Serving/150g	111	0.4	74	1.7	16.1	0.3	1.0
Saute with Onion & Bacon, Country Supper, Waitrose*	¼ Pack/100g	112	4.3	112	1.9	16.4	4.3	1.3
Saute, Deep Fried, McCain*	1oz/28g	47	2.0	167	2.6	23.3	7.0	0.0
Saute, Oven Baked, McCain*	1oz/28g	56	1.1	199	4.4	36.9	3.8	0.0
Smiles, Weighed Baked, McCain*	1 Serving/100g	237	10.1	237	3.4	33.4	10.1	3.1
Smiles, Weighed Frozen, McCain*	1 Serving/100g	191	8.0	191	2.6	27.0	8.0	2.7
Spicy with Chorizo, Tapas, Waitrose*	1 Serving/260g	512	35.6	197	6.7	11.8	13.7	1.1
Sumthings, Weighed Frozen, McCain*	1 Serving/100g	187	7.9	187	2.9	26.2	7.9	2.4
Vivaldi, Boiled in Unsalted Water, Sainsbury's*	1 Serving/200g	144	0.2	72	1.8	17.0	0.1	1.2
Wedges, Jumbo, TTD, Sainsbury's*	1 Serving/165g	279	6.8	169	2.4	30.7	4.1	3.1
White, Raw, Flesh & Skin	**1 Large/369g**	**284**	**0.3**	**77**	**2.0**	**17.5**	**0.1**	**2.2**
White, Raw, Weighed with Skin, Flesh Only, Average	**1 Med/213g**	**153**	**0.3**	**72**	**1.9**	**16.1**	**0.2**	**1.2**
White, Vivaldi, TTD, Sainsbury's*	1 Serving/100g	76	0.1	76	1.8	17.0	0.1	1.2
with Garlic Butter & Parsley Oil, Easy Steam, Tesco*	1/3 Pack/120g	90	3.2	75	0.9	11.2	2.7	1.1
POTATOES INSTANT								
Mashed, Made Up with Water, Average	**1 Serving/180g**	**118**	**0.3**	**66**	**1.7**	**14.5**	**0.2**	**1.3**
Mashed, Original, Dry Weight, Smash*	1 Serving/30g	101	0.3	343	8.3	71.8	1.0	6.7
POUSSIN								
Meat & Skin, Raw, Average	**1oz/28g**	**57**	**3.9**	**202**	**19.1**	**0.0**	**13.9**	**0.0**
Spatchcock, British, Waitrose*	½ Poussin/225g	364	20.2	162	19.0	1.2	9.0	0.0
POWERADE								
Berry & Tropical Fruit, Coca-Cola*	1 Bottle/500ml	120	0.0	24	0.0	5.6	0.0	0.0

	Measure INFO/WEIGHT	per Measure KCAL	FAT	Nutrition Values per 100g / 100ml KCAL	PROT	CARB	FAT	FIBRE
POWERADE								
Isotonic, Sports Drink, Coca-Cola*	1 Bottle/500ml	120	0.0	24	0.0	5.6	0.0	0.0
Zero, Coca-Cola*	1 Bottle/500ml	5	0.0	1	0.0	0.0	0.0	0.0
PRAWN COCKTAIL								
& Orkney Crab, M&S*	1 Serving/90g	180	13.8	200	14.2	1.8	15.3	0.6
20% More Prawns, M&S*	½ Pack/100g	330	31.6	330	8.9	2.2	31.6	0.2
BFY, Morrisons*	1 Serving/100g	149	10.3	149	4.7	9.7	10.3	0.1
BGTY, Sainsbury's*	1 Pack/200g	330	24.2	165	9.3	4.5	12.1	0.5
HL, Tesco*	1 Pack/170g	305	23.9	180	7.1	5.7	14.1	0.6
King, Sainsbury's*	1 Pack/260g	328	15.1	126	5.8	12.7	5.8	2.3
Light Choices, Tesco*	1 Pot/140g	210	16.0	150	7.5	4.3	11.4	1.3
Reduced Fat, M&S*	1 Pack/200g	260	15.0	130	11.9	3.2	7.5	0.7
Reduced Fat, Tesco*	1 Serving/200g	304	21.2	152	7.6	6.5	10.6	0.4
Tesco*	1 Tub/170g	476	39.1	280	6.6	10.2	23.0	1.0
TTD, Sainsbury's*	1 Serving/100g	333	30.6	333	11.5	2.9	30.6	0.5
PRAWN CRACKERS								
Asda*	1 Serving/25g	134	8.8	535	2.0	53.0	35.0	0.0
Food to Go, Sainsbury's*	1 Bag/40g	214	12.5	534	2.9	60.2	31.3	0.4
Green Thai Curry, M&S*	1 Pack/50g	250	12.9	500	3.2	62.2	25.8	1.6
M&S*	1 Bag/50g	262	15.6	525	2.8	57.4	31.3	0.8
Ready to Eat, Sharwood's*	1 Bag/60g	316	18.5	527	0.5	62.0	30.8	1.2
Sainsbury's*	1 Cracker/3g	16	1.0	537	2.4	60.4	31.7	0.8
Tesco*	1/3 Pack/20g	114	7.4	570	2.5	56.5	37.1	0.9
Waitrose*	1 Pack/50g	266	16.0	533	2.4	58.6	32.1	1.6
PRAWN TOAST								
Baguette from Selection, Modern Asian, M&S*	1 Toast/23g	60	3.3	270	11.0	21.3	14.9	2.1
Chinese Snack Selection, Morrisons*	1 Toast/13g	41	2.6	328	11.3	23.1	21.2	6.6
from Chinese Selection, Ken Hom, Tesco*	1 Toast/12g	48	3.8	385	13.3	11.5	30.5	4.0
Oriental Selection, Waitrose*	1 Toast/14g	38	2.4	272	11.1	18.3	17.2	2.1
Sesame Prawn, Toasted Triangles, M&S*	1 Pack/220g	616	39.6	280	12.4	17.3	18.0	2.0
Sesame, Occasions, Sainsbury's*	1 Toast/12g	34	2.2	283	9.9	19.2	18.5	2.0
Sesame, Oriental Snack Selection, Sainsbury's*	1 Toast/12g	40	2.7	335	9.3	23.0	22.9	5.1
PRAWNS								
Atlantic, Extra Large, TTD, Sainsbury's*	¼ Pack/100g	79	1.0	79	17.4	0.1	1.0	0.5
Batter Crisp, Lyons*	1 Pack/160g	350	20.3	219	8.0	18.2	12.7	1.1
Boiled	***1 Prawn/3g***	***3***	***0.0***	***99***	***22.6***	***0.0***	***0.9***	***0.0***
Chilli & Coriander, Sweet Chilli Dipping Sauce, COU, M&S*	1 Pack/120g	130	1.9	108	11.7	11.4	1.6	0.7
Cooked & Peeled, Average	***1oz/28g***	***21***	***0.2***	***77***	***17.6***	***0.2***	***0.6***	***0.0***
Crispy, with Sweet Chilli Dipping Sauce, M&S*	1 Pack/240g	490	20.2	204	8.2	23.6	8.4	0.6
Filo Wrapped & Breaded, M&S*	1 Serving/19g	45	2.5	235	9.5	20.4	13.0	1.4
Honduran & Cocktail Sauce Dipper, M&S*	1 Pack/120g	258	21.6	215	13.6	0.0	18.0	1.1
Hot & Spicy, Average	***1 Serving/170g***	***461***	***26.9***	***271***	***9.4***	***22.8***	***15.8***	***2.2***
Hot & Spicy, Whitby*	1 Portion/125g	319	16.4	255	9.3	25.0	13.1	2.2
Icelandic, Raw, Average	***1oz/28g***	***30***	***0.4***	***106***	***22.7***	***0.0***	***1.6***	***0.0***
King in Filo, Finest, Tesco*	1 Prawn/20g	38	0.6	189	13.0	27.8	2.9	1.6
King in Sweet Chilli Sauce with Noodles, COU, M&S*	1 Pack/400g	260	1.6	65	4.8	10.3	0.4	1.5
King with Chilli & Coriander, M&S*	1 Pack/140g	147	5.6	105	17.1	0.5	4.0	0.5
King with Garlic Butter, M&S*	1 Serving/100g	165	9.0	165	12.5	9.1	9.0	0.5
King with Garlic, Parsley & Lemon Butter, COOK!, M&S*	½ Pack/110g	160	11.3	145	12.9	0.8	10.2	0.5
King with Ginger & Spring Onion, Waitrose*	1 Pack/300g	207	5.1	69	6.4	7.1	1.7	1.9
King, Crevettes, Cooked & Peeled, Sainsbury's*	1 Pack/225g	205	1.1	91	21.8	0.1	0.5	0.3
King, Frozen, Morrisons*	½ Bag/100g	62	0.6	62	14.0	0.2	0.6	0.6
King, in Chilli Sauce, Inspirations, Birds Eye*	1 Portion/125g	269	20.9	215	10.0	6.1	16.7	0.1
King, Jumbo, TTD, Sainsbury's*	½ Pack/90g	63	0.6	70	15.7	0.1	0.7	0.5

	Measure INFO/WEIGHT	per Measure KCAL	FAT	Nutrition Values per 100g / 100ml KCAL	PROT	CARB	FAT	FIBRE
PRAWNS								
King, Raw, Average	*1 Bag/200g*	*145*	*1.9*	*72*	*15.8*	*0.2*	*1.0*	*0.1*
King, Raw, Peeled, Sainsbury's*	½ Pack/90g	61	0.6	68	14.3	0.8	0.7	0.5
King, Shell On, TTD, Sainsbury's*	1 Serving/100g	67	0.7	67	14.3	0.8	0.7	0.5
King, Tandoori, Average	*1 Prawn/59g*	*33*	*0.6*	*55*	*5.7*	*5.9*	*1.1*	*0.7*
Large, Wrapped, Party Food, M&S*	1 Wrap/26g	49	1.5	190	14.8	18.8	5.7	1.3
North Atlantic, Peeled, Cooked, Average	*1oz/28g*	*22*	*0.3*	*80*	*17.5*	*0.0*	*1.1*	*0.0*
North Atlantic, Raw, Average	*1oz/28g*	*17*	*0.1*	*62*	*14.4*	*0.0*	*0.4*	*0.0*
Peeled, TTD, Sainsbury's*	1 Serving/100g	65	0.9	65	14.1	0.1	0.9	0.5
Raw, Average	*1oz/28g*	*21*	*0.2*	*75*	*17.0*	*0.2*	*0.6*	*0.0*
Raw, Jumbo, TTD, Sainsbury's*	½ Pack/85g	115	2.4	135	25.5	2.0	2.8	0.5
Skewers, Sweet Chilli, King, BBQ Favourites, Asda*	1 Skewer/48g	48	0.5	100	16.6	5.4	1.1	1.0
Skewers, Sweet Chilli, Tesco*	1 Skewer/22g	26	0.2	120	20.4	6.9	0.9	0.5
Succulent King with a Sweet Chilli Sauce, Birds Eye*	1 Serving/140g	251	17.2	179	10.5	6.5	12.3	0.1
Tempura, Finest, Tesco*	1 Prawn/18g	31	1.6	175	11.5	11.0	9.1	4.0
Tiger, Cooked & Peeled, Average	*1 Pack/180g*	*151*	*2.0*	*84*	*18.4*	*0.1*	*1.1*	*0.0*
Tiger, Jumbo, Average	*1 Serving/50g*	*39*	*0.2*	*78*	*18.2*	*0.3*	*0.5*	*0.0*
Tiger, Raw, Average	*1 Prawn/30g*	*19*	*0.2*	*64*	*14.2*	*0.0*	*0.7*	*0.0*
Tiger, Wrapped, M&S*	1 Pack/190g	477	25.8	251	11.3	20.7	13.6	1.3
Wild Caught, Large, Canadian, LL, Waitrose*	1 Serving/100g	69	1.4	69	14.0	0.0	1.4	0.0
PRAWNS CHILLI								
& Coriander, King, Honduran, M&S*	½ Pack/70g	70	2.2	100	17.2	0.1	3.2	0.4
& Coriander, King, Sainsbury's*	1 Pack/140g	112	1.8	80	16.6	0.4	1.3	0.5
Sweet, Thai, King, Sainsbury's*	1 Serving/150g	177	6.1	118	6.4	13.9	4.1	1.9
with Spicy Chilli Dip, King, Sainsbury's*	½ Pack/150g	282	10.8	188	8.6	22.2	7.2	1.0
PRAWNS CREOLE								
Spicy, BGTY, Sainsbury's*	1 Pack/350g	357	8.4	102	4.8	15.6	2.4	0.4
PRAWNS IN								
Creamy Garlic Sauce, Youngs*	1 Serving/158g	261	22.9	165	8.5	0.3	14.5	0.0
PRAWNS ORIENTAL								
M&S*	1 Pack/200g	440	23.4	220	11.9	16.9	11.7	0.9
PRAWNS SZECHUAN								
Spicy, COU, M&S*	1 Pack/400g	380	3.6	95	4.5	16.9	0.9	1.5
PRAWNS WITH								
a Spicy Cajun Dip, King, Sainsbury's*	1 Pack/240g	254	4.3	106	14.8	9.1	1.8	1.4
Chilli & Coriander, Cooked & Peeled, Tesco*	1 Pack/160g	144	3.4	90	16.7	0.2	2.1	0.5
Chilli, Coriander & Lime, King, Waitrose*	1 Pack/140g	143	3.2	102	19.9	0.5	2.3	0.6
Garlic & Herb Butter, King, Fresh, M&S*	1 Serving/200g	330	18.0	165	12.5	9.1	9.0	0.5
Ginger & Spring Onion, Sainsbury's*	1 Pack/300g	198	9.3	66	4.7	4.7	3.1	0.3
Green Thai Sauce, Tiger, Waitrose*	½ Pack/117g	108	2.7	92	16.1	0.8	2.3	0.1
Lemon & Pepper, Honduran, King, M&S*	1 Pack/140g	133	3.6	95	17.4	0.4	2.6	0.7
PRESERVE								
Rhubarb & Ginger, Mackays Ltd*	1 Serving/10g	27	0.0	269	0.3	66.7	0.0	0.0
PRETZELS								
American Style, Salted, Sainsbury's*	1 Serving/50g	202	2.2	403	10.8	79.7	4.5	1.8
Cheddar Cheese, Penn State Pretzels*	1 Sm Bag/30g	124	2.8	412	10.0	71.6	9.3	3.8
Choc Full of, Cadbury*	½ Bag/55g	250	10.4	455	7.7	62.0	19.0	2.9
Giant, Penn State Pretzels*	1 Pretzel/18g	66	0.7	374	10.5	74.7	3.7	4.1
Giant, Salted, Tesco*	1 Serving/25g	99	1.1	395	12.2	75.8	4.3	3.4
Jumbo, Tesco*	1 Serving/50g	194	3.4	388	9.7	71.9	6.8	5.4
Lightly Salted, Tesco*	1 Serving/25g	99	1.8	395	9.3	73.4	7.1	5.5
Mini, M&S*	1 Pack/45g	194	6.0	430	10.4	66.6	13.4	4.9
New York Style, Salted, Mini, Shapers, Boots*	1 Bag/25g	94	0.5	375	10.0	79.0	2.1	4.2
Peanut Butter Filled, H K Anderson*	10 Pretzels/30g	140	7.0	467	6.7	50.0	23.3	6.7

INFO/WEIGHT	Measure	per Measure KCAL	FAT	Nutrition Values per 100g / 100ml KCAL	PROT	CARB	FAT	FIBRE

PRETZELS

INFO/WEIGHT	Measure	KCAL	FAT	KCAL	PROT	CARB	FAT	FIBRE
Salt & Cracked Black Pepper, COU, M&S*	1 Pack/25g	100	0.6	390	11.4	79.1	2.4	2.6
Salted, Average	*1 Serving/30g*	*114*	*0.8*	*380*	*10.3*	*79.8*	*2.6*	*3.0*
Salted, Mini, M&S*	1 Pack/25g	94	0.5	375	10.0	79.0	2.1	4.2
Salted, Sainsbury's*	1 Serving/50g	200	1.8	401	9.8	82.4	3.6	3.4
Sea Salt & Black Pepper, Penn State Pretzels*	1 Serving/25g	94	1.0	375	10.4	73.7	4.2	4.7
Soft, Almond, Auntie Anne's*	1 Pretzel/112g	350	2.0	312	7.1	66.1	1.8	1.8
Soft, Cheddar & Red Onion, New York Bakery Co*	1 Pretzel/59g	168	2.5	284	11.8	46.7	4.3	5.3
Soft, Cinnamon Sugar with Butter, Auntie Anne's*	1 Pretzel/112g	470	12.0	420	7.1	75.0	10.7	1.8
Soft, Cinnamon Sugar, Auntie Anne's*	1 Pretzel/112g	380	1.0	339	7.1	75.0	0.9	1.8
Soft, Jalapeno, Auntie Anne's*	1 Pretzel/126g	300	1.0	238	6.4	50.0	0.8	1.6
Soft, Salted, Original, Auntie Anne's*	1 Pretzel/112g	310	1.0	277	7.1	58.0	0.9	1.8
Soft, Sesame, Auntie Anne's*	1 Pretzel/112g	360	6.0	321	8.9	59.8	5.4	2.7
Sour Cream & Chive, Penn State Pretzels*	1 Serving/25g	111	3.2	443	8.9	71.8	12.9	2.0
Sour Cream & Onion, M&S*	1 Serving/30g	136	4.4	455	11.0	70.9	14.5	0.7
Sweet Thai Chilli Twists, Penn State Pretzels*	1 Serving/25g	98	2.0	393	9.8	70.1	8.2	6.8
Wheat, Gluten Free, Trufree*	1 Bag/60g	282	12.0	470	0.5	72.0	20.0	0.7
with Sea Salt, Giant, M&S*	1 Pretzel/8g	31	0.5	390	9.7	77.3	6.8	5.4

PRINGLES*

INFO/WEIGHT	Measure	KCAL	FAT	KCAL	PROT	CARB	FAT	FIBRE
Barbecue, Pringles*	1 Serving/50g	266	18.0	533	4.9	48.0	36.0	5.1
Cheese & Onion, Pringles*	1 Serving/25g	132	8.5	528	4.1	50.0	34.0	3.4
Hot & Spicy, Pringles*	1 Serving/25g	132	8.5	530	4.6	49.0	34.0	3.7
Light, Original, Pringles*	1 Serving/25g	121	6.2	484	4.3	59.0	25.0	3.6
Light, Sour Cream & Onion, Pringles*	1 Serving/25g	122	6.2	487	4.7	57.0	25.0	3.6
Margarita Pizza, Classic Takeaways, Pringles*	1 Serving/25g	134	8.0	538	3.9	53.0	32.0	2.6
Original, Pringles*	1 Serving/25g	130	8.5	522	3.8	51.0	34.0	2.6
Paprika, Pringles*	1 Serving/25g	132	8.5	529	4.9	49.0	34.0	6.5
Prawn Cocktail, Pringles*	1 Serving/25g	130	8.0	518	4.1	53.0	32.0	2.5
Salt & Vinegar, Pringles*	1 Serving/25g	128	8.0	512	3.9	52.0	32.0	2.4
Sour Cream & Onion, Pringles*	1 Serving/25g	133	8.8	531	4.5	49.0	35.0	3.6
Texas BBQ Sauce, Pringles*	1 Serving/25g	132	8.5	527	4.2	50.0	34.0	3.5

PROFITEROLES

INFO/WEIGHT	Measure	KCAL	FAT	KCAL	PROT	CARB	FAT	FIBRE
Asda*	1 Serving/64g	218	17.2	343	5.0	20.0	27.0	0.0
Chocolate Covered, Tesco*	1 Serving/72g	295	21.2	410	5.7	29.3	29.5	2.0
Chocolate, 8 Pack, Co-Op*	¼ Pack/112g	330	17.9	295	6.0	31.0	16.0	2.0
Chocolate, Sainsbury's*	1/6 Pot/95g	192	8.5	202	5.4	25.1	8.9	0.8
Chocolate, Tesco*	1 Serving/76g	293	21.8	386	5.1	26.9	28.7	0.5
Choux & Chocolate Sauce, Tesco*	1 Serving/77g	295	22.0	386	5.1	26.9	28.7	0.5
Filled with Cream, Stack, Fresh, M&S*	1 Serving/75g	281	21.4	375	5.3	23.6	28.5	1.9
in a Pot, Waitrose*	1 Pot/80g	207	11.3	259	6.3	25.6	14.1	2.9
Waitrose*	4 Profiteroles/75g	269	17.9	359	4.8	31.1	23.9	0.7

PRUNES

INFO/WEIGHT	Measure	KCAL	FAT	KCAL	PROT	CARB	FAT	FIBRE
Dried, Average	*1 Prune/7g*	*11*	*0.0*	*158*	*2.5*	*36.4*	*0.4*	*5.8*
in Apple Juice, Average	*1 Serving/90g*	*76*	*0.1*	*84*	*0.8*	*19.8*	*0.1*	*1.4*
in Fruit Juice, Average	*1oz/28g*	*24*	*0.0*	*86*	*0.9*	*20.9*	*0.2*	*2.9*
in Syrup, Average	*1oz/28g*	*25*	*0.0*	*89*	*0.9*	*21.5*	*0.2*	*2.6*
Pitted in Juice, 825g Jar, Tesco*	1 Serving/206g	165	1.0	80	0.8	17.0	0.5	3.3
Pitted, Californian, Ready to Eat, Sweetvine, Aldi*	4 Prunes/30g	48	0.1	161	2.5	34.0	0.4	5.7
Pitted, Ready to Eat, Everyday Value, Tesco*	4 Prunes/40g	66	0.2	165	2.5	34.0	0.4	5.7
Ready to Eat, Dried, Organic, LL, Waitrose*	1 Serving/30g	73	0.1	243	2.2	56.8	0.4	7.3
Ready to Eat, Wholefoods, Tesco*	1 Serving/100g	230	0.3	230	1.9	54.9	0.3	6.5
Stewed with Sugar	*1oz/28g*	*29*	*0.1*	*103*	*1.3*	*25.5*	*0.2*	*3.1*
Stewed without Sugar	*1oz/28g*	*23*	*0.1*	*81*	*1.4*	*19.5*	*0.3*	*3.3*

	Measure INFO/WEIGHT	per Measure KCAL	FAT	Nutrition Values per 100g / 100ml KCAL	PROT	CARB	FAT	FIBRE
PUDDING								
Bread, Retail Average	*1 Slice/120g*	*301*	*8.0*	*251*	*8.4*	*41.8*	*6.7*	*0.5*
Brilliant Black Forest, Graze*	1 Punnet/37g	97	3.3	262	4.0	40.0	9.0	2.0
Cherry Cobbler, GFY, Asda*	1 Pudding/100g	158	2.0	158	2.1	33.0	2.0	0.9
Chocolate & Salted Caramel, Melting, Finest, Tesco*	1 Pudding/100g	402	23.4	402	4.5	42.4	23.4	2.0
Chocolate Bombe, Cooked, Fox's*	½ Pudding/114g	435	16.9	383	4.3	57.0	14.9	1.7
Chocolate Ganache, Mini Pot, Gu*	1 Pot/45g	199	16.6	442	3.3	26.4	36.8	2.3
Chocolate Ganache, Salted Caramel, Puds, Gu*	1 Pot/45g	171	11.9	381	3.2	31.6	26.5	1.6
Chocolate Sponge with Rich Caramel Sauce, Cadbury*	1 Pudding/110g	352	16.6	320	4.0	41.1	15.1	1.2
Chocolate, M&S*	¼ Pudding/76g	265	12.0	350	4.1	48.0	15.8	2.1
Chocolate, Melting Middle, M&S*	1 Pudding/155g	510	27.8	330	5.8	36.2	18.0	3.1
Creamed Sago, Ambrosia*	1 Serving/200g	158	3.2	79	2.5	13.6	1.6	0.2
Crumble, Fruit, Hot, Weight Watchers*	1 Crumble/90g	163	4.1	181	2.2	35.0	4.6	2.4
Eve's with Custard, Less Than 5% Fat, M&S*	1 Pudding/205g	318	9.4	155	3.4	24.7	4.6	0.7
Golden Syrup, Steamed, Aunty's*	1 Pudding/100g	293	4.1	293	3.3	57.3	4.1	0.8
Hot Chocolate Melting Middle Puds, Gu*	1 Pud/100g	409	26.9	409	6.0	36.0	26.9	2.7
Jam, Roly Poly & Custard, Co-Op*	1 Serving/105g	262	7.4	250	3.0	44.0	7.0	0.8
Jam, Roly Poly, Aunt Bessie's*	1 Serving/75g	290	10.4	387	3.4	62.2	13.8	0.9
Jam, Roly Poly, Sainsbury's*	¼ Pack/81g	291	11.5	359	4.4	53.3	14.2	0.5
Lemon, Steamed, BGTY, Sainsbury's*	1 Pudding/110g	307	3.2	279	3.0	60.2	2.9	0.7
Pineapple Upside Down, Waitrose*	¼ Pudding/113g	303	12.7	269	3.3	38.0	11.3	1.2
Queen of Puddings	1oz/28g	60	2.2	213	4.8	33.1	7.8	0.2
Souffle, Hot Chocolate, Gu*	1 Pot/65g	298	23.5	458	6.0	24.1	36.2	2.5
Sponge with Golden Syrup, Individual, Mr Kipling*	1 Pudding/95g	395	16.7	366	3.1	53.1	15.5	0.6
Sticky Toffee, Co-Op*	¼ Pudding/100g	355	20.0	355	3.0	40.0	20.0	0.7
Sticky Toffee, Farmfoods*	¼ Pudding/186g	627	11.9	337	4.1	65.7	6.4	0.3
Sticky Toffee, Indulgent, Specially Selected, Aldi*	¼ Pudding/113g	380	13.5	338	2.6	53.0	12.0	2.2
Sticky Toffee, Tesco*	1 Serving/110g	287	14.7	261	3.3	31.8	13.4	0.7
Sticky Toffee, Weight Watchers*	1 Pudding/100g	172	1.1	172	3.0	27.2	1.1	20.5
Suet, Average	*1oz/28g*	*94*	*5.1*	*335*	*4.4*	*40.5*	*18.3*	*0.9*
Syrup, M&S*	1 Serving/105g	370	10.5	352	3.9	61.7	10.0	0.8
Truffle, Chocolate with Raspberry Compote, Gu*	1 Pot/80g	250	14.6	312	2.8	28.8	18.2	1.8
PUMPKIN								
Boiled in Salted Water	*1oz/28g*	*4*	*0.1*	*13*	*0.6*	*2.1*	*0.3*	*1.1*
Kabocha, Tesco*	1 Serving 50g	20	0.0	39	1.1	8.3	0.1	1.6
Potimarron, Raw, Average	*1 Serving/80g*	*21*	*0.1*	*26*	*1.0*	*6.5*	*0.1*	*1.9*
Solid Pack, 100% Pure, Canned, Libby's*	1 Can/425g	139	1.7	33	1.6	7.4	0.4	4.1

P

	Measure INFO/WEIGHT	per Measure KCAL	FAT	Nutrition Values per 100g / 100ml KCAL	PROT	CARB	FAT	FIBRE
QUAVERS								
Cheese, Walkers*	1 Bag/20g	109	6.1	534	2.7	62.5	30.1	1.1
Prawn Cocktail, Walkers*	1 Bag/16g	88	5.1	537	2.1	62.0	31.0	1.2
Salt & Vinegar, Walkers*	1 Bag/16g	86	4.9	527	1.9	62.0	30.0	1.2
QUICHE								
Asparagus & Feta, Little, Higgidy*	1 Portion/155g	369	23.4	238	8.1	17.3	15.1	1.4
Asparagus & Herby Summer Vegetable, Higgidy*	1 Quiche/400g	848	50.0	212	5.9	18.9	12.5	2.7
Asparagus & Mushroom, Tesco*	½ Quiche/200g	474	32.8	237	5.1	17.2	16.4	1.2
Baby Spinach & Gruyere, Sainsbury's*	¼ Quiche/93g	228	16.0	245	7.4	15.1	17.2	1.0
Bacon & Cheese, Pork Farms*	1 Pack/120g	378	24.0	315	11.1	20.8	20.0	0.0
Bacon & Cheese, Sainsbury's*	¼ Quiche/100g	237	15.0	237	7.0	18.6	15.0	0.7
Bacon & Leek, Individual, Tesco*	1 Quiche/175g	485	32.4	277	8.3	19.4	18.5	0.9
Bacon & Leek, Tesco*	¼ Quiche/100g	260	18.0	260	6.9	17.5	18.0	1.2
Bacon & Tomato, Asda*	1 Serving/107g	201	8.6	188	8.0	21.0	8.0	1.1
Bacon, Leek & Cheese, Weight Watchers*	1 Quiche/165g	327	15.7	198	8.2	18.0	9.5	1.8
Bacon, Leek & Mushroom, M&S*	¼ Quiche/100g	245	16.4	245	6.9	17.2	16.4	1.3
Bacon, Smoked & Mature Cheddar, Higgidy*	1 Quiche/400g	1096	74.0	274	8.4	18.6	18.5	1.5
Broccoli & Stilton, Mini, Sainsbury's*	1 Quiche/14g	52	3.0	369	8.8	35.2	21.4	3.3
Broccoli, Tesco*	1 Serving/100g	249	17.2	249	6.0	17.6	17.2	1.4
Broccoli, Tomato & Cheese, Classic, Sainsbury's*	1 Serving/100g	223	14.5	223	5.3	17.1	14.5	1.6
Broccoli, Tomato & Cheese, Deep Filled, Sainsbury's*	¼ Quiche/100g	203	12.9	203	5.2	16.9	12.9	2.3
Caramelised Onion & Roquefort, Finest, Tesco*	1 Quiche/150g	401	26.7	267	7.2	17.0	17.8	5.1
Cheese & Bacon, Crustless, Tesco*	1 Serving/85g	199	12.8	234	10.0	14.4	15.0	0.6
Cheese & Broccoli, Morrisons*	1/3 Quiche/134g	338	22.4	253	7.1	18.4	16.8	1.7
Cheese & Egg	1oz/28g	88	6.2	314	12.5	17.3	22.2	0.6
Cheese & Ham, Sainsbury's*	1 Serving/100g	266	19.0	266	9.3	14.4	19.0	1.2
Cheese & Mushroom, Budgens*	½ Quiche/170g	474	32.8	279	7.8	18.4	19.3	1.4
Cheese & Onion, 25% Reduced Fat, Asda*	½ Quiche/78g	163	7.0	209	11.0	21.0	9.0	2.4
Cheese & Onion, Asda*	½ Quiche/200g	578	39.6	289	9.0	18.6	19.8	1.5
Cheese & Onion, Co-Op*	¼ Quiche/88g	262	19.2	300	10.0	17.0	22.0	1.0
Cheese & Onion, Crustless, Asda*	1 Quiche/160g	277	15.2	173	7.6	14.3	9.5	1.3
Cheese & Onion, Crustless, Weight Watchers*	1 Quiche/160g	267	12.3	167	11.3	11.1	7.7	4.3
Cheese & Onion, Deep Filled, Sainsbury's*	¼ Quiche/100g	254	17.2	254	7.3	17.2	17.2	2.7
Cheese & Onion, Finest, Tesco*	1 Serving/130g	346	24.3	266	9.1	15.3	18.7	2.5
Cheese & Onion, HL, Tesco*	¼ Quiche/100g	180	7.8	180	9.4	17.6	7.8	1.8
Cheese & Onion, Individual, Sainsbury's*	1 Quiche/180g	542	34.9	301	9.9	21.6	19.4	1.5
Cheese & Onion, M&S*	1 Slice/100g	250	17.2	250	8.2	16.1	17.2	1.5
Cheese & Onion, Reduced Fat, Eat Smart, Morrisons*	1 Quiche/400g	824	36.8	206	7.7	16.9	9.2	0.7
Cheese & Onion, Retail, Average	**¼ Quiche/100g**	**262**	**17.8**	**262**	**8.4**	**17.1**	**17.8**	**1.3**
Cheese & Onion, Value, Tesco*	½ Quiche/200g	526	36.4	263	8.6	16.1	18.2	0.7
Cheese & Onion, Vintage, Caramelised, Finest, Tesco*	¼ Quiche/100g	300	18.6	300	9.4	22.4	18.6	1.7
Cheese & Onion, VLH Kitchens	1 Serving/80g	134	7.5	167	9.6	18.1	6.0	1.8
Cheese & Onion, Weight Watchers*	1 Quiche/165g	325	15.3	197	7.0	21.2	9.3	1.6
Cheese & Tomato, Asda*	¼ Quiche/105g	274	17.8	261	8.0	19.0	17.0	0.9
Cheese & Tomato, M&S*	1 Serving/100g	230	15.6	230	7.7	15.1	15.6	1.6
Cheese & Tomato, Retail, Average	**¼ Quiche/100g**	**268**	**17.1**	**268**	**8.0**	**20.2**	**17.1**	**1.1**
Chicken & Basil, Finest, Tesco*	1 Serving/134g	381	24.9	284	9.3	19.8	18.6	1.3
Ham & Tomato, M&S*	½ Pack/200g	440	31.0	220	8.1	12.4	15.5	2.9
Ham & Soft Cheese, Tesco*	¼ Quiche/100g	280	20.1	280	7.4	17.5	20.1	1.9
Leek & Sweet Potato, Waitrose*	½ Quiche/200g	440	29.0	220	5.3	17.0	14.5	2.3
Leek, Cheese & Chive, Sainsbury's*	1/3 Quiche/125g	292	20.2	234	7.1	14.9	16.2	1.3
Lorraine, Asda*	¼ Quiche/100g	246	16.2	246	6.6	18.5	16.2	4.2
Lorraine, BGTY, Sainsbury's*	1 Serving/128g	273	14.0	213	10.9	17.7	10.9	0.7
Lorraine, Budgens*	1 Pack/180g	520	30.8	289	8.2	25.6	17.1	0.8

	Measure INFO/WEIGHT	per Measure		Nutrition Values per 100g / 100ml				
		KCAL	FAT	KCAL	PROT	CARB	FAT	FIBRE
QUICHE								
Lorraine, Co-Op*	¼ Quiche/100g	275	20.6	275	8.1	14.9	20.6	2.6
Lorraine, Crustless, Asda*	1 Quiche/160g	259	12.6	162	9.3	13.5	7.9	1.1
Lorraine, Crustless, Light Choices, Tesco*	1 Pack/160g	280	13.4	175	12.6	11.8	8.4	2.5
Lorraine, Crustless, You Count, LL, Waitrose*	1 Quiche/160g	295	15.4	185	8.9	15.2	9.6	0.9
Lorraine, ES, Asda*	¼ Quiche/100g	270	18.0	270	8.0	19.0	18.0	2.3
Lorraine, Finest, Tesco*	1 Serving/100g	330	25.1	330	8.4	17.5	25.1	1.5
Lorraine, Light Choices, Tesco*	¼ Pack/100g	170	6.4	170	12.3	15.5	6.4	3.2
Lorraine, Quiche Selection, M&S*	1 Slice/56g	160	11.5	285	12.8	12.3	20.6	2.1
Lorraine, Reduced Fat, Eat Smart, Morrisons*	¼ Quiche/100g	209	9.8	209	9.4	17.8	9.8	0.5
Lorraine, Retail, Average	**¼ Quiche/100g**	**280**	**19.5**	**280**	**9.0**	**16.8**	**19.5**	**2.0**
Lorraine, Sainsbury's*	½ Quiche/200g	598	42.4	299	10.6	16.3	21.2	0.9
Lorraine, Small, Waitrose*	1 Pack/170g	507	35.0	298	9.8	18.4	20.6	2.3
Lorraine, Smoked Bacon & Cheese, M&S*	¼ Quiche/100g	270	18.4	270	9.7	16.4	18.4	1.6
Lorraine, Snack, Morrisons*	1 Serving/50g	142	9.4	285	10.2	19.0	18.7	2.0
Lorraine, TTD, Sainsbury's*	1/3 Quiche/158g	402	28.3	254	10.9	12.3	17.9	2.5
Mediterranean Style Vegetable, Classic, Sainsbury's*	1 Quiche/400g	868	50.4	217	6.2	19.8	12.6	2.2
Mediterranean Vegetable, Weight Watchers*	1 Quiche/165g	285	13.5	173	3.8	21.1	8.2	4.0
Mushroom	1oz/28g	80	5.5	284	10.0	18.3	19.5	0.9
Mushroom, M&S*	¼ Quiche/100g	235	16.7	235	6.1	14.6	16.7	2.8
Mushroom, Tesco*	¼ Quiche/100g	250	17.5	250	5.6	17.4	17.5	1.0
Red Pepper, Goats Cheese & Spinach, Waitrose*	1 Serving/100g	218	14.3	218	6.5	15.8	14.3	2.6
Salmon & Asparagus, HE, Tesco*	1 Quiche/345g	621	26.6	180	7.5	20.2	7.7	1.2
Salmon & Broccoli, Asda*	¼ Quiche/106g	289	18.0	273	10.0	20.0	17.0	2.6
Salmon & Broccoli, Tesco*	1 Serving/133g	311	20.1	234	7.9	16.6	15.1	0.9
Smoked Bacon & Cheddar, Little, Higgidy*	1 Quiche/155g	485	33.8	313	11.5	17.6	21.8	1.0
Smoked Salmon & Spinach, Little, Higgidy*	1 Quiche/155g	448	31.5	289	8.6	17.5	20.3	0.9
Spinach & Ricotta, Tesco*	¼ Quiche/100g	237	14.9	237	5.8	19.9	14.9	1.0
Spinach & Roast Red Pepper, Little, Higgidy*	1 Quiche/155g	397	27.3	256	9.1	15.2	17.6	1.2
Spinach, Feta & Roasted Red Pepper, Higgidy*	¼ Quiche/100g	247	17.1	247	8.4	17.1	17.1	1.1
Three Cheese & Onion, GFY, Asda*	1 Serving/73g	188	10.2	258	10.0	23.0	14.0	3.1
Tomato & Cheese, Sainsbury's*	1/3 Quiche/133g	374	24.5	281	7.9	20.9	18.4	1.5
Tomato, Cheese & Courgette, Asda*	1 Quiche/100g	333	17.0	333	11.0	34.0	17.0	5.0
Tomato, Mozzarella, & Basil, Weight Watchers*	1 Quiche/165g	300	12.2	182	6.1	22.8	7.4	1.3
Tomato, Pesto & Mozzarella, TTD, Sainsbury's*	1/3 Quiche/158g	370	25.6	234	5.5	16.5	16.2	2.1
Tuna, Tomato & Basil, Asda*	1 Serving/125g	305	20.0	244	9.0	16.0	16.0	1.5
Vegetable, Tesco*	1 Serving/100g	257	17.7	257	6.9	17.5	17.7	1.5
QUINCE								
Average	**1 fruit/209g**	**37**	**0.1**	**18**	**0.2**	**4.3**	**0.1**	**1.3**
QUINOA								
Cooked, LL, Waitrose*	1 Serving/180g	216	3.5	120	9.9	4.4	1.9	2.8
Dry Weight, Average	**1 Serving/70g**	**258**	**4.2**	**368**	**14.1**	**64.2**	**6.1**	**7.0**
Flakes, Biofair*	1 Serving/40g	155	2.3	387	11.7	72.2	5.7	8.9
Organic, Dry Weight, LL, Waitrose*	1 Serving/40g	154	2.3	384	13.1	68.9	5.8	5.9
QUORN*								
Bacon Style Rashers, Deli, Quorn*	1 Rasher/15g	30	2.3	199	11.8	3.0	15.5	5.0
Balls, Swedish Style, Frozen, Quorn*	¼ Pack/75g	88	1.9	117	12.0	9.0	2.5	5.2
Beef Style Pieces, Quorn*	½ Pack/75g	69	1.7	92	13.5	4.5	2.2	5.0
Biryani, Chicken Style, Lunch Pot, Quorn*	1 Pot/300g	300	13.0	100	3.5	10.9	4.4	1.7
Bites, Quorn*	½ Pack/70g	77	1.8	110	13.8	8.0	2.5	5.0
Burger, Frozen, Quorn*	1 Burger/50g	75	3.0	150	14.4	7.7	6.0	4.0
Burger, Smoked Chilli & Lime, Chef's Selection, Quorn*	1 Burger/90g	147	6.3	163	17.0	6.6	7.0	3.0
Burgers, Chicken Style, Quorn*	1 Burger/67g	149	8.1	222	10.5	16.0	12.0	4.0
Burgers, Quarter Pounder, Mexican Style, Quorn*	1 Burger/113g	180	6.3	159	18.3	8.9	5.6	3.8

QUORN*	Measure INFO/WEIGHT	per Measure KCAL	FAT	Nutrition Values per 100g / 100ml KCAL	PROT	CARB	FAT	FIBRE
Burgers, Quarter Pounder, Quorn*	1 Burger/114g	170	6.8	150	14.4	7.7	6.0	4.0
Burgers, Sizzling, Quorn*	1 Burger/80g	123	4.8	154	18.0	7.0	6.0	3.0
Chicken Style Dippers, Quorn*	4 Dippers/92g	195	8.0	212	11.1	21.2	8.7	2.4
Chicken Style Pieces, Frozen or Chilled, Quorn*	1 Serving/87g	77	1.2	89	14.0	1.0	1.4	8.3
Chicken Style Tikka Pieces, Quorn*	1 Pack/175g	201	5.2	115	12.5	7.0	3.0	6.0
Chilli, Vegetarian, Tesco*	1 Pack/400g	340	3.2	85	4.4	15.0	0.8	2.1
Cottage Pie, Quorn*	1 Lg Pack/500g	365	10.0	73	2.5	10.0	2.0	2.5
Curry & Rice, Quorn*	1 Pack/300g	306	8.7	102	3.7	14.4	2.9	1.9
Curry, Red Thai, Quorn*	1 Serving/250g	240	12.0	96	5.6	6.1	4.8	3.6
En Croute, Cheddar Cheese & Ham Style, Quorn*	1 Pastry/200g	486	28.0	243	7.2	22.0	14.0	3.0
En Croute, Creamy Mushroom & Garlic, Quorn*	1 Pastry/200g	460	29.0	230	5.9	19.0	14.5	3.2
Escalope, Cheese & Leek, Quorn*	1 Escalope/120g	256	13.2	213	9.0	17.0	11.0	5.0
Escalope, Creamy Garlic & Mushroom, Quorn*	1 Escalope/120g	291	15.0	243	10.5	20.5	12.5	3.0
Escalope, Garlic & Herb, Quorn*	1 Escalope/140g	293	16.5	209	8.9	16.9	11.8	3.8
Escalope, Gruyere Cheese, Quorn*	1 Escalope/110g	267	15.4	243	10.0	18.0	14.0	2.6
Escalope, Lemon & Black Pepper, Quorn*	1 Escalope/110g	256	12.9	233	9.6	20.5	11.7	2.1
Escalope, Mozzarella & Pesto, Quorn*	1 Escalope/120g	271	15.6	226	10.0	15.0	13.0	4.5
Escalope, Turkey Style, Sage & Onion, Quorn*	1 Escalope/100g	188	9.8	188	10.0	15.0	9.8	4.5
Fajita Meal Kit, Quorn*	½ Pack/214g	268	5.4	125	7.0	18.5	2.5	3.5
Fajita, Strips, Quorn*	½ Pack/70g	76	1.1	108	14.0	7.0	1.5	5.0
Fillets, Breaded, Mini, Quorn*	1 Fillet/30g	59	2.9	196	10.2	15.0	9.6	4.5
Fillets, Chicken Style, Plain, Quorn*	1 Fillet/64g	68	1.0	106	13.0	5.0	1.5	5.0
Fillets, Crispy, Quorn*	1 Fillet/100g	192	8.5	192	12.5	14.2	8.5	4.0
Fillets, Garlic & Herb, Quorn*	1 Fillet/100g	208	9.8	208	13.9	16.1	9.8	4.1
Fillets, Lemon & Pepper, Quorn*	1 Fillet/100g	195	8.5	195	13.3	16.2	8.5	3.5
Fishless Fingers, Quorn*	1 Finger/288g	66	3.0	233	10.0	22.0	10.5	5.0
Girasoli, Chorizo & Mozzarella Filled, Quorn*	½ Pack/125g	360	12.9	288	10.2	36.5	10.3	4.5
Goujons, Quorn*	1 Goujon/30g	59	2.9	196	10.2	15.0	9.6	4.5
Grills, Lamb Style, Quorn*	1 Grill/90g	126	4.0	140	16.0	5.6	4.4	5.5
Kievs, Mini, Quorn*	1 Kiev/20g	41	2.2	207	14.0	13.0	11.0	6.5
Kofta, Lamb Style, Bites, Quorn*	1 Bite/25g	47	2.4	186	5.0	20.0	9.5	3.0
Lamb Style, Strips, Quorn*	¼ Pack/75g	74	1.1	99	14.8	3.5	1.5	6.0
Lasagne, Frozen or Chilled, Quorn*	1 Pack/300g	303	8.1	101	4.8	12.5	2.7	1.6
Mexican Chilli, Chef's Selection, Quorn*	½ Pack/170g	143	4.3	84	6.6	6.5	2.5	4.5
Mince, Frozen & Chilled, Quorn*	1 Serving/87g	91	1.7	105	14.5	4.5	2.0	5.5
Mini Savoury Eggs, Quorn*	1 Egg/20g	51	2.3	257	15.0	21.0	11.5	4.6
Noodles, Sweet Chilli, Quorn*	1 Pack/400g	352	9.2	88	4.2	12.7	2.3	1.5
Nuggets, Crispy, Chicken Style, Quorn*	1 Nugget/17g	33	2.0	198	12.0	8.0	12.0	4.8
Pasty, Cornish Style, Quorn*	1 Pasty/150g	320	15.0	213	6.9	22.5	10.0	3.0
Pie, Chicken Style & Mushroom, Quorn*	1 Pie/235g	515	26.6	219	6.7	21.2	11.3	2.8
Pie, Meat Free Steak, Quorn*	1 Pie/235g	439	18.8	187	5.6	22.0	8.0	2.0
Pie, Mince & Potato, Quorn*	1 Pie/200g	388	16.0	194	6.5	22.5	8.0	3.0
Pieces, Bacon Style, Quorn*	1 Pack/100g	103	2.5	103	15.0	5.0	2.5	5.0
Pork Steaks, Quorn*	1 Steak/83g	132	7.1	159	16.6	1.4	8.5	5.3
Roast, Chicken Style, Quorn*	1/5 Roast/91g	96	1.8	106	15.0	4.5	2.0	4.9
Sausage Roll, Chilled, Quorn*	1 Roll/130g	293	12.1	225	12.3	21.2	9.3	3.8
Sausage, Best of British, Chef's Selection, Quorn*	1 Sausage/60g	111	5.7	185	11.0	12.0	9.5	3.5
Sausages, Bangers, Bramley Apple, Quorn*	1 Sausage/50g	59	2.3	117	11.5	7.5	4.6	3.0
Sausages, Bangers, Quorn*	1 Sausage/50g	58	2.4	116	11.7	6.6	4.8	3.0
Sausages, Cocktail, Quorn*	1 Sausage/15g	33	1.8	218	11.2	13.9	12.2	3.9
Sausages, Cumberland, Quorn*	1 Sausage/50g	86	3.5	172	13.5	12.0	7.0	3.5
Sausages, Frankfurter, Quorn*	1 Frankfurter/45g	92	6.3	205	13.5	4.5	14.0	3.5
Sausages, Pork & Apple Style, Quorn*	1 Sausage/50g	58	2.3	117	11.5	7.5	4.6	3.0

QUORN*

INFO/WEIGHT	Measure	per Measure KCAL	per Measure FAT	Nutrition Values per 100g / 100ml KCAL	PROT	CARB	FAT	FIBRE
Sausages, Quorn*	1 Sausage/40g	71	3.1	177	10.2	13.4	7.8	6.2
Sausages, Wild Garlic & Parsley,,Chef's Selection, Quorn*	1 Sausage/60g	104	5.4	174	12.0	9.0	9.0	4.5
Slices, Chicken Style, Deli, Quorn*	1 Slice/13g	13	0.3	107	16.3	4.5	2.6	6.0
Slices, Chicken Style, Wafer Thin, Quorn*	¼ Pack/25g	30	0.7	119	16.3	4.5	2.6	5.9
Slices, Ham Style, Quorn*	¼ Pack/25g	30	0.5	122	16.0	6.5	2.2	5.8
Slices, Ham Style, Smoky, Quorn*	¼ Pack/25g	34	0.5	136	15.5	9.0	2.0	5.0
Slices, Ham Style, Wafer Thin, Deli, Quorn*	1/3 Pack/60g	66	1.3	110	16.0	6.5	2.2	5.8
Slices, Peppered Beef Style, Quorn*	¼ Pack/25g	29	0.5	115	14.5	7.6	2.1	4.0
Slices, Pepperoni Style, Quorn*	1 Slice/5g	11	0.8	217	12.0	6.5	15.0	4.0
Slices, Roast Chicken Style, Quorn*	½ Pack/50g	54	1.1	109	16.0	6.4	2.2	5.6
Slices, Turkey Style with Stuffing, Deli, Quorn*	½ Pack/50g	60	1.2	120	16.0	8.9	2.3	4.0
Southern Style, Fried Strips, Quorn*	1 Strip/31g	62	2.9	200	9.5	19.0	9.5	3.5
Spaghetti Bolognese, Quorn*	1 Pack/300g	255	1.8	85	4.4	14.8	0.6	1.5
Steak Strips, Frozen, Quorn*	¼ Pack/75g	75	1.8	100	14.3	4.3	2.4	6.0
Steaks, Peppered, Quorn*	1 Steak/98g	123	3.9	126	13.6	5.7	4.0	6.9
Stir Fry, Spicy Chilli with Vegetables & Rice, Quorn*	½ Pack/170g	162	1.7	95	5.9	15.6	1.0	1.8
Turkey & Sage Slices, Meat Free, Quorn*	¼ Pack/25g	32	0.6	128	16.0	8.9	2.3	4.0

Q

	Measure INFO/WEIGHT	per Measure KCAL	FAT	Nutrition Values per 100g / 100ml KCAL	PROT	CARB	FAT	FIBRE
RABBIT								
Meat Only, Raw	*1oz/28g*	*38*	*1.5*	*137*	*21.9*	*0.0*	*5.5*	*0.0*
Meat Only, Raw, Weighed with Bone	*1 Serving/200g*	*164*	*6.6*	*82*	*13.1*	*0.0*	*3.3*	*0.0*
Meat Only, Stewed	*1oz/28g*	*32*	*0.9*	*114*	*21.2*	*0.0*	*3.2*	*0.0*
Meat Only, Stewed, Weighed with Bone	*1oz/28g*	*11*	*0.3*	*41*	*7.6*	*0.0*	*1.1*	*0.0*
RADISH								
Red, Unprepared, Average	*1 Radish/8g*	*1*	*0.0*	*11*	*0.6*	*1.7*	*0.2*	*0.8*
White, Mooli, Raw	*1oz/28g*	*4*	*0.0*	*13*	*0.7*	*2.5*	*0.1*	*0.0*
RAISINS								
& Apricot, The Fruit Factory*	1 Box/14g	41	0.1	290	3.5	67.9	0.5	6.3
& Sultanas, Jumbo, M&S*	1 Serving/80g	212	0.4	265	2.4	62.4	0.5	2.6
& Sultanas, The Fruit Factory*	1 Box/14g	43	0.1	305	3.0	72.3	0.5	4.0
Cherry Infused, Nak'd*	1 Pack/25g	68	0.0	272	2.1	79.0	0.0	2.0
Crazy Cola Infused, Nak'd*	1 Pack/25g	68	0.1	272	2.1	69.3	0.4	2.0
Lime Infused, Tangy, Nak'd*	1 Pack/25g	68	0.0	272	2.1	69.3	0.0	0.0
Pineapple Infused, Nak'd*	1 Pack/25g	68	0.0	272	3.0	79.0	0.0	4.0
Seedless, Average	*1 Serving/75g*	*215*	*0.4*	*287*	*2.2*	*68.5*	*0.5*	*3.2*
Sunny, Whitworths*	1 Box/43g	123	0.2	294	2.6	70.0	0.4	5.3
RAITA								
Dip, Indian, Asda*	1 Pot/70g	120	11.5	172	2.6	3.6	16.4	0.5
Plain, Average	*1oz/28g*	*16*	*0.6*	*57*	*4.2*	*5.8*	*2.2*	*0.0*
RASPBERRIES								
Freeze Dried, Simply*	1 Serving/10g	37	0.0	370	10.0	80.0	0.0	20.0
Fresh, Raw, Average	*1 Serving/80g*	*20*	*0.2*	*25*	*1.3*	*4.7*	*0.3*	*6.5*
Frozen, Average	*1 Serving/100g*	*27*	*0.3*	*27*	*1.3*	*4.7*	*0.3*	*5.2*
in Syrup, Canned	*1oz/28g*	*25*	*0.0*	*88*	*0.6*	*22.5*	*0.1*	*1.5*
RATATOUILLE								
Average	*1oz/28g*	*23*	*2.0*	*82*	*1.3*	*3.8*	*7.0*	*1.8*
Provencale, Asda*	½ Can/195g	98	3.9	50	1.0	7.0	2.0	1.0
Provencale, French Style Mixed Vegetables, Tesco*	½ Can/195g	76	3.9	39	1.1	4.2	2.0	1.9
Roasted Vegetable, Sainsbury's*	1 Pack/300g	134	3.0	45	1.4	7.5	1.0	2.3
RAVIOLI								
Beef	1 Serving/300g	501	13.7	167	6.4	25.0	4.6	1.4
Beef & Red Wine, Italiano, Tesco*	½ Pack/200g	424	13.0	212	7.3	30.0	6.5	2.3
Beef in Tomato Sauce, Canned, Great Stuff, Asda*	1 Can/200g	146	3.0	73	2.2	12.7	1.5	1.4
Beef, Tesco*	1 Serving/194g	175	5.0	90	4.3	12.3	2.6	1.5
Beef, Weight Watchers*	1 Pack/300g	258	6.3	86	4.3	12.1	2.1	0.8
Cheese in Tomato Sauce, Canned, Tesco*	1 Can/410g	328	8.2	80	2.5	13.0	2.0	0.5
Cheese, Garlic & Herb, Fresh, Organic, Tesco*	1 Serving/125g	382	19.5	306	11.3	30.1	15.6	0.9
Chicken & Mushroom, Finest, Tesco*	½ Pack/125g	268	8.9	214	11.6	25.8	7.1	1.1
Chicken, Tomato & Basil, Finest, Tesco*	1 Serving/200g	358	12.0	179	9.6	21.7	6.0	1.0
Four Cheese in Tomato Sauce, COU, M&S*	1 Pack/345g	345	7.6	100	7.5	12.3	2.2	1.5
Four Cheese, Italian Choice, Asda*	1 Pack/449g	467	26.9	104	3.4	9.0	6.0	2.1
Garlic Mushroom, Finest, Tesco*	1 Serving/250g	552	18.2	221	8.9	30.0	7.3	2.0
Goat's Cheese & Pesto, Asda*	½ Pack/150g	204	5.4	136	6.0	20.0	3.6	0.0
in Tomato Sauce, Canned, Sainsbury's*	½ Can/200g	166	2.0	83	3.1	15.5	1.0	0.5
in Tomato Sauce, Heinz*	1 Can/400g	308	6.8	77	2.4	13.2	1.7	0.9
Meat, Italian, Fresh, Asda*	½ Pack/150g	261	6.3	174	8.0	26.0	4.2	0.0
Mushroom, Fresh, Sainsbury's*	½ Pack/125g	196	5.1	157	7.4	22.6	4.1	1.9
Mushroom, Wild, Finest, Tesco*	1 Serving/200g	472	12.2	236	10.8	34.4	6.1	1.9
Pancetta & Mozzarella, Finest, Tesco*	1 Serving/125g	344	13.2	275	12.2	32.8	10.6	1.8
Rich Beef & Red Wine, Morrisons*	1 Pack/300g	813	20.7	271	12.0	42.8	6.9	2.6
Roasted Vegetable, Asda*	½ Pack/150g	218	0.8	145	6.0	29.0	0.5	0.0
Salmon & Dill, Sainsbury's*	1 Pack/300g	615	21.3	205	8.7	26.5	7.1	3.0

R

	Measure INFO/WEIGHT	per Measure KCAL	FAT	Nutrition Values per 100g / 100ml KCAL	PROT	CARB	FAT	FIBRE
RAVIOLI								
Smoked Salmon & Dill, Sainsbury's*	1 Serving/125g	256	8.9	205	8.7	26.5	7.1	0.7
Spinach & Ricotta, Waitrose*	1 Serving/125g	309	9.0	247	10.5	35.0	7.2	1.9
Tomato, Cheese & Meat, Sainsbury's*	1 Serving/125g	314	16.1	251	12.4	21.4	12.9	2.2
Vegetable, Canned, Sainsbury's*	1 Can/400g	328	2.8	82	2.6	16.3	0.7	0.7
Vegetable, Tesco*	½ Can/200g	164	1.4	82	2.6	16.3	0.7	0.7
with Minced Beef, in Rich Tomato Sauce, Corale, Aldi*	½ Can/200g	172	2.0	86	2.8	16.4	1.0	0.5
RED BULL*								
Regular, Red Bull*	1 Can/250ml	112	0.0	45	0.0	11.3	0.0	0.0
REDCURRANTS								
Raw, Average	*1oz/28g*	*6*	*0.0*	*20*	*1.1*	*4.3*	*0.0*	*3.3*
Raw, Stalks Removed	*1 Serving/100g*	*21*	*0.0*	*21*	*1.1*	*4.4*	*0.0*	*0.0*
REEF*								
Orange & Passionfruit, Reef*	1 Bottle/275ml	179	0.0	65	0.0	9.5	0.0	0.0
RELISH								
Barbeque, Sainsbury's*	1 Serving/50g	50	1.0	100	1.0	19.3	2.1	1.1
Branston, Sweet Onion, Crosse & Blackwell*	1 Serving/10g	15	0.0	153	1.0	36.3	0.4	0.7
Branston, Tomato & Red Pepper, Crosse & Blackwell*	1 Serving/15g	24	0.1	160	1.3	37.4	0.4	0.7
Burger, Juicy, Asda*	1 Tbsp/15g	17	0.1	113	1.2	25.4	0.7	0.7
Caramelised Red Onion, Tesco*	1 Serving/10g	28	0.0	280	0.6	69.1	0.1	0.7
Onion & Garlic, Spicy, Waitrose*	1 Tbsp/15g	35	0.2	232	0.8	54.2	1.1	1.7
Onion, Sainsbury's*	1 Serving/15g	23	0.1	151	0.9	36.0	0.4	0.7
Onion, Sweet, Heinz*	1 Tbsp/38g	38	0.2	102	1.0	23.5	0.4	0.6
Sweetcorn, American Style, Maryland, Tesco*	1 Serving/15g	15	0.0	101	1.1	23.9	0.1	0.9
Sweetcorn, Bick's*	1 Tbsp/22g	23	0.0	103	1.3	24.3	0.2	0.0
Tomato & Chilli Texan Style, Tesco*	1 Tbsp/14g	20	0.0	140	1.7	32.0	0.1	1.1
Tomato Spicy, Bick's*	1 Serving/28g	28	0.1	99	1.3	23.2	0.2	0.0
Tomato, Sweet, Heinz*	1 Serving/25g	34	0.0	136	0.9	32.6	0.2	0.9
REVELS								
Mars*	1 Pack/35g	168	7.3	480	5.1	68.0	20.9	0.0
RHUBARB								
in Juice, Canned, Drained, Average	*1 Serving/100g*	*46*	*0.0*	*46*	*0.5*	*10.8*	*0.0*	*0.8*
Raw, Average	*1 Stalk/51g*	*11*	*0.1*	*21*	*0.9*	*4.5*	*0.2*	*1.8*
Sliced, Frozen, Asda*	1 Serving/100g	11	0.1	11	0.9	0.8	0.1	1.4
Stewed with Sugar, Average	*1oz/28g*	*32*	*0.0*	*116*	*0.4*	*31.2*	*0.0*	*2.0*
RIBENA*								
Blackcurrant Juice Drink, Ready Made, Ribena*	1 Carton/200ml	82	0.0	41	0.0	10.6	0.0	0.0
Blackcurrant, Diluted with Water, Ribena*	1 Serving/100ml	46	0.0	46	0.0	11.4	0.0	0.0
Blackcurrant, No Added Sugar, Diluted, Ribena*	1 Serving/250ml	11	0.0	4	0.0	0.6	0.0	0.0
Blackcurrant, Original, Undiluted, Ribena*	1 Serving/50ml	108	0.0	216	0.0	53.0	0.0	0.0
Blackcurrant, Really Light, No Added Sugar, Ribena*	1 Carton/250ml	8	0.0	3	0.0	0.8	0.0	0.0
Light, Ribena*	1 Carton/288ml	26	0.0	9	0.1	2.1	0.0	0.0
Plus, Apple & Peach, Immunity Support, Ribena*	1 Carton/200ml	2	0.0	1	0.0	0.2	0.0	0.0
Really Light, Undiluted, Ribena*	1 Serving/25ml	20	0.0	80	0.0	2.5	0.0	0.0
Strawberry Juice Drink, Ribena*	1 Carton/288ml	130	0.0	45	0.0	10.9	0.0	0.0
Winter Spice, Squash, Diluted, Ribena*	1 Serving/250ml	13	0.0	5	0.0	0.7	0.0	0.0
RIBS								
Beef, BBQ, Rich Soy & Worcester Glaze, Sainsbury's*	½ Pack/113g	254	16.5	225	16.9	6.3	14.6	0.3
in a Chinese Style Coating, Tesco*	1 Serving/250g	420	21.8	168	19.5	5.3	8.7	2.5
Loin, Chinese, Sainsbury's*	1 Rib/42g	103	5.0	246	27.2	7.2	12.0	0.9
Loin, Chinese, Taste Summer, Sainsbury's*	1 Serving/30g	38	2.3	128	11.7	2.8	7.8	0.1
Pork, Barbecue, Meat Only, Cooked, Average	*1 Serving/100g*	*275*	*17.9*	*275*	*21.4*	*7.2*	*17.9*	*0.3*
Pork, Barbeque, Weighed with Bone, Cooked, Average	*1 Serving/100g*	*220*	*14.3*	*220*	*17.1*	*5.8*	*14.3*	*0.3*
Pork, Chinese Style, Average	*1 Serving/300g*	*736*	*44.7*	*245*	*17.9*	*10.0*	*14.9*	*0.7*

R

	Measure INFO/WEIGHT	per Measure KCAL	per Measure FAT	Nutrition Values per 100g / 100ml KCAL	PROT	CARB	FAT	FIBRE
RIBS								
Pork, Chops, Raw, Lean & Fat, Weighed with Bone	**1 Chop/130g**	**241**	**16.1**	**186**	**18.5**	**0.0**	**12.4**	**0.0**
Pork, Full Rack, Sainsbury's*	1 Serving/225g	567	38.7	252	18.0	6.5	17.2	0.9
Spare, Barbecue, Chinese Style, Farmfoods*	1 Pack/400g	464	25.2	116	9.3	5.6	6.3	0.1
Spare, Chinese Style, Summer Eating, Asda*	1 Serving/116g	334	18.6	288	32.0	4.1	16.0	0.8
Spare, Sweet, Sticky, Mini, M&S*	1 Pack/300g	615	34.5	205	16.6	8.6	11.5	0.2
RICE								
Arborio, Dry, Average	**1 Serving/80g**	**279**	**0.6**	**348**	**7.1**	**78.3**	**0.8**	**0.8**
Basmati & Wild, Cooked, Sainsbury's*	½ Pack/125g	150	0.8	120	3.1	25.7	0.6	1.3
Basmati & Wild, Dry Weight, Tilda*	1 Serving/70g	244	0.3	349	9.4	77.0	0.5	1.0
Basmati with Mushroom, Dine In, Veetee*	1 Pack/280g	372	6.4	133	3.3	24.4	2.3	1.2
Basmati, Boil in the Bag, Dry, Average	**1 Serving/50g**	**176**	**0.4**	**352**	**8.4**	**77.8**	**0.8**	**0.4**
Basmati, Brown, Dry, Average	**1 Serving/50g**	**177**	**1.5**	**353**	**9.5**	**71.8**	**3.0**	**2.2**
Basmati, Cooked, Average	**1 Serving/140g**	**189**	**1.0**	**135**	**3.1**	**29.0**	**0.7**	**0.4**
Basmati, Cooked, Tilda*	1 Serving/200g	214	0.2	107	2.4	24.0	0.1	1.2
Basmati, Dry Weight, Average	**1 Serving/60g**	**212**	**0.6**	**353**	**8.1**	**77.9**	**1.0**	**0.6**
Basmati, Indian, Dry, Average	**1 Serving/75g**	**260**	**0.7**	**346**	**8.4**	**76.1**	**0.9**	**0.1**
Basmati, Microwavable, Golden Sun, Lidl*	½ Pack/125g	188	2.8	150	3.4	28.7	2.2	1.0
Basmati, Microwave, Cooked, Average	**1 Serving/125g**	**182**	**2.3**	**146**	**2.7**	**30.0**	**1.8**	**0.0**
Basmati, Microwave, Quick Cups, Sun Rice*	1 Cup/120g	205	2.5	171	3.3	27.8	2.1	1.1
Basmati, Microwave, Tesco*	½ Pack/125g	185	1.1	148	3.3	31.0	0.9	1.9
Basmati, Microwaveable, Tesco*	½ Pack/125g	212	2.2	170	4.0	34.1	1.8	0.5
Basmati, Stir Fry, Kung Po, Straight to Pan, Tilda*	1 Serving/120g	151	2.5	126	2.6	24.2	2.1	2.1
Basmati, White, Dry, Average	**1 Serving/75g**	**262**	**0.4**	**349**	**8.1**	**77.1**	**0.6**	**0.4**
Basmati, Wholegrain, Cooked, Tilda*	1 Portion/180g	203	1.6	113	3.3	23.0	0.9	3.2
Beef, Savoury, Batchelors*	1 Pack/120g	431	2.8	359	8.9	75.7	2.3	2.5
Brown Basmati, Butternut Squash, Tilda*	½ Pack/125g	164	5.1	131	3.3	20.3	4.1	1.2
Brown Basmati, Wholegrain & Wild, Pouch, Tilda*	½ Pack/125g	160	2.6	128	3.0	23.4	2.1	1.7
Brown, Cooked, Average	**1 Serving/140g**	**173**	**1.5**	**123**	**2.6**	**26.6**	**1.1**	**0.9**
Brown, Dry, Average	**1 Serving/75g**	**266**	**2.3**	**355**	**7.5**	**76.2**	**3.0**	**1.4**
Brown, Long Grain, Dry, Average	**1 Serving/50g**	**182**	**1.4**	**364**	**7.6**	**76.8**	**2.8**	**2.0**
Brown, Short Grain, Dry, Average	**1 Serving/50g**	**176**	**1.4**	**351**	**6.8**	**77.6**	**2.8**	**1.0**
Brown, Whole Grain, Cooked, Average	**1 Serving/170g**	**223**	**1.9**	**132**	**2.6**	**27.8**	**1.1**	**1.2**
Brown, Whole Grain, Dry, Average	**1 Serving/40g**	**138**	**1.2**	**344**	**7.4**	**71.6**	**2.9**	**3.0**
Chicken, Savoury, Batchelors*	1 Pack/124g	455	1.9	367	8.9	79.4	1.5	2.6
Chicken, Savoury, Smart Price, Asda*	½ Pack/168g	210	1.5	125	3.2	26.0	0.9	2.4
Chinese Style, Express, Uncle Ben's*	1 Pack/250g	392	5.5	157	3.4	30.9	2.2	0.4
Coconut, Thai, Sainsbury's*	½ Pack/100g	178	9.1	178	2.6	21.3	9.1	1.9
Egg Fried, Asda*	1 Pack/229g	286	5.7	125	3.6	22.0	2.5	2.3
Egg Fried, Average	**1 Serving/300g**	**624**	**31.8**	**208**	**4.2**	**25.7**	**10.6**	**0.4**
Egg Fried, Chinese Style, Tesco*	1 Portion/250g	418	10.5	167	4.4	27.9	4.2	0.7
Egg Fried, Chinese Takeaway, Iceland*	1 Pack/340g	374	7.8	110	4.2	18.1	2.3	1.1
Egg Fried, Chinese Takeaway, Tesco*	1 Serving/200g	250	3.0	125	4.7	23.3	1.5	1.8
Egg Fried, Express, Uncle Ben's*	½ Pack/125g	216	5.2	173	4.0	29.9	4.2	0.3
Egg Fried, M&S*	½ Pack/150g	315	10.5	210	4.2	32.4	7.0	0.3
Egg Fried, Micro, Tesco*	1 Pack/250g	312	9.2	125	4.6	18.3	3.7	6.4
Egg Fried, Sainsbury's*	1 Pack/250g	432	9.5	173	4.5	30.3	3.8	0.8
Egg, Chinese Style, Morrisons*	1 Serving/250g	285	11.9	114	2.1	16.8	4.8	0.7
Express Microwave, Uncle Ben's*	1 Serving/250g	370	4.2	148	3.2	30.0	1.7	0.0
Fried, Chicken, Chinese Takeaway, Iceland*	1 Pack/340g	510	15.6	150	6.5	20.7	4.6	0.6
Fried, Duck, Chicken & Pork Celebration, Sainsbury's*	1 Pack/450g	544	16.2	121	7.9	14.2	3.6	1.5
Garlic & Coriander Flavoured, Patak's*	1 Serving/125g	186	2.8	149	2.6	28.9	2.2	0.0
Golden Savoury, Dry Weight, Batchelors*	1 Pack/120g	437	3.4	364	10.1	74.7	2.8	2.4
Golden Vegetable, Freshly Frozen, Asda*	1 Sachet/200g	238	2.6	119	3.2	23.6	1.3	1.3

RICE

INFO/WEIGHT	Measure	per Measure		Nutrition Values per 100g / 100ml				
		KCAL	FAT	KCAL	PROT	CARB	FAT	FIBRE
Golden Vegetable, Savoury, Morrisons*	1 Serving/50g	70	0.4	141	3.4	30.1	0.8	1.1
Golden Vegetable, Savoury, Newgate, Lidl*	½ Pack/60g	70	0.4	117	2.9	24.0	0.7	2.1
Ground, Whitworths*	1 Serving/28g	98	0.2	349	7.7	77.7	0.8	0.7
Long Grain, & Wild, Dry, Average	*1 Serving/75g*	*254*	*1.5*	*338*	*7.6*	*72.6*	*2.0*	*1.7*
Long Grain, American, Cooked, Average	*1 Serving/160g*	*229*	*2.8*	*143*	*3.0*	*28.8*	*1.8*	*0.2*
Long Grain, American, Dry, Average	*1 Serving/50g*	*175*	*0.5*	*350*	*7.2*	*77.8*	*1.1*	*0.6*
Long Grain, Boil in the Bag, Golden Sun, Lidl*	1 Bag/125g	440	1.4	352	7.7	77.0	1.1	1.8
Long Grain, Brown, Micro Rice, Asda*	1 Portion/100g	153	1.4	153	3.8	30.2	1.4	2.4
Long Grain, Cooked, Value, Tesco*	1 Portion/50g	175	0.4	350	7.7	78.0	0.8	0.4
Long Grain, Dry, Average	*1 Serving/50g*	*169*	*0.5*	*337*	*7.4*	*75.5*	*1.0*	*1.7*
Long Grain, Microwavable, Cooked, Average	*1 Serving/150g*	*180*	*0.9*	*120*	*2.7*	*25.8*	*0.6*	*0.7*
Mexican Style, Ainsley Harriott*	1 Pack/170g	206	1.5	121	1.7	26.5	0.9	2.3
Mexican Style, Cooked, Express, Uncle Ben's*	1 Pack/250g	385	4.8	154	3.2	31.1	1.9	0.7
Mexican Style, Old El Paso*	1 Serving/75g	268	0.8	357	9.0	78.0	1.0	0.0
Mexican, Spicy, Lidl*	½ Pack/125g	196	2.5	157	4.0	29.5	2.0	2.3
Mild Curry, Savoury, Batchelors*	1 Pack/120g	426	2.5	355	8.0	76.1	2.1	1.6
Mixed Vegetable, Savoury, Dry Weight, Tesco*	1 Pack/120g	450	3.2	375	7.8	79.1	2.7	2.9
Mushroom & Coconut, Organic, Waitrose*	1 Pack/300g	474	15.0	158	3.7	24.5	5.0	1.4
Mushroom & Pepper, Savoury, Cooked, Morrisons*	1 Serving/200g	204	1.6	102	2.3	21.5	0.8	0.0
Mushroom Pilau, Bombay Brasserie, Sainsbury's*	1 Pack/400g	672	17.2	168	3.7	28.6	4.3	0.7
Mushroom Savoury, Batchelors*	½ Pack/61g	217	1.3	356	10.7	73.6	2.1	2.8
Paella, Savoury, Tesco*	1 Serving/60g	220	2.8	367	8.4	72.7	4.7	4.5
Peshwari, Special, Uncle Ben's*	½ Pack/125g	226	4.2	181	3.0	33.6	3.4	0.0
Pilau, Cooked, Average	*1 Serving/200g*	*349*	*8.8*	*174*	*3.5*	*30.3*	*4.4*	*0.8*
Pilau, Dry, Average	*1oz/28g*	*101*	*0.7*	*362*	*8.4*	*78.2*	*2.4*	*3.4*
Pilau, Indian Mushroom, Sainsbury's*	1 Serving/100g	119	2.4	119	3.0	21.3	2.4	1.9
Pilau, Mushroom, Sainsbury's*	1 Pack/250g	400	13.8	160	3.4	24.1	5.5	2.4
Pilau, Spinach & Carrot, Waitrose*	1 Pack/350g	466	8.4	133	3.1	24.8	2.4	1.2
Pilau, Spinach, Bombay Brasserie, Sainsbury's*	1 Pack/401g	642	17.3	160	3.5	26.9	4.3	0.8
Pilau, Waitrose*	½ Pack/175g	308	7.4	176	4.2	30.4	4.2	1.2
Pudding, Dry Weight, Average	*1 Serving/100g*	*356*	*1.1*	*356*	*6.9*	*82.0*	*1.1*	*0.4*
Risotto, Dry, Average	*1 Serving/50g*	*174*	*0.6*	*348*	*7.8*	*76.2*	*1.3*	*2.4*
Saffron, Cooked, Average	*1 Serving/150g*	*208*	*4.7*	*139*	*2.6*	*25.3*	*3.2*	*0.5*
Special Fried, Cantonese, Sainsbury's*	½ Pack/250g	442	10.0	177	4.9	30.4	4.0	1.2
Special Fried, Chinese Takeaway, Iceland*	1 Pack/350g	630	17.5	180	5.5	28.2	5.0	1.2
Special Fried, Chinese, Tesco*	1 Serving/300g	618	33.3	206	6.5	19.9	11.1	0.8
Special Fried, M&S*	1 Pack/450g	922	35.1	205	6.2	27.2	7.8	0.5
Special Fried, Sainsbury's*	1 Serving/166g	272	7.6	164	5.1	25.5	4.6	0.7
Special Fried, Waitrose*	1 Serving/350g	532	22.4	152	6.1	17.6	6.4	3.2
Stir Fry, Thai Green, Tilda*	½ Pack/120g	155	4.8	129	2.9	20.3	4.0	4.0
Thai Sticky, Tesco*	1 Serving/250g	358	6.2	143	2.5	27.6	2.5	0.4
Thai, Cooked, Average	*1 Serving/100g*	*136*	*1.8*	*136*	*2.5*	*27.4*	*1.8*	*0.3*
Thai, Dry, Average	*1 Serving/50g*	*174*	*0.2*	*348*	*7.1*	*78.9*	*0.4*	*0.9*
Thai, Fragrant, Dry, Average	*1 Serving/75g*	*272*	*0.5*	*363*	*7.2*	*82.0*	*0.7*	*0.3*
Thai, Glutinous, Sticky, White, Dry, Raw	*1 Serving/100g*	*370*	*0.6*	*370*	*6.8*	*81.7*	*0.6*	*2.8*
Valencia for Paella, Asda*	1 Serving/125g	435	1.0	348	6.0	79.0	0.8	0.0
White, Cooked, Average	*1 Serving/140g*	*182*	*1.1*	*130*	*2.6*	*28.7*	*0.8*	*0.2*
White, Cooked, Frozen, Average	*1 Serving/150g*	*168*	*0.8*	*112*	*2.9*	*23.8*	*0.6*	*1.2*
White, Flaked, Dry Weight, Average	*1oz/28g*	*97*	*0.3*	*346*	*6.6*	*77.5*	*1.2*	*0.0*
White, Fried	1oz/28g	37	0.9	131	2.2	25.0	3.2	0.6
White, Long Grain, Dry Weight, Average	*1 Serving/50g*	*181*	*1.0*	*362*	*7.1*	*79.1*	*1.9*	*0.4*
White, Microwave, Cooked, Average	*½ Pack/125g*	*185*	*2.4*	*148*	*3.3*	*29.4*	*1.9*	*1.4*
Whole Grain, Dry, Average	*1 Serving/50g*	*171*	*1.2*	*342*	*8.2*	*72.0*	*2.3*	*4.0*

R

	Measure INFO/WEIGHT	per Measure		Nutrition Values per 100g / 100ml				
		KCAL	FAT	KCAL	PROT	CARB	FAT	FIBRE

RICE

	Measure INFO/WEIGHT	KCAL	FAT	KCAL	PROT	CARB	FAT	FIBRE
Wholegrain, Microwave, Eat Well, M&S*	½ Pack/125g	181	1.5	145	2.5	31.0	1.2	2.2
with Red Kidney Beans, Average	**1oz/28g**	**49**	**1.0**	**175**	**5.6**	**32.4**	**3.5**	**2.5**

RICE CAKES

	Measure INFO/WEIGHT	KCAL	FAT	KCAL	PROT	CARB	FAT	FIBRE
Apple & Cinnamon Flavour, Kallo*	1 Cake/11g	41	0.2	376	6.2	83.1	2.2	3.9
Asda*	1 Cake/8g	31	0.2	386	8.7	81.1	3.0	2.8
Barbeque, Tesco*	1 Cake/9g	28	0.2	328	9.6	66.8	2.5	6.2
Caramel Flavour, Kallo*	1 Cake/10g	38	0.5	383	6.2	78.9	4.8	3.9
Caramel, Jumbo, Snack-A-Jacks, Quaker Oats*	1 Cake/13g	51	0.3	390	5.5	87.0	2.1	1.4
Caramel, Jumbo, Tesco*	1 Cake/10g	34	0.3	340	7.0	74.0	3.0	5.0
Caramel, Large, Tesco*	1 Cake/10g	34	0.2	344	6.5	73.9	2.5	5.1
Caramel, Less Than 3% Fat, Sainsbury's*	1 Pack/35g	134	0.6	382	5.6	86.4	1.6	1.8
Caramel, Snack, Snack-A-Jacks, Quaker Oats*	1 Bag/30g	122	0.9	405	6.0	88.0	3.0	0.8
Caramel, Tesco*	1 Serving/2g	9	0.1	379	5.5	98.2	2.9	0.9
Cheese & Onion, Snack, Snack-A-Jacks, Quaker Oats*	1 Bag/30g	120	2.2	400	6.7	77.0	7.5	1.5
Cheese, Jumbo, Free From, Tesco*	1 Serving/10g	44	1.8	439	8.1	62.1	17.6	3.8
Cheese, Snack, Snack-A-Jacks, Quaker Oats*	1 Bag/26g	108	2.1	415	8.5	77.0	8.0	0.9
Chocolate Chip, Jumbo, Snack-A-Jacks, Quaker Oats*	1 Cake/15g	62	1.0	410	6.0	81.0	7.0	1.7
Dark Chocolate, Organic, Kallo*	1 Cake/12g	57	2.9	471	6.8	57.2	24.1	7.4
Honey, Kallo*	1 Cake/10g	40	0.2	388	5.4	86.6	2.2	1.6
Lightly Salted, Thick Slice, Low Fat, Kallo*	1 Cake/8g	28	0.2	372	8.0	78.7	2.8	5.1
Low Fat, Kallo*	1 Cake/10g	38	0.2	375	6.2	83.1	2.2	3.9
Mature Cheese & Chive, Kallo*	1 Cake/9g	32	0.4	374	8.2	75.2	4.5	3.1
Milk Chocolate, Organic, Kallo*	1 Cake/11g	57	3.2	509	6.5	56.2	28.7	3.5
Multigrain, Ryvita*	3 Cakes/11g	43	0.5	384	9.1	76.2	4.7	5.3
Organic, Tesco*	1 Cake/8g	29	0.2	380	7.2	80.7	2.9	3.4
Paprika, Good Food*	1 Cake/12g	50	1.1	414	7.9	73.0	9.3	3.1
Salt & Vinegar Flavour, Morrisons*	1 Bag/30g	122	2.6	407	6.7	75.8	8.6	1.2
Salt & Vinegar, Jumbo, Snack-A-Jacks, Quaker Oats*	1 Cake/10g	41	0.6	391	7.4	75.4	5.7	1.6
Salt & Vinegar, Jumbo, Tesco*	1 Cake/9g	31	0.2	347	8.4	72.7	2.5	6.0
Salt & Vinegar, Snack, Tesco*	1 Pack/35g	116	0.6	332	7.5	71.5	1.8	1.1
Sea Salt & Balsamic Vinegar, Kallo*	1 Cake/9g	32	0.2	361	6.5	78.1	2.5	3.0
Sesame Teriyaki, Clearspring*	1 Cake/7g	28	0.2	377	6.5	82.8	2.2	0.0
Sesame, No Added Salt, Thick Sliced, Organic, Kallo*	1 Cake/10g	37	0.3	373	8.0	78.0	3.2	5.4
Sesame, Slightly Salted, Thick Slice, Organic, Kallo*	1 Cake/8g	28	0.2	373	8.0	78.0	3.2	5.4
Sesame, Slightly Salted, Thin Slice, Organic, Kallo*	1 Cake/5g	17	0.1	373	8.0	78.0	3.2	5.4
Slightly Salted, Mrs Crimble's*	1 Slice/6g	21	0.2	380	7.6	80.4	3.1	3.2
Slightly Salted, Organic, Thin Slice, Kallo*	1 Cake/5g	17	0.1	372	8.0	78.7	2.8	5.1
Slightly Salted, Thick Slice, Organic, Kallo*	1 Cake/8g	28	0.2	372	8.0	78.7	2.8	5.1
Sour Cream & Chive Flavour, Sainsbury's*	1 Pack/30g	119	2.6	396	7.9	72.0	8.5	2.9
Sweet Chilli Flavour, Snack-A-Jacks, Quaker Oats*	1 Pack/26g	108	2.0	414	7.3	78.9	7.5	1.1
Thin Slice, No Added Salt, Organic, Kallo*	1 Cake/5g	19	0.1	372	8.0	78.7	2.8	5.1
Toasted Sesame, Ryvita*	1 Pack/11g	43	0.5	391	8.4	78.4	4.9	3.5
Wholegrain, Mild Chilli, Tesco*	1 Cake/10g	38	1.4	400	7.2	59.8	14.4	5.8
Wholegrain, No Added Salt, BGTY, Sainsbury's*	1 Cake/8g	30	0.2	372	8.0	78.7	2.8	5.1
Wholegrain, Salt & Vinegar, Tesco*	1 Cake/9g	28	0.2	314	8.4	61.9	2.6	6.0
with Belgian Milk Chocolate, & Caramel Pieces, Kallo*	1 Biscuit/13g	63	2.8	485	6.2	65.1	21.8	1.9
with Sea Salt, Harvest Morn, Aldi*	1 Cake/7g	27	0.2	379	8.7	78.0	2.2	5.1

RICE CRACKERS

	Measure INFO/WEIGHT	KCAL	FAT	KCAL	PROT	CARB	FAT	FIBRE
Authentic Thai Chilli, Tyrrells*	½ Pack/75g	389	20.2	519	5.0	64.0	27.0	1.0
Barbecue, Sakata*	½ Pack/50g	204	1.3	407	7.3	85.2	2.6	1.6
Black Pepperdoms & Fruity Mango Chutney, Graze*	1 Punnet/24g	80	1.2	335	2.0	71.0	5.0	1.0
Brown, Wakama*	1 Cracker/5g	19	0.0	375	8.0	84.8	0.4	0.0
Cheddar Gorge, Graze*	1 Punnet/26g	139	9.0	534	10.6	48.3	34.7	2.3

	Measure INFO/WEIGHT	per Measure KCAL	FAT	Nutrition Values per 100g / 100ml KCAL	PROT	CARB	FAT	FIBRE
RICE CRACKERS								
Cheese, Tesco*	1 Serving/25g	104	2.0	416	7.9	78.1	8.0	1.8
Chilli, Temptations, Tesco*	1 Serving/25g	128	7.2	512	4.4	58.0	28.8	0.0
Crispy, Sour Cream & Herbs, Go Ahead, McVitie's*	1 Serving/25g	106	2.0	422	7.1	78.2	8.0	1.8
Japanese Seaweed, Very Nori-sh, Graze*	1 Punnet/14g	64	1.8	454	5.9	78.8	12.7	1.0
Japanese Style, Mix, Asda*	1 Serving/25g	96	0.2	385	6.8	88.0	0.6	0.5
Japanese Style, Tesco*	1 Serving/25g	101	1.5	405	11.7	75.2	6.1	3.3
Japanese, Apollo*	1 Pack/75g	297	3.5	396	9.6	78.8	4.7	0.9
Japanese, Graze*	1 Pack/40g	159	1.9	397	9.0	79.7	4.7	0.0
Japanese, Mini, Sunrise*	1 Serving/50g	180	0.0	360	7.0	83.0	0.0	7.0
Korean Chilli, Graze*	1 Pack/19g	98	5.1	519	5.0	64.0	27.0	0.5
Sainsbury's*	1 Serving/20g	87	1.9	433	11.2	74.3	9.4	1.0
Salt & Pepper, Asda*	1 Cracker/5g	19	0.0	385	7.0	87.0	1.0	2.2
Sour Cream & Chive, Sakata*	1 Serving/25g	107	2.0	430	7.8	80.6	7.9	0.0
Thai, Sesame & Soy Sauce, M&S*	1 Pack/55g	210	2.6	385	7.6	77.8	4.8	1.4
Thin, Blue Dragon*	3 Crackers/5g	20	0.2	395	6.1	84.4	3.7	0.0
Veggie Sushi Plate, Graze*	1 Punnet/24g	107	3.1	444	11.1	68.4	12.8	3.9
RICE PUDDING								
50% Less Fat, Asda*	½ Can/212g	180	1.7	85	3.3	16.2	0.8	0.2
Banana & Toffee (Limited Edition), Muller Rice, Muller*	1 Pot/190g	207	4.2	109	3.1	19.3	2.2	0.4
Canned, Average	***1oz/28g***	***25***	***0.7***	***89***	***3.4***	***14.0***	***2.5***	***0.2***
Canned, Basics, Sainsbury's*	½ Can/213g	157	1.7	74	3.1	13.7	0.8	1.4
Canned, BGTY, Sainsbury's*	1 Can/425g	344	2.6	81	3.3	15.5	0.6	0.4
Canned, GFY, Asda*	½ Can/213g	168	1.3	79	2.8	15.5	0.6	0.1
Clotted Cream, Cornish, Waitrose*	1 Serving/150g	304	20.1	203	3.0	17.6	13.4	0.5
Clotted Cream, M&S*	1 Pudding/185g	431	30.7	233	3.0	19.2	16.6	0.2
Creamed, Canned, Ambrosia*	1 Can/425g	382	8.1	90	3.1	16.2	1.9	0.0
Creamed, Pot, Ambrosia*	1 Pot/150g	156	3.8	104	3.3	17.0	2.5	0.1
Creamed, Value, Tesco*	1 Can/425g	348	3.4	82	3.2	15.5	0.8	0.0
Creamed, Weight Watchers*	1 Pot/130g	108	0.9	83	3.2	16.0	0.7	0.3
Creamy, Ambrosia*	½ Can/212g	197	4.0	93	3.2	15.7	1.9	0.0
Low Fat, Devon, Creamed, Ambrosia*	½ Can/213g	193	2.8	91	3.2	16.5	1.3	0.0
Low Fat, Tesco*	1 Can/425g	404	5.5	95	3.2	16.9	1.3	0.1
Original, Muller Rice, Muller*	1 Pot/190g	196	4.9	103	3.6	16.3	2.6	0.3
Raspberry, Mini Pot, Muller Rice, Muller*	1 Pot/95g	101	2.2	106	3.2	18.2	2.3	0.5
Raspberry, Mullerice, Muller*	1 Pot/190g	201	4.4	106	3.2	18.2	2.3	0.5
Strawberry, Mini Pot, Muller Rice, Muller*	1 Pot/95g	102	2.2	107	3.2	18.4	2.3	0.4
Strawberry, Mullerrice, Muller*	1 Pot/200g	220	4.4	110	3.2	19.3	2.2	0.4
Thick & Creamy, Nestle*	1 Can/425g	527	23.8	124	3.1	15.4	5.6	0.2
Toffee, Smooth, Muller Rice, Muller*	1 Pot/190g	201	4.4	106	3.3	18.0	2.3	0.3
Vanilla Custard, Mullerrice, Muller*	1 Pot/200g	230	5.0	115	3.4	19.8	2.5	0.3
with Strawberry Sauce, Ambrosia*	1 Pot/160g	174	3.2	109	2.7	19.8	2.0	0.1
RICE WINE								
Sake, Average	***1 Tbsp/15ml***	***20***	***0.0***	***134***	***0.5***	***5.0***	***0.0***	***0.0***
Shaoxing, Waitrose*	1 Tbsp/15ml	21	0.0	138	1.6	3.9	0.0	0.2
RIGATONI								
Dry, Average	***1 Serving/80g***	***272***	***1.2***	***340***	***11.4***	***68.4***	***1.5***	***2.7***
RISOTTO								
Balls, Mushroom, Occasions, Sainsbury's*	1 Ball/25g	76	3.4	304	3.8	41.2	13.8	1.7
Balls, Sun Dried Tomato, Occasions, Sainsbury's*	1 Ball/25g	71	3.8	285	6.8	30.8	15.0	2.9
Beetroot & Goats Cheese, Lovely Vegetables, M&S*	1 Pack/379g	530	17.0	140	4.4	20.7	4.5	3.6
Butternut Squash, Fresh Ideas, M Kitchen, Morrisons*	1 Pot/350g	371	11.9	106	1.8	16.8	3.4	0.7
Butternut, Pearl Barely, Veg Pot, Innocent*	1 Pot/390g	285	5.1	73	2.9	12.6	1.3	3.8
Caramelised Onion & Gruyere Cheese, M&S*	1 Pack/200g	350	20.6	175	3.0	17.8	10.3	1.7

R

	Measure INFO/WEIGHT	per Measure KCAL	FAT	Nutrition Values per 100g / 100ml KCAL	PROT	CARB	FAT	FIBRE
RISOTTO								
Cheese Flavour, Made Up, Ainsley Harriott*	1 Sachet/140g	565	14.6	404	7.8	69.6	10.4	9.1
Cheese, Onion & Wine, Rice & Simple, Ainsley Harriott*	1 Pack/140g	253	7.0	181	3.1	31.0	5.0	1.6
Chicken	1 Serving/380g	494	17.4	130	7.2	15.2	4.6	1.3
Chicken & Bacon, Italiano, Tesco*	1 Pack/450g	652	20.2	145	5.9	20.2	4.5	1.5
Chicken & Lemon, Weight Watchers*	1 Pack/330g	327	6.9	99	6.3	13.7	2.1	0.5
Chicken & Mushroom, Finest, Tesco*	1 Pack/400g	496	11.2	124	7.4	17.2	2.8	0.5
Chicken & Mushroom, Waitrose*	1 Pack/350g	364	16.1	104	6.0	9.7	4.6	0.8
Chicken & Sun Dried Tomato, Waitrose*	1 Pack/350g	385	22.0	110	6.0	7.2	6.3	0.3
Chicken, BGTY, Sainsbury's*	1 Pack/327g	356	6.2	109	7.5	15.5	1.9	1.0
Chicken, Lemon & Wild Rocket, Sainsbury's*	1 Pack/360g	683	41.0	190	16.2	5.6	11.4	0.1
Chicken, Ready Meal, M&S*	1 Pack/360g	450	15.8	125	6.7	14.4	4.4	0.9
Green Bean, Asparagus & Pecorino, Finest, Tesco*	1 Pack/400g	460	15.6	115	4.4	15.0	3.9	1.5
Haddock & Mushroom, COU, M&S*	1 Pack/400g	320	3.2	80	6.4	12.1	0.8	2.0
Hot Smoked Salmon & Spinach, M&S*	½ Pack/300g	420	24.0	140	6.4	11.0	8.0	0.6
Italian Creamy Chicken & Mushroom, CBY, Asda*	1 Pack/350g	374	11.9	107	6.6	11.9	3.4	1.3
King Prawn & Snow Crab, M&S*	1 Pack/365g	402	16.4	110	4.1	12.7	4.5	0.5
King Prawn, Pea & Mint, M&S*	½ Pack/300g	405	18.6	135	3.8	15.9	6.2	0.9
Mushroom & Chestnut, Waitrose*	1 Pack/400g	496	90.0	124	14.6	58.4	22.5	7.2
Mushroom, Asda*	1 Pack/340g	340	11.6	100	2.3	15.0	3.4	0.6
Mushroom, COU, M&S*	1 Pack/375g	338	5.6	90	3.0	16.1	1.5	1.5
Mushroom, HL, Tesco*	1 Pack/400g	320	3.2	80	2.6	15.6	0.8	0.6
Mushroom, Italiano, Tesco*	1 Pack/340g	367	6.8	108	2.4	20.0	2.0	4.6
Roasted Red Pepper & Italian Cheese, M&S*	1 Pack/400g	500	13.2	125	2.9	20.4	3.3	1.0
Roasted Vegetable & Sunblush Tomato, Finest, Tesco*	½ Pack/200g	306	18.0	153	3.7	14.5	9.0	1.4
Salmon & Prawn, Eat Smart, Morrisons*	1 Pack/381g	339	5.3	89	4.9	14.1	1.4	0.8
Seafood, HL, Tesco*	1 Pack/365g	328	3.6	90	5.3	14.1	1.0	0.9
Seafood, Youngs*	1 Pack/350g	424	13.0	121	4.5	17.4	3.7	0.1
Tomato & Mascarpone, Cooked, Ainsley Harriott*	1 Sachet/346g	553	18.7	160	2.5	25.3	5.4	1.6
Tomato & Mascarpone, M&S*	1 Pack/360g	468	19.1	130	2.7	17.5	5.3	0.9
Vegetable, Average	**1oz/28g**	**41**	**1.8**	**147**	**4.2**	**19.2**	**6.5**	**2.2**
Vegetable, Brown Rice, Average	**1oz/28g**	**40**	**1.8**	**143**	**4.1**	**18.6**	**6.4**	**2.4**
Wild Mushroom & Garlic, Tesco*	1 Pack/320g	522	14.1	163	3.6	27.2	4.4	1.6
ROCK SALMON								
Raw, Flesh Only, Average	**1oz/28g**	**43**	**2.7**	**154**	**16.6**	**0.0**	**9.7**	**0.0**
ROCKET								
Baby Leaf, M&S*	½ Bag/40g	10	0.2	25	2.7	1.4	0.5	2.1
Fresh, Raw, Average	**1 Serving/80g**	**12**	**0.4**	**16**	**0.8**	**1.7**	**0.5**	**1.2**
Wild, Morrisons*	1 Serving/100g	17	0.6	17	0.9	1.7	0.6	1.4
ROE								
Cod, Average	**1 Can/100g**	**96**	**2.8**	**96**	**17.1**	**0.5**	**2.8**	**0.0**
Cod, Hard, Coated in Batter, Fried	1oz/28g	53	3.3	189	12.4	8.9	11.8	0.2
Herring, Soft, Fried in Blended Oil	1oz/28g	74	4.4	265	26.3	4.7	15.8	0.2
Herring, Soft, Raw	**1oz/28g**	**22**	**0.1**	**78**	**18.2**	**0.5**	**0.4**	**0.0**
ROGAN JOSH								
Chicken & Rice, Sainsbury's*	1 Pack/500g	675	27.0	135	6.7	14.1	5.4	2.4
Chicken Breast, Chunks, Hot, Sainsbury's*	½ Pack/114g	143	2.0	126	23.6	3.9	1.8	1.0
Chicken with Pilau Rice, Farmfoods*	1 Pack/325g	354	6.8	109	5.3	17.1	2.1	0.4
Lamb & Pilau Rice, Indian Takeaway, Asda*	1 Pack/569g	888	27.9	156	7.0	21.0	4.9	1.7
Lamb & Pilau Rice, Tesco*	1 Pack/550g	770	29.2	140	6.0	16.9	5.3	1.0
Lamb with Pilau Rice, Eastern Classics*	1 Pack/400g	604	21.6	151	5.6	19.9	5.4	1.0
Lamb, Asda*	1 Pack/450g	688	40.5	153	13.0	5.0	9.0	3.1
Lamb, Indian, Takeaway, CBY, Asda*	½ Pack/200g	218	12.0	109	8.0	5.1	6.0	1.4
Lamb, Sainsbury's*	1 Pack/400g	660	44.4	165	11.3	4.9	11.1	1.9

R

	Measure INFO/WEIGHT	per Measure KCAL	FAT	Nutrition Values per 100g / 100ml KCAL	PROT	CARB	FAT	FIBRE
ROGAN JOSH								
Lamb, Tesco*	1 Pack/350g	402	20.3	115	10.2	5.0	5.8	1.3
Lamb, Waitrose*	½ Pack/175g	242	13.3	138	12.4	5.0	7.6	1.3
Prawn & Pilau Rice, BGTY, Sainsbury's*	1 Pack/401g	353	3.2	88	4.8	15.3	0.8	1.9
Prawn, COU, M&S*	1 Pack/400g	360	2.4	90	4.9	16.2	0.6	0.8
ROLL								
All Day Breakfast, Asda*	1 Roll/220g	581	26.4	264	10.0	29.0	12.0	0.0
Brie & Grapes, M&S*	1 Roll/57g	174	10.4	306	11.1	24.5	18.2	1.4
Cheese & Chutney, M&S*	1 Roll/165g	256	1.2	155	13.9	23.1	0.7	1.2
Cheese & Onion, Asda*	1 Serving/67g	199	12.0	298	7.0	27.0	18.0	2.0
Cheese & Onion, Co-Op*	1 Roll/66g	195	11.9	295	7.0	26.0	18.0	2.0
Cheese & Onion, Iceland*	1 Roll/67g	222	13.6	332	7.5	29.6	20.4	1.5
Cheese & Onion, King Size, Pork Farms*	1 Serving/130g	443	28.6	341	7.4	28.4	22.0	0.0
Cheese & Onion, M&S*	1 Roll/25g	80	5.1	320	9.6	24.7	20.5	1.3
Cheese & Onion, Sainsbury's*	1 Roll/67g	205	13.6	306	8.0	22.9	20.3	1.9
Cheese & Onion, Tesco*	1 Roll/67g	203	12.1	305	7.3	28.0	18.1	1.9
Cheese & Pickle, Sainsbury's*	1 Roll/136g	359	13.6	264	10.6	35.1	10.0	0.0
Cheese, Tomato & Onion, Sainsbury's*	1 Pack/100g	518	28.1	518	18.4	47.9	28.1	0.0
Chicken Salad, HE, Tesco*	1 Serving/224g	289	5.8	129	10.3	16.0	2.6	1.1
Chicken Salad, HL, Tesco*	1 Serving/100g	149	2.0	149	10.6	22.3	2.0	1.2
Chicken, Bacon & Cheese, 7 Inch, Delicious, Boots*	1 Roll/197g	416	13.4	211	13.0	24.0	6.8	1.5
Chicken, Salad, Mini, Selection Pack, British, M&S*	1 Roll/61g	134	4.1	220	11.9	28.1	6.8	2.1
Chunky Cheese & Mustard, Finest, Tesco*	1 Roll/88g	260	9.0	295	10.9	40.0	10.2	2.4
Egg & Bacon, Sub, Shapers, Boots*	1 Serving/169g	320	7.3	189	11.0	27.0	4.3	1.3
Egg & Cress, HL, Tesco*	1 Pack/175g	322	6.8	184	9.6	27.7	3.9	1.2
Egg Mayo & Cress, Fullfillers*	1 Roll/125g	266	11.8	213	10.0	25.7	9.4	0.0
Egg Mayonnaise & Cress, Sub, Delicious, Boots*	1 Pack/205g	399	14.1	195	10.0	23.0	6.9	2.4
Ham & Cheese in Pastry, Pork Farms*	1 Roll/70g	216	12.5	308	8.0	28.8	17.9	0.0
Ham & Tomato, Taste!*	1 Serving/112g	211	4.8	188	10.4	27.0	4.3	0.0
Ham Salad, BGTY, Sainsbury's*	1 Roll/178g	292	3.4	164	10.8	25.9	1.9	0.0
Ham Salad, HL, Tesco*	1 Roll/203g	284	5.3	140	9.8	19.3	2.6	0.0
Ham Salad, J D Gross, Lidl*	1 Roll/154g	293	9.2	190	7.7	29.1	6.0	1.9
Ham, Darwins Deli*	1 Serving/125g	298	7.5	238	11.0	37.4	6.0	0.0
Large Ploughmans, Ginsters*	1 Pack/140g	473	33.5	338	10.2	20.5	23.9	1.8
Leicester Ham & Cheese, Sub, Waitrose*	1 Pack/206ml	582	31.2	282	12.6	24.0	15.1	13.0
Mushroom & Bacon, Crusty, M&S*	1 Roll/160g	424	20.2	265	8.7	29.0	12.6	2.3
Oak Smoked Salmon, M&S*	1 Roll/55g	139	6.2	252	14.6	23.1	11.3	1.2
Pork, Stuffing & Apple Sauce, Roast, Boots*	1 Roll/218g	602	26.2	276	10.0	32.0	12.0	1.8
Roast Chicken & Mayonnaise, Big, Sainsbury's*	1 Pack/185g	479	27.4	259	9.6	21.8	14.8	0.0
Sausage, Lincolnshire, COU, M&S*	1 Roll/175g	280	4.7	160	10.0	23.2	2.7	2.6
Steak & Onion, M&S*	1 Serving/150g	308	10.5	205	11.0	24.5	7.0	3.8
Tuna & Sweetcorn with Mayonnaise, Shell*	1 Pack/180g	536	26.3	298	13.1	28.6	14.6	0.0
Tuna Cheese Melt, Boots*	1 Roll/199g	612	35.8	308	13.0	23.0	18.0	1.2
Tuna Mayo & Cucumber, Taste!*	1 Serving/111g	274	12.5	247	9.0	27.3	11.3	0.0
Turkey Salad, Northern Bites*	1 Roll/231g	323	8.3	140	8.6	19.6	3.6	3.0
ROLO								
Chocolate, Nestle*	2 Pieces/20g	102	5.3	509	4.1	62.6	26.6	1.3
Little, Nestle*	1 Pack/40g	196	9.4	491	4.0	65.5	23.5	0.5
Nestle*	1 Sweet/5g	24	1.0	478	4.4	68.2	20.4	1.1
ROOT BEER								
Average	*1 Can/330ml*	*135*	*0.0*	*41*	*0.0*	*10.6*	*0.0*	*0.0*
ROSE WATER								
The English Provender Co.*	1 Tsp/5g	0	0.0	2	0.1	0.6	0.1	0.1

	Measure INFO/WEIGHT		per Measure KCAL	FAT	Nutrition Values per 100g / 100ml KCAL	PROT	CARB	FAT	FIBRE

ROSEMARY

	Measure INFO/WEIGHT	per Measure KCAL	FAT	KCAL	PROT	CARB	FAT	FIBRE
ROSEMARY								
Dried	*1 Tsp/1g*	*3*	*0.2*	*331*	*4.9*	*46.4*	*15.2*	*0.0*
Fresh	*1 Tsp/0.7g*	*1*	*0.0*	*99*	*1.4*	*13.5*	*4.4*	*0.0*
ROSTI								
Garlic & Mushroom, Finest, Tesco*	1 Serving/200g	346	19.6	173	5.7	15.4	9.8	1.7
Oven Baked, McCain*	1 Rosti/100g	194	9.3	194	2.6	25.0	9.3	2.3
Potato & Leek, Sainsbury's*	½ Pack/190g	296	20.9	156	4.5	9.8	11.0	0.3
Potato & Root Vegetable, COU, M&S*	1 Rosti/100g	85	2.7	85	1.6	13.3	2.7	1.5
Potato Cakes, Baby, M&S*	1 Rosti/23g	40	1.5	175	3.5	25.1	6.7	1.6
Potato, McCain*	1 Rosti/95g	161	8.6	169	2.2	19.6	9.1	0.0
Potato, Onion & Gruyere, Finest, Tesco*	½ Pack/200g	206	10.6	103	3.2	10.5	5.3	2.0
ROULADE								
Chocolate, Finest, Tesco*	1 Serving/80g	222	4.5	277	3.4	53.2	5.6	2.3
Chocolate, Sainsbury's*	1 Serving/72g	264	15.7	367	5.7	36.9	21.8	1.8
Lemon, Asda*	1 Serving/100g	343	12.0	343	2.7	56.0	12.0	0.0
Orange & Lemon Meringue, Co-Op*	1 Serving/82g	287	9.8	350	3.0	57.0	12.0	0.3
Raspberry, Finest, Tesco*	1/6 Roulade/75g	220	9.2	295	2.7	41.5	12.4	2.7
Salmon & Spinach, Tesco*	1 Serving/60g	155	14.2	258	9.5	1.7	23.7	0.2
Toffee Pecan, Finest, Tesco*	1 Serving/60g	218	8.9	363	3.6	53.8	14.8	0.5
RUM								
37.5% Volume	*1 Pub Shot/35ml*	*72*	*0.0*	*207*	*0.0*	*0.0*	*0.0*	*0.0*
40% Volume	*1 Pub Shot/35ml*	*78*	*0.0*	*222*	*0.0*	*0.0*	*0.0*	*0.0*
Captain Morgans & Cola, Premixed, Canned, Diageo*	1 Can/250ml	180	0.0	72	0.0	9.1	0.0	0.0
Malibu, 21% Volume, Pernod Ricard*	1 Pub Shot/35ml	70	0.0	200	0.0	29.0	0.0	0.0
White	*1 Pub Shot/35ml*	*72*	*0.0*	*207*	*0.0*	*0.0*	*0.0*	*0.0*
RUSKS								
Banana, Farleys*	1 Serving/17g	70	1.5	409	7.3	75.1	8.8	2.9
Original, Farleys*	1 Rusk/17g	69	1.2	406	7.1	77.6	7.1	2.4

R

	Measure INFO/WEIGHT	per Measure		Nutrition Values per 100g / 100ml				
		KCAL	FAT	KCAL	PROT	CARB	FAT	FIBRE
SAAG								
Chicken, Masala, M&S*	½ Pack/175g	228	12.4	130	13.3	3.1	7.1	5.2
Chicken, Masala, Waitrose*	1 Pack/400g	452	20.9	113	11.7	3.8	5.2	1.8
Paneer, Sainsbury's*	1 Pack/300g	441	32.7	147	7.1	3.9	10.9	2.5
SAFFRON								
Average	*1 Tsp/1g*	*2*	*0.0*	*310*	*11.4*	*61.5*	*5.9*	*0.0*
SAGE								
Dried, Ground	*1 Tsp/1g*	*3*	*0.1*	*315*	*10.6*	*42.7*	*12.7*	*0.0*
Fresh	*1oz/28g*	*33*	*1.3*	*119*	*3.9*	*15.6*	*4.6*	*0.0*
SAGO								
Raw	*1oz/28g*	*99*	*0.1*	*355*	*0.2*	*94.0*	*0.2*	*0.5*
SALAD								
3 Bean, Sainsbury's*	1 Tub/270g	281	6.2	104	7.1	13.6	2.3	5.9
5 Bean & Mint, Asda*	1 Pack/340g	408	12.9	120	6.2	12.7	3.8	5.3
Adzuki & Edamame Bean, Aromatic, Waitrose*	1/3 Pack/67g	62	1.5	93	7.5	5.7	2.2	10.3
Alfresco Style, Tesco*	1 Serving/200g	40	0.6	20	0.9	3.3	0.3	2.1
American Style, Sweet & Crispy, Morrisons*	1 Serving/25g	7	0.1	28	1.2	4.2	0.3	2.0
Aromatic Herb, Waitrose*	¼ Pack/27g	4	0.1	15	0.9	1.7	0.5	1.0
Assorted, Asda*	1 Serving/100g	22	0.6	22	2.4	1.7	0.6	0.0
Avocado & Feta, Gourmet To Go, M&S*	1 Pack/320g	512	32.0	160	5.4	12.1	10.0	3.1
Avocado & Tomato, Italian, Bowl, Sainsbury's*	1 Bowl/180g	97	4.7	54	1.0	6.7	2.6	1.3
Baby Leaf & Beetroot, Bistro, M&S*	1 Pack/165g	41	0.0	25	2.0	3.6	0.0	2.0
Baby Leaf & Herb, Asda*	1 Serving/50g	7	0.1	14	2.3	0.7	0.2	2.4
Baby Leaf with Watercress, Tesco*	1 Serving/30g	6	0.2	19	1.8	1.3	0.7	1.8
Baby Leaf, Asda*	1 Serving/80g	10	0.2	12	2.1	0.2	0.3	1.7
Baby Leaf, Florette*	1 Serving/40g	5	0.1	12	2.0	0.4	0.3	1.0
Baby Leaf, Fully Prepared, Sainsbury's*	½ Bag/63g	10	0.3	16	1.3	1.9	0.4	1.5
Baby Leaf, Italian Style, M&S*	1 Serving/55g	11	0.3	20	1.3	2.3	0.5	1.3
Baby Leaf, M&S*	1 Pack/100g	20	0.2	20	3.0	1.7	0.2	0.5
Baby Leaf, Mild, Seasonal, Tesco*	½ Pack/42g	9	0.3	21	1.5	1.6	0.6	1.8
Baby Leaf, Organic, Sainsbury's*	1 Serving/20g	3	0.1	14	1.5	1.4	0.3	1.1
Baby Leaf, Sainsbury's*	1 Serving/60g	12	1.1	20	2.8	1.1	1.9	1.9
Baby Leaf, Seasonal, Organic, Sainsbury's*	1 Serving/30g	3	0.1	10	1.6	0.4	0.3	1.2
Baby Leaf, Seasonal, Sainsbury's*	¼ Bag/63g	11	0.3	17	2.8	0.5	0.5	2.7
Baby Leaf, Sweet, Seasonal, M&S*	½ Bag/60g	9	0.2	15	2.4	0.6	0.4	1.8
Baby Tomato, Tesco*	1 Pack/205g	35	0.6	17	0.8	2.8	0.3	0.9
Bacon Caesar, Sainsbury's*	1 Pack/256g	415	32.5	162	4.7	12.0	12.7	1.4
Bag, Tesco*	1 Serving/200g	38	0.8	19	0.9	3.0	0.4	1.4
Bean & Chorizo, Tapas Selection, Sainsbury's*	1 Serving/22g	29	1.4	132	8.1	10.7	6.3	1.9
Bean & Sweetcorn, Side, M&S*	1 Serving/125g	131	9.0	105	2.5	7.0	7.2	1.3
Bean, M&S*	1 Serving/80g	72	0.7	90	6.4	14.3	0.9	3.9
Bean, Mexican, Sainsbury's*	1 Pot/260g	291	8.1	112	5.2	12.9	3.1	5.8
Bean, Mixed, Vinaigrette, Tesco*	1 Can/400g	280	2.0	70	3.2	13.1	0.5	1.9
Beans, Mixed, in Water, Essential, Waitrose*	1 Serving/80g	68	0.6	85	6.5	12.9	0.8	6.2
Beetroot	1oz/28g	28	1.9	100	2.0	8.4	6.8	1.7
Beetroot & Carrot, Continental, Iceland*	1 Serving/100g	24	0.2	24	1.2	4.3	0.2	2.1
Beetroot & Cherry Tomato, & Lemon Dressing, M&S*	1 Pack/215g	129	8.2	60	1.3	5.2	3.8	1.5
Beetroot & Lettuce, Asda*	1 Serving/30g	5	0.0	16	1.4	2.7	0.0	2.5
Beetroot with Balsamic Dressing, Finest, Tesco*	1 Portion/75g	49	1.1	65	1.1	11.9	1.5	2.4
Beetroot, Asda*	1 Carton/270g	119	1.1	44	1.3	8.8	0.4	2.4
Beetroot, Co-Op*	1 Pack/250g	100	0.8	40	0.9	8.0	0.3	2.0
Beetroot, Freshly Prepared, Tesco*	1 Pack/240g	58	0.7	24	1.9	3.3	0.3	2.7
Beetroot, Morrisons*	1 Tsp/10g	6	0.1	62	0.8	10.5	1.3	2.3
Beetroot, Roast with Quinoa & Feta, Tesco*	1 Pack/400g	452	19.6	113	4.8	12.4	4.9	2.3

	Measure INFO/WEIGHT	per Measure KCAL	FAT	Nutrition Values per 100g / 100ml KCAL	PROT	CARB	FAT	FIBRE
SALAD								
Beetroot, Sainsbury's*	1 Tub/200g	148	2.4	74	1.7	14.1	1.2	1.7
Bistro, Asda*	1 Serving/180g	29	0.0	16	1.4	2.7	0.0	2.5
Bistro, Morrisons*	1 Serving/20g	5	0.0	23	1.2	4.2	0.2	2.0
Bistro, Sainsbury's*	1 Pack/150g	26	0.3	17	1.9	2.0	0.2	2.0
Bistro, Washed Ready to Eat, Tesco*	1 Pack/140g	22	0.7	16	1.1	1.7	0.5	1.0
Black Bean Salsa, Salad Bar, Waitrose*	1 Serving/100g	118	5.8	118	0.0	0.0	5.8	0.0
Bocconcini Mozzarella with Sun Ripened Tomato, M&S*	½ Pack/100g	250	21.4	250	9.8	4.9	21.4	2.0
British Ham & Free Range Egg, M&S*	1 Pack/280g	182	6.4	65	6.1	5.3	2.3	1.0
Broccoli, Edamame & Black Bean, Sainsbury's*	1 Pack/190g	229	3.6	121	5.8	16.8	1.9	6.6
Bulgar Wheat, Lentil & Edamame Shaker, Waitrose*	1 Pack/190g	217	10.6	114	4.7	11.1	5.6	4.4
Cabbage & Leek, Crunchy Mix, Sainsbury's*	½ Pack/126g	24	0.8	19	1.2	2.1	0.6	1.9
Cabbage, Beetroot & Carrot, Mix, Florette*	½ Pack/100g	30	0.2	30	1.3	4.4	0.2	0.0
Caesar	1 Serving/200g	352	27.8	176	4.8	8.1	13.9	0.7
Caesar Pasta, Salad Bar, Waitrose*	1 Serving/100g	260	18.0	260	0.0	0.0	18.0	0.0
Caesar with Dressing, Croutons & Parmesan, M&S*	1 Serving/115g	190	15.5	165	4.3	6.4	13.5	1.4
Caesar with Parmigiano Reggiano, Tesco*	1 Bag/275g	552	49.0	201	4.1	5.8	17.8	1.3
Caesar, Bacon, M&S*	1 Serving/250g	400	31.2	160	7.1	4.1	12.5	1.3
Caesar, Chicken & Bacon, Gourmet, M&S*	1 Salad/250g	550	43.5	220	9.0	7.3	17.4	0.7
Caesar, Chicken & Bacon, Tesco*	1 Pack/200g	506	40.2	253	6.6	11.4	20.1	1.0
Caesar, Co-Op*	¼ Pack/50g	88	7.5	175	3.0	6.0	15.0	2.0
Caesar, HE, Tesco*	1 Serving/100g	101	6.2	101	3.2	8.0	6.2	0.7
Caesar, Kit, Asda*	½ Pack/113g	154	9.0	136	5.0	11.0	8.0	1.4
Caesar, Kit, Tesco*	½ Pack/138g	279	25.3	202	4.7	4.5	18.3	1.3
Caesar, Kit, Waitrose*	1 Bag/250g	436	36.1	174	4.4	6.1	14.4	1.3
Caesar, M&S*	1 Pack/268g	510	40.5	190	5.7	8.3	15.1	1.3
Caesar, Morrisons*	1 Serving/115g	194	18.1	169	3.6	5.9	15.7	0.3
Caesar, Sainsbury's*	½ Bag/128g	227	19.3	177	3.6	6.7	15.1	1.0
Cajun Chicken, David Lloyd Leisure*	1 Pack/300g	429	10.0	143	11.7	17.7	3.3	1.0
Cannellini Bean & Chicken, M&S*	1 Serving/225g	250	14.7	111	5.9	7.4	6.5	3.1
Cannellini Bean & Chorizo, Sainsbury's*	1 Pack/250g	228	8.0	91	5.3	10.2	3.2	1.6
Cannellini Bean & Tuna, M&S*	1 Serving/255g	215	11.6	84	5.3	5.4	4.5	2.1
Caponata, Organic, Florentin*	1 Serving/100g	111	12.3	111	1.5	3.7	12.3	0.0
Caribbean Chicken, Shapers, Boots*	1 Pack/220g	222	5.1	101	5.8	14.0	2.3	1.2
Carrot & Beetroot with a Balsamic Dressing, Asda*	1 Pack/160g	101	6.6	63	0.9	5.6	4.1	1.0
Carrot & Nut with French Dressing, Average	***1oz/28g***	***61***	***4.9***	***218***	***2.1***	***13.7***	***17.6***	***2.4***
Carrot & Sultana, BGTY, Sainsbury's*	½ Pack/100g	55	0.3	55	0.6	12.4	0.3	0.0
Carrot & Sultana, HL, Tesco*	1 Tub/225g	142	1.4	63	1.2	13.2	0.6	2.5
Carrot with Fresh Coriander Vinaigrette, M&S*	½ Pack/105g	126	3.6	120	3.7	19.1	3.4	6.5
Carrot, Courgette & Coriander, Salad Bar, Waitrose*	1 Serving/100g	92	7.9	92	0.0	0.0	7.9	0.0
Carrot, M&S*	1 Pack/215g	280	7.3	130	3.1	22.4	3.4	2.7
Carrot, Peanut & Sultana, Asda*	1 Serving/20g	54	4.0	272	8.0	15.0	20.0	4.5
Celery & Apple, Salad Bar, Waitrose*	1 Serving/100g	136	12.9	136	0.0	0.0	12.9	0.0
Chargrilled Chicken & Bacon, Tesco*	1 Pack/300g	657	37.8	219	7.8	18.7	12.6	0.9
Chargrilled Chicken & Pesto, Sainsbury's*	1 Pack/250g	375	15.2	150	7.9	15.8	6.1	1.3
Chargrilled Chicken Wholefood, M&S*	1 Pot/219g	230	4.2	105	10.1	11.6	1.9	4.8
Chargrilled Chicken, Snack, Tesco*	1 Pot/300g	384	14.4	128	6.1	15.0	4.8	2.4
Chargrilled Chicken, Tesco*	1 Serving/300g	384	14.4	128	6.1	15.0	4.8	2.4
Cheese & Coleslaw, Tesco*	1 Serving/125g	135	10.9	108	3.4	3.4	8.7	1.1
Cheese Layered, M&S*	½ Pack/230g	300	20.5	130	4.6	9.3	8.9	1.2
Cheese, HL, Tesco*	1 Serving/30g	32	0.9	107	18.0	2.0	3.0	0.0
Cheese, Layered, Snack, Sainsbury's*	1 Pack/190g	397	29.1	209	5.4	12.4	15.3	0.0
Cheese, Layered, Tesco*	1 Serving/225g	437	32.0	194	5.8	10.8	14.2	0.8
Cheese, Ploughmans, Asda*	1 Bowl/300g	246	10.8	82	3.6	8.9	3.6	1.0

S

SALAD

	Measure INFO/WEIGHT	per Measure KCAL	FAT	Nutrition Values per 100g / 100ml KCAL	PROT	CARB	FAT	FIBRE
Cherry Tomato, Salad bar, Waitrose*	1 Serving/100g	77	5.3	77	0.0	0.0	5.3	0.0
Cherry Tomato, Tesco*	1 Pack/210g	136	9.4	65	0.9	4.2	4.5	1.1
Chick Pea & Cous Cous, Tesco*	1 Serving/250g	245	6.5	98	3.2	15.5	2.6	0.0
Chick Pea & Spinach, M&S*	1 Serving/260g	299	10.7	115	7.3	12.5	4.1	2.7
Chick Pea & Sweet Potato, Salad Bar, Sainsbury's*	1 Serving/100g	99	1.9	99	0.0	9.6	1.9	0.0
Chicken & Bacon Layered, Tesco*	1 Pack/360g	600	39.6	167	4.6	12.1	11.0	1.8
Chicken & Bacon Ranch, Sainsbury's*	1 Pack/210g	315	15.8	150	8.4	12.1	7.5	0.9
Chicken & Bacon, Layered, Waitrose*	1 Serving/200g	246	14.8	123	6.7	7.4	7.4	2.1
Chicken & Moroccan Cous Cous, Tesco*	1 Pack/210g	252	4.2	120	7.8	16.9	2.0	3.5
Chicken Caesar Bistro, M&S*	½ Pack/135g	189	14.3	140	5.0	6.5	10.6	0.6
Chicken Caesar, Asda*	1 Pack/273g	535	43.7	196	10.0	3.0	16.0	1.9
Chicken Caesar, Eat Well, M&S*	1 Pack/397g	595	24.6	150	9.9	18.7	6.2	2.1
Chicken Caesar, Fresh, Sainsbury's*	1 Serving/200g	278	20.0	139	6.0	6.2	10.0	1.2
Chicken Caesar, M&S*	½ Pack/140g	266	20.0	190	6.7	8.7	14.3	0.8
Chicken Caesar, Shapers, Boots*	1 Pack/200g	205	5.8	102	8.2	10.0	2.9	1.0
Chicken Caesar, Snack, Sainsbury's*	1 Pack/182g	164	9.1	90	5.9	5.3	5.0	1.0
Chicken Caesar, Snack, Tesco*	1 Serving/300g	420	20.4	140	8.2	11.4	6.8	1.7
Chicken Noodle & Sweet Chilli, Shapers, Boots*	1 Pack/197g	266	5.1	135	12.0	16.0	2.6	0.9
Chicken Noodle, Thai Style, Sainsbury's*	1 Pack/260g	283	7.5	109	6.6	14.2	2.9	1.3
Chicken with Mayonnaise, Waitrose*	1 Pack/208g	406	19.8	195	10.3	17.1	9.5	2.5
Chicken, Avocado & Bacon, M&S*	1 Serving/235g	235	13.6	100	8.5	2.8	5.8	2.8
Chicken, Caesar, Tesco*	1 Pack/300g	330	13.5	110	6.8	10.6	4.5	0.8
Chicken, HE, Tesco*	1 Salad/216g	296	3.0	137	8.4	22.6	1.4	1.2
Chicken, Honey & Mustard, Bowl, Fresh, Sainsbury's*	1 Serving/300g	408	23.7	136	5.9	10.3	7.9	1.7
Chicken, Layer, HE, Tesco*	1 Pack/400g	268	4.4	67	5.8	8.4	1.1	2.1
Chicken, Roast, Snack, Tesco*	1 Pack/300g	324	21.6	108	6.0	4.8	7.2	1.9
Chicken, Sweet Chilli, BGTY, Sainsbury's*	1 Serving/200g	206	0.8	103	6.0	18.7	0.4	0.0
Chicken, Tesco*	1 Serving/300g	348	22.2	116	5.3	7.0	7.4	1.0
Chicken, Tomato Chilli, & Rice, COU, M&S*	1 Pack/340g	357	5.1	105	6.8	16.0	1.5	0.9
Chickpea & Bean, Salad Bar, Waitrose*	1 Serving/100g	165	10.2	165	0.0	2.2	10.2	0.0
Chilli Chicken & Spicy Cous Cous, HE, Tesco*	1 Serving/190g	251	4.6	132	6.5	21.1	2.4	1.5
Chilli, Tomato, Chick Pea & Butter Bean, Tesco*	1 Pack/130g	146	6.0	112	3.4	14.3	4.6	0.5
Classic Caesar, M&S*	½ Pack/112g	174	14.2	155	2.9	6.8	12.7	0.5
Classic with Chive Dressing, M&S*	½ Pack/138g	76	5.8	55	0.9	3.3	4.2	1.6
Classic with Green Herb Dressing, Co-Op*	1 Serving/90g	86	8.1	95	1.0	2.0	9.0	1.0
Classic, Complete Salad, Sainsbury's*	1 Pack/220g	112	8.4	51	1.0	3.3	3.8	1.4
Classic, Co-Op*	½ Pack/80g	16	0.2	20	0.8	2.9	0.3	2.2
Coleslaw, Bowl, Budgens*	1 Pack/163g	220	18.2	135	1.5	7.1	11.2	1.4
Coleslaw, Bowl, Tesco*	1 Bowl/300g	327	30.3	109	1.0	3.4	10.1	1.3
Coleslaw, Classics, M&S*	1 Pot/190g	124	4.4	65	1.9	8.8	2.3	1.3
Continental Four Leaf, Sainsbury's*	½ Pack/100g	13	0.2	13	1.2	1.7	0.2	1.9
Cous Cous & Roast Vegetable, GFY, Asda*	1 Serving/100g	120	1.6	120	3.5	23.0	1.6	2.7
Cous Cous & Roasted Vegetable, Waitrose*	1 Pack/220g	396	13.4	180	5.1	26.1	6.1	1.2
Cous Cous, BFY, Morrisons*	½ Pot/113g	164	4.0	145	4.6	23.8	3.5	0.5
Cous Cous, BGTY, Sainsbury's*	1 Pot/200g	236	4.4	118	4.7	19.7	2.2	2.8
Cous Cous, Waitrose*	1 Pot/200g	344	10.0	172	4.9	26.9	5.0	1.4
Crayfish & Mango, COU, M&S*	1 Pack/250g	285	5.3	114	4.1	18.6	2.1	1.9
Crayfish & Mango, Finest, Tesco*	1 Pack/270g	296	13.7	110	4.3	11.3	5.1	0.5
Crisp & Crunchy, Asda*	1 Pack/250g	55	1.5	22	0.8	3.3	0.6	1.4
Crisp & Sweet Lettuce Leaves, Florette*	¼ Pack/70g	10	0.4	14	0.8	1.7	0.5	0.9
Crisp Mixed, Tesco*	1 Pack/200g	40	0.6	20	1.1	3.2	0.3	2.0
Crisp, Mixed, Morrisons*	1 Pack/230g	39	0.7	17	1.0	2.8	0.3	0.0
Crispy Carrot & Sweetcorn, Growers Selection, Asda*	¼ Pack/82g	21	0.4	25	1.1	2.9	0.5	2.1

S

SALAD

	Measure INFO/WEIGHT	KCAL	FAT	KCAL	PROT	CARB	FAT	FIBRE
Crispy Duck & Herb, M&S*	½ Pack/140g	378	25.6	270	20.7	3.7	18.3	1.4
Crispy Green, Sainsbury's*	1 Serving/70g	8	0.1	12	0.9	1.6	0.2	0.8
Crispy Leaf, Sainsbury's*	½ Pack/68g	9	0.3	14	1.0	1.7	0.4	1.7
Crispy Medley, Waitrose*	1 Serving/50g	8	0.2	15	0.8	1.7	0.5	0.9
Crispy, Co-Op*	1 Serving/80g	13	0.2	16	0.8	3.0	0.3	1.0
Crispy, Florette*	1 Portion/100g	22	0.3	22	1.5	3.4	0.3	3.0
Crunchy Spring, Side, M&S*	1 Serving/160g	32	0.3	20	0.9	4.1	0.2	1.3
Crunchy, Basics, Sainsbury's*	1 Pack/200g	50	0.4	25	1.3	3.4	0.2	2.2
Crunchy, Everyday Essentials, Aldi*	½ Bag/100g	24	0.5	24	1.3	2.9	0.5	2.2
Crunchy, Fully Prepared, Sainsbury's*	½ Pack/150g	24	0.2	16	1.1	3.0	0.1	1.7
Crunchy, Value, Tesco*	1 Serving/56g	11	0.2	19	1.2	2.8	0.3	2.1
Crunchy, Waitrose*	½ Pack100g	18	0.4	18	1.0	2.6	0.4	1.5
Cucumber & Cherry Tomato, Fresh Tastes, Asda*	1 Serving/100g	22	0.3	22	1.6	2.4	0.3	0.0
Duo Lambs Lettuce & Ruby Chard, Florette*	1 Serving/35g	7	0.1	21	2.0	1.0	0.4	2.9
Edamame & Butter Bean, TTD, Sainsbury's*	1/3 Pack/62g	70	2.5	113	6.6	9.9	4.1	4.9
Egg & Baby Spinach, Waitrose*	1 Pack/215g	167	13.5	78	3.5	1.8	6.3	1.0
Egg & Ham with Salad Cream Dressing, M&S*	1 Pack/240g	145	7.2	60	4.9	3.2	3.0	1.2
Egg & Spinach, Protein Pot, Free Range, M&S*	1 Pot/105g	152	10.7	145	12.1	1.1	10.2	0.1
Egg, Layered, Bowl, Tesco*	1 Pack/410g	726	57.8	177	4.2	8.4	14.1	1.3
English Garden, Tesco*	1 Serving/180g	22	0.4	12	0.7	1.8	0.2	0.7
Exotic with Mango & Chilli Dressing, Co-Op*	½ Pack/65g	25	0.4	38	0.6	7.7	0.6	0.8
Falafel & Red Pepper, Tabbouleh, Tesco*	1 Pack/260g	254	9.3	98	3.3	11.7	3.6	2.6
Falafel, Bulgar Wheat & Houmous, Eat Well, M&S*	1 Pack/300g	420	16.8	140	4.7	15.7	5.6	4.0
Feta Cheese & Sunblushed Tomato, M&S*	1 Serving/190g	361	21.1	190	5.5	17.2	11.1	2.1
Feta, & Butternut Squash, Tesco*	1 Pot/245g	404	19.1	165	6.5	14.9	7.8	3.1
Fine Cut, Asda*	1 Serving/100g	24	0.3	24	1.2	4.3	0.3	2.3
Florida, Retail, Average	**1oz/28g**	**63**	**5.7**	**224**	**0.9**	**9.7**	**20.5**	**1.0**
Four Bean, Finest, Tesco*	1 Pack/225g	259	9.4	115	4.2	14.2	4.2	4.6
Four Bean, Sainsbury's*	½ Pot/113g	121	3.2	107	6.6	11.5	2.8	4.8
Four Leaf, Tesco*	1oz/28g	4	0.1	15	0.8	1.8	0.5	0.9
French Goat's Cheese, Extra Fine, Asda*	1 Pack/185g	462	35.2	250	8.4	11.4	19.0	0.8
Fresh & Crispy, Tesco*	1 Serving/230g	30	0.7	13	0.7	1.9	0.3	1.3
Fruity Moroccan Cous Cous, Waitrose*	1 Pack/90g	139	3.2	154	5.0	25.6	3.6	4.6
Fruity Tabbouleh, Salad Bar, Waitrose*	1 Serving/100g	184	6.6	184	0.0	0.0	6.6	0.0
Garden Side with Dressing, Waitrose*	1 Pack/184g	101	8.1	55	12.0	2.6	4.4	13.0
Garden with Watercress, M&S*	1 Salad/80g	10	0.1	12	1.5	1.4	0.1	1.4
Garden with Yoghurt & Mint Dressing, GFY, Asda*	1 Serving/195g	51	2.0	26	1.1	3.2	1.0	0.0
Garden, Classic, Morrisons*	1 Tray/175g	33	0.5	19	0.8	3.2	0.3	2.8
Garden, Side, Asda*	1 Pack/175g	32	0.5	18	0.9	2.8	0.3	1.3
Garden, Sweet & Crunchy, Tesco*	1 Pack/225g	54	0.9	24	1.0	4.2	0.4	1.4
Giant Green Cous Cous & Wheatberry, LL, Waitrose*	1 Pot/200g	290	11.6	145	5.0	18.1	5.8	3.5
Goat's Cheese & Cous Cous, Waitrose*	1 Pack/300g	372	14.4	124	4.8	15.3	4.8	2.2
Goats Cheese, Bowl, Sainsbury's*	1 Serving/100g	161	11.9	161	5.8	7.6	11.9	1.3
Goat's Cheese, Sainsbury's*	1 Pack/192g	242	12.9	126	5.0	10.6	6.7	1.7
Greek	1oz/28g	36	3.5	130	2.7	1.9	12.5	0.8
Greek Feta & Pepper with Cous Cous, Asda*	1 Pack/316g	262	10.4	83	3.2	10.2	3.3	0.0
Greek Style Feta, Tip & Mix, M&S*	1 Pack/195g	214	18.3	110	4.0	2.5	9.4	1.6
Greek Style with Herb Dressing, Tesco*	1 Pack/240g	305	28.3	127	3.2	2.0	11.8	1.0
Greek Style with Houmous Dip & Pitta, Sainsbury's*	1 Bowl/195g	296	17.4	152	5.4	12.5	8.9	2.6
Greek Style with White Wine Vinaigrette, Tesco*	1 Pack/235g	256	22.3	109	3.5	2.3	9.5	1.5
Greek Style, Bowl, M&S*	1 Bowl/223g	212	18.3	95	2.5	2.4	8.2	0.7
Greek Style, Fresh, Food Counter, Sainsbury's*	1 Serving/166g	247	23.2	149	1.9	2.7	14.0	0.0
Greek Style, Waitrose*	½ Pack/125g	54	2.8	43	1.9	4.0	2.2	1.2

SALAD

INFO/WEIGHT	Measure	per Measure KCAL	FAT	Nutrition Values per 100g / 100ml KCAL	PROT	CARB	FAT	FIBRE
Greek with Basil & Mint Oil Dressing, M&S*	1 Pack/200g	220	19.6	110	3.6	2.2	9.8	1.5
Greek, Side, Waitrose*	1 Pack/175g	175	15.8	100	2.1	2.2	9.0	1.1
Green Lentil, Red Pepper & Spinach, Waitrose*	1 Pack/250g	485	20.0	194	8.6	22.0	8.0	2.9
Green Side, M&S*	1 Serving/200g	30	0.4	15	0.9	2.5	0.2	0.0
Green Side, Sainsbury's*	1 Pack/200g	28	0.2	14	1.2	2.1	0.1	1.4
Green Side, Tesco*	1 Serving/100g	12	0.3	12	0.7	1.6	0.3	1.3
Green with Honey & Mustard Dressing, M&S*	1 Pack/200g	120	9.6	60	0.9	2.7	4.8	0.8
Green, Average	*1oz/28g*	*4*	*0.1*	*13*	*0.8*	*1.8*	*0.3*	*0.9*
Green, Complete, Sainsbury's*	1/3 Pack/55g	92	6.7	168	4.2	10.3	12.2	1.4
Green, Crispy, Fresh, Sainsbury's*	1 Serving/40g	5	0.1	12	0.9	1.6	0.2	0.8
Green, Mixed, Average	*1 Serving/100g*	*12*	*0.3*	*12*	*0.7*	*1.8*	*0.3*	*1.0*
Ham & Free Range Egg, Fresh Tastes, Asda*	1 Bowl/265g	167	9.3	63	5.7	2.2	3.5	0.8
Ham & Free Range Egg, Good & Balanced, Asda*	1 Pack/265g	148	6.3	56	5.3	2.8	2.4	0.9
Ham Hock, Waitrose*	1 Pack/350g	245	9.5	70	6.6	4.8	2.7	2.0
Ham, Antony Worrall Thompson's*	1 Pack/202g	257	2.6	127	9.8	19.1	1.3	2.7
Herb Garden, Morrisons*	1 Serving/28g	4	0.1	14	0.9	1.7	0.5	0.0
Herb, Asda*	1 Serving/20g	2	0.1	12	1.8	0.6	0.3	2.0
Honey Smoked Salmon & New Potato, M&S*	1 Pack/270g	270	14.3	100	5.5	7.5	5.3	1.5
Iceberg & Cabbage, Asda*	½ Pack/125g	24	0.4	19	1.0	3.1	0.3	1.5
Italian Style with Rocket & Lambs Lettuce, M&S*	½ Bag/60g	12	0.3	20	1.3	2.3	0.5	1.3
Italian Style, Asda*	1 Serving/20g	3	0.1	15	1.1	1.6	0.5	1.2
Italian Style, Tesco*	1/3 Pack/40g	6	0.2	16	1.0	1.9	0.5	1.2
Italian Wild Rocket & Parmesan, Sainsbury's*	1 Serving/50g	88	7.4	177	7.5	3.4	14.8	0.5
King Prawn, Thai Style, M&S*	1 Pack/295g	266	7.4	90	4.4	12.6	2.5	1.3
Large, Bowl, Sainsbury's*	1/6 Pack/52g	12	0.2	23	0.9	4.3	0.3	1.1
Layered, King Prawn & Mango, LL, Waitrose*	1 Pack/300g	195	4.2	65	3.9	9.2	1.4	1.7
Leaf, Crispy, Asda*	1 Serving/80g	11	0.4	14	0.8	1.6	0.5	0.9
Leafy Bistro, Florette*	1 Tub/110g	24	0.2	22	1.2	2.8	0.2	2.0
Leafy Mixed, Co-Op*	1 Bag/200g	40	0.6	20	1.0	4.0	0.3	1.0
Leaves, Oriental Mix, Waitrose*	1 Bag/100g	18	0.6	18	1.5	1.7	0.6	1.9
Lemon Cous Cous & Roasted Pepper, COU, M&S*	1 Pack/340g	306	7.8	90	3.2	14.6	2.3	1.8
Lovely Summer, Jamie Oliver*	½ Bag/60g	48	4.0	80	1.7	4.0	6.6	1.2
Luscious Leafy Tomato Trio, Steve's Leaves*	1 Pack/130g	108	7.0	83	2.0	5.1	5.4	2.0
Mediterranean Chicken, HL, Tesco*	1 Pack/263g	305	4.2	116	7.7	16.4	1.6	2.4
Mediterranean Pasta, Salad Bar, Waitrose*	1 Serving/100g	156	4.0	156	0.0	0.0	4.0	0.0
Mediterranean Style, Asda*	½ Pack/135g	22	0.0	16	1.0	3.0	0.0	0.0
Mediterranean Style, Tray, Morrisons*	1 Tray/100g	26	0.3	26	1.2	3.6	0.3	1.8
Mediterranean with Chicken, Nando's*	1 Portion/250g	395	23.6	158	15.0	3.3	9.4	1.8
Mix, Crisp & Sweet Lettuce Leaves, Florette*	1 Portion/67g	12	0.2	18	1.5	1.2	0.3	2.5
Mixed Bean, Asda*	½ Can/145g	126	3.6	87	5.0	11.0	2.5	6.0
Mixed Bean, Canned, Sainsbury's*	1 Can/270g	227	2.4	84	5.4	13.5	0.9	3.8
Mixed Bean, Tesco*	1 Serving/70g	49	0.4	70	3.2	13.1	0.5	1.9
Mixed Fish & Leaves	1 Serving/250g	203	9.5	81	5.3	6.8	3.8	0.8
Mixed Leaf & Baby Basil, a Taste of Italy, Florette*	1 Pack/155g	143	8.2	92	2.7	8.5	5.3	1.0
Mixed Leaf Medley, Waitrose*	1 Serving/25g	4	0.1	15	0.8	1.7	0.5	1.4
Mixed Leaf Tomato & Olive, Tesco*	1 Serving/170g	150	13.3	88	1.0	3.4	7.8	2.0
Mixed Leaf, Asda*	1 Serving/100g	21	0.2	21	1.5	3.2	0.2	2.1
Mixed Leaf, Tomato & Olive, Tesco*	1 Serving/170g	150	13.3	88	1.0	3.4	7.8	0.0
Mixed Leaf, Tomato, Feta, Boots*	1 Pack/179g	218	17.0	122	3.7	5.4	9.5	1.0
Mixed Leaves with Beetroot, Earthy, Waitrose*	1 Bag/140g	34	0.6	24	1.5	3.6	0.4	2.1
Mixed Leaves, Tesco*	1 Serving/20g	3	0.1	14	0.9	1.6	0.4	0.9
Mixed Pepper, Asda*	½ Pack/100g	24	0.3	24	1.0	4.3	0.3	1.7
Mixed Vegetable, Aldi*	1 Serving/200g	120	4.0	60	0.6	10.0	2.0	0.0

SALAD

INFO/WEIGHT	Measure	per Measure		Nutrition Values per 100g / 100ml				
		KCAL	FAT	KCAL	PROT	CARB	FAT	FIBRE
Mixed, (Basic Mix), Albert Heijn*	1 Pack/300g	57	0.0	19	1.0	2.5	0.0	2.5
Mixed, Bowl, Waitrose*	¼ Pack/64g	9	0.3	14	0.8	1.6	0.5	1.4
Mixed, Crisp, Mild, Tesco*	½ Pack/145g	29	0.4	20	1.2	3.0	0.3	2.1
Mixed, Florette*	1 Serving/100g	20	0.2	20	1.3	3.4	0.2	3.0
Mixed, Green Leaf, Lasting Leaf*	1 Serving/69g	12	0.3	17	0.8	1.8	0.4	1.5
Mixed, Iceland*	1 Serving/50g	12	0.1	24	1.2	4.3	0.2	2.1
Mixed, Medley, Bowl, Waitrose*	¼ Pack/60g	9	0.3	15	0.9	1.7	0.5	1.0
Mixed, Sainsbury's*	1 Serving/100g	21	0.2	21	1.4	3.4	0.2	2.1
Mixed, Sweet & Crispy, Tesco*	1 Serving/200g	48	0.6	24	1.0	4.2	0.3	2.0
Mixed, Sweet & Crunchy, Lasting Leaf*	1 Serving/62g	15	0.2	24	0.8	3.6	0.3	1.9
Mixed, Tesco*	1 Serving/100g	24	0.3	24	1.0	4.2	0.3	2.0
Mozzarella & Rocket, Asda*	1 Serving/265g	435	31.8	164	7.0	7.0	12.0	1.5
Mozzarella & Sunkissed Tomato, Tesco*	1 Bag/160g	270	22.9	169	4.6	4.3	14.3	2.1
Mozzarella & Tomato, (no dressing)	1 Serving/105g	190	14.5	182	8.0	5.9	13.8	3.3
Mozzarella & Tomato, M&S*	1 Serving/310g	400	14.8	129	5.5	15.5	4.8	0.9
Mushrooms in Tomato Sauce, Bowl, Sainsbury's*	1 Serving/100g	72	4.8	72	2.5	3.3	4.8	0.5
New Potato, Tomato & Egg with Salad Cream, M&S*	1 Pack/300g	165	7.2	55	2.9	5.4	2.4	1.3
New Potato, Tuna & Egg, M&S*	1 Pack/340g	255	12.9	75	3.8	6.7	3.8	0.7
Noodle & Sesame, Salad Bar, Waitrose*	1 Serving/100g	178	11.5	178	0.0	0.0	11.5	0.0
Noodle with Thai Style Chicken, M&S*	½ Pot/145g	160	7.1	110	5.2	11.6	4.9	1.4
Noodle, Sweet Chilli Chicken, Shapers, Boots*	1 Serving/197g	256	4.1	130	11.0	17.0	2.1	1.1
Nutty Rice, LL, Waitrose*	1 Portion/200g	368	14.4	184	4.5	25.3	7.2	3.1
Orzo & Sunbaked Tomato, BGTY, Sainsbury's*	1 Tub/276g	292	6.1	106	3.1	18.5	2.2	2.5
Pancetta, Express, Pizza Express*	1 Salad/90g	200	17.9	223	7.4	3.3	20.0	0.0
Pasta, Chicken & Sweetcorn, Morrisons*	1 Serving/220g	255	3.5	116	6.7	18.7	1.6	1.0
Pasta, Chicken with Tomato & Basil, Urban Eat*	1 Pack/280g	202	7.6	72	4.1	7.3	2.7	1.1
Pasta, Tomato, Morrisons*	1 Serving/50g	46	0.6	92	3.0	17.3	1.2	2.4
Pasta, Tuna & Sweetcorn, Morrisons*	1 Serving/100g	227	15.1	227	5.0	16.1	15.1	2.2
Pea & Ham, M&S*	1 Pack/335g	420	13.8	125	7.1	12.6	4.1	4.7
Pea Shoot, Baby Cos & Batavia Lettuce, Bagged, M&S*	1 Bag/120g	24	0.6	20	2.6	0.8	0.5	2.3
Pea Shoots & Baby Leaves, Steve's Leaves*	1 Pack/60g	14	0.4	24	2.7	2.0	0.6	2.0
Prawn & Avocado, M&S*	1 Serving/220g	176	15.0	80	3.0	2.0	6.8	3.1
Prawn Cocktail, Tesco*	1 Pack/300g	360	18.0	120	5.7	10.9	6.0	0.8
Prawn Layer, Eat Well, M&S*	1 Pack/220g	143	4.6	65	4.3	6.9	2.1	1.4
Prawn Layered, Co-Op*	1 Pack/300g	375	18.0	125	4.0	14.0	6.0	2.0
Prawn Layered, M&S*	1 Pack/455g	410	17.7	90	4.5	8.9	3.9	1.2
Prawn, Bowl, Sainsbury's*	1 Bowl/400g	632	46.8	158	3.7	9.4	11.7	1.2
Prawn, Layered, Asda*	1 Tub/380g	403	15.6	106	5.0	11.5	4.1	0.0
Prawn, Layered, Individual, Tesco*	1 Pack/180g	215	10.0	120	4.3	12.5	5.6	1.4
Prawn, Layered, Sainsbury's*	1 Pack/275g	355	21.2	129	3.6	11.2	7.7	1.1
Prawn, Layered, Tesco*	1 Pack/180g	243	13.0	135	4.2	13.1	7.2	2.0
Rainbow, Jewelled, Jamie Oliver, Boots*	1 Pack/198g	208	12.7	105	3.5	7.4	6.4	2.1
Red Cabbage & Sweetcorn, Crunchy, M&S*	1 Serving/80g	28	0.4	35	1.3	6.6	0.5	1.2
Rice, Chicken Tikka, COU, M&S*	1 Pack/390g	410	3.9	105	5.1	18.7	1.0	0.6
Rice, Coronation, Tesco*	1 Serving/50g	104	7.6	207	2.0	15.9	15.1	0.8
Rice, Mexican with Beans, COU, M&S*	1 Serving/250g	250	3.5	100	6.0	15.6	1.4	1.2
Rice, Rainbow, M&S*	1 Serving/262g	340	8.4	130	2.5	23.3	3.2	1.5
Rice, Rainbow, Waitrose*	1/3 Pack/60g	70	1.6	117	3.2	18.1	2.7	3.6
Rice, Spanish Style, with Chicken, M&S*	1 Serving/220g	319	12.8	145	5.8	17.4	5.8	0.5
Roast Butternut Squash & Fennel, TTD, Sainsbury's*	1 Pack/165g	214	7.6	130	3.4	15.2	4.6	6.9
Roast Chicken, Tesco*	1 Salad/300g	348	22.2	116	5.3	7.0	7.4	1.0
Roast Pepper Cous Cous, HL, Tesco*	1 Pot/220g	308	4.6	140	5.6	24.3	2.1	1.7
Roasted Artichoke & Pepper, M&S*	1 Serving/220g	638	53.9	290	4.1	12.8	24.5	5.1

SALAD

	Measure INFO/WEIGHT	per Measure KCAL	FAT	Nutrition Values per 100g / 100ml KCAL	PROT	CARB	FAT	FIBRE
Roasted Vegetables & Cous Cous, Sainsbury's*	1 Pot/225g	378	24.1	168	5.3	12.6	10.7	1.9
Rocket, Leafy, Asda*	1 Serving/75g	10	0.1	13	1.5	1.4	0.1	1.8
Rocket, Tesco*	1oz/28g	4	0.1	14	0.8	1.7	0.5	0.9
Salmon & Roquette, M&S*	1 Serving/255g	306	20.4	120	3.9	8.5	8.0	1.0
Salmon, Hot Smoked with Potato Salad, M&S*	1 Pack/338g	270	7.4	80	4.5	10.3	2.2	1.3
Salmon, Moroccan Style, Light Lunch, John West*	1 Pack/220g	299	11.7	136	11.7	8.8	5.3	3.4
Santini, Side, M&S*	1 Pack/195g	127	11.1	65	1.0	3.0	5.7	2.0
Satay Style Chicken & Noodle, Warm, Tesco*	1 Pack/235g	256	7.8	109	6.8	12.3	3.3	1.6
Seafood, Marinated, M&S*	1 Serving/90g	108	5.8	120	13.4	2.3	6.4	0.8
Seafood, Marinated, Waitrose*	1 Tub/160g	235	10.6	147	16.3	5.5	6.6	0.0
Seafood, Prawn & Calamari, Deli, M&S*	1 Pack/120g	132	6.1	110	14.7	1.2	5.1	0.8
Seasonal, Organic, Waitrose*	¼ Pack/25g	4	0.1	15	0.8	1.7	0.5	0.9
Selection, Side, M&S*	1 Serving/255g	153	12.8	60	1.1	2.5	5.0	1.3
Shredded Beetroot, Asda*	1 Serving/140g	29	0.4	21	1.1	3.5	0.3	1.5
Side, Fresh & Crispy, Tesco*	1 Salad/230g	30	0.7	13	0.7	1.9	0.3	1.3
Side, Garden with Cherry Tomatoes, Waitrose*	1 Pack/170g	25	0.7	15	0.8	2.0	0.4	1.3
Smoked Ham, Weight Watchers*	1 Pack/181g	233	3.6	129	11.0	16.6	2.0	3.0
Spcied Chicken, Quinoa & Cashew Nut, Tesco*	1 Pack/250g	394	19.5	158	8.4	11.9	7.8	3.1
Spiced Roast Cauliflower & Lentil, Waitrose*	1/3 Pack/63	86	4.2	136	5.1	10.2	6.7	7.3
Spicy Chickpea & Halloumi, Cranks*	1 Pack/238g	295	11.2	124	5.0	15.5	4.7	2.6
Spicy Chickpea, BGTY, Sainsbury's*	½ Pack/125g	119	2.1	95	4.7	15.3	1.7	5.5
Spicy Mexican Bean, Salad Bar, Waitrose*	1 Serving/100g	119	4.7	119	0.0	0.0	4.7	0.0
Spinach, Rocket & Watercress, Asda*	1 Serving/100g	21	0.6	21	2.8	1.2	0.6	1.9
Sprouted Pea & Bean, Mint Dressing, Eat Well, M&S*	1 Pot/165g	182	8.7	110	7.3	8.7	5.3	7.4
Sweet & Crispy, M&S*	1 Serving/140g	49	1.4	35	1.7	4.7	1.0	1.6
Sweet & Crispy, Side, Sainsbury's*	¼ Bag/93g	23	0.2	25	1.3	4.4	0.2	2.2
Sweet & Crunchy, Mixed, Prepared, Co-Op*	1 Serving/120g	42	0.4	35	1.1	5.9	0.3	1.8
Sweet & Crunchy, Morrisons*	1 Serving/100g	23	0.3	23	0.8	3.4	0.3	1.8
Sweet & Crunchy, Sainsbury's*	1 Pack/150g	22	0.2	15	0.9	2.6	0.1	1.8
Sweet Chilli Chicken Noodle, COU, M&S*	1 Pack/340g	408	7.8	120	6.8	17.4	2.3	1.2
Sweet Chilli Chicken Noodle, Tesco*	1 Pack/245g	243	4.2	99	7.5	12.7	1.7	1.4
Sweet Green, M&S*	1 Serving/150g	22	0.4	15	1.5	1.3	0.3	2.0
Sweet Leaf & Carrot, Asda*	½ Pack/164g	34	0.5	21	0.9	3.6	0.3	1.4
Sweet Leaf, Fully Prepared, Fresh, Sainsbury's*	¼ Pack/75g	12	0.1	16	0.8	3.0	0.1	2.1
Sweet Leaf, M&S*	1 Pack/110g	38	0.9	35	1.5	5.3	0.8	2.1
Sweet Leaf, Sainsbury's*	1 Serving/80g	19	0.2	24	0.8	3.6	0.3	1.9
Sweet Leafy, Organic, Tesco*	1 Serving/250g	45	1.0	18	0.8	2.7	0.4	1.9
Sweet Pepper Side, Tesco*	1 Serving/54g	22	0.2	41	1.3	8.0	0.4	2.1
Sweet Pepper with Corn, Tesco*	1 Pack/270g	103	1.4	38	1.3	7.2	0.5	1.5
Tabbouleh & Feta, Tesco*	1 Pack/225g	302	11.2	134	5.4	16.7	5.0	0.6
Tabbouleh Feta, Finest, Tesco*	1 Pack/225g	266	11.7	118	4.2	13.7	5.2	0.6
Tabbouleh, HL, Tesco*	1 Serving/200g	194	3.6	97	3.5	16.8	1.8	1.3
Tabbouleh, Salad Bar, Waitrose*	1 Serving/100g	94	1.7	94	0.0	0.0	1.7	0.0
Tenderleaf, Waitrose*	1 Serving/200g	30	1.0	15	0.9	1.6	0.5	1.1
Tenderstem Broccoli, Kale & Quinoa, Side, Waitrose*	1 Pack/165g	173	7.6	105	6.9	6.8	4.6	4.2
Three Bean & Mint, Finest, Tesco*	½ Pack/115g	155	6.9	135	6.8	7.7	6.0	11.5
Three Bean & Pesto, Italian Style, Boots*	1 Serving/290g	374	12.5	129	8.3	14.0	4.3	1.8
Three Bean with Mint Vinaigrette, M&S*	1 Pack/250g	250	6.0	100	5.9	8.2	2.4	11.1
Three Bean, Sainsbury's*	1 Serving/125g	108	6.3	86	4.2	6.0	5.0	0.0
Three Bean, Tinned, Tesco*	1 Tin/160g	176	1.6	110	7.7	17.6	1.0	5.3
Tomato & Basil, Bowl, M&S*	1 Serving/225g	225	22.7	100	0.8	3.7	10.1	1.1
Tomato & Cucumber, Ready To eat, Morrisons*	¼ Pack/81g	17	0.2	21	0.9	3.7	0.3	2.0
Tomato & Mozzarella, Finest, Tesco*	1 Pack/175g	254	21.4	145	5.6	3.3	12.2	0.7

	Measure INFO/WEIGHT	per Measure KCAL	FAT	Nutrition Values per 100g / 100ml KCAL	PROT	CARB	FAT	FIBRE
SALAD								
Tomato & Mozzarella, M&S*	1 Pack/220g	264	16.5	120	9.8	2.8	7.5	1.1
Tomato & Onion	1oz/28g	20	1.7	72	0.8	4.0	6.1	1.0
Tomato, Avocado & Rocket, M&S*	1 Pack/350g	508	46.9	145	1.7	4.1	13.4	0.2
Tomato, Lettuce & Cucumber, Classics, M&S*	1 Serving/275g	151	11.6	55	0.9	3.3	4.2	1.6
Tortellini & Chargrilled Vegetable, Tesco*	1 Serving/300g	492	23.1	164	5.1	18.7	7.7	1.7
Tuna & Mixed Bean	1 Serving/220g	287	14.4	131	9.5	11.2	6.6	3.7
Tuna & Three Bean, Healthily Balanced, M&S*	1 Serving/350g	332	10.2	95	8.7	8.8	2.9	4.6
Tuna & Tomato, Boots*	1 Pack/171g	150	10.3	88	6.5	2.0	6.0	1.0
Tuna Layer, COU, M&S*	1 Pack/340g	272	8.8	80	6.2	7.5	2.6	1.5
Tuna Layered, Waitrose*	1 Bowl/300g	636	58.8	212	4.0	4.8	19.6	1.0
Tuna Nicoise, Finest, Tesco*	1 Serving/250g	430	23.5	172	8.5	13.3	9.4	0.8
Tuna, Bowl, Fresh, Asda*	1 Serving/160g	184	11.2	115	8.0	5.0	7.0	0.0
Tuna, Bowl, Sainsbury's*	1 Serving/200g	336	21.4	168	6.1	11.7	10.7	1.5
Tuna, French Style, Light Lunch, John West*	1 Pack/220g	218	6.2	99	7.5	9.8	2.8	2.5
Tuna, Italian Style, Light Lunch, John West*	1 Pack/220g	205	5.7	93	7.3	9.8	2.6	0.5
Tuna, Layered, Tesco*	1 Serving/370g	466	29.2	126	4.4	9.4	7.9	1.0
Tuna, Mediterranean Style, Light Lunch, John West*	1 Pack/220g	211	4.2	96	8.5	10.0	1.9	2.4
Tuna, Mediterranean Style, Nixe, Lidl*	1 Pack/220g	255	5.5	116	10.0	12.0	2.5	2.8
Tuna, Mexican Style, Nixe, Lidl*	1 Tub/220g	293	11.0	133	11.0	9.4	5.0	3.0
Tuna, Pasta, Layered, Asda*	1 Serving/100g	98	2.8	98	5.4	12.7	2.8	1.9
Tuna, Snack, HL, Tesco*	1 Serving/300g	237	3.3	79	7.2	10.1	1.1	1.7
Tuna, Tomato Salsa Style, Light Lunch, John West*	1 Pack/220g	187	2.9	85	7.6	10.8	1.3	0.8
Waldorf, Average	**1 Serving/100g**	**193**	**17.7**	**193**	**1.4**	**7.5**	**17.7**	**1.3**
Waldorf, TTD, Sainsbury's*	¼ Pot/69g	203	19.5	296	1.9	8.1	28.4	4.7
Waldorf, with a Creamy Lemon Dressing, M&S*	1 Pack/125g	151	8.6	121	2.6	9.6	6.9	5.1
Wasabi Rocket & Cooler Leaves, Steve's Leaves*	1 Bag/60g	16	0.2	26	3.0	1.2	0.4	3.0
Watercress, Spinach & Rocket, Tesco*	1 Serving/30g	7	0.2	22	3.0	0.8	0.8	1.9
Watercress, Spinach & Rocket, Waitrose*	1 Bag/145g	30	1.2	21	2.2	1.2	0.8	1.5
Wheatberries, Spelt & Haricot, Good & Balanced, Asda*	½ Pack/125g	193	2.9	153	4.6	26.0	2.3	4.8
Wheatberry & Bean Refreshing, Waitrose*	1 Pack/220g	297	13.2	135	4.7	11.9	6.0	7.2
Wholefood, Super, Nutritionally Balanced, M&S*	1 Pack/285g	271	8.0	95	2.6	14.7	2.8	3.5
Wild Red Rocket & Milder Leaves, Steve's Leaves*	1 Bag/500g	10	0.2	19	2.8	0.8	0.5	2.6
Wild Rice, Salad Bar, Waitrose*	1 Serving/100g	159	6.6	159	0.0	0.0	6.6	0.0
Wild Rocket & Chard, Waitrose*	½ Bag/53g	8	0.3	15	0.8	1.7	0.5	1.4
with Crunchy Coleslaw, Bowl, M&S*	1 Pack/325g	455	44.8	140	1.0	2.5	13.8	2.0
with Salmon, Superfood, Leggera, Pizza Express*	1 Plate/480g	451	29.3	94	6.7	3.2	6.1	1.2
with Sweetcorn, Side, Tesco*	1 Serving/135g	51	0.7	38	1.3	7.2	0.5	1.5
SALAD CREAM								
Average	**1 Tsp/5g**	**17**	**1.4**	**335**	**1.7**	**18.6**	**27.8**	**0.1**
Heinz*	1 Tbsp/15g	50	4.0	332	1.4	20.0	26.8	0.0
Reduced Calorie, Average	**1 Tsp/5g**	**6**	**0.4**	**130**	**1.0**	**12.9**	**7.9**	**0.2**
Weight Watchers*	1 Serving/14g	16	0.6	115	1.5	16.2	4.4	0.0
SALAMI								
Average	**1 Slice/5g**	**18**	**1.3**	**360**	**28.4**	**1.8**	**26.2**	**0.0**
Danish, Average	**1 Serving/17g**	**89**	**8.8**	**524**	**13.2**	**1.3**	**51.7**	**0.0**
German, Average	**1 Serving/60g**	**200**	**16.4**	**333**	**20.3**	**1.6**	**27.3**	**0.1**
German, Peppered, Average	**3 Slices/25g**	**86**	**6.8**	**342**	**22.2**	**2.5**	**27.1**	**0.2**
Healthy Range, Average	**4 Slices/25g**	**55**	**3.6**	**220**	**22.4**	**0.6**	**14.3**	**0.0**
La Rougelle, Deluxe, Lidl*	1 Slice/5g	19	1.6	386	21.0	1.0	33.0	0.5
Meatster, Alpenmark, Aldi*	1 Serving/25g	124	11.0	497	24.0	1.0	44.0	0.5
Milano, Average	**1 Serving/70g**	**278**	**22.6**	**397**	**25.9**	**0.9**	**32.2**	**0.0**
Napoli, Average	**1 Slice/5g**	**17**	**1.3**	**342**	**27.1**	**0.8**	**25.5**	**0.0**
Pepperoni, Italian, Morrisons*	1 Slice/6g	23	1.9	406	24.0	0.9	34.0	0.0

S

INFO/WEIGHT	Measure	per Measure		Nutrition Values per 100g / 100ml				
		KCAL	FAT	KCAL	PROT	CARB	FAT	FIBRE
SALAMI								
Spanish, Wafer Thin, Tesco*	1 Pack/80g	273	18.8	341	25.5	6.8	23.5	0.0
SALMON								
Alaskan Pink, Canned, Crown Prince*	¼ Cup/55g	90	4.0	164	20.0	0.0	7.3	0.0
Alaskan, Wild, TTD, Sainsbury's*	1 Fillet/115g	173	8.3	150	21.2	0.1	7.2	0.1
Cooked, Prepacked, Average	*1 Fillet/93g*	*180*	*11.1*	*194*	*21.8*	*0.0*	*11.9*	*0.0*
Fillets with Lemon & Herb Butter, Asda*	1 Fillet/125g	305	22.5	244	20.0	0.4	18.0	0.0
Fillets with Sicilian Citrus Glaze, Sainsbury's*	1 Fillet/145g	371	25.8	256	21.9	2.3	17.8	0.0
Fillets, Alaskan, Wild, Sockeye, As Sold, Waitrose*	1 Serving/110g	165	7.3	150	21.8	0.4	6.6	0.5
Fillets, BBQ, Kiln Roasted, Waitrose*	1 Fillet/79g	208	12.3	263	25.3	5.3	15.6	0.0
Fillets, Black Pepper, Kiln Roasted, Fishmonger, Aldi*	1 Fillet/93g	226	15.8	243	22.0	0.5	17.0	0.5
Fillets, Boneless, Wild Alaskan, Keta, LL, Waitrose*	1 Fillet/110g	170	6.2	155	25.9	0.2	5.6	0.3
Fillets, Cajun, Waitrose*	1 Serving/150g	214	9.8	143	20.6	0.4	6.5	0.0
Fillets, Chargrilled, Sainsbury's*	1 Serving/270g	270	19.5	243	20.9	0.2	17.6	0.0
Fillets, Ginger, Chilli & Lime, Kiln Roasted, Aldi*	1 Pack/185g	416	25.9	225	23.0	0.5	14.0	0.5
Fillets, Honey Roast, Co-Op*	1 Fillet/100g	250	13.8	250	26.7	4.7	13.8	0.1
Fillets, Kiln Roasted, Tesco*	1 Fillet/88g	202	12.8	230	22.7	1.1	14.5	0.5
Fillets, Lemon & Dill Sauce, Pink, Inspirations, Birds Eye*	1 Fillet/225g	349	20.5	155	17.9	0.3	9.1	0.1
Fillets, Lightly Smoked, TTD, Sainsbury's*	1 Serving/100g	201	13.2	201	20.2	0.3	13.2	0.6
Fillets, Lime & Coriander Marinade, Pacific, Sainsbury's*	1 Serving/100g	139	4.1	139	24.4	1.3	4.1	0.9
Fillets, Raw, Average	*1 Sm Fillet/120g*	*227*	*14.0*	*189*	*20.9*	*0.1*	*11.7*	*0.1*
Fillets, Skin On, TTD, Sainsbury's*	1 Fillet/126g	249	14.3	197	23.5	0.2	11.3	0.1
Fillets, Smoked, Sweet & Smoky Barbecue Sauce, M&S*	½ Pack/119g	277	17.5	233	18.9	6.3	14.7	0.5
Fillets, Sweet Chilli & Ginger Sauce, Gastro, Youngs*	1 Serving/137g	174	5.6	127	20.5	1.9	4.1	0.2
Fillets, Sweet Chilli, Kiln Roasted, Tesco*	1 Fillet/93g	241	15.4	259	23.3	3.4	16.6	1.4
Fillets, Watercress & Creme Fraiche, The Saucy Fish Co.*	2 Fillets/230g	428	26.9	186	20.1	0.1	11.7	0.0
Fillets, with Orange & Dill Dressing, Tesco*	1 Serving/300g	540	30.9	180	17.7	4.1	10.3	0.7
Flakes, Honey Roast, Average	*1oz/28g*	*56*	*3.0*	*198*	*24.0*	*1.9*	*10.7*	*0.2*
Flakes, Honey Roast, Sainsbury's*	½ Pack/60g	115	5.4	192	25.4	2.0	9.0	0.6
Gravadlax with Mustard Sauce, Waitrose*	1 Pack/200g	382	22.2	191	21.8	1.0	11.1	0.4
Gravadlax, Cured with Salt, Sugar & Herbs	1 Serving/100g	119	3.3	119	18.3	3.1	3.3	0.4
Gravadlax, Finest, Tesco*	1 Serving/70g	125	6.9	178	22.1	0.2	9.9	0.0
Gravadlax, M&S*	1 Serving/140g	294	16.0	210	18.4	5.3	11.4	0.5
Gravadlax, Scottish, M&S*	1 Serving/70g	147	8.0	210	18.4	5.3	11.4	0.5
Grilled	*1oz/28g*	*60*	*3.7*	*215*	*24.2*	*0.0*	*13.1*	*0.0*
Hot Smoked, Average	*1 Serving/62g*	*103*	*4.4*	*166*	*24.0*	*0.9*	*7.2*	*0.1*
Hot Smoked, Kiln Baked, TTD, Sainsbury's*	½ Pack/63g	121	6.4	193	24.6	0.7	10.2	0.5
Juniper & Birch Smoked, TTD, Sainsbury's*	½ Pack/60g	132	8.4	220	23.3	0.3	14.0	0.1
Mild Oak Smoked, Average	*1 Slice/25g*	*46*	*2.5*	*182*	*22.6*	*0.1*	*10.2*	*0.0*
Mornay, with Broccoli, Weight Watchers*	1 Pack/320g	231	9.6	72	4.5	6.5	3.0	0.5
Mousse, Tesco*	1 Mousse/57g	100	7.0	177	13.5	2.9	12.4	0.2
Mousse, with Lemon & Dill, Hot Smoked, Waitrose*	1 Mousse/60g	146	12.6	244	11.3	2.5	21.0	0.0
Pink in Brine, Average	*1 Sm Can/105g*	*129*	*5.5*	*122*	*18.8*	*0.0*	*5.3*	*0.0*
Pink, Canned, Average	*1 Serving/125g*	*162*	*7.2*	*130*	*19.5*	*0.1*	*5.8*	*0.1*
Poached, Average	*1 Serving/90g*	*176*	*10.5*	*195*	*22.5*	*0.2*	*11.7*	*0.3*
Potted, M&S*	1 Serving/75g	184	14.5	245	17.1	0.5	19.4	1.2
Red in Brine, Average	*1oz/28g*	*42*	*2.2*	*149*	*19.7*	*0.0*	*7.8*	*0.0*
Red, Average	*½ Can/90g*	*141*	*7.4*	*156*	*20.4*	*0.1*	*8.2*	*0.1*
Roasted, Slices, Tesco*	1 Slice/33g	71	3.5	215	26.7	2.7	10.5	1.9
Skewers, Teriyaki, Sweet,,,M&S*	1 Skewer/48g	96	5.9	201	17.1	5.8	12.2	0.0
Smoked, & Cucumber Parcel, TTD, Sainsbury's*	1 Parcel/57g	118	8.7	206	14.2	2.4	15.2	1.2
Smoked, Appetisers, Tesco*	1/3 Pack/33g	80	6.2	240	16.3	1.1	18.5	0.0
Smoked, Average	*1 Serving/70g*	*126*	*7.0*	*179*	*21.9*	*0.5*	*10.0*	*0.1*
Smoked, Hot, with Dill, Kiln Roasted, Fishmonger, Aldi*	1 Fillet/93g	193	11.2	208	24.0	0.5	12.0	0.5

S

	Measure INFO/WEIGHT	per Measure KCAL	FAT	Nutrition Values per 100g / 100ml KCAL	PROT	CARB	FAT	FIBRE
SALMON								
Smoked, Irish, Organic, Specially Selected, Aldi*	1 Serving/50g	78	3.5	155	23.0	0.5	7.0	0.5
Smoked, Kiln Roasted, Scottish, Waitrose*	½ Pack/75g	162	9.9	216	24.2	0.0	13.2	0.4
Smoked, Parcels, TTD, Sainsbury's*	1 Serving/58g	144	11.1	250	13.4	5.7	19.3	1.0
Smoked, Pieces, Waitrose*	½ Pack/50g	87	4.3	174	23.9	0.3	8.6	0.1
Smoked, Slices, Value, Tesco*	1 Serving/100g	180	9.7	180	22.9	0.1	9.7	0.0
Smoked, Sockeye, Wild, TTD, Sainsbury's*	½ Pack/60g	82	1.9	137	26.3	0.7	3.2	0.6
Smoked, Trimmings, Average	**1 Serving/55g**	**101**	**5.7**	**184**	**22.8**	**0.2**	**10.3**	**0.0**
Smoked, Trimmings, Value, Tesco*	1 Serving/50g	89	5.0	178	22.1	0.2	9.9	0.0
Smoked, Wild Alaskan, TTD, Sainsbury's*	¼ Pack/25g	34	0.8	137	26.3	0.7	3.2	0.6
Steaks	**1 Serving/100g**	**180**	**11.0**	**180**	**20.2**	**0.0**	**11.0**	**0.0**
Steamed	**1oz/28g**	**55**	**3.6**	**197**	**20.1**	**0.0**	**13.0**	**0.0**
Wild Alaskan, Keta, Fillets, Sainsbury's*	1 Fillet/115g	178	6.4	155	25.9	0.2	5.6	0.3
SALMON EN CROUTE								
Frozen, Tesco*	1 Serving/166g	365	18.4	220	10.1	19.1	11.1	1.1
M&S*	½ Pack/185g	574	40.5	310	10.4	17.3	21.9	0.6
Retail, Average	**1oz/28g**	**81**	**5.3**	**288**	**11.8**	**18.0**	**19.1**	**0.0**
Wild Alaskan, Inspired To Cook, Sainsbury's*	1 Parcel/173g	476	24.4	275	12.5	24.7	14.1	10.8
with Lemon & Dill, Easy to Cook, Waitrose*	½ Pack/185g	487	31.5	263	10.7	16.9	17.0	2.7
SALMON IN								
a Creamy Horseradish Sauce, Fillets, Wonnemeyer*	1 Serving/300g	459	31.5	153	9.4	5.3	10.5	0.0
Chilli Lime & Ginger Dressing, The Saucy Fish Co.*	1 Fillet/140g	273	15.8	195	16.7	5.5	11.3	0.0
Creamy Watercress Sauce, Fillets, Scottish, Seafresh*	1 Pack 300g	528	38.7	176	13.7	1.2	12.9	0.1
Dill Sauce, Youngs*	1 Pack/435g	265	10.0	61	6.1	4.2	2.3	0.1
Lime & Coriander, Fillets, Good Choice, Iceland*	½ Pack/150g	189	4.4	126	19.8	5.1	2.9	0.8
Tomato & Mascarpone Sauce, Fillets, Asda*	½ Pack/181g	279	19.9	154	13.0	0.8	11.0	0.6
White Wine & Cream Sauce, Tesco*	1 Serving/170g	279	19.2	164	13.5	2.0	11.3	1.2
White Wine & Parsley Dressing, Fillets, Tesco*	1 Fillet/150g	291	20.4	194	17.5	0.3	13.6	0.6
SALMON WITH								
a Cream Sauce, Scottish Fillets, M&S*	1 Serving/200g	360	26.0	180	13.8	1.0	13.0	0.1
a Dill & Orange Crust, Cooked, Waitrose*	½ Pack/105g	259	17.3	247	21.3	3.0	16.5	0.6
Garlic & Herb Butter, Tesco*	1 Fillet/112g	291	23.1	260	17.6	0.0	20.6	0.0
Sweet Chilli Lime & Ginger, Simply Fish, Tesco*	½ Pack/98g	235	17.2	240	17.4	3.2	17.5	0.0
Sweet Chilli, Hot Smoked, Scottish, Tesco*	1 Fillet/120g	252	12.7	210	26.1	1.7	10.6	0.6
SALSA								
Bottled, M&S*	½ Jar/136g	95	3.3	70	1.2	12.0	2.4	1.5
Cool, Sainsbury's*	1 Serving/100g	31	0.5	31	1.0	5.6	0.5	1.2
GFY, Asda*	½ Pot/236g	85	0.9	36	1.1	7.0	0.4	0.7
Hot, Fresh, Chilled, Tesco*	1 Tub/200g	120	4.8	60	1.4	7.5	2.4	1.2
Medium Hot, Discovery*	1 Serving/30g	17	0.1	56	1.4	11.7	0.4	0.8
Mild, Original, Old El Paso*	1 Sachet/144g	60	0.7	42	1.6	9.0	0.5	0.0
Original from Dinner Kit, Old El Paso*	1 Jar/226g	71	0.7	32	1.2	6.0	0.3	0.0
Red Onion & Tomato, Tapas Selection, Sainsbury's*	1 Serving/22g	17	1.0	77	3.0	6.0	4.5	0.9
Smokey BBQ, Weight Watchers*	1 Serving/56g	20	0.1	36	1.1	7.6	0.1	2.3
Spiced Mango, Ginger & Chilli, Weight Watchers*	½ Pot/50g	42	0.1	85	1.0	19.9	0.2	2.6
Spicy Mango & Lime, Morrisons*	½ Pot/85g	62	0.3	73	1.0	15.9	0.4	1.3
Spicy, Less Than 3% Fat, M&S*	½ Pot/85g	30	0.7	35	1.3	5.6	0.8	0.8
Sweetcorn, Fresh, Sainsbury's*	¼ Pot/51g	32	0.9	63	1.1	10.5	1.8	1.3
Tomato & Avocado, Chunky, COU, M&S*	½ Pack/86g	30	1.2	35	0.8	5.4	1.4	1.4
Tomato, Chunky, Tesco*	1 Pot/170g	68	2.2	40	1.1	5.9	1.3	1.1
Tomato, Mexican Style, Dip, Morrisons*	½ Pack/50g	26	0.9	51	1.2	7.6	1.8	0.8
Tomato, Onion, Coriander & Chilli, Fresh, Waitrose*	1 Tub/170g	110	5.3	65	1.3	8.0	3.1	1.2
Tomato, Spicy, Worldwide Sauces*	1 Serving/25g	8	0.0	30	1.2	5.9	0.2	1.2
Tomato, Sun Ripened, Tesco*	1 Serving/40g	46	1.7	115	5.0	14.2	4.2	4.6

	Measure INFO/WEIGHT	per Measure KCAL	FAT	Nutrition Values per 100g / 100ml KCAL	PROT	CARB	FAT	FIBRE
SALSA								
Tomato, Vine Ripened, Tesco*	½ Tub/100g	47	1.8	47	1.0	6.7	1.8	1.1
with Jalapeño Chilli, M&S*	1 Tbsp/15g	15	0.6	100	1.0	14.0	4.0	2.0
SALT								
Alternative, Reduced Sodium, Losalt*	10g	0	0.0	0	0.0	0.0	0.0	0.0
Rock, Average	*¼ Tsp/1g*	*0*	*0.0*	*0*	*0.0*	*0.0*	*0.0*	*0.0*
Rock, Natural, Tidmans*	1 Serving/100g	0	0.0	0	0.0	0.0	0.0	0.0
Table, Average	*1 Tsp/5g*	*0*	*0.0*	*0*	*0.0*	*0.0*	*0.0*	*0.0*
SAMBUCA								
Average	*1 Pub Shot/35ml*	*122*	*0.0*	*348*	*0.0*	*37.2*	*0.0*	*0.0*
SAMOSAS								
Chicken Tikka, Indian, Sainsbury's*	1 Samosa/55g	131	5.5	237	9.4	25.0	10.0	4.6
Chicken, Mumtaz*	1 Serving/105g	177	8.3	169	19.6	4.9	7.9	0.0
Lamb, Morrisons*	1 Samosa/50g	144	7.8	288	9.8	27.0	15.7	1.5
Vegetable Lightly Spiced, Sainsbury's*	1 Samosa/50g	112	6.3	223	4.0	23.5	12.5	1.2
Vegetable, Indian Starter Selection, M&S*	1 Samosa/21g	60	3.5	290	5.0	29.0	16.9	3.3
Vegetable, Indian, Takeaway, CBY, Asda*	1 Samosa/50g	126	5.2	250	5.2	32.5	10.3	3.3
Vegetable, Large, Individual, Sainsbury's*	1 Samosa/110g	254	16.5	231	3.3	20.7	15.0	2.1
Vegetable, Large, Tesco*	1 Samosa/64g	148	7.9	231	4.8	25.2	12.4	3.4
Vegetable, M&S*	1 Samosa/45g	115	6.9	255	5.1	24.8	15.3	2.8
Vegetable, Mini, Asda*	1 Samosa/23g	52	2.0	233	6.0	32.0	9.0	2.6
Vegetable, Mini, Indian Snack Selection, Sainsbury's*	1 Samosa/25g	70	4.0	280	4.7	29.8	15.8	3.2
Vegetable, Mini, Indian Snack Selection, Tesco*	1 Samosa/32g	76	4.2	238	4.7	25.5	13.0	3.3
Vegetable, Mini, Indian, Party Selection, Tesco*	1 Samosa/30g	58	1.5	195	3.6	33.9	5.0	2.2
Vegetable, Mini, Waitrose*	1 Samosa/29g	70	3.8	242	3.6	27.1	13.2	3.1
Vegetable, Morrisons*	1 Samosa/60g	101	3.5	169	4.9	24.1	5.8	2.0
Vegetable, Retail, Average	*1 Samosa/110g*	*239*	*10.2*	*217*	*5.1*	*30.0*	*9.3*	*2.5*
Vegetable, Waitrose*	1 Samosa/58g	129	6.6	223	4.5	23.8	11.4	3.8
SANDWICH								
All Day Breakfast, Deep Filled, Morrisons*	1 Pack/480g	1138	50.4	237	11.9	22.4	10.5	2.5
All Day Breakfast, Finest, Tesco*	1 Pack/275g	660	41.5	240	9.7	16.4	15.1	1.6
All Day Breakfast, HL, Tesco*	1 Pack/223g	328	8.0	147	11.9	16.8	3.6	2.7
All Day Breakfast, Tesco Classic*	1 Pack/374g	636	29.9	170	8.0	14.5	8.0	3.0
Argi Bhaji, Cranks*	1 Pack/204g	401	10.6	197	5.2	31.3	5.2	2.2
Avocado, Mozzarella & Tomato, M&S*	1 Pack/273g	655	36.0	240	8.8	21.7	13.2	2.3
Bacon & Brie, Finest, Tesco*	1 Pack/201g	571	33.6	284	14.1	19.4	16.7	2.1
Bacon & Egg, Co-Op*	1 Pack/188g	536	32.0	285	13.0	20.0	17.0	2.0
Bacon & Egg, HL, Tesco*	1 Serving/178g	328	9.3	184	11.5	22.7	5.2	1.7
Bacon & Egg, Sainsbury's*	1 Pack/160g	384	17.8	240	13.0	22.0	11.1	1.8
Bacon & Egg, Tesco*	1 Pack/213g	494	19.6	232	14.8	21.6	9.2	1.8
Bacon, Brie & Mango Chutney, Daily Bread*	1 Serving/213g	555	22.7	261	12.7	28.6	10.7	0.0
Bacon, Cheese & Chicken, Triple, BGTY, Sainsbury's*	1 Serving/266g	506	16.8	190	12.7	20.7	6.3	2.6
Bacon, Lettuce & Tomato, Deep Fill, Ginsters*	1 Pack/197g	439	18.1	223	10.3	24.7	9.2	2.7
Bacon, Lettuce & Tomato, LBU, Co-Op*	1 Pack/195g	410	14.2	210	10.2	25.1	7.3	2.3
Bacon, Lettuce & Tomato, Malted Bread, Sainsbury's*	1 Pack/190g	417	16.6	219	11.2	22.7	8.7	2.7
Bacon, Lettuce & Tomato, Weight Watchers*	1 Pack/153g	237	2.4	155	9.4	25.8	1.6	2.4
Bap, Ham & Salad, Co-Op*	1 Bap/164g	295	4.9	180	8.0	30.0	3.0	2.0
Bap, Tuna & Sweetcorn, Malted, Co-Op*	1 Bap/212g	530	27.6	250	9.0	24.0	13.0	2.0
Beef & Horseradish, Sainsbury's*	1 Pack/187g	389	13.3	208	12.0	24.1	7.1	0.0
Beef & Pate, M&S*	1 Pack/188g	310	7.3	165	11.2	21.6	3.9	2.4
Beef & Salad, Roast, Daily Bread*	1 Pack/202g	319	8.3	158	9.0	21.4	4.1	0.0
Beef, Roast, Daily Bread*	1 Pack/199g	281	5.4	141	8.7	20.0	2.7	0.0
Beef, Roast, Finest, Tesco*	1 Sandwich/222g	464	15.8	209	14.8	19.6	7.1	3.8
Beef, Roast, Handmade, Tesco*	1 Pack/223g	439	15.8	197	12.5	20.7	7.1	1.6

S

SANDWICH

INFO/WEIGHT	Measure	per Measure KCAL	FAT	Nutrition Values per 100g / 100ml KCAL	PROT	CARB	FAT	FIBRE
Beef, Roast, Plain, From Restaurant, Average	**1 Sandwich/139g**	**346**	**13.8**	**249**	**15.5**	**24.1**	**9.9**	**0.0**
Beef, Roast, Sainsbury's*	1 Pack/174g	426	17.4	245	9.4	29.3	10.0	0.0
Beef, Salt with Gherkins & Mustard Mayo, Sainsbury's*	1 Pack/242g	486	18.2	201	9.3	24.1	7.5	3.1
Big Breakfast on White Bread, Sainsbury's*	1 Pack/241g	509	20.2	211	12.1	20.5	8.4	2.7
Bloomer, BLT, Freshly Prepared, M&S*	1 Pack/210g	430	19.5	205	8.2	21.8	9.3	1.8
BLT, Asda*	1 Sandwich/172g	325	11.9	189	9.9	21.8	6.9	4.6
BLT, BGTY, Sainsbury's*	1 Pack/196g	331	4.4	169	10.4	27.0	2.2	0.0
BLT, COU, M&S*	1 Pack/174g	278	4.7	160	9.5	25.6	2.7	2.5
BLT, HE, Tesco*	1 Pack/175g	364	8.8	208	13.0	27.8	5.0	2.0
BLT, HL, Tesco*	1 Pack/190g	287	2.7	151	10.1	24.5	1.4	1.6
BLT, M&S*	1 Serving/181g	381	14.7	210	10.7	23.8	8.1	1.8
BLT, Salt Controlled, Shapers, Boots*	1 Pack/180g	290	6.1	161	9.3	23.0	3.4	3.0
BLT, Tesco*	1 Pack/203g	520	29.2	256	11.9	19.5	14.4	1.5
BLT, Waitrose*	1 Pack/184g	398	16.4	216	9.5	24.5	8.9	2.3
Brie & Grape, Finest, Tesco*	1 Pack/209g	527	31.6	252	8.5	20.6	15.1	1.5
Brie & Wild Cranberry, Delicious, Boots*	1 Pack/168g	413	18.5	246	9.1	27.0	11.0	3.3
Brie LT, Cranks*	1 Pack/192g	383	16.9	199	7.7	21.5	8.8	1.7
Brie with Apple & Grapes, Sainsbury's*	1 Pack/220g	473	24.2	215	8.2	20.8	11.0	0.0
British Chicken & Sweetcorn, Eat Well, M&S*	1 Pack/194g	340	10.5	175	11.4	19.6	5.4	3.1
Cheddar & Celery, Good to Go, Waitrose*	1 Pack/198g	435	20.6	220	9.6	20.8	10.4	2.4
Cheddar & Celery, M&S*	1 Pack/200g	540	31.8	270	9.7	22.4	15.9	1.5
Cheddar & Coleslaw, Simply, Boots*	1 Pack/185g	538	33.3	291	9.2	23.0	18.0	1.8
Cheddar & Ham with Pickle, Smoked, Finest, Tesco*	1 Pack/217g	532	24.7	245	11.9	23.7	11.4	3.9
Cheddar & Ham, M&S*	1 Pack/165g	396	18.6	240	15.1	20.0	11.3	1.7
Cheddar & Ham, Smoked, Deep Filled, Tesco*	1 Serving/203g	573	33.1	282	14.3	19.5	16.3	1.2
Cheddar & Pickle, Mature, Sainsbury's*	1 Pack/171g	588	27.0	344	14.3	38.7	15.8	7.0
Cheddar & Tomato, Mature, Big, Sainsbury's*	1 Pack/233g	596	25.6	256	12.9	26.3	11.0	0.0
Cheddar Gorge, Cranks*	1 Pack/190g	454	23.2	239	11.5	19.4	12.2	3.0
Cheddar, Oldfields*	1 Pack/121g	384	17.3	317	12.8	33.2	14.3	1.5
Cheddar, Red Leicester & Onion, Tesco*	1 Pack/182g	604	38.9	332	11.0	23.8	21.4	2.5
Cheese & Coleslaw, M&S*	1 Pack/186g	498	32.4	268	10.2	17.6	17.4	3.2
Cheese & Ham, Smoked, Co-Op*	1 Pack/167g	334	8.4	200	15.0	24.0	5.0	2.0
Cheese & Marmite, No Mayonnaise, Boots*	1 Pack/156g	420	20.0	269	12.2	26.3	12.8	1.7
Cheese & Onion, Deep Fill, Tesco*	1 Pack/212g	742	51.9	350	12.3	20.2	24.5	1.3
Cheese & Onion, Ginsters*	1 Pack/172g	491	26.8	286	11.1	25.4	15.6	1.8
Cheese & Onion, HL, Tesco*	1 Pack/168g	314	9.9	187	10.3	23.2	5.9	1.7
Cheese & Onion, M&S*	1 Serving/188g	460	24.2	245	11.2	21.3	12.9	2.9
Cheese & Onion, Morrisons*	1 Pack/142g	260	2.4	183	14.1	27.8	1.7	2.9
Cheese & Onion, Reduced Fat, NUME, Morrisons*	1 Pack/142g	348	13.6	245	11.8	26.1	9.6	3.5
Cheese & Onion, Tesco*	1 Pack/178g	573	37.9	322	11.6	21.0	21.3	3.5
Cheese & Onion, Waitrose*	1 Pack/176g	579	38.7	329	12.5	20.2	22.0	2.8
Cheese & Pickle, Tesco*	1 Pack/140g	400	19.3	286	12.7	27.8	13.8	1.4
Cheese & Pickle, Virgin Trains*	1 Pack/158g	444	19.6	281	11.5	31.1	12.4	0.0
Cheese & Salad, Budgens*	1 Pack/169g	250	3.0	148	10.9	21.9	1.8	1.6
Cheese & Salad, COU, M&S*	1 Pack/188g	244	3.0	130	12.1	17.0	1.6	2.4
Cheese & Salad, Tesco*	1 Serving/188g	429	22.4	228	10.1	20.2	11.9	2.1
Cheese & Spring Onion, Asda*	1 Pack/160g	576	39.9	361	13.0	21.0	25.0	1.9
Cheese & Spring Onion, Co-Op*	1 Pack/164g	607	42.6	370	12.0	21.0	26.0	3.0
Cheese & Spring Onion, Sainsbury's*	1 Serving/177g	605	39.5	342	11.4	24.0	22.3	1.1
Cheese & Tomato, Asda*	1 Pack/154g	388	19.7	252	11.0	23.2	12.8	3.7
Cheese & Tomato, Co-Op*	1 Pack/155g	365	18.5	235	10.6	21.8	11.9	1.9
Cheese & Tomato, Freshmans*	1 Pack/111g	248	18.6	223	11.0	8.0	16.8	0.0
Cheese & Tomato, Organic, M&S*	1 Pack/165g	559	35.3	339	11.8	24.8	21.4	1.9

S

SANDWICH

	Measure INFO/WEIGHT	per Measure KCAL	FAT	Nutrition Values per 100g / 100ml KCAL	PROT	CARB	FAT	FIBRE
Cheese & Tomato, Sainsbury's*	1 Pack/216g	542	26.3	251	12.9	22.8	12.2	0.0
Cheese & Tomato, Tesco*	1 Pack/182g	582	38.9	320	9.2	22.6	21.4	1.1
Cheese Ploughman's, Deep Fill, Ginsters*	1 Pack/213g	491	24.2	231	8.4	23.8	11.4	2.2
Cheese, Ham & Pickle, Co-Op*	1 Serving/185g	370	7.4	200	13.0	27.0	4.0	3.0
Cheese, Ham & Pickle, HL, Tesco*	1 Pack/201g	312	4.2	155	13.1	21.0	2.1	1.7
Cheese, Ham & Pickle, Simply, Boots*	1 Pack/225g	551	29.2	245	11.0	21.0	13.0	2.4
Cheese, Ham & Pickle, Tesco*	1 Serving/215g	497	24.7	231	11.7	20.3	11.5	1.8
Cheese, Ham, & Pickle, Healthy Range, Average	*1 Pack/185g*	*299*	*5.1*	*162*	*13.6*	*20.6*	*2.8*	*2.5*
Cheese, Ham, BLT, Triple Pack, Asda*	1 Pack/260g	614	31.2	236	12.2	20.3	12.0	3.0
Cheese, Savoury, Sandwich King*	1 Pack/135g	328	11.2	243	11.6	30.2	8.3	0.0
Cheese, Three & Onion, Boots*	1 Pack/169g	566	33.8	335	11.0	28.0	20.0	1.9
Cheese, Three & Spring Onion, Shell*	1 Pack/168g	672	50.9	400	11.1	20.8	30.3	0.0
Chicken & Bacon, Deep Fill, Ginsters*	1 Pack/200g	435	15.7	224	12.4	25.3	8.1	2.4
Chicken & Bacon, Deep Filled, Co-Op*	1 Pack/166g	556	33.2	335	16.0	23.0	20.0	3.0
Chicken & Bacon, HE, Tesco*	1 Pack/155g	240	2.6	155	10.4	24.6	1.7	1.7
Chicken & Bacon, HL, Tesco*	1 Pack/193g	318	6.2	165	13.5	19.5	3.2	2.7
Chicken & Bacon, M&S*	1 Pack/185g	509	27.2	275	15.9	20.2	14.7	2.1
Chicken & Bacon, Roast, Boots*	1 Pack/175g	413	14.0	236	15.4	26.3	8.0	2.2
Chicken & Bacon, Tesco*	1 Pack/195g	486	24.2	249	14.3	20.0	12.4	2.7
Chicken & Bacon, Waitrose*	1 Serving/191g	495	23.5	259	11.8	25.3	12.3	2.2
Chicken & Bacon, with Ranch Dressing, LL, Waitrose*	1 Pack/196g	300	4.7	153	10.4	21.4	2.4	1.9
Chicken & Balsamic Roasted Tomatoes, COU, M&S*	1 Pack/200g	280	4.6	140	11.6	18.1	2.3	2.6
Chicken & Coleslaw, Tesco*	1 Pack/160g	305	7.1	191	12.0	25.7	4.4	2.4
Chicken & Ham, Healthy Living, Co-Op*	1 Pack/150g	285	6.0	190	12.0	28.0	4.0	3.0
Chicken & Ham, Roast, Tesco*	1 Pack/228g	561	31.9	246	13.3	16.6	14.0	1.2
Chicken & Mayo, The Sandwich Company*	1 Pack/72g	251	10.7	348	17.8	35.9	14.8	0.0
Chicken & Mayo, Wholemeal, Sodhexo*	1 Pack/128g	346	17.4	270	13.1	24.0	13.6	3.6
Chicken & Mayonnaise, Country Harvest*	1 Pack/120g	268	9.0	223	13.1	27.6	7.5	0.0
Chicken & Pepperonata, COU, M&S*	1 Pack/171g	240	2.9	140	10.4	20.9	1.7	1.3
Chicken & Pesto, on Malted Bread, Sainsbury's*	1 Pack/202g	373	13.3	185	10.8	19.3	6.6	2.7
Chicken & Salad, Co-Op*	1 Pack/195g	448	21.4	230	10.0	24.0	11.0	2.0
Chicken & Salad, COU, M&S*	1 Pack/194g	262	3.7	135	9.8	19.0	1.9	1.6
Chicken & Salad, Deep Filled, Tesco*	1 Pack/238g	440	19.5	185	13.1	14.6	8.2	2.8
Chicken & Salad, GFY, Asda*	1 Pack/194g	252	2.9	130	12.0	17.0	1.5	2.6
Chicken & Salad, Ham & Cheese, Twin, Tesco*	1 Pack/189g	434	21.5	230	10.8	21.1	11.4	2.3
Chicken & Salad, Healthy Living, Co-Op*	1 Pack/196g	265	3.5	135	10.4	19.1	1.8	3.9
Chicken & Salad, HL, Tesco*	1 Pack/207g	290	3.9	140	13.9	16.8	1.9	2.7
Chicken & Salad, Low Fat, Waitrose*	1 Pack/188g	291	8.1	155	10.4	18.6	4.3	2.1
Chicken & Salad, Roast, COU, M&S*	1 Pack/196g	265	4.5	135	8.9	19.6	2.3	2.2
Chicken & Salad, Roast, Healthy Selection, Budgens*	1 Pack/168g	244	3.2	145	11.7	21.1	1.9	1.0
Chicken & Salad, Roast, Waitrose*	1 Pack/217g	482	24.1	222	9.4	21.1	11.1	2.0
Chicken & Salad, Roast, Weight Watchers*	1 Pack/186g	266	8.0	143	10.3	15.8	4.3	2.8
Chicken & Salad, Sainsbury's*	1 Pack/240g	425	14.2	177	12.1	18.8	5.9	0.0
Chicken & Salad, Tesco*	1 Pack/193g	386	17.6	200	11.9	17.6	9.1	1.5
Chicken & Salad, Waitrose*	1 Pack/208g	406	19.8	195	10.3	17.1	9.5	2.5
Chicken & Salad with Mayo, BGTY, Sainsbury's*	1 Serving/200g	314	4.8	157	12.0	21.9	2.4	0.0
Chicken & Salad with Mayonnaise, Woolworths*	1 Serving/183g	337	12.4	184	11.3	19.3	6.8	0.0
Chicken & Stuffing, Light Choices, Tesco*	1 Pack/172g	275	4.8	160	14.4	18.7	2.8	6.9
Chicken & Stuffing, HL, Tesco*	1 Serving/171g	270	5.5	158	13.7	23.8	3.2	2.1
Chicken & Stuffing, M&S*	1 Pack/166g	398	17.1	240	13.9	23.1	10.3	5.6
Chicken & Stuffing, Roast, Tesco*	1 Sandwich/200g	450	14.4	225	15.0	24.8	7.2	1.9
Chicken & Stuffing, Shapers, Boots*	1 Serving/185g	327	5.2	177	13.0	25.0	2.8	2.2
Chicken & Stuffing, Waitrose*	1 Pack/183g	450	18.8	246	12.8	25.6	10.3	1.5

S

SANDWICH	Measure INFO/WEIGHT	per Measure KCAL	FAT	Nutrition Values per 100g / 100ml KCAL	PROT	CARB	FAT	FIBRE
Chicken & Tomato Relish, Chargrilled, Shapers, Boots*	1 Pack/190g	294	5.7	155	12.0	20.0	3.0	3.1
Chicken & Watercress, COU, M&S*	1 Pack/164g	266	2.8	162	12.8	23.9	1.7	2.1
Chicken Jalfrezi, Deep Fill, Ginsters*	1 Pack/171g	389	14.6	227	8.4	29.3	8.5	1.7
Chicken Mayo, Simply, Delicious, Boots*	1 Pack/148g	318	8.6	215	14.0	25.0	5.8	2.2
Chicken Salad with Tomato & Basil, HL, Tesco*	1 Pack/188g	279	3.4	148	13.1	18.8	1.8	1.9
Chicken Salad, Deep Fill, Ginsters*	1 Pack/203g	364	12.4	179	10.3	20.8	6.1	2.1
Chicken Salad, HL, Tesco*	1 Serving/190g	247	3.4	130	12.3	15.8	1.8	4.5
Chicken Salad, Light Choices, Tesco*	1 Pack/207g	290	3.9	140	13.9	16.8	1.9	2.7
Chicken Triple, LBU, Co-Op*	1 Pack/290g	566	15.4	195	13.8	21.8	5.3	2.2
Chicken with Honey Mustard Mayo, Chargrilled, Spar*	1 Pack/168g	428	19.2	255	13.1	25.0	11.4	0.0
Chicken with Mayo on Thick Softgrain, Tasties*	1 Pack/192g	338	15.2	176	9.5	16.1	7.9	0.0
Chicken with Pork Sage & Onion Stuffing, Tesco*	1 Pack/136g	376	17.0	276	12.1	28.1	12.5	1.4
Chicken, Bacon & Salad, Big, Sainsbury's*	1 Pack/249g	610	31.6	245	11.1	21.7	12.7	0.0
Chicken, Bacon, & Avocado, M&S*	1 Pack/242g	508	28.3	210	10.7	15.8	11.7	3.2
Chicken, Bacon, & Cheese, Club, M&S*	1 Pack/383g	805	37.2	210	11.9	18.5	9.7	1.9
Chicken, BLT, Deli Continental*	1 Pack/224g	509	26.9	227	12.4	17.3	12.0	0.0
Chicken, British, & Chorizo, Finest, Tesco*	1 Pack/186g	391	12.6	210	15.7	21.2	6.8	2.7
Chicken, Caesar, Boots*	1 Pack/226g	531	27.1	235	9.8	22.0	12.0	1.7
Chicken, Caesar, Finest, Tesco*	1 Pack/199g	454	19.9	228	15.4	19.2	10.0	1.4
Chicken, Chargrilled, Pitta Pocket, M&S*	1 Pack/208g	279	7.3	134	11.2	14.5	3.5	1.6
Chicken, Coronation, Indulgence, Taste!*	1 Pack/159g	396	18.8	249	9.1	26.5	11.8	0.0
Chicken, Coronation, M&S*	1 Pack/210g	420	20.4	200	11.2	20.2	9.7	3.1
Chicken, Coronation, Sainsbury's*	1 Pack/212g	411	14.4	194	9.7	21.5	6.8	4.1
Chicken, Flame Grilled, Rustlers*	1 Pack/150g	346	14.2	231	16.3	20.1	9.5	0.0
Chicken, Mexican, Healthy Choices, Shell*	1 Serving/168g	376	11.8	224	12.2	28.1	7.0	0.0
Chicken, No Mayo, M&S*	1 Pack/142g	248	3.3	175	16.6	20.6	2.3	3.2
Chicken, No Mayonnaise, Waitrose*	1 Pack/173g	332	9.5	192	11.6	24.0	5.5	2.1
Chicken, Pesto, Shapers, Boots*	1 Pack/181g	311	4.2	172	12.0	26.0	2.3	1.7
Chicken, Roast, & Salad, Shapers, Boots*	1 Pack/183g	274	4.4	150	12.0	20.0	2.4	3.4
Chicken, Roast, Salad, BGTY, Sainsbury's*	1 Pack/182g	268	4.0	147	11.9	19.9	2.2	2.7
Chicken, Roast, Tesco*	1 Pack/162g	378	11.8	233	14.7	26.0	7.3	2.1
Chicken, Rolls, Slider Selection, Tesco*	1 Pack/160g	365	7.5	230	10.6	35.7	4.7	1.0
Chicken, Salad on Malted Bread, BGTY, Sainsbury's*	1 Pack/216g	346	7.3	160	12.7	19.7	3.4	2.7
Chicken, Salad, Aldi*	1 Pack/195g	338	4.5	173	11.5	23.8	2.3	2.0
Chicken, Salad, M&S*	1 Pack/226g	350	9.3	155	10.6	18.8	4.1	3.0
Chicken, Southern Fried, Tesco*	1 Pack/174g	365	13.9	210	9.8	24.2	8.0	1.6
Chicken, Stuffing & Red Onion, Co-Op*	1 Pack/180g	360	10.6	200	13.0	22.4	5.9	2.7
Chicken, Tikka on Pepper Chilli Bread, Shapers, Boots*	1 Pack/172g	296	4.5	172	13.0	25.0	2.6	2.5
Chicken, with Lemon Dressing, British, COU, M&S*	1 Pack/151g	264	4.1	175	13.4	22.2	2.7	3.0
Chicken, Working Lunch*	1 Pack/169g	298	7.7	176	14.0	19.9	4.5	1.8
Classic Feast, M&S*	1 Serving/295g	841	51.6	285	10.6	21.3	17.5	4.7
Club, New York Style, Sainsbury's*	1 Serving/212g	608	33.5	287	13.3	22.8	15.8	2.7
Corned Beef on White, Simply, Brambles*	1 Pack/126g	325	10.8	258	14.2	30.8	8.6	1.4
Corned Beef, Tomato & Onion, Salad Garden*	1 Pack/137g	338	14.8	247	14.2	23.0	10.8	0.0
Crayfish & Rocket, Bistro, Waitrose*	1 Pack/193g	422	19.5	219	11.5	20.4	10.1	2.4
Cream Cheese & Ham, Tesco*	1 Pack/212g	655	36.7	309	11.0	27.2	17.3	1.2
Cream Cheese & Salad, Sandwich Box*	1 Pack/138g	250	8.0	181	5.6	26.3	5.8	0.0
Cream Cheese, & Salad, Choice*	1 Serving/156g	294	7.4	188	7.8	28.1	4.7	0.0
Cream Cheese, Red Pepper & Spinach, Daily Bread*	1 Pack/156g	273	8.1	175	7.4	24.0	5.2	0.0
Cumberl& Sausage, Ginsters*	1 Pack/210g	564	29.5	268	9.3	26.0	14.0	2.4
Curried Chickpea, Raynors Sandwiches*	1 Pack/166g	320	7.6	193	6.3	32.5	4.6	0.0
Deep Fill, All Day Breakfast, Ginsters*	1 Pack/200g	484	18.4	242	11.4	27.6	9.2	1.5
Egg & Bacon Mayo, Delifresh*	1 Pack/129g	310	12.6	240	10.1	29.7	9.8	2.1

S

SANDWICH

INFO/WEIGHT	Measure	per Measure		Nutrition Values per 100g / 100ml				
		KCAL	FAT	KCAL	PROT	CARB	FAT	FIBRE
Egg & Bacon, Deep Fill, Ginsters*	1 Pack/216g	503	21.8	233	14.5	21.0	10.1	2.3
Egg & Cress, BGTY, Sainsbury's*	1 Pack/145g	268	7.5	185	9.1	25.4	5.2	2.7
Egg & Cress, COU, M&S*	1 Pack/192g	240	5.2	125	9.8	15.5	2.7	2.8
Egg & Cress, Free Range, M&S*	1 Pack/192g	307	9.0	160	10.7	17.8	4.7	3.0
Egg & Cress, Free Range, Sainsbury's*	1 Pack/204g	404	16.9	198	10.5	20.3	8.3	3.3
Egg & Cress, M&S*	1 Pack/182g	331	17.7	182	10.1	13.6	9.7	3.2
Egg & Cress, on Wholemeal Bread, Refectory*	1 Pack/140g	323	14.7	231	9.8	24.7	10.5	0.0
Egg & Cress, Reduced Fat, Waitrose*	1 Pack/162g	262	10.4	162	9.7	16.5	6.4	6.4
Egg & Cress, No Mayo, Light Choices, Tesco*	1 Pack/160g	280	7.2	175	9.4	23.7	4.5	3.0
Egg & Cress, on Wheat Germ Bread, Tesco*	1 Pack/150g	255	6.9	169	9.5	21.7	4.6	1.4
Egg & Cress, with Mayo, Oatmeal Bread, Heinz*	1 Pack/150g	304	10.8	203	9.6	25.0	7.2	2.7
Egg & Salad, Co-Op*	1 Pack/190g	285	7.6	150	7.0	22.0	4.0	4.0
Egg & Salad, Deep Filled, Asda*	1 Pack/231g	395	16.2	171	8.0	19.0	7.0	1.0
Egg & Salad, Free Range, Waitrose*	1 Pack/180g	281	11.5	156	7.6	16.9	6.4	3.3
Egg & Cress, Reduced Fat, Asda*	1 Pack/164g	290	8.7	177	9.8	22.4	5.3	0.0
Egg & Salad, Shapers, Boots*	1 Pack/184g	304	8.5	165	6.9	24.0	4.6	1.1
Egg & Tomato, Deep Fill, Spar*	1 Serving/183g	348	13.6	190	8.2	22.8	7.4	0.0
Egg & Ham, Deli Club, Tesco*	1 Pack/220g	433	15.4	197	11.4	20.5	7.0	2.7
Egg & Salad with Mayonnaise, Wholemeal, Waitrose*	1 Pack/180g	257	8.8	143	8.3	16.5	4.9	3.6
Egg & Tomato, Delicious, Boots*	1 Pack/218g	362	10.0	166	8.2	22.0	4.6	2.0
Egg Mayo Salad, You Count, LL, Waitrose*	1 Pack/196g	314	10.2	160	8.8	18.5	5.2	2.2
Egg Mayo, Free Range, Asda*	1 Sandwich/178g	311	10.1	175	9.3	21.5	5.7	2.1
Egg Mayo, Free Range, on Oatmeal Bread, M&S*	1 Pack/180g	315	12.2	175	9.4	18.2	6.8	2.8
Egg Mayonnaise & Cress, Delicious, Boots*	1 Pack/195g	343	12.3	176	8.7	21.0	6.3	3.9
Egg Mayonnaise, & Cress, BHS*	1 Serving/188g	462	23.9	246	10.0	24.7	12.7	1.9
Egg Mayonnaise, & Cress, Co-Op*	1 Serving/159g	405	23.8	255	9.0	21.0	15.0	2.0
Egg Mayonnaise, & Cress, Co-Op*	1 Pack/159g	405	24.0	255	8.8	20.8	15.1	1.9
Egg Mayonnaise, & Cress, Reduced Fat, Waitrose*	1 Pack/162g	300	12.8	185	10.4	18.1	7.9	3.4
Egg Mayonnaise, & Cress, Shapers, Boots*	1 Pack/156g	292	7.6	187	11.0	25.0	4.9	2.6
Egg Mayonnaise, & Cress, Wheatgerm Bread, Asda*	1 Pack/158g	371	19.6	235	9.7	21.3	12.4	1.9
Egg Mayonnaise, & Cress, Wholemeal Bread, Oldfields*	1 Pack/128g	301	14.3	235	9.7	24.0	11.2	3.6
Egg Mayonnaise, & Gammon Ham, Strollers*	1 Pack/170g	400	19.3	236	13.0	20.5	11.4	0.0
Egg Mayonnaise, Boots*	1 Pack/184g	448	23.9	244	9.7	22.0	13.0	2.3
Egg Mayonnaise, Deep Fill, Benedicts*	1 Pack/195g	560	21.6	287	9.6	36.3	11.1	0.0
Egg Mayonnaise, Free Range, Finest, Tesco*	1 Pack/217g	412	19.1	190	10.9	16.8	8.8	2.3
Egg Mayonnaise, HL, Tesco*	1 Pack/162g	253	6.0	156	9.3	21.4	3.7	2.8
Egg Mayonnaise, on Malted Wheatgrain, Taste!*	1 Serving/169g	394	20.8	233	10.6	20.0	12.3	0.0
Egg Mayonnaise, Shell*	1 Pack/189g	522	29.1	276	9.8	24.7	15.4	0.0
Egg Mayonnaise, Waitrose*	1 Pack/180g	396	20.5	220	10.1	19.1	11.4	3.4
Egg Salad, on Softgrain Bread, HL, Tesco*	1 Sandwich/197g	290	4.7	147	7.0	23.6	2.4	1.7
Egg, Co-Op*	1 Pack/190g	285	7.0	150	6.8	22.1	3.7	3.7
Egg, Tomato & Salad Cream, M&S*	1 Pack/216g	400	14.9	185	7.4	21.7	6.9	2.3
Goat's Cheese, Sunblush Tomato, Deli Continental*	1 Pack/179g	480	29.4	268	9.5	20.5	16.4	0.0
Ham & Cheese, Ginsters*	1 Sandwich/170g	434	20.9	256	14.1	22.1	12.3	2.5
Ham & Cheese, Morrisons*	1 Serving/183g	273	4.6	149	12.5	19.2	2.5	4.1
Ham & Cheese Salad, Pick of the Pantry, on a Roll*	1 Pack/228g	431	22.6	189	10.9	13.5	9.9	2.6
Ham & Coleslaw, Smoked, Brambles*	1 Pack/166g	283	4.1	171	8.2	28.8	2.5	1.8
Ham & Edam, Smoked, Shapers, Boots*	1 Pack/183g	315	11.9	172	9.3	19.0	6.5	2.7
Ham & Emmental, Tesco*	1 Pack/179g	305	6.8	170	10.7	22.1	3.8	1.3
Ham & Mustard Mayo on White, Urban Eat*	1 Pack/130g	299	11.2	230	11.0	27.2	8.6	1.4
Ham & Mustard, Ginsters*	1 Pack/140g	307	9.4	219	11.8	28.0	6.7	2.5
Ham & Mustard, LBU, Co-Op*	1 Pack/162g	310	7.9	191	13.2	22.4	4.9	1.8
Ham & Mustard, Salad, BGTY, Sainsbury's*	1 Pack/183g	261	3.8	143	8.7	22.4	2.1	2.6

SANDWICH

	Measure INFO/WEIGHT	per Measure KCAL	FAT	Nutrition Values per 100g / 100ml KCAL	PROT	CARB	FAT	FIBRE
Ham & Mustard, Smoked, Tesco*	1 Pack/131g	315	11.4	240	11.5	28.0	8.7	1.4
Ham & Mustard, Tesco*	1 Pack/147g	437	27.9	297	10.6	20.8	19.0	1.2
Ham & Philadelphia Light, Dry Cured, Boots*	1 Pack/172g	339	9.3	197	12.8	24.4	5.4	2.5
Ham & Salad with Mustard, Finest, Tesco*	1 Pack/200g	466	21.0	233	15.3	19.3	10.5	1.3
Ham & Salad, British, COU, M&S*	1 Pack/204g	255	4.3	125	6.7	19.9	2.1	2.9
Ham & Salad, Ginsters*	1 Pack/179g	287	6.2	160	8.8	23.6	3.4	0.0
Ham & Salad, Healthy, Spar*	1 Serving/181g	286	6.7	158	8.4	22.7	3.7	0.0
Ham & Salad, Shapers, Boots*	1 Pack/195g	269	2.7	138	9.4	22.0	1.4	1.8
Ham & Swiss Cheese, Big, Sainsbury's*	1 Pack/218g	652	36.4	299	11.6	25.4	16.7	0.5
Ham & Swiss Cheese, M&S*	1 Pack/159g	393	20.0	247	14.7	18.9	12.6	3.3
Ham & Tomato, Brambles*	1 Pack/159g	288	7.3	181	11.1	24.1	4.6	3.3
Ham & Tomato, GFY, Asda*	1 Pack/173g	254	2.9	147	10.0	23.0	1.7	1.4
Ham & Pickle, Simple, EAT*	1 Pack/233g	354	11.6	152	7.3	20.5	5.0	1.6
Ham & Turkey with Salad, Co-Op*	1 Serving/181g	290	5.4	160	10.0	24.0	3.0	3.0
Ham & Turkey with Salad, Co-Op*	1 Pack/188g	263	5.6	140	9.0	21.0	3.0	2.0
Ham Salad, Light Choices, HL, Tesco*	1 Pack/190g	266	5.3	140	11.0	19.8	2.8	2.1
Ham, Cheese & Mayo, Brown Bread, Mattessons*	1 Pack/172g	439	18.1	255	13.8	27.0	10.5	2.2
Ham, Cheese, & Pickle, Average	**1 Pack/220g**	**524**	**25.1**	**238**	**12.2**	**21.6**	**11.4**	**2.5**
Ham, Cheese, & Pickle, BGTY, Sainsbury's*	1 Sandwich/198g	325	5.0	164	14.0	21.3	2.5	2.1
Ham, Cheese, & Pickle, Healthy Living, Co-Op*	1 Pack/185g	370	7.4	200	13.0	27.0	4.0	3.0
Ham, Cheese, & Pickle, Heinz*	1 Pack/188g	466	24.2	248	11.3	21.7	12.9	4.8
Ham, Cheese, & Pickle, Leicester, Waitrose*	1 Pack/205g	512	24.4	250	11.9	23.7	11.9	2.1
Ham, Cheese, & Pickle, Platter, M&S*	1 Sandwich/224g	582	33.4	260	11.9	19.3	14.9	5.3
Ham, Cheese, Pickle & Lettuce, No Mayo, Tesco*	1 Pack/207g	435	16.2	210	12.2	23.0	7.8	2.7
Ham, Tomato, & Lettuce, Oldfields*	1 Pack/216g	393	17.5	182	12.3	19.0	8.1	3.5
Houmous, & Crunchy Salad, Oldfields*	1 Pack/180g	256	7.6	142	6.3	20.0	4.2	0.0
Houmungously Crunchy, Cranks*	1 Pack/199g	353	14.2	177	5.6	21.3	7.1	2.8
Indian Summer, Cranks*	1 Pack/224g	477	20.2	213	9.5	21.8	9.0	3.3
Italian Salami & Mozzarella, Toasted Focaccia, Costa*	1 Pack/157g	430	20.1	274	10.8	27.9	12.8	0.0
Just Cheese, Go Eat*	1 Pack/132g	413	22.4	313	14.0	25.0	17.0	3.2
Just Chicken, No Mayo, Tesco*	1 Pack/120g	246	3.8	205	15.9	28.1	3.2	3.8
Just Ham, No Mayo, Tesco*	1 Pack/122g	250	4.9	205	11.6	30.4	4.0	2.1
Just Ham, Tesco*	1 Pack/114g	240	4.8	210	12.1	29.2	4.2	1.5
King Prawn & Avocado, Finest, Tesco*	1 Pack/185g	370	16.6	200	9.1	19.6	9.0	2.5
King Prawn, Sainsbury's*	1 Pack/204g	424	16.3	208	11.6	22.3	8.0	0.0
Lemon Chicken & Mangetout Salad, COU, M&S*	1 Pack/186g	260	5.0	140	10.6	19.0	2.7	3.7
Mozzarella, & Pepperoni, Sainsbury's*	1 Pack/171g	380	12.2	222	10.5	29.0	7.1	0.0
Mozzarella, & Tomato Calzone, Waitrose*	1 Pack/175g	410	19.4	234	10.8	22.7	11.1	2.2
Mozzarella, & Tomato, Waitrose*	1 Pack/193g	359	18.1	186	9.7	15.7	9.4	2.3
Mozzarella, Pesto & Pine Nuts, Sainsbury's*	1 Pack/180g	423	17.5	235	10.2	26.8	9.7	2.8
New York Deli, Boots*	1 Pack/245g	397	12.5	162	10.0	19.0	5.1	1.7
New York Deli, CBY, Asda*	1 Pack/200g	320	7.3	160	9.8	20.1	3.6	0.0
New York Deli, ES, Asda*	1 Pack/201g	403	15.4	201	12.4	20.6	7.7	3.8
Pastrami, & Emmental, New York, Boots*	1 Sandwich/169g	340	8.8	201	11.0	27.0	5.2	2.2
Philadelphia Salad, The Classic Sandwich Co*	1 Pack/135g	264	12.3	196	6.2	22.1	9.1	0.0
Pitta, Falafel, Houmous & Salad, Benedicts*	1 Pack/220g	405	13.0	184	6.8	26.1	5.9	0.0
Ploughman in a Pickle, Cranks*	1 Pack/241g	604	21.7	250	10.5	30.7	9.0	2.2
Ploughman's, Cheddar Cheese, Deep Fill, Asda*	1 Pack/229g	471	22.9	206	9.0	20.0	10.0	4.3
Ploughman's, Cheddar Cheese, Gibsons*	1 Sandwich/198g	469	22.8	237	9.8	23.7	11.5	0.0
Ploughman's, Cheddar, Mature Vintage, Sainsbury's*	1 Pack/204g	439	20.2	215	9.3	22.3	9.9	0.0
Ploughman's, Cheese, Deep Fill, Sutherland*	1 Pack/220g	558	32.3	254	9.2	21.4	14.7	0.0
Ploughman's, Deep Fill, Tesco*	1 Pack/245g	551	27.4	225	10.9	20.2	11.2	1.4
Poached Salmon & Watercress, Lochmuir, M&S*	1 Pack/192g	355	11.7	185	10.3	22.3	6.1	1.6

S

SANDWICH	Measure INFO/WEIGHT	per Measure KCAL	per Measure FAT	Nutrition Values per 100g / 100ml KCAL	PROT	CARB	FAT	FIBRE
Pork & Apple Sauce, Bells*	1 Pack/180g	341	8.1	190	11.5	26.1	4.5	0.0
Pork, & Autumn Chutney, Shapers, Boots*	1 Pack/160g	275	6.4	172	9.5	23.0	4.0	2.4
Pork, BBQ, Pulled, & Slaw, Skinny Hog, Shapers, Boots*	1 Pack/192g	338	5.4	176	11.0	26.0	2.8	2.1
Prawn & Rocket, Lemon Dressing, TTD, Sainsbury's*	1 Pack/203g	430	20.9	212	9.9	18.7	10.3	2.3
Prawn Cocktail, HE, Tesco*	1 Pack/154g	245	4.2	159	11.0	22.0	2.7	1.8
Prawn Cocktail, Platter, M&S*	1 Sandwich/200g	460	25.6	230	8.1	22.3	12.8	2.2
Prawn Cocktail, Waitrose*	1 Pack/196g	300	8.0	153	8.3	20.7	4.1	2.5
Prawn Mayonnaise on Oatmeal Bread, Sainsbury's*	1 Pack/150g	278	10.0	185	9.7	20.3	6.7	2.1
Prawn Mayonnaise, COU, M&S*	1 Pack/155g	240	3.6	155	10.2	22.9	2.3	2.8
Prawn Mayonnaise, GFY, Asda*	1 Pack/160g	251	4.5	157	10.0	23.0	2.8	2.8
Prawn Mayonnaise, Ginsters*	1 Pack/160g	397	21.1	248	9.1	23.3	13.2	2.4
Prawn Mayonnaise, M&S*	1 Pack/156g	328	12.0	210	10.0	24.7	7.7	2.2
Prawn Mayonnaise, Malted Bread, Tesco*	1 Pack/181g	369	14.3	204	9.4	22.9	7.9	2.0
Prawn Mayonnaise, Morrisons*	1 Pack/157g	234	3.9	149	9.0	22.7	2.5	3.0
Prawn Mayonnaise, Oatmeal Bread, Waitrose*	1 Pack/180g	463	27.0	257	10.2	20.4	15.0	3.2
Prawn Mayonnaise, Shapers, Boots*	1 Pack/160g	293	7.5	183	9.4	25.6	4.7	2.5
Prawn Mayonnaise, Tesco*	1 Pack/152g	350	16.3	230	10.2	22.2	10.7	2.6
Prawn, Crayfish & Rocket, Tesco*	1 Pack/193g	425	17.4	220	11.4	22.3	9.0	2.0
Prawn, Marie Rose, Waitrose*	1 Pack/164g	226	5.6	138	8.8	18.0	3.4	1.9
Rare Roast Beef & Horseradish, Eat Well, M&S*	1 Serving/200g	360	9.2	180	13.1	21.9	4.6	2.7
Rib, BBQ, Pork, Rustlers*	1 Pack/170g	459	22.1	270	14.3	22.9	13.0	2.0
Roast Chicken Salad, Light Choices, Tesco*	1 Pack/194g	300	4.3	155	11.2	22.0	2.2	1.2
Roast Chicken, Ginsters*	1 Pack/160g	313	10.1	196	13.6	21.2	6.3	2.6
Rokafeta, Cranks*	1 Pack/185g	377	18.1	204	6.9	21.1	9.8	1.9
Salmon & Black Pepper, Smoked, Fulfilled*	1 Pack/120g	293	10.3	244	13.8	29.0	8.6	0.0
Salmon & Cucumber, Brown Bread, Waitrose*	1 Pack/150g	296	10.6	197	10.5	22.7	7.1	1.4
Salmon & Cucumber, Light Choices, Tesco*	1 Pack/178g	330	5.7	185	10.1	26.8	3.2	2.3
Salmon & Cucumber, M&S*	1 Pack/168g	329	13.9	196	11.0	19.5	8.3	2.6
Salmon & Cucumber, Red, Healthy Choice, Asda*	1 Pack/149g	285	11.5	191	10.6	19.9	7.7	2.1
Salmon & Cucumber, Red, Tesco*	1 Pack/144g	284	9.2	197	11.1	23.8	6.4	1.9
Salmon & Cucumber, White Bread, Waitrose*	1 Pack/161g	305	8.6	189	9.8	25.5	5.3	1.7
Salmon & Egg, Smoked, Delicious, Boots*	1 Pack/170g	343	10.7	202	9.9	25.0	6.3	3.0
Salmon & Rocket, Poached, M&S*	1 Pack/180g	495	26.8	275	13.5	21.2	14.9	2.1
Salmon & Soft Cheese, Smoked, Waitrose*	1 Pack/154g	300	10.0	195	14.8	19.2	6.5	4.2
Salmon & Spinach, Poached, Shapers, Boots*	1 Pack/168g	284	7.6	169	9.2	23.0	4.5	3.1
Salmon, Red, Wild & Cucumber, Eat Well, M&S*	1 Pack/208g	385	14.4	185	10.7	18.0	6.9	3.3
Salmon, Smoked & Soft Cheese, Sainsbury's*	1 Pack/165g	383	15.2	232	11.9	25.1	9.2	2.4
Salmon, Smoked, Daily Bread*	1 Pack/122g	296	10.6	243	13.5	28.0	8.7	0.0
Sausage, Speedy Snacks*	1 Serving/93g	258	9.4	279	11.6	35.2	10.2	0.0
Seafood Medley, M&S*	1 Pack/227g	468	28.1	206	7.2	16.3	12.4	3.5
Spicy Falafel & Houmous Salad, Delifresh*	1 Pack/209g	429	19.7	205	6.1	24.0	9.4	2.6
Spinach Feta, Amy's Kitchen*	1 Roll/128g	262	9.0	205	8.6	27.0	7.0	2.3
Steak, Hot, M&S*	1 Roll/190g	513	15.2	270	11.9	37.0	8.0	3.2
Sub, Beef & Onion, M&S*	1 Pack/207g	611	31.7	295	13.3	25.6	15.3	1.5
Sub, Beef & Onion, Roast, Sainsbury's*	1 Serving/174g	426	17.4	245	9.4	29.3	10.0	0.0
Sub, Chicken & Bacon, Sainsbury's*	1 Pack/190g	554	27.0	291	13.4	27.4	14.2	0.8
Sub, Chicken, & Salad, Asda*	1 Sub/200g	460	27.2	230	9.4	17.4	13.6	0.9
Sub, Ham, & Tomato Salad, Shapers, Boots*	1 Pack/170g	286	3.9	168	9.2	28.0	2.3	1.4
Sub, Turkey, Stuffing, & Cranberry, Sainsbury's*	1 Sub/265g	603	19.1	227	10.6	29.2	7.2	1.9
Tikka Chicken & Mango Chutney, Tesco*	1 Pack/201g	352	4.8	175	11.6	25.4	2.4	2.6
Tuna Mayonnaise, & Cucumber, Classic*	1 Serving/185g	429	22.8	232	10.6	19.8	12.3	0.0
Tuna Mayonnaise, & Cucumber, Daily Bread*	1 Pack/190g	392	16.6	206	12.1	19.8	8.7	0.0
Tuna Mayonnaise, & Cucumber, Simply, Boots*	1 Pack/200g	498	26.0	249	12.0	21.0	13.0	2.4

S

SANDWICH

	Measure INFO/WEIGHT	per Measure KCAL	FAT	Nutrition Values per 100g / 100ml KCAL	PROT	CARB	FAT	FIBRE
Tuna Nicoise, Tesco*	1 Pack/215g	395	12.2	184	10.3	22.2	5.7	1.3
Tuna & Cucumber on Oatmeal Bread, Ginsters*	1 Pack/175g	290	7.2	166	11.7	20.7	4.1	2.4
Tuna & Cucumber, BGTY, Sainsbury's*	1 Pack/178g	268	3.2	151	11.3	22.3	1.8	3.1
Tuna & Cucumber, Co-Op*	1 Serving/268g	510	13.4	190	12.0	25.0	5.0	2.0
Tuna & Cucumber, Finest, Tesco*	1 Pack/169g	380	16.7	225	10.2	23.4	9.9	2.7
Tuna & Cucumber, Healthy Living, Co-Op*	1 Pack/192g	250	3.5	130	10.9	17.9	1.8	3.0
Tuna & Cucumber, Less Than 350 Cals, Ginsters*	1 Serving/193g	298	7.5	154	10.8	19.0	3.9	3.1
Tuna & Cucumber, on a Roll, M&S*	1 Roll/160g	320	12.0	200	11.8	21.6	7.5	3.2
Tuna & Cucumber, Weight Watchers*	1 Pack/173g	279	2.9	161	11.4	25.1	1.7	1.4
Tuna & Cucumber, You Count, LL, Waitrose*	1 Pack/195g	321	5.3	165	13.0	21.4	2.7	1.4
Tuna & Lemon Mayo, Shapers, Boots*	1 Pack/206g	318	9.7	154	10.0	18.0	4.7	1.7
Tuna & Salad, Bloomer, M&S*	1 Pack/231g	600	36.9	260	11.8	17.8	16.0	2.6
Tuna & Salad, Classic*	1 Pack/230g	449	15.9	195	8.7	27.3	6.9	2.1
Tuna & Sweetcorn, BGTY, Sainsbury's*	1 Pack/187g	309	5.1	165	10.8	24.7	2.7	2.8
Tuna & Sweetcorn, COU, M&S*	1 Pack/180g	270	4.3	150	12.6	19.0	2.4	3.8
Tuna & Sweetcorn, Ginsters*	1 Pack/169g	348	11.4	205	9.6	26.4	6.7	2.4
Tuna & Sweetcorn, LBU, Co-Op*	1 Pack/200g	380	9.2	190	11.7	24.1	4.6	2.4
Tuna & Sweetcorn, Light Choices, HL, Tesco*	1 Pack/168g	285	3.2	170	11.2	25.9	1.9	2.8
Tuna & Sweetcorn, on Malt Bread, Tesco*	1 Pack/175g	350	8.2	200	11.6	27.5	4.7	2.2
Tuna & Sweetcorn, Sainsbury's*	1 Pack/183g	392	15.6	214	12.1	22.3	8.5	0.0
Tuna & Tomato, & Onion, COU, M&S*	1 Pack/177g	250	4.2	141	11.1	18.8	2.4	2.2
Tuna, Crunch, HL, Tesco*	1 Pack/180g	261	4.3	145	11.0	19.9	2.4	0.5
Tuna, Healthy Options, Spar*	1 Pack/150g	268	3.6	179	14.3	24.9	2.4	0.0
Tuna, Mayonnaise & Cucumber, Finest, Tesco*	1 Pack/225g	484	19.1	215	11.6	23.1	8.5	1.7
Turkey with All the Christmas Trimmings, Tesco*	1 Pack/189g	425	14.2	225	10.8	28.0	7.5	1.9
Turkey & Bacon, COU, M&S*	1 Pack/165g	256	4.0	155	12.0	21.0	2.4	1.7
Turkey & Cranberry, COU, M&S*	1 Pack/180g	279	3.1	155	12.1	22.8	1.7	2.9
Turkey & Lettuce & Tomato, Shapers, Boots*	1 Pack/217g	310	4.8	143	9.8	21.0	2.2	2.9
Turkey & Mustard Slaw, Smoked, Good to Go, Waitrose*	1 Pack/201g	440	19.3	219	12.6	19.4	9.6	2.3
Turkey & Salad, Brambles*	1 Pack/170g	248	2.0	146	9.3	24.5	1.2	2.0
Turkey & Salt Beef, Smoked, LL, Waitrose*	1 Pack/180g	290	4.7	161	11.9	21.1	2.6	2.6
Turkey & Stuffing, M&S*	1 Pack/190g	352	9.3	185	12.3	23.1	4.9	1.9
Turkey, Bacon & Cranberry, Christmas, Waitrose*	1 Pack/211g	411	12.4	195	12.2	21.5	5.9	3.4
Turkey, Smoked on Wholemeal, Sodhexo*	1 Pack/128g	259	6.1	202	16.1	23.8	4.8	3.6
Vegetable, Roasted, Open, COU, M&S*	1 Pack/150g	260	2.2	173	8.4	31.3	1.5	4.4
Veggie Threesome, Cranks*	1 Pack/227g	500	20.5	220	9.0	24.3	9.0	3.0
Wensleydale & Carmelised Carrot Chutney, Brambles*	1 Pack/181g	445	21.5	246	10.8	24.4	11.9	1.9
Wensleydale & Carrot, M&S*	1 Pack/183g	430	22.5	235	9.9	21.4	12.3	2.8

SANDWICH FILLER

	Measure INFO/WEIGHT	per Measure KCAL	FAT	Nutrition Values per 100g / 100ml KCAL	PROT	CARB	FAT	FIBRE
Cheese & Bacon, Tesco*	1 Serving/50g	199	18.8	398	12.2	2.6	37.6	1.2
Cheese & Onion, 35% Less Fat, CBY, Asda*	1 Serving/50g	122	9.8	244	12.8	3.5	19.6	1.2
Cheese & Onion, CBY, Asda*	1 Serving/60g	214	19.7	356	11.3	3.0	32.8	1.8
Cheese & Onion, GFY, Asda*	1 Serving/50g	114	9.5	227	11.5	2.6	19.0	2.6
Cheese & Onion, Reduced Fat, Supermarket, Average	**1 Serving/100g**	**227**	**18.1**	**227**	**11.8**	**4.4**	**18.1**	**1.7**
Cheese & Onion, Sainsbury's*	1 Tub/200g	632	59.6	316	8.7	3.2	29.8	2.2
Cheese & Onion, Supermarket, Average	**1 Serving/100g**	**405**	**38.6**	**405**	**10.2**	**4.1**	**38.6**	**1.3**
Cheese & Onion, Tesco*	1 Pack/170g	721	72.4	424	10.0	0.2	42.6	1.5
Chicken & Bacon with Sweetcorn, Sainsbury's*	1 Serving/60g	123	9.4	205	12.0	4.0	15.7	0.9
Chicken & Stuffing, Sainsbury's*	½ Tub/120g	397	37.8	331	6.5	5.3	31.5	1.7
Chicken & Sweetcorn, Sainsbury's*	1 Tub/170g	396	33.7	233	11.0	2.7	19.8	1.9
Chicken & Sweetcorn, Asda*	1 Serving/60g	187	16.8	312	11.0	4.0	28.0	2.0
Chicken Tikka, BGTY, Sainsbury's*	½ Pot/85g	99	2.6	117	16.5	6.0	3.0	1.0
Chicken Tikka, HE, Tesco*	1 Serving/100g	110	3.6	110	7.1	12.4	3.6	1.0

S

	Measure INFO/WEIGHT	per Measure KCAL	FAT	Nutrition Values per 100g / 100ml KCAL	PROT	CARB	FAT	FIBRE
SANDWICH FILLER								
Chicken Tikka, Mild, Heinz*	1 Serving/52g	102	7.3	196	5.2	12.3	14.0	0.7
Chicken, Sweetcorn & Bacon, Tesco*	1 Serving/50g	167	14.8	334	12.3	4.3	29.7	1.6
Chunky Seafood Cocktail, Tesco*	1 Serving/100g	308	27.8	308	6.0	8.3	27.8	2.0
Corned Beef & Onion, Deli, Asda*	1 Serving/50g	170	15.5	340	12.0	3.3	31.0	0.7
Coronation Chicken, 50 % Less Fat, Tesco*	1 Serving/50g	102	6.3	205	11.5	9.7	12.6	2.7
Coronation Chicken, BGTY, Sainsbury's*	1 Portion/50g	73	3.5	146	11.9	8.9	7.0	1.4
Coronation Chicken, Sainsbury's*	¼ Tub/60g	183	14.8	305	12.1	8.9	24.6	1.2
Coronation Chicken, Tesco*	1 Tbsp/30g	88	7.0	293	11.4	9.2	23.2	0.7
Egg & Bacon, Fresh, Tesco*	1 Serving/45g	112	9.0	248	12.7	4.2	20.1	0.6
Egg & Salad Cream, CBY, Asda*	1 Serving/100g	165	10.4	165	10.3	7.2	10.4	0.5
Egg Mayonnaise 50% Less Fat, Tesco*	1 Serving/50g	65	3.8	130	10.2	3.8	7.6	0.5
Egg Mayonnaise, 50% Less Fat, CBY, Asda*	1 Serving/50g	67	4.2	134	10.3	4.2	8.3	0.5
Egg Mayonnaise, BGTY, Sainsbury's*	1 Serving/63g	71	4.1	113	10.2	3.4	6.5	0.1
Egg Mayonnaise, Country Fresh, Aldi*	¼ Pack/50g	106	8.9	211	9.8	2.9	17.8	0.0
Egg Mayonnaise, Deli, Asda*	1 Serving/50g	114	10.0	227	11.0	0.8	20.0	0.3
Egg Mayonnaise, Morrisons*	1 Serving/50g	71	5.3	142	10.0	1.7	10.6	0.0
Egg Mayonnaise, Tesco*	1 Serving/50g	100	7.8	199	10.9	3.5	15.6	0.5
Egg Mayonniase, Reduced Fat, Tesco*	1 Serving/50g	50	2.6	100	11.0	1.0	5.3	3.5
Poached Salmon & Cucumber, Deli, M&S*	1 Pot/170g	348	27.7	205	14.0	1.0	16.3	0.5
Prawn Marie Rose, Sainsbury's*	1 Serving/60g	121	10.6	201	8.1	2.5	17.6	0.9
Prawn Mayonnaise, Deli, Asda*	1 Serving/50g	170	16.5	339	9.0	1.6	33.0	0.4
Prawn Mayonnaise, GFY, Asda*	1 Serving/57g	101	7.4	177	12.0	3.0	13.0	0.1
Prawn Mayonnaise, M&S*	½ Pack/170g	502	47.6	295	10.6	0.6	28.0	0.3
Prawn Mayonnaise, Waitrose*	1 Pot/170g	537	52.9	316	8.9	0.2	31.1	0.0
Smoked Salmon & Soft Cheese, M&S*	1 Pack/170g	450	40.6	265	11.1	4.9	23.9	0.0
Three Cheese & Onion, Premier Deli*	1 Serving/100g	540	54.8	540	10.8	1.0	54.8	2.0
Tuna & Sweetcorn, 30% Less Fat, CBY, Asda*	1 Serving/100g	131	7.1	131	10.3	6.0	7.1	0.7
Tuna & Sweetcorn, CBY, Asda*	1 Serving/100g	223	17.6	223	10.3	5.5	17.6	0.9
Tuna & Sweetcorn, Deli, Asda*	1 Serving/50g	148	13.0	296	12.0	3.4	26.0	1.4
Tuna & Sweetcorn, Morrisons*	1 Tub/170g	382	28.4	225	15.3	7.0	16.7	3.4
Tuna & Sweetcorn, Reduced Fat, Average	**1 Serving/100g**	**119**	**5.4**	**119**	**11.5**	**5.8**	**5.4**	**1.2**
Tuna & Sweetcorn, Reduced Fat, HL, Tesco*	1 Serving/50g	68	3.2	136	11.4	8.0	6.3	0.8
Tuna & Sweetcorn, Reduced Fat, Tesco*	1 Serving/100g	140	6.3	140	11.4	8.0	6.3	0.8
Tuna & Sweetcorn, Supermarket, Average	**1 Serving/100g**	**228**	**17.8**	**228**	**11.6**	**5.7**	**17.8**	**1.4**
Tuna & Sweetcorn, Tesco*	1 Serving/54g	127	9.8	235	8.6	8.1	18.1	0.6
Tuna Mayonnaise & Cucumber, Choice, Tesco*	1 Serving/200g	463	22.8	232	12.8	23.2	11.4	1.6
Tuna Mayonnaise, BGTY, Sainsbury's*	1 Serving/100g	114	3.4	114	17.6	3.5	3.4	0.1
SANDWICH SPREAD								
Beef, Classic, Shippam*	1 Pot/75g	133	8.8	177	15.5	2.2	11.8	0.0
Chicken & Bacon, Asda*	¼ Jar/43g	153	13.2	359	18.0	2.0	31.0	1.0
Chicken, Classic, Shippam*	1 Serving/35g	64	4.4	182	15.5	1.8	12.5	0.0
Crab, Classic, Shippam*	1 Jar/35g	60	3.8	170	13.1	4.6	10.9	0.0
Heinz*	1 Tbsp/10ml	22	1.3	220	1.0	24.0	13.0	1.0
Light, Heinz*	1 Tbsp/10g	16	0.9	161	1.1	18.2	9.2	0.9
Salmon, Classic, Shippam*	1 Serving/35g	70	4.9	200	14.7	4.2	14.1	0.0
Tuna & Mayonnaise, Shippam*	1 Pot/75g	189	13.9	252	18.3	3.1	18.5	0.0
SARDINES								
Boneless, in Tomato Sauce, John West*	1 Can/120g	197	12.0	164	17.0	1.5	10.0	0.0
Grilled	**1oz/28g**	**55**	**2.9**	**195**	**25.3**	**0.0**	**10.4**	**0.0**
Grilled, No Added Brine, Canned, John West*	1 Can/100g	198	11.9	198	22.8	0.0	11.9	0.1
in Brine, Canned, Drained	**1oz/28g**	**38**	**2.1**	**136**	**17.0**	**0.0**	**7.6**	**0.0**
in Oil, Canned, Drained	**1oz/28g**	**51**	**3.2**	**180**	**19.1**	**0.0**	**11.6**	**0.0**
in Spring Water, Portuguese, Sainsbury's*	1 Can/90g	165	9.3	183	22.4	0.0	10.3	0.0

S

	Measure INFO/WEIGHT	per Measure KCAL	FAT	Nutrition Values per 100g / 100ml KCAL	PROT	CARB	FAT	FIBRE
SARDINES								
in Tomato Sauce, Canned	1oz/28g	45	2.8	162	17.0	1.4	9.9	0.0
Raw, Whole with Head	*1oz/28g*	*22*	*1.2*	*78*	*9.7*	*0.0*	*4.3*	*0.0*
SATAY								
Chicken & Turkey, Co-Op*	1 Pack/120g	264	16.8	220	20.0	4.0	14.0	0.0
Chicken & Turkey, Sainsbury's*	1 Stick/20g	44	2.8	222	20.0	4.0	14.0	1.9
Chicken with Peanut Sauce, Waitrose*	1 Pack/250g	492	27.0	197	18.9	6.0	10.8	0.5
Chicken, Breast, Party Bites, Sainsbury's*	1 Stick/10g	16	0.1	157	34.1	2.7	0.9	0.1
Chicken, Indonesian, Charlie Bigham's*	½ Pack/300g	555	36.6	185	14.2	4.9	12.2	1.5
Chicken, Indonesian, Mini, Sainsbury's*	1 Stick/10g	17	0.7	171	23.0	4.0	7.0	0.7
Chicken, Kebab, Waitrose*	½ Pack/125g	246	13.5	197	18.9	6.0	10.8	0.5
Chicken, M&S*	1 Satay/43g	90	5.5	210	19.1	4.4	12.7	0.7
Chicken, Sticks, Asda*	1 Stick/20g	43	2.8	216	18.0	4.5	14.0	0.0
Chicken, Taste Original*	1 Stick/20g	33	1.3	164	23.0	2.5	6.5	0.7
Chicken, Tikka, Mini, Asda*	1 Pack/80g	178	12.4	222	15.5	5.2	15.5	2.4
SATSUMAS								
Fresh, Raw, Flesh Only, Average	*1 Sm Fruit/56g*	*21*	*0.0*	*37*	*0.9*	*8.6*	*0.1*	*1.3*
Weighed with Peel, Average	*1 Sm Fruit/60g*	*16*	*0.0*	*26*	*0.6*	*6.1*	*0.1*	*0.6*
SAUCE								
Apple, Bramley, M&S*	1 Tbsp/15g	21	0.0	140	0.2	32.6	0.3	0.4
Apple, Bramley, Sainsbury's*	1 Tsp/15g	17	0.0	111	0.2	27.2	0.1	1.8
Apple, Everyday Value, Tesco*	1 Tbsp/15g	15	0.0	105	0.1	24.8	0.1	0.5
Apple, Smart Price, Asda*	1 Tsp/5g	5	0.0	101	0.3	25.0	0.0	0.9
Arrabbiata, Italian, Tesco*	½ Pot/175g	72	0.5	41	1.3	8.3	0.3	1.1
Balti Cooking, CBY, Asda*	1 Jar/570g	473	27.9	83	1.7	6.9	4.9	2.3
Balti Curry, Tesco*	1 Serving/200g	126	9.2	63	1.7	4.3	4.6	1.7
Balti, Asda*	¼ Jar/125g	155	12.5	124	1.6	7.0	10.0	1.7
Balti, Cooking, BGTY, Sainsbury's*	¼ Jar/129g	98	4.0	76	1.1	10.9	3.1	0.6
Balti, Cooking, Sharwood's*	¼ Jar/140g	120	8.3	86	1.2	7.1	5.9	1.4
Balti, Cooking, Tesco*	1 Serving/500g	395	20.0	79	1.5	9.2	4.0	2.2
Balti, Kanpur Garden, Lidl*	1 Jar/350g	388	21.7	111	1.6	11.3	6.2	1.9
Balti, Loyd Grossman*	½ Jar/175g	180	11.7	103	1.3	8.4	6.7	1.7
Balti, Ready Made, Average	*1 Serving/100g*	*98*	*6.1*	*98*	*2.0*	*8.3*	*6.1*	*1.8*
Balti, Tomato & Coriander, Canned, Patak's*	1 Can/283g	235	17.0	83	0.8	6.5	6.0	1.2
Barbecue, Asda*	1 Serving/135g	128	0.3	95	1.2	22.0	0.2	0.6
Barbeque, Cook in, Homepride*	1 Can/500g	375	7.5	75	0.7	14.6	1.5	0.6
Barbeque, Simply Sausages Ranch, Colman's*	1 Serving/130g	96	0.1	74	1.8	16.6	0.1	1.1
BBQ, Bick's*	1 Serving/100g	119	0.3	119	1.6	27.5	0.3	0.0
BBQ, Heinz*	1 Serving/20g	28	0.1	139	1.1	31.7	0.3	0.5
BBQ, HP*	1 Serving/20ml	29	0.0	143	0.8	33.1	0.2	0.0
BBQ, Spicy Mayhem, HP*	1 Serving/2g	3	0.0	156	0.9	36.7	0.1	0.0
Bearnaise, Mary Berry*	1 Serving/100g	435	39.8	435	1.7	17.3	39.8	0.4
Bearnaise, Sainsbury's*	1 Tbsp/15g	59	6.2	393	0.6	5.0	41.0	0.0
Bechamel for Lasagne, Loyd Grossman*	1 Jar/400g	396	33.2	99	0.6	5.4	8.3	0.1
Beef Bolognese, Weight Watchers*	1 Pot/300g	171	8.4	57	4.3	3.6	2.8	1.4
Beef in Ale, Cooking, Asda*	1 Jar/500g	160	1.0	32	1.6	6.0	0.2	0.0
Bhuna, Cooking, Sharwood's*	1/3 Jar/140g	116	7.6	83	1.2	7.6	5.4	1.6
Biryani, Medium & Aromati, Oven Bake, Patak's*	½ Jar/175g	135	9.3	77	1.1	6.1	5.3	1.7
Black Bean & Red Pepper, Sharwood's*	½ Jar/213g	132	3.0	62	1.9	10.5	1.4	1.2
Black Bean & Roasted Garlic, Stir Fry, Tesco*	½ Pack/90g	95	4.4	105	2.3	12.9	4.9	0.6
Black Bean Garlic, Lee Kum Kee*	1 Serving/19g	30	1.0	157	10.5	15.8	5.3	0.0
Black Bean, Asda*	1 Serving/55g	55	0.8	100	2.9	19.0	1.4	0.0
Black Bean, Canton, Stir Fry, Blue Dragon*	½ Pack/60g	53	1.2	88	2.8	14.8	2.0	1.5
Black Bean, Cantonese, Sharwood's*	½ Jar/212g	131	3.0	62	1.9	10.5	1.4	1.2

S

SAUCE

INFO/WEIGHT	Measure	per Measure		Nutrition Values per 100g / 100ml				
		KCAL	FAT	KCAL	PROT	CARB	FAT	FIBRE
Black Bean, Crushed, Stir Fry Sensations, Amoy*	1 Pouch/150g	150	4.4	100	2.4	16.9	2.9	1.0
Black Bean, Ready to Stir Fry, M&S*	1 Sachet/120g	78	1.1	65	2.5	11.5	0.9	1.4
Black Bean, Stir Fry, Fresh Ideas, Tesco*	½ Sachet/25g	33	0.7	132	4.2	22.6	2.8	0.8
Black Bean, Stir Fry, Fresh Tastes, Asda*	1 Pack/180ml	149	5.2	83	3.7	10.4	2.9	1.4
Black Bean, Stir Fry, Fresh, M&S*	1 Pot/120g	120	0.7	100	2.6	20.3	0.6	1.4
Black Bean, Stir Fry, Morrisons*	1 Serving/50g	92	5.4	185	4.1	17.3	10.8	1.5
Black Bean, Stir Fry, Sharwood's*	1 Jar/195g	127	0.6	65	2.3	12.9	0.3	0.0
Black Pepper, Stir Fry, Blue Dragon*	½ Sachet/60g	47	2.6	79	1.6	8.4	4.4	0.1
Bolognese, Italiano, Tesco*	1 Serving/175g	194	13.1	111	5.9	4.8	7.5	0.8
Bolognese, Loyd Grossman*	¼ Jar/106g	80	3.1	75	2.0	10.2	2.9	1.4
Bolognese, Smooth, Dolmio*	1 Serving/125g	61	1.0	49	1.5	8.0	0.8	0.0
Bolognese, Waitrose*	1 Serving/175g	150	8.6	86	5.4	5.3	4.9	2.0
Bramley Apple, Colman's*	1 Tbsp/15ml	16	0.0	107	0.2	26.5	0.0	1.3
Branston, Brown, Crosse & Blackwell*	1 Serving/15g	18	0.0	121	0.7	29.0	0.2	0.7
Branston, Rich & Fruity, Crosse & Blackwell*	1 Serving/15g	20	0.1	134	0.5	30.0	0.5	1.6
Bread, Christmas, Tesco*	1 Serving/60g	64	3.2	107	3.3	11.8	5.3	0.5
Bread, Luxury, M&S*	1 Serving/115g	196	16.2	170	3.2	8.1	14.1	2.2
Bread, M&S*	1 Serving/85g	153	12.4	180	3.1	8.7	14.6	0.2
Bread, Made with Semi-Skimmed Milk	1 Serving/45g	42	1.4	93	4.3	12.8	3.1	0.3
Brown, Asda*	1 Serving/10g	10	0.0	97	0.7	23.0	0.2	0.4
Brown, Bottled	1 Tsp/6g	6	0.0	99	1.1	25.2	0.0	0.7
Brown, Original, HP*	1 Tbsp/15g	18	0.0	122	0.9	28.3	0.1	0.4
Brown, Reduced Salt & Sugar, HP*	1 Tbsp/15g	13	0.0	87	0.7	20.0	0.1	0.3
Brown, Tesco*	1 Tsp/10g	10	0.0	104	0.7	25.1	0.1	0.6
Brown, Tiptree, Wilkin & Sons*	1 Serving/100g	104	0.0	104	1.1	42.0	0.0	0.0
Brown, Value, Tesco*	1 Serving/15g	13	0.0	86	0.7	18.8	0.1	0.3
Burger, Hellmann's*	1 Tbsp/15g	36	3.2	240	1.1	12.0	21.0	0.0
Butter & Tarragon, Chicken Tonight, Knorr*	¼ Jar/125g	132	13.0	106	1.0	2.1	10.4	0.7
Butter Chicken, Patak's*	1 Jar/500g	725	60.0	145	1.2	7.6	12.0	1.4
Butter Chicken, Simmer, Passage To India*	½ Pack/100g	188	11.7	188	2.2	18.9	11.7	3.2
Butter Chicken, TTD, Sainsbury's*	½ Pack/174g	272	23.5	156	1.8	6.7	13.5	0.9
Cantonese, Sizzling, Uncle Ben's*	½ Jar/270g	416	16.5	154	0.7	24.0	6.1	0.0
Caramelised Onion & Red Wine, M&S*	1 Serving/52g	31	1.6	60	1.9	6.7	3.1	0.6
Caramelised Orange, The Bay Tree*	1 Serving/168g	188	0.2	112	0.8	28.1	0.1	0.5
Chasseur, Classic, Chicken Tonight, Knorr*	¼ Jar/125g	61	3.6	49	0.6	5.3	2.9	0.7
Chasseur, Cook in, Homepride*	1 Can/390g	160	0.4	41	0.7	9.2	0.1	0.4
Cheese, Basics, Sainsbury's*	¼ Pot/124g	71	3.1	57	2.5	6.1	2.5	0.5
Cheese, Dry, Asda*	1 Serving/27g	101	3.0	373	4.4	64.0	11.0	7.0
Cheese, Fresh, Italiano, Tesco*	½ Tub/175g	236	16.1	135	6.8	6.2	9.2	0.0
Cheese, Fresh, Waitrose*	1 Pot/350g	458	34.3	131	5.1	5.7	9.8	0.0
Cheese, Instant, Morrisons*	1 Serving/14g	38	2.8	272	7.9	14.3	20.3	0.0
Cheese, Italian Style, Finest, Tesco*	½ Pot/175g	355	20.8	203	10.1	14.0	11.9	0.0
Cheese, Italian, Tesco*	½ Carton/175g	238	15.6	136	5.8	8.3	8.9	0.0
Cheese, Italiano, Tesco*	1 Pot/350g	368	20.0	105	5.3	8.0	5.7	0.0
Cheese, Made with Semi-Skimmed Milk	1 Serving/60g	107	7.6	179	8.1	9.1	12.6	0.2
Cheese, Made with Whole Milk	1 Serving/60g	118	8.8	197	8.0	9.0	14.6	0.2
Cherry Tomato & Fresh Basil, M&S*	1 Serving/175g	131	9.3	75	1.2	5.5	5.3	1.1
Chickpea & Spinach, Asda*	1 Jar/500g	365	14.0	73	3.5	8.4	2.8	2.0
Chilli & Garlic, Blue Dragon*	1 Serving/30ml	26	0.1	85	1.1	19.7	0.2	0.0
Chilli & Garlic, Lea & Perrins*	1 Tsp/6g	4	0.0	60	1.0	14.9	0.0	0.0
Chilli & Garlic, Stir Fry, M&S*	1 Serving/83g	120	1.0	145	0.7	32.4	1.2	1.1
Chilli Con Carne, Classic, Loyd Grossman*	1 Jar/350g	242	10.5	69	2.2	7.6	3.0	1.3
Chilli Con Carne, Cook in, BGTY, Sainsbury's*	¼ Jar/125g	69	0.6	55	1.7	11.0	0.5	2.5

S

	Measure INFO/WEIGHT	per Measure KCAL	FAT	Nutrition Values per 100g / 100ml KCAL	PROT	CARB	FAT	FIBRE

SAUCE

	Measure INFO/WEIGHT	KCAL	FAT	KCAL	PROT	CARB	FAT	FIBRE
Chilli Con Carne, Hot, Uncle Ben's*	1 Jar/500g	295	3.0	59	2.3	10.9	0.6	1.7
Chilli Con Carne, Homepride*	½ Jar/250g	145	1.2	58	1.6	11.1	0.5	1.6
Chilli Men, Spicy, Wagamama*	½ Jar/125g	138	5.9	110	2.0	14.9	4.7	0.6
Chilli with Kidney Beans, Old El Paso*	1 Serving/115g	92	0.5	80	4.3	14.8	0.4	0.0
Chilli, Amoy*	1 Tsp/6g	2	0.0	25	1.0	5.2	0.0	1.0
Chilli, Barbeque, Encona*	1 Tbsp/15ml	19	0.0	129	1.3	30.7	0.1	0.0
Chilli, Hot, Asda*	1 Jar/570g	319	2.3	56	2.1	11.0	0.4	1.9
Chilli, Hot, Blue Dragon*	1 Tbsp/15ml	14	0.0	96	0.5	23.0	0.2	0.0
Chilli, Hot, Mexican, Morrisons*	¼ Jar/125g	72	0.6	58	2.2	11.2	0.5	2.0
Chilli, Linghams*	1 Tsp/5g	4	0.0	79	0.0	17.3	0.8	0.0
Chilli, Sweet, Thai, Dipping, Original, Blue Dragon*	1 Serving/30ml	69	0.2	229	0.6	55.1	0.7	1.6
Chilli, Tesco*	1 Tsp/5ml	4	0.2	90	1.3	14.0	3.2	1.1
Chilli, Tomato Based, Bottled, Average	*1 Tbsp/15g*	*16*	*0.0*	*104*	*2.5*	*19.8*	*0.3*	*5.9*
Chinese Stir Fry, Sainsbury's*	½ Sachet/75g	61	1.9	81	0.4	14.1	2.5	1.0
Chinese Style Curry, Cooking, Asda*	1 Jar/560g	465	24.1	83	1.5	9.6	4.3	1.7
Chinese Style, Stir Fry, Fresh, Asda*	½ Sachet/50ml	93	6.0	186	1.5	18.0	12.0	0.0
Chinese, Curry, Farmfoods*	1 Sachet/200g	220	17.6	110	0.6	7.1	8.8	0.7
Chinese, Stir Fry, Sachet, Fresh, Sainsbury's*	½ Sachet/51ml	83	5.7	163	1.7	14.1	11.1	1.8
Chip Shop Curry, Knorr*	1 Sachet/150ml	146	6.9	97	1.7	12.4	4.6	0.7
Chip Shop Curry, Prepared, CBY, Asda*	1 Serving/62ml	50	3.0	80	0.5	8.6	4.8	0.2
Chocolate, Dessert, M&S*	1 Dtsp/11g	35	1.0	330	2.1	59.3	9.4	1.9
Chocolate, Sainsbury's*	1 Serving/25g	81	1.6	323	1.8	64.7	6.3	2.7
Chop Suey, Cantonese, Sharwood's*	1 Serving/200g	146	2.8	73	0.6	14.4	1.4	0.4
Chow Mein, Stir Fry, Asda*	½ Jar/98g	97	1.0	99	1.6	21.0	1.0	0.1
Chow Mein, Stir Fry, Blue Dragon*	1 Sachet/120g	110	3.5	92	1.1	15.4	2.9	0.4
Chow Mein, Stir Fry, Morrisons*	½ Sachet/50g	85	2.6	170	1.3	29.0	5.1	0.7
Chow Mein, Stir Fry, Straight to Wok, Amoy*	1 Pack/120g	172	7.0	143	0.9	21.9	5.8	0.5
Coconut, Ginger & Lemon Grass, Stir Fry, Wagamama*	½ Jar/125g	144	7.1	115	1.2	14.7	5.7	0.4
Coconut, Lime & Coriander, Cooking, Nando's*	1 Serving/65g	88	6.5	135	1.5	12.2	10.0	1.2
Cooking, Fiesta, Chilli, Aldi*	¼ Jar/124g	87	0.6	70	2.5	12.5	0.5	2.6
Coronation Chicken, Schwartz*	1 Pack/35g	124	5.1	354	14.9	29.1	14.5	23.8
Country French, Chicken Tonight, Knorr*	¼ Jar/125g	110	8.8	89	0.4	5.3	7.1	0.8
Country French, Low Fat, Chicken Tonight, Knorr*	¼ Jar/125g	56	3.6	45	0.4	4.4	2.9	0.7
Cranberry & Port, M&S*	1 Serving/75g	71	0.3	95	2.3	20.2	0.4	2.1
Cranberry Jelly, Baxters*	1 Tsp/15g	40	0.0	268	0.0	67.0	0.0	0.0
Cranberry Jelly, Morrisons*	1 Tsp/12g	23	0.0	189	0.2	47.0	0.0	0.1
Cranberry, Sainsbury's*	1 Tsp/15g	23	0.0	154	0.8	37.1	0.3	1.3
Cranberry, Tesco*	1 Tsp/15g	23	0.0	156	0.1	38.8	0.0	1.3
Cranberry, Waitrose*	1 Tbsp/20g	31	0.0	156	0.2	38.5	0.2	14.0
Cream, Graddsås, Ikea*	1 Serving/60ml	72	6.6	120	1.0	4.0	11.0	0.0
Creamy Leek & Bacon, Gastro, Loyd Grossman*	½ Pouch/165g	193	15.7	117	2.6	4.9	9.5	0.5
Creamy Mushroom, Cooking, M&S*	1 Jar/510g	663	57.6	130	1.3	5.4	11.3	0.5
Creamy Mushroom, Knorr*	1 Serving/125g	111	9.6	89	0.4	4.5	7.7	0.4
Curry, Asda*	1 Tbsp/15g	62	2.1	414	13.0	59.0	14.0	1.3
Curry, Basics, Sainsbury's*	¼ Jar/110g	70	2.8	64	0.7	9.7	2.5	0.9
Curry, Chinese Style, Cooking, CBY, Asda*	1 Serving/140g	89	4.3	64	1.5	7.4	3.1	3.5
Curry, Cook in, Homepride*	½ Can/250g	140	4.8	56	1.1	8.6	1.9	0.5
Curry, Green Thai, Finest, Tesco*	1 Serving/350g	420	37.1	120	1.4	4.8	10.6	0.7
Curry, Green Thai, Sharwood's*	1 Serving/403g	431	30.6	107	1.1	8.4	7.6	0.1
Curry, Kashmiri, Bibijis*	¼ Pack/119g	51	1.7	43	2.1	7.1	1.4	1.5
Curry, Medium, Uncle Ben's*	1 Jar/500g	330	10.0	66	0.9	10.9	2.0	0.0
Curry, Red Thai, Finest, Tesco*	1 Jar/350g	388	31.5	111	1.3	6.2	9.0	0.9
Curry, Red Thai, Sainsbury's*	½ Pouch/250g	390	35.8	156	1.7	5.0	14.3	1.5

S

	Measure INFO/WEIGHT	per Measure		Nutrition Values per 100g / 100ml				
		KCAL	FAT	KCAL	PROT	CARB	FAT	FIBRE
Curry, Smart Price, Asda*	¼ Jar/110g	73	2.0	66	1.4	11.0	1.8	0.6
Curry, Sweet	1 Serving/115g	105	6.4	91	1.2	9.6	5.6	1.4
Curry, Thai Coconut, Uncle Ben's*	1 Serving/125g	128	6.0	102	1.4	13.2	4.8	0.0
Dark Soy, Sesame & Ginger, for Fish, Schwartz*	1 Pack/300g	279	4.2	93	1.3	18.8	1.4	0.5
Dill & Lemon, Delicate for Fish, Schwartz*	1 Pack/300g	387	34.2	129	1.1	5.6	11.4	0.5
Fish Pie, Fresh, The Saucy Fish Co.*	1 Pack/230g	179	12.9	78	2.4	4.6	5.6	0.0
Fish, Nuoc Mam, Thai, Blue Dragon*	1 Tsp/5ml	7	0.0	145	5.9	30.9	0.1	0.0
for Fajitas, Original Smoky BBQ, Cooking, Old El Paso*	1 Jar/395g	222	5.1	56	1.5	9.6	1.3	0.0
for Lasagne, White, Tesco*	1 Jar/430g	452	35.7	105	2.2	5.3	8.3	0.6
Four Cheese for Pasta, Asda*	½ Jar/155g	242	21.7	156	3.5	3.9	14.0	0.1
Four Cheese for Pasta, Waitrose*	1 Pot/300g	392	24.8	112	6.6	5.5	7.1	0.5
Four Cheese, Reduced Fat, Morrisons*	½ Tub/175g	161	9.4	92	6.1	4.8	5.4	0.5
Fruity, HP*	1 Tsp/6g	8	0.0	141	1.2	35.1	0.1	0.0
Garlic & Chive, Heinz*	1 Serving/10ml	35	3.3	350	1.0	11.3	33.2	0.1
Garlic & Chive, Table & Dip, Heinz*	1 Serving/10ml	32	3.0	323	1.0	12.1	29.9	0.2
Garlic & Herb, Cooking, Simply Stir, Philadelphia *	1 Serving/60g	81	7.2	135	2.5	4.6	12.0	0.4
Garlic, Creamy, Sainsburys*	1 Tbsp/15g	44	4.3	296	0.5	7.6	29.0	1.5
Garlic, Heinz*	1 Serving/10ml	32	3.0	323	1.0	12.1	29.9	1.2
Gastro Chicken & Chorizo,,Loyd Grossman*	½ Pouch/175g	178	10.7	102	3.4	7.0	6.1	2.7
Green Peppercorn, Dry, Sainsbury's*	1 Tbsp/15ml	68	7.3	455	0.4	3.8	48.5	0.1
Green Thai Curry, Asda*	1 Jar/340g	309	27.2	91	0.5	4.3	8.0	0.2
Green Thai Curry, Express, Uncle Ben's*	1 Pack/170g	131	9.9	77	1.1	5.4	5.8	0.0
Green Thai Curry, M&S*	½ Jar/175g	175	13.3	100	1.1	7.4	7.6	0.8
Green Thai, Loyd Grossman*	½ Jar/175g	182	11.2	104	1.6	10.0	6.4	0.8
Green Thai, Stir Fry, Asda*	1 Pack/180ml	344	27.4	191	2.4	11.1	15.2	1.0
Green Thai, Stir Fry, Sainsbury's*	½ Pack/75g	112	8.0	149	1.2	11.9	10.7	1.0
Hoisin & Garlic, Blue Dragon*	1 Serving/60g	80	1.6	133	1.2	26.1	2.6	0.0
Hoisin & Plum, Dipping, Finest, Tesco*	1 Serving/50g	78	0.3	156	2.3	35.3	0.6	1.4
Hoisin & Plum, Stir Fry, HL, Tesco*	1 Serving/250g	148	3.2	59	2.1	9.7	1.3	1.3
Hoisin & Plum, Sweet & Fruity, Stir Fry, Sharwood's*	1 Serving/136g	128	1.8	94	0.7	19.9	1.3	0.9
Hoisin & Spring Onion, Stir Fry, Sharwood's*	1 Jar/165g	196	1.5	119	1.3	26.5	0.9	0.8
Hoisin, Lee Kum Kee*	1 Serving/35g	80	0.5	230	1.2	53.3	1.3	0.8
Hoisin, Sharwood's*	1 Tbsp/15g	32	0.0	211	2.7	49.5	0.3	0.1
Hoisin, Stir Fry, CBY, Asda*	1 Jar/210g	296	2.3	141	0.8	31.3	1.1	1.4
Hoisin, Stir Fry, Fresh Tastes, Asda*	½ Sachet/90ml	122	0.8	135	1.8	29.7	0.9	0.0
Hoisin, Stir Fry, Tesco*	½ Sachet/60g	87	2.9	145	1.1	23.9	4.9	0.5
Hollandaise, Atkins & Potts*	1 Serving/30g	144	15.0	480	1.2	6.2	50.0	0.3
Hollandaise, Classic, for Fish, Schwartz*	1 Sachet/300g	456	49.2	152	0.7	0.4	16.4	2.0
Hollandaise, Dry, Maille*	1 Serving/30g	148	15.2	495	1.0	10.8	50.6	0.0
Hollandaise, Finest, Tesco*	1 Serving/98g	473	44.5	485	1.4	17.2	45.6	0.3
Hollandaise, Fresh, Average	**1 Pack/150g**	**342**	**32.4**	**228**	**2.4**	**6.1**	**21.6**	**0.0**
Hollandaise, Homemade, Average	**1oz/28g**	**198**	**21.3**	**707**	**4.8**	**0.0**	**76.2**	**0.0**
Hollandaise, M&S*	1 Serving/10g	41	4.4	410	0.9	3.6	43.6	0.5
Hollandaise, Mary Berry*	1 Serving/100g	472	43.8	472	1.4	17.8	43.8	0.3
Hollandaise, Sainsbury's*	1 Tbsp/15g	72	7.6	478	0.2	5.9	50.4	0.4
Honey & Mustard, Chicken Tonight, Knorr*	¼ Jar/125g	132	6.6	106	1.0	12.6	5.3	1.8
Honey & Mustard, for Cooking, Asda*	1 Serving/200g	234	14.0	117	0.6	13.0	7.0	0.0
Honey & Mustard, Low Fat, Chicken Tonight, Knorr*	¼ Jar/131g	105	3.0	80	1.0	13.8	2.3	0.8
Horseradish Cream, Tesco*	1 Serving/15g	29	1.8	195	2.3	18.7	11.9	2.1
Horseradish, Colman's*	1 Tbsp/15ml	17	0.9	112	1.9	9.8	6.2	2.6
Horseradish, Creamed, Colman's*	1 Tsp/16g	37	2.1	229	4.3	21.4	13.3	0.0
Horseradish, Creamed, M&S*	1 Tsp/5g	16	1.5	325	2.4	12.1	29.3	2.5
Horseradish, Creamed, Waitrose*	1 Tbsp/16g	30	1.6	185	2.4	19.6	9.9	2.3

S

SAUCE

INFO/WEIGHT	Measure	per Measure KCAL	FAT	Nutrition Values per 100g / 100ml KCAL	PROT	CARB	FAT	FIBRE
Horseradish, Creamy, Sainsbury's*	1 Tsp/5g	11	0.6	223	2.8	28.9	11.8	1.6
Horseradish, Hot, Morrisons*	1 Serving/20g	22	1.1	110	1.6	10.9	5.6	1.1
Horseradish, Hot, Tesco*	1 Tsp/5g	9	0.5	185	2.3	19.7	10.6	2.3
Horseradish, Mustard, Sainsbury's*	1 Tsp/5g	8	0.3	163	7.9	18.2	6.6	3.5
Horseradish, Sainsbury's*	1 Dtsp/10g	14	0.7	145	1.5	17.8	6.6	2.4
Hot Chilli, Sharwood's*	1 fl oz/30ml	36	0.2	120	0.5	29.4	0.6	1.3
Hot Pepper	1 Tsp/5g	1	0.1	26	1.6	1.7	1.5	0.0
Hot Pepper, Encona*	1 Tsp/5ml	3	0.1	52	0.5	10.5	1.2	0.0
Hot, Cholula Hot Sauce*	1 Tbsp/12g	3	0.1	22	1.0	2.5	1.0	0.0
Italian Hot Chilli, Dolmio*	½ Pack/150g	104	5.8	69	1.3	7.1	3.9	0.0
Italian Tomato & Herb, for Pasta, BGTY, Sainsbury's*	½ Jar/250g	138	0.8	55	2.1	10.9	0.3	0.0
Italian Tomato & Mascarpone, Sainsbury's*	½ Tub/175g	158	10.2	90	2.6	6.8	5.8	1.2
Italian, Tomato & Mascarpone, Tesco*	½ Tub/175g	159	11.0	91	2.7	5.9	6.3	0.7
Jalfrezi, Average	*1 Sm Jar/350g*	*326*	*23.7*	*93*	*1.3*	*6.7*	*6.8*	*1.6*
Jalfrezi, Cooking, CBY, Asda*	1 Jar/570g	445	27.4	78	1.1	7.2	4.8	0.9
Jalfrezi, Cooking, Kanpur Garden, Lidl*	½ Jar/250g	232	14.0	93	1.6	8.3	5.6	1.6
Jalfrezi, Cooking, Sainsbury's*	1 Serving/250g	160	6.0	64	1.0	9.6	2.4	1.7
Jalfrezi, Loyd Grossman*	½ Jar/175g	159	10.3	91	1.4	7.3	5.9	1.6
Jalfrezi, Piri Piri, Finest, Tesco*	1 Serving/175g	145	10.8	83	1.2	5.7	6.2	1.5
Jalfrezi, Tesco*	1 Jar/500g	450	32.5	90	1.3	6.6	6.5	2.4
Jerk/BBQ, Levi Roots*	¼ Bottle/78g	94	0.1	121	1.1	28.8	0.1	0.5
Korma, Asda*	1 Serving/225g	434	33.8	193	2.5	12.0	15.0	2.2
Korma, Authentic, VLH Kitchens	1 Serving/118g	180	11.0	152.7	1.9	6.7	13.0	0.8
Korma, Coconut & Cream, Mild in Glass Jar, Patak's*	1 Jar/540g	940	79.4	174	1.3	9.1	14.7	0.8
Korma, Cooking, GFY, Asda*	¼ Jar/143g	110	4.4	77	2.0	10.2	3.1	0.6
Korma, Cooking, HE, Tesco*	¼ Jar/125g	120	8.0	96	1.9	7.4	6.4	0.6
Korma, Cooking, Light Choices, Tesco*	¼ Jar/125g	100	4.0	80	1.6	10.2	3.2	1.6
Korma, Cooking, Patak's*	¼ Jar/125g	211	17.5	169	1.3	9.3	14.0	2.4
Korma, Cooking, Sharwood's*	1 Jar/420g	680	42.8	162	1.7	15.9	10.2	2.2
Korma, Curry, Average	*1 Sm Jar/350g*	*584*	*42.3*	*167*	*2.3*	*11.7*	*12.1*	*1.3*
Korma, Curry, Loyd Grossman*	½ Jar/175g	224	14.5	128	1.5	11.3	8.3	0.8
Korma, Curry, Uncle Ben's*	1 Jar/500g	630	42.0	126	1.4	11.1	8.4	0.0
Korma, Mild Curry, BFY, Morrisons*	¼ Jar/118g	150	7.2	127	1.3	16.8	6.1	1.5
Korma, Tesco*	¼ Jar/125g	192	14.6	154	2.4	9.9	11.7	1.3
Korma, with Flaked Almonds, Weight Watchers*	1 Serving/175g	107	3.7	61	2.0	8.5	2.1	1.6
Lasagne, Creamy, Light, Dolmio*	¼ Jar/118g	101	7.4	86	0.4	6.7	6.3	0.0
Lemon & Ginger, Stir Fry, Finest, Tesco*	¼ Jar/85g	144	0.2	169	0.2	41.7	0.2	0.2
Lime & Coriander, Tangy for Fish, Schwartz*	1 Pack/300g	381	37.2	127	1.1	2.7	12.4	1.3
Lime Honey & Ginger, Stir Fry, Sharwood's*	1 Serving/50g	34	0.0	69	0.3	16.6	0.1	0.2
Madras, Aldi*	1 Serving/113g	68	2.3	60	1.5	9.0	2.0	0.0
Madras, Average	*1 Sm Jar/350g*	*355*	*24.2*	*102*	*1.7*	*8.0*	*6.9*	*1.7*
Madras, Cooking, Kanpur Garden, Lidl*	½ Jar/175g	158	8.8	90	2.0	8.0	5.0	2.0
Madras, Cooking, Sharwood's*	1 Tsp/2g	2	0.1	86	1.5	6.9	5.8	1.3
Madras, Cooking, Tesco*	1/3 Jar/161g	145	9.2	90	1.9	6.9	5.7	2.5
Madras, Cumin & Chilli, Original, in Glass Jar, Patak's*	1 Jar/540g	648	38.3	120	2.1	11.9	7.1	1.8
Madras, Indian, Sharwood's*	1 Jar/420g	433	26.5	103	1.8	9.7	6.3	1.9
Madras, Sharwood's*	1 Jar/420g	466	28.1	111	1.8	10.9	6.7	2.5
Madras, Tesco*	½ Jar/200g	168	13.0	84	1.1	5.2	6.5	1.3
Mango, Kashmiri Style, Finest, Tesco*	½ Jar/175g	285	23.8	163	2.4	7.7	13.6	0.9
Marie Rose, Fresh, The Saucy Fish Co.*	1 Pack/150g	590	59.7	393	1.6	7.0	39.8	0.0
Mint Garden, Fresh, Tesco*	1 Tsp/5g	2	0.0	40	2.6	3.6	0.4	1.5
Mint, Bramwells, Aldi*	1 Serving/30g	28	0.2	93	0.5	21.0	0.5	0.0
Mint, Sainsbury's*	1 Dtsp/10g	13	0.0	126	2.5	28.7	0.1	4.0

	Measure INFO/WEIGHT	per Measure KCAL	FAT	Nutrition Values per 100g / 100ml KCAL	PROT	CARB	FAT	FIBRE
SAUCE								
Mint, Value, Tesco*	1 Serving/10g	4	0.0	41	1.1	9.0	0.1	1.8
Mornay, Cheese, Asda*	¼ Pot/71g	114	9.0	161	6.8	6.6	12.7	0.4
Moroccan Chicken, Chicken Tonight, Knorr*	¼ Jar/125g	91	1.6	73	0.4	14.7	1.3	1.4
Mushroom, Creamy, Asda*	1 Serving/125g	76	4.6	61	0.8	6.0	3.7	0.5
Mushroom, Creamy, Chicken Tonight, Knorr*	¼ Jar/125g	99	7.1	79	0.5	6.0	5.7	1.0
Onion, Made with Semi-Skimmed Milk	1 Serving/60g	52	3.0	86	2.9	8.4	5.0	0.4
Onion, Made with Skimmed Milk	1 Serving/60g	46	2.4	77	2.9	8.4	4.0	0.4
Orange & Dill for Fish, Zesty, Schwartz*	1 Pack/300g	180	1.5	60	0.4	13.5	0.5	0.5
Oriental, Cantonese, Uncle Ben's*	¼ Jar/125g	108	0.2	86	0.8	20.3	0.2	1.2
Oyster, Blue Dragon*	1 Tsp/5ml	6	0.0	121	3.4	26.9	0.0	0.0
Parsley Lemon Caper, NCG Food Co*	¼ Carton/65ml	137	12.1	211	2.5	8.7	18.6	0.8
Parsley, Fresh, Sainsbury's*	½ Pot/150g	117	7.6	78	2.0	5.9	5.1	0.5
Parsley, Instant, Dry, Asda*	1 Serving/23g	82	1.6	355	7.0	66.0	7.0	4.4
Parsley, Made Up, Bisto*	1 Serving/50ml	41	2.4	82	0.6	9.2	4.8	0.0
Parsley, Tesco*	½ Pack/89g	85	5.1	95	2.8	8.1	5.7	1.1
Pasta Bake, Creamy Tomato & Bacon, Homepride*	1 Serving/110g	99	6.9	90	1.9	6.5	6.3	0.0
Pasta Bake, Creamy Tomato & Herb, Homepride*	1 Serving/125g	128	8.8	102	1.5	8.3	7.0	0.9
Pasta Bake, Tomato & Cheese, Dolmio*	¼ Jar/125g	70	1.5	56	2.1	9.1	1.2	1.2
Pasta Bake, Tuna, Homepride*	½ Jar/250g	208	13.0	83	1.4	7.6	5.2	0.9
Pasta, Tomato & Mushroom, Cucina, Aldi*	1 Jar/500g	165	1.0	33	1.1	5.7	0.2	1.9
Peanut, Sainsbury's*	1 Sachet/70g	185	9.2	264	1.9	34.7	13.1	1.6
Peking Lemon, Stir Fry, Blue Dragon*	1 Serving/35g	47	0.2	134	0.0	31.6	0.7	0.5
Pepper & Tomato, Spicy, Stir Through, M&S*	½ Jar/95g	166	14.6	175	1.6	7.5	15.4	0.0
Pepper, Creamy, Schwartz*	1 Pack/170g	116	9.2	68	1.5	3.4	5.4	1.0
Pepper, Creamy, Tesco*	1 Serving/85ml	128	11.4	151	1.2	6.4	13.4	0.5
Peppercorn, Creamy, Asda*	¼ Jar/137g	137	11.0	100	1.1	6.0	8.0	0.2
Peppercorn, Creamy, Chicken Tonight, Knorr*	¼ Jar/125g	110	9.8	88	0.3	3.8	7.8	0.4
Peppercorn, M&S*	1 Pack/200g	220	16.4	110	3.0	5.6	8.2	0.0
Peri-Peri, Garlic, Nando's*	1 Serving/15g	9	0.5	59	0.5	6.6	3.4	0.8
Peri-Peri, Hot & Zingy, Heinz*	1 Tbsp/15g	10	0.5	70	0.5	8.3	3.1	0.0
Peri-Peri, Hot, Nando's*	1 Serving/5g	4	0.2	75	0.6	9.6	3.8	1.3
Peri-Peri, Sweet, Nando's*	1 Tbsp/25g	36	0.5	142	0.5	30.7	2.1	0.0
Plum, Spiced, Heinz*	1 Serving/25g	32	0.0	128	0.5	31.1	0.1	1.0
Prawn Cocktail, Frank Cooper*	1 Tbsp/15g	47	4.0	316	0.8	18.3	26.7	0.1
Prawn Cocktail, Morrisons*	1 Portion/15ml	81	8.5	540	1.4	5.5	56.9	1.1
Pulled Pork, Apple Bourbon, Campbells*	1 fl oz/30ml	30	0.0	100	0.0	25.0	0.0	1.7
Puttanesca, Fresh, Waitrose*	½ Pot/176g	118	7.7	67	1.8	6.2	4.4	1.2
Raspberry, Dessert, M&S*	1 Serving/20g	24	0.1	120	0.5	28.7	0.3	2.6
Red Pepper, Fresh, Asda*	¼ Pot/82g	35	1.0	43	1.4	6.8	1.2	1.1
Red Thai Curry, Stir Fry, Blue Dragon*	1 Sachet/120g	112	9.6	93	0.9	4.4	8.0	0.5
Red Thai, Cooking, Asda*	½ Jar/160g	136	9.1	85	0.9	6.8	5.7	1.5
Red Thai, Loyd Grossman*	1Jar/350g	438	22.8	125	2.8	13.7	6.5	1.5
Red Wine, Cook in, Homepride*	¼ Can/98g	47	0.6	48	0.5	10.1	0.6	0.0
Red Wine, Cooking, BGTY, Sainsbury's*	1 Serving/125g	52	0.6	42	0.5	8.8	0.5	0.8
Redcurrant, Colman's*	1 Tsp/12g	44	0.0	368	0.7	90.0	0.0	0.0
Reggae Reggae, Cooking, Levi Roots*	½ Jar/175g	215	0.9	123	1.3	28.5	0.5	0.7
Reggae Reggae, Jerk BBQ, Levi Roots*	1 Jar/310g	375	0.3	121	1.1	28.8	0.1	0.5
Rich Hoisin, Stir Fry, Straight to Wok, Amoy*	½ Sachet/60g	68	1.4	114	1.8	21.4	2.3	0.7
Roast Peanut Satay, Stir Fry, Straight to Wok, Amoy*	½ Pack/60g	106	6.4	176	4.0	16.3	10.6	1.3
Roasted Peanut Satay, Stir Fry Sensations, Amoy*	1 Pouch/160g	354	19.8	221	4.7	21.9	12.4	1.0
Rogan Josh, Curry, The Curry Sauce Company*	1 Serving/235g	310	23.7	132	1.9	8.4	10.1	1.5
Rogan Josh, Medium, Sharwood's*	½ Jar/210g	151	7.6	72	1.4	8.6	3.6	0.5
Rogan Josh, Sharwood's*	½ Jar/210g	220	16.8	105	1.2	7.0	8.0	1.5

S

SAUCE

INFO/WEIGHT	Measure	per Measure		Nutrition Values per 100g / 100ml				
		KCAL	FAT	KCAL	PROT	CARB	FAT	FIBRE
Rogan Josh, Tesco*	½ Can/220g	156	10.3	71	1.3	5.9	4.7	1.4
Rogan Josh, VLH Kitchens	1 Serving/460g	374	1.2	81.5	1.4	6.1	5.3	1.4
Satay, Stir Fry, Asian Fusion, Waitrose*	½ Pack/70g	118	9.7	168	3.4	6.7	13.8	1.9
Satay, with Peanuts & Chillies, Cooking, Blue Dragon*	1 Serving/110g	198	10.7	180	4.3	18.0	9.7	1.5
Sausage Casserole, Cook in, Homepride*	½ Jar/250g	92	0.5	37	0.7	8.0	0.2	0.6
Seafood, Average	*1 Tsp/5g*	*20*	*1.9*	*410*	*1.4*	*15.4*	*38.0*	*0.2*
Seafood, Colman's*	1 Tbsp/15g	44	3.4	296	0.9	21.5	22.9	0.4
Seafood, GFY, Asda*	1 Dstp/10ml	31	2.7	313	0.6	17.0	27.0	0.0
Seafood, Sainsbury's*	1 Tbsp/15g	50	4.2	330	0.7	17.6	28.2	0.1
Seafood, Tesco*	1 Serving/10g	46	4.4	465	1.8	15.6	43.5	0.3
Smoked Bacon & Tomato, Stir in, Dolmio*	½ Tub/75g	74	4.2	98	4.6	7.2	5.6	1.3
Smoked Paprika & Tomato, M&S*	1 Serving/300g	135	5.1	45	1.3	6.1	1.7	0.9
Soy & Garlic, Stir Fry, Fresh Tastes, Asda*	1 Pack/180g	175	6.7	97	1.7	14.1	3.7	0.5
Soy & Plum, Stir Fry Additions, COOK!, M&S*	½ Sachet/60g	48	0.2	80	1.5	17.5	0.3	1.5
Soy, Average	*1 Tsp/5ml*	*3*	*0.0*	*64*	*8.7*	*8.3*	*0.0*	*0.0*
Soy, Dark, Amoy*	1 Tsp/5ml	5	0.0	106	0.9	25.6	0.0	0.0
Soy, Dark, Average	*1 Tsp/5g*	*4*	*0.0*	*84*	*4.0*	*16.7*	*0.1*	*0.2*
Soy, Light, Amoy*	1 Tsp/5ml	3	0.0	52	2.5	10.5	0.0	0.0
Soy, Naturally Brewed, Kikkoman*	1 Tbsp/15g	11	0.0	74	10.3	8.1	0.0	0.0
Soy, Reduced Salt, Amoy*	1 Tsp/5ml	3	0.0	56	4.0	10.0	0.0	0.0
Soy, Rich, Sharwood's*	1 Tsp/5ml	4	0.0	79	3.1	16.6	0.4	0.0
Soy, Wasabi & Lemon Grass, Stir Fry, Finest, Tesco*	1 Pack/125g	119	2.8	95	1.5	16.3	2.2	0.9
Soya, Japanese, Waitrose*	1 Tbsp/15ml	11	0.1	74	7.7	9.4	0.6	0.8
Spaghetti Bolognese, Dolmio*	1 Serving/100g	33	0.2	33	1.5	6.3	0.2	1.3
Spanish Chicken, Batts, Lidl*	½ Jar/250g	122	4.8	49	1.3	5.9	1.9	1.4
Spanish Chicken, Chicken Tonight, Knorr*	¼ Jar/125g	68	2.0	55	1.6	7.3	1.6	2.3
Spiced Tomato Tagine, Sainsbury's*	1 Jar/355g	227	5.7	64	1.7	10.6	1.6	4.3
Spicy Pepperoni & Tomato, Stir in, Dolmio*	½ Pack/75g	116	8.7	154	3.3	9.3	11.6	0.8
Spicy Sweet & Sour, Sharwood's*	1 Serving/138g	142	0.7	103	0.7	23.8	0.5	0.4
Sri Lankan Devil Curry, Sharwood's*	1 Jar/380g	220	11.4	58	0.5	7.2	3.0	2.1
Sticky BBQ, Spread & Bake, Heinz*	¼ Jar/78g	131	0.5	168	1.0	39.6	0.6	1.2
Sticky Plum, Stir Fry, Blue Dragon*	1 Serving/60g	145	0.2	242	0.1	35.6	0.3	0.0
Stir Fry, Chinese with Soy, Ginger & Garlic, Tesco*	1 Pack/150g	180	8.4	120	2.1	14.2	5.6	0.8
Stir Fry, Chinese, Tesco*	1 Serving/90g	86	3.2	95	1.3	14.3	3.5	0.6
Stir Fry, Pad Thai, Amoy*	1 Pack/120g	179	5.4	149	2.5	24.7	4.5	1.3
Stir Fry, Pad Thai, Tesco*	1 Pack/125g	112	2.9	90	1.3	15.8	2.3	0.8
Stir Fry, Sweet Soy with Ginger & Garlic, Blue Dragon*	½ Pack/60g	52	0.0	87	0.8	20.6	0.0	0.1
Stir Fry, Sweet Thai Chilli, Straight to Wok, Amoy*	1 Serving/60g	68	1.1	113	0.3	23.8	1.8	0.3
Stroganoff, Cooking, CBY, Asda*	¼ Jar/125g	95	5.2	76	1.6	7.7	4.2	0.5
Stroganoff, Mushroom, Creamy, M&S*	1 Serving/75g	86	6.9	115	3.3	4.8	9.2	0.6
Sweet & Sour with Mango, Sharwood's*	1/3 Jar/138g	134	0.1	97	0.7	23.3	0.1	1.3
Sweet & Sour, Chinese, Sainsbury's*	½ Jar/150g	222	0.2	148	0.2	36.6	0.1	0.1
Sweet & Sour, Cook In, Glass Jar, Homepride*	1 Jar/500g	335	0.5	67	0.3	16.2	0.1	0.5
Sweet & Sour, Cooking, Chinese, Sainsbury's*	¼ Jar/125g	155	0.1	124	0.6	30.1	0.1	0.7
Sweet & Sour, Cooking, Light Choices, Tesco*	1 Jar/510g	357	0.5	70	0.3	16.1	0.1	0.5
Sweet & Sour, Extra Pineapple, Asda*	¼ Jar/148g	138	0.4	93	0.5	22.0	0.3	0.3
Sweet & Sour, Extra Pineapple, Uncle Ben's*	1 Serving/165g	147	0.3	89	0.3	21.2	0.2	0.7
Sweet & Sour, Fresh, Sainsbury's*	1 Sachet/50ml	102	4.3	205	0.8	31.2	8.6	0.3
Sweet & Sour, GFY, Asda*	½ Jar/164g	77	0.3	47	0.4	11.0	0.2	0.3
Sweet & Sour, HL, Tesco*	1 Jar/510g	326	0.5	64	0.4	15.4	0.1	0.5
Sweet & Sour, Light, Uncle Ben's*	¼ Jar/125g	71	0.1	57	0.4	12.6	0.1	0.9
Sweet & Sour, Organic, Seeds of Change*	1 Jar/350g	350	0.4	100	0.4	24.4	0.1	0.6
Sweet & Sour, Oriental, Chicken Tonight, Knorr*	½ Jar/262g	217	2.6	83	0.4	20.8	1.0	0.5

S

SAUCE

	Measure INFO/WEIGHT	per Measure KCAL	FAT	Nutrition Values per 100g / 100ml KCAL	PROT	CARB	FAT	FIBRE
Sweet & Sour, Original, Uncle Ben's*	1 Pack/300g	264	0.6	88	0.4	21.9	0.2	0.8
Sweet & Sour, Peking Style, Finest, Tesco*	1 Serving/175g	147	0.2	84	0.6	20.1	0.1	0.5
Sweet & Sour, Spicy, Uncle Ben's*	1 Jar/400g	364	0.4	91	0.6	22.1	0.1	0.0
Sweet & Sour, Stir Fry, Asda*	1 Serving/63g	146	3.2	232	0.8	46.0	5.0	0.0
Sweet & Sour, Stir Fry, M&S*	1 Pack/120g	150	0.5	125	0.7	29.8	0.4	1.3
Sweet & Sour, Stir Fry, Pouch, Average	**1 Serving/100g**	**124**	**1.9**	**124**	**0.8**	**25.7**	**1.9**	**1.0**
Sweet & Sour, Stir Fry, Sachet, Blue Dragon*	1 Sachet/120g	145	0.1	122	0.2	29.7	0.1	0.3
Sweet & Sour, Stir Fry, Sharwood's*	1 Jar 160g	168	0.8	105	0.6	24.5	0.5	0.8
Sweet & Sour, Stir Fry, Tesco*	½ Jar/222g	164	0.4	74	0.6	17.0	0.2	0.4
Sweet & Sour, Stir Fry, Waitrose*	1 Serving/50ml	94	2.2	187	1.2	35.6	4.4	1.8
Sweet & Sour, Take-Away	1oz/28g	44	1.0	157	0.2	32.8	3.4	0.0
Sweet & Sour, Value, Tesco*	1 Serving/100g	83	0.2	83	0.3	20.0	0.2	1.0
Sweet Chilli & Lemon Grass, Stir Fry, Sharwood's*	1 Serving/155g	127	0.2	82	0.3	19.7	0.1	0.3
Sweet Chilli, Dipping, M&S*	1 Tbsp/15g	34	0.1	225	0.9	53.2	0.7	0.6
Sweet Chilli, Dipping, Sharwood's*	1 Bottle/150ml	339	3.9	226	0.6	51.5	2.6	1.6
Sweet Chilli, Dipping, Thai, Amoy*	1 Serving/10g	14	0.3	142	0.5	34.2	2.8	0.3
Sweet Chilli, Garlic, Stir Fry, Blue Dragon*	1 Pack/120g	142	0.1	118	0.2	28.8	0.1	0.3
Sweet Chilli, Heinz*	1 Serving/25g	38	0.1	150	0.3	36.5	0.4	6.4
Sweet Chilli, Stir Fry, Additions, Tesco*	1 Serving/50g	106	3.8	211	0.3	35.2	7.6	0.6
Sweet Chilli, Stir Fry, BGTY, Sainsbury's*	1 Pack/150ml	178	2.8	119	0.6	25.0	1.9	1.1
Sweet Chilli, Vitasia, Lidl*	1 Tbsp/15ml	24	0.1	158	0.6	39.0	0.6	0.0
Sweet Curry, Eazy Squirt, Heinz*	1 Serving/10ml	12	0.0	124	0.7	29.0	0.3	0.5
Sweet Pepper, Stir in, Dolmio*	½ Pot/75g	77	4.6	103	1.4	9.6	6.2	1.6
Sweet Thai Chilli, Uncle Ben's*	¼ Jar/125g	131	0.4	105	0.8	23.6	0.3	1.1
Szechuan, Spicy Tomato, Stir Fry, Blue Dragon*	½ Sachet/60g	59	1.8	98	1.3	15.8	3.0	0.9
Szechuan, Tomato, Spicy, Stir Fry, Sharwoods*	½ Jar/98g	56	0.3	57	1.1	12.0	0.3	0.8
Tabasco, Tabasco*	1 Tsp/5ml	1	0.0	12	1.3	0.8	0.8	0.6
Tamarind & Lime, Stir Fry, Sainsbury's*	1 Serving/75g	88	5.6	117	1.1	11.4	7.4	0.8
Tartare	1oz/28g	84	6.9	299	1.3	17.9	24.6	0.0
Tartare, Colman's*	1 Tbsp/15g	45	3.7	290	1.5	17.0	24.0	0.6
Tartare, Mild & Creamy, Heinz*	1 Tbsp/15g	47	4.2	312	0.9	13.4	28.3	0.1
Tartare, Rich, Colman's*	1 Tsp/5ml	14	1.2	284	1.2	17.0	23.0	0.6
Tartare, Sainsbury's*	1 Serving/20ml	94	9.8	469	0.4	5.8	49.0	1.0
Tartare, Tesco*	1 Tbsp/15g	43	3.3	287	1.5	19.6	21.8	0.3
Teriyaki, Asda*	1 Serving/98g	99	0.1	101	2.1	23.0	0.1	0.0
Teriyaki, Japanese Grill, Kikkoman*	1 Serving/15ml	24	0.0	158	4.5	30.8	0.1	0.0
Teriyaki, Lee Kum Kee*	1 Serving/15g	27	0.0	178	2.2	42.4	0.0	0.5
Teriyaki, Stir Fry, Blue Dragon*	1 Sachet/120g	124	0.0	103	0.5	25.0	0.0	0.0
Teriyaki, Stir Fry, Fresh Ideas, Tesco*	1 Serving/25g	33	0.6	133	1.1	26.9	2.3	0.0
Teriyaki, Stir Fry, Sharwood's*	1 Jar/150g	144	0.4	96	0.9	22.5	0.3	0.3
Thai Chilli, Dipping, Sainsbury's*	1 Tbsp/15g	30	0.0	201	0.2	49.8	0.0	5.0
Thai Curry, Yellow, Loyd Grossman*	1 Serving/100g	111	7.5	111	1.7	9.1	7.5	1.0
Thai Fish, Nuoc Mam, Amoy*	1 Tbsp/15ml	12	0.0	80	13.4	6.7	0.0	0.0
Thai Green Curry, Stir Fry, Blue Dragon*	1 Sachet/120g	74	4.8	62	0.9	5.7	4.0	0.5
Thai Green, Sainsbury's*	¼ Pack/125g	170	11.9	136	1.8	10.8	9.5	2.1
Thai Kaffir Lime, Chilli & Basil, Stir Fry, Sainsbury's*	½ Jar/175g	166	10.3	95	1.3	9.2	5.9	1.1
Thai, Sweet Chilli, Blue Dragon*	1 Serving/15g	28	0.1	188	0.5	45.5	0.6	0.0
Tikka Masala for One, Express, Uncle Ben's*	1 Sachet/170g	168	10.7	99	1.5	9.0	6.3	0.0
Tikka Masala with Coriander, Weight Watchers*	½ Jar/175g	130	3.7	74	2.6	11.2	2.1	0.7
Tikka Masala, Cooking, HL, Tesco*	¼ Jar/125g	78	3.1	62	0.4	9.0	2.5	0.7
Tikka Masala, COU, M&S*	½ Pack/100g	80	2.6	80	4.5	9.9	2.6	1.7
Tikka Masala, GFY, Asda*	½ Jar/250g	190	8.0	76	2.9	9.0	3.2	0.5
Tikka Masala, Hot & Spicy in Glass Jar, Patak's*	1 Jar/350g	332	23.8	95	1.7	6.5	6.8	1.7

S

	Measure INFO/WEIGHT	per Measure KCAL	FAT	KCAL	PROT	CARB	FAT	FIBRE
SAUCE								
Tikka Masala, Medium, Cooking, Sharwood's*	1/3 Jar/140g	150	9.7	107	1.3	9.7	6.9	0.5
Tikka Masala, Ready Made, Average	*1 Sm Jar/350g*	*422*	*28.8*	*121*	*2.0*	*9.6*	*8.2*	*1.2*
Toffee Fudge, Sainsbury's*	1 Serving/40g	134	1.5	336	1.9	73.9	3.7	0.4
Toffee, Luxury, Rowse*	1 Serving/20g	67	0.7	336	1.9	73.9	3.7	0.4
Toffee, Old English, Dessert, Asda*	1 Serving/28g	99	1.7	355	2.3	73.0	6.0	0.0
Tomato & Basil for Pasta Stir & Serve, Homepride*	1 Jar/480g	278	13.9	58	1.2	6.7	2.9	0.0
Tomato & Basil Sauce, Fresh, Tesco*	1 Pot/500g	245	9.0	49	1.5	6.8	1.8	0.8
Tomato & Basil, for Meatballs, Dolmio*	¼ Jar/125g	48	0.2	38	1.5	6.9	0.2	1.3
Tomato & Basil, Fresh, Asda*	½ Tub/175g	100	3.7	57	1.5	7.9	2.1	0.5
Tomato & Basil, Fresh, Organic, Waitrose*	¼ Pot/175g	77	3.0	44	1.0	6.2	1.7	0.8
Tomato & Basil, Italian, Sainsbury's*	½ Pot/175g	102	4.4	58	1.6	7.0	2.5	0.7
Tomato & Basil, Tesco*	½ Jar/175g	84	5.8	48	0.7	3.8	3.3	0.8
Tomato & Chilli, Waitrose*	1 Pot/350g	182	9.1	52	10.0	6.2	2.6	3.2
Tomato & Creme Fraiche, Less Than 3% Fat, Asda*	1 Pot/300g	168	8.4	56	0.7	7.0	2.8	0.5
Tomato & Garlic for Pasta, Asda*	¼ Jar/125g	80	2.9	64	2.7	8.0	2.3	1.1
Tomato & Garlic, for Meatballs, Dolmio*	1 Portion/125g	46	0.1	37	1.6	6.5	0.1	0.0
Tomato & Marscapone, Finest, Tesco*	1 Serving/350g	270	17.5	77	2.7	5.4	5.0	0.8
Tomato & Marscapone, Italiano, Tesco*	1 Serving/175g	194	15.2	111	2.8	5.4	8.7	0.6
Tomato & Mascarpone, Asda*	½ Tub/175g	152	10.2	87	1.8	7.0	5.8	0.5
Tomato & Mascarpone, Fresh, Tesco*	½ Pot/175g	206	15.2	118	2.8	7.1	8.7	0.6
Tomato & Roasted Garlic, Stir in, Dolmio*	½ Pack/75g	94	7.6	125	1.2	7.7	10.2	0.0
Tomato, Heinz*	1 Tbsp/17g	18	0.0	103	0.9	24.1	0.1	0.7
Tomato, Pizza Topping, Napolina*	1 Serving/70g	34	1.5	49	0.9	6.3	2.2	0.6
Vindaloo, Hot, Patak's*	1 Jar/540g	643	46.4	119	1.7	8.5	8.6	2.1
Watercress & Creme Fraiche, COU, M&S*	½ Pack/154g	100	2.8	65	3.2	9.2	1.8	0.5
Watercress, & Stilton, Creamy for Fish, Schwartz*	1 Pack/300g	141	12.3	47	0.6	2.0	4.1	0.7
Watercress, Fresh, The Saucy Fish Co.*	1 Pack/150g	170	14.5	113	2.2	5.8	9.7	0.0
White Wine & Cream, Cook in, Classic, Homepride*	¼ Can/125g	101	5.1	81	1.0	8.0	4.1	0.4
White Wine & Mushroom, BGTY, Sainsbury's*	¼ Jar/125g	81	2.5	65	2.8	9.0	2.0	0.3
White Wine & Parsley, Pour Over, Loyd Grossman*	½ Sachet/85g	94	7.9	111	1.0	5.6	9.3	0.5
White Wine & Tarragon, French for Fish, Schwartz*	1 Pack/300g	372	33.3	124	1.1	5.0	11.1	0.8
White Wine, Chardonnay, M&S*	1 Serving/160ml	184	16.0	115	1.4	4.6	10.0	0.9
White, Savoury, Made with Semi-Skimmed Milk	1oz/28g	36	2.2	128	4.2	11.1	7.8	0.2
White, Savoury, Made with Whole Milk	1oz/28g	42	2.9	150	4.1	10.9	10.3	0.2
Wild Mushroom, Finest, Tesco*	½ Pack/175g	158	11.9	90	1.9	5.2	6.8	0.4
Worcester, Morrisons*	1 Serving/5ml	6	0.0	120	0.0	28.0	0.0	0.0
Worcestershire, Average	*1 Tsp/5g*	*3*	*0.0*	*65*	*1.4*	*15.5*	*0.1*	*0.0*
Worcestershire, Lea & Perrins*	1 Tsp/5ml	5	0.0	96	0.8	21.0	0.9	0.0
Yellow Bean & Cashew, Tesco*	½ Jar/210g	170	6.1	81	1.6	11.9	2.9	0.3
Yellow Bean, Stir Fry, Sainsbury's*	½ Jar/100g	126	1.3	126	1.8	26.7	1.3	0.8
SAUCE MIX								
Beef Bourguignon, Colman's*	1 Pack/40g	136	0.8	340	7.0	72.0	2.0	3.0
Beef Stroganoff, Colman's*	1 Pack/40g	140	3.6	350	11.6	56.1	8.9	2.7
Bombay Potatoes, Schwartz*	1 Pack/33g	84	4.0	254	16.1	20.1	12.1	31.1
Bread, Colman's*	1 Pack/40g	131	0.4	327	11.4	67.9	1.1	3.2
Bread, Luxury as Sold, Schwartz*	1 Pack/40g	148	1.5	369	11.5	70.3	3.8	3.7
Bread, Made Up, Colman's*	1 Serving/75ml	70	1.5	95	5.0	14.0	2.0	0.6
Cajun Chicken, Schwartz*	1 Pack/38g	108	0.5	285	6.4	61.9	1.3	0.5
Cheddar Cheese, Colman's*	1 Pack/40g	164	6.0	410	19.0	51.0	15.0	2.0
Cheddar Cheese, Dry Mix, Schwartz*	1 Pack/40g	144	3.0	361	18.4	55.1	7.4	2.3
Cheese Flavour, Dairy Free, Free & Easy*	4 Teasp/15g	4	0.1	26	0.6	4.9	0.4	0.3
Cheese, Made Up with Skimmed Milk	1 Serving/60g	47	1.4	78	5.4	9.5	2.3	0.0
Chicken Chasseur, Colman's*	1 Pack/45g	128	0.7	284	8.0	59.2	1.6	3.8

	Measure INFO/WEIGHT	per Measure KCAL	per Measure FAT	Nutrition Values per 100g / 100ml KCAL	PROT	CARB	FAT	FIBRE
SAUCE MIX								
Chicken Chasseur, Schwartz*	1 Pack/40g	126	1.8	316	9.6	59.1	4.6	6.8
Chicken Supreme, Colman's*	1 Pack/40g	143	3.7	358	12.1	56.7	9.2	2.4
Chilli Con Carne, Asda*	1 Sachet/50g	157	0.8	314	7.0	68.0	1.6	2.5
Chilli Con Carne, Hot, Colman's*	1 Pack/37g	122	1.1	330	12.0	60.0	3.0	9.0
Chilli Con Carne, Recipe Mix, Bramwells, Aldi*	1 Pack/38g	130	1.1	341	6.2	70.0	2.8	5.3
Chilli Con Carne, Recipe Mix, Schwartz*	1 Pack/41g	133	1.5	324	8.2	60.8	3.6	0.0
Chip Shop Curry, Dry Weight, Bisto*	1 Dtsp/9g	38	1.6	427	3.4	63.5	17.7	1.3
Coq Au Vin, Colman's*	1 Pack/50g	150	0.9	301	5.6	65.6	1.8	3.3
Cream, for Meatballs, Ikea*	1 Pack/40g	179	9.4	448	9.6	49.2	23.6	0.0
for Garlic Mushrooms, Creamy, Schwartz*	1 Pack/35g	109	1.6	311	7.6	59.7	4.7	4.2
Four Cheese, Colman's*	1 Pack/35g	127	3.9	362	17.1	48.4	11.1	1.8
Hollandaise, Colman's*	1 Pack/28g	104	3.1	372	6.4	61.6	11.1	1.8
Hollandaise, Schwartz*	1 Pack/25g	98	3.2	394	10.6	59.2	12.8	3.7
Lamb Hotpot, Colman's*	1 Pack/40g	119	0.7	297	6.9	63.3	1.7	2.1
Lemon Butter for Fish, Schwartz*	1 Pack/38g	136	3.0	357	6.1	65.3	8.0	5.8
Mixed Herbs for Chicken, So Juicy, Maggi*	1 Pack/34g	97	1.0	285	8.3	53.8	2.8	5.5
Paprika For Chicken, So Juicy, Maggi*	1 Pack/34g	91	1.4	267	8.8	45.5	4.0	7.1
Parsley & Chive for Fish, Schwartz*	1 Pack/38g	132	3.2	348	9.0	58.9	8.5	7.7
Parsley, Creamy, Made Up, Schwartz*	1 Serving/79g	59	2.0	75	4.2	8.7	2.5	0.3
Parsley, Dry, Colman's*	1 Pack/20g	63	0.3	313	7.2	67.9	1.4	3.8
Pepper, Creamy, Colman's*	1 Pack/25g	88	2.8	352	13.0	50.0	11.0	0.0
Pepper, Creamy, Schwartz*	1 Pack/25g	86	1.7	342	17.9	52.0	6.9	7.0
Peppercorn, Mild, Creamy, Schwartz*	1 Pack/25g	88	2.2	352	13.8	55.0	8.6	5.0
Savoury Mince, Schwartz*	1 Pack/35g	108	0.7	310	14.6	58.3	2.0	1.8
Shepherds Pie, Bramwells*	1 Pack/50g	168	3.0	336	8.6	62.0	6.0	6.9
Shepherd's Pie, Schwartz*	1 Pack/38g	118	0.9	311	8.2	60.3	2.3	11.1
Spaghetti Bolognese, Colman's*	1 Pack/40g	120	0.4	300	8.9	64.1	0.9	5.2
Spaghetti Bolognese, Schwartz*	1 Pack/40g	114	0.6	285	9.2	59.0	1.6	7.0
Stroganoff, Beef, Schwartz*	1 Pack/35g	125	3.6	358	15.6	50.8	10.3	4.4
Sweet & Sour for Chicken, So Juicy, Maggi*	½ Pack/15g	42	0.3	279	7.1	55.8	2.3	3.5
Thickening Granules, McDougalls*	1 Tbsp/10g	46	1.9	463	0.0	73.7	18.7	0.0
Tuna Napolitana, Schwartz*	1 Pack/30g	107	3.9	357	10.3	49.6	13.1	0.5
White Wine with Herbs, Creamy, Schwartz*	1 Pack/26g	86	1.7	330	8.0	60.0	6.5	9.1
White, Dry Weight, Bisto*	1 Dtsp/9g	45	2.5	496	3.2	57.4	28.2	0.4
White, Instant, Made Up, Sainsbury's*	1 Serving/90ml	65	2.5	72	0.8	10.9	2.8	0.1
White, Made Up with Semi-Skimmed Milk	1oz/28g	20	0.7	73	4.0	9.6	2.4	0.0
White, Made Up with Skimmed Milk	1oz/28g	17	0.3	59	4.0	9.6	0.9	0.0
White, Savoury, Colman's*	1 Pack/25g	105	3.8	420	9.0	63.0	15.0	2.0
White, Savoury, Schwartz*	1 Pack/25g	108	5.7	434	11.5	45.6	22.9	5.9
SAUERKRAUT								
Average	*1oz/28g*	*3*	*0.0*	*11*	*1.1*	*1.6*	*0.0*	*0.9*
SAUSAGE								
Beef with Onion & Red Wine, Finest, Tesco*	1 Sausage/63g	117	6.9	185	13.2	8.5	10.9	1.2
Beef, Average	*1 Sausage/60g*	*151*	*11.1*	*252*	*14.5*	*7.0*	*18.5*	*0.6*
Bockwurst, Average	*1 Sausage/45g*	*114*	*10.4*	*253*	*10.8*	*0.8*	*23.0*	*0.0*
Bratwurst, Frozen, Lidl*	1 Sausage/80g	235	21.4	294	12.8	0.5	26.8	0.0
Bratwurst, Linessa, Lidl*	1 Sausage/65g	170	14.3	262	16.0	0.0	22.0	0.1
Cheese & Leek, Tesco*	1 Sausage/55g	135	7.9	245	6.6	21.3	14.4	3.9
Chicken & Tarragon, Butchers Choice, Sainsbury's*	1 Sausage/47g	106	6.8	225	18.1	5.8	14.4	0.2
Chicken, Manor Farm*	1 Sausage/65g	126	8.1	194	13.7	6.6	12.5	1.2
Chipolata, Average	*1 Sausage/28g*	*81*	*6.5*	*291*	*12.1*	*8.7*	*23.1*	*0.7*
Chipolata, Lamb & Rosemary, Tesco*	1 Sausage/32g	69	4.9	218	11.3	8.3	15.5	0.0
Chipolata, Pork & Honey, Finest, Tesco*	2 Sausages/64g	170	12.3	265	14.0	8.7	19.2	0.7

SAUSAGE

INFO/WEIGHT	Measure	per Measure		Nutrition Values per 100g / 100ml				
		KCAL	FAT	KCAL	PROT	CARB	FAT	FIBRE
Chipolata, Pork, Extra Lean, BGTY, Sainsbury's*	1 Sausage/24g	46	2.1	189	16.9	10.9	8.6	0.5
Chipolata, Pork, Free Range, Duchy Originals, Waitrose*	2 Chipolatas/46g	104	6.4	227	21.7	3.5	14.0	0.1
Chipolata, Pork, Rosemary & Honey, Duchy, Waitrose*	2 Chipolatas/49g	133	8.7	271	20.8	6.0	17.7	2.1
Chipolata, Premium, Average	*1 Serving/80g*	*187*	*13.8*	*234*	*14.8*	*4.7*	*17.3*	*1.2*
Chipolata, TTD, Sainsbury's*	1 Sausage/27g	79	6.0	294	20.3	3.0	22.3	0.6
Chorizo, Average	*1 Serving/80g*	*250*	*19.4*	*313*	*21.1*	*2.6*	*24.2*	*0.2*
Chorizo, Iberico, Bellota, TTD, Sainsbury's*	1 Slice/3g	17	1.5	498	27.0	1.0	42.9	0.0
Chorizo, Lean, Average	*1 Sausage/67g*	*131*	*9.2*	*195*	*15.7*	*2.3*	*13.7*	*0.8*
Chorizo, Spanish, Ring, Ocado*	1 Ring/225g	1199	111.4	533	19.3	1.6	49.5	1.9
Cocktail, Average	*1 Sausage/7g*	*23*	*1.9*	*323*	*12.1*	*8.6*	*26.7*	*0.9*
Cocktail, Wrapped in Bacon, Pork, Finest, Tesco*	1 Sausage/18g	60	4.6	343	23.4	3.4	26.3	0.6
Cocktail, Wrapped in Bacon, Pork, Raw, Finest, Tesco*	1 Sausage/21g	61	5.3	292	15.8	0.6	25.1	0.5
Cumberland, Average	*1 Sausage/57g*	*167*	*13.0*	*293*	*13.8*	*8.6*	*22.8*	*0.8*
Cumberland, Healthy Range, Average	*1 Sausage/53g*	*75*	*2.1*	*142*	*17.4*	*9.0*	*4.0*	*0.9*
Cumberland, Weight Watchers*	1 Sausage/39g	55	1.3	140	18.6	8.3	3.4	1.1
Debrecziner, Spicy Smoked, Gebirgsjager*	1 Sausage/37g	118	10.4	320	16.0	1.0	28.0	0.0
Extrawurst, German, Waitrose*	1 Slice/28g	80	7.1	281	13.0	1.0	25.0	0.0
Free From Wheat & Gulten, Sainsbury's*	1 Serving/23g	61	4.8	268	15.2	4.5	21.0	1.8
French Saucisson, Tesco*	1 Slice/5g	19	1.4	379	26.7	4.1	28.4	0.0
Garlic, Average	*1 Slice/11g*	*25*	*2.0*	*227*	*15.7*	*0.8*	*18.2*	*0.0*
Garlic, British, M&S*	1 Pack/113g	220	17.0	195	15.0	0.0	15.0	0.0
Garlic, German, Sliced, Waitrose*	2 Slices/10g	22	1.7	215	15.5	0.0	16.9	0.2
Garlic, Sliced, Mattessons*	1 Slice/13g	22	1.4	172	16.0	2.1	11.0	0.0
Garlic, Tesco*	1 Slice/13g	23	1.5	175	15.2	3.0	11.4	0.0
German, Bierwurst, Selection, Sainsbury's*	1 Slice/4g	8	0.6	224	15.0	1.0	17.8	0.1
German, Extrawurst, Selection, Sainsbury's*	1 Slice/3g	9	0.8	279	13.1	0.5	25.0	0.1
German, Schinkenwurst, Selection, Sainsbury's*	1 Slice/3g	8	0.7	251	13.1	0.3	21.9	0.1
Irish Recipe, Asda*	1 Sausage/57g	120	6.8	212	12.1	14.0	12.0	2.7
Irish, Average	*1 Sausage/40g*	*119*	*8.3*	*298*	*10.7*	*17.2*	*20.7*	*0.7*
Lamb, Spiced & Mint, Morrisons*	1 Sausage/34g	79	4.5	233	22.9	5.1	13.2	1.1
Lincolnshire, Average	*1 Sausage/42g*	*122*	*9.1*	*291*	*14.6*	*9.2*	*21.8*	*0.6*
Lincolnshire, Healthy Range, Average	*1 Sausage/50g*	*89*	*4.3*	*177*	*15.8*	*9.0*	*8.6*	*0.8*
Lincolnshire, Thick, Grilled, Signature, Morrisons*	1 Sausage/55g	124	7.3	225	22.2	3.0	13.2	2.5
Lorne, Average	*1 Sausage/25g*	*78*	*5.8*	*312*	*10.8*	*16.0*	*23.1*	*0.6*
Lorne, Simon Howie*	1 Slice/75g	160	13.0	213	15.0	13.1	17.3	0.0
Mediterranean Style Paprika, Waitrose*	1 Sausage/67g	190	16.1	283	12.1	4.6	24.0	1.9
Merguez	1 Merguez/55g	165	14.3	300	16.0	0.6	26.0	0.0
Mortadella, Sainsbury's*	1 Slice/13g	34	2.8	261	17.3	0.1	21.2	0.1
Perfect Bake, Cooked, Richmond*	1 Sausage/46g	108	6.5	234	12.0	17.0	14.0	0.0
Pigs in Blankets, Cooked, Morrisons*	1 Roll/22g	52	2.9	235	22.9	5.2	13.3	1.5
Polish Kabanos, Sainsbury's*	1 Sausage/25g	92	7.6	366	23.0	0.1	30.4	0.1
Pork & Apple, Average	*1 Sausage/57g*	*146*	*10.7*	*256*	*14.5*	*7.5*	*18.8*	*1.9*
Pork & Apple, TTD, Sainsbury's*	1 Sausage/44g	132	9.9	297	16.5	7.7	22.2	1.3
Pork & Beef, Average	*1 Sausage/45g*	*133*	*10.2*	*295*	*8.7*	*13.6*	*22.7*	*0.5*
Pork & Bramley Apple, Grilled, Finest, Tesco*	2 Sausages/123g	345	22.8	280	16.4	11.7	18.5	1.5
Pork & Chilli, Grilled, Finest, Tesco*	2 Sausage/108g	275	17.3	255	19.9	7.2	16.0	1.3
Pork & Herb, Average	*1 Sausage/75g*	*231*	*19.5*	*308*	*13.2*	*5.4*	*26.0*	*0.4*
Pork & Herb, Grilled, TTD, Sainsbury's*	1 Sausage/51g	152	12.1	298	19.1	1.7	23.8	0.7
Pork & Herb, Healthy Range, Average	*1 Sausage/59g*	*75*	*1.4*	*126*	*16.0*	*10.8*	*2.4*	*1.1*
Pork & Leek, Average	*1oz/28g*	*73*	*5.6*	*262*	*14.6*	*6.0*	*20.0*	*1.1*
Pork & Leek, Mini Meal, 092, Wiltshire Farm Foods*	1 Serving/210g	276	16.3	131	3.7	11.6	7.8	1.0
Pork & Leek, The Best, Morrisons*	1 Sausage/63g	158	10.9	251	17.9	5.8	17.3	1.0
Pork & Leek, Thick, Signature, Morrisons*	1 Sausage/55g	127	8.6	231	20.5	1.5	15.6	1.4

S

SAUSAGE

Measure INFO/WEIGHT	per Measure KCAL	FAT	Nutrition Values per 100g / 100ml KCAL	PROT	CARB	FAT	FIBRE
Pork & Onion, Gluten Free, Asda* — 1 Sausage/41g	105	7.0	257	20.0	6.0	17.0	1.8
Pork & Red Onion, TTD, Sainsbury's* — 1 Sausage/48g	138	8.8	288	18.5	12.4	18.3	1.4
Pork & Sweet Chilli, Waitrose* — 1 Sausage/67g	151	10.1	226	15.5	6.9	15.1	2.7
Pork & Tomato, Grilled, Average — *1 Sausage/47g*	*127*	*9.7*	*273*	*13.9*	*7.5*	*20.8*	*0.4*
Pork, & Fresh Herb, Uncooked, TTD, Sainsbury's* — 1 Sausage/50g	132	10.0	269	20.0	1.1	20.4	0.5
Pork, 30% Less Fat, Butcher's Choice, Sainsbury's* — 1 Sausage/50g	99	5.4	198	15.9	9.5	10.7	0.5
Pork, Average — *1 Sausage/45g*	*139*	*11.2*	*309*	*11.9*	*9.8*	*25.0*	*0.8*
Pork, Bacon & Cheese, Asda* — ¼ Pack/114g	329	23.9	289	18.0	7.0	21.0	0.4
Pork, Bacon & Maple Syrup, Grilled, ES, Asda* — 2 Sausages/108g	280	24.4	259	11.5	2.0	22.6	1.0
Pork, Battered, Thick, Average — *1oz/28g*	*126*	*10.2*	*448*	*17.3*	*21.7*	*36.3*	*2.0*
Pork, Casserole, Diet Chef Ltd* — 1 Portion/300g	303	18.3	101	6.6	4.9	6.1	1.4
Pork, Chipolata, M&S* — 2 Chipolatas/62g	180	15.3	290	16.3	0.6	24.7	0.5
Pork, Cumberland, Deluxe, Lidl* — 1 Sausage/54g	137	9.5	254	19.4	3.5	17.6	1.1
Pork, Cumberland, TTD, Sainsbury's* — 1 Sausage/46g	132	9.7	288	21.4	3.1	21.1	0.6
Pork, Extra Lean, Average — *1 Sausage/54g*	*84*	*3.7*	*155*	*17.3*	*6.1*	*6.8*	*0.8*
Pork, Fresh, Ultimate, Outdoor Bred, TTD, Sainsbury's* — 1 Sausage/46g	138	10.5	300	22.3	1.3	22.8	0.5
Pork, Frozen, Fried — *1oz/28g*	*88*	*6.9*	*316*	*13.8*	*10.0*	*24.8*	*0.0*
Pork, Garden herb, 97%, Debbie & Andrews* — 1 Sausage/67g	141	5.1	211	21.3	0.5	7.6	1.0
Pork, Garlic & Herb, Average — *1 Sausage/76g*	*203*	*16.5*	*268*	*12.0*	*6.0*	*21.8*	*1.2*
Pork, Gluten Free, Premium, The Black Farmer's Daughter* — 2 Sausage/133g	321	26.2	241	14.8	1.0	19.7	0.6
Pork, Gourmet, Waitrose* — 2 Sausages/133g	285	20.1	214	14.1	5.6	15.1	0.4
Pork, Outdoor Bred, Irish, Rankin Selection* — 1 Sausage/67g	161	12.5	241	14.9	3.9	18.7	1.5
Pork, Premium, Average — *1 Sausage/74g*	*191*	*13.6*	*258*	*14.9*	*8.3*	*18.4*	*1.0*
Pork, Reduced Fat, Asda* — 1 Sausage/54g	76	1.9	140	15.3	11.8	3.5	1.9
Pork, Reduced Fat, Chilled, Grilled — *1 Sausage/45g*	*104*	*6.2*	*230*	*16.2*	*10.8*	*13.8*	*1.5*
Pork, Reduced Fat, Healthy Range, Average — *1 Sausage/57g*	*86*	*3.4*	*151*	*15.6*	*9.0*	*6.0*	*0.9*
Pork, Skinless, Average — *1oz/28g*	*81*	*6.6*	*291*	*11.7*	*8.2*	*23.6*	*0.6*
Pork, Skinless, Sizzling, Classics, Grilled, Wall's* — 1 Sausage/24g	48	5.9	201	11.5	8.9	24.6	1.4
Pork, Smoked, Reduced Fat, Mattessons* — ½ Pack/113g	288	21.5	255	14.0	7.0	19.0	0.9
Pork, Thick, Average — *1 Sausage/39g*	*115*	*8.7*	*296*	*13.3*	*10.0*	*22.4*	*1.0*
Pork, Thick, Reduced Fat, Healthy Range, Average — *1 Sausage/52g*	*90*	*3.8*	*172*	*14.0*	*12.3*	*7.4*	*0.8*
Pork, Thin, Grilled, Richmond* — 1 Sausage/23g	58	3.7	254	12.0	16.0	16.0	2.6
Premium, Chilled, Fried — *1oz/28g*	*77*	*5.8*	*275*	*15.8*	*6.7*	*20.7*	*0.0*
Premium, Chilled, Grilled — *1oz/28g*	*82*	*6.3*	*292*	*16.8*	*6.3*	*22.4*	*0.0*
Premium, Pork, (8 Pack), Weight Watchers* — 1 Sausage/39g	60	1.6	155	20.0	7.8	4.2	1.7
Red Onion & Rosemary, Linda McCartney* — 2 Sausages/100g	128	3.7	128	14.2	9.7	3.7	5.8
Saucisson Montagne, Waitrose* — 1 Slice/5g	21	1.8	421	20.7	1.9	36.7	0.0
Saveloy, The Delicatessen, Tesco* — 1 Saveloy/65g	185	14.9	285	9.5	8.3	23.0	2.3
Sicilian Style, Grilled, TTD, Sainsbury's* — 2 Sausage/89g	257	20.5	290	18.8	1.1	23.1	1.0
Smoked, Average — *1 Sausage/174g*	*588*	*52.2*	*338*	*13.0*	*4.0*	*30.0*	*0.0*
Spicy Pork & Pepper, Summer Selection, Sainsbury's* — 1 Sausage/33g	86	5.7	260	20.1	6.0	17.3	1.6
Spicy, Pork, Polenta & Sun Dried Tomato, Waitrose* — 1 Sausage/67g	165	11.9	247	11.8	9.8	17.8	0.9
Thick, Irish, Fresh, Grilled, Richmond* — 2 Sausages/80g	203	12.7	254	11.7	16.0	15.9	2.6
Thuringian Rostbratwurst, Wolf* — 1 Sausage/100g	265	22.5	265	14.0	1.0	22.5	0.0
Toulouse, M&S* — 1 Sausage/57g	123	8.9	215	12.4	5.8	15.6	1.3
Toulouse, TTD, Sainsbury's* — 1 Sausage/45g	146	11.5	324	21.4	2.3	25.5	0.8
Turkey & Chicken, Average — *1 Sausage/57g*	*126*	*8.2*	*222*	*14.4*	*8.2*	*14.6*	*1.8*
Turkey, Average — *1 Sausage/57g*	*90*	*4.6*	*157*	*15.7*	*6.3*	*8.0*	*0.0*
Tuscan, M&S* — 1 Sausage/66g	145	10.6	220	14.9	4.6	16.0	0.6
Venison & Pork, Waitrose* — 1 Sausage/64g	93	4.0	146	16.5	5.3	6.3	1.1
Venison & Red Wine, TTD, Sainsbury's* — 1 Sausage/39g	88	5.2	228	20.7	5.8	13.6	1.7
Venison, Grilled, Finest, Tesco* — 1 Sausage/41g	86	5.5	215	16.6	6.3	13.7	0.6
Wiejska, Polish, Sainsbury's* — 1/8 Pack/50g	78	4.5	157	18.7	0.4	9.0	0.5

S

	Measure INFO/WEIGHT	per Measure KCAL	FAT	Nutrition Values per 100g / 100ml KCAL	PROT	CARB	FAT	FIBRE
SAUSAGE								
Wild Boar	1 Sausage/85g	220	17.0	259	16.5	1.2	20.0	0.0
SAUSAGE & MASH								
2 British Pork & Rich Onion Gravy, M&S*	1 Pack/400g	340	6.8	85	5.7	12.2	1.7	1.3
Bangers, Morrisons*	1 Pack/300g	306	14.7	102	3.0	12.3	4.9	0.8
British Classic, Tesco*	1 Pack/450g	675	42.8	150	5.1	11.1	9.5	0.9
Chef Select, Lidl*	1 Pack/450g	472	26.6	105	4.7	7.6	5.9	1.4
Iceland*	1 Pack/440g	484	26.0	110	3.8	10.4	5.9	1.6
in Cider Gravy with Apple & Onion, Weight Watchers*	1 Pack/400g	332	11.6	83	5.5	7.5	2.9	2.2
Light Choices, Tesco*	1 Pack/400g	360	8.8	90	4.4	11.8	2.2	1.4
with Red Wine & Onion Gravy, BGTY, Sainsbury's*	1 Pack/380g	315	7.2	83	5.0	11.4	1.9	2.0
Average	*1 Serving/231g*	*285*	*16.1*	*123*	*4.5*	*10.4*	*7.0*	*1.0*
SAUSAGE MEAT								
Pork, Average	*1oz/28g*	*96*	*8.2*	*344*	*9.9*	*10.2*	*29.4*	*0.6*
SAUSAGE ROLL								
Buffet, HE, Tesco*	1 Roll/30g	83	3.8	278	9.6	31.2	12.8	1.5
Cocktail, Average	*1 Roll/15g*	*57*	*3.7*	*378*	*8.9*	*29.4*	*24.9*	*1.9*
Cumberland, CBY, Asda*	1 Roll/66g	201	10.9	304	8.3	28.9	16.5	3.1
Frozen, Greggs Iceland Exclusive*	1 Roll/103g	371	26.3	360	8.0	22.0	25.5	1.5
HE, Tesco*	1 Roll/70g	195	9.0	278	9.6	31.2	12.8	1.5
Jumbo, Sainsbury's*	1 Roll/145g	492	34.4	339	8.2	23.2	23.7	1.5
Large, Freshbake*	1 Roll/52g	153	9.5	294	6.6	25.9	18.3	4.6
Mini, Tesco*	1 Roll/15g	53	3.7	356	9.0	23.9	24.9	1.5
Mini, Waitrose*	1 Roll/35g	124	9.2	353	13.0	16.1	26.3	1.0
Party Size, Tesco*	1 Roll/14g	49	3.5	350	5.9	25.0	24.9	1.1
Pork, Morrisons*	1 Roll/70g	195	9.0	278	9.6	31.2	12.8	1.5
Pork, Snack, 30% Less Fat, CBY, Asda*	1 Serving/33g	85	4.2	258	11.1	22.5	12.8	4.0
Puff Pastry	1 Med/60g	230	16.6	383	9.9	25.4	27.6	1.0
Puff Pastry, Sainsbury's*	1 Roll/65g	250	18.1	384	8.3	25.0	27.9	0.9
Snack Size, Tesco*	1 Roll/32g	118	8.8	369	9.1	21.7	27.4	2.3
Snack, GFY, Asda*	1 Roll/34g	112	7.0	329	9.4	26.5	20.6	0.9
Snack, Sainsbury's*	1 Roll/34g	130	8.5	383	9.7	29.9	25.0	2.1
TTD, Sainsbury's*	1 Roll/115g	440	31.9	383	11.9	21.3	27.8	2.0
SAUSAGE ROLL VEGETARIAN								
Linda McCartney*	1 Roll/52g	145	7.1	278	13.1	26.0	13.7	1.6
Mini, Linda McCartney*	1 Roll/14g	41	2.2	293	11.3	23.7	15.8	5.2
SAUSAGE VEGETARIAN								
Asda*	1 Sausage/43g	81	3.9	189	20.0	7.0	9.0	2.9
Barbecue, Taifun*	1 Sausage/63g	160	10.9	256	21.4	2.3	17.5	0.0
Braai Flavour, Fry's Special Vegetarian*	1 Sausage/63g	86	4.4	138	16.5	10.0	7.0	4.0
Cheese & Sundried Tomato, Tesco*	1 Sausage/50g	82	3.4	165	17.4	7.7	6.8	6.5
Chilli & Coriander, Secret Sausages*	1 Sausage/40g	60	0.6	150	4.6	27.8	1.4	4.0
Cumberland, Cauldron Foods*	1 Sausage/46g	75	4.0	163	14.0	6.5	8.6	2.0
Glamorgan Leek & Cheese, Sainsbury's*	1 Sausage/50g	98	5.2	197	4.3	21.3	10.5	2.7
Glamorgan, Cooked, Asda*	1 Sausage/50g	113	6.2	226	5.3	21.8	12.4	2.8
Glamorgan, Leek & Cheese, Goodlife*	1 Sausage/50g	94	4.9	188	4.9	20.0	9.8	2.3
Italian, Linda McCartney*	1 Sausage/50g	76	2.8	152	16.8	6.9	5.6	3.4
Italian, Tofurky*	1 Sausage/63g	167	8.2	270	29.0	12.0	13.0	8.0
Leek & Cheese, Organic, Cauldron Foods*	1 Sausage/41g	80	4.1	194	14.4	11.3	10.1	1.7
Lincolnshire, Asda*	1 Sausage/56g	96	4.5	172	17.0	8.0	8.0	1.4
Lincolnshire, Chilled, Cauldron Foods*	1 Sausage/46g	76	4.1	165	14.0	6.5	8.8	2.0
Lincolnshire, Frozen, Tesco*	1 Sausage/50g	78	2.5	155	15.5	10.8	5.0	3.0
Linda McCartney*	1 Sausage/50g	101	4.4	202	22.5	8.3	8.8	1.6
Realeat*	1 Sausage/40g	66	3.9	165	17.2	2.0	9.8	8.1

S

	Measure INFO/WEIGHT	per Measure KCAL	per Measure FAT	Nutrition Values per 100g / 100ml KCAL	PROT	CARB	FAT	FIBRE
SAUSAGE VEGETARIAN								
Spinach, Leek & Cheese, Gourmet, Wicken Fen*	1 Sausage/46g	92	4.7	201	10.3	17.0	10.2	1.9
Sun Dried Tomato & Herb, Linda McCartney*	1 Sausage/35g	93	5.4	266	21.8	10.1	15.4	1.7
SCALLOPS								
Breaded, Thai Style with Plum Sauce, Finest, Tesco*	1 Serving/210g	401	14.7	191	11.5	20.6	7.0	0.8
Canadian, Finest, Tesco*	½ Pack/100g	80	0.2	80	16.4	2.6	0.2	0.1
Lemon Grass & Ginger, Tesco*	½ Pack/112g	90	1.1	80	15.2	2.5	1.0	0.6
Peruvian, with Smokey Chipotle Butter, Waitrose*	½ Pack/82g	129	4.2	158	20.8	6.9	5.1	0.5
Raw, Bay or Sea with Roe, Average	*1 Lge Scallop/15g*	*13*	*0.1*	*88*	*16.8*	*2.4*	*0.8*	*0.0*
Steamed, Average	*1oz/28g*	*33*	*0.4*	*118*	*23.2*	*3.4*	*1.4*	*0.0*
with Roasted Garlic Butter, Finest, Tesco*	1 Serving/100g	201	14.3	201	16.2	1.8	14.3	0.4
SCAMPI								
& Chips, Chunky, Finest, Tesco*	1 Pack/280g	420	15.4	150	5.9	18.3	5.5	1.4
& Chips, with Peas	1 Serving/490g	822	43.6	168	10.1	11.3	8.9	1.2
Bites, Everyday, Value, Tesco*	½ pack/125g	262	10.0	210	9.4	23.4	8.0	1.2
Breaded & Chips, Oakhouse Foods Ltd*	1 Meal/300g	456	16.5	152	4.6	21.5	5.5	2.3
Breaded, Baked, Average	*½ Pack/255g*	*565*	*27.4*	*222*	*10.7*	*20.5*	*10.7*	*1.0*
Breaded, Fried in Oil, Average	*1 Serving/100g*	*237*	*13.6*	*237*	*9.4*	*20.5*	*13.6*	*0.0*
Wholetail with a Hint of Lemon, Youngs*	1 Pack/228g	505	20.5	202	9.6	22.4	8.2	1.2
Wholetail, Breaded, Frozen, CBY, Asda*	1 Serving/93g	197	8.7	212	9.7	21.4	9.4	1.3
Wholetail, in Crunchy Crumb, Morrisons*	1 Pack/250g	508	21.7	203	9.6	19.9	8.7	1.7
Wholetail, Lemon & Herb Tempura Battered, Youngs*	½ Pack/101g	215	10.0	213	10.4	18.9	9.9	3.3
Wholetail, Oven Baked, Gastro, Youngs*	½ Pack/99g	226	10.0	228	9.6	23.9	10.1	1.5
Wholetail, Premium, Youngs*	1 Serving/125g	256	11.4	205	29.5	21.6	9.1	2.1
SCHNAPPS								
Vodkat, Intercontinental Brands Ltd*	1 Serving/25ml	31	0.0	124	0.0	0.8	0.0	0.0
SCONE								
3% Fat, M&S*	1 Scone/65g	179	1.6	275	7.2	55.1	2.5	2.3
All Butter, CBY, Asda*	1 Serving/100g	377	14.5	377	7.2	54.3	14.5	1.7
All Butter, Sultana, Duchy Originals*	1 Scone/78g	276	9.8	353	7.3	52.9	12.5	2.6
All Butter, Tesco*	1 Scone/60g	225	8.2	375	8.2	53.5	13.7	0.9
Cheese & Black Pepper, Mini, M&S*	1 Scone/18g	67	3.3	370	10.2	41.1	18.3	1.7
Cheese, Average	*1 Scone/40g*	*145*	*7.1*	*363*	*10.1*	*43.2*	*17.8*	*1.6*
Cheese, Cornish, TTD, Sainsbury's*	1 Scone/74g	267	13.8	361	12.3	36.1	18.6	2.3
Cheese, ES, CBY, Asda*	1 Serving/100g	315	8.7	315	0.0	18.9	8.7	0.0
Cheese, Sainsbury's*	1 Scone/70g	250	13.0	357	10.6	36.9	18.6	2.0
Cherry, Double Butter, Genesis Crafty*	1 Scone/63g	198	4.8	314	6.8	54.5	7.6	1.4
Cherry, Genesis Crafty*	1 Scone/81g	226	5.8	279	4.9	50.5	7.1	0.0
Cherry, M&S*	1 Scone/60g	202	7.3	337	6.9	49.7	12.2	1.9
Clotted Cream, Cornish, TTD, Sainsbury's*	1 Scone/70g	269	12.7	384	8.4	46.6	18.2	2.1
Devon, Asda*	1 Scone/59g	208	6.3	353	7.3	55.5	10.6	3.0
Devon, M&S*	1 Scone/59g	225	9.6	380	7.1	50.8	16.2	1.5
Devon, Sainsbury's*	1 Scone/54g	201	8.4	372	7.1	51.1	15.5	1.6
Devon, Waitrose*	1 Scone/72g	268	9.5	373	7.5	56.0	13.2	2.3
Fresh Cream with Strawberry Jam, Tesco*	1 Scone/83g	290	15.6	352	4.7	40.7	18.9	1.1
Fresh Cream, Finest, Tesco*	1 Serving/133g	469	23.2	354	4.6	44.5	17.5	1.7
Fresh Cream, Tesco*	1 Scone/80g	242	9.9	304	15.8	32.3	12.5	0.9
Fruit, Average	*1 Scone/40g*	*126*	*3.9*	*316*	*7.3*	*52.9*	*9.8*	*0.0*
Fruit, Breakfast Griddle, Genesis Crafty*	1 Scone/65g	192	5.5	296	6.2	50.7	8.5	1.9
Fruit, Genesis Crafty*	1 Scone/78g	231	6.6	296	6.2	50.7	8.5	0.0
Fruit, Smart Price, Asda*	1 Scone/41g	139	4.1	338	7.0	55.0	10.0	3.0
Fruit, Waitrose*	1 Scone/59g	190	4.8	325	6.3	56.5	8.2	2.2
Mix, Fruit, Asda*	1 Scone/48g	143	2.4	301	7.0	57.0	5.0	3.7
Plain, Average	*1 Scone/40g*	*145*	*5.8*	*362*	*7.2*	*53.8*	*14.6*	*1.9*

S

	Measure INFO/WEIGHT	per Measure KCAL	FAT	Nutrition Values per 100g / 100ml KCAL	PROT	CARB	FAT	FIBRE
SCONE								
Plain, CBY, Asda*	1 Serving/100g	364	14.8	364	0.0	5.9	14.8	0.0
Plain, Genesis Crafty*	1 Scone/74g	227	7.4	307	6.8	49.1	10.0	0.0
Potato, Average	*1 Scone/40g*	*118*	*5.7*	*296*	*5.1*	*39.1*	*14.3*	*1.6*
Potato, Mother's Pride*	1 Scone/37g	77	0.8	207	4.7	42.0	2.2	4.3
Red Berry, Mixed, Finest, Tesco*	1 Scone/110g	344	9.5	313	7.8	50.1	8.6	1.9
Strawberry Jam with Cream, CBY, Asda*	1 Serving/100g	332	16.7	332	5.2	40.1	16.7	2.8
Strawberry, Fresh Cream, Sainsbury's*	1 Scone/60g	218	11.2	363	6.5	42.5	18.6	1.4
Sultana, Finest, Tesco*	1 Scone/70g	238	7.6	340	8.9	50.9	10.9	2.1
Sultana, GFY, Asda*	1 Scone/59g	192	2.6	324	7.0	64.0	4.4	2.0
Sultana, M&S*	1 Scone/66g	231	8.2	350	6.5	53.0	12.5	2.0
Sultana, Reduced Fat, Waitrose*	1 Scone/65g	187	3.4	287	6.6	53.2	5.3	2.6
Sultana, Sainsbury's*	1 Scone/54g	176	5.9	327	6.9	50.2	11.0	6.5
Sultana, Tesco*	1 Scone/60g	189	5.0	315	7.1	52.5	8.4	2.6
Sultana, TTD, Sainsbury's*	1 Scone/70g	239	8.1	341	6.5	52.9	11.5	2.6
Sultana, Value, Tesco*	1 Scone/40g	134	4.0	335	6.5	53.8	10.1	2.7
Tattie, Scottish, Nick Nairn's*	1 Scone/21g	42	0.3	199	4.0	34.7	1.6	0.7
Wholemeal	1 Scone/40g	130	5.8	326	8.7	43.1	14.4	5.2
Wholemeal, Fruit	1 Scone/40g	130	5.1	324	8.1	47.2	12.8	4.9
SEA BASS								
Butterflied, M&S*	½ Pack/159g	258	14.5	162	19.2	0.7	9.1	0.6
Cooked, Dry Heat, Average	*1 Fillet/100g*	*124*	*2.6*	*124*	*23.6*	*0.0*	*2.6*	*0.0*
Fillets, Pan Fried, CBY, Asda*	½ Pack/90g	173	11.2	192	18.1	1.3	12.5	1.0
Fillets, Skinless, Boneless, TTD, Sainsbury's*	1 Serving/100g	162	9.2	162	19.4	0.5	9.2	0.5
Raw, Fillet, Average	*1 Fillet/95g*	*108*	*3.4*	*113*	*20.3*	*0.0*	*3.5*	*0.1*
SEA BREAM								
Fillet, Cooked, Dry Heat, Average	*1 Serving/100g*	*124*	*3.0*	*124*	*24.0*	*0.0*	*3.0*	*0.0*
Fillets, Pea & Mint,,M&S*	1 Fillet/140g	291	21.7	208	14.3	2.6	15.5	0.5
Fillets, Raw, Average	*1oz/28g*	*27*	*0.8*	*96*	*17.5*	*0.0*	*2.9*	*0.0*
SEAFOOD								
Cocktail, Average	*1oz/28g*	*24*	*0.4*	*87*	*15.6*	*2.9*	*1.5*	*0.0*
Cocktail, Frozen, CBY, Asda*	1 Bag/300g	213	1.5	71	15.3	1.0	0.5	0.6
Selection, Asda*	1 Pack/240g	173	1.9	72	13.4	2.9	0.8	0.0
Selection, Fresh, Tesco*	1 Pack/234g	187	2.3	80	17.7	0.1	1.0	0.0
Selection, M&S*	1 Serving/200g	170	2.0	85	17.4	1.6	1.0	0.5
Selection, Sainsbury's*	½ Pack/125g	85	1.2	68	14.6	0.8	1.0	2.5
SEAFOOD STICKS								
Average	*1 Stick/15g*	*16*	*0.0*	*106*	*8.0*	*18.4*	*0.2*	*0.2*
Chilled or Frozen, Youngs*	1 Stick/14g	15	0.2	108	9.0	15.4	1.2	0.6
SEASONING MIX								
Aromat, Knorr*	1oz/28g	45	1.0	161	11.7	15.1	3.7	0.9
Blackened Cajun Spice for Chefs, Schwartz*	1 Serving/100g	234	6.4	234	0.1	34.4	6.4	0.0
Cajun, Perfect Shake, As Sold, Schwartz*	1 Tbsp/1g	2	0.1	249	9.9	27.2	7.0	19.0
Chicken Fajitas, Schwartz*	1 Pack/35g	99	0.9	283	10.9	54.1	2.5	10.8
Chicken Provencal, Schwartz*	1 Pack/35g	104	0.7	296	9.3	55.3	2.0	9.9
Chilli, Old El Paso*	1 Pack/39g	117	2.0	301	7.0	57.0	5.0	0.0
Garlic, For Chicken, So Juicy, Maggi*	1 Pack/30g	95	0.8	316	9.4	58.9	2.8	8.7
Garlic, Papyrus Sheets, SoTender, Maggi*	1 Sheet/6g	25	1.9	438	6.3	24.4	32.5	11.4
Italian Herb, Schwartz*	1 Tsp/1g	3	0.0	338	11.0	64.5	4.0	0.0
Italian Herbs, Papyrus Sheets, SoTender, Maggi*	1 Sheet/6g	26	2.0	440	7.3	22.1	34.1	7.7
Jamaican Jerk Chicken, Recipe, Schwartz*	1 Pack/27g	75	0.8	276	9.8	69.8	3.0	17.2
Lamb, Simply Shake, Schwartz*	1oz/28g	54	0.9	193	12.1	53.1	3.1	23.9
Lemon & Herb, for Chicken, Cook in Bag, Average	*1 Bag/34g*	*121*	*1.9*	*356*	*10.8*	*63.7*	*5.5*	*4.1*
Mediterranean Chicken, Season & Shake, Colman's*	1 Pack/33g	99	0.7	300	10.3	56.8	2.1	5.9

S

	Measure INFO/WEIGHT	per Measure KCAL	FAT	Nutrition Values per 100g / 100ml KCAL	PROT	CARB	FAT	FIBRE
SEASONING MIX								
Mediterranean Roasted Vegetable, Schwartz*	1 Pack/30g	86	1.2	288	6.9	56.1	4.0	10.3
Mediterranean, for Chicken, Cook in Bag, Average	*1 Bag/33g*	*99*	*0.7*	*302*	*10.6*	*56.6*	*2.0*	*7.0*
One Pan Rice Meal, for Chicken, Old El Paso*	¼ Pack/89g	203	4.3	228	4.4	40.9	4.8	1.7
Paprika, for Chicken, Cook in Bag, Average	*1 Bag/34g*	*96*	*1.3*	*283*	*12.3*	*45.8*	*4.0*	*8.1*
Paprika, Papyrus Sheets, SoTender, Maggi*	1 Sheet/6g	25	2.0	431	9.1	12.2	35.2	14.5
Piri Piri, Perfect Shake, Special Blend, Schwartz*	100g	328	2.0	328	11.4	66.2	2.0	0.0
Potato Roasties, Rosemary & Garlic, Crispy, Schwartz*	1 Pack/33g	88	2.6	267	13.0	36.1	7.8	21.1
Potato Roasties, Southern Fried, Crispy, Schwartz*	1 Pack/35g	78	1.5	222	9.2	36.2	4.4	25.1
Potato Wedges, Garlic & Herb, Schwartz*	1 Pack/38g	106	1.9	278	11.4	47.1	4.9	11.7
Red Wine & Shallots, for Beef, as Sold, So Juicy, Maggi*	1 Bag/35g	106	0.6	304	10.8	60.6	1.8	1.1
Season-All, Schwartz*	1 Tsp/6g	4	0.1	72	2.3	11.6	1.8	0.0
Shepherd's Pie, Colman's*	1 Pack/50g	170	1.0	340	13.0	60.0	2.0	5.0
Shotz, Smoky BBQ Pork, Seasoning, Schwartz*	1oz/28g	64	0.3	228	1.0	53.8	1.0	0.0
Singapore Curry Chicken Noodles, So Stir Fry, Maggi*	1 Pack/185g	796	37.6	430	8.2	51.9	20.3	3.3
Spicy Cajun, Bags Better Chicken*	1 Pack/30g	94	3.2	313	7.7	58.0	10.7	11.7
Sticky Spare Ribs, Season & Shake, Colman's*	1 Pack/52g	179	1.5	344	5.1	72.7	2.8	4.0
Taco, Old El Paso*	¼ Pack/9g	30	0.4	334	5.5	69.0	4.0	0.0
Thai Seven Spice, Schwartz*	1 Serving/10g	24	0.4	243	7.5	44.1	4.1	0.0
SEAWEED								
Crispy, Average	*1oz/28g*	*182*	*17.3*	*651*	*7.5*	*15.6*	*61.9*	*7.0*
Nori, Dried, Raw	*1oz/28g*	*38*	*0.4*	*136*	*30.7*	*0.0*	*1.5*	*44.4*
Wakame, Dried, Raw	*1oz/28g*	*20*	*0.7*	*71*	*12.4*	*0.0*	*2.4*	*47.1*
SEED & NUT MIX								
Sunflower & Pumpkin Seeds, M&S*	1 Pack/200g	1150	98.8	575	26.9	6.1	49.4	10.7
SEED MIX								
Fennel Seed & Honey Peanuts, Graze*	1 Punnet/35g	184	12.2	526	16.6	44.9	34.8	5.6
Granola, Graze*	1 Pack/25g	122	7.4	490	12.0	43.7	29.7	0.0
Omega, Graze*	1 Pack/25g	153	12.4	613	28.4	13.1	49.7	0.0
Omega, Morrisons*	¼ Pack/25g	138	11.4	554	20.9	15.0	45.6	6.4
Omega, Munchy Seeds*	1 Bag/30g	184	14.9	613	28.4	13.1	49.7	2.2
Original, The Food Doctor*	1 Serving/30g	157	13.3	522	28.2	3.7	44.4	17.7
Roasted, Graze*	1 Pack/25g	160	12.9	640	27.1	4.8	51.5	0.0
Salad Sprinkle, Nature's Harvest*	1 Serving/8g	48	4.1	598	20.0	14.6	51.1	4.9
Savoury Roasted Seeds, Graze*	1 Pack/34g	203	16.2	595	21.4	17.8	47.5	5.5
Snacking, CBY, Asda*	1 Serving/25g	145	10.9	581	33.1	10.9	43.5	6.7
Toasted, Asda*	1 Serving/28g	132	9.0	470	34.4	10.6	32.2	11.6
Wholesome, LL, Waitrose*	1 Serving/30g	166	13.6	554	21.3	15.5	45.2	8.0
SEEDS								
Chia, Black, The Chia Company*	1 Tbsp/15g	69	4.6	458	20.4	37.0	30.4	36.0
Chia, White, The Chia Company*	1 Tbsp/15g	69	5.1	458	20.4	37.0	34.0	36.0
Fenugreek, Average	*1 Tsp/4g*	*12*	*0.2*	*323*	*23.0*	*58.4*	*6.4*	*24.6*
Fiery, Graze*	1 Pack/34g	173	14.8	510	21.8	17.3	43.5	7.9
Flaxseed, Sunflower & Pumpkin, Milled, Linwoods*	1 Scoop/10g	54	4.9	542	22.7	2.4	49.1	16.2
Hemp, Shelled, Linwoods*	2 Tbsps/30g	178	14.8	593	35.1	7.6	49.5	5.9
Mustard, Average	*1 Tsp/3g*	*15*	*0.9*	*469*	*34.9*	*34.9*	*28.8*	*14.7*
Nigella, Average	*1 Tsp/5g*	*20*	*1.7*	*392*	*21.3*	*1.9*	*33.3*	*8.4*
Poppy, Average	*1 Tbsp/9g*	*47*	*3.9*	*533*	*18.0*	*23.7*	*44.7*	*10.0*
Pumpkin, Average	*1 Tbsp/10g*	*57*	*4.6*	*568*	*27.9*	*13.0*	*45.9*	*3.8*
Pumpkin, LL, Waitrose*	1 Serve/30g	171	13.7	569	24.4	15.2	45.6	5.3
Pumpkin, Sainsbury's*	1 Pack/90g	490	37.6	545	36.7	5.5	41.8	5.7
Pumpkin, Whole, Roasted, Salted, Average	*1 Serving/50g*	*261*	*21.1*	*522*	*33.0*	*13.4*	*42.1*	*3.9*
Sesame, Average	*1oz/28g*	*171*	*15.8*	*610*	*22.3*	*3.6*	*56.4*	*7.8*
Sesame, LL, Waitrose*	1 Serving/100g	598	58.0	598	18.2	0.9	58.0	11.8

S

	Measure INFO/WEIGHT	per Measure KCAL	FAT	Nutrition Values per 100g / 100ml KCAL	PROT	CARB	FAT	FIBRE

SEEDS

	Measure INFO/WEIGHT	KCAL	FAT	KCAL	PROT	CARB	FAT	FIBRE
Sesame, Tesco*	1 Tsp/4g	24	2.3	598	18.2	0.9	58.0	7.9
Sunflower, Average	*1 Tbsp/10g*	*59*	*4.9*	*585*	*23.4*	*15.0*	*48.7*	*5.7*

SEMOLINA

Average	*1oz/28g*	*98*	*0.5*	*348*	*11.0*	*75.2*	*1.8*	*2.1*
Pudding, Creamed, Ambrosia*	1 Can/425g	344	7.2	81	3.3	13.1	1.7	0.2
Pudding, Creamed, Co-Op*	1 Can/425g	382	8.5	90	4.0	15.0	2.0	0.0

SHALLOTS

Pickled in Hot & Spicy Vinegar, Tesco*	1 Onion/18g	14	0.0	77	1.0	18.0	0.1	1.9
Raw, Average	*1 Serving/80g*	*16*	*0.2*	*20*	*1.5*	*3.3*	*0.2*	*1.4*

SHANDY

Bavaria*	1 Can/300ml	109	0.0	36	0.0	0.0	0.0	0.0
Bitter, Original, Ben Shaws*	1 Can/330ml	89	0.0	27	0.0	6.0	0.0	0.0
Canned, Morrisons*	1 Can/330ml	36	0.0	11	0.0	1.8	0.0	0.0
Homemade, Average	*1 Pint/568ml*	*148*	*0.0*	*26*	*0.2*	*2.9*	*0.0*	*0.0*
Lemonade, Schweppes*	1 Can/330ml	76	0.0	23	0.0	5.1	0.0	0.0

SHARK

Raw	*1oz/28g*	*29*	*0.3*	*102*	*23.0*	*0.0*	*1.1*	*0.0*

SHARON FRUIT

Average	*1oz/28g*	*19*	*0.0*	*68*	*0.7*	*17.3*	*0.0*	*1.5*

SHERRY

Dry, Average	*1 Glass/120ml*	*139*	*0.0*	*116*	*0.2*	*1.4*	*0.0*	*0.0*
Medium	*1 Serving/50ml*	*58*	*0.0*	*116*	*0.1*	*5.9*	*0.0*	*0.0*
Sweet	*1 Serving/50ml*	*68*	*0.0*	*136*	*0.3*	*6.9*	*0.0*	*0.0*

SHORTBREAD

All Butter, Deans*	1 Biscuit/15g	77	3.8	511	4.9	65.7	25.4	1.2
All Butter, Fingers, Highland, Sainsbury's*	2 Biscuits/40g	208	11.5	521	4.8	59.4	28.8	2.7
All Butter, Fingers, McVitie's*	1 Finger/20g	106	5.4	530	6.5	64.7	27.2	0.0
All Butter, Fingers, Royal Edinburgh Bakery*	1 Biscuit/17g	88	4.8	519	5.8	60.3	28.3	1.8
All Butter, Fingers, Scottish, M&S*	1 Finger/18g	90	4.9	510	5.7	58.9	27.8	4.7
All Butter, Petticoat Tails, Co-Op*	1 Biscuit/13g	68	3.8	520	5.0	60.0	29.0	2.0
All Butter, Petticoat Tails, Gardiners of Scotland*	1 Biscuit/12g	64	3.4	514	5.2	62.1	27.2	0.0
All Butter, Round, Luxury, M&S*	1 Biscuit/20g	105	5.8	525	6.2	60.0	29.0	2.0
All Butter, Royal Edinburgh, Asda*	1 Biscuit/18g	93	5.1	519	5.8	60.3	28.3	1.8
All Butter, Scottish, M&S*	1 Biscuit/34g	173	9.5	510	5.7	58.9	27.8	2.3
All Butter, Thins, M&S*	1 Biscuit/10g	50	2.2	485	5.8	68.4	21.1	3.5
All Butter, Trufree*	1 Biscuit/11g	58	3.1	524	2.0	66.0	28.0	0.9
Average	*1oz/28g*	*139*	*7.3*	*498*	*5.9*	*63.9*	*26.1*	*1.9*
Belgian Chocolate Chunk, Asda*	1 Biscuit/20g	106	6.2	531	7.0	56.0	31.0	1.8
Caramel, Millionaires, Fox's*	1 Serving/16g	75	3.9	483	6.1	57.9	25.3	0.1
Choc Chip, Fair Trade, Co-Op*	1 Biscuit/19g	100	6.0	526	5.3	57.9	31.6	2.6
Chocolate Chip, Jacob's*	1 Biscuit/17g	87	4.7	513	5.2	61.2	27.5	1.8
Chocolate Chip, Tesco*	1 Serving/20g	105	6.1	525	7.5	55.0	30.6	3.0
Chocolate Chunk, Belgian, TTD, Sainsbury's*	1 Biscuit/19g	101	5.7	521	5.1	59.1	29.4	2.0
Clotted Cream, Finest, Tesco*	1 Biscuit/20g	109	6.4	543	5.2	58.0	32.2	1.7
Crawfords*	1 Biscuit/13g	67	3.4	533	6.6	65.0	27.4	2.0
Demerara, Rounds, TTD, Sainsbury's*	1 Biscuit/22g	113	5.9	508	5.1	62.2	26.5	1.8
Double Choc Chip, Petit Four, Scottish, Tesco*	1 Serving/50g	266	15.0	531	5.1	60.4	30.0	1.7
Dutch, M&S*	1 Biscuit/17g	90	5.1	540	5.4	59.0	30.8	2.5
Fingers, Asda*	1 Finger/18g	93	5.1	519	5.8	60.3	28.3	18.0
Fingers, Cornish Cookie*	1 Finger/25g	124	6.4	498	6.4	61.0	25.5	0.0
Fingers, Deans*	1 Finger/24g	115	5.9	488	5.1	60.1	24.8	1.4
Fingers, Highland, Organic, Sainsbury's*	1 Finger/16g	84	4.8	527	5.8	58.7	29.9	1.9
Fingers, Scottish, Finest, Tesco*	1 Biscuit/21g	104	5.0	498	5.1	65.5	23.9	2.0

	Measure INFO/WEIGHT	per Measure KCAL	per Measure FAT	Nutrition Values per 100g / 100ml KCAL	PROT	CARB	FAT	FIBRE
SHORTBREAD								
Highland, Organic, Duchy Originals*	1 Biscuit/16g	80	4.2	515	5.2	61.8	27.4	1.7
Mini Bites, Co-Op*	1 Biscuit/10g	53	3.0	530	7.0	59.0	30.0	2.0
Mini Bites, Country Table*	1 Biscuit/10g	52	3.0	525	7.1	59.3	29.5	1.5
Orange Marmalade & Oatflake, Deans*	1 Biscuit/20g	105	5.9	524	6.7	59.3	29.6	3.2
Organic, Waitrose*	1 Biscuit/13g	62	3.0	495	5.8	63.0	24.4	1.8
Petticoat Tails, All Butter, Highland, Sainsbury's*	1 Biscuit/13g	64	3.6	516	6.3	58.0	28.8	2.2
Pure Butter, Jacob's*	1 Biscuit/20g	105	5.9	525	5.7	58.6	29.7	1.8
Rings, Handbaked, Border*	1 Biscuit/17g	86	4.9	520	6.2	61.2	29.5	0.0
Stem Ginger, Waitrose*	1 Biscuit/15g	71	3.3	487	4.7	66.0	22.7	1.6
Wheat & Gluten Free, Free From Range, Tesco*	1 Biscuit/20g	98	5.2	490	6.0	58.0	26.0	6.0
SHRIMP								
Boiled, Average	*1 Serving/60g*	*70*	*1.4*	*117*	*23.8*	*0.0*	*2.4*	*0.0*
Frozen, Average	*1oz/28g*	*20*	*0.2*	*73*	*16.5*	*0.0*	*0.8*	*0.0*
in Brine, Canned, Drained, Average	*1oz/28g*	*17*	*0.2*	*61*	*13.5*	*0.0*	*0.8*	*0.0*
SKATE								
Grilled	*1oz/28g*	*22*	*0.1*	*79*	*18.9*	*0.0*	*0.5*	*0.0*
in Batter, Fried in Blended Oil	1oz/28g	47	2.8	168	14.7	4.9	10.1	0.2
Raw, Edible Portion	*1oz/28g*	*18*	*0.1*	*64*	*15.1*	*0.0*	*0.4*	*0.0*
SKIPS								
Cheesy, KP Snacks*	1 Bag/17g	89	5.0	524	6.2	58.5	29.5	1.0
Prawn Cocktail, KP Snacks*	1 Bag/15g	82	4.7	532	6.0	58.7	30.1	1.0
SKITTLES								
Mars*	1 Pack/55g	223	2.4	406	0.0	90.6	4.4	0.0
SLICES								
Bacon & Cheese, Pastry, Tesco*	1 Slice/165g	480	32.0	291	7.4	21.7	19.4	1.0
Beef, Minced Steak & Onion, Tesco*	1 Slice/150g	424	27.2	283	8.7	21.3	18.1	1.6
Cheddar Cheese & Onion, Ginsters*	1 Slice/180g	583	40.9	324	7.1	22.8	22.7	1.0
Cheese & Ham, Pastry, Sainsbury's*	1 Slice/118g	352	23.2	298	7.8	22.5	19.7	1.8
Cheese & Onion, Pastry, Tesco*	1 Slice/150g	502	37.0	335	8.0	20.1	24.7	1.4
Cheese, Leek & Red Onion Plait, Linda McCartney*	1 Plait/170g	473	28.1	278	6.7	25.9	16.5	2.4
Cheese, Potato & Onion, Pastry, Taste!*	1 Slice/155g	501	30.4	323	8.6	28.1	19.6	0.0
Chicken & Ham, Taste!*	1 Slice/155g	356	15.3	230	10.8	24.2	9.9	0.0
Chicken & Mushroom, Ginsters*	1 Slice/180g	439	26.8	244	8.3	19.1	14.9	1.8
Chicken & Mushroom, Tesco*	1 Slice/165g	457	28.9	277	9.2	20.6	17.5	0.9
Chicken Lattice, Ginsters*	1 Lattice/400g	1060	66.8	265	10.6	18.0	16.7	1.5
Chicken, Spicy, Deep Fill, Ginsters*	1 Slice/180g	499	30.6	277	9.2	21.8	17.0	1.4
Custard, Pastry, Tesco*	1 Slice/108g	275	11.1	255	2.8	37.2	10.3	1.3
Fresh Cream, Tesco*	1 Slice/75g	311	21.0	414	3.5	37.4	27.9	1.0
Goats Cheese & Spinach, Crisp & Creamy, Waitrose*	1 Slice/100g	351	22.7	351	7.6	28.3	22.7	1.8
Ham & Cheese, Ginsters*	1 Pack/180g	511	33.7	284	8.5	20.4	18.7	2.5
Meat Feast, Ginsters*	1 Slice/180g	468	32.0	260	8.0	17.2	17.8	2.2
Minced Beef & Onion, Crestwood, Aldi*	1 Slice/165g	543	40.1	329	6.3	19.7	24.3	3.1
Peppered Steak, Asda*	1 Slice/164g	483	31.1	295	9.0	22.0	19.0	1.2
Pork & Egg, Gala, Tesco*	1 Slice/105g	333	24.2	317	10.3	17.2	23.0	3.4
Raisin, Crispy, Light Choices, Tesco*	1 Biscuit/15g	56	0.6	370	6.0	76.6	3.9	5.5
Steak & Onion, Aberdeen Angus, Tesco*	1 Slice/165g	444	27.7	269	8.7	20.7	16.8	1.3
Steak, Peppered, Deep Fill, Ginsters*	1 Slice/180g	513	36.2	285	9.4	16.1	20.1	3.1
Steak, Peppered, Ginsters*	1 Slice/180g	457	27.0	254	8.4	21.3	15.0	1.6
Westcountry Cheddar & Onion, Ginsters*	1 Slice/180g	486	32.6	270	6.7	20.8	18.1	2.2
SLIM FAST*								
Bars, Chocolate Caramel Treat, Snack, Slim Fast*	1 Bar/26g	95	2.6	360	3.5	63.0	10.0	1.5
Bars, Chocolate Peanut, Meal, Slim Fast*	1 Bar/56g	210	7.2	380	24.0	50.0	13.0	5.0
Bars, Chocolate, Nutty, Nougat, Snack, Slim Fast*	1 Bar/25g	95	3.0	380	4.0	63.0	12.0	1.5

S

INFO/WEIGHT	Measure	per Measure		Nutrition Values per 100g / 100ml				
		KCAL	FAT	KCAL	PROT	CARB	FAT	FIBRE

SLIM FAST*

	INFO/WEIGHT	KCAL	FAT	KCAL	PROT	CARB	FAT	FIBRE
Bars, Heavenly Chocolate Delight, Snack, Slim Fast*	1 Bar/24g	95	3.2	390	5.0	58.0	13.0	7.0
Bars, Summer Berry, Meal, Slim Fast*	1 Bar/60g	210	5.0	350	23.3	51.7	8.3	5.8
Crackers, Cheddar Flavour Bites, Snack Bag, Slim Fast*	1 Pack/22g	92	2.0	417	9.6	72.8	9.2	2.5
Milk Shake, Blissful Banana, Powder, Dry, Slim Fast*	2 Scoops/37g	131	2.4	359	13.4	60.2	6.7	11.0
Milk Shake, Blissful Banana, Slim Fast*	1 Bottle/325ml	206	5.6	63	4.3	6.6	1.7	2.3
Milk Shake, Café Latte, Ready to Drink, Slim Fast*	1 Bottle/325ml	206	5.6	63	4.3	6.6	1.7	2.3
Milk Shake, Chunky Chocolate, Powder, Dry, Slim Fast*	2 Scoops/37g	132	2.7	363	13.9	59.0	7.5	10.9
Milk Shake, Chunky Chocolate, Slim Fast*	1 Bottle/325ml	126	3.4	63	4.3	6.6	1.7	2.3
Milk Shake, Simply Vanilla, Powder, Dry, Slim Fast*	2 Scoops/37g	131	2.4	360	13.4	60.9	6.5	11.0
Milk Shake, Simply Vanilla, Slim Fast*	1 Bottle/325ml	206	5.6	63	4.3	6.6	1.7	2.3
Milk Shake, Summer Strawberry, Powder, Dry, Slim Fast*	2 Scoops/37g	139	2.4	380	13.5	60.1	6.6	11.1
Milk Shake, Summer Strawberry, Slim Fast*	1 Bottle/325ml	206	5.6	63	4.3	6.6	1.7	2.3
Pretzels, Sour Cream & Chive, Snack Bag, Slim Fast*	1 Pack/23g	99	2.2	432	9.7	74.9	9.5	4.1
Tortillas, Barbecue Flavour, Snack Bag, Slim Fast*	1 Bag/22g	96	2.6	435	6.5	73.9	11.8	3.6

SMARTIES

	INFO/WEIGHT	KCAL	FAT	KCAL	PROT	CARB	FAT	FIBRE
Mini Eggs, Nestle*	1 Lge Bag/100g	496	20.4	496	3.9	72.9	20.4	2.8
Mini, Treat Size, Smarties, Nestle*	1 Carton/14g	68	2.8	471	5.0	68.1	19.6	1.0
Nestle*	1 Tube/40g	188	7.1	469	3.9	72.5	17.7	2.4
Tree Decoration, Nestle*	1 Chocolate/18g	95	5.4	529	5.6	58.9	30.1	0.8

SMOOTHIE

	INFO/WEIGHT	KCAL	FAT	KCAL	PROT	CARB	FAT	FIBRE
Apple, Cucumber & Lemon, LL, Waitrose*	1 Bottle/250ml	102	0.2	41	0.3	9.0	0.1	1.3
Apples & Blackcurrants for Kids, Innocent*	1 Carton/180ml	104	0.2	58	0.3	14.1	0.1	0.1
Banana & Mango, Juice, Calypso*	1 Carton/200ml	106	0.0	53	0.0	12.8	0.0	1.0
Banana, Dairy, Tesco*	1 Bottle/250ml	165	1.0	66	1.6	14.0	0.4	0.4
Banana, M&S*	1 Bottle/500ml	400	2.0	80	1.8	16.8	0.4	1.2
Berry Blast, Pret a Manger*	1 Pack/362g	186	2.4	51	0.6	10.9	0.7	1.7
Berry, Prepacked, Average	*1 Serving/250ml*	*133*	*0.5*	*53*	*0.7*	*11.6*	*0.2*	*0.9*
Blackberries, Strawberries & Blackcurrants, Innocent*	1 Serving/200ml	108	0.0	54	0.6	11.9	0.0	1.5
Blueberry, Berrie Smoothie, Roberts*	1 Pot/200g	110	1.0	55	0.3	11.0	0.5	2.7
Blueberry, Blackberry & Strawberry, COU, M&S*	1 Bottle/250ml	150	0.8	60	0.8	13.1	0.3	0.3
Cherries & Strawberries, Innocent*	1 Bottle/250ml	122	0.2	49	0.6	12.6	0.1	0.0
Coconut Crush, Pret a Manger*	1 Pack/218g	102	2.3	47	0.5	8.6	1.1	1.6
Cranberries, Blueberries, Cherries, Innocent*	1 Serving/250ml	138	0.0	55	0.3	12.8	0.0	1.3
Fruit, Cranberry & Raspberry, Juice Republic*	1 Bottle/250mls	182	1.0	73	0.5	16.0	0.4	0.0
Gold Machine, Naked Juice Co*	1 Bottle/450ml	262	0.0	58	0.8	13.3	0.0	0.0
Guavas, Mangoes & Goji Berries, Innocent*	1 Bottle/250ml	112	0.2	45	0.6	12.0	0.1	2.1
Kiwi, Apples & Limes, Innocent*	1 Bottle/250ml	125	0.2	50	0.5	11.0	0.1	1.8
Mango & Orange, Smoothie Smile*	1 Bottle/250ml	130	1.0	52	0.4	11.7	0.4	0.0
Mango & Passionfruit, Prepacked, Average	*1 Serving/250ml*	*145*	*0.3*	*58*	*0.6*	*12.7*	*0.1*	*1.5*
Mango & Passionfruit, Tesco*	1 Glass/250ml	150	0.2	60	0.5	12.7	0.1	1.8
Mango & West Indian Cherry, Plus, Tesco*	1 Serving/250ml	133	0.6	53	0.6	12.2	0.2	0.5
Mangoes & Passion Fruits, Pure Fruit, Innocent*	1 Bottle/250ml	142	0.5	57	0.6	12.5	0.2	1.6
Mixed Berry, CBY, Asda*	1 Glass/250ml	143	0.5	57	0.6	12.6	0.0	1.6
Orange, Mango & Pineapple, Prepacked, Average	*1 Serving/250ml*	*131*	*0.2*	*52*	*0.6*	*11.9*	*0.1*	*0.7*
Orange, Mango, Banana & Passion Fruit, Asda*	1 Serving/100ml	55	0.2	55	0.8	12.0	0.2	1.1
Oranges, Mangoes & Pineapples For Kids, Innocent*	1 Carton/180ml	94	0.2	52	0.7	11.7	0.1	0.9
Peaches & Passionfruit, for Kids, Innocent*	1 Carton/180ml	95	0.0	53	0.6	14.7	0.0	0.9
Peaches & Passionfruits, Innocent For Kids*	1 Carton/180ml	95	0.0	53	0.6	14.7	0.0	0.9
Pineapple & Passion Fruit, Sweetbird*	1 Serving/330ml	175	0.3	53	0.8	12.3	0.1	0.0
Pineapple, Banana & Coconut, CBY, Asda*	1 Glass/250ml	178	2.8	71	0.7	13.6	1.1	1.0
Pineapple, Banana & Coconut, Prepacked, Average	*1 Serving/250ml*	*163*	*3.0*	*65*	*0.6*	*12.8*	*1.2*	*0.9*
Pineapple, Banana & Pear, Asda*	1 Bottle/250ml	147	0.3	59	0.5	13.6	0.1	0.3
Pineapple, Mango & Passion Fruit, ES, Asda*	½ Bottle/250ml	100	0.5	40	0.5	9.0	0.2	1.3

	Measure INFO/WEIGHT	per Measure KCAL	FAT	Nutrition Values per 100g / 100ml KCAL	PROT	CARB	FAT	FIBRE
SMOOTHIE								
Pineapples, Bananas & Coconuts, Innocent*	1 Bottle/250ml	172	2.8	69	0.7	13.6	1.1	1.0
Pomegranates, Blueberries & Acai, Special, Innocent*	1 Serving/250ml	170	0.5	68	0.6	15.6	0.2	0.8
Raspberry & Bio Yoghurt, M&S*	1 Bottle/500ml	275	1.5	55	2.0	10.8	0.3	0.9
Raspberry & Blueberry, Plus, Tesco*	1 Serving/100ml	59	0.3	59	2.6	11.6	0.3	0.5
Raspberry, Banana & Peach, Sainsbury's*	1 Bottle/251ml	138	0.3	55	0.8	12.8	0.1	1.5
Strawberry & Banana, Fruit, Serious Food Company*	1 Bottle/250ml	135	0.0	54	0.5	12.7	0.0	1.3
Strawberry & Banana, Juice, Calypso*	1 Carton/200ml	100	0.0	50	0.0	11.9	0.0	0.0
Strawberry & Banana, Morrisons*	1 Bottle/250ml	135	0.0	54	0.5	13.0	0.0	0.6
Strawberry & Banana, PJ Smoothies*	1 Bottle/250ml	118	0.2	47	0.4	11.0	0.1	0.0
Strawberry & Banana, Prepacked, Average	**1 Serving/250ml**	**131**	**0.2**	**53**	**0.6**	**11.9**	**0.1**	**0.9**
Strawberry & Banana, Pure Fruit, Innocent*	1 Bottle/250ml	132	0.2	53	0.7	13.1	0.1	1.3
Strawberry & Banana, Tesco*	1 Sm Bottle/250ml	112	0.5	45	0.6	10.1	0.2	0.8
SMOOTHIE MIX								
Strawberry & Spinach, As Consumed, Tesco*	1 Smoothie/257g	95	0.5	37	0.5	7.7	0.2	1.4
SNAILS								
in Garlic Butter, Average	**6 Snails/50g**	**219**	**20.8**	**438**	**9.7**	**8.0**	**41.5**	**1.0**
SNAPPER								
Red, Fried in Blended Oil	**1oz/28g**	**35**	**0.9**	**126**	**24.5**	**0.0**	**3.1**	**0.0**
Red, Weighed with Bone, Raw	**1oz/28g**	**12**	**0.2**	**42**	**9.2**	**0.0**	**0.6**	**0.0**
SNICKERS								
& Hazelnut, Snickers*	1 Bar/49g	240	11.7	489	8.1	59.5	23.9	0.0
Mars*	1 Snacksize/41g	208	11.5	511	9.4	54.3	28.2	1.3
SOPOCKA								
Sliced, Cured, Pork Loin	1 Serving/100g	101	2.9	101	17.8	0.8	2.9	0.0
SORBET								
Exotic Fruit, Sainsbury's*	1 Serving/75g	90	1.5	120	1.2	24.1	2.0	0.0
Lemon	1 Scoop/60g	79	0.0	131	0.9	34.2	0.0	0.0
Lemon Harmony, Haagen-Dazs*	1 Serving/90ml	214	10.2	238	1.5	32.5	11.3	0.0
Lemon, Asda*	1 Serving/100g	120	0.0	120	0.0	30.0	0.0	0.0
Lemon, Sainsbury's*	¼ Pot/89g	100	0.0	112	0.0	28.1	0.0	0.1
Lemon, Tesco*	1 Serving/75g	80	0.0	106	0.0	26.2	0.0	0.4
Lemon, The Real Ice Company*	1 Serving/100g	117	0.1	117	0.1	29.1	0.1	0.4
Mango, Tesco*	1 Serving/100g	107	0.0	107	0.1	26.5	0.0	0.3
Mango, Waitrose*	1 Pot/100g	90	0.0	90	0.1	22.1	0.0	0.6
Orange, Del Monte*	1 Sorbet/500g	625	0.5	125	0.2	32.1	0.1	0.0
Raspberry & Blackberry, Fat Free, M&S*	1 Sorbet/125g	140	0.0	112	0.4	27.5	0.0	0.6
Raspberry, Haagen-Dazs*	½ Cup/105g	120	0.0	114	0.0	28.6	0.0	1.9
Raspberry, Tesco*	1 Serving/70ml	97	0.0	138	0.5	34.0	0.0	0.0
Sicilian Lemon, Seriously Fruity, Waitrose*	1/5 Pot/100ml	77	0.1	77	18.8	13.5	0.1	0.2
Strawberry & Champagne, Sainsbury's*	¼ Pot/89g	95	0.0	107	0.2	25.5	0.0	0.6
Strawberry, Fruit Ice, Starburst, Mars*	1 Stick/93ml	99	0.1	106	0.1	26.7	0.1	0.0
SOUFFLE								
Cheese	1oz/28g	71	5.4	253	11.4	9.3	19.2	0.3
Cheese, Alizonne*	1 Serving/33g	129	3.4	392	60.5	14.5	10.2	0.2
Cheese, Mini, Waitrose*	1 Souffle/14g	32	2.4	232	16.0	2.9	17.4	2.4
Chocolate, Gu*	1 Pot/70g	307	24.9	439	6.3	24.4	35.6	2.9
Lemon, Finest, Tesco*	1 Pot/80g	270	20.5	338	2.9	24.1	25.6	0.2
Plain	1oz/28g	56	4.1	201	7.6	10.4	14.7	0.3
Strawberry, M&S*	1 Serving/95g	171	10.1	180	1.6	19.5	10.6	0.9
SOUP								
Asian Tomato Rice & Ginger, Skinny Soup, Glorious!*	½ Pot/300g	159	5.4	53	1.0	8.2	1.8	0.8
Asparagus & Chicken, Waitrose*	1 Can/415g	166	4.6	40	2.1	5.3	1.1	0.7
Asparagus & Creme Fraiche, Morrisons*	½ Pot/300g	186	11.7	62	1.3	5.4	3.9	0.5

S

SOUP

	Measure INFO/WEIGHT	per Measure KCAL	FAT	Nutrition Values per 100g / 100ml KCAL	PROT	CARB	FAT	FIBRE
Asparagus in a Cup, You Count, LL, Waitrose*	1 Serving/200ml	57	1.6	28	0.5	4.8	0.8	0.3
Asparagus, Cream of, Canned, M&S*	½ Can/200g	108	7.2	54	0.9	4.3	3.6	0.2
Asparagus, Fresh, Finest, Tesco*	½ Pot/300g	153	8.1	51	1.6	5.0	2.7	1.0
Asparagus, Fresh, M&S*	1 Serving/300g	135	10.8	45	1.1	2.5	3.6	0.9
Asparagus, NCG Food Co*	½ Carton/300g	132	7.2	44	1.5	4.1	2.4	0.9
Asparagus, Slimline, Cup, Waitrose*	1 Sachet/204ml	51	1.4	25	0.4	4.3	0.7	0.7
Asparagus, Waitrose*	1 Serving/300g	60	3.6	20	0.9	1.5	1.2	0.9
Autumn Vegetable & Lentil, Heinz*	1 Can/400g	184	1.2	46	2.3	8.6	0.3	1.0
Bacon & Lentil, CBY, Asda*	½ Pot/300g	177	4.2	59	3.8	7.2	1.4	1.2
Bean & Vegetable, Chunky, CBY, Asda*	1 Can/400g	224	1.2	56	2.6	9.7	0.3	1.9
Beef & Ale, Canned, M&S*	1 Can/400g	150	4.0	38	1.0	5.4	1.0	1.4
Beef & Mushroom, Big Soup, Heinz*	1 Can/515g	216	2.6	42	2.3	7.0	0.5	0.7
Beef & Tomato in a Cup, Sainsbury's*	1 Serving/210ml	61	1.1	29	0.6	5.6	0.5	0.2
Beef & Tomato, Cup a Soup, Made Up, Batchelors*	1 Serving/252g	83	1.6	33	0.6	6.3	0.6	0.4
Beef & Vegetable Broth, Chunky, Canned, M&S*	1 Can/415g	166	3.3	40	1.9	6.4	0.8	0.6
Beef & Vegetable, Big Soup, Heinz*	1 Can/400g	212	4.0	53	3.5	7.5	1.0	0.9
Beef & Vegetable, Chunky, Asda*	1 Can/400g	212	8.4	53	1.7	5.7	2.1	2.2
Beef & Vegetable, Chunky, Meal, Tesco*	1 Can/400g	140	2.0	35	3.3	4.2	0.5	1.0
Beef Broth, Big Soup, Heinz*	1 Can/400g	184	2.8	46	2.5	7.0	0.7	0.9
Beef Broth, Classic, Heinz*	1 Can/400g	180	2.0	45	1.9	7.6	0.5	0.8
Beetroot with Chopped Dill, Duchy Originals*	½ Pot/298g	152	7.4	51	1.1	5.9	2.5	0.9
Beetroot, Tomato & Buckwheat, Stay Full, Baxters*	1 Can/400g	264	4.8	66	3.4	8.7	1.2	2.9
Big Red Tomato, Heinz*	½ Can/210g	63	0.8	30	0.5	6.4	0.4	0.0
Blended Sweetcorn & Yellow Pepper, Heinz*	½ Can/200g	98	4.2	49	0.9	6.6	2.1	0.6
Boston Bean & Ham, NCG Food Co*	½ Carton/300g	171	0.6	57	2.4	7.8	0.2	1.6
Brazilian Beef & Black Bean, Glorious!*	½ Pot/300g	144	6.9	48	2.0	4.8	2.3	0.8
British Beef, & Yorkshire Ale, Hearty, Duchy Originals*	1 Pack/350g	186	8.4	53	2.3	5.6	2.4	0.6
Broccoli & Cauliflower, Cup, BFY, Morrisons*	1 Sachet/15g	56	2.1	376	4.9	57.2	14.2	4.9
Broccoli & Cheddar, Heinz*	1 Can/430g	340	24.1	79	2.6	4.4	5.6	0.6
Broccoli & Stilton, Canned, Sainsbury's*	½ Can/200g	84	4.0	42	1.5	4.2	2.0	0.6
Broccoli & Stilton, Canned, Tesco*	1 Can/400g	240	14.0	60	1.7	5.0	3.5	0.4
Broccoli & Stilton, Classics, Fresh, Tesco*	½ Pot/300g	180	8.4	60	2.9	5.8	2.8	1.1
Broccoli & Stilton, Cup Soup, Ainsley Harriott*	1 Satchet/229ml	87	1.8	38	1.0	7.0	0.8	1.3
Broccoli & Stilton, Farmers Market, Heinz*	½ Can/200g	108	7.4	54	1.5	3.2	3.7	0.9
Broccoli & Stilton, Fresh, Sainsbury's*	½ Pot/300ml	141	9.9	47	2.7	1.8	3.3	1.5
Broccoli & Stilton, NCG Food Co*	1 Carton/600ml	240	14.4	40	2.2	1.9	2.4	1.1
Broccoli & Stilton, Tesco*	1 Can/400g	192	10.4	48	1.9	4.2	2.6	1.2
Broccoli, Pea & Mint, LL, Waitrose*	1 Pot/400g	200	9.6	50	2.7	4.3	2.4	2.1
Broccoli, Salmon & Watercress, Stay Full, Baxters*	1 Can/400g	244	8.8	61	3.3	5.8	2.2	2.4
Broth, Wholegrain Farro & Ham Hock, LL, Waitrose*	1 Pot/398g	247	8.4	62	4.3	6.4	2.1	1.6
Burmese Chicken, with Coconut & Rice, Waitrose*	½ Pot/300g	268	12.9	89	4.2	7.7	4.3	1.3
Butter Bean & Chorizo, Meal, Sainsbury's*	1 Pot/400g	257	9.6	64	3.9	5.6	2.4	2.3
Butternut Squash & Red Pepper, Vegetarian, Baxters*	1 Can/415g	149	2.5	36	0.9	6.6	0.6	0.5
Butternut Squash & Tarragon, Waitrose*	½ Pot/300g	123	6.6	41	0.8	4.5	2.2	1.0
Butternut Squash, Diet Chef Ltd*	1 Pack/300g	135	5.4	45	0.8	6.5	1.8	1.6
Butternut Squash, Fresh, Waitrose*	½ Pot/300g	153	8.7	51	0.5	5.8	2.9	0.8
Butternut Squash, Spiced, HL, Tesco*	½ Pack/300g	123	5.1	41	0.9	5.3	1.7	0.6
Carrot & Butter Bean, Diet Chef Ltd*	1 Pack/300g	174	2.1	58	2.7	10.3	0.7	2.8
Carrot & Butter Bean, Vegetarian, Baxters*	1 Can/415g	237	7.9	57	1.5	7.2	1.9	2.2
Carrot & Coriander, Average	**1 Serving/200g**	**83**	**4.3**	**42**	**0.6**	**4.8**	**2.2**	**1.0**
Carrot & Coriander, Blended, Heinz*	½ Can/200g	104	5.4	52	0.7	6.2	2.7	0.6
Carrot & Coriander, Canned, BGTY, Sainsbury's*	½ Can/200g	62	2.0	31	0.8	4.8	1.0	0.9
Carrot & Coriander, Canned, GFY, Asda*	1 Can/400g	116	2.4	29	0.7	5.3	0.6	0.6

SOUP

Measure INFO/WEIGHT	per Measure KCAL	FAT	Nutrition Values per 100g / 100ml KCAL	PROT	CARB	FAT	FIBRE
Carrot & Coriander, Canned, M&S* ½ Can/210g	94	5.0	45	0.4	5.9	2.4	0.9
Carrot & Coriander, Canned, Tesco* 1 Can/400g	220	11.6	55	0.7	5.7	2.9	0.8
Carrot & Coriander, Classic, Classic, Heinz* 1 Can/400g	164	6.4	41	0.4	5.8	1.6	0.9
Carrot & Coriander, Fresh, Healthy Living, Co-Op* 1 Pot/600g	180	6.0	30	0.6	4.7	1.0	1.0
Carrot & Coriander, Fresh, LL, Waitrose* ½ Pot/300g	141	9.6	47	0.7	3.6	3.2	1.0
Carrot & Coriander, Fresh, M&S* ½ Pot/300g	90	4.5	30	0.4	4.2	1.5	0.5
Carrot & Coriander, Low Calorie, Average **1 Serving/200g**	**45**	**1.3**	**22**	**0.6**	**3.5**	**0.6**	**1.1**
Carrot & Coriander, Warming Moroccan Spices, Heinz* 1 Can/400g	196	7.6	49	0.5	6.7	1.9	1.2
Carrot & Coriander, Weight Watchers* 1 Pouch/300g	102	3.9	34	0.4	5.1	1.3	0.6
Carrot & Ginger, Fresh, Sainsbury's* 1 Pot/600g	150	5.4	25	0.4	3.9	0.9	1.0
Carrot & Lentil, Microwave, Heinz* 1 Can/303g	94	0.3	31	1.5	6.1	0.1	0.8
Carrot & Lentil, Weight Watchers* 1 Can/295g	87	0.3	29	1.3	5.5	0.1	0.7
Carrot & Orange 1oz/28g	6	0.1	20	0.4	3.7	0.5	1.0
Carrot & Orange, Fresh, Finest, Tesco* ½ Tub/300g	150	5.7	50	0.7	7.5	1.9	1.1
Carrot & Parsnip, Spiced, Duchy Originals, Waitrose* ½ Pot/300g	145	9.7	48	0.8	3.6	3.2	1.1
Carrot, Coriander & Ginger, So Organic, Sainsbury's* ½ Can/197g	75	3.3	38	0.3	5.3	1.7	0.7
Carrot, Onion & Chickpea, Healthy, Baxters* 1 Can/415ml	170	0.8	41	1.9	8.0	0.2	1.2
Carrot, Orange & Ginger, Go Organic* 1 Jar/495g	119	4.0	24	0.5	3.6	0.8	1.4
Carrot, Red Lentil & Cumin, Organic, Waitrose* 1 Pack/350g	175	8.8	50	0.2	6.7	2.5	0.6
Carrot, Thai, Skinny, Aldi* ½ Pot/300g	90	4.8	30	0.5	3.3	1.6	0.6
Cauliflower Cheese, with Ham, Yorkshire Provender* 1 Pot/600g	438	28.2	73	4.1	2.9	4.7	0.0
Celeriac & Truffle, NCG Food Co* 1 Serving/300g	225	17.7	75	1.1	4.3	5.9	0.7
Chantenay Carrot & Parsnip, Fresh, ES, Asda* ½ Pot/300g	153	8.4	51	1.2	4.8	2.8	0.8
Chicken & Black Eyed Pea, Gumbo, Hearty, Baxters* 1 Can/400g	184	2.0	46	2.6	6.7	0.5	1.5
Chicken & Chunky Vegetable, Hearty, Baxters* 1 Can/400g	184	1.6	46	2.3	7.6	0.4	1.4
Chicken & Leek, Big Soup, Heinz* ½ Can/258g	162	5.2	63	3.0	8.2	2.0	0.6
Chicken & Leek, Cup a Soup, Made Up, Batchelors* 1 Serving/259g	96	4.7	37	0.5	4.7	1.8	0.7
Chicken & Leek, Instant, Cup, Average **1 Pack/19g**	**73**	**2.7**	**382**	**5.0**	**58.2**	**14.4**	**8.5**
Chicken & Leek, Soup in a Cup, Made Up, Sainsbury's* 1 Serving/200ml	82	3.3	41	0.4	6.2	1.6	0.1
Chicken & Mushroom, Extra, Slim a Soup, Batchelors* 1 Serving/257g	90	1.5	35	1.4	5.9	0.6	0.3
Chicken & Mushroom, Kitchen Creations, Soupreme, Aldi* ½ Can/200g	186	4.8	93	3.0	14.3	2.4	1.1
Chicken & Noodle Laksa, Fuller Longer, M&S* 1 Pot/385g	289	7.7	75	7.0	7.1	2.0	0.9
Chicken & Pasta Big, Heinz* ½ Can/200g	68	0.8	34	1.8	5.9	0.4	0.8
Chicken & Spelt Broth, Duchy Originals, Waitrose* ½ Pot/300g	135	3.6	45	3.5	4.9	1.2	0.5
Chicken & Sweetcorn, Asda* 1 Pot/600g	246	8.4	41	2.2	4.9	1.4	1.6
Chicken & Sweetcorn, Canned, BGTY, Sainsbury's* ½ Can/200g	56	0.8	28	1.5	4.5	0.4	0.2
Chicken & Sweetcorn, Canned, HL, Tesco* ½ Can/200g	70	0.6	35	1.6	6.4	0.3	0.3
Chicken & Sweetcorn, Canned, Tesco* 1 Can/400g	240	6.0	60	1.6	8.2	1.5	0.7
Chicken & Sweetcorn, Cantonese, Fresh, Sainsbury's* ½ Pot/300ml	135	1.5	45	2.1	7.9	0.5	0.5
Chicken & Sweetcorn, CBY, Asda* 1 Pot/600g	294	9.6	49	4.4	4.1	1.6	0.5
Chicken & Sweetcorn, Fresh, Asda* 1 Pack/500g	260	9.5	52	2.6	6.0	1.9	0.0
Chicken & Sweetcorn, Fresh, Average **1 Serving/300g**	**146**	**3.1**	**48**	**2.4**	**7.3**	**1.0**	**0.6**
Chicken & Sweetcorn, Light Choice, Tesco* ½ Can/200g	84	0.8	42	1.7	7.9	0.4	0.2
Chicken & Sweetcorn, NCG Food Co* 1 Carton/600g	282	5.4	47	1.0	8.7	0.9	0.5
Chicken & Vegetable, Big Soup, Heinz* ½ Can/200g	104	2.8	52	3.3	6.7	1.4	0.8
Chicken & Vegetable, Broth, Peas & Spinach, LL, Waitrose* ½ Pot/300g	135	5.1	45	3.1	4.0	1.7	0.8
Chicken & Vegetable, Canned, Average **1 Can/400g**	**192**	**8.5**	**48**	**2.5**	**4.6**	**2.1**	**0.8**
Chicken & Vegetable, Chunky, Canned, Eat Well, M&S* ½ Can/213g	138	4.0	65	4.6	6.9	1.9	1.0
Chicken & Vegetable, Chunky, Canned, Soupreme, Aldi* 1 Can/400g	184	2.4	46	3.0	6.4	0.6	1.3
Chicken & Vegetable, Classic, Heinz* 1 Can/400g	132	1.6	33	1.2	6.2	0.4	0.6
Chicken & Vegetable, Country Kitchen* ½ Pot/250g	93	3.0	37	1.7	4.6	1.2	0.5
Chicken & Vegetable, Cully & Sully* ½ Pot200g	98	6.8	49	1.9	3.0	3.4	0.8
Chicken & Vegetable, Fresh, M&S* ½ Pot/300g	123	5.1	41	3.5	2.3	1.7	1.2

S

SOUP

INFO/WEIGHT	Measure	per Measure KCAL	per Measure FAT	Nutrition Values per 100g / 100ml KCAL	PROT	CARB	FAT	FIBRE
Chicken & Vegetable, Healthy, Baxters*	1 Can/415g	170	2.1	41	1.9	6.3	0.5	1.8
Chicken & Vegetable, Hearty, Heat Eat & Enjoy, Lidl*	1 Pack/400g	240	7.2	60	0.9	2.3	1.8	0.5
Chicken & Vegetable, Soup to Go, Asda*	1 Pot/330g	145	5.0	44	2.4	5.1	1.5	0.7
Chicken Arrabiata, Meal, Fresh, Sainsbury's*	1 Pot/400g	232	6.0	58	4.1	5.3	1.5	1.5
Chicken Balti, Meal, Sainsbury's*	1 Pack/400g	242	7.1	61	3.9	6.3	1.8	1.8
Chicken Broth, Favourites, Baxters*	1 Can/400g	140	1.2	35	1.7	5.9	0.3	1.0
Chicken Curry & Brown Rice, Sainsbury's*	1 Can/400g	208	4.4	52	3.1	6.3	1.1	2.1
Chicken Curry, CBY, Asda*	½ Pot/300g	216	5.4	72	5.0	8.6	1.8	0.5
Chicken Leek & Potato Soup, Weight Watchers*	1 Tin/295g	80	1.2	27	0.9	5.0	0.4	0.3
Chicken Miso, Noodle, Waitrose*	1 Pot/400g	268	8.8	67	5.9	5.9	2.2	0.9
Chicken Noodle & Vegetable, Slim a Soup, Batchelors*	1 Serving/203g	55	1.0	27	0.8	4.8	0.5	0.6
Chicken Noodle in a Cup, You Count, LL, Waitrose*	1 Cup/205ml	43	0.2	21	0.7	4.5	0.1	0.1
Chicken Noodle, Canned, Sainsbury's*	½ Can/217g	78	0.7	36	1.7	7.4	0.3	0.7
Chicken Noodle, Chunky, Campbell's*	½ Can/200g	86	1.2	43	2.8	6.5	0.6	0.0
Chicken Noodle, Classic, Heinz*	1 Can/400g	124	1.2	31	1.2	6.0	0.3	0.2
Chicken Noodle, Clear, Weight Watchers*	1 Can/295g	51	0.6	17	0.8	3.1	0.2	0.2
Chicken Noodle, Cup Soup, Dry, Heinz*	1 Sachet/20g	48	0.5	240	8.0	46.0	2.5	1.5
Chicken Noodle, Cup Soup, Eat Smart, Morrisons*	1 Sachet/216g	41	0.2	19	0.6	4.1	0.1	0.2
Chicken Noodle, Cup Soup, Made Up, Heinz*	1 Serving/218ml	48	0.4	22	0.7	4.3	0.2	0.1
Chicken Noodle, Cup, Asda*	1 Sachet/13g	40	0.2	305	9.0	63.0	1.9	3.6
Chicken Noodle, Cup, GFY, Asda*	1 Sachet/215ml	43	0.2	20	0.6	4.2	0.1	0.1
Chicken Noodle, Dry, Nissin*	1 Pack/85g	364	14.1	428	9.5	62.0	16.6	3.3
Chicken Noodle, Fresh, CBY, Asda*	½ Pot/297g	98	1.2	33	2.5	4.3	0.4	0.9
Chicken Noodle, in a Cup, BGTY, Sainsbury's*	1 Sachet/59g	14	0.3	23	1.4	4.2	0.4	0.4
Chicken Noodle, Soup in a Cup, Made Up, Sainsbury's*	1 Serving/200ml	44	0.2	22	0.7	4.7	0.1	0.2
Chicken, & Barley, Broth, Heinz*	1 Can/400g	128	1.2	32	1.3	5.9	0.3	0.8
Chicken, & Country Vegetable, Farmers Market, Heinz*	½ Can/200g	106	4.6	53	2.2	5.3	2.3	1.3
Chicken, Barley & Vegetable, Fuller Longer, M&S*	1 Pack/400g	200	6.0	50	4.9	4.5	1.5	1.6
Chicken, Chardonnay Wine & Tarragon, Finest, Tesco*	½ Pot/300g	171	9.6	57	3.1	3.7	3.2	0.3
Chicken, Classic, New Covent Garden*	½ Pack/213g	151	9.6	71	2.9	4.8	4.5	0.5
Chicken, Coconut & Lemon Grass, Fresh, Waitrose*	½ Pot/300g	303	24.9	101	2.6	4.1	8.3	0.8
Chicken, Condensed, 99% Fat Free, Campbell's*	1 Can/295g	77	2.1	26	1.0	3.8	0.7	0.1
Chicken, Courgette & Orzo Pasta, Meal Soup, Glorious!*	½ Pot/300g	141	4.2	47	3.5	5.1	1.4	0.8
Chicken, Cream of, Canned, Happy Shopper*	½ Can/200g	106	6.2	53	1.9	4.4	3.1	0.0
Chicken, Cream of, Canned, Morrisons*	½ Can/202g	105	5.3	52	2.3	4.7	2.6	0.5
Chicken, Cream of, Canned, Tesco*	1 Can/400g	260	15.2	65	1.2	5.5	3.8	0.0
Chicken, Cream of, Reduced Salt, Heinz*	1 Can/400g	216	12.0	54	1.7	4.9	3.0	0.1
Chicken, Cream of, Soupreme, Aldi*	1 Can/400g	228	15.2	57	1.8	3.8	3.8	0.4
Chicken, Creamed, Basics, Sainsbury's*	1 Can/400ml	120	6.0	30	0.6	3.5	1.5	0.1
Chicken, Cup, Calorie Counter, Dry, Co-Op*	1 Sachet/13g	40	1.4	320	6.0	49.0	11.0	7.0
Chicken, Fresh, Sainsbury's*	½ Carton/300g	126	5.7	42	2.2	4.0	1.9	0.3
Chicken, Green Thai, Sainsbury's*	1 Pot/600g	366	19.8	61	1.9	5.8	3.3	0.3
Chicken, Green Thai, Spiced, M&S*	½ Pot/300g	195	11.4	65	2.0	6.3	3.8	0.6
Chicken, Green Thai, Waitrose*	1 Pot/600g	462	30.0	77	4.4	3.5	5.0	1.6
Chicken, in a Cup, Sainsbury's*	1 Serving/221ml	86	3.8	39	0.7	5.3	1.7	0.1
Chicken, Jamaican Jerk & Pumpkin, Sainsbury's*	½ Pot/300g	141	5.1	47	2.7	5.1	1.7	0.2
Chicken, Leek & White Wine, Fresh, Finest, Tesco*	1 Pack/300g	216	12.6	72	2.8	5.7	4.2	0.3
Chicken, Low Fat, Condensed, Batchelors*	1 Can/295g	148	4.1	50	1.9	7.5	1.4	0.2
Chicken, Morrocan Spiced, Skinny Soup, Glorious!*	½ Pot/300g	135	4.2	45	1.9	5.9	1.4	0.0
Chicken, Mulligatawny, Finest, Tesco*	½ Pot/300g	216	7.8	72	5.2	6.5	2.6	0.9
Chicken, Mushroom & Rice, M&S*	1 Pack/350g	206	7.7	59	2.7	6.6	2.2	0.9
Chicken, Potato & Bacon, Big Soup, Heinz*	1 Can/515g	294	11.3	57	3.0	6.1	2.2	0.5
Chicken, Potato & Leek, Weight Watchers*	1 Can/295g	97	2.4	33	1.1	5.1	0.8	0.3

SOUP

INFO/WEIGHT	Measure	per Measure KCAL	FAT	Nutrition Values per 100g / 100ml KCAL	PROT	CARB	FAT	FIBRE
Chicken, Red Thai, Covent Garden Soup Co*	½ Carton/300g	177	9.9	59	2.8	3.6	3.3	1.6
Chicken, Red Thai, Waitrose*	1 Pot/6400g	316	14.8	79	6.5	5.1	3.7	0.7
Chicken, Thai Style, GFY, Asda*	½ Can/200g	66	2.2	33	1.3	4.4	1.1	0.8
Chicken, Thai, Fresh, Finest, Tesco*	½ Tub/300g	255	16.2	85	4.1	4.2	5.4	1.1
Chicken, Thai, GFY, Asda*	1 Serving/200g	85	3.0	42	1.7	5.5	1.5	0.5
Chilli Bean, Mexican, Tesco*	1 Carton/600g	270	6.6	45	2.2	6.4	1.1	1.9
Chilli Pumpkin, Fresh, Sainsbury's*	½ Carton/300g	120	7.2	40	0.6	4.0	2.4	1.3
Chilli, Meal, Chunky, Canned, Tesco*	½ Can/200g	120	2.4	60	5.0	6.3	1.2	1.6
Chowder, Bacon & Corn, M&S*	½ Pot/300g	195	10.8	65	2.5	6.0	3.6	1.8
Chowder, Clam, New England, Select, Campbell's*	1 Cup/240ml	221	14.4	92	2.5	6.0	6.0	0.8
Chowder, Prawn, Manhattan, Fresh, Sainsbury's*	1 Serving/300g	177	6.9	59	1.6	7.9	2.3	0.1
Chunky Chilli Beef, Asda*	1 Can/400g	212	4.0	53	4.2	5.7	1.0	2.4
Chunky Minestrone, LL, Waitrose*	1 Can/400g	166	0.4	42	1.3	8.7	0.1	1.9
Chunky Vegetable, Fresh, CBY, Asda*	½ Pot/300g	117	2.1	39	1.6	5.9	0.7	1.1
Chunky Winter Vegetable, M&S*	1 Can/400g	140	0.8	35	1.2	6.3	0.2	1.5
Chunky, Chicken & Vegetable Meal Soup, Tesco*	1 Can/400g	184	7.2	46	2.5	4.6	1.8	1.0
Chunky, Lentil & Bacon, Canned, M&S*	1 Can/400g	180	2.4	45	3.3	5.8	0.6	2.1
Cock-A-Leekie, Favourites, Baxters*	1 Can/400g	116	2.4	29	1.1	4.7	0.6	0.3
Country Garden, Canned, Vegetarian, Baxters*	1 Can/400g	144	2.0	36	1.0	6.2	0.5	1.0
Country Mushroom, Selection, Campbell's*	1 Serving/250ml	80	4.5	32	0.6	3.4	1.8	0.5
Country Vegetable, Asda*	1 Serving/125g	59	3.6	47	0.6	4.5	2.9	0.8
Country Vegetable, Canned, Heinz, Weight Watchers*	1 Can/295g	97	0.6	33	1.2	5.9	0.2	1.0
Country Vegetable, Chunky, Baxters*	1 Can/400g	188	2.4	47	1.6	7.2	0.6	2.0
Country Vegetable, Fresh, Asda*	1 Carton/500g	195	2.0	39	1.9	7.0	0.4	0.0
Country Vegetable, Fresh, Sainsbury's*	½ Pot/300g	123	2.7	41	1.6	6.6	0.9	2.5
Country Vegetable, Knorr*	1 Pack/500ml	160	3.5	32	0.9	5.5	0.7	1.2
Country Vegetable, Weight Watchers*	1 Can/295g	97	0.3	33	1.2	6.3	0.1	1.0
Courgette & Parmesan, Fresh, Sainsbury's*	1 Pack/300ml	198	16.8	66	1.5	2.5	5.6	0.4
Cream of, Tomato, Reduced Salt, Heinz*	½ Can/200g	117	6.1	58	0.9	6.7	3.0	0.4
Cup, Chicken & Vegetable with Croutons, Campbell's*	1 Sachet/222ml	100	4.0	45	0.7	5.9	1.8	0.9
Egg, Drop, Average	**1 Bowl/500g**	**470**	**30.0**	**94**	**6.0**	**4.0**	**6.0**	**0.0**
English Broccoli & Stilton, Dry, Knorr*	1 Pack/65g	331	24.6	509	11.7	30.3	37.9	1.6
Farmhouse Vegetable, Canned, BGTY, Sainsbury's*	½ Can/200ml	52	1.6	26	0.5	4.4	0.8	0.9
Farmhouse Vegetable, Fresh, Avonmore*	½ Carton/250g	138	5.0	55	1.9	7.4	2.0	0.8
Farmhouse Vegetable, Soup-A-Cup, GFY, Asda*	1 Sachet/219ml	59	1.1	27	0.6	4.9	0.5	0.4
Farmhouse Vegetable, Thick, Co-Op*	1 Can/400g	140	1.6	35	1.0	7.0	0.4	0.3
Fire Roasted Tomato & Red Pepper, Asda*	½ Tub/265g	114	6.9	43	0.7	4.1	2.6	1.0
Fish, Bouillabaise, Bistro, M&S*	1 Pack/820g	2665	18.0	325	10.0	4.3	2.2	1.3
Fish, Frozen, Findus*	1 Serving/85g	128	4.7	150	11.0	13.0	5.5	0.0
Florida Spring Vegetable, Dry, Knorr*	1 Pack/36g	104	2.0	290	7.8	52.2	5.6	5.2
Fragrant Thai Carrot, Skinny Soup, Glorious!*	½ Tub/298g	119	5.4	40	0.3	3.5	1.8	1.6
French Onion	1oz/28g	11	0.6	40	0.2	5.7	2.1	1.0
French Onion, Chilled, M&S*	½ Pot/300g	150	4.5	50	2.0	7.2	1.5	1.0
French Onion, Favourites, Baxters*	½ Can/200g	68	1.2	34	0.6	6.0	0.6	0.6
French Onion, Knorr*	1 Pack/40g	118	1.0	296	6.0	62.5	2.5	6.6
Garden Pea, Cream of, Jeremy's Soups Ltd*	1 Serving/300g	138	9.3	46	1.6	2.9	3.1	1.2
Garden Vegetable with Barley, Co-Op*	1 Pot/600g	240	0.6	40	2.1	7.4	0.1	0.7
Garden Vegetable, Heinz*	1 Can/400g	160	3.2	40	0.9	7.2	0.8	0.9
Gazpacho, Traditional, Chef Select, Lidl*	¼ Carton/250ml	92	5.5	37	0.9	2.9	2.2	0.0
Goa Carnival, NCG Food Co*	½ Carton/300g	144	8.4	48	1.6	4.9	2.8	1.4
Goan Spiced Tomato & Lentil, Skinny Soup, Glorious!*	½ Pot/300g	153	3.3	51	2.1	8.1	1.1	1.2
Golden Vegetable, Calorie Counter, Cup, Co-Op*	1 Sachet/12g	40	1.2	335	7.0	54.0	10.0	5.0
Golden Vegetable, Cup, GFY, Asda*	1 Sachet/217ml	52	1.1	24	0.5	4.4	0.5	0.2

S

SOUP

INFO/WEIGHT	Measure	per Measure		Nutrition Values per 100g / 100ml				
		KCAL	FAT	KCAL	PROT	CARB	FAT	FIBRE
Golden Vegetable, Dry, Knorr*	1 Pack/76g	299	14.4	394	10.4	45.4	19.0	3.3
Golden Vegetable, Slim a Soup, Batchelors*	1 Sachet/207g	58	1.7	28	0.5	4.7	0.8	0.7
Green Thai Curry, Chicken Noodle, M&S*	1 Pack/256g	333	9.0	130	5.3	18.9	3.5	1.1
Green Vegetables & Lentil, Lima*	1 Serving/300g	96	3.6	32	1.6	3.7	1.2	0.5
Greens & Grains, Skinny Souper, NCG Food Co*	1 Pack/400g	192	4.4	48	2.2	6.8	1.1	2.5
Haddock, Smoked, Chowder, M&S*	½ Pot/300g	180	7.2	60	3.1	6.4	2.4	0.8
Ham Hock, Leek & Potato, Chunky, Soup Pot, Tesco*	1 Pot/350g	174	6.3	50	2.5	5.5	1.8	1.0
Heart of West Africa, Meal Soup, Glorious!*	½ Carton/300g	219	11.1	73	1.9	7.5	3.7	1.2
Hearty Vegetable, 99% Fat Free, Prepared, Campbell's*	1 Can/295g	91	1.2	31	0.8	6.1	0.4	0.0
Highlander's Broth, Favourites, Baxters*	1 Can/400g	192	5.6	48	1.7	6.3	1.4	0.9
Indian Chicken, Glorious!*	½ Pot/300g	201	7.5	67	3.4	7.6	2.5	0.7
Italian Bean & Pasta, Healthy, Baxters*	1 Can/415g	208	1.2	50	2.1	8.6	0.3	2.4
Italian Bean, Fresh, LL, Waitrose*	½ Pot/300g	165	7.2	55	1.6	6.0	2.4	1.7
Italian Meatball Meal, Tesco*	1 Pot/379g	265	6.8	70	2.5	9.6	1.8	0.8
Italian Minestrone, M&S*	1 Can/425g	191	2.1	45	2.2	9.0	0.5	0.8
Italian Plum Tomato & Mascarpone, Finest, Tesco*	1 Pot/600g	360	13.8	60	1.3	7.2	2.3	0.6
Italian Style Tomato & Basil, Co-Op*	1 Pack/500g	200	10.0	40	1.0	4.0	2.0	0.6
Italian Tomato & Basil, Canned, Organic, Suma*	½ Can/200g	82	2.4	41	1.4	5.2	1.2	1.7
Italian Tomato with Basil, Vegetarian, Baxters*	1 Can/415g	170	3.7	41	1.4	5.7	0.9	0.6
Italian Wedding, Deli Inspired, Baxters*	1 Can/400g	199	5.4	48	2.1	6.9	1.3	0.9
Kale & Nutmeg with Ground Black Pepper, NCG Food Co*	½ Carton/300g	99	3.9	33	1.0	3.9	1.3	1.0
Keralan Spiced Chicken, Waitrose*	½ Pot/300g	222	14.1	74	3.9	4.0	4.7	2.2
Lamb & Vegetable, Big Soup, Heinz*	½ Can/200g	120	2.6	60	3.0	9.1	1.3	1.3
Leek & Chicken, Knorr*	1 Serving/300ml	82	5.2	27	0.6	2.4	1.7	0.1
Leek & Maris Piper Potato, Chilled, M&S*	1 Serving/300g	165	11.4	55	0.6	4.5	3.8	0.9
Leek & Potato in a Cup, BGTY, Sainsbury's*	1 Serving/218ml	59	1.5	27	0.3	4.9	0.7	0.2
Leek & Potato in a Mug, Light Choices, Tesco*	1 Sachet/220g	55	0.9	25	0.5	4.9	0.4	0.6
Leek & Potato, Chunky, Meal, Canned, Tesco*	½ Can/200g	60	2.6	30	1.0	3.5	1.3	1.0
Leek & Potato, Creamy, Fresh, Asda*	1 Serving/300g	106	2.4	35	1.0	5.4	0.8	1.2
Leek & Potato, Cup a Soup, Batchelors*	1 Sachet/28g	121	4.9	432	5.2	63.2	17.6	1.8
Leek & Potato, Fresh with Cream, Tesco*	½ Tub/300g	180	7.2	60	1.5	8.0	2.4	0.9
Leek & Potato, Fresh, Chilled, CBY, Asda*	½ Pot/300g	105	2.4	35	1.0	5.4	0.8	1.2
Leek & Potato, Fresh, Sainsbury's*	½ Pot/300ml	141	7.2	47	1.0	5.3	2.4	0.4
Leek & Potato, Fresh, Waitrose*	½ Pot/300g	108	5.1	36	0.7	4.6	1.7	0.9
Leek & Potato, Mix, Asda*	½ Pack/100g	25	0.0	25	0.6	5.7	0.0	1.5
Leek & Potato, Slim a Soup, Batchelors*	1 Serving/204g	57	1.4	28	0.4	5.0	0.7	0.2
Leek & Potato, Soup in a Cup, Made Up, Waitrose*	1 Sachet/204ml	47	1.0	23	0.3	4.3	0.5	0.5
Leek & Potato, Soup in a Mug, HL, Tesco*	1 Serving/16g	54	0.9	336	4.3	67.1	5.6	7.4
Leek & Potato, Weight Watchers*	1 Sachet/215ml	58	1.1	27	0.5	5.1	0.5	0.1
Leek, Cream of, Favourites, Baxters*	1 Can/400g	228	16.8	57	1.1	3.8	4.2	0.7
Lentil & Bacon, Canned, Tesco*	1 Serving/200g	96	1.4	48	3.2	7.2	0.7	0.5
Lentil & Bacon, Classic, Heinz*	1 Can/400g	232	5.6	58	2.7	8.4	1.4	0.7
Lentil & Bacon, Favourites, Baxters*	1 Can/400g	216	4.4	54	3.3	7.4	1.1	0.8
Lentil & Bacon, Morrisons*	1 Can/400g	188	2.0	47	3.1	7.4	0.5	1.1
Lentil & Bacon, Sainsbury's*	½ Pot/300g	199	5.4	66	4.3	8.2	1.8	1.3
Lentil & Smoked Bacon, NCG Food Co*	½ Carton/300g	153	3.0	51	3.7	8.9	1.0	4.3
Lentil & Tomato, NCG Food Co*	½ Pack/284g	162	3.1	57	3.6	8.1	1.1	0.7
Lentil & Tomato, Spicy, Chunky, Fresh, Tesco*	½ Pot/300g	195	5.4	65	2.6	9.7	1.8	1.3
Lentil & Vegetable Soup, Healthy, Baxters*	1 Can/415g	174	1.2	42	1.9	7.4	0.3	1.2
Lentil & Vegetable with Bacon, Organic, Baxters*	½ Can/211g	93	1.5	44	1.9	7.6	0.7	1.0
Lentil & Vegetable, Diet Chef Ltd*	1 Pack/300g	156	0.9	52	2.6	9.6	0.3	2.1
Lentil with Red Lentils, Carrots, Potato & Onion, Asda*	1 Can/400g	192	0.8	48	1.4	10.2	0.2	1.2
Lentil, Asda*	½ Can/202g	89	0.4	44	2.6	8.0	0.2	0.7

S

SOUP

Measure INFO/WEIGHT	per Measure KCAL	FAT	Nutrition Values per 100g / 100ml KCAL	PROT	CARB	FAT	FIBRE
Lentil, Average	*1 Carton/600g*	*594*	*22.8*	*99*	*4.4*	*12.7*	*3.8*	*1.1*
Lentil, Bacon & Mixed Bean, Low Fat, Aldi*	1 Serving/400g	260	3.6	65	4.7	9.5	0.9	1.6
Lentil, Canned	1 Serving/220g	86	0.4	39	3.1	6.5	0.2	1.2
Lentil, Carrot & Cumin, Canned, BGTY, Sainsbury's*	1 Can/400g	204	3.6	51	2.3	8.4	0.9	0.1
Lentil, Classic, Heinz*	1 Can/400g	192	0.8	48	2.3	8.7	0.2	0.8
Lentil, Tomato & Vegetable, M&S*	1 Can/415g	170	3.4	41	2.0	6.3	0.8	1.4
Lobster Bisque, Luxury, with Brandy & Cream, Baxters*	1 Can/400g	272	17.2	68	2.6	4.8	4.3	0.2
Lobster Bisque, NCG Food Co*	½ Carton/300g	108	1.8	36	3.2	4.4	0.6	0.4
Lobster Bisque, Waitrose*	½ Carton/300g	201	13.8	67	0.9	5.5	4.6	0.6
Malaysian Chicken & Sweetcorn, Dry, Knorr*	1 Pack/57g	211	6.5	370	10.6	56.3	11.4	1.8
Mediterranean Fish, Waitrose*	½ Pot/300g	108	2.7	36	3.4	3.5	0.9	0.7
Mediterranean Minestrone, Campbell's*	½ Carton/250ml	95	2.8	38	0.9	6.1	1.1	0.6
Mediterranean Tomato & Vegetable, Fresh, Tesco*	½ Pot/300g	105	2.1	35	1.0	6.2	0.7	0.7
Mediterranean Tomato, Fresh, Organic, Sainsbury's*	1 Serving/250ml	78	3.5	31	1.3	3.3	1.4	1.0
Mediterranean Tomato, Slim a Soup, Cup, Batchelors*	1 Serving/208g	56	1.2	27	0.5	4.8	0.6	0.4
Mediterranean Tomato, Vegetarian, Baxters*	1 Can/400g	126	0.4	32	0.9	5.6	0.1	0.8
Mediterranean Vegetable, GFY, Asda*	½ Pot/250g	80	4.2	32	0.5	3.6	1.7	1.6
Mexican Bean, Safe To Eat*	1 Pouch/400g	140	1.2	35	2.4	4.7	0.3	1.8
Mexican Beef Chilli, Mighty, Asda*	1 Can/400g	192	2.8	48	3.3	7.0	0.7	0.9
Mexican Black Bean, ES, Asda*	½ Pot/263g	194	10.8	74	2.3	7.0	4.1	1.7
Mexican Chilli Beef & Bean, Soups of the World, Heinz*	1 Can/515g	360	9.3	70	4.5	9.0	1.8	1.6
Mexican Chipotle Chicken, NCG Food Co*	½ Carton/300g	186	3.3	62	3.9	8.0	1.1	2.3
Minestrone in a Cup, BGTY, Sainsbury's*	1 Serving/200ml	54	0.2	27	0.8	6.0	0.1	0.6
Minestrone Verde, NCG Food Co*	½ Carton/300g	123	2.4	41	1.8	6.1	0.8	1.2
Minestrone with Basil & Parmesan, Stay Full, Baxters*	1 Can/400g	276	5.2	69	3.5	9.2	1.3	2.6
Minestrone with Croutons in a Cup, Sainsbury's*	1 Sachet/225ml	72	0.9	32	0.9	6.3	0.4	0.5
Minestrone with Croutons in a Mug, Tesco*	1 Sachet/23g	83	1.9	360	9.0	62.6	8.1	2.7
Minestrone with Croutons, Dry, Soupreme, Aldi*	1 Serving/27g	94	1.7	349	7.6	65.3	6.4	4.4
Minestrone with Ditalini Pasta, NCG Food Co*	½ Carton/300g	102	2.1	34	1.2	5.3	0.7	1.0
Minestrone with Meatballs, Fuller Longer, M&S*	1 Pack/400g	260	10.0	65	5.2	5.8	2.5	1.2
Minestrone with Pancetta, NCG Food Co*	1 Carton/600g	306	11.4	51	2.3	5.6	1.9	1.2
Minestrone with Pasta, Chunky, Co-Op*	1 Pack/400g	140	2.4	35	1.0	6.0	0.6	0.7
Minestrone, Canned	1oz/28g	9	0.2	32	1.4	5.1	0.8	0.6
Minestrone, Canned, Average	*1 Can/400g*	*252*	*12.0*	*63*	*1.8*	*7.6*	*3.0*	*0.9*
Minestrone, CBY, Asda*	½ Can/200g	70	1.0	35	0.4	6.4	0.5	1.6
Minestrone, Chilled, M&S*	½ Pot/300g	135	3.9	45	2.0	5.8	1.3	1.9
Minestrone, Chunky, Asda*	½ Tub/300g	111	4.2	37	1.4	4.7	1.4	1.8
Minestrone, Chunky, Classic, Fresh, Tesco*	½ Pot/300g	126	2.1	42	1.2	7.8	0.7	1.2
Minestrone, Chunky, Fresh, Baxters*	1 Serving/250g	95	1.8	38	1.5	6.5	0.7	1.1
Minestrone, Chunky, Fresh, Sainsbury's*	½ Pot/300g	93	0.6	31	1.4	6.1	0.2	2.3
Minestrone, Chunky, Waitrose*	1 Can/415g	195	3.3	47	1.6	8.3	0.8	1.1
Minestrone, Classic, Heinz*	1 Can/400g	128	0.8	32	1.0	6.2	0.2	0.8
Minestrone, Diet Chef Ltd*	1 Pack/300g	123	1.8	41	1.4	7.5	0.6	1.2
Minestrone, Favourites, Baxters*	1 Can/400g	156	2.4	39	1.5	5.5	0.6	1.3
Minestrone, Fresh, Asda*	½ Pot/300g	138	2.1	46	1.8	8.2	0.7	1.2
Minestrone, Fresh, Average	*1 Carton/600g*	*244*	*4.9*	*41*	*1.7*	*6.8*	*0.8*	*1.2*
Minestrone, Fresh, Morrisons*	1 Pot/506ml	182	2.0	36	1.9	6.4	0.4	0.2
Minestrone, Fresh, Tesco*	½ Carton/300g	150	3.3	50	1.6	7.7	1.1	1.3
Minestrone, Fresh, Waitrose*	1 Pack/600g	240	8.4	40	1.1	5.8	1.4	0.8
Minestrone, Instant, Cup, Average	*1 Pack/23g*	*79*	*0.7*	*351*	*7.7*	*72.1*	*3.3*	*3.4*
Minestrone, Packet, Dry, Knorr*	1 Pack/61g	204	2.4	335	12.0	58.8	4.0	6.9
Minestrone, Sainsbury's*	½ Can/200g	66	0.8	33	1.1	6.3	0.4	0.9
Minestrone, Squeeze & Stir, Heinz*	1 Made up/196g	59	1.4	30	0.8	5.0	0.7	0.4

SOUP

	Measure INFO/WEIGHT	per Measure KCAL	FAT	Nutrition Values per 100g / 100ml KCAL	PROT	CARB	FAT	FIBRE
Minestrone, Tuscan, Weight Watchers*	1 Can/295g	121	3.2	41	1.0	6.9	1.1	0.8
Minted Lamb Hot Pot, Big Soup, Heinz*	1 Can/400g	228	5.2	57	2.9	8.1	1.3	1.0
Miso with Tofu, Instant, Kikkoman*	1 Sachet/10g	35	1.0	350	30.0	30.0	10.0	0.0
Miso, Instant, Blue Dragon*	1 Sachet/18g	25	0.7	139	10.0	14.4	3.9	0.0
Miso, Instant, Dry, Sanchi*	1 Sachet/8g	27	0.6	336	18.4	48.6	7.6	0.0
Miso, Japanese, Made Up, Yutaka*	1 Serving/250ml	24	0.7	10	0.6	1.1	0.3	0.0
Miso, Wakama*	1 Sachet/8g	27	0.6	336	18.7	48.6	7.6	0.0
More Bangalore, Skinnylicious, Skinny Soup, Glorious!*	½ Pot/300g	147	4.2	49	2.0	6.1	1.4	2.2
Moreish Mushroom, NCG Food Co*	1 Carton/300g	90	3.0	30	1.3	2.9	1.0	1.4
Moroccan Chicken & Vegetable, LL, Waitrose*	½ Pot/300g	192	5.7	64	3.7	7.9	1.9	1.9
Moroccan Chicken, Finest, Tesco*	½ Pot/300g	180	5.1	60	3.6	6.8	1.7	1.2
Moroccan Chicken, NCG Food Co*	1 Serving/300g	108	5.7	36	2.1	2.7	1.9	0.4
Moroccan Lentil, Waitrose*	½ Pot/300g	153	1.5	51	3.5	8.2	0.5	3.4
Moroccan Style, Spiced Chicken, Eat Well, M&S*	1 Portion/300g	195	9.9	65	4.0	5.3	3.3	4.4
Moroccan Vegetable Harira, Meal Soup, Glorious!*	1 Pot/600g	288	3.6	48	2.0	8.7	0.6	1.1
Mulligatawny	1 Serving/220g	213	15.0	97	1.4	8.2	6.8	0.9
Mulligatawny, Canned, Tesco*	1 Can/400g	188	4.0	47	1.3	8.1	1.0	0.3
Mulligatawny, Classic, Heinz*	1 Can/400g	232	7.6	58	1.9	8.0	1.9	0.5
Mushroom & Chestnut, Fresh, Finest, Tesco*	1 Serving/250g	130	8.2	52	1.1	4.7	3.3	0.7
Mushroom & Chicken, Co-Op*	1 Pack/400g	220	16.0	55	0.9	5.0	4.0	0.0
Mushroom & Crouton, Cup Soup, Made Up, Heinz*	1 Cup/200ml	80	4.2	40	0.7	4.5	2.1	0.0
Mushroom & Garlic, Slimming Cup a Soup, Tesco*	1 Serving/16g	58	1.6	360	5.8	61.1	10.3	3.2
Mushroom Potage, Woodl& Mushrooms, Baxters*	1 Can/415g	328	20.8	79	1.6	6.9	5.0	0.3
Mushroom with Croutons in a Cup, Waitrose*	1 Sachet/212g	102	4.2	48	0.6	6.8	2.0	0.5
Mushroom with Croutons, Soup in a Mug, Tesco*	1 Serving/226ml	115	4.7	51	1.0	6.8	2.1	0.4
Mushroom, Cream of, Canned	1 Serving/220g	101	6.6	46	1.1	3.9	3.0	0.1
Mushroom, Cream of, Canned, Happy Shopper*	½ Can/200g	98	5.0	49	1.2	5.4	2.5	0.0
Mushroom, Cream of, Canned, Tesco*	½ Can/200g	94	5.8	47	0.7	4.8	2.9	0.2
Mushroom, Cream of, Classics, Heinz*	1 Can/400g	208	11.2	52	1.5	5.2	2.8	0.1
Mushroom, Cream of, Condensed, Batchelors*	1 Can/295g	330	25.1	112	1.3	7.5	8.5	0.2
Mushroom, Cream of, Crosse & Blackwell*	1 Can/400g	186	9.9	47	1.3	4.7	2.5	0.0
Mushroom, Cream of, Favourites, Baxters*	1 Can/400g	244	15.2	61	1.0	5.6	3.8	0.2
Mushroom, Cream of, Fresh, Tesco*	½ Tub/300g	96	2.4	32	1.4	4.8	0.8	0.5
Mushroom, Cream of, Porcini, Black Label, Heinz*	1 Can/400g	220	10.8	55	1.7	5.8	2.7	0.2
Mushroom, Cully & Sully*	1 Carton/400g	192	17.6	48	0.8	1.3	4.4	1.0
Mushroom, Diet Chef Ltd*	1 Pack/300g	105	5.1	35	1.9	3.2	1.7	0.9
Mushroom, Dry, Symingtons*	1 Serving/23g	80	2.1	348	17.8	48.4	9.2	6.7
Mushroom, Fresh, Average	***1 Serving/300g***	***146***	***9.3***	***49***	***1.3***	***4.0***	***3.1***	***0.8***
Mushroom, Fresh, M&S*	½ Pack/300g	165	11.7	55	1.8	3.5	3.9	0.9
Mushroom, in a Cup, Sainsbury's*	1 Serving/200ml	96	3.8	48	0.5	7.0	1.9	0.2
Mushroom, Low Fat, Fresh, Sainsbury's*	½ Pot/300g	132	8.7	44	0.7	3.7	2.9	0.6
Mushroom, Thick & Creamy, Mug, Asda*	1 Sachet/226ml	106	2.7	47	0.8	8.0	1.2	0.5
Mushroom, Weight Watchers*	1 Can/295g	83	2.1	28	1.1	4.5	0.7	0.1
Mushroom, Wild, NCG Food Co*	1 Carton/600g	222	7.2	37	1.5	4.1	1.2	0.9
Oriental Spiced Tomato, Skinny Soup, Glorious!*	1 Pot/600g	258	10.8	43	1.0	5.8	1.8	1.1
Oxtail, Average	***1 Can/400g***	***163***	***4.5***	***41***	***2.0***	***5.8***	***1.1***	***0.4***
Oxtail, Canned	1 Serving/220g	97	3.7	44	2.4	5.1	1.7	0.1
Oxtail, Chunky, Meaty, Fresh, M Kitchen, Morrisons*	½ Pot/300g	128	4.2	43	1.9	5.6	1.4	0.0
Oxtail, Classic, Heinz*	1 Can/400g	168	2.0	42	1.9	7.3	0.5	0.3
Oxtail, Cup Soup, Co-Op*	1 Sachet/19g	67	1.7	355	7.0	63.0	9.0	1.0
Oxtail, Diet Chef Ltd*	1 Pack/300g	144	3.6	48	1.8	7.5	1.2	0.5
Oxtail, Favourites, Baxters*	1 Can/400g	192	4.4	48	1.8	6.8	1.1	0.5
Oxtail, For One, Heinz*	1 Can/300g	126	1.5	42	1.9	7.3	0.5	0.3

SOUP

INFO/WEIGHT	Measure	per Measure		Nutrition Values per 100g / 100ml				
		KCAL	FAT	KCAL	PROT	CARB	FAT	FIBRE
Oxtail, Hearty, Canned, Crosse & Blackwell*	1 Can/400g	180	7.6	45	2.1	4.6	1.9	0.3
Oxtail, Soupreme, Aldi*	1 Can/400g	152	2.0	38	2.2	6.0	0.5	0.5
Parsnip & Apple, COU, M&S*	1 Can/415g	187	10.4	45	0.7	5.4	2.5	1.2
Parsnip & Chilli, Diet Chef Ltd*	1 Serving/300g	102	4.2	34	0.8	5.4	1.4	1.3
Parsnip & Honey, Fresh, Sainsbury's*	½ Carton/300g	192	12.6	64	1.1	5.4	4.2	1.5
Parsnip & Orchard Apple, Duchy Originals*	1 Pack/350g	116	3.2	33	0.7	5.4	0.9	1.0
Parsnip, Creamy, NCG Food Co*	½ Carton/300g	174	9.0	58	1.2	6.6	3.0	1.6
Parsnip, Fresh, Morrisons*	½ Pot/250g	100	3.8	40	0.9	5.8	1.5	1.4
Parsnip, Fresh, VLH Kitchens	1 Serving/400g	180	0.4	45	0.9	5.8	1.6	1.4
Parsnip, Mr Bean's*	1 Tin/400g	208	7.6	52	1.9	6.7	1.9	0.0
Parsnip, Spicy, Average	*1 Serving/400g*	*212*	*11.2*	*53*	*0.9*	*6.0*	*2.8*	*1.6*
Parsnip, Spicy, Fresh, Tesco*	1 Serving/300g	123	6.3	41	0.8	4.6	2.1	1.9
Pasta, Tomato & Basil, Bertolli*	1 Serving/100g	47	1.1	47	1.5	7.9	1.1	1.6
Pea & Ground Sesame, NCG Food Co*	1 Serving/300g	144	5.9	48	3.1	3.4	2.0	1.9
Pea & Ham, Canned, Favourites, Baxters*	1 Can/400g	218	4.0	55	3.3	7.1	1.0	2.0
Pea & Ham, Canned, Tesco*	1 Can/400g	240	4.4	60	2.6	9.0	1.1	0.8
Pea & Ham, CBY, Asda*	1 Pot/600g	282	6.6	47	2.9	5.6	1.1	1.4
Pea & Ham, Classic, Heinz*	1 Can/400g	252	3.2	63	2.8	10.1	0.8	1.1
Pea & Ham, Diet Chef Ltd*	1 Portion/300g	138	3.3	46	3.2	5.8	1.1	2.6
Pea & Ham, Diet Chef Ltd*	1 Pack/300g	138	3.3	46	3.2	5.8	1.1	2.6
Pea & Ham, Eat Well, M&S*	½ Can/207g	93	2.1	45	3.7	5.1	1.0	2.2
Pea & Ham, Fresh, Sainsbury's*	½ Pack/300ml	120	1.5	40	1.9	7.0	0.5	0.3
Pea & Ham, Fresh, Waitrose*	1 Serving/300g	196	10.0	65	2.9	6.2	3.3	1.6
Pea & Ham, TTD, Sainsbury's*	1 Bowl/300g	188	7.2	63	3.7	6.0	2.4	1.2
Pea & Mint, Fresh, CBY, Asda*	½ Pot/300g	111	0.6	37	2.1	6.0	0.2	1.3
Pea & Mint, Fresh, Co-Op*	½ Tub/300g	105	1.7	35	1.7	4.8	0.6	1.8
Pea & Mint, Fresh, Finest, Tesco*	1 Serving/300g	165	7.2	55	1.3	6.0	2.4	1.5
Pea & Mint, Fresh, M&S*	1 Serving/164g	49	0.2	30	1.8	6.3	0.1	1.5
Pea & Mint, Fresh, Sainsbury's*	½ Pot/300g	102	2.7	34	1.4	5.0	0.9	1.9
Pea & Mint, with Leek, Fresh, Waitrose*	1 Serving/300g	123	4.5	41	1.7	4.4	1.5	1.5
Pepper, Sweetcorn & Chilli, Mexican, TTD, Sainsbury's*	½ Pot/300g	190	6.6	63	2.4	7.2	2.2	3.0
Pepper, with Chilli, Italiamo, Lidl*	1 Can/390ml	222	9.4	57	0.6	7.6	2.4	1.3
Perfect Pea, NCG Food Co*	1 Carton/300g	93	0.9	31	1.7	4.6	0.3	1.7
Plum Tomato & Basil, NCG Food Co*	½ Carton/300g	132	6.0	44	1.3	5.2	2.0	1.3
Potato & Leek	1oz/28g	15	0.7	52	1.5	6.2	2.6	0.8
Potato & Leek with Peppers & Chicken, Stockmeyer*	½ Can/200g	118	4.8	59	2.6	6.7	2.4	0.8
Potato & Leek, Canned, Sainsbury's*	½ Can/200g	92	3.2	46	1.0	6.7	1.6	0.3
Potato & Leek, Classics, Canned, Heinz*	1 Can/400g	184	7.2	46	0.8	6.7	1.8	0.6
Potato & Leek, Favourites, Baxters*	1 Can/400g	192	7.2	48	1.0	6.6	1.8	0.9
Potato & Leek, Instant, Cup, Average	*1 Pack/22g*	*83*	*1.9*	*379*	*5.0*	*70.0*	*8.7*	*4.0*
Potato & Leek, Thick & Tasty, Cup Soup, Morrisons*	1 Sachet/226ml	97	2.0	43	0.4	8.4	0.9	0.5
Potato, Leek & Bacon, Fresh, Baxters*	½ Pot/300g	249	16.8	83	2.0	6.1	5.6	0.7
Potato, Leek & Chicken, Canned, BGTY, Sainsbury's*	½ Can/200g	62	0.8	31	1.6	5.3	0.4	0.4
Pumpkin Ghoulash, NCG Food Co*	1 Carton/600g	186	1.2	31	1.3	5.2	0.2	1.2
Pumpkin, Creamy, Very Special, Heinz*	1 Sm Can/290g	188	5.5	65	1.3	9.9	1.9	1.1
Pumpkin, Spicy, Fresh, Sainsbury's*	½ Pot/300g	87	3.0	29	0.9	4.2	1.0	1.3
Puy Lentil & Vine Ripened Tomato, Finest, Tesco*	1 Pot/600g	360	7.8	60	2.8	9.2	1.3	1.5
Red Lentil & Chilli, Fresh, LL, Waitrose*	½ Pot/300g	138	4.5	46	1.7	6.4	1.5	1.3
Red Lentil & Ham, Waitrose*	½ Pot/300g	147	3.3	49	3.9	5.8	1.1	2.0
Red Lentil & Smoked Bacon, M&S*	½ Pot/300g	225	9.6	75	4.3	6.6	3.2	1.9
Red Lentil & Tomato, Canned, Tesco*	½ Can/300g	189	3.9	63	4.0	8.9	1.3	1.1
Red Lentil & Vegetable, Favourites, Baxters*	1 Can/400g	192	2.0	48	2.6	8.3	0.5	1.2
Red Pepper & Wensleydale, Asda*	1 Carton/600g	306	12.6	51	2.5	5.0	2.1	0.8

S

SOUP

INFO/WEIGHT	Measure	per Measure		Nutrition Values per 100g / 100ml				
		KCAL	FAT	KCAL	PROT	CARB	FAT	FIBRE
Red Pepper, Tomato & Basil, M&S*	1 Can/415g	83	1.2	20	1.3	2.7	0.3	0.8
Rice & Noodle, Instant, Thai Kitchen*	1 Pack/45g	190	3.0	422	6.7	82.2	6.7	0.0
Roast Sweet Potato, Quinoa & Corn, Coles*	1 Bag/430g	150	1.7	35	1.2	5.9	0.4	1.2
Roasted Red Pepper & Tomato, Canned, Sainsbury's*	1 Can/400g	196	6.0	49	1.0	7.5	1.5	0.9
Roasted Red Pepper & Tomato, M&S*	1 Serving/150g	105	7.4	70	1.4	5.0	4.9	0.6
Roasted Red Pepper & Tomato, Weight Watchers*	1 Can/400g	136	0.4	34	0.7	7.7	0.1	0.6
Roasted Red Pepper, Finest, Tesco*	1 Pot/600g	290	12.6	48	1.4	5.4	2.1	1.1
Roasted Red Pepper, Fresh, Waitrose*	1 Pack/600g	172	9.0	29	0.8	3.0	1.5	1.0
Roasted Vegetable, Chunky, M&S*	1 Can/400g	140	2.4	35	1.3	5.8	0.6	1.1
Roasted Vegetable, Fresh, Sainsbury's*	½ Pot/300ml	78	1.5	26	0.5	4.8	0.5	1.2
Root Vegetable & Barley, Broth, Special, Heinz*	1 Can/400g	188	6.0	47	0.9	7.4	1.5	1.1
Root Vegetable, Medley, NCG Food Co*	1 Pot/600ml	168	4.8	28	0.7	4.9	0.8	1.1
Royal Game, Favourites, Baxters*	1 Can/400g	152	0.8	38	1.8	6.9	0.2	0.3
Scotch Broth, British, Sainsbury's*	1 Can/415g	149	2.9	36	1.9	5.4	0.7	0.9
Scotch Broth, Canned, Tesco*	½ Can/200g	85	2.6	42	1.3	5.9	1.3	0.8
Scotch Broth, Classic, Heinz*	1 Can/400g	156	2.4	39	1.4	6.7	0.6	0.6
Scotch Broth, Co-Op*	1 Can/400g	220	5.2	55	2.7	7.9	1.3	2.3
Scotch Broth, Favourites, Baxters*	1 Can/400g	196	6.0	49	1.8	6.2	1.5	1.5
Scotch Broth, Fresh, Baxters*	1 Serving/300g	108	2.1	36	1.6	5.9	0.7	0.6
Scotch Broth, Fresh, Tesco*	½ Pack/300g	129	5.4	43	1.7	5.0	1.8	1.4
Scotch Broth, M&S*	1 Serving/300g	150	7.2	50	2.1	5.1	2.4	1.1
Scotch Vegetable with Lamb, Favourites, Baxters*	1 Can/400g	172	2.0	43	2.0	7.6	0.5	1.7
Seafood Chowder, Waitrose*	1 Can/404g	226	11.3	56	2.2	5.6	2.8	0.6
Seven Vegetable, Canned, Farmers Market, Heinz*	1 Can/400g	228	8.0	57	0.7	8.2	2.0	1.4
Shrimp Dumpling Udon, Abokado*	1 Pot/730g	356	8.4	49	2.9	10.4	1.2	0.2
Sicilian Tomato & Balsamic, Skinny Soup, Glorious!*	½ Pot/300g	90	3.0	30	1.1	2.9	1.0	0.0
Smoked Bacon & Bean, Diet Chef Ltd*	1 Pack/300g	162	3.3	54	2.8	8.2	1.1	2.1
Smoked Bacon & Three Bean, Chunky, Baxters*	1 Can/400g	232	4.8	58	2.9	8.8	1.2	1.8
Smoked Haddock Chowder, NCG Food Co*	½ Carton/300g	125	4.2	42	1.9	4.8	1.4	1.4
Smoked Salmon & Dill, Fresh, Finest, Tesco*	½ Carton/300g	240	16.5	80	2.2	5.3	5.5	0.6
Smokey Plum Tomato & Black Bean Soup, NCG Food Co*	½ Carton/302g	124	1.8	41	2.0	7.0	0.6	1.7
Smoky Tomato, Atkins & Potts*	1 Pack/400g	336	23.2	84	1.1	6.1	5.8	0.6
Soup, Leek & Potato, Fresh, Sainsbury's*	½ Pot/300g	114	3.6	38	0.7	6.1	1.2	1.3
Spiced Spinach & Green Lentil, Asda*	½ Pot/250g	122	5.0	49	2.7	5.0	2.0	0.0
Spicy Butternut Squash & Sweet Potato, NCG Food Co*	½ Carton/300g	120	3.6	40	0.8	6.0	1.2	1.0
Spicy Corn Chowder, NCG Food Co*	½ Carton/300g	132	5.4	44	1.6	4.3	1.8	2.2
Spicy Lentil & Vegetable, Chilled, M&S*	½ Serving/300g	150	2.4	50	2.7	8.0	0.8	1.1
Spicy Lentil, in a Mug, Light Choices, Tesco*	1 Sachet/221ml	62	0.0	28	1.1	5.9	0.0	0.0
Spicy Parsnip, NCG Food Co*	½ Box/297g	116	3.9	39	0.9	5.8	1.3	1.8
Spicy Parsnip, Vegetarian, Baxters*	1 Can/425g	212	10.6	50	0.7	5.3	2.5	1.7
Spicy Sweetcorn, Fresh, NCG Food Co*	½ Carton/300g	159	4.8	53	1.4	7.8	1.6	0.7
Spicy Tomato & Rice with Sweetcorn, Healthy, Baxters*	1 Can/414g	211	0.8	51	1.6	9.2	0.2	1.0
Spicy Tomato & Vegetable, Healthy Living, Co-Op*	1 Can/400g	180	3.2	45	2.0	8.0	0.8	2.0
Spicy Tomato, Cup a Soup, Batchelors*	1 Sachet/23g	74	0.7	322	7.6	65.8	3.2	3.2
Spicy, Three Bean, Tesco*	½ Carton/300g	165	4.5	55	2.8	7.3	1.5	2.1
Spinach & Watercress, NCG Food Co*	½ Carton/298g	60	1.2	20	1.3	2.8	0.4	0.8
Spirulina Greens, Super Boost, Soupologie*	1 Serving/300g	81	4.8	27	1.1	1.4	1.6	0.8
Split Pea & Ham, Asda*	1 Serving/300g	129	0.6	43	3.5	6.9	0.2	0.7
Split Peas, Yellow, Simply Organic*	1 Pot/600g	354	3.0	59	4.3	10.4	0.5	2.6
Spring Vegetable, Classic, Heinz*	1 Can/400g	148	1.6	37	0.8	7.0	0.4	0.8
Spring Vegetable, Sainsbury's*	½ Can/200g	72	0.8	36	0.8	7.4	0.4	0.6
Squash, Butternut & Ginger, Waitrose*	½ Pot/300g	210	17.4	70	0.9	3.5	5.8	1.0
Squash, Butternut, Curried, & Lentil, Seeds of Change*	1 Pack/400g	164	1.2	41	2.3	7.2	0.3	1.9

SOUP

INFO/WEIGHT	Measure	per Measure		Nutrition Values per 100g / 100ml				
		KCAL	FAT	KCAL	PROT	CARB	FAT	FIBRE
Starry Thai Sky, SkinnyLicious, Skinny Soup, Glorious!*	1 Pot/600g	192	8.4	32	1.0	3.5	1.4	0.8
Steak & Onion, Angus, Big Soup, Heinz*	½ Can/250g	135	2.1	54	3.3	7.7	0.8	0.9
Steak & Potato, Angus, Big Soup, Heinz*	½ Can/250g	120	2.0	48	3.1	6.8	0.8	0.6
Stilton, Celery & Watercress, Morrisons*	1 Serving/250g	272	23.0	109	3.9	3.1	9.2	0.3
Summer Vegetable, NCG Food Co*	1 Carton/600g	336	14.4	56	1.7	6.5	2.4	0.7
Sun Dried Tomato & Basil, Heinz*	1 Serving/275ml	124	5.2	45	0.6	6.5	1.9	0.1
Sunny Thai Chicken, Glorious!*	½ Pot/300g	201	6.6	67	3.6	8.3	2.2	1.0
Super Chicken Noodle, Dry, Knorr*	1 Pack/56g	182	2.7	325	14.3	56.0	4.9	1.8
Super Sweet Potato & Black Bean, M&S*	½ Pot/300g	189	4.5	63	2.6	8.2	1.5	3.3
Super Vegetable, M&S*	½ Pot/300g	120	4.2	40	1.0	5.0	1.4	1.2
Superbean, Lentil & Barley, M&S*	1 Pack/600g	270	9.0	45	1.8	5.1	1.5	2.1
Sweet Green Pea, with Mint, Duchy Originals, Waitrose*	½ Pot/300g	168	7.8	56	2.2	5.2	2.6	1.4
Sweet Potato & Coconut, COU, M&S*	1 Can/415g	166	5.4	40	0.7	6.7	1.3	0.8
Sweetcorn & Chilli, COU, M&S*	½ Can/275g	138	6.6	50	0.9	6.1	2.4	0.4
Sweetcorn, Cream of, Campbell's*	1 Serving/80g	41	2.2	51	0.6	6.2	2.7	0.5
Tangy Tomato, Slim a Soup, Batchelors*	1 Serving/230ml	81	1.0	35	1.1	6.7	0.4	0.5
Thai Chicken, Cully & Sully*	1 Pack/400g	204	7.2	51	2.7	6.4	1.8	0.6
Thai Chicken, NCG Food Co*	½ Carton/300g	174	10.5	58	2.6	4.1	3.5	0.8
Thai Chicken, Whole & Hearty, CBY, Asda*	1 Pot/400g	265	8.4	66	4.3	7.1	2.1	0.9
Thai Pumpkin Coconut, NCG Food Co*	1 Carton/568ml	182	7.4	32	1.3	3.5	1.3	1.1
Three Bean & Vegetable, HL, Tesco*	1 Portion/200g	90	0.6	45	2.1	7.5	0.3	1.9
Three Bean & Vegetable, Light Choices, Tesco*	½ Can/200g	110	0.6	55	2.6	9.7	0.3	1.9
Timeless Tuscany, Meal Soup, Glorious!*	½ Carton/300g	120	1.2	40	2.8	6.2	0.4	0.7
Tomato & Basil, CBY, Asda*	½ Pot/297g	89	2.4	30	1.0	4.3	0.8	0.7
Tomato & Basil, Creamy, Cully & Sully*	1 Pack/400g	216	18.5	54	0.8	2.5	4.6	0.5
Tomato & Basil, Cup a Soup, Made Up, GFY, Asda*	1 Serving/250ml	50	0.2	20	0.4	4.4	0.1	0.2
Tomato & Basil, Cup, Co-Op*	1 Sachet/45g	158	1.8	350	2.0	76.0	4.0	4.0
Tomato & Basil, Fresh, Avonmore*	1 Sm Carton/250g	135	7.5	54	1.2	5.5	3.0	0.2
Tomato & Basil, Fresh, Finest, Tesco*	½ Pot/300g	219	14.7	73	1.0	6.3	4.9	0.6
Tomato & Basil, Fresh, Low Fat, Sainsbury's*	½ Carton/300ml	75	1.8	25	1.1	4.1	0.6	0.7
Tomato & Basil, Fresh, M Kitchen, Morrisons*	½ Pot/300g	115	3.6	38	1.0	5.5	1.2	0.7
Tomato & Basil, Fresh, M&S*	½ Pot/300g	120	5.1	40	1.0	5.0	1.7	1.3
Tomato & Basil, Fresh, Sainsbury's*	½ Pot/300g	114	3.0	38	1.1	5.9	1.0	0.7
Tomato & Basil, Fresh, The Fresh Soup Company*	½ Pot/250g	85	2.2	34	1.3	5.1	0.9	0.6
Tomato & Basil, Fresh, Waitrose*	½ Pot/300g	109	3.9	36	1.0	4.9	1.3	0.7
Tomato & Basil, GFY, Asda*	1 Serving/250ml	100	3.5	40	0.9	6.0	1.4	1.6
Tomato & Basil, Instant, Cup, Average	**1 Pack/22g**	**76**	**1.2**	**346**	**6.1**	**67.8**	**5.4**	**4.2**
Tomato & Basil, Soup-A-Slim, Asda*	1 Sachet/16g	52	0.3	326	7.0	70.0	2.0	3.9
Tomato & Basil, Squeeze & Stir, Heinz*	1 Made Up/196g	114	5.7	58	0.9	6.8	2.9	0.4
Tomato & Basil, Weight Watchers*	1 Serving/295g	77	1.8	26	0.6	4.4	0.6	0.5
Tomato & Lentil, Organic, Tideford*	1 Carton/300g	120	2.7	40	2.3	8.1	0.9	0.9
Tomato & Lentil, Truly Irresistible, Co-Op*	½ Pot/300g	165	2.1	55	3.1	8.0	0.7	1.2
Tomato & Orange, HE, Tesco*	1 Pack/400g	132	0.8	33	0.6	7.1	0.2	0.4
Tomato & Red Pepper, Cream of, Sainsbury's*	½ Can/200g	125	6.0	63	1.0	7.9	3.0	1.0
Tomato & Spinach, Organic, Waitrose*	1 Serving/300g	126	5.7	42	1.4	4.9	1.9	0.7
Tomato & Three Bean, Canned, BGTY, Sainsbury's*	½ Can/200g	120	2.2	60	2.8	8.4	1.1	2.4
Tomato & Three Bean, Co-Op*	½ Can/200g	130	1.8	65	3.7	10.2	0.9	2.0
Tomato & Vegetable, Cup a Soup, Batchelors*	1 Serving/218g	107	2.6	49	1.1	8.5	1.2	0.6
Tomato & Vegetable, Organic, Baxters*	1 Can/400g	200	3.2	50	1.6	9.2	0.8	0.8
Tomato, & Basil, Canned, M&S*	1 Can/400g	140	2.8	35	0.7	5.8	0.7	0.5
Tomato, & Fire Roasted Pepper, Mexican, Skinny, Glorious!*	½ Pot/300g	93	5.7	31	0.9	2.4	1.9	0.0
Tomato, Canned, HL, Tesco*	½ Can/200g	110	4.0	55	0.7	7.4	2.0	0.5
Tomato, Canned, Light Choices, Tesco*	½ Can/200g	90	3.8	45	0.9	5.9	1.9	0.4

S

	Measure INFO/WEIGHT	per Measure KCAL	FAT	Nutrition Values per 100g / 100ml KCAL	PROT	CARB	FAT	FIBRE

SOUP

	Measure INFO/WEIGHT	KCAL	FAT	KCAL	PROT	CARB	FAT	FIBRE
Tomato, Chunky, Organic, Canned, Amy's Kitchen*	1 Can/400g	212	5.6	53	1.2	8.6	1.4	1.2
Tomato, Co-Op*	½ Can/200g	80	2.6	40	0.7	6.9	1.3	0.2
Tomato, Cream of with a Hint of Basil, Heinz*	½ Can/200g	114	6.0	57	0.9	6.6	3.0	0.4
Tomato, Cream of with Red Pepper, Classic, Heinz*	1 Can/400g	232	11.6	58	0.9	7.0	2.9	0.6
Tomato, Cream of, Asda*	½ Can/200g	122	6.4	61	0.7	7.3	3.2	0.7
Tomato, Cream of, Canned, Average	*1 Can/400g*	*208*	*12.0*	*52*	*0.8*	*5.9*	*3.0*	*0.7*
Tomato, Cream of, Canned, Crosse & Blackwell*	1 Can/400g	228	10.0	57	0.9	7.4	2.5	0.8
Tomato, Cream of, Canned, Tesco*	½ Can/192g	115	4.8	60	0.9	7.4	2.5	0.8
Tomato, Cream of, Classic, Heinz*	½ Can/200g	118	6.0	59	0.9	6.7	3.0	0.4
Tomato, Cream of, Classics, Soupreme, Aldi*	1 Can/400g	192	8.0	48	0.8	6.4	2.0	0.8
Tomato, Cream of, Condensed, Batchelors*	1 Can/295g	454	19.5	154	1.7	21.9	6.6	0.6
Tomato, Cream of, for One, Heinz*	1 Can/300g	189	10.8	63	0.8	6.9	3.6	0.4
Tomato, Cream of, Fresh, Sainsbury's*	1 Pot/600g	318	19.2	53	0.8	5.2	3.2	1.3
Tomato, Cream of, Fresh, Waitrose*	½ Pot/300g	99	2.1	33	1.1	5.6	0.7	1.5
Tomato, Cream of, in a Cup, Sainsbury's*	1 Sachet/233ml	112	2.1	48	0.7	9.3	0.9	0.1
Tomato, Cream of, Kick of Chilli, Black Label, Heinz*	1 Can/400g	232	12.0	58	0.9	6.6	3.0	0.4
Tomato, Cream of, Mexican Spices, Black Label, Heinz*	1 Can/400g	244	12.0	61	1.0	7.1	3.0	0.5
Tomato, Cream of, Morrisons*	1 Serving/205g	141	6.2	69	1.2	9.4	3.0	0.6
Tomato, Cream of, Organic, Heinz*	1 Can/400g	220	10.4	55	1.0	7.0	2.6	0.4
Tomato, Cream of, Prepared, Campbell's*	½ Can/295g	195	9.4	66	0.8	8.5	3.2	0.0
Tomato, Cream of, Sainsbury's*	1 Can/400g	244	12.8	61	0.7	7.3	3.2	0.7
Tomato, Cream of, with Spanish Chorizo, Heinz*	1 Can/400g	244	12.0	61	1.4	6.9	3.0	0.3
Tomato, Cup a Soup, Made Up, Batchelors*	1 Sachet/256g	92	2.3	36	0.3	6.7	0.9	0.3
Tomato, Diet Chef Ltd*	1 Pack/300g	159	5.4	53	1.3	7.7	1.8	1.2
Tomato, Fresh, Tesco*	1 Serving/100g	44	2.3	44	0.7	5.2	2.3	0.4
Tomato, Lighter Life*	1 Pack/36g	125	2.6	347	34.7	33.9	7.2	7.5
Tomato, Mediterranean, Rich, Fresh, Baxters*	1 Carton/600g	318	10.2	53	1.8	7.7	1.7	1.1
Tomato, Original, Cup a Soup, Batchelors*	1 Sachet/24g	90	2.1	387	3.9	70.5	9.0	3.4
Tomato, Red Pepper & Basil, Thick & Creamy, Asda*	1 Sachet/24g	89	2.3	370	5.6	65.7	9.4	5.5
Tomato, Red Pepper & Pesto, 99 Calories, NCG Food Co*	1 Pack/300g	99	3.9	33	1.0	4.3	1.3	1.0
Tomato, Singapore Crushed, Skinny Soup, Glorious!*	½ Pot/300g	129	5.4	43	1.0	5.8	1.8	1.1
Tomato, Slow Roasted, NCG Food Co*	½ Carton/300g	96	1.5	32	0.9	5.5	0.5	1.1
Tomato, Smart Price, Asda*	1 Can/400g	184	7.6	46	0.6	6.5	1.9	0.9
Tomato, Vegetable & Lentils, Warming, NCG Food Co*	1 Serving/300g	138	2.4	46	2.2	6.6	0.8	1.6
Tomato, Weight Watchers*	1 Can/295g	76	1.5	26	0.7	4.6	0.5	0.3
Traditional Vegetable, Knorr*	1 Serving/200ml	42	0.2	21	1.0	3.2	0.1	1.0
Turkey Broth, Canned, Baxters*	½ Can/208g	79	1.5	38	1.3	6.5	0.7	0.7
Turkey Broth, Favourites, Baxters*	1 Can/400g	152	2.8	38	1.3	6.5	0.7	0.7
Tuscan Bean, Canned, HL, Tesco*	½ Can/200ml	140	3.6	70	3.5	10.3	1.8	1.3
Tuscan Bean, Chunky, LL, Waitrose*	½ Can/200g	101	1.0	50	2.6	7.6	0.5	2.3
Tuscan Bean, NCG Food Co*	½ Carton/300g	84	2.4	28	1.6	3.7	0.8	1.0
Tuscan Chicken & Orzo, Glorious!*	½ Pot/300g	120	1.2	40	2.8	6.2	0.4	0.7
Vegetable & Barley Broth, Canned, Organic, Sainsbury's*	½ Can/200g	48	0.8	24	1.4	3.7	0.4	0.9
Vegetable & Lentil, Waitrose*	½ Pot/300g	138	4.5	46	2.9	5.2	1.5	3.5
Vegetable Broth, Canned, HL, Tesco*	½ Can/200g	74	0.4	37	1.2	7.4	0.2	1.0
Vegetable Broth, Hearty, Weight Watchers*	1 Can/295g	135	0.6	46	2.0	8.2	0.2	1.4
Vegetable Curry, CBY, Asda*	½ Pot/300g	240	2.1	80	4.5	13.3	0.7	1.1
Vegetable Mulligatawny, Tesco*	½ Pack/300g	210	7.5	70	1.9	9.0	2.5	1.1
Vegetable with Croutons, Soup in a Mug, Tesco*	1 Pack/23g	90	3.7	392	6.2	55.2	16.3	8.0
Vegetable, Asda*	1 Can/400g	144	1.6	36	1.1	7.0	0.4	0.8
Vegetable, Batchelors*	1 Can/400g	168	3.6	42	1.0	5.3	0.9	4.4
Vegetable, Canned	1oz/28g	13	0.2	48	1.4	9.9	0.6	1.5
Vegetable, Canned, Average	*1 Can/400g*	*208*	*16.0*	*52*	*0.9*	*3.2*	*4.0*	*0.9*

S

	Measure INFO/WEIGHT	KCAL	FAT	KCAL	PROT	CARB	FAT	FIBRE
SOUP								
Vegetable, Canned, Essential, Waitrose*	½ Can/200g	103	1.0	52	1.9	9.2	0.5	1.4
Vegetable, Canned, Tesco*	½ Can/200g	70	1.0	35	1.1	5.9	0.5	1.0
Vegetable, Chunky, Canned, Sainsbury's*	1 Can/400g	184	2.8	46	1.5	8.3	0.7	1.2
Vegetable, Chunky, Canned, Soupreme, Aldi*	1 Can/400g	172	4.0	43	1.1	6.4	1.0	2.3
Vegetable, Chunky, Fresh, Organic, Simply Organic*	½ Tub/300g	153	4.5	51	1.9	9.0	1.5	1.4
Vegetable, Chunky, Fresh, Tesco*	1 Serving/300g	123	5.7	41	0.6	5.5	1.9	1.0
Vegetable, Chunky, Organic, Tesco*	½ Pot/300g	150	3.6	50	1.7	8.0	1.2	2.1
Vegetable, Classic, Heinz*	1 Can/400g	188	3.2	47	1.1	8.3	0.8	0.9
Vegetable, Cream of, Cup a Soup, Batchelors*	1 Sachet/33g	134	5.3	406	5.8	59.8	16.0	6.2
Vegetable, Cream of, Cup a Soup, Soupreme, Aldi*	1 Pack/21g	73	2.2	356	4.9	59.5	10.7	6.3
Vegetable, Cream of, Cup Soup, Soupreme, Aldi*	1 Serving/27g	95	2.8	352	4.8	59.6	10.5	6.3
Vegetable, Cream of, Fresh, Sainsbury's*	1 Pot/600g	216	12.6	36	0.5	3.8	2.1	1.2
Vegetable, Cream of, Velouté De Légumes, Liebig*	1 Portion/200ml	84	4.0	42	0.7	5.3	2.0	1.0
Vegetable, Cully & Sully*	1 Pack/400g	204	14.4	51	0.6	4.2	3.6	0.9
Vegetable, Cup Soup, Dry, Heinz*	1 Sachet/16g	54	1.1	348	5.8	64.5	7.1	3.2
Vegetable, Cup Soup, Eat Smart, Morrisons*	1 Pack/213ml	51	1.1	24	0.4	4.4	0.5	0.4
Vegetable, Cup Soup, Made Up, Heinz*	1 Cup/200g	50	1.0	25	0.4	4.7	0.5	0.2
Vegetable, Cup, Soupreme, Aldi*	1 Sachet/26g	115	6.1	444	8.1	49.7	23.6	2.3
Vegetable, Extra Thick, Canned, Sainsbury's*	1 Can/400g	184	2.4	46	1.5	8.6	0.6	1.4
Vegetable, for One, Heinz*	1 Can/300g	129	2.1	43	1.1	8.1	0.7	0.9
Vegetable, Fresh, Average	**1 Serving/300g**	**118**	**4.1**	**40**	**1.4**	**5.4**	**1.4**	**1.3**
Vegetable, From Heinz, Canned, Weight Watchers*	1 Can/295g	86	0.9	29	0.9	5.6	0.3	0.8
Vegetable, in a Cup, BGTY, Sainsbury's*	1 Sachet/200g	52	1.6	26	0.5	4.4	0.8	0.9
Vegetable, in a Cup, HL, Tesco*	1 Sachet/18g	66	1.4	367	7.2	66.1	7.8	2.8
Vegetable, Instant, Cup, Average	**1 Pack/19g**	**69**	**2.0**	**362**	**8.7**	**57.1**	**10.5**	**5.5**
Vegetable, Lentil & Pearl Barley, Rootiful, NCG Food Co*	½ Carton/300g	162	3.9	54	2.4	7.2	1.3	1.6
Vegetable, Moroccan, LL, Waitrose*	1 Pack/300g	172	3.3	57	1.9	9.7	1.1	0.5
Vegetable, Soup in a Mug, As Consumed, HL, Tesco*	1 Serving/218ml	70	1.2	30	0.7	5.5	0.5	0.4
Vegetable, Soup-A-Cups, Asda*	1 Sachet/200ml	59	1.1	30	0.6	5.5	0.6	0.4
Vegetable, Soupreme, Aldi*	½ Can/200g	62	0.8	31	1.2	4.8	0.4	1.6
Vegetable, Tesco*	½ Carton/200g	78	2.6	39	0.9	5.8	1.3	1.0
Vegetable, Wholesome, Heat Eat & Enjoy, Lidl*	1 Carton/400g	208	14.4	52	0.9	3.6	3.6	1.0
Veloute de Cresson, Knorr*	1 Bowl/250ml	50	1.8	20	0.3	3.0	0.7	0.2
Vine Ripened Tomato & Basil, Fresh, Avonmore*	1 Serving/300g	141	8.1	47	1.0	4.7	2.7	0.3
West Indian Chicken, Bowl, Bowl Soups*	1 Bowl/400g	240	4.8	60	2.4	8.1	1.2	1.4
Wild Mushroom & Maderia, Fresh, Finest, Tesco*	½ Tub/300g	250	16.8	85	2.1	5.2	5.7	0.7
Winter Vegetable, Broth, Classic, Heinz*	1 Serving/200g	56	0.2	28	0.8	5.3	0.1	0.8
Winter Vegetable, NCG Food Co*	½ Pack/300g	117	2.1	39	2.0	5.1	0.7	2.3
Wonton, Blue Dragon*	1 Can/410g	102	5.3	25	1.2	2.0	1.3	0.2
SOUP MIX								
Leek & Potato, As Sold, Good & Balanced, Asda*	¼ Pack/125g	69	0.4	55	1.7	10.5	0.3	1.7
Leek & Potato, Made Up, Sainsbury's*	½ Pack/204g	39	0.4	19	0.6	3.6	0.2	0.5
Pea & Ham, Traditional, King	1 Serving/200ml	66	0.4	33	2.2	5.9	0.2	0.0
Soup & Broth Mix, Dry, Wholefoods, Tesco*	¼ Pack/125g	456	2.4	365	14.7	71.4	1.9	7.3
SOUTHERN COMFORT								
37.5% Volume	**1 Pub Shot/35ml**	**72**	**0.0**	**207**	**0.0**	**0.0**	**0.0**	**0.0**
SOYA								
Barbeque Chilli, Vegelicious, Tesco*	1 Portion/450g	450	15.8	100	3.1	12.9	3.5	2.7
Chunks, Protein, Natural, Nature's Harvest*	1 Serving/50g	172	0.5	345	50.0	35.0	1.0	4.0
Mince, Dry Weight, Sainsbury's*	1 Serving/50g	164	0.4	328	47.2	33.2	0.8	3.6
Mince, Granules	**1oz/28g**	**74**	**1.5**	**263**	**43.2**	**11.0**	**5.4**	**0.0**
SPAGHETTI								
Brown Rice, Gluten Free, Organic, Dove's Farm*	1 Serving/70g	237	1.0	338	7.9	70.3	1.5	4.1

S

	Measure INFO/WEIGHT	per Measure KCAL	FAT	Nutrition Values per 100g / 100ml KCAL	PROT	CARB	FAT	FIBRE
SPAGHETTI								
Cooked, Average	*1oz/28g*	*33*	*0.2*	*119*	*4.1*	*24.8*	*0.6*	*1.1*
Dried, Waitrose*	1 Serving/75g	256	1.0	341	11.5	70.7	1.3	3.7
Dry, Average	*1oz/28g*	*98*	*0.4*	*350*	*12.1*	*72.1*	*1.5*	*2.4*
Durum Wheat, Dry, Average	*1oz/28g*	*97*	*0.1*	*348*	*12.4*	*71.8*	*0.4*	*1.4*
Egg, Fresh, Cooked, Tesco*	½ Pack/150g	480	3.7	320	9.7	62.7	2.5	3.4
Fresh, Cooked, Average	*1 Serving/125g*	*182*	*2.2*	*146*	*6.1*	*26.9*	*1.7*	*1.8*
Fresh, Dry, Average	*1 Serving/100g*	*278*	*3.0*	*278*	*10.8*	*53.0*	*3.0*	*2.2*
Hoops, & Sausages, Tesco*	1 Serving/205g	184	6.8	90	3.1	11.9	3.3	0.2
Hoops, Canned, Smart Price, Asda*	½ Can/205g	127	0.6	62	1.7	13.0	0.3	0.4
Hoops, in Tomato Sauce, Heinz*	½ Can/200g	106	0.4	53	1.7	11.1	0.2	0.5
Hoops, in Tomato Sauce, Multigrain, Snap Pot, Heinz*	1 Pot/190g	112	0.6	59	1.6	12.7	0.3	1.5
Hoops, in Tomato Sauce, Snap Pot, Heinz*	1 Pot/192g	113	0.6	59	1.6	12.7	0.3	1.5
Hoops, Tesco*	½ Can/205g	123	0.4	60	1.6	12.9	0.2	0.5
in Tomato Sauce with Parsley, Weight Watchers*	1 Sm Can/200g	100	0.4	50	1.8	9.9	0.2	0.6
in Tomato Sauce, Basics, Sainsbury's*	1 Can/410g	197	1.2	48	1.4	10.0	0.3	0.7
in Tomato Sauce, Canned	1oz/28g	18	0.1	64	1.9	14.1	0.4	0.7
in Tomato Sauce, Heinz*	½ Can/200g	120	0.6	60	1.7	12.7	0.3	2.4
in Tomato Sauce, HP*	1 Can/410g	247	0.8	60	1.5	13.1	0.2	0.4
Marinara	1 Serving/450g	675	18.9	150	8.0	19.0	4.2	0.9
Rings, in Tomato Sauce, Canned, Sainsbury's*	1 Serving/213g	136	0.8	64	1.9	13.3	0.4	0.5
TTD, Sainsbury's*	1 Serving/90g	321	1.5	357	12.3	73.1	1.7	2.5
Wheat Free, Tesco*	1 Serving/100g	340	2.0	340	8.0	72.5	2.0	2.5
Whole Wheat, Cooked, Average	*1oz/28g*	*32*	*0.3*	*113*	*4.7*	*23.2*	*0.9*	*3.5*
Whole Wheat, Dry, Average	*1 Serving/100g*	*324*	*2.6*	*324*	*13.5*	*62.2*	*2.6*	*8.0*
with Sausages, in Tomato Sauce, Heinz*	1 Can/400g	352	14.0	88	3.4	10.8	3.5	0.5
with Tomato & Cheese, Tesco*	½ Pack/250g	280	6.5	112	4.0	18.1	2.6	1.1
SPAGHETTI & MEATBALLS								
COU, M&S*	1 Pack/400g	360	8.0	90	6.0	12.3	2.0	2.6
GFY, Asda*	1 Pack/400g	344	6.0	86	7.0	11.0	1.5	1.5
Ready Meal, Healthy Range, Average	*1 Serving/400g*	*375*	*8.3*	*94*	*5.7*	*12.9*	*2.1*	*1.7*
Italian, Sainsbury's*	1 Pack/450g	495	21.2	110	5.0	11.9	4.7	2.7
Little Dish*	1 Pack/200g	227	9.6	114	6.2	10.6	4.8	1.6
Tesco*	1 Serving/475g	641	30.9	135	5.1	14.1	6.5	0.9
SPAGHETTI BOLOGNESE								
Al Forno, Sainsbury's*	1 Pack/400g	460	19.6	115	7.8	10.0	4.9	1.1
As Consumed, Savers, Morrisons*	1 Pack/300g	338	10.4	120	4.5	16.3	3.7	1.6
BGTY, Sainsbury's*	1 Pack/400g	416	9.2	104	6.3	14.4	2.3	1.1
Canned, Asda*	½ Can/205g	174	5.7	85	4.2	10.7	2.8	0.6
CBY, Asda*	1 Pack/100g	108	2.0	108	6.0	15.6	2.0	2.0
Cook*	1 Portion/430g	636	24.9	148	7.6	16.2	5.8	1.0
Co-Op*	1 Pack/300g	285	12.0	95	4.0	11.0	4.0	1.0
Egg Pasta in Rich Beef Sauce, Waitrose*	1 Pack/400g	404	10.4	101	7.6	11.7	2.6	1.0
Italian, Chilled, Tesco*	1 Pack/400g	520	17.2	130	6.5	15.9	4.3	1.5
M&S*	1 Pack/400g	380	8.4	95	7.5	11.7	2.1	1.7
Quick Pasta, Dry, Sainsbury's*	1 Serving/63g	231	2.8	367	10.8	71.0	4.4	3.3
Sainsbury's*	1 Pack/400g	525	18.8	131	6.1	16.0	4.7	2.2
Weight Watchers*	1 Pack/320g	293	6.1	91	5.7	12.6	1.9	0.8
SPAGHETTI CARBONARA								
Chicken & Asparagus, Sainsbury's*	1 Pack/450g	657	27.4	146	6.6	16.2	6.1	1.1
Chicken, Mushroom & Ham, Asda*	1 Pack/700g	686	14.0	98	10.0	10.0	2.0	1.5
COU, M&S*	1 Pack/330g	346	7.2	105	6.1	15.7	2.2	0.8
Creamy, Mini Meals, Heinz*	1 Sm Can/200g	130	2.7	65	3.8	9.0	1.4	0.6
Italian, Chilled, Sainsbury's*	1 Pack/400g	492	15.6	123	5.5	16.1	3.9	1.4

S

	Measure INFO/WEIGHT	per Measure KCAL	per Measure FAT	Nutrition Values per 100g / 100ml KCAL	PROT	CARB	FAT	FIBRE
SPAGHETTI CARBONARA								
Italian, Fresh, Chilled, Tesco*	1 Pack/430g	606	26.2	141	7.6	13.9	6.1	1.3
Light Choices, Tesco*	1 Pack/400g	460	9.6	115	6.9	15.7	2.4	1.2
M&S*	1 Pack/400g	560	27.2	140	5.2	14.0	6.8	0.9
M&S*	1 Pack/400g	660	36.0	165	6.5	14.2	9.0	0.6
Ready Meal, Average	***1 Pack/400g***	***524***	***21.5***	***131***	***5.9***	***14.4***	***5.4***	***1.1***
SPAGHETTI WITH								
King Prawn, Italian, Cooked, Finest, Tesco*	1 Pack/390g	485	22.9	125	5.0	12.2	5.9	1.3
SPAM*								
Fritters, Hormel Foods*	1 Fritter/80g	221	14.5	276	10.2	18.1	18.1	2.2
Pork & Ham, Chopped, Spam*	1 Serving/100g	289	24.3	289	15.0	3.2	24.3	0.0
SPELT								
Organic, Easy Grain, The Food Doctor*	1 Pack/225g	326	4.0	145	5.2	26.6	1.8	5.9
SPICE MIX								
for Fajitas, Old El Paso*	1 Pack/35g	107	2.1	306	9.0	54.0	6.0	0.0
for Mexican Fajitas, Discovery*	½ Pack/15g	34	1.0	230	8.0	35.0	6.5	17.5
Ras El Hanout, Al'fez*	1 Tsp/2g	4	0.2	217	9.8	25.7	8.3	17.5
SPINACH								
Baby, Average	***1 Serving/90g***	***22***	***0.7***	***25***	***2.8***	***1.6***	***0.8***	***2.1***
Boiled or Steamed, Average	***1 Serving/80g***	***17***	***0.6***	***21***	***2.6***	***0.9***	***0.8***	***2.1***
Canned, Average	***1 Serving/80g***	***16***	***0.4***	***20***	***2.8***	***1.3***	***0.5***	***2.7***
Chopped, Frozen, Waitrose*	1 Serving/80g	20	0.6	25	2.8	1.6	0.8	2.7
Creamed with Marscarpone Sauce, Sainsbury's*	½ Pack/147g	110	6.3	75	4.2	5.0	4.3	3.4
Creamed, Frozen, Weight Watchers*	1 Portion/112g	48	1.1	43	2.5	5.0	1.0	1.5
Frozen, Leaf, GutBio*	1 Portion/50g	13	0.2	26	3.0	1.0	0.5	2.8
Leaf, Frozen, Organic, Waitrose*	1 Serving/80g	20	0.6	25	2.8	1.6	0.8	2.1
Mornay, Waitrose*	½ Pack/125g	112	8.6	90	3.3	3.6	6.9	1.6
Raw, Average	***1 Serving/80g***	***19***	***0.6***	***24***	***2.9***	***1.4***	***0.7***	***2.2***
SPIRALI								
Dry, Average	***1 Serving/50g***	***176***	***0.8***	***352***	***12.2***	***72.6***	***1.6***	***2.8***
SPIRITS								
37.5% Volume	***1 Pub Shot/35ml***	***72***	***0.0***	***207***	***0.0***	***0.0***	***0.0***	***0.0***
40% Volume	***1 Shot/35ml***	***78***	***0.0***	***222***	***0.0***	***0.0***	***0.0***	***0.0***
SPLIT PEAS								
Dried, Average	***1oz/28g***	***89***	***0.5***	***319***	***22.1***	***57.4***	***1.7***	***3.2***
Green, Dried, Boiled, Average	***1 Tbsp/35g***	***40***	***0.2***	***115***	***8.3***	***19.8***	***0.6***	***3.9***
Yellow, Wholefoods, Tesco*	1 Serving/15g	52	0.4	345	22.1	58.2	2.4	6.3
SPONGE FINGERS								
Boudoir, Sainsbury's*	1 Finger/5g	20	0.2	396	8.1	82.8	3.6	0.4
Tesco*	1 Finger/5g	19	0.2	386	7.6	80.6	3.7	1.0
Trifle, Average	***1 Sponge/24g***	***77***	***0.5***	***319***	***5.2***	***69.9***	***2.2***	***0.8***
Trifle, Sainsbury's*	1 Sponge/24g	77	0.4	323	5.3	71.9	1.6	1.1
Trifle, Tesco*	1 Sponge/24g	75	0.6	311	5.3	66.6	2.6	1.1
SPONGE PUDDING								
Average	***1 Portion/170g***	***578***	***27.7***	***340***	***5.8***	***45.3***	***16.3***	***1.1***
Blackberry & Apple, HE, Tesco*	1 Pot/103g	159	1.4	155	3.1	32.6	1.4	0.7
Blackcurrant, BGTY, Sainsbury's*	1 Serving/110g	155	1.0	141	2.5	30.7	0.9	3.2
Canned, Average	***1 Serving/75g***	***214***	***8.6***	***285***	***3.1***	***45.4***	***11.4***	***0.8***
Chocolate & Sauce, Co-Op*	1 Pack/225g	608	29.2	270	5.0	34.0	13.0	0.6
Chocolate, Less Than 3% Fat, BGTY, Sainsbury's*	1 Pudding/105g	180	2.0	171	4.5	34.0	1.9	0.9
Chocolate, M&S*	¼ Pudding/131g	524	32.2	400	6.1	38.6	24.6	1.8
Chocolate, M&S*	1 Pudding/105g	401	24.3	382	5.7	36.0	23.1	3.5
Chocolate, Waitrose*	1 Pudding/110g	400	22.5	363	3.6	41.4	20.4	1.7
Golden Syrup, Co-Op*	1 Can/300g	945	39.0	315	2.0	47.0	13.0	0.6

S

	Measure INFO/WEIGHT	per Measure KCAL	FAT	Nutrition Values per 100g / 100ml KCAL	PROT	CARB	FAT	FIBRE
SPONGE PUDDING								
Honey& Fig, M&S*	¼ Pudding/73g	225	12.0	310	3.6	34.8	16.6	3.4
Lemon Curd, Heinz*	¼ Can/78g	236	9.1	302	2.6	46.7	11.7	0.6
Lemon, M&S*	1 Pudding/105g	326	16.0	310	4.3	39.4	15.2	2.3
Lemon, Waitrose*	1 Serving/105g	212	2.5	202	3.4	41.7	2.4	1.4
Mixed Berry, BGTY, Sainsbury's*	1 Pudding/110g	189	2.6	172	2.4	33.3	2.4	3.8
Raspberry Jam, Asda*	½ Pudding/147g	481	16.2	327	3.1	54.0	11.0	4.1
Strawberry Jam, Heinz*	¼ Can/82g	230	6.2	281	2.6	50.4	7.6	0.6
Sultana with Toffee Sauce, HL, Tesco*	1 Serving/80g	280	2.2	350	3.2	60.2	2.8	1.0
Summer Fruits, BGTY, Sainsbury's*	1 Serving/110g	243	4.7	221	2.7	42.9	4.3	1.0
Syrup & Custard, Morrisons*	1 Serving/125g	290	8.6	232	3.4	39.1	6.9	0.8
Syrup, BGTY, Sainsbury's*	1 Pudding/110g	338	4.5	307	2.8	64.6	4.1	0.4
Syrup, Individual, Tesco*	1 Pudding/110g	390	14.5	355	3.1	55.6	13.2	0.5
Syrup, Sainsbury's*	¼ Pudding/110g	408	13.0	371	2.7	63.5	11.8	0.4
Treacle with Custard, Farmfoods*	1 Serving/145g	539	33.1	372	3.2	38.4	22.8	0.8
Treacle, Heinz*	1 Serving/160g	445	13.0	278	2.5	48.9	8.1	0.6
Treacle, Waitrose*	1 Pudding/105g	385	13.8	367	2.8	59.5	13.1	0.5
with Dried Fruit	1oz/28g	93	4.0	331	5.4	48.1	14.3	1.2
with Jam or Treacle	1oz/28g	93	4.0	333	5.1	48.7	14.4	1.0
SPOTTED DICK								
Average	*1 Serving/105g*	*343*	*17.5*	*327*	*4.2*	*42.7*	*16.7*	*1.0*
Individual, Tesco*	1 Pudding/121g	417	14.5	345	3.2	55.2	12.0	1.2
with Custard	1 Serving/210g	438	15.6	209	3.4	31.5	7.4	1.3
SPRATS								
Fried	*1oz/28g*	*116*	*9.8*	*415*	*24.9*	*0.0*	*35.0*	*0.0*
Raw	*1oz/28g*	*33*	*2.1*	*117*	*12.4*	*0.0*	*7.5*	*0.0*
SPREAD								
Butter Me Up, Light, Tesco*	1 Thin Spread/7g	24	2.7	350	0.3	0.5	38.0	0.0
Butter Me Up, Tesco*	1 Thin Spread/7g	38	4.1	540	0.8	1.2	59.0	0.0
Butterlicious, Vegetable, Sainsbury's*	1 Thin Spread/7g	44	4.8	628	0.6	1.1	69.0	0.0
Buttersoft, Light, Reduced Fat, Sainsbury's*	1 Thin Spread/7g	38	4.2	544	0.4	0.5	60.0	0.0
Buttery Taste, Benecol*	1 Thin Spread/7g	40	4.4	575	0.0	0.8	63.3	0.0
Clover, Light, Dairy Crest Ltd*	1 Serving/7g	32	3.4	455	0.7	2.9	49.0	0.0
Dairy Free, Organic, Pure Spreads*	1 Thin Spread/7g	37	4.1	533	0.5	0.0	59.0	0.0
Enriched Olive, Tesco*	1 Thin Spread/7g	38	4.1	540	0.2	1.2	59.0	0.0
From Soya, Kallo*	1 Thin Spread/7g	27	2.6	380	7.0	6.0	37.0	0.0
Gold, Low Fat, Omega 3, St Ivel*	1 Thin Spread/7g	25	2.7	360	0.5	3.1	38.0	0.0
Heart, Cholesterol Reducing, Dairygold	1 Thin Spread/7g	24	2.5	338	0.7	2.8	36.0	0.0
Irish, Dairy, Original, LowLow*	1 Thin Spread/7g	24	2.7	346	0.4	0.5	38.0	0.0
Lactofree Spreadable, Lactofree, Arla*	1 Serving/10g	68	7.5	679	0.5	0.5	75.0	0.0
Light, Benecol*	1 Thin Spread/7g	23	2.4	333	2.5	0.0	35.0	0.0
Lighter Than Light, Flora*	1 Serving/10g	19	1.8	188	5.0	1.6	18.0	0.0
Low Fat, Average	*1 Thin Spread/7g*	*27*	*2.8*	*390*	*5.8*	*0.5*	*40.5*	*0.0*
Low Fat, Better By Far, Morrisons*	1 Thin Spread/7g	44	4.8	627	0.5	1.0	69.0	0.0
Olive Light, GFY, Asda*	1 Thin Spread/7g	24	2.7	345	0.8	0.0	38.0	0.0
Olive Light, Low Fat, BGTY, Sainsbury's*	1 Thin Spread/7g	19	2.0	265	0.1	0.8	29.0	0.0
Olive Light, Sainsbury's*	1 Thin Spread/7g	24	2.7	348	1.5	0.0	38.0	0.0
Olive Oil, 55% Reduced Fat, Benecol*	1 Thin Spread/7g	35	3.8	498	0.3	0.5	55.0	0.0
Olive Oil, Bertolli*	1 Thin Spread/7g	38	4.1	536	0.2	1.0	59.0	0.0
Olive, Light, Low Fat, HL, Tesco*	1 Thin Spread/7g	24	2.7	348	1.5	0.0	38.0	0.0
Olive, Low Fat, Morrisons*	1 Thin Spread/7g	24	2.7	346	0.9	0.0	38.0	0.0
Olive, Reduced Fat, Asda*	1 Thin Spread/7g	38	4.1	536	0.2	1.1	59.0	0.0
Olive, Reduced Fat, M&S*	1 Thin Spread/7g	38	4.1	536	0.2	1.1	59.0	0.0
Olive, Reduced Fat, So Organic, Sainsbury's*	1 Thin Spread/7g	38	4.2	537	0.1	0.4	59.5	0.0

S

	Measure INFO/WEIGHT	per Measure KCAL	per Measure FAT	Nutrition Values per 100g / 100ml KCAL	PROT	CARB	FAT	FIBRE
SPREAD								
Olive, Waitrose*	1 Thin Spread/7g	37	4.1	534	0.2	0.5	59.0	0.0
Olivite, Low Fat, Weight Watchers*	1 Thin Spread/7g	25	2.7	351	0.0	0.2	38.9	0.0
Orange, Thick Cut, St Dalfour*	1 Spread/11g	23	0.0	211	0.6	52.0	0.1	1.6
Pure Gold, Light, 65% Less Fat, Asda*	1 Thin Spread/7g	17	1.8	239	2.5	1.0	25.0	0.0
Soft, Reduced Fat, Smart Price, Asda*	1 Thin Spread/7g	32	3.5	455	0.2	1.0	50.0	0.0
Soft, Value, Tesco*	1 Thin Spread/7g	30	3.4	433	0.0	0.0	48.1	0.0
Sunflower, Asda*	1 Thin Spread/7g	44	4.9	635	0.2	1.0	70.0	0.0
Sunflower, Average	**1 Thin Spread/7g**	**42**	**4.6**	**595**	**0.1**	**0.4**	**65.9**	**0.4**
Sunflower, Enriched, Tesco*	1 Thin Spread/7g	37	4.1	535	0.1	0.2	59.0	0.0
Sunflower, Light, BFY, Morrisons*	1 Thin Spread/7g	24	2.7	342	0.0	0.0	38.0	0.0
Sunflower, Light, BGTY, Sainsbury's*	1 Thin Spread/7g	19	2.0	265	0.1	0.8	29.0	0.0
Sunflower, Light, Reduced Fat, Asda*	1 Thin Spread/7g	24	2.7	347	0.3	1.0	38.0	0.1
Sunflower, Low Fat, Aldi*	1 Thin Spread/7g	26	2.7	366	0.2	5.7	38.0	0.0
Sunflower, Low Fat, M&S*	1 Thin Spread/7g	24	2.7	342	0.0	0.0	38.0	1.0
Sunflower, M&S*	1 Thin Spread/7g	44	4.9	630	0.0	0.0	70.0	3.0
Sunflower, Morrisons*	1 Thin Spread/7g	37	4.1	531	0.0	0.2	59.0	0.0
Sunflower, Sainsbury's*	1 Thin Spread/7g	37	4.1	532	0.1	0.2	59.0	0.0
Sunflower, Waitrose*	1 Thin Spread/7g	44	4.9	631	0.0	0.2	70.0	0.0
Vegetable with Buttermilk, Beautifully Butterfully*	1 Spread/10g	49	5.4	488	0.4	0.0	54.0	0.0
Vegetable, Dairy Free, Free From, Sainsbury's*	1 Thin Spread/7g	44	4.9	630	0.0	0.0	70.0	3.0
Vitalite, St Ivel*	1 Thin Spread/7g	35	3.9	503	0.0	0.0	56.0	0.0
with Soya, Dairy Free, Pure Spreads*	1 Thin Spread/7g	34	3.8	490	0.5	1.0	54.0	0.0
with Sunflower, Dairy Free, Organic, Pure Spreads*	1 Thin Spread/7g	42	4.7	603	0.0	0.0	67.0	0.0
SPRING ROLLS								
Char Sui Pork & Bacon, M&S*	1 Pack/220g	528	20.7	240	4.8	33.9	9.4	0.6
Chicken, & Chilli, Cantonese, Sainsbury's*	1 Roll/51g	85	2.8	166	9.7	19.4	5.5	0.6
Chicken, & Chilli, Sainsbury's*	1 Roll/50g	92	4.6	185	9.6	15.6	9.3	2.8
Chicken, Asda*	1 Roll/58g	115	5.2	199	4.6	25.0	9.0	3.4
Chinese Takeaway, Tesco*	1 Roll/50g	100	4.3	201	4.4	26.4	8.6	1.5
Dim Sum, Sainsbury's*	1 Roll/12g	26	1.2	216	4.1	28.2	9.6	2.9
Duck with Sweet Chilli Sauce, Waitrose*	1 Roll/72g	66	1.4	92	5.1	14.0	1.9	0.9
Duck, M&S*	1 Roll/30g	75	3.4	250	9.8	27.7	11.2	1.5
Duck, Mini, Asda*	1 Roll/18g	47	1.9	259	8.7	32.8	10.3	1.9
Duck, Morrisons*	1 Roll/65g	147	6.7	226	6.2	27.2	10.3	1.2
Duck, Party Bites, Sainsbury's*	1 Roll/20g	49	1.8	245	10.1	31.4	8.8	1.0
Mini Vegetable, Co-Op*	1 Roll/18g	40	1.6	220	4.1	30.9	9.1	2.7
Mini, Asda*	1 Roll/20g	35	0.6	175	3.5	33.6	3.0	1.9
Mini, Sainsbury's*	1 Roll/12g	27	1.2	221	4.2	28.7	9.9	1.6
Oriental Vegetable, Tesco*	1 Roll/68g	152	7.6	225	4.0	25.9	11.3	1.6
Prawn, Cantonese, Sainsbury's*	1 Roll/28g	46	1.7	162	6.8	20.3	6.0	2.5
Prawn, Crispy, M&S*	1 Roll/34g	75	3.4	220	10.0	22.2	9.9	1.3
Thai Prawn, Waitrose*	1 Roll/50g	110	4.8	219	8.0	25.4	9.5	2.4
Thai, Sainsbury's*	1 Roll/30g	69	3.4	229	2.9	28.8	11.3	3.5
Vegetable, Asda*	1 Roll/62g	126	5.6	203	3.5	27.0	9.0	2.7
Vegetable, Cantonese, Large, Sainsbury's*	1 Roll/63g	130	6.3	205	3.6	25.3	9.9	1.5
Vegetable, Cantonese, Sainsbury's*	1 Roll/36g	84	4.2	233	3.6	28.1	11.7	1.4
Vegetable, Chilled, Tesco*	1 Roll/68g	149	7.6	221	4.0	25.9	11.3	1.6
Vegetable, Chinese Takeaway, Sainsbury's*	1 Roll/59g	100	3.7	170	4.0	24.4	6.3	2.8
Vegetable, Frozen, Tesco*	1 Roll/60g	123	6.4	205	3.5	23.0	10.6	1.3
Vegetable, M&S*	1 Roll/37g	80	3.6	215	4.3	27.8	9.6	2.0
Vegetable, Mini, Occasions, Sainsbury's*	1 Roll/24g	52	2.3	216	4.1	28.2	9.6	2.9
Vegetable, Mini, Oriental Selection, Waitrose*	1 Roll/18g	35	1.2	192	4.2	28.6	6.8	1.7
Vegetable, Mini, Party Food, M&S*	1 Roll/20g	40	1.6	200	3.7	26.2	8.1	2.7

	Measure INFO/WEIGHT	per Measure KCAL	FAT	Nutrition Values per 100g / 100ml KCAL	PROT	CARB	FAT	FIBRE
SPRING ROLLS								
Vegetable, Mini, Tesco*	1 Roll/18g	36	1.5	205	4.4	26.4	8.6	1.5
Vegetable, Oriental Selection, Party, Iceland*	1 Roll/15g	36	1.4	241	4.3	34.1	9.7	2.1
Vegetable, Oriental, Sainsbury's*	1 Roll/61g	137	7.2	224	3.8	24.3	11.8	2.9
Vegetable, Tempura, M&S*	1 Pack/140g	280	12.0	200	2.8	27.9	8.6	1.8
Vegetable, Waitrose*	1 Roll/57g	107	5.3	187	3.7	22.1	9.3	3.4
SPRITE*								
Sprite*	1 Bottle/500ml	215	0.0	43	0.0	10.5	0.0	0.0
Zero, Lemon & Lime, Sprite*	1 Bottle/500ml	6	0.0	1	0.0	0.0	0.0	0.0
Zero, Sprite*	1 Can/330ml	3	0.0	1	0.0	0.0	0.0	0.0
SPRITZER								
Red Grape, Non-Alcoholic, ES, Asda*	1 Lge Bottle/750ml	330	0.0	44	0.0	11.0	0.0	0.0
Rose & Grape, Non Alcoholic, ES, Asda*	1 Bottle/750ml	90	0.0	12	0.0	3.0	0.0	0.0
White Wine, Echo Falls*	1 Serving/125ml	78	0.0	39	0.0	0.0	0.0	0.0
with White Zinfadel, Echo Falls*	1 Serving/200ml	216	0.0	108	0.0	0.0	0.0	0.0
SPROUTS								
Radish, China Rose, Aconbury Sprouts*	½ Pack/65g	52	1.0	80	7.5	8.9	1.6	0.0
SQUASH								
Apple & Blackcurrant, No Added Sugar, Tesco*	1 Serving/30mls	4	0.0	15	0.2	2.0	0.0	0.0
Apple & Blackcurrant, Special R, Diluted, Robinson's*	1 fl oz/30ml	2	0.0	8	0.1	1.1	0.1	0.0
Apple & Blackcurrant, Special R, Robinson's*	1 Serving/30ml	2	0.0	8	0.1	1.1	0.0	0.0
Apple & Strawberry High Juice, Sainsbury's*	1 Serving/250ml	82	0.2	33	0.1	8.2	0.1	0.1
Apple, Hi Juice, Tesco*	1 fl oz/30ml	52	0.0	173	0.0	42.5	0.0	0.0
Blackcurrant, High Juice, M&S*	1 Glass/250ml	50	0.0	20	0.1	5.2	0.0	0.1
Blackcurrant, High Juice, Tesco*	1 Serving/75ml	215	0.0	287	0.3	70.0	0.0	0.0
Blackcurrant, No Added Sugar, Tesco*	1 Serving/25ml	4	0.0	14	0.4	1.7	0.0	0.0
Cherries & Berries, Tesco*	1 Serving/25mls	5	0.0	21	0.2	3.2	0.0	0.0
Cranberry, Light, Classic, Undiluted, Ocean Spray*	1 Serving/50ml	32	0.0	63	0.2	14.1	0.0	0.0
Fruit & Barley Orange, Diluted, Robinson's*	1 Serving/50ml	6	0.0	12	0.2	1.7	0.0	0.1
Fruit & Barley, No Added Sugar, Robinson's*	1 fl oz/30ml	4	0.0	14	0.3	2.0	0.0	0.0
Fruit & Barley, Tropical, No Added Sugar, Robinson's*	1 Serving/60ml	7	0.0	12	0.2	1.6	0.0	0.0
Grapefruit, High Juice, No Added Sugar, Sainsbury's*	1 Serving/25ml	2	0.0	6	0.1	1.1	0.0	0.0
Lemon Barley Water, Made Up, Robinson's*	1 Serving/250ml	48	0.0	19	0.1	4.4	0.0	0.0
Lemon, Double Concentrate, Value, Tesco*	1 Serving/25mls	3	0.0	11	0.2	0.3	0.0	0.0
Lemon, No Added Sugar, Double Concentrate, Tesco*	1 Serving/25ml	4	0.0	16	0.3	0.7	0.0	0.0
Mixed Fruit, Diluted, Kia Ora*	1 Serving/250ml	5	0.0	2	0.0	0.3	0.0	0.0
Orange & Mango, No Added Sugar, Robinson's*	1 Serving/25ml	2	0.0	8	0.2	0.9	0.0	0.0
Orange & Mango, Special R, Diluted, Robinson's*	1 Serving/250ml	20	0.0	8	0.2	0.9	0.0	0.0
Orange & Pineapple, No Sugar Added, Robinson's*	1 Serving/25ml	2	0.0	8	0.2	0.7	0.0	0.2
Orange, Hi Juice, Tesco*	1 Serving/75ml	140	0.1	187	0.3	45.0	0.1	0.0
Orange, No Added Sugar, High Juice, Sainsbury's*	1 Serving/100ml	6	0.1	6	0.1	1.1	0.1	0.1
Pink Grapefruit, High Juice, Undiluted, Robinson's*	1 Glass/250ml	455	0.2	182	0.2	43.3	0.1	0.0
Spaghetti, Baked	*1oz/28g*	*6*	*0.1*	*23*	*0.7*	*4.3*	*0.3*	*2.1*
Spaghetti, Including Pips & Rind, Raw	*1oz/28g*	*5*	*0.1*	*20*	*0.4*	*3.4*	*0.4*	*1.7*
Summer Fruits, High Juice, Undiluted, Robinson's*	1 fl oz/30ml	61	0.0	203	0.1	49.0	0.1	0.0
Summer Fruits, High Juice, Waitrose*	1 Serving/250ml	102	0.0	41	0.0	10.0	0.0	0.0
Summer Fruits, No Added Sugar, Made Up, Morrisons*	1 Glass/200ml	3	0.0	2	0.0	0.2	0.0	0.0
Summer, All Varieties	1 Sm Squash/118g	19	0.2	16	1.2	3.4	0.2	1.1
Summerfruits, High Juice, Tesco*	1 Serving/50ml	12	0.0	23	0.2	4.5	0.0	0.0
Winter, Acorn, Baked, Average	*1oz/28g*	*16*	*0.0*	*56*	*1.1*	*12.6*	*0.1*	*3.2*
Winter, Acorn, Raw, Average	*1oz/28g*	*9*	*0.0*	*30*	*0.6*	*6.8*	*0.1*	*1.7*
Winter, All Varieties, Flesh Only, Raw, Average	*1oz/28g*	*10*	*0.0*	*34*	*1.0*	*8.6*	*0.1*	*1.5*
Winter, Butternut, Baked, Average	*1oz/28g*	*9*	*0.0*	*32*	*0.9*	*7.4*	*0.1*	*1.4*
Winter, Butternut, Raw, Prepared, Average	*1 Serving/80g*	*29*	*0.1*	*36*	*1.1*	*8.3*	*0.1*	*1.6*

S

	Measure INFO/WEIGHT	per Measure KCAL	FAT	Nutrition Values per 100g / 100ml KCAL	PROT	CARB	FAT	FIBRE
SQUASH								
Winter, Butternut, Raw, Unprepared, Average	*1 Serving/80g*	*24*	*0.1*	*30*	*0.9*	*6.8*	*0.1*	*1.3*
SQUID								
Calamari, Battered with Tartar Sauce Dip, Tesco*	1 Pack/210g	573	41.0	273	8.9	15.4	19.5	0.6
Calamari, Chargrilled, Red Pepper Seasoning, Deli, M&S*	1 Pack/115g	115	2.3	100	20.8	0.4	2.0	0.5
in Batter, Fried in Blended Oil, Average	*1oz/28g*	*55*	*2.8*	*195*	*11.5*	*15.7*	*10.0*	*0.5*
Raw, Average	*1oz/28g*	*23*	*0.5*	*81*	*15.4*	*1.2*	*1.7*	*0.0*
with Sweet Chilli Sauce, Pan Fried, CBY, Asda*	1 Serving/125g	229	9.3	183	9.6	19.0	7.4	0.9
STARBAR								
Cadbury*	1 Bar/53g	260	14.8	491	10.7	49.0	27.9	0.0
STARBURST								
Mars*	1 Pack/45g	185	3.4	411	0.3	85.3	7.6	0.0
STEAK & KIDNEY PUDDING								
M&S*	1 Pudding/121g	260	13.4	215	9.2	19.4	11.1	3.2
Sainsbury's*	1 Pudding/435g	1135	62.6	261	10.5	22.3	14.4	0.8
Waitrose*	1 Pudding/223g	497	26.1	223	8.9	20.4	11.7	1.2
STEW								
Beef & Dumplings	1 Serving/652g	766	32.7	117	7.4	10.7	5.0	0.8
Beef & Dumplings, Countryside*	1 Pack/300g	246	6.9	82	8.1	7.3	2.3	0.5
Beef & Dumplings, Farmfoods*	1 Pack/300g	312	13.2	104	4.0	12.0	4.4	1.1
Beef & Dumplings, Frozen, Asda*	1 Pack/400g	392	13.2	98	6.0	11.0	3.3	0.8
Beef & Dumplings, Morrisons*	1 Pack/400g	440	18.4	110	6.0	11.1	4.6	1.5
Beef with Dumplings, Classic British, Sainsbury's*	1 Pack/450g	531	23.4	118	7.7	10.2	5.2	0.5
Beef with Dumplings, COU, M&S*	1 Pack/454g	431	11.8	95	8.9	9.1	2.6	0.8
Beef with Dumplings, Sainsbury's*	1 Pack/450g	603	27.4	134	9.3	10.5	6.1	0.7
Beef, Asda*	½ Can/196g	178	4.9	91	10.0	7.0	2.5	1.5
Beef, Meal for One, M&S*	1 Pack/440g	350	8.4	80	7.0	8.7	1.9	2.0
Beef, Value, Tesco*	1 Serving/200g	170	9.8	85	4.0	6.2	4.9	1.0
Chicken & Dumplings, Birds Eye*	1 Pack/320g	282	8.6	88	7.0	8.9	2.7	0.5
Chicken & Dumplings, Tesco*	1 Serving/450g	567	29.7	126	7.6	9.1	6.6	0.7
Chicken, Morrisons*	1 Pack/400g	492	7.6	123	17.6	8.9	1.9	0.5
Chickpea, Roast Sweet Potato, & Feta, Stewed!*	½ Pot/250g	188	7.2	75	3.3	8.8	2.9	2.7
Irish, Asda*	¼ Can/196g	172	7.8	88	6.0	7.0	4.0	1.0
Irish, Morrisons*	1 Can/392g	243	4.7	62	3.8	8.9	1.2	0.0
Lentil & Vegetable, Organic, Simply Organic*	1 Pack/400g	284	6.0	71	3.5	11.0	1.5	1.3
Lentil & Winter Vegetable, Organic, Pure & Pronto*	1 Pack/400g	364	9.6	91	3.6	14.0	2.4	4.0
Mixed Vegetable Topped with Herb Dumplings, Tesco*	1 Pack/420g	508	26.0	121	1.9	14.5	6.2	1.3
Pearl Barley Gumbo, CBY, Asda*	1 Pack/350g	336	6.6	96	3.0	14.5	1.9	4.4
Tuscan Bean, Tasty Veg Pot, Innocent*	1 Pot/400g	320	7.6	80	3.1	12.5	1.9	3.6
STIR FRY								
Baby Vegetable & Pak Choi, Two Step, Tesco*	½ Pack/95g	29	0.8	31	2.1	4.0	0.8	2.3
Bean Sprout & Vegetable with Red Peppers, Asda*	1 Pack/350g	126	3.9	36	1.8	4.7	1.1	2.3
Bean Sprout, Chinese, Sainsbury's*	1 Pack/300g	144	8.4	48	1.9	5.1	2.8	1.5
Bean Sprout, Ready to Eat, Washed, Sainsbury's*	1 Serving/150g	82	5.8	55	1.5	3.3	3.9	1.8
Bean Sprouts & Vegetables, Asda*	½ Pack/173g	107	6.9	62	2.0	4.5	4.0	1.8
Bean Sprouts, Chinese, Asda*	½ Pack/155g	54	0.8	35	2.9	4.0	0.5	1.5
Beef, BGTY, Sainsbury's*	½ Pack/125g	156	5.1	125	22.0	0.1	4.1	0.0
Cabbage, Carrot, Broccoli & Onion, Vegetable, Tesco*	1 Serving/100g	31	0.4	31	1.9	4.9	0.4	2.6
Chicken Chow Mein, Fresh, HL, Tesco*	1 Pack/400g	312	4.8	78	5.7	11.4	1.2	1.3
Chicken Chow Mein, Orient Express, Oriental Express*	1 Pack/400g	384	10.8	96	7.3	10.7	2.7	2.2
Chinese Chicken, As Consumed, Iceland*	½ Pack/371g	353	2.6	95	6.5	15.2	0.7	1.0
Chinese Chicken, Sizzling, Oriental Express*	1 Pack/400g	400	8.0	100	6.6	13.8	2.0	1.7
Chinese Exotic Vegetable, Sainsbury's*	1 Pack/350g	133	7.7	38	1.7	2.8	2.2	1.8
Chinese Leaf & Mixed Peppers, Cook Asian, M&S*	1 Pack/260g	65	1.3	25	1.4	3.4	0.5	1.8

S

STIR FRY

	Measure INFO/WEIGHT	per Measure KCAL	FAT	Nutrition Values per 100g / 100ml KCAL	PROT	CARB	FAT	FIBRE
Chinese Mushroom, Sainsbury's*	1 Serving/175g	66	4.2	38	1.7	2.4	2.4	1.7
Chinese Prawn, Asda*	1 Serving/375g	345	2.2	92	3.6	18.0	0.6	1.8
Chinese Style Chicken, GFY, Asda*	1 Pack/338g	362	5.8	107	6.0	17.0	1.7	1.5
Chinese Style Rice with Vegetables, Tesco*	1 Serving/550g	495	13.8	90	2.2	14.8	2.5	0.3
Chinese Style, Co-Op*	1 Pack/300g	105	1.2	35	3.0	6.0	0.4	2.0
Chinese Vegetable & Oyster Sauce, Asda*	1 Serving/150g	93	3.8	62	1.9	8.0	2.5	0.4
Chinese Vegetables with Chinese Style Sauce, Tesco*	1 Serving/350g	133	3.5	38	1.4	5.6	1.0	1.2
Chinese Vegetables with Oyster Sauce, Tesco*	1 Pack/350g	98	0.7	28	2.0	4.6	0.2	1.1
Chinese Vegetables, Oriental Express*	½ Pack/200g	44	0.4	22	1.4	3.7	0.2	2.2
Chinese Vegetables, Tesco*	1 Serving/175g	93	0.7	53	1.6	10.8	0.4	1.3
Chinese with Soy, Garlic & Ginger, Tesco*	1 Pack/150g	90	0.2	60	1.5	12.6	0.1	0.5
Family Pack, Vegetables & Beansprouts, Fresh, Tesco*	1 Pack/600g	108	0.6	18	2.0	2.2	0.1	2.1
Green Vegetable, M&S*	1 Pack/220g	165	13.0	75	3.1	2.5	5.9	2.2
Mixed Pepper & Vegetable, Asda*	½ Pack/150g	42	1.5	28	1.6	3.2	1.0	2.6
Mixed Pepper, Crisp & Sweet, Waitrose*	½ Pack/150g	51	0.6	34	1.9	4.8	0.4	1.9
Mixed Pepper, HL, Tesco*	1 Pack/325g	62	0.3	19	1.9	2.6	0.1	1.5
Mixed Pepper, Sainsbury's*	1 Pack/300g	188	12.9	70	1.5	4.6	4.8	1.2
Mixed Pepper, Tesco*	1/3 Pack/100g	23	0.1	23	1.9	3.7	0.1	1.9
Mixed Pepper, Tesco*	½ Bag/140g	48	0.6	34	2.0	4.6	0.4	2.0
Mixed Vegetable, Asda*	1 Serving/200g	96	5.0	48	1.7	4.7	2.5	3.0
Mushroom, Just Stir Fry, Sainsbury's*	1 Pack/350g	172	9.4	49	2.8	3.3	2.7	2.8
Mushroom, Tesco*	1 Portion/100g	34	0.5	34	2.6	3.9	0.5	2.0
Mushroom, Waitrose*	½ Pack/165g	43	0.7	26	2.3	3.3	0.4	1.6
Noodles & Bean Sprouts, Tesco*	½ Pack/125g	131	2.6	105	4.2	16.1	2.1	0.7
Oriental Mix, Quick & Easy, Frozen, Cooked, CBY, Asda*	1 Pack/500g	130	1.0	26	1.1	3.5	0.2	3.0
Oriental Style Pak Choi, M&S*	1 Pack/220g	165	12.5	75	2.2	3.5	5.7	2.4
Oriental Style, Vegetables, Sainsbury's*	1 Pack/300g	195	14.4	65	1.5	4.1	4.8	2.1
Oriental Vegetable, Frozen, Asda*	1 Serving/150g	116	6.8	77	2.1	7.0	4.5	1.7
Sweet & Sour, Co-Op*	½ Pack/187g	103	1.7	55	2.0	10.0	0.9	3.0
Sweet Pepper, M&S*	1 Pack/400g	160	7.2	40	2.3	3.5	1.8	0.6
Vegetable & Beansprout, Tesco*	1 Pack/380g	129	1.9	34	2.0	5.4	0.5	2.2
Vegetable & Beansprout, Waitrose*	1 Pack/300g	78	0.9	26	1.4	4.5	0.3	2.1
Vegetable & Broccoli, Fresh Tastes, Asda*	½ Bag/175g	88	3.5	50	2.5	3.7	2.0	3.7
Vegetable & Mushroom, Asda*	½ Pack/160g	59	2.4	37	2.4	3.4	1.5	3.4
Vegetable & Noodle, Asda*	1 Pack/330g	465	14.8	141	4.0	21.0	4.5	3.0
Vegetable Noodles, BGTY, Sainsbury's*	1 Pack/455g	391	9.1	86	3.2	14.0	2.0	1.4
Vegetable, Asda*	1 Pack/300g	132	6.9	44	1.6	4.2	2.3	3.1
Vegetable, Basics, Sainsbury's*	½ Bag/325g	101	2.9	31	2.1	3.5	0.9	2.2
Vegetable, Cantonese, Sainsbury's*	1 Serving/150g	90	5.2	60	2.8	4.2	3.5	2.7
Vegetable, Chinese Style, Tesco*	1 Pack/360g	79	0.7	22	1.9	3.2	0.2	1.4
Vegetable, Chinese, Mixed, Amoy*	1 Serving/110g	27	0.3	25	1.8	3.7	0.3	0.0
Vegetable, Crunchy, Sainsbury's*	½ Pack/150g	86	5.8	57	1.4	4.1	3.9	2.1
Vegetable, Crunchy, Waitrose*	1 Pack/300g	81	0.3	27	1.6	4.8	0.1	2.4
Vegetable, Mixed, Frozen, Everyday Value, Tesco*	3 Heap Tbsp/80g	80	3.4	100	2.3	10.0	4.3	4.7
Vegetable, Oriental, Frozen, Freshly, Asda*	1 Serving/100g	25	0.3	25	2.2	3.4	0.3	2.0
Vegetable, Oriental, Just Stir Fry, Sainsbury's*	½ Pack/135g	94	7.2	70	2.2	3.4	5.3	1.9
Vegetable, Rainbow, Fresh Tastes, Asda*	½ Pack/225g	119	5.0	53	1.8	4.6	2.2	3.8
Vegetable, Ready Prepared, M&S*	½ Pack/150g	38	0.4	25	2.2	3.5	0.3	2.2
Vegetable, Sweet & Crunchy, Waitrose*	1 Pack/300g	69	0.3	23	1.8	3.6	0.1	1.4
Vegetable, Tesco*	¼ Bag/100g	35	0.4	35	1.8	4.7	0.4	2.5
Vegetables & Bean Sprout, M&S*	1 Pack/350g	105	1.4	30	1.8	4.6	0.4	2.0
Vegetables with Oyster Sauce, Asda*	1 Serving/150g	93	3.8	62	1.9	8.0	2.5	0.0
Vegetables, Family, Sainsbury's*	1 Serving/300g	123	6.6	41	1.6	3.8	2.2	2.1

S

	INFO/WEIGHT	KCAL	FAT	KCAL	PROT	CARB	FAT	FIBRE
STIR FRY								
Vegetables, Fresh, Asda*	½ Pack/150g	106	7.5	71	1.7	4.9	5.0	1.7
Vegetables, Mixed Pepper, M&S*	½ Pack/150g	52	0.6	35	1.9	4.9	0.4	1.9
Vegetables, Mixed with Slices of Pepper, Tesco*	1 Pack/300g	102	1.2	34	2.0	4.6	0.4	2.0
STOCK								
Beef, Fresh, Sainsbury's*	¼ Pot/113g	27	0.6	24	5.1	0.5	0.5	0.5
Beef, Fresh, Tesco*	1 Serving/300ml	54	0.9	18	2.1	1.6	0.3	0.5
Beef, Made Up, Stock Pot, Knorr*	1 Serving/100ml	10	0.4	10	0.2	1.0	0.4	0.0
Beef, Rich, Stock Pot, Knorr*	1 Pot/28g	42	1.1	150	3.0	27.0	4.0	0.8
Beef, Simply Stock, Knorr*	1 Serving/100ml	6	0.0	6	1.4	0.1	0.0	0.0
Chicken, As Sold, Stock Pot, Knorr*	1 Pot/28g	45	12.6	160	4.0	26.0	45.0	0.8
Chicken, Cooks' Ingredients, Waitrose*	1 Pack/500ml	75	0.5	15	3.2	0.3	0.1	0.2
Chicken, Fresh, Sainsbury's*	½ Pot/142ml	23	0.1	16	3.7	0.1	0.1	0.3
Chicken, Fresh, Tesco*	1 Serving/300ml	27	0.3	9	1.6	0.5	0.1	0.5
Chicken, Granules, Knorr*	1 Tsp/5g	10	0.2	232	13.1	36.5	3.7	0.4
Chicken, Home Prepared, Average	*1 fl oz/30ml*	*7*	*0.3*	*24*	*3.8*	*0.7*	*0.9*	*0.3*
Chicken, Made Up, Stock Pot, Knorr*	1 Serving/125ml	15	0.3	12	0.2	1.6	0.2	0.0
Chicken, Prepared, Tesco*	1 Serving/300ml	54	0.3	18	2.4	1.8	0.1	0.5
Fish, Fresh, Finest, Tesco*	1 Serving/100g	10	0.0	10	0.6	1.8	0.0	0.5
Fish, Home Prepared, Average	*1 Serving/250ml*	*42*	*2.0*	*17*	*2.3*	*0.0*	*0.8*	*0.0*
Vegetable, 3 Peppercorn, Flavour Pot,Knorr*	1 Pot/9g	14	0.6	160	0.9	22.0	7.0	4.5
Vegetable, As Sold, Stock Pot, Knorr*	1 Serving/100ml	9	0.5	180	6.0	19.0	9.0	1.5
Vegetable, Made Up, Stock Pot, Knorr*	1 Serving/100ml	10	0.5	10	0.4	1.0	0.5	0.1
STOCK CUBES								
Beef Flavour, Made Up, Oxo*	1 Cube/189ml	17	0.4	9	0.6	1.3	0.2	0.1
Beef, Dry Weight, Bovril*	1 Cube/6g	12	0.2	197	10.8	29.3	4.1	0.0
Beef, Dry Weight, Oxo*	1 Cube/6g	15	0.3	265	17.3	38.4	4.7	1.5
Beef, Knorr*	1 Cube/10g	31	2.3	310	5.0	19.0	23.0	0.0
Beef, Organic, Kallo*	1 Cube/12g	25	1.0	208	16.7	16.7	8.3	0.0
Beef, Value, Tesco*	1 Cube/10g	14	0.4	135	11.1	12.9	3.9	6.6
Chicken	1 Cube/6g	14	0.9	237	15.4	9.9	15.4	0.0
Chicken, Dry, Average	*1 Cube/10g*	*29*	*1.8*	*293*	*7.3*	*25.5*	*18.0*	*0.4*
Chicken, Dry, Oxo*	1 Cube/7g	17	0.2	249	10.9	44.0	3.3	0.9
Chicken, Just Bouillon, Kallo*	1 Cube/12g	30	1.3	247	11.8	26.1	10.6	1.0
Chicken, Knorr*	1 Cube/10g	31	2.0	310	4.0	29.0	20.0	0.0
Chicken, Made Up, Average	*1 Pint/568ml*	*43*	*1.0*	*8*	*0.4*	*1.1*	*0.2*	*0.1*
Chicken, Prepared, Oxo*	1 Cube/100ml	9	0.1	9	0.4	1.5	0.1	0.1
Chicken, Tesco*	1 Cube/11g	32	2.5	290	10.5	11.1	22.6	0.7
Fish, Knorr*	1 Cube/10g	32	2.4	321	8.0	18.0	24.0	1.0
Fish, Sainsbury's*	1 Cube/11g	31	2.2	282	19.1	7.3	20.0	0.9
Ham, Knorr*	1 Cube/10g	31	1.9	313	11.8	24.4	18.7	0.0
Lamb, Made Up, Knorr*	1 Serving/100ml	5	0.6	5	0.3	0.3	0.6	0.1
Vegetable Bouillon, Vegetarian, Amoy*	1 Cube/10g	30	2.0	300	0.0	20.0	20.0	0.0
Vegetable Bouillon, Yeast Free, Made Up, Marigold*	1 Serving/250ml	19	1.6	8	0.0	0.5	0.6	0.0
Vegetable, Average	*1 Cube/7g*	*18*	*1.2*	*253*	*13.5*	*11.6*	*17.3*	*0.0*
Vegetable, Dry, Oxo*	1 Cube/6g	17	0.3	251	10.4	41.4	4.9	1.4
Vegetable, Knorr*	1 Cube/10g	33	2.4	330	10.0	25.0	24.0	1.0
Vegetable, Low Salt, Organic, Made Up, Kallo*	1 Serving/500ml	50	3.5	10	0.3	0.7	0.7	0.2
Vegetable, Made Up, Organic, Kallo*	2 Cubes/100ml	7	0.4	7	0.1	0.5	0.4	0.1
Vegetable, Made up, Oxo*	1 Cube/100ml	9	0.2	9	0.4	1.4	0.2	0.1
Vegetable, Organic, Yeast Free, Dry, Kallo*	1 Cube/11g	37	3.1	334	11.4	8.2	27.8	2.3
Vegetable, Smart Price, Asda*	1 Cube/11g	27	2.1	243	6.0	12.0	19.0	0.0
Vegetable, Value, Tesco*	1 Cube/10g	14	0.3	145	10.6	17.4	3.3	3.6

S

Measure INFO/WEIGHT	per Measure KCAL	FAT	Nutrition Values per 100g / 100ml KCAL	PROT	CARB	FAT	FIBRE

STRAWBERRIES

	Measure INFO/WEIGHT	KCAL	FAT	KCAL	PROT	CARB	FAT	FIBRE
Dried, Urban Fresh Fruit*	1 Pack/35g	111	0.1	318	1.6	77.0	0.4	5.9
Fresh, Raw, Average	*1 Strawberry/12g*	*3*	*0.0*	*28*	*0.8*	*6.0*	*0.1*	*1.4*
Frozen, Average	*1 Serving/100g*	*30*	*0.2*	*30*	*0.8*	*6.3*	*0.2*	*1.0*
in Fruit Juice, Canned, Average	*1/3 Can/127g*	*58*	*0.0*	*46*	*0.4*	*11.0*	*0.0*	*1.0*
in Light Syrup, Canned, Drained, Tesco*	1 Can/149g	100	0.1	67	0.5	16.0	0.1	0.7
in Syrup, Canned, Average	*1 Serving/100g*	*63*	*0.0*	*63*	*0.4*	*15.2*	*0.0*	*0.6*
Yoghurt Coated, Lightly, Bites, Yu!*	1 Bag/18g	70	1.8	389	3.0	61.3	9.9	10.2

STROGANOFF

	Measure INFO/WEIGHT	KCAL	FAT	KCAL	PROT	CARB	FAT	FIBRE
Beef & Rice, TTD, Sainsbury's*	1 Pack/410g	595	20.9	145	9.6	15.2	5.1	1.7
Beef with Rice 'n' Peppers, Tesco*	1 Pack/450g	562	19.8	125	7.5	13.1	4.4	0.4
Beef with White & Wild Rice, Classic, Tesco*	1 Pack/500g	770	29.6	154	9.5	15.5	5.9	2.3
Beef, 115, Oakhouse Foods Ltd*	1 Meal/400g	428	19.6	107	5.0	10.8	4.9	0.6
Beef, Asda*	1 Serving/120g	276	20.4	230	16.0	3.3	17.0	0.6
Beef, Eat Smart, Morrisons*	1 Pack/400g	344	9.2	86	5.0	11.2	2.3	0.9
Beef, Finest, Tesco*	½ Pack/200g	330	13.4	165	9.4	16.2	6.7	0.7
Beef, Weight Watchers*	1 Pack/330g	297	7.6	90	4.3	13.0	2.3	0.1
Beef, with White & Wild Rice, You Count, LL, Waitrose*	1 Pack/370g	418	9.0	113	6.0	16.3	2.4	1.0
Chicken with Rice, BGTY, Sainsbury's*	1 Pack/415g	448	5.4	108	7.0	17.1	1.3	1.1
Pork with Rice, HE, Tesco*	1 Pack/450g	482	8.1	107	7.0	15.8	1.8	0.5

STRUDEL

	Measure INFO/WEIGHT	KCAL	FAT	KCAL	PROT	CARB	FAT	FIBRE
Apple & Mincemeat, Tesco*	1 Serving/100g	322	16.7	322	3.3	39.6	16.7	2.0
Apple with Sultanas, Tesco*	1/6 Strudel/100g	245	12.0	245	2.9	30.9	12.0	0.7
Apple, Co-Op*	1 Slice/100g	225	12.0	225	3.0	28.0	12.0	3.0
Apple, Frozen, Sainsbury's*	1 Serving/100g	283	15.4	283	3.2	32.8	15.4	1.9
Apple, Ovenbaked, CBY, Asda*	1 Slice/100g	249	12.0	249	2.7	31.6	12.0	1.7
Apple, Sainsbury's*	1/6 Strudel/90g	255	13.9	283	3.2	32.8	15.4	1.9
Apple, Tesco*	1 Serving/150g	432	21.6	288	3.3	36.4	14.4	2.8
Woodland Fruit, Sainsbury's*	1/6 Strudel/95g	276	14.8	290	3.7	34.0	15.5	2.0
Woodland Fruit, Tesco*	1 Serving/100g	257	13.1	257	3.2	31.5	13.1	1.8

STUFFING

	Measure INFO/WEIGHT	KCAL	FAT	KCAL	PROT	CARB	FAT	FIBRE
Parsley & Thyme, Co-Op*	1 Serving/28g	95	0.8	340	10.0	67.0	3.0	6.0
Pork, Chestnut & Onion, Cooked, Finest, Tesco*	1/8 Pack/41g	108	6.9	263	12.9	13.6	16.8	2.4
Sage & Onion with Lemon, Paxo*	1 Serving/50g	61	0.6	122	3.4	24.2	1.2	1.9
Sage & Onion, for Chicken, Paxo*	1 Serving/50g	62	0.9	123	3.6	23.0	1.8	1.7
Sausagemeat & Thyme, Made Up, Celebrations, Paxo*	1 Serving/50g	80	1.8	160	6.3	25.8	3.5	4.0
Sausagemeat, Sainsbury's*	1 Serving/100g	175	4.2	175	7.0	27.0	4.2	2.3

STUFFING BALLS

	Measure INFO/WEIGHT	KCAL	FAT	KCAL	PROT	CARB	FAT	FIBRE
British Pork, Sage & Onion, Cooked, Finest, Tesco*	2 Balls/49g	110	5.0	224	13.9	17.4	10.2	2.2
Pork, Sausagemeat, Aunt Bessie's*	1 Ball/26g	55	2.1	212	7.2	27.3	8.2	3.0
Sage & Onion, Aunt Bessie's*	1 Ball/26g	63	2.3	243	6.4	34.4	8.9	3.1
Sage & Onion, Meat-Free, Aunt Bessie's*	1 Ball/28g	54	1.9	193	5.4	28.0	6.7	1.7
Tesco*	1 Ball/21g	65	4.1	315	9.6	23.5	20.0	1.4

STUFFING MIX

	Measure INFO/WEIGHT	KCAL	FAT	KCAL	PROT	CARB	FAT	FIBRE
Apple & Herb, Special Recipe, Sainsbury's*	1 Serving/41g	68	0.9	165	3.8	32.4	2.2	2.2
Apricot & Walnut, Made Up, Celebrations, Paxo*	1 Serving/50g	80	1.8	161	4.3	28.0	3.5	2.8
Sage & Onion, Asda*	1 Serving/27g	29	0.2	107	3.4	22.0	0.6	1.3
Sage & Onion, Co-Op*	1 Serving/28g	94	0.6	335	10.0	68.0	2.0	6.0
Sage & Onion, Dry Weight, Tesco*	1 Pack/170g	578	4.1	340	10.3	69.3	2.4	6.3
Sage & Onion, Made Up, Paxo*	1 Serving/50g	72	0.6	143	3.2	29.9	1.2	1.9
Sage & Onion, Made Up, Paxo*	1 Serving/60g	74	1.1	123	3.6	23.0	1.8	1.7
Sage & Onion, Prepared, Tesco*	1 Serving/100g	50	0.4	50	1.5	10.1	0.4	0.9
Sage & Onion, Value, Tesco*	1 Ball/38g	133	1.1	350	10.2	70.7	2.9	5.1
Sage & Onion, with Apple, Made Up, Paxo*	1 Serving/50g	69	0.8	138	3.8	26.0	1.6	2.2

	Measure INFO/WEIGHT	per Measure KCAL	FAT	Nutrition Values per 100g / 100ml KCAL	PROT	CARB	FAT	FIBRE
STUFFING MIX								
Sausage Meat, Morrisons*	1 Serving/20g	35	0.5	174	6.8	30.8	2.6	2.9
SUET								
Beef, Tesco*	1 Serving/100g	854	91.9	854	0.6	6.2	91.9	0.1
Vegetable, Average	*1oz/28g*	*234*	*24.6*	*836*	*1.2*	*10.1*	*87.9*	*0.0*
SUGAR								
Brown, Soft, Average	*1 Tsp/4g*	*15*	*0.0*	*382*	*0.0*	*96.5*	*0.0*	*0.0*
Brown, Soft, Light, Average	*1 Tsp/5g*	*20*	*0.0*	*393*	*0.2*	*97.8*	*0.1*	*0.0*
Caster, Average	*1 Tsp/5g*	*20*	*0.0*	*399*	*0.0*	*99.8*	*0.0*	*0.0*
Castor, White, Fairtrade, Sainsbury's*	1 Serving/100g	401	0.2	401	0.5	99.9	0.2	0.0
Dark Brown, Muscovado, Average	*1 Tsp/7g*	*27*	*0.0*	*380*	*0.2*	*94.8*	*0.0*	*0.0*
Dark Brown, Soft, Average	*1 Tsp/5g*	*18*	*0.0*	*369*	*0.1*	*92.0*	*0.0*	*0.0*
Demerara, Average	*1 Tsp/5g*	*18*	*0.0*	*368*	*0.2*	*99.2*	*0.0*	*0.0*
Fructose, Fruit Sugar, Tate & Lyle*	1 Tsp/4g	16	0.0	400	0.0	100.0	0.0	0.0
Golden, Unrefined, Average	*1 Tsp/4g*	*16*	*0.0*	*399*	*0.0*	*99.8*	*0.0*	*0.0*
Granulated, Organic, Average	*1 Tsp/4g*	*16*	*0.0*	*398*	*0.2*	*99.7*	*0.0*	*0.0*
Icing, Average	*1 Tsp/4g*	*16*	*0.0*	*394*	*0.0*	*102.2*	*0.0*	*0.0*
Light Or Diet, Average	*1 Tsp/4g*	*16*	*0.0*	*394*	*0.0*	*98.5*	*0.0*	*0.0*
Maple, Average	*1 Tsp/5g*	*18*	*0.0*	*354*	*0.1*	*90.9*	*0.2*	*0.0*
Vanilla, Fiddes Payne*	1 Serving/100g	397	0.1	397	0.1	99.2	0.1	0.5
White Plus Stevia Blend, Light at Heart, Tate & Lyle*	1 Serving/2g	8	0.0	398	0.0	99.6	0.0	0.0
White, Granulated, Average	*1 Tsp/5g*	*20*	*0.0*	*398*	*0.0*	*100.0*	*0.0*	*0.0*
SULTANAS								
Average	*1oz/28g*	*82*	*0.1*	*291*	*2.8*	*69.2*	*0.4*	*2.0*
SUNDAE								
Blackcurrant, M&S*	1 Sundae/53g	212	10.2	400	3.0	54.2	19.2	1.9
Chocolate & Cookie, Weight Watchers*	1 Pot/82g	128	2.8	156	2.5	30.3	3.4	2.2
Chocolate & Vanilla, Tesco*	1 Sundae/70g	140	6.0	199	2.8	27.5	8.6	0.5
Chocolate Brownie, Finest, Tesco*	1 Serving/215g	778	56.5	362	2.7	28.7	26.3	2.3
Chocolate Mint, COU, M&S*	1 Pot/90g	108	2.3	120	5.4	17.8	2.6	0.5
Chocolate, Sainsbury's*	1 Pot/140g	393	29.8	281	2.5	19.3	21.3	0.6
Hot Fudge, Two Scoop, Baskin Robbins*	1 Serving/203g	530	29.0	261	3.9	30.5	14.3	0.0
Ice Cream	1 Serving/170g	482	15.4	284	5.9	45.3	9.1	0.3
Strawberry & Vanilla, Weight Watchers*	1 Pot/105g	148	2.2	141	1.2	29.1	2.1	0.3
Strawberry, Burger King*	1 Sundae/150g	223	6.5	149	7.1	25.8	4.3	0.1
Strawberry, M&S*	1 Sundae/45g	173	8.0	385	3.4	53.3	17.8	1.0
Strawberry, Tesco*	1 Sundae/48g	194	8.7	408	3.3	57.6	18.3	1.3
Toffee & Vanilla, Tesco*	1 Serving/70g	133	4.5	189	2.1	30.7	6.4	0.1
Toffee, Good Puds, M Kitchen, Morrisons*	1 Pot/138g	268	13.4	194	3.6	22.9	9.7	0.4
SUNNY DELIGHT*								
Florida Style, Sunny Delight*	1 Serving/200ml	70	0.2	35	0.4	7.4	0.1	0.2
SUSHI								
California Roll Box, M&S*	1 Pack/230g	391	12.0	170	7.0	22.0	5.2	1.1
California Roll Selection, Classics, M&S*	1 Pack/225g	326	6.1	145	7.0	23.2	2.7	1.1
California Rolls 8 Pack	1 Pack/206g	354	9.3	172	5.1	27.5	4.5	1.4
California Set, Waitrose*	1 Pack/120g	223	9.1	186	3.8	25.2	7.6	1.7
Californian Roll & Nigiri, Selection, M&S*	1 Pack/215g	355	5.8	165	7.1	28.0	2.7	1.1
Californian Roll, Nigiri & Maki Selection, M&S*	1 Pack/210g	294	4.4	140	4.4	25.9	2.1	2.2
Chicken, M&S*	1 Pack/186g	260	4.1	140	6.0	24.4	2.2	1.0
Chicken, Tesco*	1 Pack/147g	243	3.5	165	5.2	30.0	2.4	1.0
Classic, Finest, Tesco*	1 Pack/232g	330	0.9	142	6.6	27.6	0.4	0.6
Fish & Veg Selection, Tesco*	1 Pack/150g	248	3.4	165	6.7	29.2	2.3	0.4
Fish Nigiri, Adventurous, Tesco*	1 Pack/200g	270	4.4	135	7.1	21.7	2.2	0.5
Fish Roll, Nigiri & Maki Selection, M&S*	1 Pack/210g	315	4.8	150	6.5	25.8	2.3	1.0

S

	Measure INFO/WEIGHT	per Measure KCAL	FAT	Nutrition Values per 100g / 100ml KCAL	PROT	CARB	FAT	FIBRE
SUSHI								
Fish, Large Pack, Tesco*	1 Pack/284g	469	11.1	165	5.5	27.0	3.9	1.5
Fish, Selection, Medium, Sainsbury's*	1 Pack/157g	256	3.9	163	5.6	28.6	2.5	1.9
Fish, Snack, Tesco*	1 Pack/104g	159	2.6	153	4.5	28.0	2.5	1.5
Fusion, M&S*	1 Pack/186g	260	3.3	140	5.1	23.8	1.8	2.9
GFY, Asda*	1 Pack/220g	352	3.1	160	4.9	32.0	1.4	0.0
Hana Set, Waitrose*	1 Serving/175g	324	4.0	185	5.4	35.7	2.3	1.4
Irodori Set with Fish, Cucumber & Avocado, Waitrose*	1 Pack/281g	472	12.4	168	5.2	26.7	4.4	1.3
Komachi Set with Salmon, Whiting & Handroll, Waitrose*	1 Pack/257g	447	13.9	174	5.3	25.8	5.4	1.2
Maki Rolls Box, Sainsbury's*	1 Pack/127g	197	2.2	155	4.5	30.5	1.7	0.8
Maki Selection, Shapers, Boots*	1 Pack/158g	225	2.1	142	3.5	29.0	1.3	1.1
Medium Pack, Tesco*	1 Pack/139g	211	3.2	152	6.3	26.6	2.3	2.3
Nigiri Set, Taiko, Salmon & Tuna, Waitrose*	1 Pack/113g	174	2.3	154	6.3	26.0	2.0	0.6
Prawn & Salmon Selection, M&S*	1 Serving/175g	255	2.9	146	5.5	27.4	1.7	0.6
Roll Selection, Sainsbury's*	1 Pack/217g	363	8.0	167	5.0	28.4	3.7	0.5
Salmon & Roll Set, Sainsbury's*	1 Serving/101g	167	2.6	165	4.9	30.4	2.6	0.8
Salmon, Smoked, Snack Pack, Tesco*	1 Pack/69g	114	1.9	165	5.0	29.1	2.7	0.9
Selection, Boots*	1 Pack/268g	434	9.6	162	5.5	27.0	3.6	1.6
Selection, Shapers, Boots*	1 Pack/162g	245	2.6	151	5.6	29.0	1.6	1.7
Snack Selection, Eat Well, M&S*	1 Pack/96g	134	0.7	140	5.3	28.7	0.7	0.8
Taiko, Fuji Set, Waitrose*	1 Pack/332g	515	10.0	155	5.0	28.0	3.0	1.0
to Share, Tesco*	1 Pack/385g	616	6.2	160	5.7	30.6	1.6	0.7
Vegetable Selection Pack, M&S*	1 Pack/154g	215	2.8	140	2.8	28.1	1.8	1.3
Vegetable, Mixed, Pick & Mix, Snack Pack, Tesco*	1 Pack/85g	132	2.0	155	3.7	28.6	2.4	1.4
Vegetarian with Pickled Vegetables, Waitrose*	1 Pack/135g	244	4.9	181	5.0	27.8	3.6	1.7
Vegetarian, Japanese Style, Shapers, Boots*	1 Pack/145g	218	3.2	150	2.9	29.0	2.2	1.3
Vegetarian, Selection, M&S*	1 Pack/171g	248	2.4	145	3.0	28.5	1.4	2.4
Vegetarian, Snack Selection, Tesco*	1 Pack/85g	106	2.8	125	3.7	20.1	3.3	0.6
Yasai Roll Set, Vegetarian, Wasabi Co Ltd*	1 Pack/392g	647	14.5	165	5.2	27.6	3.7	0.0
Yo!, Bento Box, Sainsbury's*	1 Pack/208g	530	6.2	255	8.4	48.7	3.0	0.9
SWEDE								
Boiled, Average	**1oz/28g**	**3**	**0.0**	**11**	**0.3**	**2.3**	**0.1**	**0.7**
Raw, Flesh Only, Peeled	**1 Serving/100g**	**24**	**0.3**	**24**	**0.7**	**5.0**	**0.3**	**1.6**
Raw, Unprepared, Average	**1oz/28g**	**5**	**0.1**	**18**	**0.7**	**3.8**	**0.3**	**1.6**
SWEET & SOUR								
Chicken Balls, Chinese Takeaway, Iceland*	1 Pack/255g	311	3.3	122	9.9	17.5	1.3	6.0
Chicken with Egg Fried Rice, GFY, Asda*	1 Pack/400g	500	7.6	125	6.0	20.3	1.9	1.8
Chicken with Egg Fried Rice, M Kitchen, Morrisons*	1 Pack/450g	706	16.2	157	8.1	22.2	3.6	1.9
Chicken with Long Grain Rice, Weight Watchers*	1 Pack/330g	300	1.6	91	5.4	15.5	0.5	1.4
Chicken with Vegetable Rice, COU, M&S*	1 Pack/400g	400	5.6	100	6.9	14.9	1.4	1.1
Chicken, & Rice, Chilled, Tesco*	1 Pack/450g	540	5.8	120	4.9	21.9	1.3	0.9
Chicken, Chinese Takeaway, Sainsbury's*	1 Pack/264g	515	16.9	195	13.1	21.3	6.4	1.0
Chicken, Diet Chef Ltd*	1 Pack/270g	270	4.9	100	8.9	12.1	1.8	1.1
Chicken, Healthy Options, Birds Eye*	1 Meal/348g	390	3.8	112	4.8	20.7	1.1	0.6
Chicken, in Batter, Cantonese, Chilled, Sainsbury's*	1 Pack/350g	560	21.0	160	8.9	22.4	6.0	0.9
Chicken, in Crispy Batter, Morrisons*	1 Pack/350g	511	13.6	146	10.1	17.6	3.9	1.2
Chicken, M&S*	1 Pack/300g	465	10.8	155	6.6	24.4	3.6	0.8
Chicken, Oriental, Tesco*	1 Pack/350g	340	4.0	97	9.3	12.2	1.1	0.8
Chicken, Take It Away, M&S*	1 Pack/200g	200	1.6	100	9.4	13.2	0.8	1.2
Chicken, Waitrose*	1 Serving/400g	372	3.2	93	9.8	11.7	0.8	1.4
Chicken, with Rice, Be Light, Aldi*	1 Pack/400g	436	2.0	109	8.8	17.0	0.5	1.2
Pork	1oz/28g	48	2.5	172	12.7	11.3	8.8	0.6
Pork, Battered, Sainsbury's*	½ Pack/175g	306	8.8	175	7.3	25.1	5.0	0.6
Pork, Cantonese, & Egg Fried Rice, Farmfoods*	1 Pack/327g	520	19.0	159	4.8	22.0	5.8	0.1

	Measure INFO/WEIGHT	per Measure KCAL	FAT	Nutrition Values per 100g / 100ml KCAL	PROT	CARB	FAT	FIBRE
SWEET & SOUR								
Roasted Vegetables, Cantonese, Sainsbury's*	1 Pack/348g	327	4.2	94	1.1	19.6	1.2	0.9
with Long Grain Rice, Rice Time, Uncle Ben's*	1 Pot/300g	393	2.4	131	1.9	28.4	0.8	0.7
SWEET POTATO								
Baked, Flesh Only, Average	*1 Med/130g*	*150*	*0.5*	*115*	*1.6*	*27.9*	*0.4*	*3.3*
Boiled in Salted Water, Average	*1 Med/200g*	*168*	*0.6*	*84*	*1.1*	*20.5*	*0.3*	*2.3*
Organic, Tesco*	1 Serving/100g	93	0.3	93	1.2	21.3	0.3	2.4
Raw, Peeled, Average	*1 Sm/130g*	*112*	*0.1*	*86*	*1.6*	*20.1*	*0.0*	*3.0*
Raw, Unprepared, Average	*1 Potato/200g*	*146*	*0.5*	*73*	*1.0*	*17.9*	*0.3*	*2.0*
Steamed, Average	*1 Med/200g*	*168*	*0.6*	*84*	*1.1*	*20.4*	*0.3*	*2.3*
Wedges, Eat Well, M&S*	½ Pack/150g	123	2.2	82	1.4	14.5	1.5	2.6
Wedges, Spicy & Zesty Chilli & Lime, Waitrose*	½ Pack/195g	205	7.0	105	1.3	15.2	3.6	3.5
SWEETBREAD								
Lamb, Fried	*1oz/28g*	*61*	*3.2*	*217*	*28.7*	*0.0*	*11.4*	*0.0*
SWEETCORN								
Baby, Frozen, Average	*1oz/28g*	*7*	*0.1*	*24*	*2.5*	*2.7*	*0.4*	*1.7*
Boiled, Average	*1oz/28g*	*31*	*0.6*	*111*	*4.2*	*19.6*	*2.3*	*2.2*
Canned with Sugar & Salt, Average	*1 Lge Can/340g*	*369*	*4.0*	*108*	*3.2*	*21.5*	*1.2*	*1.9*
Canned, Value, Tesco*	1 Can/260g	213	2.9	82	2.4	15.5	1.1	2.2
Frozen, Average	*1 Serving/80g*	*84*	*1.7*	*105*	*3.8*	*17.9*	*2.1*	*1.8*
No Sugar & Salt, Canned, Average	*½ Can/125g*	*99*	*1.3*	*79*	*2.7*	*15.0*	*1.1*	*1.6*
Supersweet, Field Fresh, Birds Eye*	1 Portion/80g	67	0.6	84	2.6	16.9	0.7	2.4
with Peppers, Canned, Average	*1 Serving/50g*	*40*	*0.2*	*79*	*2.6*	*16.4*	*0.3*	*0.6*
SWEETENER								
Calorie Free, Truvia*	1 Sachet/2g	0	0.0	0	0.0	99.0	0.0	0.0
Canderel*	1 Tbsp/2g	8	0.0	379	24.7	7.0	0.0	5.3
Canderel, Spoonful, Canderel*	1 Tsp/0.5g	2	0.0	384	2.9	93.0	0.0	0.0
Granulated, Low Calorie, Splenda*	1 Tsp/0.5g	2	0.0	391	0.0	97.7	0.0	0.0
Granulated, Silver Spoon*	1 Tsp/0.5g	2	0.0	387	1.0	96.8	0.0	0.0
Granulated, Tesco*	1 Tsp/1g	4	0.0	383	1.8	94.0	0.0	0.0
Lucuma Powder, Navitas*	1 Tbsp/15g	60	0.0	400	6.7	86.7	0.0	0.0
Natural Syrup, Fruit, Dark, Sweet Freedom*	1 Tsp/5g	13	0.0	292	0.0	79.0	0.0	0.0
Silver Spoon*	1 Tablet/0.05g	0	0.0	325	10.0	71.0	0.0	0.0
Slendasweet, Sainsbury's*	1 Tsp/1g	4	0.0	395	1.8	97.0	0.0	0.1
Sweetex*	1oz/28g	0	0.0	0	0.0	0.0	0.0	0.0
Tablet, Average	*1 Tablet/0.1g*	*0*	*0.0*	*355*	*8.7*	*73.0*	*0.0*	*0.8*
Tablets, Low Calorie, Canderel*	1 Tablet/0.1g	0	0.0	342	13.0	72.4	0.0	0.0
Tablets, Splenda*	1 Tablet/0.1g	0	0.0	345	10.0	76.2	0.0	1.6
Tablets, Tesco*	1 Tablet/1g	0	0.0	20	2.0	2.0	0.5	0.0
Xylosweet, Xylitol*	1 Serving/4g	10	0.0	240	0.0	100.0	0.0	0.0
SWEETS								
Almonds, Sugared, Dragee*	1 Sweet/4g	17	0.6	472	10.0	68.3	17.9	2.5
Banana, Baby Foam, M&S*	1/3 Pack/34g	131	0.0	385	4.1	92.7	0.0	0.0
Big Purple One, Quality Street, Nestle*	1 Sweet/39g	191	9.9	490	4.7	60.5	25.5	0.7
Black Jacks & Fruit Salad, Bassett's*	1 Serving/190g	760	11.8	400	0.7	84.9	6.2	0.0
Bon Bons, Strawberry, Classic Favourites, Asda*	1 Sweet/5g	20	0.3	402	0.0	88.0	5.6	0.0
Butter Candies, Original, Werther's*	1 Sweet/5g	21	0.4	424	0.1	85.7	8.9	0.1
Butterscotch Candies, Weight Watchers*	1 Box/42g	95	0.0	226	0.0	81.9	0.0	14.5
Candy Cane, Average	*1oz/28g*	*100*	*0.0*	*357*	*3.6*	*85.7*	*0.0*	*0.0*
Candy Corn, Brachs*	19 Pieces/39g	140	0.0	359	0.0	92.3	0.0	0.0
Candy Floss, Asda*	1 Tub/75g	292	0.0	390	0.0	100.0	0.0	0.0
Candy Foam Shapes, Fun Fruits, Value, Tesco*	1 Serving/25g	94	0.0	374	3.1	90.3	0.1	0.5
Cherry Lips, Chewits*	1 Serving/100g	319	0.2	319	5.6	72.1	0.2	0.0
Chew	1oz/28g	107	1.6	381	1.0	87.0	5.6	1.0

S

SWEETS

INFO/WEIGHT	Measure	per Measure		Nutrition Values per 100g / 100ml				
		KCAL	FAT	KCAL	PROT	CARB	FAT	FIBRE
Chewits, Blackcurrant	1 Pack/33g	125	0.9	378	0.3	86.9	2.7	0.0
Chewits, Blackcurrant, Leaf*	1 Chew/3g	12	0.1	385	0.2	87.5	3.0	0.0
Chewits, Fruit Salad, Leaf*	1 Chew/3g	12	0.1	385	0.2	87.5	3.0	0.0
Chewits, Strawberry, Leaf*	1 Chew/3g	12	0.1	385	0.2	87.5	3.0	0.0
Chews, Calcium, Ellactiva*	1 Sweet/7g	24	1.1	350	1.4	51.4	15.7	0.0
Chews, Just Fruit, Fruit-tella*	1 Serving/43g	170	2.8	400	0.9	79.5	6.5	0.0
Chews, Spearmint, Victoria, Aldi*	1 Sweet/10g	40	0.8	405	0.3	83.8	7.6	0.0
Chews, Strawberry Mix, Starburst*	1 Sweet/4g	15	0.3	401	0.0	83.9	7.3	0.0
Choco & Mint, Mentos*	1 Pack/38g	156	3.2	410	2.8	79.0	8.5	0.0
Chocolate Caramels, Milk, Tesco*	1 Sweet/3g	15	0.5	444	2.7	72.1	16.1	0.1
Chocolate Eclairs, Cadbury*	1 Sweet/8g	36	1.4	455	4.5	68.9	17.9	0.0
Chocolate Eclairs, Co-Op*	1 Sweet/8g	38	1.6	480	3.0	71.0	20.0	0.6
Chocolate Limes, Pascall*	1 Sweet/8g	27	0.2	333	0.3	77.2	2.5	0.0
Cola Bottles, Asda*	1 Serving/100g	329	0.2	329	9.0	73.0	0.2	0.0
Cola Bottles, Fizzy, M&S*	1 Pack/200g	650	0.0	325	6.4	75.0	0.0	0.0
Cream Caramel, Sula*	1 Sweet/3g	10	0.0	297	0.4	86.1	0.0	0.0
Crunchies, Fruit, Fruit-tella*	1 Box/23g	90	1.2	390	0.7	86.0	5.0	0.0
Dolly Mix, Bassett's*	1 Bag/45g	171	1.4	380	3.0	85.1	3.1	0.4
Double Lolly, Swizzels Matlow*	1 Lolly/10g	41	0.3	407	0.0	92.4	3.4	0.0
Drumstick, Matlow's*	1 Pack/40g	164	2.2	409	0.4	88.3	5.5	0.0
Edinburgh Rock, Gardiners of Scotland*	1 Piece/2g	8	0.0	380	0.1	94.4	0.3	0.8
Fizzy Mix, Tesco*	½ Bag/50g	166	0.0	332	5.2	75.2	0.0	0.0
Flumps, Bassett's*	1 Serving/5g	16	0.0	325	4.0	77.0	0.0	0.0
Flumps, Fluffy Mallow Twists, Fat Free, Bassett's*	1 Twist/13g	30	0.0	230	4.1	77.1	0.0	0.0
Foamy Mushrooms, Chewy, Asda*	1 Sweet/3g	9	0.0	347	4.2	82.0	0.2	0.0
Fruit Gums & Jellies	1 Tube/33g	107	0.0	324	6.5	79.5	0.0	0.0
Fruit, Mentos*	1 Sweet/3g	10	0.0	333	0.0	100.0	0.0	0.0
Fruities, Lemon & Lime, Weight Watchers*	1 Sweet/2g	3	0.0	134	0.0	54.0	0.0	33.0
Fruity Chews, Starburst*	1 Sweet/8g	34	0.6	404	0.0	83.4	7.4	0.0
Fruity Frogs, Rowntree's*	1 Serving/40g	128	0.1	321	4.7	74.5	0.2	0.0
Gummy Bears	10 Bears/22g	85	0.0	386	0.0	98.9	0.0	98.9
Gummy Mix, Tesco*	1 Pack/100g	327	0.1	327	5.9	75.7	0.1	0.0
Gummy Worms	10 Worms/74g	286	0.0	386	0.0	98.9	0.0	98.9
Gummy Zingy Fruits, Bassett's*	1 Sm Bag/40g	135	0.0	337	5.1	79.2	0.0	0.0
Jellies, Fruit, Ringtons*	4 Jellies/44g	150	0.2	341	0.1	84.0	0.4	0.7
Jellies, Very Berry, Rowntrees*	1 Sweet/4g	12	0.0	326	5.0	74.8	0.2	0.1
Jelly Babies, Morrisons*	1 Serving/227g	781	0.0	344	5.3	80.7	0.0	0.0
Jelly Beans, Tesco*	¼ Bag/63g	243	0.2	385	0.1	94.5	0.3	0.3
Jelly Squirms, Sour, The Natural Confectionery Co.*	1 Sweet/6g	20	0.0	325	2.8	78.2	0.1	0.0
Kisses, Hershey*	1 Sweet/5g	28	1.6	561	7.0	59.0	32.0	0.0
Laces, Apple Flavour, Tesco*	5 Laces/15g	52	0.5	347	3.6	74.8	3.2	2.1
Laces, Strawberry, Sainsbury's*	1 Serving/25g	94	1.2	377	3.3	76.3	4.6	0.1
Laces, Strawberry, Tesco*	1 Serving/75g	260	2.4	347	3.6	74.8	3.2	2.1
Lances, Strawberry & Cream Flavour, Tesco*	1 Bag/75g	276	0.9	368	3.2	86.1	1.2	2.1
Lances, Strawberry Flavour, Fizzy, Tesco*	½ Pack/50g	177	1.3	354	2.8	79.8	2.6	1.8
Lemon Mint Flavour, Herb Drops, Sugar Free, Ricola*	1 Sweet/3g	7	0.0	235	0.0	96.0	0.0	0.0
Liquorice Torpedoes, Sweets For Life*	1 Serving/100g	368	0.3	368	4.1	87.1	0.3	1.4
Lovehearts, Swizzels*	1oz/28g	100	0.0	359	0.7	88.2	0.0	0.0
Maoam Sour, Haribo*	1 Pack/22g	85	1.4	386	1.2	80.0	6.5	0.1
Maynards Sours, Bassett's*	1 Pack/52g	169	0.0	325	6.1	75.0	0.0	0.0
Midget Gems, Maynards*	1 Sweet/1g	3	0.0	340	8.7	76.2	0.0	0.0
Milk Chocolate Eclairs, Sainsbury's*	1 Sweet/8g	33	1.1	442	2.1	75.7	14.5	0.5
Milk Chocolate Eclairs, Value, Tesco*	1 Bag/200g	918	32.6	459	2.6	75.2	16.3	1.0

S

	Measure INFO/WEIGHT	per Measure KCAL	FAT	Nutrition Values per 100g / 100ml KCAL	PROT	CARB	FAT	FIBRE
SWEETS								
Milk Duds, Hershey*	13 Pieces/33g	170	6.0	510	3.0	84.0	18.0	0.0
Mini Marti, Mushrooms, Asda*	1 Sweet/3g	10	0.0	340	3.8	81.1	0.1	0.0
Original, Chocolate Soft Caramel, Speciality, Werther's*	1 Piece/6g	30	1.5	480	5.1	61.5	23.5	1.0
Paradise Fruits, Dominion, Aldi*	1 Sweet/6g	23	0.0	382	0.0	95.5	0.0	0.0
Parma Violets, Swizzlers*	1 Sm Tube/10g	41	0.0	406	0.9	99.1	0.0	0.0
Percy Pig & Pals, Soft, M&S*	1 Sweet/8g	30	0.0	344	5.8	80.0	0.1	0.0
Pic 'n' Mix, Woolworths*	1 Serving/180g	750	6.0	417	0.0	96.7	3.3	0.0
Randoms, Rowntree's*	1 Pack/50g	164	0.2	328	4.9	75.7	0.3	0.6
Refreshers, Bassett's*	1oz/28g	106	0.0	377	4.3	78.1	0.0	0.0
Rhubarb & Custard, Sainsbury's*	1 Sweet/8g	28	0.0	351	0.1	87.7	0.0	0.0
Rhubarb & Custards, Tesco*	1 Sweet/9g	36	0.0	396	0.3	97.6	0.5	0.1
Rotella, Haribo*	1 Sweet/13g	43	0.0	343	1.5	84.0	0.2	0.0
Sherbert Dib Dab with Strawberry Lolly, Barratt*	1 Pack/23g	90	0.0	385	0.1	95.6	0.1	0.0
Sherbert Lemons, M&S*	1 Serving/20g	76	0.0	380	0.0	93.9	0.0	0.0
Shrimps & Bananas, Sainsbury's*	½ Pack/50g	188	0.0	376	2.5	91.3	0.1	0.5
Soft Fruits, Trebor*	1 Roll/45g	165	0.0	367	0.0	90.9	0.0	0.0
Sour Apple Sticks, Fizzy Wizzy, Woolworths*	1 Sweet/5g	18	0.1	358	2.8	79.8	2.7	0.0
Strawberry & Cream, Sugar Free, Sula*	1 Sweet/3g	9	0.2	267	0.2	90.5	5.4	0.0
Tic Tac, Cool Cherry, Ferrero*	1 Pack/18g	69	0.1	382	0.2	92.2	0.7	0.0
Tootsie Roll, Small Midgees, Tootsie*	1 Sweet/7g	23	0.5	350	2.5	70.0	7.5	0.0
Tooty Frooties, Rowntree's*	1 Bag/28g	111	1.0	397	0.1	91.5	3.5	0.0
Wine Gummies, Matlow, Swizzels*	1 Pack/16g	52	0.0	324	0.0	58.7	0.0	0.0
Yo Yo's, All Flavours, 100% Fruit, We Are Bear*	1 Roll/10g	28	0.0	275	1.9	63.4	0.2	12.0
Yo Yo's, Strawberry 100% Fruit, We Are Bear*	1 Roll/10g	28	0.0	275	1.9	63.4	0.2	12.0
York Fruits, Terry's*	1 Sweet/9g	29	0.0	320	0.0	78.5	0.0	0.5
SWORDFISH								
Grilled, Average	*1oz/28g*	*39*	*1.5*	*139*	*22.9*	*0.0*	*5.2*	*0.0*
Raw, Average	*1oz/28g*	*42*	*2.0*	*149*	*21.1*	*0.0*	*7.2*	*0.0*
SYRUP								
Balsamic, Merchant Gourmet*	1 Tsp/5g	12	0.0	232	0.4	60.0	0.1	0.0
Butterscotch, Monin*	1 Serving/30ml	100	0.0	333	0.0	80.0	0.0	0.0
Caramel, for Coffee, Lyle's*	2 Tsps/10ml	33	0.0	329	0.0	83.0	0.0	0.0
Caramel, Sugar Free, Monin*	1 Serving/30ml	0	0.0	0	0.0	13.3	0.0	0.0
Chocolate Mint, Monin*	1 Serving/30ml	100	0.0	333	0.0	80.0	0.0	0.0
Cinnamon, Monin*	1 Serving/30ml	100	0.0	333	0.0	80.0	0.0	0.0
Corn, Dark, Average	*1 Tbsp/20g*	*56*	*0.0*	*282*	*0.0*	*76.6*	*0.0*	*0.0*
Gingerbread, Monin*	1 Serving/30ml	90	0.0	300	0.0	76.7	0.0	0.0
Golden, Average	*1 Tbsp/20g*	*61*	*0.0*	*304*	*0.4*	*78.2*	*0.0*	*0.0*
Hazelnut, Monin*	1 Serving/30ml	90	0.0	300	0.0	73.3	0.0	0.0
Maple, Average	*1 Tbsp/20g*	*52*	*0.0*	*262*	*0.0*	*67.2*	*0.2*	*0.0*
Organic Rice Malt, Clearspring*	2 Tbsp/42g	133	0.2	316	1.5	76.8	0.4	0.0
Peppermint, Monin*	1 Serving/30ml	96	0.0	320	0.0	80.0	0.0	0.0
Praline, Monin*	1 Serving/30ml	94	0.0	313	0.0	76.7	0.0	0.0
Sugar	1Tbsp/20g	64	0.0	319	0.0	83.9	0.0	0.0
Vanilla, Monin*	1 Shot/35ml	119	0.0	340	0.0	84.4	0.0	0.0
Vanilla, Sugar Free, Monin*	1 Serving/30ml	0	0.0	0	0.0	13.3	0.0	0.0

S

	Measure INFO/WEIGHT	per Measure KCAL	FAT	Nutrition Values per 100g / 100ml KCAL	PROT	CARB	FAT	FIBRE
TABOULEH								
Average	**1oz/28g**	**33**	**1.3**	**119**	**2.6**	**17.2**	**4.6**	**0.0**
TACO KIT								
Chicken Tinga, as Sold, Restaurante, Old El Paso*	1 Taco/39g	94	1.6	237	7.2	42.3	4.0	1.7
Garlic & Paprika, Crunchy, As Sold, Old El Paso *	1 Taco/26g	77	3.6	296	3.8	37.3	13.8	2.7
Smoky BBQ, Soft, As Sold, St& n Stuff, Old El Paso*	1 Taco/44g	94	1.8	213	5.6	37.1	4.2	2.0
TACO SHELLS								
Corn, Crunchy, Old El Paso*	1 Taco/10g	51	2.6	506	7.0	61.0	26.0	0.0
Old El Paso*	1 Taco/12g	57	2.7	478	7.4	60.8	22.8	0.0
Traditional, Discovery*	1 Taco/11g	55	3.2	489	5.7	53.4	28.1	6.0
TAGINE								
Lamb, Moroccan Style with Cous Cous, COU, M&S*	1 Pack/400g	340	5.6	85	8.9	8.3	1.4	1.6
Spicy Chermoula, Tasty Veg Pot, Innocent*	1 Pot/400g	356	9.6	89	3.4	13.8	2.4	5.0
TAGLIATELLE								
Carbonara, Italiano, Tesco*	1 Serving/325g	757	37.4	233	8.6	23.8	11.5	1.2
Carbonara, Ready Meal, Average	**1 Serving/400g**	**460**	**13.4**	**115**	**5.5**	**15.8**	**3.3**	**1.0**
Carbonara, TTD, Sainsbury's*	1 Pack/405g	644	25.9	159	7.8	17.6	6.4	1.6
Chicken & Tomato, Italiano, Tesco*	1 Pack/400g	416	8.4	104	6.6	14.8	2.1	0.8
Creamy Mushroom, CBY, Asda*	1 Pak/400g	428	10.8	107	3.7	16.3	2.7	1.4
Dry, Average	**1 Serving/100g**	**356**	**1.8**	**356**	**12.6**	**72.4**	**1.8**	**1.0**
Egg, Dry, Average	**1 Serving/75g**	**272**	**2.5**	**362**	**14.2**	**68.8**	**3.3**	**2.3**
Egg, Fresh, Cooked, Tesco*	½ Pack/150g	415	3.1	277	9.6	52.8	2.1	3.2
Egg, Fresh, Dry, Average	**1 Serving/125g**	**345**	**3.5**	**276**	**10.6**	**53.0**	**2.8**	**2.1**
Fresh, Dry, Average	**1 Serving/75g**	**211**	**2.0**	**281**	**11.4**	**53.3**	**2.6**	**2.6**
Garlic & Herb, Fresh, Tesco*	1 Serving/125g	361	4.6	289	12.0	51.8	3.7	1.5
Garlic & Herbs, Cooked, Pasta Reale*	1 Pack/250g	390	2.8	156	6.2	30.4	1.1	1.0
Garlic Mushroom, Italiano, Tesco*	1 Pack/450g	738	41.0	164	5.2	15.2	9.1	0.6
Ham & Mushroom, Asda*	1 Pack/340g	469	12.9	138	6.0	20.0	3.8	0.2
Ham & Mushroom, BGTY, Sainsbury's*	1 Pack/400g	368	4.8	92	4.2	15.5	1.2	1.1
Ham & Mushroom, Italian, Sainsbury's*	1 Pack/400g	548	19.6	137	5.0	17.5	4.9	1.3
Ham & Mushroom, Italian, Waitrose*	1 Pack/400g	556	22.0	139	7.0	14.5	5.5	1.5
Lamb Ragu, Slow Cooked, Finest, Tesco*	1 Pack/400g	560	19.2	140	8.5	14.9	4.8	1.1
Multigrain, BGTY, Uncooked, Sainsbury's*	1 Serving/190g	294	4.8	155	7.0	26.0	2.5	3.0
Mushroom & Bacon, Sainsbury's*	1 Pack/450g	585	23.4	130	7.1	13.8	5.2	0.5
Salmon & King Prawn, HL, Tesco*	1 Pack/400g	480	9.6	120	6.5	17.2	2.4	1.7
Smoked Salmon, Ready Meals, M&S*	1 Pack/360g	612	40.3	170	6.2	10.6	11.2	0.9
Sundried Tomato, Fresh, Morrisons*	1 Pack/250g	748	8.2	299	11.1	56.4	3.3	3.5
Tricolore, Waitrose*	½ Pack/125g	351	3.6	281	12.0	51.6	2.9	1.6
Verdi, Fresh, Average	**1 Serving/125g**	**171**	**1.8**	**137**	**5.5**	**25.5**	**1.5**	**1.8**
TAHINI PASTE								
Average	**1 Tsp/6g**	**36**	**3.5**	**607**	**18.5**	**0.9**	**58.9**	**8.0**
TANGERINES								
Fresh, Raw	**1oz/28g**	**10**	**0.0**	**35**	**0.9**	**8.0**	**0.1**	**1.3**
Fresh, Raw, Weighed with Peel, Average	**1 Med/70g**	**13**	**0.1**	**18**	**0.5**	**4.2**	**0.1**	**0.7**
TANGO*								
Cherry, Britvic*	1 Bottle/500ml	55	0.0	11	0.0	2.4	0.0	0.0
Orange, Britvic*	1 Can/330ml	63	0.0	19	0.1	4.4	0.0	0.0
TAPAS								
Basque Beef, (Estofado Vasco), Tapas at, Tesco*	½ Pack/80g	80	3.1	100	9.5	6.4	3.9	1.5
Champinones Al Ajillo, Tapas at, Tesco*	½ Pack/85g	123	11.6	145	2.3	2.5	13.6	1.5
Chorizo & Cheese Croquettes, Tapas at, Tesco*	½ Pack/117g	263	11.1	225	5.4	28.6	9.5	2.6
Patatas Bravas, Tapas at, Tesco*	½ Pack/125g	169	6.4	135	2.5	18.7	5.1	3.0
Pollo Con Salsa, Tapas at, Tesco*	½ Pack/75g	94	6.5	125	9.4	2.1	8.7	0.7

	Measure INFO/WEIGHT	per Measure KCAL	FAT	Nutrition Values per 100g / 100ml KCAL	PROT	CARB	FAT	FIBRE
TAPIOCA								
Creamed, Ambrosia*	½ Can/213g	159	3.4	75	2.6	12.6	1.6	0.2
Raw	*1oz/28g*	*101*	*0.0*	*359*	*0.4*	*95.0*	*0.1*	*0.4*
TARAMASALATA								
Average	*1 Tbsp/30g*	*143*	*14.4*	*478*	*4.2*	*7.9*	*47.9*	*1.1*
HE, Tesco*	1 Pot/170g	430	34.3	253	4.3	13.5	20.2	0.7
M&S*	1 Serving/100g	480	48.9	480	4.9	6.4	48.9	0.7
Reduced Fat, Waitrose*	1 Pack/170g	522	48.3	307	4.0	8.9	28.4	1.5
Sainsbury's*	¼ Tub/50g	236	24.0	472	4.0	7.5	48.1	0.0
Smoked Salmon, Tesco*	1 Serving/95g	474	48.2	499	3.0	7.7	50.7	0.3
Supreme, Waitrose*	1 Serving/20g	84	8.1	421	7.4	6.3	40.7	2.9
Tesco*	1/8 Tub/25g	115	11.2	460	2.9	10.5	44.8	1.0
TARRAGON								
Dried, Ground	*1 Tsp/2g*	*5*	*0.1*	*295*	*22.8*	*42.8*	*7.2*	*0.0*
Fresh, Average	*1 Tbsp/4g*	*2*	*0.0*	*49*	*3.4*	*6.3*	*1.1*	*0.0*
TART								
Apple & Fresh Cream, Asda*	½ Tart/50g	134	8.0	267	3.4	33.0	16.0	0.8
Apricot Lattice, Sainsbury's*	1 Slice/125g	321	14.2	257	3.4	35.3	11.4	2.6
Aubergine & Feta, Roast Marinated, Sainsbury's*	1 Serving/105g	227	15.2	216	4.8	16.6	14.5	1.7
Bakewell, Average	*1 Tart/50g*	*228*	*14.8*	*456*	*6.3*	*43.5*	*29.7*	*1.9*
Bakewell, Cherry, Morrisons*	1 Tart/46g	198	9.8	430	4.6	54.9	21.4	1.3
Bakewell, Free From, Tesco*	1 Tart/50g	170	4.6	340	1.6	63.0	9.2	4.8
Bakewell, Lemon, Easter, Morrisons*	1 Tart/45g	186	7.1	413	3.1	64.8	15.7	1.8
Bakewell, M&S*	¼ Tart/75g	345	20.0	460	7.5	48.1	26.7	2.1
Bakewell, Toffee, Morrisons*	1 Tart/47g	201	7.4	422	3.0	67.2	15.5	0.9
Cherry Tomato & Mascarpone, ES, Asda*	1 Tart/153g	290	18.3	190	4.6	16.0	12.0	1.1
Chocolate, Co-Op*	1 Tart/22g	102	6.8	465	4.0	42.0	31.0	0.7
Custard, Individual, Average	*1 Tart/94g*	*260*	*13.6*	*277*	*6.3*	*32.4*	*14.5*	*1.2*
Date Pecan & Almond, Sticky, Sainsbury's*	1/8 Tart/75g	298	10.3	397	5.0	63.5	13.7	1.7
Egg Custard, Asda*	1 Tart/80g	215	10.4	269	9.0	29.0	13.0	1.2
Egg Custard, Tesco*	1 Tart/82g	214	10.0	261	6.2	31.5	12.2	1.1
Egg Custard, Twin Pack, Tesco*	1 Tart/90g	240	11.4	270	5.6	31.6	12.8	0.9
Feta Cheese & Spinach, Puff Pastry, Tesco*	1 Tart/108g	306	19.2	283	7.1	23.5	17.8	0.9
Filo Asparagus Tartlette, M&S*	1 Serving/15g	45	3.1	300	4.4	25.2	20.4	2.1
Frangipane, Chocolate & William Pear, Waitrose*	1/6 Pack/80g	219	12.4	274	3.5	29.9	15.5	2.5
Gruyere Pancetta & Balsamic Onion, Finest, Tesco*	¼ Tart/106g	320	21.9	301	7.7	21.3	20.6	3.3
Italian Lemon & Almond, Sainsbury's*	1 Slice/49g	182	11.6	371	7.4	31.9	23.7	4.1
Jam, Assorted, Asda*	1 Tart/30g	122	4.8	407	2.7	63.0	16.0	2.4
Jam, Assorted, Tesco*	1 Tart/35g	123	5.0	351	3.4	51.9	14.4	1.2
Jam, Assorted, VLH Kitchens	1 Serving/34g	44.2	42.4	130	3.4	56.0	14.4	1.3
Jam, Average	*1 Slice/90g*	*342*	*13.4*	*380*	*3.3*	*62.0*	*14.9*	*1.6*
Jam, Real Fruit, Mr Kipling*	1 Tart/35g	136	5.2	388	3.8	67.9	14.9	1.7
Jam, Real Fruit, Sainsbury's*	1 Tart/37g	142	5.2	383	3.4	60.9	14.0	1.4
Leek & Stilton, Morrisons*	1 Serving/125g	392	26.9	314	6.9	23.1	21.5	0.3
Lemon & Raspberry, Finest, Tesco*	1 Tart/120g	360	16.8	300	5.2	38.4	14.0	2.9
Lemon Curd, Asda*	1 Tart/30g	121	4.5	402	2.8	64.0	15.0	2.2
Lemon, M&S*	1/6 Tart/50g	208	14.6	415	5.0	32.7	29.3	0.9
Lemon, Sainsbury's*	1/8 Tart/56g	258	15.8	459	4.4	47.0	28.1	0.6
Lemon, Sicilian, Individual, Finest, Tesco*	1 Tart/110g	410	20.0	373	5.0	47.0	18.2	0.7
Mixed Fruit, Fresh, Waitrose*	1 Tart/129g	351	17.4	272	4.2	32.8	13.5	1.5
Normandy Apple & Calvados, Finest, Tesco*	1/6 Tart/100g	256	7.6	256	3.2	41.4	7.6	1.9
Pineapple, Individual, Waitrose*	1 Tart/54g	216	6.1	400	2.2	77.2	11.3	0.5
Raspberry & Blueberry, Tesco*	1 Serving/85g	168	7.5	198	2.7	27.0	8.8	2.8
Red Pepper, Serrano Ham & Goats Cheese, Waitrose*	1 Serving/100g	293	19.2	293	8.7	21.3	19.2	3.2

T

	Measure INFO/WEIGHT	per Measure		Nutrition Values per 100g / 100ml				
		KCAL	FAT	KCAL	PROT	CARB	FAT	FIBRE
TART								
Roasted Vegetable, Finest, Tesco*	¼ Tart/113g	226	13.2	200	3.1	20.6	11.7	2.3
Spinach & Ricotta, Individual, TTD, Sainsbury's*	1 Quiche/170g	466	33.7	274	7.5	16.5	19.8	1.4
Strawberry & Fresh Cream, Finest, Tesco*	1 Tart/129g	350	19.1	271	3.3	31.1	14.8	1.2
Strawberry Custard, Asda*	1 Tart/100g	335	15.0	335	3.1	47.0	15.0	0.0
Strawberry, Fresh, M&S*	1 Tart/120g	305	18.4	255	3.1	26.4	15.4	2.4
Strawberry, Reduced Sugar, Asda*	1 Tart/37g	141	3.7	380	4.6	67.5	10.1	1.2
Strawberry, Sainsbury's*	1 Serving/206g	521	26.2	253	2.6	32.0	12.7	0.7
Strawberry, Waitrose*	1 Serving/101g	241	12.0	239	3.8	29.2	11.9	1.2
Summer Fruit Crumble, Morrisons*	1 Tart/128g	379	15.1	296	3.6	43.8	11.8	1.3
Toffee Apple, Co-Op*	1 Tart/20g	69	3.2	345	3.0	47.0	16.0	0.7
Toffee Pecan, M&S*	1 Tart/91g	414	24.1	455	6.0	48.5	26.5	2.0
Tomato, Mozzarella & Basil Puff, Sainsbury's*	1/3 Tart/120g	318	25.0	265	9.2	10.2	20.8	0.9
Treacle Lattice, Mr Kipling*	1/6 Tart/70g	256	8.5	365	4.4	59.8	12.1	1.1
Treacle with Custard	1 Serving/251g	586	23.5	233	3.1	36.1	9.4	0.8
Treacle, Average	**1 Portion/125g**	**460**	**17.6**	**368**	**3.7**	**60.4**	**14.1**	**1.1**
Treacle, Sainsbury's*	1 Serving/100g	369	12.1	369	4.3	60.6	12.1	1.2
Treacle, Tesco*	1 Slice/63g	228	7.6	362	3.9	58.5	12.1	1.7
Treacle, Waitrose*	¼ Tart/106g	302	11.0	285	2.8	45.0	10.4	0.6
Vegetable & Feta, Deli, M&S*	½ Tart/115g	315	18.4	274	5.0	20.0	16.0	6.0
Zesty Lemon, Tesco*	1/6 Tart/64g	260	15.5	405	5.3	41.0	24.2	0.7
TARTE								
Au Citron, Frozen, Tesco*	1/6 Tarte/81g	255	11.8	315	5.4	39.4	14.6	0.7
Au Citron, Frozen, TTD, Sainsbury's*	1/6 Tarte/80g	232	13.4	290	4.7	40.7	16.8	7.7
Au Citron, Seriously Lemony, Large, Waitrose*	1 Tarte/470g	1589	81.8	338	4.6	40.8	17.4	0.5
Au Citron, Waitrose*	1 Tarte/100g	325	18.1	325	4.9	35.7	18.1	1.0
Aux Cerises, Finest, Tesco*	1 Serving/98g	219	7.0	225	4.9	35.4	7.2	0.6
Bacon, Leek & Roquefort, Bistro, Waitrose*	¼ Tarte/100g	277	18.2	277	8.4	19.8	18.2	0.6
Normande, French Style, M&S*	1/6 Tarte/85g	245	16.1	290	3.3	26.8	19.0	0.7
Spinach & Goats Cheese, Flamme, TTD, Sainsbury's*	1/3 Quiche/77g	227	16.7	296	6.9	18.1	21.8	5.0
Tatin, Sainsbury's*	1 Serving/120g	244	8.0	203	2.9	32.8	6.7	1.9
TARTLETS								
Butternut Squash & Goats Cheese, Linda McCartney*	1 Tartlet/150g	405	25.0	270	6.3	24.2	16.7	1.2
Cheddar, Vintage, Potato & Leek, Waitrose*	1 Tartlet/130g	391	25.0	301	7.7	23.3	19.2	2.2
Mushroom Medley, BGTY, Sainsbury's*	1 Serving/80g	134	8.0	167	4.7	14.5	10.0	3.4
Red Onion & Goats Cheese, Sainsbury's*	1 Tartlet/113g	335	21.8	297	7.0	23.7	19.3	1.5
Salmon & Watercress, Hot Smoked, Waitrose*	1 Serving/130g	315	19.9	242	8.1	18.0	15.3	3.0
Tomato & Goats Cheese, Waitrose*	1 Tartlet/130g	295	19.0	227	6.6	17.4	14.6	2.0
TEA								
Assam, Blended, TTD, Sainsbury's*	1 Serving/2g	0	0.0	0	0.0	0.0	0.0	0.0
Blackberry & Nettle, Twinings*	1 Cup/250ml	5	0.0	2	0.0	0.3	0.0	0.0
Blackcurrant, Fruit Creations, Typhoo*	1 Sm Cup/100ml	5	0.0	5	0.2	0.8	0.0	0.2
Camomile, Pure, Classic Herbal, Twinings*	1 Serving/200ml	4	0.0	2	0.0	0.3	0.0	0.0
Chai, Twinings*	1 Cup/200ml	2	0.0	1	0.1	0.0	0.0	0.0
Chamomile & Spiced Apple, Warming, Twinings*	1 Cup/100ml	2	0.0	2	0.0	0.3	0.0	0.0
Damask, Rose, Chinese, Choi Time*	1 Mug/500ml	0	0.3	0	0.0	0.0	0.1	0.0
Decaf, Tetley*	1 Cup/100ml	1	0.0	1	0.0	0.3	0.0	0.0
Earl Grey, Black, Pret a Manger*	1 Serving/360ml	14	0.5	4	0.3	0.4	0.1	0.0
Earl Grey, Green, Twinings*	1 Cup/200ml	2	0.0	1	0.0	0.2	0.0	0.0
Earl Grey, Infusion with Water, Average	**1 Mug/250ml**	**2**	**0.0**	**1**	**0.0**	**0.2**	**0.0**	**0.0**
Fennel, Sweet, Twinings*	1 fl oz/30ml	1	0.0	2	0.0	0.3	0.0	0.0
Fruit Or Herbal, Made with Water, Twinings*	1 Mug/200ml	8	0.0	4	0.0	1.0	0.0	0.0
Fruit, Green, Infusion, Eat Well, M&S*	½ Pack/150g	80	1.2	53	1.4	9.8	0.8	0.6
Fruit, Twinings*	1 Mug/227ml	4	0.0	2	0.0	0.4	0.0	0.0

T

	Measure INFO/WEIGHT	per Measure		Nutrition Values per 100g / 100ml				
		KCAL	FAT	KCAL	PROT	CARB	FAT	FIBRE
TEA								
Fruits of the Forest, Westminster Tea*	1 Bag/250ml	5	0.0	2	0.0	0.6	0.0	0.0
Green Tea Pure, Twinings*	1 Serving/100g	1	0.0	1	0.0	0.2	0.0	0.0
Green with Citrus, Twinings*	1 Serving/200ml	2	0.0	1	1.0	0.2	0.0	0.0
Green with Jasmine, Twinings*	1 Serving/100ml	1	0.0	1	0.0	0.2	0.0	0.0
Green with Jasmine, Wellbeing Selection, Flavia*	1 Cup/200ml	0	0.0	0	0.0	0.0	0.0	0.0
Green with Mango, Brewed with Water, Twinings*	1 Cup/200ml	2	0.0	1	0.0	0.2	0.0	0.0
Green with Mint, Whittards of Chelsea*	1 Cup/100ml	1	0.0	1	0.2	0.1	0.0	0.0
Ice with Lemon, Lipton*	1 Bottle/325ml	91	0.0	28	0.0	6.9	0.0	0.0
Ice with Mango, Lipton*	1 Bottle/500ml	165	0.0	33	0.0	8.1	0.0	0.0
Ice with Peach, Lipton*	1 Bottle/500ml	140	0.0	28	0.0	6.8	0.0	0.0
Iced, Peach, Twinings*	1 Serving/200ml	60	0.2	30	0.1	7.3	0.1	0.0
Jasmine, Twinings*	1 fl oz/30ml	0	0.0	1	0.0	0.2	0.0	0.0
Lemon & Ginger, Lipton*	1 Cup/200ml	8	0.0	4	0.5	0.5	0.0	0.0
Lemon, Instant, Original, Lift*	1 Serving/15g	53	0.0	352	0.0	87.0	0.0	0.0
Light & Delicate, Green with Lemon, Twinings*	1 Cup/100ml	1	0.1	1	0.1	0.2	0.1	0.1
Made with Water	1 Mug/227ml	0	0.0	0	0.1	0.0	0.0	0.0
Made with Water with Semi-Skimmed Milk, Average	*1 Cup/200ml*	*14*	*0.4*	*7*	*0.5*	*0.7*	*0.2*	*0.0*
Made with Water with Skimmed Milk, Average	*1 Mug/270ml*	*16*	*0.5*	*6*	*0.5*	*0.7*	*0.2*	*0.0*
Made with Water with Whole Milk, Average	*1 Cup/200ml*	*16*	*0.8*	*8*	*0.4*	*0.5*	*0.4*	*0.0*
Morning Detox, Twinings*	1 Serving/200ml	5	0.0	2	0.0	0.3	0.0	0.0
Nettle & Peppermint, Twinings*	1 Cup/200ml	2	0.0	1	0.0	0.2	0.0	0.0
Nettle & Sweet Fennel, Twinings*	1 Cup/200ml	4	0.0	2	0.0	0.3	0.0	0.0
Peppermint, Made with Water, Average	*1 Serving/200ml*	*3*	*0.0*	*2*	*0.0*	*0.2*	*0.0*	*0.0*
Red Bush, Made with Water, Tetley*	1 Mug/250ml	2	0.0	1	0.0	0.1	0.0	0.0
TEACAKES								
Average	*1 Teacake/60g*	*178*	*4.5*	*296*	*8.0*	*52.5*	*7.5*	*0.0*
Caramel, Highlights, Mallows, Cadbury*	1 Teacake/15g	61	1.9	408	6.2	69.1	12.4	3.6
Currant, Sainsbury's*	1 Teacake/72g	204	2.9	284	8.2	53.7	4.0	2.5
Fruit, Lidl*	1 Teacake/62g	166	2.7	267	10.6	46.3	4.4	2.2
Fruited, Co-Op*	1 Teacake/62g	160	2.0	258	9.7	46.8	3.2	3.2
Fruited, M&S*	1 Teacake/60g	156	0.6	260	8.9	53.4	1.0	2.0
Fruity, Warburton's*	1 Teacake/63g	160	2.2	256	8.7	48.0	3.5	2.7
Hovis*	1 Teacake/60g	155	1.5	258	9.0	49.9	2.5	3.0
Jam, Biscuit & Mallow, Chocolate Covered, Burton's*	1 Teacake/13g	57	2.4	455	3.8	66.9	19.3	1.1
Large, Sainsbury's*	1 Teacake/100g	291	6.8	291	8.3	49.1	6.8	3.4
Large, TTD, Sainsbury's*	1 Teacake/90g	264	3.5	293	7.5	57.0	3.9	2.6
Lees*	1 Teacake/19g	81	2.9	426	4.2	67.7	15.4	0.0
Mallow, Tesco*	1 Teacake/14g	63	2.7	450	4.1	65.4	19.1	1.0
Mallow, Value, Tesco*	1 Teacake/14g	60	2.3	425	3.6	65.8	16.2	1.4
Marshmallow, Milk Chocolate, Tunnock's*	1 Teacake/24g	106	4.6	440	4.9	61.9	19.2	2.4
Mini Bites, M&S*	1 Bite/6g	29	1.2	484	3.2	72.6	20.3	2.1
Morrisons*	1 Teacake/64g	172	1.9	268	9.9	50.7	2.9	2.8
Richly Fruited, Waitrose*	1 Teacake/72g	205	2.7	285	7.8	55.0	3.7	2.2
Sainsbury's*	1 Teacake/70g	171	2.5	244	8.0	45.0	3.6	2.6
Tesco*	1 Teacake/61g	163	2.1	267	7.8	51.1	3.5	2.4
Toasted, Average	*1 Teacake/60g*	*197*	*5.0*	*329*	*8.9*	*58.3*	*8.3*	*0.0*
with Fruit, Morning Fresh, Aldi*	1 Teacake/65g	155	2.2	239	7.4	44.6	3.4	2.3
with Orange Filling, M&S*	1 Teacake/20g	80	2.8	410	4.5	66.6	14.2	0.9
TEMPEH								
Average	*1oz/28g*	*46*	*1.8*	*166*	*20.7*	*6.4*	*6.4*	*4.3*
TEQUILA								
Average	*1 Pub Shot/35ml*	*78*	*0.0*	*224*	*0.0*	*0.0*	*0.0*	*0.0*

T

INFO/WEIGHT	Measure	per Measure KCAL	FAT	Nutrition Values per 100g / 100ml KCAL	PROT	CARB	FAT	FIBRE
TERRINE								
Ham Hock, M&S*	1 Slice/70g	98	4.1	140	22.5	0.1	5.8	0.5
Salmon & Crayfish, Slice, Finest, Tesco*	1 Serving/110g	148	5.7	135	21.9	0.1	5.2	0.1
Salmon & King Prawn, Waitrose*	1 Serving/75g	98	4.0	130	19.3	1.3	5.3	0.0
Salmon & Lemon, Luxury, Tesco*	1 Serving/50g	98	7.8	196	10.6	3.2	15.7	0.8
Salmon, Poached, Tesco*	1 Pack/113g	349	30.6	309	15.5	0.8	27.1	0.0
Salmon, Three, M&S*	1 Serving/80g	168	12.2	210	17.6	0.8	15.3	0.9
THYME								
Dried, Average	*1 Tsp/1g*	*3*	*0.1*	*276*	*9.1*	*45.3*	*7.4*	*0.0*
Fresh, Average	*1 Tsp/1g*	*1*	*0.0*	*95*	*3.0*	*15.1*	*2.5*	*0.0*
TIA MARIA								
Original	*1 Pub Shot/35ml*	*105*	*0.0*	*300*	*0.0*	*0.0*	*0.0*	*0.0*
TIC TAC								
Fresh Mint, Ferrero*	2 Tic Tacs/1g	4	0.0	390	0.0	97.5	0.0	0.0
Lime & Orange, Ferrero*	2 Tic Tacs/1g	4	0.0	386	0.0	95.5	0.0	0.0
Orange, Ferrero*	2 Tic Tacs/1g	4	0.0	385	0.0	95.5	0.0	0.0
Spearmint, Ferrero*	1 Box/16g	62	0.0	390	0.0	97.5	0.0	0.0
TIKKA MASALA								
Chicken, & Pilau Basmati Rice, Frozen, Patak's*	1 Pack/400g	580	20.0	145	9.9	15.1	5.0	0.2
Chicken, & Pilau Rice, Asda*	1 Serving/500g	720	20.0	144	6.2	20.7	4.0	0.9
Chicken, & Pilau Rice, Asda*	1 Pack/400g	608	19.6	152	7.0	20.0	4.9	1.5
Chicken, & Pilau Rice, BGTY, Sainsbury's*	1 Pack/400g	380	4.8	95	8.1	13.0	1.2	1.1
Chicken, & Pilau Rice, GFY, Asda*	1 Pack/450g	495	9.0	110	6.0	17.0	2.0	0.8
Chicken, & Pilau Rice, Takeaway, Asda*	1 Pack/561g	852	27.5	152	7.0	20.0	4.9	1.5
Chicken, & Rice, Be Light, Aldi*	1 Pack/400g	516	10.0	129	9.8	16.0	2.5	1.5
Chicken, & Rice, Light Choices, Tesco*	1 Pack/450g	472	7.2	105	7.9	14.6	1.6	1.3
Chicken, & Vegetable, HL, Tesco*	1 Pack/450g	360	12.2	80	6.8	6.9	2.7	1.8
Chicken, Asda*	1 Pack/340g	388	20.4	114	9.0	6.0	6.0	1.5
Chicken, Breast, GFY, Asda*	1 Pack/380g	486	14.4	128	19.0	4.5	3.8	0.2
Chicken, Canned, Morrisons*	1 Can/400g	436	19.6	109	12.0	3.9	4.9	0.6
Chicken, COU, M&S*	½ Pack/175g	245	13.0	140	12.5	5.6	7.4	1.6
Chicken, COU, M&S*	1 Pack/400g	400	6.8	100	7.6	14.1	1.7	1.3
Chicken, Hot, Sainsbury's*	1 Pack/400g	604	37.2	151	13.2	3.6	9.3	1.5
Chicken, Hot, Tesco*	1 Pack/400g	588	34.4	147	8.7	8.6	8.6	1.0
Chicken, Indian Takeaway, Tesco*	1 Serving/125g	100	3.2	80	8.9	4.9	2.6	2.1
Chicken, Indian, Medium, Sainsbury's*	1 Pack/400g	848	61.2	212	13.2	5.3	15.3	0.1
Chicken, Indian, Takeaway, CBY, Asda*	½ Pack/225g	256	11.0	114	8.6	8.3	4.9	1.2
Chicken, Indian, Tesco*	1 Pack/350g	560	32.6	160	11.6	7.2	9.3	0.6
Chicken, Large, Sainsbury's*	1 Pack/650g	1105	68.9	170	11.7	7.0	10.6	0.3
Chicken, M&S*	½ Pack/175g	245	13.0	140	12.5	5.6	7.4	1.6
Chicken, Morrisons*	1 Pack/340g	561	34.7	165	12.4	5.9	10.2	1.7
Chicken, Ocado*	1 Pack/350g	592	35.0	169	11.0	7.9	10.0	1.8
Chicken, Waitrose*	½ Pack/200g	298	19.4	149	12.8	2.6	9.7	1.6
Chicken, with Fragrant Pilau Rice, Heated, Finest, Tesco*	1 Pack/417g	651	22.5	156	8.4	17.8	5.4	1.5
Chicken, with Fruit & Nut Pilau Rice, Sainsbury's*	1 Pack/500g	885	45.5	177	7.6	16.1	9.1	2.8
Chicken, with Pilau Rice, Frozen, Waitrose*	1 Pack/400g	676	32.4	169	9.3	14.6	8.1	2.1
Chicken, with Pilau Rice, Hot, Tesco*	1 Pack/550g	798	31.9	145	7.4	15.0	5.8	1.4
Chicken, with Pilau Rice, You Count, LL, Waitrose*	1 Pack/400g	445	5.2	111	7.8	15.9	1.3	2.4
Chicken, with Rice & Naan, Big Dish, Tesco*	1 Pack/600g	960	40.4	160	6.7	18.1	6.7	1.2
Chicken, with Rice, Ready Meal, Healthy Range	*1 Pack/400g*	*390*	*6.4*	*98*	*6.6*	*14.3*	*1.6*	*1.1*
Chicken, with Rice, Sainsbury's*	1 Pack/500g	960	41.0	192	8.3	21.2	8.2	0.1
Chicken, with Yellow Rice, Light Choices, Tesco*	1 Pack/441g	485	8.8	110	4.9	17.4	2.0	1.0
King Prawn & Rice, Finest, Tesco*	1 Pack/475g	618	30.4	130	6.0	16.6	6.4	1.2

T

	Measure INFO/WEIGHT	per Measure KCAL	FAT	Nutrition Values per 100g / 100ml KCAL	PROT	CARB	FAT	FIBRE
TIKKA MASALA								
Prawn, COU, M&S*	1 Pack/400g	400	6.4	100	6.9	14.7	1.6	1.9
Spicy, with Long Grain Rice, Rice Time, Uncle Ben's*	1 Tub/300g	399	11.7	133	2.3	21.7	3.9	0.9
Vegetable with Rice, Tesco*	1 Pack/450g	500	19.4	111	2.6	15.5	4.3	0.9
Vegetable, & Wholegrain Rice, Rice Time, Uncle Ben's*	1 Pack/285g	299	5.7	105	2.2	18.8	2.0	1.4
Vegetable, Indian, Tesco*	1 Pack/225g	234	13.5	104	2.4	10.4	6.0	2.4
Vegetable, Waitrose*	1 Serving/196g	149	4.3	76	3.6	10.5	2.2	3.8
TILAPIA								
Raw, Average	*100g*	*95*	*1.0*	*95*	*20.0*	*0.0*	*1.0*	*0.0*
TIME OUT								
Break Pack, Cadbury*	1 Serving/20g	108	6.3	530	6.2	58.3	30.7	0.0
Chocolate Fingers, Cadbury*	2 Fingers/35g	186	10.6	530	7.1	57.3	30.3	1.1
Orange, Snack Size, Cadbury*	1 Finger/11g	61	3.6	555	5.0	59.4	32.9	0.0
TIRAMISU								
Asda*	1 Pot/100g	252	11.0	252	4.3	34.0	11.0	0.5
BGTY, Sainsbury's*	1 Pot/90g	140	2.4	156	4.5	28.3	2.7	0.3
Dine in Dessert, M&S*	½ Tiramisu/145g	515	36.7	355	2.6	28.8	25.3	0.7
Family Size, Tesco*	1 Serving/125g	356	18.1	285	4.3	34.5	14.5	4.3
Italian, Co-Op*	1 Pack/90g	230	9.0	255	5.0	37.0	10.0	0.4
Morrisons*	1 Pot/90g	248	9.9	276	4.0	38.0	11.0	0.0
Raspberry, M&S*	1 Serving/84g	197	12.1	235	3.8	22.9	14.4	0.2
Sainsbury's*	1 Serving/100g	263	10.0	263	4.4	40.2	10.0	0.1
Single Size, Tesco*	1 Pot/100g	290	12.9	290	3.8	35.1	12.9	4.5
Trifle, Sainsbury's*	1 Serving/100g	243	15.7	243	2.3	23.2	15.7	0.6
Waitrose*	1 Pot/90g	221	11.2	246	6.4	27.2	12.4	0.0
TOAD IN THE HOLE								
Average	*1 Serving/231g*	*640*	*40.2*	*277*	*11.9*	*19.5*	*17.4*	*1.1*
Mini, Aunt Bessie's*	1 Serving/62g	118	6.8	191	11.0	12.0	11.0	3.6
Tesco*	1 Serving/188g	461	28.4	245	8.5	18.7	15.1	2.6
Vegetarian, Aunt Bessie's*	1 Pack/190g	502	19.4	264	15.6	27.5	10.2	2.7
with Three Sausages, Asda*	1 Pack/150g	435	27.0	290	10.0	22.0	18.0	1.0
TOASTIE								
All Day Breakfast, M&S*	1 Serving/174g	375	13.8	215	11.2	25.0	7.9	1.7
Cheese & Onion, Ginsters*	1 Toastie/122g	330	12.3	269	10.9	33.1	10.0	1.5
Cheese & Pickle, M&S*	1 Toastie/136g	320	9.1	235	10.4	33.5	6.7	2.6
Ham & Cheddar, British, M&S*	1 Pack/128g	269	8.6	210	15.5	22.3	6.7	1.3
Ham & Cheese, Tesco*	1 Serving/138g	388	18.2	281	11.5	29.1	13.2	1.0
Ham & Cheese, White Bread	1 Toastie/150g	409	14.9	273	14.5	31.3	9.9	0.9
TOFFEE APPLE								
Average	*1 Apple/141g*	*188*	*3.0*	*133*	*1.2*	*29.2*	*2.1*	*2.3*
TOFFEE CRISP								
Biscuit, Nestle*	1 Original/44g	228	12.1	519	3.7	62.8	27.6	1.4
Bitesize, Nestle*	1 Serving/20g	101	5.4	518	3.8	63.0	27.6	1.3
TOFFEES								
Assorted, Bassett's*	1 Toffee/8g	35	1.1	434	3.8	73.1	14.0	0.0
Assorted, Sainsbury's*	1 Sweet/8g	37	1.3	457	2.2	76.5	15.8	0.2
Brazil Nut, Diabetic, Thorntons*	1 Serving/20g	93	7.0	467	3.2	49.0	35.1	0.5
Chewy, Werther's*	1 Toffee/5g	22	0.8	436	3.5	71.3	15.2	0.1
Dairy, Smart Price, Asda*	1 Sweet/9g	37	1.3	407	1.3	68.4	14.2	0.0
Dairy, Waitrose*	1 Toffee/8g	37	1.1	458	2.0	80.2	14.3	0.5
Devon Butter, Thorntons*	1 Sweet/9g	40	1.5	444	1.7	72.2	16.7	0.0
English Butter, Co-Op*	1 Toffee/8g	38	1.6	470	2.0	71.0	20.0	0.0
Everyday Value, Tesco*	3 Toffees/23g	101	3.3	450	2.1	77.3	14.8	0.3
Liquorice, Thorntons*	1 Bag/100g	506	29.4	506	1.9	58.8	29.4	0.0

T

	Measure INFO/WEIGHT	per Measure KCAL	FAT	Nutrition Values per 100g / 100ml KCAL	PROT	CARB	FAT	FIBRE
TOFFEES								
Milk Chocolate Covered, Thorntons*	1 Bag/215g	1120	66.0	521	4.1	57.2	30.7	0.9
Mixed, Average	*1oz/28g*	*119*	*5.2*	*426*	*2.2*	*66.7*	*18.6*	*0.0*
Original, Hard Butter Candies, Sugar Free, Werther's*	1 Pack/80g	231	7.0	289	0.2	86.8	8.8	0.1
Original, Thorntons*	1 Bag/100g	514	30.1	514	1.8	59.3	30.1	0.0
TOFU								
Average	*1 Pack/250g*	*297*	*16.5*	*119*	*13.4*	*1.4*	*6.6*	*0.1*
Beech Smoked, Organic, Cauldron Foods*	½ Pack/110g	124	7.8	113	10.9	1.0	7.1	0.5
Firm Silken Style, Blue Dragon*	1 Pack/216g	134	5.8	62	6.9	2.4	2.7	0.0
Fried, Average	*1oz/28g*	*75*	*4.0*	*268*	*28.6*	*9.3*	*14.1*	*0.0*
Original, Organic, Cauldron Foods*	¼ Pack/99g	84	4.2	85	10.0	1.9	4.2	0.9
Pieces, Marinated, Organic, Cauldron Foods*	1 Pack/160g	363	27.2	227	17.5	1.0	17.0	2.7
TOMATILLOS								
Raw	*1 Med/34g*	*11*	*0.3*	*32*	*1.0*	*5.8*	*1.0*	*1.9*
TOMATO PASTE								
Average	*1 Tbsp/20g*	*19*	*0.0*	*96*	*5.0*	*19.2*	*0.2*	*1.5*
Sun Dried, Average	*1 Hpd Tsp/10g*	*38*	*3.5*	*385*	*3.2*	*13.8*	*35.2*	*0.0*
TOMATO PUREE								
Average	*1 Tsp/5g*	*4*	*0.0*	*76*	*4.5*	*14.1*	*0.2*	*2.3*
Double Concentrate, Average	*1 Tbsp/15g*	*13*	*0.0*	*85*	*4.9*	*14.9*	*0.2*	*3.6*
Sun Dried, & Olive Oil & Herbs, GIA*	1 Serving/20g	41	4.3	204	2.6	0.5	21.6	0.0
TOMATOES								
Baby, Everyday Value, Tesco*	6 Tomatoes/100g	20	0.3	20	0.7	3.1	0.3	1.0
Cherry, Average	*1 Tomato/15g*	*3*	*0.0*	*18*	*0.7*	*3.0*	*0.3*	*0.5*
Cherry, Canned, TTD, Sainsbury's*	½ Can/204g	47	0.4	23	1.4	4.0	0.2	0.9
Cherry, on the Vine, Average	*1 Serving/80g*	*15*	*0.3*	*18*	*0.7*	*3.1*	*0.3*	*1.2*
Cherry, Piccolo, on the Vine, Finest, Tesco*	1 Pack/220g	44	0.7	20	0.7	3.1	0.3	1.0
Cherry, Tinned, Napolina*	1 Can/400g	92	2.4	23	1.2	3.3	0.6	0.0
Chopped, Canned, Average	*1 Can/400g*	*77*	*0.6*	*19*	*1.1*	*3.3*	*0.2*	*0.9*
Chopped, Canned, Branded Average	*1 Serving/130g*	*27*	*0.2*	*21*	*1.1*	*3.8*	*0.1*	*0.8*
Chopped, Canned, Parioli, Cucina*	½ Can/200g	50	0.4	25	1.4	4.0	0.2	0.9
Chopped, Italian, Average	*½ Can/200g*	*47*	*0.2*	*23*	*1.3*	*4.4*	*0.1*	*0.9*
Chopped, with Garlic, Average	*½ Can/200g*	*43*	*0.3*	*21*	*1.2*	*3.8*	*0.1*	*0.8*
Chopped, with Herbs, Average	*½ Can/200g*	*42*	*0.3*	*21*	*1.1*	*3.8*	*0.1*	*0.8*
Chopped, with Olive Oil & Roasted Garlic, Sainsbury's*	1 Pack/390g	187	8.2	48	1.3	5.9	2.1	1.0
Fresh, Raw, Average	*1 Medium/123g*	*22*	*0.2*	*18*	*0.9*	*3.9*	*0.2*	*1.2*
Fried in Blended Oil	1 Med/85g	77	6.5	91	0.7	5.0	7.7	1.3
Green Tiger, Raw, M&S*	1 Serving/80g	16	0.2	20	0.7	3.1	0.3	1.0
Grilled, Average	*1 Medium/85g*	*17*	*0.3*	*20*	*0.8*	*3.5*	*0.3*	*1.5*
in Tomato Juice, with Chilli & Peppers, Chopped, Asda*	1 Pack/400g	92	1.2	23	1.0	4.0	0.3	0.0
Plum, Baby, Average	*1 Serving/50g*	*9*	*0.2*	*18*	*1.5*	*2.3*	*0.3*	*1.0*
Plum, in Tomato Juice, Average	*1 Can/400g*	*71*	*0.4*	*18*	*1.0*	*3.3*	*0.1*	*0.7*
Plum, in Tomato Juice, Premium, Average	*1 Can/400g*	*93*	*1.2*	*23*	*1.3*	*3.8*	*0.3*	*0.7*
Pomodorino, TTD, Sainsbury's*	1 Tomato/8g	1	0.0	17	0.7	3.1	0.4	1.3
Ripened on the Vine, Average	*1 Medium/123g*	*22*	*0.4*	*18*	*0.7*	*3.1*	*0.3*	*0.7*
Roasted, Starter, Pizza Express*	1 Serving/60g	97	6.0	162	4.7	14.3	10.0	7.7
Santini, M&S*	1 Serving/80g	16	0.2	20	0.7	3.1	0.3	1.0
Stuffed with Rice Based Filling, Average	*1oz/28g*	*59*	*3.8*	*212*	*2.1*	*22.2*	*13.4*	*1.1*
Sugardrop, Finest, Tesco*	1 Tomato/14g	3	0.0	20	0.7	3.1	0.3	1.0
Sun Dried in Oil	100g	301	24.8	301	5.8	13.5	24.8	7.0
Sun Dried, Average	*3 Pieces/20g*	*43*	*3.2*	*214*	*4.7*	*13.0*	*15.9*	*3.3*
Sun Dried, in Oil, GIA*	1 Serving/10g	15	1.4	153	1.9	7.5	13.9	0.0
Sun Dried, in Olive Oil, M&S*	1 Jar/280g	644	57.1	230	3.9	7.9	20.4	6.7
Sun Dried, Moist, Waitrose*	1 Serving/25g	44	0.5	175	11.8	27.4	2.0	7.2

	Measure INFO/WEIGHT	per Measure KCAL	FAT	Nutrition Values per 100g / 100ml KCAL	PROT	CARB	FAT	FIBRE
TOMATOES								
Sunblush, TTD, Sainsbury's*	¼ Pack/30g	42	3.2	140	2.4	8.8	10.6	5.8
Sundried, Cooks Ingredients, Waitrose*	4 Pieces/15g	26	0.1	175	7.3	35.2	0.4	13.9
Sundried, in Vegetable Oil, Aldi*	1 Serving/50g	76	3.0	153	5.8	15.9	6.0	9.0
Sundried, Italian, Merchant Gourmet*	1 Serving/50g	56	0.4	111	5.7	20.4	0.7	1.3
Sweet, Aromatico, ES, ES, Asda*	1 Serving/100g	21	0.5	21	0.7	3.1	0.5	1.3
Sweet, Baby, Mixed, Finest, Tesco*	½ Pack/125g	25	0.4	20	0.7	3.1	0.3	1.0
Vine, Large, TTD, Sainsbury's*	1 Tomato/78g	13	0.2	17	0.7	3.1	0.3	1.3
TONGUE								
Lunch, Average	*1oz/28g*	*51*	*3.0*	*181*	*20.1*	*1.8*	*10.6*	*0.0*
Ox from Deli Counter, Sainsbury's*	1 Serving/100g	195	13.3	195	18.3	0.5	13.3	0.1
Slices, Average	*1oz/28g*	*56*	*3.9*	*201*	*18.7*	*0.0*	*14.0*	*0.0*
TONIC WATER								
Average	*1 Glass/250ml*	*82*	*0.0*	*33*	*0.0*	*8.8*	*0.0*	*0.0*
Diet, Asda*	1 Glass/200ml	2	0.0	1	0.0	0.0	0.0	0.0
Indian with Lime, Low Calorie, Tesco*	1 Glass/250ml	5	0.0	2	0.0	0.0	0.0	0.0
Indian, Britvic*	1 Mini Can/150ml	39	0.2	26	0.1	6.2	0.1	0.1
Indian, Diet, Schweppes*	1 Glass/100ml	1	0.0	1	0.0	0.0	0.0	0.0
Indian, Fever-Tree*	1 Bottle/200ml	76	0.0	38	0.0	9.0	0.0	0.0
Indian, Sainsbury's*	1 Can/150ml	46	0.0	31	0.0	7.4	0.0	0.0
Indian, Schweppes*	1 Serving/500ml	110	0.0	22	0.0	5.1	0.0	0.0
Indian, Slimline, Schweppes*	1 Serving/188ml	3	0.0	2	0.4	0.0	0.0	0.0
Indian, Sugar Free, Essential, Waitrose*	1 Serving/50ml	1	0.0	2	0.0	0.0	0.0	0.0
Indian, with a Hint of Lemon, Low Calorie, Asda*	1 Serving/300ml	3	0.3	1	0.0	0.0	0.1	0.0
Low Calorie, Tesco*	1 Serving/200ml	4	0.0	2	0.0	0.5	0.0	0.0
Soda Stream*	1 Glass/100ml	15	0.0	15	0.0	3.2	0.0	0.0
TOPIC								
Mars*	1 Bar/47g	234	12.3	498	6.2	59.6	26.2	1.7
TORTE								
Chocolate & Pecan Brownie, Gu*	1/6 Torte/67g	292	17.7	436	5.3	45.1	26.4	3.1
Chocolate Brownie, Belgian, TTD, Sainsbury's*	1 Slice/90g	360	24.6	400	5.6	32.5	27.3	0.8
Chocolate Fondant, Gu*	1/8 Torte/63g	264	18.9	423	5.7	32.0	30.2	1.8
Chocolate Orange & Almond, Gu*	1 Serving/65g	273	19.8	420	5.0	28.2	30.5	2.7
Chocolate Truffle, Waitrose*	1 Serving/116g	359	20.1	309	4.6	30.1	17.3	1.4
Chocolate, Tesco*	1 Serving/50g	126	6.0	251	3.6	32.3	11.9	1.0
Raspberry, BGTY, Sainsbury's*	1 Serving/100g	154	3.9	154	2.6	27.0	3.9	1.2
TORTELLINI								
3 Cheese, Sainsbury's*	1 Serving/50g	196	4.4	391	14.4	63.8	8.7	3.0
Beef & Red Wine, Italian, Asda*	½ Pack/150g	242	4.2	161	9.0	25.0	2.8	0.0
Beef & Red Wine, Italiano, Tesco*	1 Serving/150g	324	4.8	216	11.7	35.3	3.2	3.3
Beef Bolognese, Rich, Italian, Giovanni Rana*	½ Pack/125g	222	9.0	178	7.6	20.6	7.2	4.1
Cheese & Ham, Italiano, Tesco*	½ Pack/150g	396	12.3	264	12.8	34.8	8.2	3.0
Cheese, Tomato & Basil, Cooked, Tesco*	1 Serving/270g	551	15.1	204	6.7	30.5	5.6	2.5
Four Cheese & Tomato, Italian, Asda*	1 Serving/150g	249	5.7	166	8.0	25.0	3.8	0.0
Four Cheese with Tomato & Basil Sauce, Tesco*	1 Pack/400g	500	14.8	125	6.1	16.9	3.7	0.6
Four Cheese, Italian, Asda*	1 Serving/150g	296	7.5	197	8.0	30.0	5.0	3.4
Garlic & Herb, Fresh, Sainsbury's*	½ Pack/150g	364	11.7	243	11.1	32.2	7.8	1.8
Garlic, Basil & Ricotta, Asda*	½ Pack/175g	318	10.5	182	6.0	26.0	6.0	2.6
Ham & Cheese, Fresh, Asda*	½ Pack/150g	255	9.0	170	6.0	23.0	6.0	1.7
Meat, Italian, Tesco*	1 Serving/125g	332	9.5	266	10.6	38.9	7.6	2.3
Mushroom, Asda*	1 Serving/125g	218	5.2	174	6.0	28.0	4.2	2.3
Pesto & Goats Cheese, Fresh, Sainsbury's*	½ Pack/150g	310	12.2	207	8.9	24.6	8.1	2.6
Ricotta & Spinach, Giovanni Rana*	½ Pack/125g	319	10.0	255	9.0	35.5	8.0	10.0
Sausage & Ham, Italiano, Tesco*	1 Pack/300g	816	27.9	272	13.1	34.0	9.3	3.7

T

	Measure INFO/WEIGHT	per Measure KCAL	FAT	Nutrition Values per 100g / 100ml KCAL	PROT	CARB	FAT	FIBRE
TORTELLINI								
Spicy Pepperoni, Asda*	½ Pack/150g	252	6.0	168	7.0	26.0	4.0	0.0
Spicy Pepperoni, Fresh, Asda*	½ Pack/150g	249	6.0	166	7.0	26.0	4.0	0.0
Spinach & Ricotta, Italian, Asda*	½ Pack/150g	189	3.6	126	5.0	21.0	2.4	0.6
Tomato & Mozzarella, Fresh, Sainsbury's*	½ Pack/150g	291	12.0	194	7.5	23.0	8.0	3.4
Trio, Fresh, Tesco*	½ Pack/125g	322	8.9	258	12.8	35.8	7.1	2.0
TORTELLONI								
Arrabbiata, Sainsbury's*	½ Pack/210g	407	11.8	194	7.1	28.8	5.6	2.6
Beef & Chianti, TTD, Sainsbury's*	½ Pack/125g	300	8.0	240	11.3	34.3	6.4	1.9
Cheese & Smoked Ham, As Consumed, Tesco*	½ Pack/270g	535	17.3	198	8.4	25.8	6.4	1.8
Chicken & Bacon, As Consumed, Italiano, Tesco*	½ Pack/280g	567	14.0	202	6.8	30.7	5.0	3.7
Four Cheese, Asda*	½ Pack/150g	312	13.0	208	7.6	24.9	8.7	1.6
Fresh, Ham & Cheese, Asda*	½ Pack/150g	315	11.4	210	8.8	26.7	7.6	1.4
Goats Cheese & Red Pepper, Morrisons*	1 Pack/150g	450	16.6	300	11.5	38.4	11.1	3.8
Pasta, Fresh, Cream Cheese, Garlic & Herb, Morrisons*	1 Serving/150g	400	9.0	267	10.3	46.1	6.0	3.2
Sausage & Ham, As Consumed, Italiano, Tesco*	½ Pack/270g	515	18.9	191	8.5	22.5	7.0	1.8
Spinach & Ricotta Cheese, Co-Op*	½ Pack/126g	315	6.3	250	10.0	41.0	5.0	4.0
Spinach & Ricotta, Chilled, Italiano, Tesco*	½ Pack/150g	412	12.8	275	10.4	38.1	8.5	3.3
Spinach & Ricotta, Emma Giordani*	1 Pack/250g	685	15.0	274	10.0	45.0	6.0	0.0
Spinach & Ricotta, Fresh, Waitrose*	½ Pack/150g	239	5.3	159	6.3	24.4	3.5	2.5
Spinach & Ricotta, Sainsbury's*	½ Pack/150g	326	10.8	217	7.8	30.2	7.2	2.4
Walnut & Gorgonzola, Fresh, Sainsbury's*	½ Pack/210g	414	12.2	197	8.4	27.8	5.8	2.4
Wild Mushroom, Italian, Sainsbury's*	½ Pack/150g	309	12.3	206	7.7	25.4	8.2	2.3
TORTIGLIONI								
Dry, Average	***1 Serving/75g***	***266***	***1.4***	***355***	***12.5***	***72.2***	***1.9***	***2.1***
TORTILLA CHIPS								
Blue, Organic, Sainsbury's*	1 Serving/50g	252	11.7	504	7.7	65.8	23.4	5.6
Classic Mexican, Phileas Fogg*	1 Serving/35g	162	6.7	464	5.9	67.2	19.1	3.8
Cool Flavour, BGTY, Sainsbury's*	1 Pack/22g	94	2.7	425	7.1	71.4	12.3	4.5
Cool Flavour, Sainsbury's*	1 Serving/50g	232	9.4	463	5.7	68.1	18.7	3.7
Cool, Salted, Sainsbury's*	1 Serving/50g	253	13.6	506	6.5	58.6	27.3	4.3
Cool, Tesco*	1 Serving/40g	190	9.9	474	6.3	56.7	24.7	7.8
Easy Cheesy!, Sainsbury's*	1 Serving/50g	249	13.0	498	7.1	58.7	26.1	4.5
Lightly Salted, M&S*	1 Serving/20g	98	4.8	490	7.2	61.5	24.1	4.5
Lightly Salted, Tesco*	1 Serving/50g	248	13.8	495	4.8	56.8	27.6	7.5
Lightly Salted, Waitrose*	1 Serving/40g	187	8.6	468	7.1	61.2	21.6	6.5
Lighty Salted, Basics, Sainsbury's*	½ Pack/50g	242	11.9	483	6.5	60.7	23.8	5.3
Mexicana Cheddar, Kettle Chips*	1 Serving/50g	249	13.3	498	7.9	56.7	26.6	5.1
Mexican Cheese, Phileas Fogg*	1 Pack/278g	1404	72.3	505	6.5	61.4	26.0	3.0
Nacho Cheese Flavour, M&S*	1 Serving/30g	144	6.7	480	7.5	62.0	22.4	4.2
Nacho Cheese Flavour, Mexican Style, Co-Op*	1 Serving/50g	248	13.5	495	7.0	58.0	27.0	4.0
Nacho Cheese Flavour, Morrisons*	1 Serving/25g	126	6.6	504	7.2	59.4	26.4	3.6
Nacho Cheese Flavour, Weight Watchers*	1 Pack/18g	83	3.3	459	5.2	66.6	18.2	4.1
Pita, Multigrain, Stacy's*	9 Chips/28g	140	5.0	500	10.7	67.9	17.9	0.0
Plain	1 Serving/100g	486	21.1	486	6.8	62.0	21.1	4.2
Salsa, M&S*	½ Bag/75g	364	18.8	485	5.7	59.1	25.1	6.1
Slightly Salted, Organic, Sainsbury's*	1 Serving/50g	226	6.6	453	10.0	73.3	13.3	13.3
with Guacamole	1 Serving/100g	515	30.8	515	6.0	53.0	30.8	6.3
TORTILLAS								
Corn, Gluten Free, Discovery*	1 Tortilla/22g	53	0.5	243	5.4	53.8	2.3	3.8
Corn, Soft, Mexican, Discovery*	1 Tortilla/40g	119	2.8	297	7.4	51.0	7.1	2.3
Corn, Soft, Old El Paso*	1 Tortilla/38g	129	2.6	343	10.0	60.0	7.0	0.0
Flour, 10 Pack, Asda*	1 Tortilla/30g	94	2.1	315	9.0	54.0	7.0	2.5
Flour, American Style, Sainsbury's*	1 Tortilla/35g	108	2.4	313	8.6	53.9	7.0	2.5

T

	Measure INFO/WEIGHT	per Measure KCAL	FAT	Nutrition Values per 100g / 100ml KCAL	PROT	CARB	FAT	FIBRE
TORTILLAS								
Flour, Bakery, Asda*	1 Tortilla/43g	129	3.0	303	9.1	50.9	7.1	2.6
Flour, From Dinner Kit, Old El Paso*	1 Tortilla/42g	144	4.9	344	8.7	51.1	11.7	0.0
Flour, Salsa, Old El Paso*	1 Tortilla/41g	132	3.7	323	9.0	52.0	9.0	0.0
Flour, Soft, Chilli & Jalapeno, Discovery*	1 Tortilla/40g	131	5.2	328	7.8	44.8	13.1	2.2
Flour, Soft, Discovery*	1 Tortilla/40g	119	2.8	298	8.0	49.6	7.1	2.4
Made with Wheat Flour	*1oz/28g*	*73*	*0.3*	*262*	*7.2*	*59.7*	*1.0*	*2.4*
Plain, Wheat, Waitrose*	1 Tortilla/43g	134	3.5	311	8.1	51.5	8.1	3.0
Wholewheat, Asda*	1 Tortilla/35g	88	2.7	252	9.8	35.7	7.8	7.1
Wrap, Morrisons*	1 Serving/60g	132	2.1	220	6.2	42.0	3.5	1.7
Wrap, Plain, Mini, Morrisons*	1 Tortilla/34g	91	1.4	267	8.1	48.9	4.0	2.8
Wrap, Plain, Nannak*	1 Wrap/80g	134	3.5	167	8.9	62.2	4.4	0.0
Wrap, Weight Watchers*	1 Wrap/42g	107	0.4	254	7.1	50.7	1.0	6.7
Wraps, Deli, Multigrain, Mission Deli*	1 Tortilla/61g	202	6.1	330	7.9	50.5	10.0	3.0
TREACLE								
Black, Average	*1 Tbsp/20g*	*51*	*0.0*	*257*	*1.2*	*67.2*	*0.0*	*0.0*
TRIFLE								
Average	*1 Portion/170g*	*272*	*10.7*	*160*	*3.6*	*22.3*	*6.3*	*0.5*
Black Forest, Asda*	1 Serving/100g	237	9.0	237	3.1	36.0	9.0	0.0
Cherry, Finest, Tesco*	¼ Trifle/163g	340	19.3	209	2.6	22.9	11.9	0.3
Chocolate, Asda*	1 Serving/125g	272	16.3	217	4.1	21.0	13.0	0.5
Chocolate, BGTY, Sainsbury's*	1 Pot/100g	137	2.7	137	4.8	23.4	2.7	1.6
Chocolate, Tesco*	1 Serving/125g	312	19.0	250	4.3	24.0	15.2	0.7
Fruit Cocktail, COU, M&S*	1 Trifle/140g	175	3.2	125	2.8	23.1	2.3	0.5
Fruit Cocktail, Individual, M&S*	1 Pot/135g	205	9.2	150	2.7	19.3	6.7	0.7
Fruit Cocktail, Individual, Shape, Danone*	1 Trifle/115g	136	3.1	118	3.2	19.6	2.7	1.6
Fruit Cocktail, Individual, Tesco*	1 Pot/113g	175	8.8	155	1.7	19.6	7.8	0.6
Fruit Cocktail, Low Fat, Danone*	1 Pot/115g	140	2.1	122	2.2	24.0	1.8	0.4
Fruit Cocktail, Sainsbury's*	1 Trifle/150g	241	9.0	161	1.8	24.8	6.0	0.4
Fruit, Sainsbury's*	1 Serving/125g	232	12.5	186	2.3	21.7	10.0	0.3
Mix, Strawberry Flavour, Bird's*	1oz/28g	119	2.9	425	2.7	78.0	10.5	1.2
Peach & Zabaglione, COU, M&S*	1 Glass/130g	150	3.0	115	2.8	20.6	2.3	0.8
Raspberry, Asda*	1 Serving/100g	175	8.0	175	1.8	24.0	8.0	0.1
Raspberry, Co-Op*	1 Trifle/125g	206	10.0	165	2.0	22.0	8.0	0.3
Raspberry, Sainsbury's*	1 Pot/135g	286	17.7	212	3.2	19.9	13.1	0.7
Raspberry, Tesco*	1 Pot/150g	210	9.8	140	1.7	18.5	6.5	1.0
Sherry, BGTY, Sainsbury's*	1 Pot/135g	146	2.3	108	3.0	20.2	1.7	0.5
Strawberry, Co-Op*	1 Serving/120g	175	9.1	146	1.7	16.7	7.6	1.4
Strawberry, Everyday Value, Tesco*	¼ Trifle/118g	157	6.4	133	1.4	18.5	5.4	2.4
Strawberry, Individual, Waitrose*	1 Pot/150g	206	8.6	137	1.8	19.7	5.7	1.0
Strawberry, Sainsbury's*	¼ Tub/150g	261	15.4	174	2.2	18.1	10.3	1.0
Strawberry, Tesco*	1 Trifle/605g	998	55.7	165	1.5	19.1	9.2	0.8
Summer Fruit, Sainsbury's*	¼ Trifle/125g	196	9.4	157	1.8	20.1	7.5	0.9
Summerfruit, BGTY, Sainsbury's*	1 Trifle/125g	151	5.5	121	1.2	19.2	4.4	0.5
TRIPE								
& Onions, Stewed	1oz/28g	26	0.8	93	8.3	9.5	2.7	0.7
TROMPRETTI								
Fresh, Waitrose*	1 Serving/125g	339	3.0	271	11.7	50.6	2.4	2.0
TROUT								
Brown, Steamed, Average	*1 Serving/120g*	*162*	*5.4*	*135*	*23.5*	*0.0*	*4.5*	*0.0*
Fillets, Scottish, Hot Smoked, TTD, Sainsbury's*	½ Pack/63g	85	3.4	136	20.8	1.0	5.4	0.5
Fillets, Skinless, Chunky, TTD, Sainsbury's*	½ Pack/123g	227	13.0	185	22.4	0.1	10.6	0.6
Fillets, with Juniper Berries, Ocean Sea, Lidl*	1 Serving/63g	87	3.5	138	22.0	0.0	5.5	0.0
Grilled, Weighed with Bones & Skin	1 Serving/100g	98	3.9	98	15.7	0.0	3.9	0.0

T

	Measure INFO/WEIGHT	per Measure KCAL	FAT	Nutrition Values per 100g / 100ml KCAL	PROT	CARB	FAT	FIBRE
TROUT								
Rainbow, Grilled, Average	*1 Serving/120g*	*162*	*6.5*	*135*	*21.5*	*0.0*	*5.4*	*0.0*
Rainbow, Raw, Average	*1oz/28g*	*33*	*1.3*	*118*	*19.1*	*0.0*	*4.7*	*0.0*
Rainbow, Smoked, Average	*1 Pack/135g*	*190*	*7.6*	*140*	*21.7*	*0.8*	*5.6*	*0.0*
Raw, Average	*1 Serving/120g*	*159*	*6.5*	*132*	*20.6*	*0.0*	*5.4*	*0.0*
Smoked, Average	*2 Fillets/135g*	*187*	*7.1*	*138*	*22.7*	*0.3*	*5.2*	*0.1*
TUNA								
Albacore, in Olive Oil, TTD, Sainsbury's*	1 Serving/80g	162	8.7	203	26.1	0.0	10.9	0.0
Bluefin, Cooked, Dry Heat, Average	*1 Serving/100g*	*184*	*6.3*	*184*	*29.9*	*0.0*	*6.3*	*0.0*
Chunks, in Brine, Average, Drained	*1 Can/130g*	*141*	*0.7*	*108*	*25.9*	*0.0*	*0.5*	*0.0*
Chunks, in Brine, Drained, Average	*1 Can/130g*	*141*	*0.7*	*108*	*25.9*	*0.0*	*0.5*	*0.0*
Chunks, in Brine, Drained, Value, Morrisons*	1 Can/120g	122	0.6	102	23.1	1.0	0.5	0.0
Chunks, in Spring Water, Average, Drained	*1 Sm Can/56g*	*60*	*0.4*	*108*	*25.4*	*0.0*	*0.6*	*0.1*
Chunks, in Sunflower Oil, Average, Drained	*1 Can/138g*	*260*	*12.6*	*188*	*26.5*	*0.0*	*9.2*	*0.0*
Chunks, Skipjack, in Brine, Average	*1 Can/138g*	*141*	*0.8*	*102*	*24.3*	*0.0*	*0.6*	*0.0*
Chunks, with a Little Brine, No Drain, 120g, John West*	1 Can/120g	130	1.1	108	25.0	0.0	0.9	0.0
Chunks, with a Little Brine, No Drain, 60g, John West*	1 Can/60g	55	0.5	91	21.0	0.0	0.8	0.0
Coronation Style, Canned, Average	*1 Can/80g*	*122*	*7.6*	*152*	*10.2*	*6.5*	*9.5*	*0.6*
Coronation, BGTY, Sainsbury's*	1 Can/80g	90	2.1	112	16.5	5.7	2.6	1.0
Fillets, in Tomato Sauce, Princes*	1 Can/120g	131	3.0	109	19.0	2.5	2.5	0.0
Flakes, in Brine, Average	*1oz/28g*	*29*	*0.2*	*104*	*24.8*	*0.0*	*0.6*	*0.0*
Flakes, in Tikka Mayo Dressing, Sainsburys*	1 Pack/85g	126	4.9	148	21.0	2.9	5.7	0.5
in a Light Lemon Mayonnaise, Slimming World, Princes*	1 Can/80g	99	3.8	124	16.8	3.5	4.8	0.0
in a Light Mayonnaise, Slimming World, Princes*	1 Can/80g	96	3.3	120	17.3	3.6	4.1	0.0
in a Tomato & Herb Dressing, Weight Watchers*	1 Can/80g	79	2.9	99	11.6	5.1	3.6	0.5
in Coronation Style Dressing, Weight Watchers*	1 Can/80g	75	2.0	94	9.3	8.7	2.5	0.4
in Thousand Island Dressing, Weight Watchers*	1 Can/79g	67	1.7	85	8.3	7.8	2.2	0.4
in Water, Average	*1 Serving/120g*	*126*	*1.0*	*105*	*24.0*	*0.1*	*0.8*	*0.0*
Light Lunch, Nicoise Style, John West*	1 Pack/250g	245	5.7	98	10.3	9.0	2.3	2.7
Lime & Black Pepper, John West*	1 Serving/85g	133	7.8	156	15.6	2.8	9.2	0.0
Steaks, Chargrilled, Italian, Sainsbury's*	1 Serving/125g	199	8.0	159	25.1	0.2	6.4	0.5
Steaks, in Brine, Average	*1 Sm Can/99g*	*106*	*0.5*	*107*	*25.6*	*0.0*	*0.6*	*0.0*
Steaks, in Olive Oil, Average	*1 Serving/111g*	*211*	*10.7*	*190*	*25.8*	*0.0*	*9.6*	*0.0*
Steaks, in Sunflower Oil, Average	*1 Can/150g*	*269*	*12.6*	*179*	*26.0*	*0.0*	*8.4*	*0.0*
Steaks, in Water, Average	*1 Serving/200g*	*215*	*0.8*	*107*	*25.6*	*0.0*	*0.4*	*0.0*
Steaks, John West*	1 Can/130g	140	0.4	108	26.2	0.0	0.3	0.0
Steaks, Lemon & Herb Marinade, Seared, Sainsbury's*	½ Pack/119g	191	8.8	161	23.4	0.1	7.4	0.0
Steaks, Marinated, Sainsbury's*	1 Serving/100g	153	5.3	153	25.1	1.3	5.3	0.5
Steaks, Raw, Average	*1 Serving/140g*	*179*	*2.7*	*128*	*27.6*	*0.1*	*1.9*	*0.2*
Steaks, Skipjack, in Brine, Average	*½ Can/75g*	*73*	*0.4*	*98*	*23.2*	*0.0*	*0.6*	*0.0*
Steaks, with a Little Brine, No Drain, John West*	1 Can/130g	140	0.4	108	26.2	0.0	0.3	0.0
Steaks, with a Little Olive Oil, No Drain, John West*	1 Can/130g	209	7.0	161	28.2	0.0	5.4	0.0
Steaks, with Lime & Coriander Dressing, Tesco*	1 Serving/150g	156	0.6	104	21.6	3.6	0.4	0.6
with a Twist, French Dressing, John West*	1 Pack/85g	135	8.2	159	15.2	2.8	9.7	0.1
with a Twist, Oven Dried Tomato & Herb, John West*	1 Pack/85g	112	5.1	132	18.0	2.0	6.0	0.0
Yellowfin, Cooked, Dry Heat, Average	*1 Serving/100g*	*139*	*1.2*	*139*	*30.0*	*0.0*	*1.2*	*0.0*
TUNA MAYONNAISE								
& Sweetcorn, Canned, BGTY, Sainsbury's*	1 Can/80g	78	1.8	97	15.2	4.0	2.3	0.7
Garlic & Herb, John West*	½ Can/92g	243	20.4	264	12.0	4.0	22.2	0.2
Light, Slimming World*	1 Serving/80g	96	3.3	120	17.3	3.6	4.1	0.0
with Sweetcorn & Green Peppers, GFY, Asda*	1 Pack/100g	103	3.0	103	14.0	5.0	3.0	0.8
with Sweetcorn, From Heinz, Weight Watchers*	1 Can/80g	114	6.3	142	11.5	6.2	7.9	0.1
with Sweetcorn, John West*	½ Can/92g	231	19.0	251	12.0	4.5	20.6	0.2

INFO/WEIGHT	Measure	per Measure KCAL	per Measure FAT	Nutrition Values per 100g / 100ml KCAL	PROT	CARB	FAT	FIBRE
TURBOT								
Grilled	*1oz/28g*	*34*	*1.0*	*122*	*22.7*	*0.0*	*3.5*	*0.0*
Raw	*1oz/28g*	*27*	*0.8*	*95*	*17.7*	*0.0*	*2.7*	*0.0*
TURKEY								
Breast Slices, Bernard Matthews*	1 Slice/20g	21	0.5	103	19.2	0.9	2.5	0.5
Breast, Butter Basted, Average	**1 Serving/75g**	**110**	**3.6**	**146**	**23.7**	**1.9**	**4.9**	**0.4**
Breast, Chunks, Bernard Matthews*	1 Serving/55g	64	0.5	116	26.1	0.9	0.9	1.6
Breast, Diced, Healthy Range, Average	**1oz/28g**	**30**	**0.4**	**108**	**23.8**	**0.0**	**1.3**	**0.0**
Breast, Honey Roast, Sliced, Average	**1 Serving/50g**	**57**	**0.7**	**114**	**24.0**	**1.6**	**1.4**	**0.2**
Breast, Joint, Raw, Average	**1 Serving/125g**	**134**	**2.6**	**108**	**21.3**	**0.7**	**2.1**	**0.6**
Breast, Joint, Ready to Roast, Ovenbaked, CBY, Asda*	1 Serving/150g	278	11.4	185	28.6	0.2	7.6	0.5
Breast, Joint, Sage & Onion Stuffed, LBU, Co-Op*	½ Pack/346g	536	24.2	155	20.2	2.8	7.0	0.5
Breast, Joint, with Sage & Onion Stuffing, Waitrose*	1 Serving/325g	377	13.3	116	19.2	1.4	4.1	0.1
Breast, Raw, Average	**1oz/28g**	**33**	**0.6**	**117**	**24.1**	**0.5**	**2.0**	**0.1**
Breast, Roasted, Average	**1oz/28g**	**37**	**0.9**	**131**	**24.6**	**0.7**	**3.3**	**0.1**
Breast, Roll, Cooked, Average	**1 Slice/10g**	**9**	**0.1**	**92**	**17.6**	**3.5**	**0.8**	**0.0**
Breast, Slices, Cooked, Average	**1 Slice/20g**	**23**	**0.3**	**114**	**24.0**	**1.2**	**1.4**	**0.3**
Breast, Smoked, Sliced, Average	**1 Slice/20g**	**23**	**0.4**	**113**	**23.4**	**0.7**	**2.0**	**0.0**
Breast, Steaks, Raw, Average	**1oz/28g**	**30**	**0.3**	**107**	**24.3**	**0.0**	**1.1**	**0.0**
Breast, Strips, Chinese Style, Sainsbury's*	¼ Pack/163g	318	7.3	196	26.4	12.5	4.5	0.5
Breast, Strips, for Stir Fry, Average	**1 Serving/175g**	**205**	**2.7**	**117**	**25.6**	**0.1**	**1.6**	**0.0**
Butter Roast, TTD, Sainsbury's*	1 Slice/28g	36	0.3	127	28.1	0.9	1.2	1.0
Butter Roasted, Carvery, Morrisons*	1 Slice/22g	25	0.3	113	24.0	1.2	1.3	0.0
Dark Meat, Raw, Average	**1oz/28g**	**29**	**0.7**	**104**	**20.4**	**0.0**	**2.5**	**0.0**
Drummers, Golden, Bernard Matthews*	1 Drummer/57g	147	10.3	258	13.1	11.0	18.0	1.1
Drumsticks, Tesco*	1 Serving/200g	272	12.6	136	19.9	0.0	6.3	0.0
Escalope, Average	**1 Escalope/138g**	**341**	**19.3**	**247**	**13.5**	**16.7**	**14.0**	**0.6**
Escalope, Spicy Mango, Bernard Matthews*	1 Escalope/136g	354	17.4	260	11.6	24.6	12.8	0.0
Goujons, Cooked, Bernard Matthews*	4 Goujons/128g	355	23.3	277	11.8	16.6	18.2	1.1
Leg, Dark Meat, Raw, Average, Weighed with Bone	**1 Serving/100g**	**73**	**1.8**	**73**	**14.3**	**0.0**	**1.8**	**0.0**
Light Meat, Raw, Average	**1oz/28g**	**29**	**0.2**	**105**	**24.4**	**0.0**	**0.8**	**0.0**
Light Meat, Roasted	**1 Cup/140g**	**163**	**3.3**	**116**	**22.1**	**0.0**	**2.4**	**0.0**
Mince, 7%, Sainsburys*	1 Serving/150g	210	10.5	140	18.9	0.5	7.0	0.0
Mince, Average	**1oz/28g**	**45**	**2.0**	**161**	**23.9**	**0.0**	**7.2**	**0.0**
Mince, Breast, 2% Fat, British, Sainsbury's*	1 Serving/100g	164	2.0	164	36.0	0.5	2.0	0.0
Mince, Lean, Healthy Range, Average	**1oz/28g**	**33**	**1.1**	**118**	**20.3**	**0.0**	**4.1**	**0.0**
Mince, Thigh, Essential, Waitrose*	1 Serving/100g	118	3.5	118	20.9	0.5	3.5	0.5
Rashers, Average	**1 Rasher/26g**	**26**	**0.4**	**101**	**19.1**	**2.3**	**1.6**	**0.0**
Rashers, Smoked, Average	**1 Serving/75g**	**76**	**1.4**	**101**	**19.8**	**1.5**	**1.8**	**0.0**
Ready to Roast, with Stuffing & Bacon, M&S*	1/3 Pack/169g	245	10.5	145	20.2	2.1	6.2	1.1
Roast, Breast, Wafer Thin, M&S*	½ Pack/50g	52	0.6	105	23.2	0.1	1.2	0.1
Roast, Meat & Skin, Average	**1oz/28g**	**48**	**1.8**	**171**	**28.0**	**0.0**	**6.5**	**0.0**
Roast, Meat Only, Average	**1 Serving/100g**	**157**	**3.2**	**157**	**29.9**	**0.0**	**3.2**	**0.0**
Roast, Sugar Marinade, Slices, M&S*	½ Pack/120g	156	1.9	130	29.0	0.2	1.6	0.5
Roast, Wafer Thin, Tesco*	1 Slice/8g	8	0.2	105	20.0	1.5	2.0	0.0
Schnitzel, Lidl*	1 Schnitzel/115g	210	8.0	183	19.0	11.0	7.0	0.0
Steaks, Breaded, Bernard Matthews*	1 Steak/110g	319	20.0	290	11.0	20.5	18.2	1.5
Steaks, in BBQ Marinade, Asda*	1 Serving/225g	356	5.2	158	30.0	4.4	2.3	0.9
Thigh, Diced, Average	**1oz/28g**	**33**	**1.2**	**117**	**19.6**	**0.0**	**4.3**	**0.0**
Wafer Thin, Cooked, Average	**1 Slice/10g**	**12**	**0.4**	**122**	**19.0**	**3.2**	**3.7**	**0.0**
Wafer Thin, Honey Roast, Average	**1 Slice/10g**	**11**	**0.2**	**109**	**19.2**	**4.2**	**1.7**	**0.2**
Wafer Thin, Smoked, Average	**1 Slice/10g**	**12**	**0.4**	**119**	**18.1**	**3.6**	**3.7**	**0.0**
TURKEY DINNER								
Roast, Asda*	1 Pack/400g	344	6.4	86	7.0	11.0	1.6	2.0

	Measure INFO/WEIGHT	per Measure KCAL	FAT	Nutrition Values per 100g / 100ml KCAL	PROT	CARB	FAT	FIBRE
TURKEY DINNER								
Roast, Meal for One, M&S*	1 Pack/370g	462	16.3	125	9.1	12.4	4.4	2.7
TURKEY HAM								
Average	*1 Serving/75g*	*81*	*2.9*	*108*	*15.6*	*2.8*	*3.9*	*0.0*
TURKEY KIEV								
Cheese & Herb, Mini, Bernard Matthews*	1 Kiev/23g	46	2.3	199	15.7	12.1	9.8	0.0
Mini, Baked, Bernard Matthews*	1 Kiev/23g	50	2.7	221	17.5	11.2	11.8	1.1
TURKISH DELIGHT								
Assorted Flavours, Julian Graves*	1 Square/30g	110	0.0	366	0.5	91.1	0.1	0.0
Dark Chocolate Covered, Thorntons*	1 Chocolate/10g	39	1.1	390	2.7	69.0	11.0	2.0
Fry's*	1 Bar/51g	185	3.4	365	1.4	74.6	6.7	1.3
Milk Chocolate, M&S*	1 Pack/55g	220	4.7	400	1.6	79.0	8.5	0.0
Sultans*	1 Serving/16g	58	0.0	360	0.0	90.0	0.0	0.0
with Mixed Nuts, Hazer Baba*	1 Piece/12g	47	0.2	389	1.6	88.5	1.7	0.0
with Rose, Hazer Baba*	1 Square/18g	70	0.3	389	1.6	88.6	1.7	0.0
TURMERIC								
Powder	*1 Tsp/3g*	*11*	*0.3*	*354*	*7.8*	*58.2*	*9.9*	*0.0*
TURNIP								
Baby, Tesco*	1 Serving/80g	24	0.2	30	0.9	6.3	0.2	1.8
Boiled, Average	*1oz/28g*	*3*	*0.1*	*12*	*0.6*	*2.0*	*0.2*	*1.9*
Mashed, Mash Direct*	1 Pack/400g	148	2.3	37	0.8	6.0	0.6	2.5
Raw, Unprepared, Average	*1oz/28g*	*5*	*0.1*	*17*	*0.7*	*3.5*	*0.2*	*1.8*
TURNOVER								
Apple, Bramley, Tesco*	1 Turnover/88g	304	22.8	346	2.7	25.4	25.9	0.9
Apple, Co-Op*	1 Turnover/77g	308	20.8	400	4.0	35.0	27.0	1.0
Apple, Fresh Cream, Sainsbury's*	1 Turnover/84g	292	20.9	347	4.1	26.9	24.8	2.5
Apple, Tesco*	1 Turnover/88g	294	19.7	334	3.2	29.8	22.4	0.9
Raspberry, Fresh Cream, Asda*	1 Turnover/100g	411	23.0	411	6.0	45.0	23.0	2.1
Raspberry, Tesco*	1 Turnover/84g	290	20.2	345	4.0	27.2	24.1	2.1
TWIGLETS								
Original, Jacob's*	1 Bag/30g	115	3.5	383	12.7	57.0	11.6	11.8
TWIRL								
Cadbury*	1 Finger/22g	118	6.8	535	7.6	56.0	30.9	0.8
Treat Size, Cadbury*	1 Bar/21g	115	6.6	535	7.6	56.0	30.9	0.8
TWIX								
Fun Size, Mars*	1 Bar/20g	99	4.8	495	4.5	64.6	24.0	1.5
Standard, Mars*	1 Pack/58g	284	13.7	490	4.7	65.5	23.7	1.5
Top, Mars*	1 Bar/28g	143	7.8	511	5.2	60.2	27.7	0.0
Twixels, Mars*	1 Finger/6g	31	1.6	513	5.0	64.0	26.1	0.0
Xtra, Mars*	1 Pack/85g	416	20.1	490	4.7	65.5	23.7	1.5
TZATZIKI								
Asda*	1 Serving/50g	54	4.2	108	3.8	4.6	8.5	1.2
Average	*1 Tbsp/15g*	*10*	*0.7*	*66*	*3.7*	*2.0*	*4.9*	*0.2*
Fresh, Sainsbury's*	1/5 Pot/46g	59	4.8	129	4.4	4.4	10.4	0.2
Greek, Authentic, Total, Fage*	1 Serving/50g	50	3.5	99	4.9	4.1	7.0	1.0
Morrisons*	½ Pot/85g	82	5.4	97	3.6	6.4	6.3	0.5
Tesco*	¼ Pack/50g	72	6.0	145	4.0	5.1	12.0	0.2
Waitrose*	1 Serving/50g	54	2.6	108	6.7	8.4	5.3	0.8

T

	Measure INFO/WEIGHT	per Measure		Nutrition Values per 100g / 100ml				
		KCAL	FAT	KCAL	PROT	CARB	FAT	FIBRE
VANILLA								
Bean, Average	**1 Pod/2g**	**6**	**0.0**	**288**	**0.0**	**13.0**	**0.0**	**0.0**
VANILLA EXTRACT								
Average	**1 Tbsp/13g**	**37**	**0.0**	**288**	**0.1**	**12.6**	**0.1**	**0.0**
Pure, Nielsen Massey Vanillas*	1 Tsp/5mls	8	0.0	160	0.1	39.5	0.2	0.1
VEAL								
Chop, Loin, Raw, Weighed with Bone, Average	**1 Chop/195g**	**317**	**17.8**	**163**	**18.9**	**0.0**	**9.1**	**0.0**
Diced, Lean, British, Waitrose*	1 Pack/275g	300	7.4	109	21.1	0.0	2.7	0.0
Escalope, Breaded, M&S*	1 Escalope/130g	292	13.9	225	13.6	18.7	10.7	0.4
Escalope, Fried, Average	**1oz/28g**	**55**	**1.9**	**196**	**33.7**	**0.0**	**6.8**	**0.0**
Mince, Raw, Average	**1oz/28g**	**40**	**2.0**	**144**	**20.3**	**0.0**	**7.0**	**0.0**
Shoulder, Lean & Fat, Roasted, Average	**1oz/28g**	**41**	**1.8**	**145**	**20.1**	**0.0**	**6.5**	**0.0**
Shoulder, Lean Only, Roasted, Average	**1oz/28g**	**35**	**1.3**	**125**	**19.9**	**0.0**	**4.4**	**0.0**
Sirloin, Lean & Fat, Roasted, Average	**1oz/28g**	**43**	**2.2**	**152**	**18.9**	**0.0**	**7.8**	**0.0**
Sirloin, Lean Only, Roasted, Average	**1oz/28g**	**33**	**1.2**	**118**	**18.4**	**0.0**	**4.4**	**0.0**
VEGEMITE								
Australian, Kraft*	1 Tsp/5g	9	0.0	173	23.5	19.7	0.0	0.0
VEGETABLE CHIPS								
Beetroot, Carrot & Parsnips, Hand Fried, Tyrrells*	½ Pack/25g	103	7.0	413	3.9	36.0	28.1	11.5
Cassava, Average	**1oz/28g**	**99**	**0.1**	**353**	**1.8**	**91.4**	**0.4**	**4.0**
Parsnip, Golden, Kettle Chips*	½ Pack/50g	258	18.8	515	4.6	39.5	37.6	8.4
Sweet Potato, Kettle Chips*	½ Pack/50g	242	16.4	483	2.4	44.4	32.8	9.3
VEGETABLE FINGERS								
Crispy, Birds Eye*	2 Fingers/60g	107	4.8	179	3.2	23.5	8.0	2.3
Sweetcorn, Tesco*	1 Finger/28g	66	3.5	236	7.7	23.0	12.6	3.0
VEGETABLE MEDLEY								
& New Potato, Asda*	½ Pack/175g	102	3.9	58	2.5	7.0	2.2	5.0
Asda*	1 Pack/300g	84	0.6	28	2.8	3.9	0.2	2.9
Buttered, Sainsbury's*	½ Pack/175g	122	6.8	70	1.7	7.0	3.9	1.8
Carrot, Courgette, Fine Bean & Baby Corn, Tesco*	1 Serving/100g	36	2.4	36	1.1	2.4	2.4	3.0
Crunchy, M&S*	1 Pack/250g	75	2.0	30	3.1	2.8	0.8	2.5
Green, Sainsbury's*	1 Pack/220g	178	14.3	81	3.0	2.5	6.5	2.9
Roasted, Waitrose*	½ Pack/200g	282	15.6	141	1.2	16.4	7.8	3.7
VEGETABLES								
& Bean, Stew Mix, Cooks' Ingredients, Waitrose*	½ Pack/200g	166	3.8	83	4.2	10.2	1.9	4.3
& Feta Cheese, Roasted, BGTY, Sainsbury's*	1 Pack/200g	264	4.4	132	6.4	21.7	2.2	0.0
Asparagus & Tenderstem Broccoli, Finest, Tesco*	½ Pack/95g	28	0.4	29	3.7	2.7	0.4	2.7
Broccoli, Leek & Cabbage, Fresh, LL, Waitrose*	1 Serving/100g	26	0.4	26	1.5	3.1	0.4	1.8
Butternut Squash, Broccoli & Spinach, Eat Well, M&S*	½ Pack/138g	55	0.7	40	2.3	5.0	0.5	2.3
Carrot & Sprouts, Microwaved, Fresh Tastes, Asda*	1 Pack/300g	150	0.9	50	1.9	8.7	0.3	2.3
Carrot, Broccoli & Cauliflower, Organic, Sainsbury's*	1 Serving/250g	62	1.5	25	1.9	3.0	0.6	2.2
Carrots, Peas & Sweetcorn, Steam, Tesco*	½ Pack/150g	150	4.2	100	3.4	15.0	2.8	3.2
Casserole, Cooks' Ingredients, Waitrose*	¼ Pack/125g	38	0.4	30	1.0	5.9	0.3	4.0
Chargrilled with Tomato Sauce, GFY, Asda*	1 Serving/260g	164	7.3	63	1.4	8.0	2.8	0.0
Crush, Potato & Pea with Minted Butter, M&S*	½ Pack/200g	180	6.8	90	3.9	9.6	3.4	3.9
Green Pea & Bean, Layer, M&S*	½ Pack/136g	75	3.5	55	3.4	4.3	2.6	3.6
Green, Minted, LL, Waitrose*	1 Pack/265g	154	6.9	58	3.0	4.1	2.6	3.2
Grilled Mix, Frozen, Essential, Waitrose*	1 Serving/80g	34	0.2	42	1.8	8.1	0.3	2.4
Italiano Marinated, Roasted, Tesco*	½ Tub/100g	121	8.6	121	1.7	9.2	8.6	0.8
Julienne, Tesco*	1 Serving/100g	30	0.3	30	1.1	5.7	0.3	1.9
Layered, with Butter, Waitrose*	1 Pack/280g	207	16.2	74	1.7	3.6	5.8	2.4
Mediterranean Roasted, Sainsbury's*	1 Serving/150g	118	5.4	79	2.2	9.5	3.6	3.4
Mediterranean Style, Asda*	½ Pack/205g	113	3.7	55	1.7	7.9	1.8	1.3
Mediterranean Style, COOK!, M&S*	½ Pack/200g	60	1.8	30	1.2	5.5	0.9	1.0

V

	Measure INFO/WEIGHT	per Measure KCAL	FAT	Nutrition Values per 100g / 100ml KCAL	PROT	CARB	FAT	FIBRE
VEGETABLES								
Mediterranean Style, M&S*	½ Pack/214g	75	1.9	35	1.2	5.5	0.9	1.0
Mediterranean Style, Ready to Roast, Sainsbury's*	½ Pack/200g	138	4.4	69	2.3	9.9	2.2	2.2
Mediterranean Style, Roasting, Tesco*	1 Serving/200g	72	2.0	36	1.1	5.7	1.0	1.3
Mediterranean, Ready to Roast, Sainsbury's*	½ Pack/182g	111	4.2	61	1.8	6.8	2.3	2.8
Mediterranean, Ready to Roast, Waitrose*	1 Serving/200g	128	8.0	64	1.3	5.6	4.0	1.6
Mix, Steamer, LL, Waitrose*	1 Bag/160g	83	1.8	52	2.8	7.7	1.1	2.8
Mixed, Baby, Steam, Fresh, Tesco*	1 Pack/160g	72	1.3	45	2.7	6.7	0.8	3.8
Mixed, Bag, M&S*	1 Serving/200g	70	0.4	35	2.9	5.6	0.2	0.0
Mixed, Broccoli, Peas & Green Beans, Co-Op*	1 Serving/80g	36	0.3	45	4.8	3.8	0.4	3.6
Mixed, Carrot, Cauliflower & Broccoli, Prepared, Co-Op*	1 Pack/250g	100	1.5	40	2.4	5.0	0.6	2.7
Mixed, Carrot, Cauliflower, & Broccoli, Fresh, Tesco*	1 Serving/80g	26	0.2	32	2.6	3.9	0.2	2.8
Mixed, Casserole with Baby Potatoes, Fresh, M&S*	½ Pack/350g	140	1.0	40	1.2	7.8	0.3	2.1
Mixed, Casserole, Frozen, Tesco*	1 Serving/100g	26	0.4	26	0.8	4.8	0.4	2.0
Mixed, Chef's Style, Ready Prepared, M&S*	1 Pack/240g	72	1.2	30	2.6	4.5	0.5	2.9
Mixed, Chunky, Frozen, Sainsbury's*	1 Serving/85g	31	0.6	37	2.9	4.7	0.7	3.1
Mixed, Crunchy, Tesco*	1 Pack/210g	63	0.8	30	1.7	5.0	0.4	2.4
Mixed, Freshly Frozen, Asda*	1 Serving/80g	42	0.6	52	3.2	8.0	0.8	3.0
Mixed, Freshly Frozen, Iceland*	1 Serving/100g	54	0.8	54	3.3	8.3	0.8	3.7
Mixed, Frozen, Aldi*	1 Serving/100g	34	0.7	34	2.8	4.3	0.7	0.0
Mixed, Frozen, Boiled in Salted Water	1oz/28g	12	0.1	42	3.3	6.6	0.5	0.0
Mixed, Frozen, Sainsbury's*	1 Serving/100g	50	0.7	50	2.9	7.9	0.7	3.5
Mixed, Frozen, Waitrose*	1 Serving/80g	43	0.6	54	3.1	8.7	0.8	3.5
Mixed, Gourmet, Frozen, Green Grocers, Lidl*	1 Serving/100g	60	2.9	60	2.7	5.8	2.9	3.9
Mixed, in Salt Water, Tesco*	1/3 Can/65g	34	0.4	53	2.6	9.2	0.6	2.7
Mixed, Italian, SteamFresh, Birds Eye*	1 Bag/150g	80	4.7	53	1.7	3.5	3.1	1.9
Mixed, Layered, Classics, M&S*	½ Pack/160g	112	6.2	70	1.2	7.3	3.9	1.2
Mixed, Macedoine de Legumes, Canned, Saint Eloi*	1 Sm Can/130g	56	0.6	43	2.1	6.7	0.5	2.5
Mixed, Minted, Buttery, Layers, Waitrose*	½ Pack/143g	158	12.4	111	3.0	3.6	8.7	3.0
Mixed, Peas & Carrots Crinkle Cut, D'Aucy*	1 Serving/265g	138	1.3	52	3.2	6.5	0.5	4.3
Mixed, Peas & Carrots, Buttery & Tender, Tesco*	½ Pack/150g	138	6.1	92	3.7	7.9	4.1	4.5
Mixed, Ready to Roast, Asda*	½ Pack/362g	315	11.6	87	1.6	13.0	3.2	2.4
Mixed, Roast, Four Seasons*	1 Serving/187g	79	0.4	42	1.2	8.8	0.2	0.0
Mixed, Seasonal Selection, Tesco*	1 Serving/100g	37	0.4	37	1.1	7.2	0.4	2.2
Mixed, Special, Sainsbury's*	1 Serving/120g	68	1.2	57	3.2	8.9	1.0	2.9
Oriental Soup, TTD, Sainsbury's*	1 Pack/200g	64	0.6	32	1.9	4.3	0.3	2.0
Ribbon, Pan Stir Fry, LL, Waitrose*	½ Pack/134g	47	0.5	35	1.3	5.4	0.4	2.4
Roast, M&S*	1 Pack/420g	273	17.6	65	1.4	4.9	4.2	0.4
Roasted, Italian, M&S*	1 Serving/95g	218	20.0	230	1.8	7.1	21.0	1.7
Roasted, Mediterranean, Tesco*	½ Pack/173g	95	3.1	55	1.3	7.6	1.8	2.0
Roasted, Mediterranean, The Best*	1 Serving/125g	100	5.7	80	2.3	7.0	4.6	3.6
Roasted, Root, ES, Asda*	½ Pack/205g	160	3.1	78	1.1	15.0	1.5	6.0
Roasted, Winter, HL, Tesco*	½ Pack/200g	160	5.0	80	1.9	12.7	2.5	3.6
Root, for Mashing, Eat Fresh, Tesco*	1 Pack/720g	238	2.9	33	0.7	5.4	0.4	2.7
Root, Honey Roast, BGTY, Sainsbury's*	½ Pack/150g	174	2.2	116	2.5	23.1	1.5	5.5
Sea, Dried, Average	**1 Serving/15g**	**14**	**0.3**	**94**	**11.0**	**8.0**	**2.0**	**48.1**
Seasonal, Pack, Sainsbury's*	1 Serving/261g	60	0.8	23	0.7	4.6	0.3	2.0
Selection, Roasted, COU, M&S*	1 Pack/250g	88	2.0	35	1.2	6.1	0.8	0.6
Sliced Carrots & Broccoli Florets, Fresh, Morrisons*	1 Portion/100g	37	0.7	37	2.2	4.1	0.7	2.5
Soup Mix, Fresh, Classic, Prepared, Tesco*	1/3 Pack/163g	60	1.0	37	1.1	5.3	0.6	2.8
Soup Mix, Prepared & Washed, Morrisons*	½ Pack/300g	117	1.2	39	1.1	7.3	0.4	1.1
Steam & Serve, Morrisons*	1 Serving/120g	66	1.3	55	2.4	8.8	1.1	2.6
Stew Pack, Budgens*	1 Serving/80g	32	0.2	40	0.9	8.4	0.3	1.2
Stir Fry, Frozen, Market, Value, Tesco*	1 Pack/750g	675	32.2	90	2.3	10.0	4.3	4.7

	Measure INFO/WEIGHT	per Measure KCAL	FAT	Nutrition Values per 100g / 100ml KCAL	PROT	CARB	FAT	FIBRE
VEGETABLES								
Stir Fry, Frozen, Morrisons*	1 Portion/80g	26	1.3	33	1.1	3.6	1.6	4.4
Stir Fry, Frozen, Sainsbury's*	1 Serving/80g	19	0.2	24	1.3	3.9	0.3	2.0
Stir Fry, Tesco*	1 Serving/150g	38	0.2	25	0.9	5.0	0.1	1.4
Summer, Roasted, TTD, Sainsbury's*	½ Pack/200g	160	2.2	80	1.8	14.5	1.1	2.6
Summer, Roasting, Tesco*	½ Pack/175g	105	6.6	60	1.0	5.1	3.8	1.6
Winter Soup Mix, Sainsbury's*	1 Portion/149g	61	0.3	41	1.1	7.9	0.2	1.7
Wok, Chinese, Stir Fry, Classic, Findus*	1 Pack/500g	150	2.5	30	1.0	5.0	0.5	3.5
VEGETARIAN								
Chicken Style, Strips, Meat Free, Fry's*	1 Serving/95g	226	12.3	238	20.4	10.0	13.0	5.6
Fingers, Fish Style, Breaded, The Redwood Co*	1 Finger/36g	94	5.2	262	16.5	16.0	14.5	0.0
Schnitzel, Breaded, Tivall*	1 Schnitzel/100g	172	8.0	172	16.0	9.0	8.0	5.0
Slices, Sage & Onion, Vegi Deli, The Redwood Co*	1 Slice/10g	23	1.4	233	21.4	5.0	14.1	0.5
Slices, Vegetable, Tesco*	1 Slice/165g	452	30.5	274	5.6	21.4	18.5	3.3
VEGETARIAN KIEV								
Cheesy Garlic, Meat Free, Sainsbury's*	1 Kiev/123g	274	15.1	223	13.8	14.3	12.3	3.5
Chicken Style, Cheesy, Garlic, Made with Soya, Tesco*	1 Kiev/113g	262	12.5	232	14.9	17.0	11.1	2.5
Garlic, Meat Free, Tesco*	1 Kiev/125g	244	11.2	195	15.0	12.5	9.0	2.6
Sweet Potato, Spinach & Quinoa, Linda McCartney*	1 Kiev/145g	319	13.5	220	3.8	28.7	9.3	3.4
Vegetable, M&S*	1 Kiev/155g	287	16.0	185	3.5	18.2	10.3	2.9
VEGETARIAN MINCE								
Frozen, Meatfree, Improved Recipe, Sainsbury's*	1Pack/454g	799	31.8	176	18.3	10.7	7.0	6.7
VENISON								
Grill Steak, Average	*1 Steak/150g*	*178*	*3.8*	*119*	*19.0*	*5.0*	*2.5*	*1.0*
in Red Wine & Onion Sauce, Fuller Longer, M&S*	1 Pack/400g	320	2.8	80	8.7	8.3	0.7	2.0
in Red Wine & Port, Average	*1oz/28g*	*21*	*0.7*	*76*	*9.8*	*3.5*	*2.6*	*0.4*
Minced, Cooked, Average	*1 Serving/100g*	*187*	*8.2*	*187*	*26.4*	*0.0*	*8.2*	*0.0*
Minced, Raw, Average	*1 Serving/100g*	*157*	*7.1*	*157*	*21.8*	*0.0*	*7.1*	*0.0*
Raw, Haunch, Meat Only, Average	*1 Serving/100g*	*103*	*1.6*	*103*	*22.2*	*0.0*	*1.6*	*0.0*
Roasted, Average	*1oz/28g*	*46*	*0.7*	*165*	*35.6*	*0.0*	*2.5*	*0.0*
Steak, Raw, Average	*1oz/28g*	*30*	*0.5*	*108*	*22.8*	*0.0*	*1.9*	*0.0*
VERMICELLI								
Dry	*1oz/28g*	*99*	*0.1*	*355*	*8.7*	*78.3*	*0.4*	*0.0*
Egg, Cooked, Average	*1 Serving/185g*	*239*	*2.6*	*129*	*5.0*	*24.0*	*1.4*	*1.0*
VERMOUTH								
Dry	*1 Shot/50ml*	*54*	*0.0*	*109*	*0.1*	*3.0*	*0.0*	*0.0*
Sweet	*1 Shot/50ml*	*76*	*0.0*	*151*	*0.0*	*15.9*	*0.0*	*0.0*
VIMTO*								
Cordial, No Added Sugar, Diluted, Vimto Soft Drinks*	1 Glass/250ml	6	0.2	2	0.1	0.4	0.1	0.0
Cordial, No Added Sugar, Undiluted, Vimto Soft Drinks*	1 Serving/50ml	2	0.0	4	0.0	0.7	0.0	0.0
Cordial, Original, Diluted, Vimto Soft Drinks*	1 Serving/200ml	60	0.0	30	0.0	7.4	0.0	0.0
Cordial, Original, Undiluted, Vimto Soft Drinks*	1 Serving/50ml	49	0.0	98	0.0	23.6	0.0	0.0
Fizzy, Vimto Soft Drinks*	1 Can/330ml	147	0.0	44	0.0	11.0	0.0	0.0
VINAIGRETTE								
Balsamic Vinegar & Pistachio, Finest, Tesco*	1 Tbsp/15ml	56	5.9	370	0.2	2.8	39.2	0.0
Balsamic, Hellmann's*	1 Tbsp/15ml	12	0.4	82	0.1	9.6	2.7	0.6
Fat Free, Hellmann's*	1 Serving/15ml	8	0.0	50	0.1	11.0	0.0	0.3
French Style, Finest, Tesco*	1 Tbsp/15ml	93	9.8	620	0.6	6.3	65.3	0.2
French, Real, Briannas*	2 Tbsp/30ml	150	17.0	500	0.0	0.0	56.7	0.0
Olive Oil & Lemon, Amoy*	½ Sachet/15ml	38	3.6	250	0.3	3.0	24.0	0.0
with Mustard, Delhaize*	1 Serving/20g	93	10.2	464	0.8	0.7	50.9	0.0
VINE LEAVES								
Stuffed with Rice	1oz/28g	73	5.0	262	2.8	23.8	18.0	0.0
Stuffed with Rice & Mixed Herbs, Sainsbury's*	1 Leaf/37g	44	1.8	120	2.6	16.3	4.9	1.2

	Measure INFO/WEIGHT	per Measure KCAL	FAT	Nutrition Values per 100g / 100ml KCAL	PROT	CARB	FAT	FIBRE
VINE LEAVES								
Stuffed, Mediterranean Deli, M&S*	1 Leaf/37g	39	1.5	105	2.6	14.2	4.1	1.2
Stuffed, Sainsbury's*	1 Parcel/38g	46	2.1	124	2.9	15.3	5.7	3.1
VINEGAR								
Aged, Balsamic, Finest, Tesco*	1 Tbsp/15ml	34	0.0	230	0.5	51.4	0.0	0.0
Balsamic, Average	*1 Tsp/5ml*	*6*	*0.0*	*115*	*0.9*	*26.0*	*0.0*	*0.0*
Balsamic, of Modena, So Organic, Sainsbury's*	1 Tsp/5g	6	0.0	111	1.4	26.3	0.1	0.1
Cider	*1 Tbsp/15ml*	*2*	*0.0*	*14*	*0.0*	*5.9*	*0.0*	*0.0*
Cyder, Aspall*	1 fl oz/30ml	5	0.0	18	0.0	0.1	0.0	0.0
Malt, Average	*1 Tbsp/15g*	*1*	*0.0*	*4*	*0.4*	*0.6*	*0.0*	*0.0*
Red Wine, Average	*1 Tbsp/15ml*	*3*	*0.0*	*19*	*0.0*	*0.3*	*0.0*	*0.0*
VODKA								
& Tonic, Ready Mixed, M&S*	1 Can/250ml	202	0.0	81	0.0	6.3	0.0	0.0
37.5% Volume	*1 Pub Shot/35ml*	*72*	*0.0*	*207*	*0.0*	*0.0*	*0.0*	*0.0*
40% Volume	*1 Pub Shot/35ml*	*78*	*0.0*	*222*	*0.0*	*0.0*	*0.0*	*0.0*
Smirnoff & Cranberry, Premixed, Canned, Diageo*	1 Can/250ml	175	0.0	70	0.0	8.5	0.0	0.0
Smirnoff & Diet Cola, Premixed, Canned, Diageo*	1 Can/250ml	100	0.0	40	0.0	0.0	0.0	0.0
Smirnoff & Tonic, Premixed, Canned, Diageo*	1 Can/250ml	158	0.0	63	0.0	6.4	0.0	0.0
VOL AU VENTS								
Garlic Mushroom, Mini, Asda*	1 Serving/17g	59	4.6	347	5.0	21.0	27.0	0.0
Mushroom & Roast Garlic, M&S*	1 Serving/19g	65	4.6	345	6.2	25.2	24.3	1.9
Mushroom, Sainsbury's*	1 Serving/14g	49	3.1	350	6.9	30.8	22.1	1.4
Seafood, Party, Youngs*	1 Serving/17g	60	4.2	354	8.3	26.0	24.8	1.0

	Measure INFO/WEIGHT	per Measure KCAL	per Measure FAT	Nutrition Values per 100g / 100ml KCAL	PROT	CARB	FAT	FIBRE
WAFERS								
Cafe Curls, Rolled, Askeys*	1 Wafer/5g	21	0.4	422	5.8	80.3	8.6	0.0
Caramel Log, Tunnock's*	1 Wafer/32g	150	6.7	468	4.2	65.7	21.0	3.4
Caramel Mallow, Weight Watchers*	1 Mallow/17g	55	0.4	329	5.5	63.9	2.1	17.8
Caramel, Dark Chocolate, Tunnock's*	1 Wafer/26g	128	6.6	492	5.2	60.7	25.4	0.0
Caramel, Milk Chocolate Coated, Value, Tesco*	1 Wafer/23g	110	4.7	475	5.6	67.6	20.2	0.6
Caramel, Tunnock's*	1 Wafer/26g	116	4.5	448	3.6	69.2	17.4	2.5
Cheese Footballs, Jacob's*	1 Serving/25g	139	9.2	556	11.8	43.9	36.7	1.5
Cream, Tunnock's*	1 Wafer/20g	103	5.6	513	6.6	63.2	28.0	0.0
Crema Cacao, Balocco, Costa*	1 Portion/45g	224	11.6	503	6.9	58.0	26.0	0.0
for Ice Cream, Askeys*	1 Wafer/2g	6	0.0	388	11.4	79.0	2.9	0.0
Hazelnut, Elledi*	1 Wafer/8g	38	1.9	493	6.3	62.4	24.3	0.0
WAFFLES								
Belgian, TTD, Sainsbury's*	1 Waffle/25g	122	7.3	490	6.0	50.6	29.3	1.2
Caramel, Asda*	1 Waffle/8g	37	1.8	459	3.3	62.0	22.0	1.1
Milk Chocolate, Tregroes*	1 Waffle/49g	220	20.5	450	4.5	57.0	42.0	0.5
Sweet, American Style, Sainsbury's*	1 Waffle/35g	160	8.9	457	7.2	50.6	25.3	1.1
Toasting, McVitie's*	1 Waffle/25g	118	6.3	474	6.0	52.6	25.5	0.6
Toffee, Tregroes, Aldi*	1 Waffle/35g	160	6.2	463	3.5	71.7	18.0	2.2
WAGON WHEEL								
Chocolate, Burton's*	1 Biscuit/39g	165	5.7	424	5.3	67.4	14.6	1.9
Jammie, Burton's*	1 Biscuit/40g	168	5.6	420	5.1	67.7	14.1	1.9
WALNUT WHIP								
Nestle*	1 Whip/35g	173	8.8	494	5.3	61.3	25.2	0.7
The, Classics, M&S*	1 Whip/26g	127	7.1	490	7.2	54.9	27.4	1.1
Vanilla, Nestle*	1 Whip/34g	165	8.4	486	5.7	60.5	24.6	0.0
WALNUTS								
Average	*1 Nut/7g*	*48*	*4.8*	*691*	*15.6*	*3.2*	*68.5*	*3.5*
Halves, Asda*	2 Halves/7g	48	4.8	689	14.7	3.3	68.5	3.5
Halves, Average	*1 Half/3g*	*23*	*2.3*	*669*	*17.4*	*6.3*	*65.0*	*4.7*
Wholesome, Organic, Kernels, LL, Waitrose*	1 Serving/30g	207	20.6	689	14.7	3.3	68.5	6.8
WASABI								
Paste, Ready Mixed, Japanese, Yutaka*	1 Tsp/5g	14	0.4	286	2.7	53.0	7.0	0.0
WATER								
Apple & Raspberry Flavour, Sparkling, Spar*	1 Glass/250ml	2	0.0	1	0.0	0.0	0.0	0.0
Apple & Strawberry Flavoured, Morrisons*	1 Serving/200ml	3	0.0	2	0.2	0.1	0.0	0.0
Blackberry & Strawberry, Sparkling, Strathmore*	1 Glass/250ml	45	0.0	18	0.0	4.3	0.0	0.0
Cranberry & Raspberry Flavoured, Morrisons*	1 Serving/200ml	3	0.0	2	0.2	0.1	0.0	0.0
Elderflower Presse, Bottle Green*	1 Serving/250ml	88	0.0	35	0.0	8.9	0.0	0.0
Elderflower, Presse, Sparkling, M&S*	1 Bottle/330ml	99	0.3	30	0.1	7.4	0.1	0.5
Juicy Spring, Blackcurrant & Apple, Drench*	1 Serving/250ml	98	0.0	39	0.0	9.2	0.0	0.0
Lemon & Lime Flavour Sparkling Spring, Co-Op*	1 Serving/200ml	2	0.0	1	0.0	0.0	0.0	0.0
Lemon & Lime Flavoured, Strathmore*	1 Bottle/500g	85	0.0	17	0.0	4.0	0.0	0.0
Lemon & Lime, Sparkling, M&S*	1 Bottle/500ml	15	0.0	3	0.0	0.4	0.0	0.0
Lemon & Lime, Still, M&S*	1 Bottle/500ml	5	0.0	1	0.0	0.2	0.0	0.0
Lemon & Lime, Sugar Free, Touch of Fruit, Volvic*	1 Bottle/150ml	2	0.0	1	0.0	0.0	0.0	0.0
Lemon, Vittel*	1 Bottle/500ml	6	0.0	1	0.0	0.0	0.0	0.0
Lemons & Limes, Spring Water, This Juicy Water*	1 Bottle/420ml	160	0.4	38	0.2	9.5	0.1	0.0
Mineral Or Tap	*1 Glass/200ml*	*0*	*0.0*	*0*	*0.0*	*0.0*	*0.0*	*0.0*
Peach & Raspberry, Still, M&S*	1 Bottle/500ml	10	0.0	2	0.0	0.0	0.0	0.0
Peach, Slightly Sparkling, Tesco*	1 Serving/200ml	4	0.0	2	0.0	0.2	0.0	0.0
Sparkling, San Pellegrino*	1 Glass/200ml	0	0.0	0	0.0	0.0	0.0	0.0
Sparkling, Smart Price, Asda*	1 Glass/300ml	0	0.0	0	0.0	0.0	0.0	0.0
Spring, Apple & Raspberry Flavoured, Sainsbury's*	1 fl oz/30ml	1	0.0	2	0.1	0.1	0.1	0.1

W

	Measure INFO/WEIGHT	per Measure KCAL	FAT	Nutrition Values per 100g / 100ml KCAL	PROT	CARB	FAT	FIBRE
WATER								
Spring, Apple & Raspberry, Sparkling, Tesco*	1 Tall Glass/330ml	7	0.0	2	0.0	0.5	0.0	0.0
Spring, Cranberry & Raspberry, Drench*	1 Bottle/440ml	146	0.4	33	0.1	7.7	0.1	0.0
Spring, Lemon & Lime, Slightly Sparkling, Tesco*	1 Serving/200ml	4	0.2	2	0.1	0.2	0.1	0.1
Spring, Orange & Passionfruit, Drench*	1 Serving/250ml	95	0.5	38	0.1	9.0	0.2	0.0
Spring, White Grape & Blackberry, Tesco*	1 Glass/200ml	4	0.0	2	0.0	0.5	0.0	0.0
Strawberry & Guava, Still, M&S*	1 Glass/250ml	5	0.0	2	0.0	0.1	0.0	0.0
Strawberry, Original, Touch of Fruit, Volvic*	1 Bottle/500ml	99	0.0	20	0.0	4.8	0.0	0.0
Strawberry, Sugar Free, Touch of Fruit, Volvic*	1 Bottle/500ml	7	0.0	1	0.0	0.1	0.0	0.0
Vitamin, XXX, Triple Berry, Glaceau, Coca-Cola*	1 Bottle/500ml	65	0.0	13	0.0	3.0	0.0	0.0
WATER CHESTNUTS								
Raw, Average	*1oz/28g*	*8*	*0.0*	*29*	*0.8*	*6.6*	*0.0*	*0.1*
Whole, in Water, Drained, Sainsbury's*	1 Can/140g	25	0.1	18	0.8	3.4	0.1	0.4
WATERCRESS								
Baby, Steve's Leaves*	1 Bag/40g	10	0.2	25	2.6	2.5	0.5	2.1
Morrisons*	1 Pack/85g	19	0.8	22	3.0	0.4	1.0	1.5
Raw, Trimmed, Average	*1 Sprig/3g*	*1*	*0.0*	*22*	*3.0*	*0.4*	*1.0*	*1.5*
WATERMELON								
Flesh Only, Average	*1 Serving/250g*	*75*	*0.8*	*30*	*0.4*	*7.0*	*0.3*	*0.4*
Raw	*1 Wedge/286g*	*48*	*0.6*	*17*	*0.3*	*3.7*	*0.2*	*0.3*
Raw, Weighed with Skin, Average	*1 Serving/100g*	*17*	*0.2*	*17*	*0.2*	*4.0*	*0.2*	*0.2*
WHEAT								
Whole Grain, Split, Average	*1 Serving/60g*	*205*	*1.0*	*342*	*11.3*	*75.9*	*1.7*	*12.2*
WHEAT BRAN								
Average	*1 Tbsp/7g*	*14*	*0.4*	*206*	*14.1*	*26.8*	*5.5*	*36.4*
Coarse, Holland & Barrett*	1 Tbsp/4g	8	0.2	206	14.1	26.8	5.5	36.4
Natural, Jordans*	1 Tbsp/7g	13	0.4	188	16.3	17.4	5.9	44.5
WHEAT GERM								
Average	*1oz/28g*	*100*	*2.6*	*357*	*26.7*	*44.7*	*9.2*	*15.6*
Natural, Jordans*	2 Tbsp/16g	54	1.5	340	28.0	36.0	9.3	13.1
WHELKS								
Boiled, Weighed without Shell	*1oz/28g*	*25*	*0.3*	*89*	*19.5*	*0.0*	*1.2*	*0.0*
WHISKEY								
Irish, Jameson*	1 Shot/25ml	58	0.0	233	0.0	0.0	0.0	0.0
Jack Daniel's*	1 Pub Shot/35ml	78	0.0	222	0.0	0.0	0.0	0.0
WHISKY								
37.5% Volume	*1 Pub Shot/35ml*	*72*	*0.0*	*207*	*0.0*	*0.0*	*0.0*	*0.0*
40% Volume	*1 Pub Shot/35ml*	*78*	*0.0*	*222*	*0.0*	*0.0*	*0.0*	*0.0*
Bells & Ginger Ale, Premixed, Canned, Diageo*	1 Can/250ml	170	0.0	68	0.0	7.6	0.0	0.0
Scots, 37.5% Volume	*1 Pub Shot/35ml*	*72*	*0.0*	*207*	*0.0*	*0.0*	*0.0*	*0.0*
Scots, 40% Volume	*1 Pub Shot/35ml*	*78*	*0.0*	*224*	*0.0*	*0.0*	*0.0*	*0.0*
Teacher's*	1 Pub Shot/35ml	78	0.0	222	0.0	0.0	0.0	0.0
WHITE PUDDING								
Average	*1oz/28g*	*126*	*8.9*	*450*	*7.0*	*36.3*	*31.8*	*0.0*
WHITEBAIT								
in Flour, Fried	*1oz/28g*	*147*	*13.3*	*525*	*19.5*	*5.3*	*47.5*	*0.2*
Raw, Average	*1 Serving/100g*	*172*	*11.0*	*172*	*18.3*	*0.0*	*11.0*	*0.0*
WHITING								
Raw	*1oz/28g*	*23*	*0.2*	*81*	*18.7*	*0.0*	*0.7*	*0.0*
Steamed	*1 Serving/85g*	*78*	*0.8*	*92*	*20.9*	*0.0*	*0.9*	*0.0*
WIENER SCHNITZEL								
Average	*1oz/28g*	*62*	*2.8*	*223*	*20.9*	*13.1*	*10.0*	*0.4*
WINE								
Cherry, Lambrini*	1 Glass/125ml	80	0.0	64	0.0	0.0	0.0	0.0

W

	Measure INFO/WEIGHT	per Measure KCAL	FAT	Nutrition Values per 100g / 100ml KCAL	PROT	CARB	FAT	FIBRE
WINE								
Elderberry & Lemon, Ame*	1 Glass/125ml	46	0.0	37	0.0	6.4	0.0	0.0
Fruit, Average	*1 Glass/125ml*	*115*	*0.0*	*92*	*0.0*	*5.5*	*0.0*	*0.0*
Grape & Apricot, Ame*	1 Glass/125ml	49	1.2	39	1.3	6.7	1.0	0.0
Madeira, Henriques & Henriques*	1 Glass/100ml	130	0.0	130	0.0	0.0	0.0	0.0
Mulled, Homemade, Average	*1 Glass/125ml*	*245*	*0.0*	*196*	*0.1*	*25.2*	*0.0*	*0.0*
Mulled, Sainsbury's*	1 Glass/125ml	112	0.0	90	0.0	8.6	0.0	0.0
Original, Lambrini*	1 Glass/125ml	88	0.0	70	0.0	0.0	0.0	0.0
Red, Amarone, Average	*1 Glass/125ml*	*120*	*0.0*	*96*	*0.1*	*3.0*	*0.0*	*0.0*
Red, Average	*1 Glass/125ml*	*104*	*0.0*	*83*	*0.0*	*2.0*	*0.0*	*0.0*
Red, Burgundy, 12.9% Abv, Average	*1 Glass/125ml*	*110*	*0.0*	*88*	*0.1*	*3.7*	*0.0*	*0.0*
Red, Cabernet Sauvignon, 13.1% Abv, Average	*1 Glass/125ml*	*105*	*0.0*	*84*	*0.1*	*2.6*	*0.0*	*0.0*
Red, Cabernet Sauvigon, Non Alcoholic, Ariel*	1 Serving/240ml	50	0.0	21	0.0	4.8	0.0	0.0
Red, California, Blossom Hill*	1 Glass/175ml	132	0.0	75	0.0	0.9	0.0	0.0
Red, Claret, 12.8% Abv, Average	*1 Glass/125ml*	*105*	*0.0*	*84*	*0.1*	*3.0*	*0.0*	*0.0*
Red, Gamay, 12.3% Abv, Average	*1 Glass/125ml*	*99*	*0.0*	*79*	*0.1*	*2.4*	*0.0*	*0.0*
Red, Merlot, 13.3% Abv, Average	*1 Glass/125ml*	*105*	*0.0*	*84*	*0.1*	*2.5*	*0.0*	*0.0*
Red, Petit Sirah, 13.5% Abv, Average	*1 Glass/125ml*	*108*	*0.0*	*86*	*0.1*	*2.7*	*0.0*	*0.0*
Red, Pinot Noir, 13% Abv, Average	*1 Glass/125ml*	*104*	*0.0*	*83*	*0.1*	*2.3*	*0.0*	*0.0*
Red, Sangiovese, 13.6% Abv, Average	*1 Glass/125ml*	*109*	*0.0*	*87*	*0.1*	*2.6*	*0.0*	*0.0*
Red, Syrah, 13.1% Abv, Average	*1 Glass/125ml*	*105*	*0.0*	*84*	*0.1*	*2.6*	*0.0*	*0.0*
Red, Zinfandel, 13.9% Abv, Average	*1 Glass/125ml*	*111*	*0.0*	*89*	*0.1*	*2.9*	*0.0*	*0.0*
Rose, Medium, Average	*1 Glass/125ml*	*98*	*0.0*	*79*	*0.0*	*2.1*	*0.0*	*0.0*
Rose, Refreshing, Weight Watchers*	1 Glass/125ml	80	0.0	64	0.0	1.6	0.0	0.0
Rose, Sparkling, Average	*1 Glass/125ml*	*102*	*0.0*	*82*	*0.0*	*2.5*	*0.0*	*0.0*
Rose, The Pink Chill, Co-Op*	1 Glass/125ml	85	0.0	68	0.0	0.0	0.0	0.0
Rose, Weight Watchers*	1 Mini Bottle/187ml	112	0.2	60	0.1	1.8	0.1	0.1
Rose, White Grenache, Blossom Hill*	1 Glass/125ml	105	0.0	84	0.0	3.2	0.0	0.0
Rose, White Zinfandel, Ernest & Julio Gallo*	1 Glass/125ml	101	0.0	81	0.2	2.7	0.0	0.0
Sangria, Average	*1 Glass/125ml*	*95*	*0.0*	*76*	*0.1*	*9.9*	*0.0*	*0.1*
Strong Ale Barley	1 Can/440ml	290	0.0	66	0.7	6.1	0.0	0.0
Vie, Rose, Low Alcohol, Blossom Hill*	1 Glass/175ml	93	0.0	53	0.0	3.9	0.0	0.0
White, Average	*1 Glass/125ml*	*95*	*0.0*	*76*	*0.0*	*2.4*	*0.0*	*0.0*
White, Chardonnay, Southern Australia, Kissing Tree*	1 Bottle/185ml	85	0.0	46	0.0	0.0	0.0	0.0
White, Chenin Blanc, 12% Abv, Average	*1 Glass/125ml*	*101*	*0.0*	*81*	*0.1*	*3.3*	*0.0*	*0.0*
White, Dry, Average	*1 Glass/125ml*	*88*	*0.0*	*70*	*0.1*	*0.6*	*0.0*	*0.0*
White, Fume Blanc, 13.1% Abv, Average	*1 Glass/125ml*	*104*	*0.0*	*83*	*0.1*	*2.3*	*0.0*	*0.0*
White, Gewurztraminer, 12.6% Abv, Average	*1 Glass/125ml*	*102*	*0.0*	*82*	*0.1*	*2.6*	*0.0*	*0.0*
White, Late Harvest, 10.6% Abv, Average	*1 Glass/125ml*	*141*	*0.0*	*113*	*0.1*	*13.4*	*0.0*	*0.0*
White, Medium, Average	*1 Glass/125ml*	*92*	*0.0*	*74*	*0.1*	*3.0*	*0.0*	*0.0*
White, Muller-Thurgau, 11.3% Abv, Average	*1 Glass/125ml*	*96*	*0.0*	*77*	*0.1*	*3.5*	*0.0*	*0.0*
White, Muscat, 11% Abv, Average	*1 Glass/125ml*	*104*	*0.0*	*83*	*0.1*	*5.2*	*0.0*	*0.0*
White, Pinot Blanc, 13.3% Abv, Average	*1 Glass/125ml*	*102*	*0.0*	*82*	*0.1*	*0.0*	*0.0*	*0.0*
White, Pinot Grigio, 13.4% Abv, Average	*1 Glass/125ml*	*105*	*0.0*	*84*	*0.1*	*2.1*	*0.0*	*0.0*
White, Riesling, 11.9% Abv, Average	*1 Glass/125ml*	*101*	*0.0*	*81*	*0.1*	*3.7*	*0.0*	*0.0*
White, Sauvignon Blanc, 13.1% Abv, Average	*1 Glass/125ml*	*102*	*0.0*	*82*	*0.1*	*2.0*	*0.0*	*0.0*
White, Semillon, 12.5% Abv, Average	*1 Glass/125ml*	*104*	*0.0*	*83*	*0.1*	*3.1*	*0.0*	*0.0*
White, Sparkling, Average	*1 Glass/125ml*	*92*	*0.0*	*74*	*0.3*	*5.1*	*0.0*	*0.0*
White, Sweet, Average	*1 Glass/120ml*	*113*	*0.0*	*94*	*0.2*	*5.9*	*0.0*	*0.0*
WINE GUMS								
Average	*1 Sweet/6g*	*19*	*0.0*	*315*	*5.0*	*73.4*	*0.2*	*0.1*
Haribo*	1 Pack/175g	609	0.4	348	0.1	86.4	0.2	0.4
WISPA								
Bite, with Biscuit in Caramel, Cadbury*	1 Bar/47g	240	13.4	510	6.4	56.9	28.6	0.0

W

	Measure INFO/WEIGHT	per Measure KCAL	FAT	Nutrition Values per 100g / 100ml KCAL	PROT	CARB	FAT	FIBRE
WISPA								
Cadbury*	1 Bar/40g	210	12.9	525	6.8	53.0	32.2	0.8
Gold, Cadbury*	1 Bar/52g	265	15.1	510	5.3	56.0	29.0	0.7
WONTON								
Prawn, Crispy from Selection, Modern Asian, M&S*	1 Wonton/25g	65	3.3	250	9.5	23.4	12.7	2.0
Prawn, Dim Sum Selection, Sainsbury's*	1 Wonton/10g	26	1.2	259	11.3	26.8	11.8	1.3
Prawn, Oriental Selection, Waitrose*	1 Wonton/18g	45	2.0	252	9.1	29.2	11.0	1.1
Prawn, Oriental Snack Selection, Sainsbury's*	1 Wonton/20g	53	2.7	265	10.6	25.6	13.4	2.0
WOTSITS								
Baked, Really Cheesy, Walkers*	1 Bag/23g	123	7.4	546	5.5	56.0	33.0	1.1
BBQ, Walkers*	1 Bag/21g	108	6.3	515	4.5	57.0	30.0	1.3
Flamin' Hot, Walkers*	1 Bag/19g	101	5.7	532	5.5	60.0	30.0	1.1
Really Cheesy, Big Eat, Walkers*	1 Bag/36g	197	11.9	547	5.5	56.0	33.0	1.1
WRAP								
3 Bean & Cheese, Co-Op*	1 Pack/201g	392	11.3	195	8.1	26.7	5.6	3.4
Bean, Mexican, GFY, Asda*	1 Pack/173g	303	5.9	175	5.0	31.0	3.4	2.3
Beef, Fajita, Boots*	1 Pack/200g	352	8.4	176	9.5	25.5	4.2	3.2
Cajun Chicken, Sandwich King*	1 Pack/138g	386	19.9	279	12.3	25.0	14.4	0.0
Cheese, & Bean, Average	***1 Pack/200g***	***365***	***13.5***	***182***	***7.4***	***22.6***	***6.8***	***2.5***
Cheese, & Roasted Beetroot, Wensleydale, Boots*	1 Pack/229g	373	11.7	163	4.8	23.0	5.1	2.9
Cheesy Gonzales, Cranks*	1 Pack/209g	501	22.3	240	8.0	27.3	10.7	1.1
Chicken Caesar, Weight Watchers*	1 Pack/158g	234	2.4	148	10.4	22.2	1.5	2.1
Chicken Fajita, Morrisons*	1 Pack/214g	430	16.5	201	9.5	22.5	7.7	1.9
Chicken Fajita, VLH Kitchens	1 Serving/170g	311	3.1	183	10.6	25.0	5.2	0.0
Chicken Tikka, Average	***1 Wrap/200g***	***403***	***15.1***	***202***	***9.5***	***23.6***	***7.6***	***4.4***
Chicken, & Bacon, Caesar Salad, Asda*	1 Pack/160g	565	35.2	353	18.0	20.8	22.0	0.9
Chicken, & Bacon, Caesar, COU, M&S*	1 Pack/170g	260	4.2	153	10.6	22.0	2.5	2.1
Chicken, & Bacon, Simple Solutions, Tesco*	1 Pack/300g	474	23.4	158	20.7	1.2	7.8	0.5
Chicken, & Sweetfire Pepper, Light Choices, Tesco*	1 Wrap/175g	350	7.9	200	10.2	28.5	4.5	1.4
Chicken, BBQ Steak, & Hoisin Duck, Selection, M&S*	1 Pack/334g	685	23.7	205	10.9	24.3	7.1	1.7
Chicken, BBQ, Shapers, Boots*	1 Wrap/156g	278	4.5	178	11.0	26.0	2.9	1.8
Chicken, Caesar, HE, Tesco*	1 Pack/170g	296	4.0	174	12.0	26.2	2.4	2.6
Chicken, Caesar, HL, Tesco*	1 Pack/200g	296	4.0	148	10.2	22.3	2.0	2.2
Chicken, Caesar, Tesco*	1 Pack/175g	480	27.4	275	10.2	22.4	15.7	1.8
Chicken, Caesar, Tesco*	1 Pack/215g	516	24.3	240	11.6	23.0	11.3	1.2
Chicken, Cajun, Tesco*	1 Pack/175g	357	13.8	204	9.4	22.6	7.9	2.3
Chicken, Chilli, GFY, Asda*	1 Pack/194g	277	4.3	143	9.1	21.6	2.2	2.3
Chicken, Chilli,,BGTY, Sainsbury's*	1 Pack/180g	313	4.3	174	10.2	28.0	2.4	0.0
Chicken, Coronation,,Waitrose*	1 Pack/164g	283	8.3	173	10.1	21.3	5.1	2.2
Chicken, Fajita, Asda*	1 Pack/180g	369	16.9	205	9.4	20.6	9.4	0.4
Chicken, Fajita, Finest, Tesco*	1 Pack/213g	422	15.6	198	9.0	24.0	7.3	1.9
Chicken, Fajita, Shapers, Boots*	1 Pack/216g	291	5.2	135	14.0	15.0	2.4	3.1
Chicken, Fajita, Tesco*	1 Pack/220g	407	11.7	185	10.6	23.2	5.3	1.8
Chicken, Fillets, with Cheese, & Bacon, Asda*	1 Pack/164g	366	21.3	223	25.0	1.4	13.0	0.0
Chicken, Italian, Sainsbury's*	½ Pack/211g	395	23.2	187	15.7	6.2	11.0	0.9
Chicken, Lemon, & Herb, Delicious, Boots*	1 Pack/173g	351	13.1	203	7.9	24.0	7.6	3.0
Chicken, M&S*	1 Pack/247g	530	24.9	215	8.2	23.4	10.1	1.6
Chicken, Mediterranean Style, Waitrose*	1 Pack/183g	296	11.0	162	8.3	18.6	6.0	2.3
Chicken, Mexican Style, Co-Op*	1 Pack/163g	367	14.7	225	11.0	26.0	9.0	3.0
Chicken, Mexican, M&S*	1 Serving/218g	447	22.5	205	8.6	19.7	10.3	1.3
Chicken, Moroccan, BGTY, Sainsbury's*	1 Pack/207g	315	3.1	152	9.4	25.3	1.5	0.0
Chicken, Moroccan, Shapers, Boots*	1 Serving/154g	251	2.3	163	10.0	27.0	1.5	1.9
Chicken, Nacho, COU, M&S*	1 Pack/175g	280	4.2	160	10.2	24.4	2.4	2.0

WRAP

INFO/WEIGHT	Measure	per Measure		Nutrition Values per 100g / 100ml				
		KCAL	FAT	KCAL	PROT	CARB	FAT	FIBRE
Chicken, Red Thai, Shapers, Boots*	1 Pack/172g	234	3.6	136	9.5	20.0	2.1	2.4
Chicken, Salad, Free From Gluten, CBY, Asda*	1 Pack/187g	352	11.0	188	9.6	23.0	5.9	2.3
Chicken, Salad, Roast, Sainsbury's*	1 Pack/214g	443	19.9	207	10.0	20.9	9.3	2.5
Chicken, Salsa, Light Choices, Tesco*	1 Pack/219g	340	5.9	155	9.7	22.6	2.7	1.9
Chicken, Spiced, & Mango with Lettuce, LL, Waitrose*	1 Wrap/139g	125	3.8	90	5.5	11.0	2.7	1.2
Chicken, Sweet Chilli, Sainsburys *	1 Pack/209g	434	11.5	208	8.5	30.1	5.5	1.8
Chicken, Sweet Chilli, Shapers, Boots*	1 Pack/195g	302	3.7	155	10.0	24.0	1.9	3.0
Chicken, Sweet Chilli, Waitrose*	1 Pack/200g	390	14.7	195	10.2	22.0	7.4	2.4
Chicken, Tandoori, GFY, Asda*	1 Pack/167g	281	4.5	168	10.0	26.0	2.7	1.7
Chilli Beef, Co-Op*	1 Pack/163g	310	9.8	190	10.0	26.0	6.0	2.0
Duck, Hoisin, Delicious, Boots*	1 Pack/160g	295	4.3	184	11.0	28.0	2.7	2.0
Duck, Hoisin, M&S*	1 Pack/225g	405	8.3	180	8.4	27.7	3.7	1.5
Duck, Hoisin, No Mayo, Triple, Tesco*	1 Pack/270g	620	18.6	230	9.3	30.7	6.9	2.3
Duck, Peking, Asda*	1 Pack/195g	406	11.1	208	10.3	27.9	5.7	2.1
Egg Mayonnaise, Tomato, & Cress, Sainsbury's*	1 Pack/255g	592	38.2	232	7.3	17.7	15.0	0.0
Feta Cheese, Flat Bread, COU, M&S*	1 Pack/180g	225	4.0	125	6.3	20.6	2.2	1.9
Feta Cheese, GFY, Asda*	1 Pack/165g	256	7.1	155	7.0	22.0	4.3	2.1
Feta, Salad, Greek, Shapers, Boots*	1 Pack/158g	241	5.7	153	6.4	24.0	3.6	1.2
Goats Cheese, & Grilled Pepper, Asda*	1 Serving/75g	194	11.2	259	5.0	26.0	15.0	2.1
Ham, Cheese & Pickle Tortilla, Weight Watchers*	1 Pack/170g	296	4.8	174	10.9	26.4	2.8	1.2
Ham, Cheese, & Pickle, Sainsbury's*	1 Pack/195g	503	23.2	258	10.9	26.8	11.9	0.9
Houmous, & Chargrilled Vegetables, Shapers, Boots*	1 Pack/186g	301	5.0	162	5.8	29.0	2.7	3.2
Mexican Bean & Potato in Spinach Tortilla, Daily Bread*	1 Pack/196g	329	10.6	168	4.9	25.0	5.4	0.0
Minted Lamb, Darwins Deli*	1 Pack/250g	287	6.3	115	3.2	19.9	2.5	0.0
Roasted Vegetable, & Feta, BGTY, Sainsbury's*	1 Serving/200g	318	8.0	159	5.8	25.0	4.0	0.0
Salad, Greek, Sainsbury's*	1 Pack/167g	242	6.2	145	6.7	21.2	3.7	1.8
Salmon, & Cucumber, Sushi, Waitrose*	1 Pack/180g	299	6.5	166	6.3	27.2	3.6	1.6
Salmon, Smoked, & Prawn, Finest, Tesco*	1 Serving/59g	84	5.3	143	14.3	1.0	9.1	0.0
Salmon, Smoked, Finest, Tesco*	1 Pack/58g	113	8.4	194	15.5	0.6	14.4	0.3
Sausage, & Bacon, Cooked, Sainsbury's*	1 Wrap/12g	38	2.6	315	17.7	12.1	21.7	0.0
Sicilian Lemon, & Roasted Vegetable, COU, M&S*	1 Pack/178g	240	3.7	135	4.9	23.8	2.1	1.9
Soft Cheese & Spinach, to Go*	1 Serving/250g	278	6.7	111	4.5	17.4	2.7	0.0
Steak, Fajita, Delicatessen, Waitrose*	1 Pack/232g	489	21.1	211	10.5	22.7	9.1	2.7
Sunny Side Up, Cranks*	1 Pack/195g	423	18.9	217	7.8	23.3	9.7	1.7
Tuna Nicoise, BGTY, Sainsbury's*	1 Pack/181g	273	7.1	151	11.0	18.0	3.9	0.0
Tuna Salsa, Healthy Eating, Wild Bean Cafe*	1 Pack/159g	245	2.7	154	11.3	23.5	1.7	1.5
Tuna, Mediterranean Style, Shapers, Boots*	1 Pack/170g	274	4.6	161	7.9	25.0	2.7	2.0
Tuna, Nicoise, HE, Tesco*	1 Pack/117g	160	2.7	137	8.3	20.6	2.3	0.5
Tuna, Sweetcorn & Red Pepper, BGTY, Sainsbury's*	1 Pack/178g	306	8.2	172	11.5	21.2	4.6	2.1
Turkey, Bacon & Cranberry, COU, M&S*	1 Pack/144g	230	2.2	160	9.6	27.1	1.5	2.3

	Measure INFO/WEIGHT	per Measure KCAL	per Measure FAT	Nutrition Values per 100g / 100ml KCAL	PROT	CARB	FAT	FIBRE
YAM								
Baked	1oz/28g	43	0.1	153	2.1	37.5	0.4	1.7
Boiled, Average	1oz/28g	37	0.1	133	1.7	33.0	0.3	1.4
Raw	1oz/28g	26	0.1	92	1.2	22.8	0.2	1.1
YEAST								
Extract	1 Tsp/9g	16	0.0	180	40.7	3.5	0.4	0.0
YOGHURT								
0.1% Fat, Lidl*	1 Pot/150g	118	0.2	79	4.0	15.6	0.1	0.0
Activia, Danone*	1 Pot/132g	125	4.2	94	3.5	12.8	3.2	2.0
Apple & Berry Pie, Dessert Recipe, Weight Watchers*	1 Pot/120g	58	0.1	49	4.1	6.8	0.1	0.3
Apple & Cinnamon, COU, M&S*	1 Pot/150g	68	0.2	45	4.2	6.1	0.1	0.2
Apple & Cinnamon, Jubileum, Tine*	1 Pot/125g	166	6.5	133	3.2	18.5	5.2	0.0
Apple & Lingonberry, Strained, Fat Free, Skyr, Arla*	1 Pot/150g	110	0.3	74	9.4	7.7	0.2	0.2
Apple & Peach, Oatie Breakfast, Moma Foods*	1 Pot/234g	309	5.6	132	4.3	24.3	2.4	1.7
Apple & Prune, Fat Free, Yeo Valley*	1 Pot/125g	98	0.1	78	5.1	14.1	0.1	0.2
Apple & Spice Bio, Virtually Fat Free, Shape, Danone*	1 Pot/120g	67	0.1	56	5.6	7.3	0.1	0.2
Apple Pie, Corner, Muller*	1 Pot/135g	193	5.5	143	3.1	22.8	4.1	0.5
Apple, & Quince, Spiced, Yeo Valley*	¼ Pot/113g	115	4.3	102	4.6	12.3	3.8	0.0
Apple, Lidl*	1 Pot/250g	228	3.5	91	3.8	15.2	1.4	0.3
Apple, Light, Muller*	1 Pot/175g	94	0.2	54	4.4	9.0	0.1	0.0
Apricot & Mango, 25% Extra Fruit, Low Fat, Asda*	1 Pot/125g	120	1.4	96	4.6	17.0	1.1	0.0
Apricot & Mango, Best There Is, Yoplait*	1 Pot/125g	130	2.0	104	4.7	17.4	1.6	0.0
Apricot & Mango, Thick & Creamy, Sainsbury's*	1 Pot/150g	178	5.4	119	4.3	17.3	3.6	0.2
Apricot & Mango, Tropical Fruit, Activ8, Ski, Nestle*	1 Pot/120g	112	2.0	93	4.3	15.1	1.7	0.2
Apricot & Nectarine, Sunshine Selection, Sainsbury's*	1 Pot/125g	115	1.9	92	4.4	15.3	1.5	0.1
Apricot & Passion Fruit, Fat Free, Yeo Valley*	1 Pot/125g	94	0.1	75	5.3	13.2	0.1	0.1
Apricot, Bio Activia, Danone*	1 Pot/125g	121	4.0	97	3.7	13.3	3.2	1.7
Apricot, Bio, Low Fat, Benecol*	1 Pot/125g	98	0.8	78	3.9	14.3	0.6	0.0
Apricot, Fat Free, Activ8, Ski, Nestle*	1 Pot/120g	88	0.8	73	4.5	13.6	0.7	0.2
Apricot, Fat Free, Weight Watchers*	1 Pot/150g	62	0.2	42	4.1	4.9	0.1	0.2
Apricot, Fruity, Mullerlight, Muller*	1 Pot/175g	88	0.2	50	4.2	7.5	0.1	0.1
Apricot, Light, Fat Free, Muller*	1 Pot/190g	93	0.2	49	4.1	7.3	0.1	0.1
Apricot, Low Fat, Tesco*	1 Pot/125g	112	2.2	90	4.3	14.1	1.8	0.0
Apricot, Pro Activ, Flora*	1 Pot/125ml	70	0.6	56	4.0	7.9	0.5	1.8
Apricot, Smooth Set French, Sainsbury's*	1 Pot/125g	100	1.5	80	3.5	13.6	1.2	0.0
Banana & Custard, Smooth, Mullerlight, Muller*	1 Pot/175g	94	0.2	54	4.1	8.6	0.1	0.6
Banana & Mango, Oatie Breakfast, Moma Foods*	1 Pot/235g	314	4.7	134	4.2	26.0	2.0	1.7
Banana & Orange, Low Fat, 25% Extra Fruit, Asda*	1 Pot/125g	125	1.4	100	4.6	18.0	1.1	0.0
Banana Choco Flakes, Crunch Corner, Muller*	1 Pot/135g	193	6.9	143	4.3	19.3	5.1	0.3
Banana, Low Fat, Average	1 Serving/100g	98	1.4	98	4.6	16.7	1.4	0.1
Black Cherry, Average	1 Serving/100g	96	2.2	96	3.4	16.5	2.2	0.1
Black Cherry, Extremely Fruity, Bio, M&S*	1 Pot/150g	165	2.2	110	4.9	18.4	1.5	0.2
Black Cherry, Fat Free, Benecol*	1 Pot/120g	78	0.6	65	3.0	11.0	0.5	2.1
Black Cherry, Greek Style, Corner, Muller*	1 Pot/150g	172	4.5	115	5.0	16.2	3.0	0.1
Black Cherry, Low Fat, Value, Tesco*	1 Pot/125g	95	0.9	76	3.0	14.2	0.7	0.6
Black Cherry, Swiss, Finest, Tesco*	1 Pot/150g	195	8.8	130	3.5	15.7	5.9	0.5
Black Cherry, Thick & Creamy, Waitrose*	1 Pot/125g	139	3.1	111	3.7	18.3	2.5	0.4
Black Cherry, VLH Kitchens	1 Serving/150g	188	2.5	125.3	3.7	19.6	3.7	1.0
Blackberry & Raspberry, Fruit Corner, Muller*	1 Pot/150g	158	5.8	105	3.8	13.1	3.9	0.9
Blackberry, Boysenberry & William Pear, M&S*	1 Pot/150g	188	9.8	125	4.0	13.6	6.5	2.4
Blackberry, Fat Free, Danone, Shape*	1 Pot/120g	74	0.2	62	6.7	8.4	0.2	2.4
Blackberry, Soya, Alpro Soya*	1 Pot/125g	91	2.6	73	3.7	9.2	2.1	1.2
Blackcurrant & Elderflower, Yeo Valley*	1 Lge Pot/450g	482	17.1	107	4.8	13.2	3.8	0.2
Blackcurrant, Bio Live, Rachel's Organic*	1 Serving/225g	166	3.8	74	3.6	11.0	1.7	0.0

YOGHURT

INFO/WEIGHT		per Measure KCAL	FAT	Nutrition Values per 100g / 100ml KCAL	PROT	CARB	FAT	FIBRE
Blackcurrant, ES, Asda*	1 Pot/100g	163	9.0	163	2.6	18.0	9.0	0.0
Blackcurrant, Fruity, Mullerlight, Muller*	1 Pot/175g	89	0.2	51	4.1	7.9	0.1	0.8
Blackcurrant, Garden Fruits, Low Fat, Tesco*	1 Pot/125g	120	2.4	95	3.8	15.1	1.9	0.3
Blackcurrant, Longley Farm*	1 Pot/150g	168	5.6	112	4.9	14.7	3.7	0.0
Blackcurrant, Low Fat, CBY, Asda*	1 Pot/125g	104	1.6	83	3.6	14.2	1.3	0.0
Blackcurrant, Low Fat, Sainsbury's*	1 Pot/125g	116	1.8	93	4.2	15.9	1.4	0.6
Blackcurrant, Probiotic, Organic, Yeo Valley*	1 Pot/150g	152	5.8	101	4.1	12.4	3.9	0.2
Blackcurrant, Thick & Creamy, Sainsbury's*	1 Pot/150g	171	5.4	114	4.3	15.9	3.6	0.4
Blackcurrant, Virtually Fat Free, Morrisons*	1 Pot/200g	114	0.4	57	5.4	8.4	0.2	0.2
Blueberries & Cream, Made Up, Easiyo*	1 Serving/100g	105	4.1	105	3.9	13.7	4.1	0.0
Blueberry Flip, Morrisons*	1 Pot/175g	201	8.0	115	3.1	15.1	4.6	0.5
Blueberry, Extremely Fruity, Low Fat, Probiotic, M&S*	1 Pot/150g	142	2.1	95	4.7	14.7	1.4	1.5
Blueberry, Fat Free, Probiotic, Organic, Yeo Valley*	1 Serving/100g	73	0.1	73	5.1	12.9	0.1	0.4
Blueberry, Fruit Corner, Muller*	1 Pot/150g	156	5.7	104	3.8	12.9	3.8	0.4
Blueberry, Greek Style, Intensely Creamy, Activia, Danone*	1 Pot/110g	112	3.3	102	5.0	13.4	3.0	0.0
Blueberry, Oatie Breakfast, Moma Foods*	1 Pot/235g	318	6.0	135	4.5	24.6	2.6	1.9
Blueberry, Probiotic, Natural Balance, Asda*	1 Pot/125g	102	2.9	82	2.1	13.1	2.3	2.6
Blueberry, Soya, with Cultures, Alpro*	1 Pot/125g	94	2.5	75	3.6	9.9	2.0	1.2
Blueberry, Specially Selected, Aldi*	1 Pot/150g	200	10.2	133	2.2	15.0	6.8	0.8
Bramble & Apple, Virtually Fat Free, Longley Farm*	1 Pot/150g	118	0.2	79	5.5	13.9	0.1	0.0
Bramley Apple & Gooseberry, M&S*	1 Pot/150g	186	10.6	124	2.8	12.3	7.1	0.5
Breakfast Crunch, Strawberry, Corner, Muller*	1 Pot/135g	163	3.5	121	5.5	0.0	2.6	0.0
British Rhubarb, Yeo Valley*	1 Serving/100g	102	3.8	102	4.6	12.3	3.8	0.0
Cereals, Fibre, Bio Activia, Danone*	1 Pot/120g	119	4.1	99	3.7	13.5	3.4	3.0
Champagne Rhubarb & Vanilla, M&S*	1 Pot/150g	195	8.7	130	3.8	15.7	5.8	0.8
Champagne Rhubarb, Finest, Tesco*	1 Pot/150g	212	11.6	141	3.4	14.1	7.7	0.7
Cherry & Wholegrain, Fat Free, Onken*	1 Serving/150g	134	0.4	89	4.8	15.0	0.3	0.0
Cherry Bakewell Tart Flavour, Muller*	1 Pot/175g	119	0.4	68	4.8	11.8	0.2	0.2
Cherry, 0.1% Fat, Shape, Danone*	1 Pot/120g	56	0.1	47	4.6	6.8	0.1	2.1
Cherry, Bio, Low Fat, Benecol*	1 Pot/150g	122	0.9	81	3.8	15.2	0.6	0.0
Cherry, Fat Free, Activia, Danone*	1 Pot/125g	76	0.1	61	4.8	9.8	0.1	0.9
Cherry, Fat Free, Optifit, Aldi*	1 Pot/125g	67	1.0	54	4.0	8.8	0.8	0.0
Cherry, Fruit, Biopot, Onken*	1 Serving/100g	107	2.7	107	3.7	16.7	2.7	0.2
Cherry, Fruity, Mullerlight, Muller*	1 Pot/175g	86	0.2	49	4.3	7.0	0.1	0.2
Cherry, Greek Style, Fruitopolis, Mullerlight, Muller*	1 Pot/130g	90	0.1	68	4.8	11.4	0.1	0.0
Cherry, Light, Fat Free, Muller*	1 Pot/175g	88	0.2	50	3.9	7.9	0.1	0.2
Cherry, Low Fat, Asda*	1 Pot/125g	120	1.4	96	4.6	17.0	1.1	0.0
Cherry, Low Fat, CBY, Asda*	1 Pot/125g	90	1.6	72	3.6	11.4	1.3	0.3
Cherry, Luscious, Intensely Creamy, Activia, Danone*	1 Pot/110g	109	3.3	99	5.0	12.8	3.0	0.2
Cherry, Pots, Probiotic, Yeo Valley*	1 Pot/119g	124	4.4	104	4.9	12.8	3.7	0.1
Chocolate, Seriously Smooth, Waitrose*	1 Pot/125g	158	3.0	126	6.0	20.1	2.4	0.1
Chocolate, Vitaline*	1 Pot/125g	102	0.6	82	3.5	15.8	0.5	0.0
Coconut & Vanilla, Greek Style, Brooklea, Aldi*	1 Pot/125g	70	0.6	56	4.9	7.8	0.5	0.5
Coconut, Low Fat, CBY, Asda*	1 Pot/125g	126	3.2	102	5.5	14.0	2.6	0.5
Cranberry, Bio Activia, Danone*	1 Pot/125g	115	4.0	92	3.6	12.3	3.2	1.7
Devon Toffee, Low Fat, Sainsbury's*	1 Pot/126g	137	1.9	109	4.3	19.6	1.5	0.0
Devonshire Fudge, 0.06% Fat, TTD, Sainsbury's*	1 Pot/150g	219	9.0	146	3.5	19.5	6.0	0.0
Eton Mess, British Classic, Corner, Muller*	1 Pot/135g	171	3.0	127	2.8	23.5	2.2	0.3
Fat Free, Vanilla, Onken*	½ Pot/225g	166	0.2	74	4.4	12.6	0.1	0.3
Fig, Bio, Activia, Danone*	1 Pot/125g	124	4.2	99	3.6	13.4	3.4	0.2
Forest Fruits, 0.1% Fat, Shape, Danone*	1 Pot/120g	55	0.1	46	4.6	6.7	0.1	2.1
Forest Fruits, Bio, Fat Free, Activia, Danone*	1 Pot/125g	72	0.1	58	4.5	8.9	0.1	1.1
Forest Fruits, Farmhouse, Twekkelo, De Zuivelhoeve*	1 Pot/500g	555	16.5	111	4.2	16.0	3.3	0.5

YOGHURT

	Measure INFO/WEIGHT	per Measure KCAL	per Measure FAT	KCAL	PROT	CARB	FAT	FIBRE
				Nutrition Values per 100g / 100ml				
Forest Fruits, M&S*	1 Pot/150g	148	2.4	99	4.7	16.8	1.6	0.5
Forest Fruits, Soya, Dairy Free, Alpro*	1 Serving/100g	79	2.2	79	3.8	10.1	2.2	1.2
French Set, Low Fat, Iceland*	1 Pot/125g	100	1.5	80	3.6	13.6	1.2	0.0
Fruit Whole Milk	1 Pot/150g	158	4.2	105	5.1	15.7	2.8	0.0
Fruit, Low Fat, Average	*1 Pot/125g*	*112*	*0.9*	*90*	*4.1*	*17.9*	*0.7*	*0.0*
Fruit, Luscious, Bio Live, Low Fat, Rachel's Organic*	1 Pot/125g	115	2.0	92	4.0	15.3	1.6	0.0
Fruits of the Forest, Iced, Linessa, Lidl*	1 Pot/170g	168	3.9	99	2.5	17.0	2.3	0.0
Fruits with Cherries, Bio, 0% Fat, Danone*	1 Pot/125g	65	0.1	52	3.6	9.1	0.1	0.0
Fruity Favourites, Organic, Yeo Valley*	1 Pot/125g	126	4.9	101	4.1	12.4	3.9	0.2
Fudge, Devonshire Style, Finest, Tesco*	1 Pot/150g	281	13.8	187	3.7	22.4	9.2	0.0
Ginger, Greek Style, Bio, Live, Rachel's Organic*	1 Serving/100g	134	7.1	134	3.2	14.3	7.1	0.0
Goats Whole Milk	*1 Carton/150g*	*94*	*5.7*	*63*	*3.5*	*3.9*	*3.8*	*0.0*
Gooseberry, Bio Live, Rachel's Organic*	1 Pot/450g	450	15.3	100	4.0	13.3	3.4	0.2
Gooseberry, Custard Style, Shapers, Boots*	1 Pot/151g	106	1.1	70	3.9	12.0	0.7	0.2
Gooseberry, Garden Fruits, Low Fat, Tesco*	1 Pot/125g	115	2.4	90	3.3	14.9	1.9	0.3
Gooseberry, Low Fat, Average	*1 Serving/100g*	*90*	*1.4*	*90*	*4.5*	*14.5*	*1.4*	*0.2*
Gooseberry, Low Fat, CBY, Asda*	1 Pot/125g	102	1.8	82	3.6	13.7	1.4	0.0
Gooseberry, Luxury Farmhouse, Stapleton*	1 Pot/150g	132	3.8	88	3.3	13.7	2.5	0.7
Gooseberry, Virtually Fat Free, Longley Farm*	1 Pot/150g	122	0.2	81	4.2	15.7	0.1	0.0
Greek 'n Coconut, Made Up, Easiyo*	1 Serving/100g	113	4.7	113	4.0	14.1	4.7	0.1
Greek Style, & Granola, Sainsbury's*	1 Pot/140g	262	7.6	187	5.8	29.0	5.4	0.6
Greek Style, & Nectarines, Food to Go, M&S*	1 Pack/200g	100	4.2	50	2.9	6.3	2.1	1.0
Greek Style, Low Fat, M&S*	1 Serving/100g	75	2.7	75	6.1	6.9	2.7	0.5
Greek Style, Luxury, Loseley*	1 Pot/175g	226	17.8	129	4.8	4.5	10.2	0.0
Greek Style, Strained, 0%, Glenisk Organic Dairy Co*	1 Pot/150g	84	0.0	56	10.0	4.0	0.0	0.0
Greek Style, with Honey, Asda*	1 Pot/150g	237	12.6	158	3.8	16.9	8.4	0.0
Greek Style, with Honey, Morrisons*	1/3 Pot/150g	236	14.3	157	4.1	13.5	9.5	0.7
Greek Style, with Strawberries, Asda*	1 Pot/125g	159	8.2	127	3.2	13.6	6.6	0.2
Greek Style, with Tropical Fruits, Asda*	1 Pot/125g	164	8.2	131	3.3	14.5	6.6	0.3
Greek, 0% Fat, Strained, Authentic, Total, Fage*	¼ Pot/125g	71	0.0	57	10.3	4.0	0.0	0.0
Greek, 0%, Mevgal*	1 Serving/100g	52	0.0	52	8.0	5.0	0.0	0.0
Greek, 2% Fat, Strained, Authentic, Total, Fage*	1 Pot/170g	124	3.4	73	9.9	3.8	2.0	0.0
Greek, Authentic, Natural, Strained, Waitrose*	1 Serving/125g	164	12.8	131	5.9	3.7	10.2	0.3
Greek, Lemon, 0% Fat, Dale Farm*	1 Serving/120g	95	0.4	79	6.4	12.2	0.3	0.7
Greek, with Honey, Strained, Authentic, Total, Fage*	1 Pot/150g	255	12.0	170	5.4	19.0	8.0	0.0
Greek, with Mango & Nectarine, 0% Fat, M&S*	1 Pot/140g	87	0.3	62	4.9	10.2	0.2	0.5
Greek, with Strawberry, 2% Fat, Total, Fage*	1 Pot/150g	140	2.4	93	6.7	12.9	1.6	0.0
Hazelnut, Longley Farm*	1 Pot/150g	201	8.5	134	5.5	16.0	5.7	0.0
Hazelnut, Sainsbury's*	1 Serving/150g	183	3.4	122	5.0	20.3	2.3	0.2
Hazelnut, Yoplait*	1 Pot/125g	166	5.0	133	4.6	19.6	4.0	0.0
Honey & Ginger, Waitrose*	1 Pot/150g	240	12.9	160	3.8	16.8	8.6	0.1
Honey & Muesli, Breakfast Break, Tesco*	1 Pot/170g	207	4.6	122	3.9	20.5	2.7	0.6
Honey Breakfast Pot, Activia, Danone*	1 Pot/160g	192	4.2	120	4.9	18.8	2.6	0.7
Honey, Greek Style, Co-Op*	1 Pot/150g	228	12.8	152	4.0	13.8	8.5	0.0
Honey, Icelandic, Strained, Fat Free, Skyr, Arla*	1 Serving/150g	110	0.2	73	9.4	7.8	0.1	0.0
Honeyed Apricot, Greek Style, Corner, Muller*	1 Pot/150g	168	4.5	112	5.0	15.5	3.0	0.1
Honeyed Peach, Greek Style, Mullerlight, Muller*	1 Pot/120g	85	0.2	71	6.3	10.3	0.2	0.2
Juicy Raspberry, Intensely Creamy, Activia, Danone*	1 Pot/110g	109	3.3	99	4.8	12.7	3.0	0.6
Kiwi, Bio, Activia, Danone*	1 Pot/125g	122	4.2	98	3.6	12.9	3.4	0.3
Lemon & Lime, BGTY, Sainsbury's*	1 Pot/125g	66	0.1	53	4.6	8.3	0.1	1.1
Lemon & Lime, Fat Free, Shape, Danone*	1 Pot/120g	61	0.1	51	4.5	7.3	0.1	0.1
Lemon Bliss, Greek Style, Lemon Layer, Strained, Liberte*	1 Pot/100g	108	2.1	108	7.4	13.7	2.1	0.2
Lemon Cheesecake, Inspired, Corner, Muller*	1 Pot/135g	201	6.2	149	3.6	22.7	4.6	0.0

Y

YOGHURT

INFO/WEIGHT	Measure	per Measure KCAL	FAT	Nutrition Values per 100g / 100ml KCAL	PROT	CARB	FAT	FIBRE
Lemon Curd with West Country Cream, Morrisons*	1 Pot/150g	244	12.7	163	3.4	17.9	8.5	0.5
Lemon Curd, Indulgent, Dessert, Waitrose*	1 Pot/150g	278	13.8	185	4.1	21.5	9.2	0.0
Lemon Curd, West Country, TTD, Sainsbury's*	1 Pot/150g	243	10.0	162	3.7	21.6	6.7	0.5
Lemon Curd, Whole Milk, Yeo Valley*	1 Pot/120g	153	5.3	128	4.8	17.2	4.4	0.2
Lemon, Greek Style, 0% Fat, Yeo Valley*	1 Pot/120g	96	0.0	80	6.7	12.7	0.0	0.0
Lemon, Greek Style, Shape, Danone*	1 Pot/125g	140	3.4	112	5.9	15.9	2.7	0.0
Lemon, Greek Style, Whipped, Bliss Corner, Muller*	1 Pot/110g	177	6.5	161	4.0	22.2	5.9	0.0
Lemon, Longley Farm*	1 Pot/150g	159	5.6	106	5.0	13.4	3.7	0.0
Lemon, Low Fat, Average	**1 Serving/100g**	**95**	**0.9**	**95**	**4.6**	**17.3**	**0.9**	**0.1**
Lemon, Soya, Sojade*	1 Pot/125g	98	2.6	78	3.8	11.0	2.1	0.1
Lemon, Summer, Biopot, Onken*	1 Pot/150g	154	3.9	103	3.9	15.9	2.6	0.1
Lemon, Thick & Fruity, Citrus Fruits, Weight Watchers*	1 Pot/120g	47	0.1	39	4.1	4.9	0.1	0.9
Low Calorie	1 Pot/120g	49	0.2	41	4.3	6.0	0.2	0.5
Madagascan Vanilla, West Country, TTD, Sainsbury's*	1 Pot/149g	224	12.5	150	3.4	14.9	8.4	0.5
Mandarin, Fat Free, Mullerlight, Muller*	1 Pot/175g	95	0.2	54	4.2	8.5	0.1	0.0
Mandarin, Longley Farm*	1 Pot/150g	141	5.7	94	4.9	13.3	3.8	0.0
Mango & Apple, Fat Free, Onken*	1 Serving/150g	132	0.2	88	4.4	16.0	0.1	0.2
Mango & Passion Fruit, Tropical Fruit, Activ8, Ski, Nestle*	1 Pot/120g	114	2.0	95	4.3	15.6	1.7	0.2
Mango & Passionfruit, Fruit Corner, Muller*	1 Pot/150g	160	5.8	107	3.8	13.5	3.9	0.3
Mango 0% Fat, Shape Delights*	1 Pot/120g	80	0.1	67	5.5	10.9	0.1	0.9
Mango Layer, Greek Style, Strained, 0% fat, Liberte*	1 Pot/100g	90	0.1	90	7.7	13.5	0.1	0.2
Mango, Bio, Activia, Danone*	1 Pot/125g	124	4.2	99	3.5	13.5	3.4	0.2
Mango, Fat Free, Shape Danone*	1 Pot/120g	74	0.1	62	6.6	8.6	0.1	2.2
Mango, Light, Muller*	1 Pot/175g	96	0.2	55	4.3	9.2	0.1	0.0
Maple & Cinnamon Granola, Low Fat, Natural, Asda*	1 Pot/140g	196	4.6	140	6.1	21.5	3.3	0.8
Mixed Berries, Jogood, Imlek*	1 Pot/200g	172	4.4	86	2.9	13.4	2.2	0.0
Mixed Berry, Icelandic, Strained, Fat Free, Skyr, Arla*	1 Pot/150g	114	0.3	76	9.4	8.0	0.2	0.2
Muesli Nut, Low Fat	1 Pot/120g	134	2.6	112	5.0	19.2	2.2	0.0
Natural with Honey, Greek Style, Sainsbury's*	1 Pot/150g	243	14.1	162	4.0	15.4	9.4	0.0
Natural, 0.1% Fat, Stirred, Biopot, Onken*	1 Serving/100g	48	0.1	48	5.4	6.4	0.1	0.0
Natural, Bio Activia, Individual Pots, Danone*	1 Pot/125g	86	4.2	69	4.2	5.5	3.4	0.0
Natural, Bio Life, Easiyo*	1 Pot/150g	95	2.7	63	5.0	6.7	1.8	0.0
Natural, Bio Live, Low Fat, Organic, Waitrose*	¼ Pot/125g	81	1.2	65	5.8	8.3	1.0	0.0
Natural, Bio Live, Very Low Fat, Ann Forshaw's*	1 Pot/125g	52	0.1	42	5.0	5.5	0.1	0.0
Natural, Bio, BFY, Morrisons*	1 Serving/100g	65	0.2	65	6.5	9.4	0.2	0.0
Natural, Bio, Co-Op*	1 Pot/150g	117	5.4	78	4.8	5.5	3.6	0.0
Natural, Bio, HL, Tesco*	1 Serving/100g	55	0.1	55	5.4	7.6	0.1	0.0
Natural, Bio, Light Choices, Tesco*	1 Serving/100g	55	0.1	55	5.4	7.6	0.1	0.0
Natural, Bio, Low Fat, Sainsbury's*	1 Serving/100g	48	1.5	48	4.0	4.6	1.5	0.0
Natural, Bio, Virtually Fat Free, HL, Tesco*	1 Serving/100g	47	0.2	47	5.5	5.8	0.2	0.1
Natural, Danone*	1 Pot/125g	71	3.6	57	3.2	3.8	2.9	0.0
Natural, Fat Free, Biopot, Dr Oetker*	¼ Pot/125g	60	0.1	48	5.4	6.4	0.1	0.0
Natural, Fat Free, Eat Smart, Morrisons*	1 Pot/150g	88	0.3	59	7.0	7.2	0.2	0.0
Natural, Fat Free, Onken*	1 Serving/100g	46	0.1	46	5.4	4.3	0.1	0.0
Natural, Fat Free, Probiotic, Essential, Waitrose*	¼ Pot/125g	68	0.0	54	5.5	7.8	0.0	0.0
Natural, Fat Free, Rachel's Organic*	1 Pot/500g	180	0.5	36	3.9	4.8	0.1	0.0
Natural, Greek Style, Average	**1 Serving/100g**	**138**	**10.6**	**138**	**4.7**	**6.1**	**10.6**	**0.0**
Natural, Greek Style, BGTY, Sainsbury's*	1 Serving/50g	39	1.4	78	5.5	7.9	2.7	0.0
Natural, Greek Style, Bio Live, Rachel's Organic*	1 Pot/450g	518	40.5	115	3.6	4.9	9.0	0.0
Natural, Greek Style, Bio Live, Tims Dairy*	1 Serving/50g	65	5.0	130	5.7	4.9	10.0	0.0
Natural, Greek Style, Fat Free, CBY, Asda*	1 Pot/200g	114	0.4	57	7.9	5.8	0.2	0.1
Natural, Greek Style, Fat Free, Tesco*	½ Pot/100g	55	0.2	55	7.5	4.8	0.2	0.4
Natural, Greek Style, HL, Tesco*	1 Serving/100g	80	2.7	80	5.7	8.2	2.7	0.0

YOGHURT

INFO/WEIGHT	per Measure KCAL	FAT	KCAL	PROT	CARB	FAT	FIBRE
Natural, Greek Style, Low Fat, Asda*	1 Serving/30g	24	0.8	80	5.7	8.2	2.7	0.0
Natural, Greek Style, Low Fat, Average	*1 Serving/100g*	*77*	*2.7*	*77*	*6.1*	*7.3*	*2.7*	*0.2*
Natural, Greek Style, Organic, Tesco*	1 Pot/500g	665	50.0	133	4.5	6.2	10.0	0.0
Natural, Greek Style, Probiotic, Unsweetened, M&S*	1 Serving/150g	195	15.2	130	5.5	4.6	10.1	0.1
Natural, Icelandic, Strained, Fat Free, Skyr, Arla*	1 Serving/150g	98	0.3	65	11.0	4.0	0.2	0.0
Natural, Longley Farm*	1 Pot/150g	118	5.2	79	4.8	7.0	3.5	0.0
Natural, Low Fat, Average	*1 Pot/125g*	*75*	*1.6*	*60*	*5.4*	*7.0*	*1.3*	*0.0*
Natural, Low Fat, Bio, Sainsbury's*	1 Pot/125g	85	1.9	68	5.6	7.9	1.5	0.0
Natural, Low Fat, Live, Waitrose*	1 Pot/175g	114	1.8	65	5.8	8.2	1.0	0.0
Natural, Low Fat, Organic, Average	*1 Serving/100g*	*87*	*1.2*	*87*	*5.7*	*7.7*	*1.2*	*0.0*
Natural, Low Fat, Value, Tesco*	1 Pot/125g	81	1.9	65	5.0	7.2	1.5	0.0
Natural, Pouring, Activia, Danone*	1 Carton/950g	484	16.2	51	4.1	4.9	1.7	0.0
Natural, Probiotic, 2% Fat, Sainsbury's*	¼ Pot/125g	76	1.9	61	4.9	7.0	1.5	0.0
Natural, Probiotic, Fat Free, Organic, Yeo Valley*	1 Pot/150g	87	0.2	58	5.9	8.4	0.1	0.0
Natural, Probiotic, Organic, Yeo Valley*	1 Pot/120g	98	5.0	82	4.6	6.5	4.2	0.0
Natural, Set, Asda*	1 Pot/450g	256	4.5	57	5.1	6.8	1.0	0.0
Natural, Set, Low Fat, Waitrose*	1 Pot/150g	99	1.8	66	5.7	8.1	1.2	0.0
Natural, Soya, Sojade*	1 Serving/100g	50	2.5	50	4.5	2.4	2.5	0.0
Natural, Whole Milk, Set, Biopot, Onken*	1 Serving/125g	85	4.4	68	4.5	4.1	3.5	0.0
Natural, Wholemilk, Live Bio, Organic, Waitrose*	1 Serving/100g	88	4.4	88	5.1	7.1	4.4	0.0
Natural, with Cow's Milk, Greek Style, Sainsbury's*	½ Pot/100g	143	10.9	143	4.5	6.6	10.9	0.0
Nectarine & Passion Fruit, 0.1% Fat, Shape, Danone*	1 Pot/120g	55	0.1	46	4.6	6.7	0.1	2.1
Nectarine, Fat Free, Weight Watchers*	1 Pot/120g	48	0.1	40	4.1	4.7	0.1	0.4
Orange & Mango, Thick & Fruity, Probiotic, COU, M&S*	1 Pot/145g	65	0.1	45	4.2	6.5	0.1	0.5
Orange & Pineapple, Tropical Fruit, Activ8, Ski, Nestle*	1 Pot/120g	112	2.0	93	4.4	15.1	1.7	0.2
Orange Blossom Honey, Finest, Tesco*	1 Pot/150g	237	10.6	158	3.5	20.1	7.1	0.0
Orange with Chocolate Flakes, Fat Free, Brooklea, Aldi*	1 Pot/165g	84	0.8	51	3.5	8.3	0.5	0.5
Orange, Low Fat, Tesco*	1 Pot/125g	114	2.2	91	4.3	14.5	1.8	0.0
Orange, Sprinkled with Dark Chocolate, Light, Muller*	1 Pot/165g	91	0.8	55	4.3	7.4	0.5	0.1
Passion Fruit, Greek Style, Luxury, Oykos, Danone*	1 Pot/110g	163	9.1	148	2.9	15.4	8.3	0.1
Peach & Apricot, 0.1% Fat, Shape, Danone*	1 Pot/120g	55	0.1	46	4.6	6.7	0.1	2.1
Peach & Apricot, Fruit Corner, Muller*	1 Pot/150g	160	5.7	107	3.9	13.5	3.8	0.5
Peach & Apricot, HL, Tesco*	1 Pot/92g	42	0.1	46	4.0	7.4	0.1	1.0
Peach & Apricot, Light, HL, Tesco*	1 Pot/200g	82	0.2	41	3.9	6.2	0.1	1.0
Peach & Mango, Thick & Creamy, Waitrose*	1 Pot/125g	136	3.1	109	3.7	17.8	2.5	0.3
Peach & Mango, Truly Fruity, Brooklea, Aldi*	1 Pot/200g	162	2.8	81	4.6	12.4	1.4	0.0
Peach & Nectarine, Bio, Fat Free, Activia, Danone*	1 Pot/125g	70	0.1	56	4.5	9.3	0.1	1.0
Peach & Passion Fruit, 0% fat,,Shape Delights*	1 Pot/120g	80	0.1	67	5.6	10.8	0.1	0.6
Peach & Passion Fruit, Average	*1 Serving/100g*	*66*	*0.7*	*66*	*4.5*	*10.6*	*0.7*	*0.4*
Peach & Passion Fruit, BGTY, Sainsbury's*	1 Pot/125g	69	0.1	55	4.9	8.6	0.1	0.1
Peach & Passion Fruit, Fat Free, Shape, Danone*	1 Pot/120g	74	0.1	62	6.6	8.6	0.1	2.3
Peach & Passion Fruit, Greek, Fruitopolis, Light, Muller*	1 Pot/130g	84	0.1	65	4.8	10.7	0.1	0.0
Peach & Passion Fruit, Layers, Mullerlight, Muller*	1 Pot/175g	94	0.2	54	3.1	9.7	0.1	0.2
Peach & Pear, Seriously Fruity, Low Fat, Waitrose*	1 Pot/125g	110	1.2	88	4.5	15.3	1.0	0.3
Peach & Pineapple, Fat Free, Mullerlight, Muller*	1 Pot/175g	89	0.2	51	4.3	7.7	0.1	0.2
Peach & Vanilla Flip, Morrisons*	1 Pot/175g	212	8.0	121	3.4	16.5	4.6	0.6
Peach & Vanilla, Average, Tesco*	1 Serving/100g	44	0.2	44	4.4	6.2	0.2	0.6
Peach & Vanilla, Thick & Creamy, Co-Op*	1 Pot/150g	180	6.9	120	3.6	16.0	4.6	0.1
Peach Melba, Low Fat, Average	*1 Serving/100g*	*75*	*0.7*	*75*	*2.6*	*14.5*	*0.7*	*0.0*
Peach, BGTY, Sainsbury's*	1 Pot/125g	61	0.2	49	4.7	7.2	0.2	0.2
Peach, Bio, Activia, Fat Free, Danone*	1 Pot/125g	71	0.1	57	4.7	9.3	0.1	1.0
Peach, Bio, Fat Free, Snackpot, Activia, Danone*	1 Pot/165g	99	0.2	60	4.6	10.2	0.1	1.0
Peach, Biopot, Wholegrain, Onken*	1 Serving/100g	114	2.8	114	4.0	17.8	2.8	0.5

YOGHURT

INFO/WEIGHT	Measure	per Measure KCAL	FAT	Nutrition Values per 100g / 100ml KCAL	PROT	CARB	FAT	FIBRE
Peach, Dairy Free, Organic, Yofu, Soya, Provamel*	1 Serving/125g	100	2.8	80	3.9	10.3	2.2	0.8
Peach, Fat Free, Probiotic, CBY, Asda*	1 Pot/125g	88	0.1	70	3.9	12.1	0.1	2.6
Peach, Forbidden Fruits, Rachel's Organic*	1 Pot/125g	156	7.6	125	3.4	14.0	6.1	0.0
Peach, Greek Style, Luxury, Oykos, Danone*	1 Pot/110g	153	8.9	140	3.1	13.4	8.1	0.3
Peach, Honeyed, Greek Style, Mullerlight, Muller*	1 Pot/120g	85	0.2	71	6.3	10.3	0.2	0.2
Peach, Low Fat, Average	*1 Serving/100g*	*86*	*1.1*	*86*	*4.5*	*14.6*	*1.1*	*0.2*
Peach, Luscious, Low Fat, Rachel's Organic*	1 Pot/125g	112	2.0	90	4.0	14.9	1.6	0.2
Peach, Smooth Style, Mullerlight, Muller*	1 Pot/125g	59	0.1	47	4.1	6.9	0.1	0.2
Peaches & Cream, Intensely Creamy, Activia, Danone*	1 Pot/120g	118	3.6	98	4.8	13.0	3.0	0.3
Pear, Greek Style, Luxury, Oykos, Danone*	1 Pot/110g	160	8.8	145	3.1	14.9	8.0	0.5
Pear, Lidl*	1 Pot/125g	108	0.1	86	4.3	16.1	0.1	0.0
Pineapple & Passion Fruit, Soya, Light, Alpro*	1 Pot/120g	94	2.3	78	3.6	10.3	1.9	0.8
Pineapple & Peach, Fruity, Mullerlight, Muller*	1 Pot/175g	89	0.2	51	4.2	7.7	0.1	0.2
Pineapple, Bio Activia, Fat Free, Danone*	1 Pot/125g	62	0.1	50	4.7	7.5	0.1	1.7
Pineapple, Low Fat, Average	*1 Serving/100g*	*89*	*1.2*	*89*	*4.6*	*14.7*	*1.2*	*0.0*
Plain, Low Fat, Average	*1 Serving/100g*	*63*	*1.6*	*63*	*5.2*	*7.0*	*1.6*	*0.0*
Plain, with Almond, Alpro*	1 Serving/125g	68	3.5	54	3.9	2.3	2.8	1.1
Plum, Probiotic, Summer Selection, Yeo Valley*	1 Pot/125g	126	4.9	101	4.1	12.4	3.9	0.1
Prune, Bifidus, Activo, Mercadona*	1 Pot/125g	70	0.1	56	4.5	6.8	0.1	3.0
Prune, Bio, Activia, Danone*	1 Pot/125g	122	4.1	98	3.6	13.1	3.3	0.8
Prune, Vitality, Low Fat, with Omega 3, Muller*	1 Pot/150g	144	2.8	96	4.7	15.0	1.9	1.1
Raspberry & Cranberry, Fat Free, Mullerlight, Muller*	1 Pot/175g	91	0.2	52	4.3	7.8	0.1	0.5
Raspberry & Vanilla, Soya, Dairy Free, Alpro*	1 Pot/125g	98	2.8	78	3.9	10.2	2.2	1.2
Raspberry, Bio Live, Low Fat, Rachel's Organic*	1 Pot/125g	114	2.0	91	4.1	15.1	1.6	0.1
Raspberry, Bio, Activia, Danone*	1 Pot/125g	112	3.5	90	3.5	12.8	2.8	2.0
Raspberry, Bio, Activia, Fat Free, Danone*	1 Pot/125g	68	0.1	54	4.7	7.2	0.1	2.6
Raspberry, Bio, Fat Free, Snackpot, Activia, Danone*	1 Pot/165g	91	0.2	54	4.7	7.2	0.1	2.6
Raspberry, Bio, Low Fat, Benecol*	1 Pot/125g	99	0.8	79	3.8	14.5	0.6	0.0
Raspberry, Bio, Low Fat, Sainsbury's*	1 Pot/150g	146	1.7	97	4.7	17.0	1.1	0.7
Raspberry, Bio, Pur Natur*	1 Pot/150g	150	4.6	100	1.4	14.5	3.1	0.0
Raspberry, Extremely Fruity, M&S*	1 Pot/200g	190	3.0	95	5.0	15.6	1.5	0.5
Raspberry, Fat Free, Probiotic, Organic, Yeo Valley*	1 Pot/125g	98	0.1	78	5.2	14.0	0.1	0.4
Raspberry, Forbidden Fruit, Rachel's Organic*	1 Pot/125g	155	7.6	124	3.4	13.8	6.1	0.1
Raspberry, Lactose Free, Lactofree, Arla*	1 Pot/125g	130	3.4	104	3.3	16.5	2.7	0.7
Raspberry, Low Fat, Average	*1 Serving/100g*	*83*	*1.1*	*83*	*4.1*	*14.1*	*1.1*	*0.8*
Raspberry, Low Fat, Stapleton*	1 Serving/150g	105	0.8	70	3.3	13.6	0.5	2.0
Raspberry, Organic, Yeo Valley*	1 Pot/150g	152	5.8	101	4.2	12.3	3.9	0.4
Raspberry, Probiotic, Live, Yeo Valley*	1 Pot/125g	106	1.2	85	5.1	14.0	1.0	0.4
Raspberry, Scottish, The Best, Morrisons*	1 Pot/150g	208	10.4	139	3.6	15.6	6.9	1.3
Raspberry, Smooth, Activ8, Ski, Nestle*	1 Pot/120g	113	2.0	94	4.6	14.8	1.7	0.7
Raspberry, Smooth, Mullerlight, Muller*	1 Pot/125g	64	0.1	51	4.2	7.8	0.1	0.6
Raspberry, Soya, Alpro*	1 Pot/125g	99	2.4	79	3.7	10.4	1.9	1.2
Raspberry, Summer, Biopot, Onken*	1/5 Pot/90g	91	2.4	101	3.8	15.0	2.7	0.6
Raspberry, Thick & Fruity, Probiotic, COU, M&S*	1 Pot/170g	76	0.2	45	4.2	6.9	0.1	0.6
Raspberry, Vitality, Low Fat, with Omega 3, Muller*	1 Pot/125g	115	2.5	92	4.3	13.4	2.0	1.3
Raspberry, with Fruit Layer, Bio Activia, Danone*	1 Pot/125g	116	3.5	93	3.4	12.5	2.8	2.0
Red Berry, Vitality, Low Fat, with Omega 3, Muller*	1 Pot/150g	138	2.8	92	4.3	13.8	1.9	0.7
Red Cherry, Fat Free, Ski, Nestle*	1 Pot 120g	97	0.1	81	4.5	15.6	0.1	0.1
Red Cherry, Fruit Corner, Muller*	1 Pot/150g	158	5.8	105	3.8	13.0	3.9	0.5
Red Cherry, Very Cherry, Activ8, Ski, Nestle*	1 Pot/120	115	2.0	96	4.5	15.7	1.7	0.1
Rhubarb & Champagne, Truly Irresistible, Co-Op*	1 Pot/150g	195	8.2	130	3.5	16.6	5.5	0.2
Rhubarb & Vanilla, Summer, Biopot, Onken*	1/5 Pot/90g	94	2.4	104	3.7	16.0	2.7	0.3
Rhubarb Crumble, Crunch Corner, Muller*	1 Pot/150g	238	8.4	159	3.6	23.5	5.6	0.5

YOGHURT

INFO/WEIGHT	Measure	per Measure KCAL	FAT	Nutrition Values per 100g / 100ml KCAL	PROT	CARB	FAT	FIBRE
Rhubarb, Eat Smart, Morrisons*	1 Pot/190g	79	0.2	42	4.1	6.1	0.1	1.4
Rhubarb, Extremely Fruity, Probiotic, Low Fat, M&S*	1 Pot/170g	153	1.7	90	4.4	15.5	1.0	0.7
Rhubarb, Greek Style, Corner, Muller*	1 Pot/150g	170	4.5	113	5.0	15.8	3.0	0.1
Rhubarb, Longley Farm*	1 Pot/150g	165	5.6	110	4.9	14.3	3.7	0.0
Rhubarb, Low Fat, Garden Fruits, Tesco*	1 Pot/125g	119	2.4	95	3.0	15.5	1.9	0.3
Rhubarb, Luxury, Aldi*	1 Pot/150g	196	9.9	131	2.3	15.0	6.6	0.9
Rhubarb, Natural, Live, Glenilen Farm*	1 Pot/160g	133	4.6	83	3.5	12.6	2.9	0.0
Rhubarb, Spiced, Thick & Creamy, COU, M&S*	1 Pot/170g	68	0.2	40	4.3	5.8	0.1	0.5
Sheep's Milk, Total, Fage*	1 Pot/200g	180	12.0	90	4.8	4.3	6.0	0.0
Sheep's, Organic, Unsweetened, Vrai*	1 Pot/125g	109	7.2	87	4.8	3.8	5.8	0.0
Sour Cherry, Icelandic, Strained, Fat Free, Skyr, Arla*	1 Pot/150g	118	0.3	79	9.4	9.0	0.2	0.1
Sticky Toffee Pudding, Dessert Style, Mullerlight, Muller*	1 Pot/175g	108	0.4	62	4.4	9.9	0.2	0.2
Strawberries & Cream, 0.06% Fat, TTD, Sainsbury's*	1 Pot/150g	183	8.2	122	3.5	14.7	5.5	0.4
Strawberries & Cream, Finest, Tesco*	1 Pot/150g	206	10.4	137	3.4	15.4	6.9	0.5
Strawberries & Cream, Signature, Morrisons*	1 Pot/150g	196	9.4	131	3.0	15.5	6.3	0.0
Strawberries & Jersey Cream, Rich & Creamy, Loseley*	1 Pot/150g	200	7.6	133	5.2	16.1	5.1	0.0
Strawberry & Banana, Oatie Breakfast, Moma Foods*	1 Pot/235g	320	5.6	136	4.3	25.4	2.4	1.7
Strawberry & Clotted Cream, Luxury, Stapleton Farm*	1 Pot/150g	147	5.7	98	3.2	13.2	3.8	0.6
Strawberry & Cornish Clotted Cream, M&S*	1 Pot/150g	218	11.6	145	3.2	15.4	7.7	0.5
Strawberry & Raspberry, HL, Tesco*	1 Pot/125g	58	0.1	46	4.2	7.0	0.1	0.0
Strawberry & Raspberry, Low Fat, Asda*	1 Pot/150g	142	1.5	95	4.6	17.4	1.0	0.2
Strawberry & Redcurrant, Farmhouse, Ann Forshaw's*	1 Pot/150g	194	7.4	129	3.8	17.4	4.9	0.2
Strawberry & Rhubarb, Onken*	1 Serving/100g	85	0.1	85	4.6	16.2	0.1	0.4
Strawberry Cheesecake, Dessert Recipe, Weight Watchers*	1 Pot/120g	57	0.1	48	4.1	6.6	0.1	0.2
Strawberry Cheesecake, Inspired by, Mullerlight, Muller*	1 Pot/165g	99	0.2	60	4.2	10.0	0.1	0.2
Strawberry Cheesecake, Inspired, Corner, Muller*	1 Pot/135g	209	6.2	155	3.6	24.3	4.6	0.1
Strawberry Crumble, Crunch Corner, Muller*	1 Pot/150g	234	8.4	156	3.6	22.9	5.6	0.5
Strawberry Rice, Low Fat, Muller*	1 Pot/190g	203	4.4	107	3.2	18.4	2.3	0.4
Strawberry Shortcake, Crunch Corner, Muller*	1 Pot/135g	212	8.0	157	4.1	21.2	5.9	0.1
Strawberry, Active, Fat Free, Optifit, Aldi*	1 Pot/125g	54	0.5	43	3.0	7.1	0.4	0.4
Strawberry, Bettabuy, Morrisons*	1 Pot/115g	91	1.5	79	4.4	12.8	1.3	0.3
Strawberry, Bio, Activia, Danone*	1 Pot/125g	124	4.1	99	3.6	13.6	3.3	0.2
Strawberry, Bio, Fat Free, Snackpot, Activia, Danone*	1 Pot/165g	101	0.2	61	5.0	10.0	0.1	0.2
Strawberry, Biopot, Wholegrain, Onken*	1 Serving/100g	111	2.9	111	4.1	17.2	2.9	0.5
Strawberry, Duo, Co-Op*	1 Pot/175g	219	8.8	125	3.0	17.0	5.0	0.7
Strawberry, Eat Smart, Morrisons*	1 Pot/200g	116	0.6	58	5.7	8.5	0.3	0.3
Strawberry, Everyday Low Fat, Co-Op*	1 Pot/125g	88	0.9	70	3.0	13.0	0.7	0.0
Strawberry, Fat Free, Average	*1 Serving/100g*	*66*	*0.1*	*66*	*4.9*	*11.1*	*0.1*	*0.6*
Strawberry, Fat Free, Greek Style, Brooklea, Aldi*	1 Pot/125g	72	0.3	57	4.9	8.8	0.2	0.2
Strawberry, Fat Free, Probiotic, Organic, Yeo Valley*	1 Pot/125g	108	1.2	86	5.1	14.1	1.0	0.1
Strawberry, Fruit 'n' Creamy, Ubley*	1 Pot/151g	167	4.4	111	4.3	16.9	2.9	0.3
Strawberry, Fruity, Mullerlight, Muller*	1 Pot/175g	89	0.2	51	4.1	7.9	0.1	0.0
Strawberry, Greek Style, Fat Free,,Mullerlight, Muller*	1 Pot/120g	83	0.2	69	6.3	9.8	0.2	0.1
Strawberry, Greek Style, Fruitopolis, Mullerlight, Muller*	1 Pot/130g	84	0.1	65	4.8	10.8	0.1	0.0
Strawberry, Greek Style, Luxury, Oykos, Danone*	1 Pot/110g	159	8.9	145	3.2	14.6	8.1	0.3
Strawberry, Happy Shopper*	1 Pot/150g	130	0.4	87	3.0	18.5	0.3	0.0
Strawberry, Healthy Balance, Corner, Muller*	1 Pot/135g	161	3.5	119	5.4	17.9	2.6	0.8
Strawberry, Icelandic, Strained, Fat Free, Skyr, Arla*	1 Pot/150g	112	0.3	75	9.4	8.0	0.2	0.2
Strawberry, Lactose Free, Lactofree, Arla*	1 Pot/125g	126	3.2	101	3.5	15.9	2.6	0.4
Strawberry, Light, Brooklea, Aldi*	1 Pot/200g	154	0.2	77	6.1	12.9	0.1	0.4
Strawberry, Light, HL, Tesco*	1 Pot/200g	80	0.2	40	3.5	6.4	0.1	0.8
Strawberry, Low Fat, Average	*1 Serving/100g*	*81*	*1.0*	*81*	*4.5*	*13.6*	*1.0*	*0.2*
Strawberry, Milbona, Lidl*	1 Pot/175g	175	5.2	100	3.0	15.0	3.0	0.0

Y

YOGHURT	Measure INFO/WEIGHT	per Measure KCAL	FAT	Nutrition Values per 100g / 100ml KCAL	PROT	CARB	FAT	FIBRE
Strawberry, Naturally Creamy, Nom Dairy UK*	1 Pot/175g	186	6.6	106	3.1	15.0	3.8	0.3
Strawberry, Organic, Yeo Valley*	1 Pot/150g	159	5.7	106	4.7	13.2	3.8	0.1
Strawberry, Pouring, Activia, Danone*	1 Serving/100g	59	1.6	59	3.9	7.3	1.6	0.1
Strawberry, Probiotic, Organic, Yeo Valley*	1 Pot/125g	125	5.0	100	4.4	11.7	4.0	0.1
Strawberry, Smooth Set French, Low Fat, Sainsbury's*	1 Pot/125g	112	4.0	90	3.7	11.8	3.2	0.0
Strawberry, Smooth, Activ8, Ski, Nestle*	1 Pot/120g	113	2.0	94	4.6	14.8	1.7	0.7
Strawberry, Soya, Dairy Free, Alpro*	1 Pot/125g	98	2.8	78	3.8	10.0	2.2	0.8
Strawberry, Thick & Creamy, Co-Op*	1 Pot/150g	182	6.9	121	3.6	16.4	4.6	0.1
Strawberry, Thick & Fruity, Probiotic, COU, M&S*	1 Pot/170g	76	0.2	45	4.1	7.3	0.1	0.4
Strawberry, Totally, Low Fat, CBY, Asda*	1 Pot/125g	104	1.2	83	4.1	14.2	1.0	0.4
Strawberry, Very Berry, Activ8, Ski, Nestle*	1 Pot/120g	110	2.0	92	4.3	15.0	1.7	0.3
Strawberry, Vitality, Low Fat, with Omega 3, Muller*	1 Pot/150g	140	2.8	93	4.3	14.0	1.9	0.8
Strawberry, White Choc Balls, Goodies, Mullerlight, Muller*	1 Pot/100g	92	2.3	92	4.1	13.1	2.3	0.0
Strawberry, Yoplait*	1 Pot/125g	61	0.2	49	4.2	7.6	0.2	0.9
Summer Berries, Fat Free, Mullerlight, Muller*	1 Pot/175g	88	0.2	50	4.1	7.6	0.1	0.4
Summer Berry Compote, Greek Style, & Granola, M&S*	1 Pot/205g	336	16.4	164	5.6	17.3	8.0	0.1
Summer Fruits, Greek Style, Corner, Muller*	1 Pot/150g	165	4.5	110	5.1	15.0	3.0	0.5
Summer Fruits, Light, Limited Edition, Muller*	1 Pot/175g	88	0.2	50	4.1	7.6	0.1	0.4
Summerfruits, Bio Live, Fat Free, Rachel's Organic*	1 Pot/125g	120	2.2	96	4.7	15.3	1.8	0.0
Sweet Treat, Low Fat, Tesco*	1 Pot/125g	131	2.9	105	3.1	18.0	2.3	0.3
Tempting Toffee, Greek Style, Muller Light *	1 Pot/120g	84	0.1	70	6.3	10.1	0.1	0.0
Timperley Rhubarb, TTD, Sainsbury's*	1 Pot/150g	168	7.4	112	3.4	13.6	4.9	0.4
Toffee & Apple, Low Fat, Co-Op*	1 Pot/125g	150	1.2	120	6.0	22.0	1.0	0.1
Toffee & Vanilla, Fat Free, Multipack, Weight Watchers*	1 Pot/120g	53	0.1	45	4.2	6.0	0.1	0.6
Toffee Popcorn, McEnnedy American Way, Lidl*	1 Pot/150g	174	5.6	116	4.0	16.0	3.7	0.0
Toffee, Benecol*	1 Pot/125g	124	0.9	99	3.8	19.3	0.7	0.0
Toffee, Chocolate Balls, Goodies, Mullerlight, Muller*	1 Pot/107g	96	2.6	90	4.0	12.0	2.4	0.0
Toffee, Chocolate Hoops, Crunch Corner, Muller*	1 Pot/135g	209	7.8	155	4.2	20.8	5.8	0.2
Toffee, COU, M&S*	1 Pot/145g	65	0.3	45	4.2	7.7	0.2	0.0
Toffee, Fat Free, Brooklea, Aldi*	1 Pot/80g	37	0.4	46	3.0	8.0	0.5	0.5
Toffee, Fat Free, Mullerlight, Muller*	1 Pot/175g	89	0.2	51	4.1	7.9	0.1	0.0
Toffee, Smooth & Creamy, Fat Free, Weight Watchers*	1 Pot/120g	48	0.1	40	3.9	5.9	0.1	0.8
Toffee, with Milk Chocolate Balls, Mullerlight, Muller*	1 Serving/100g	90	2.4	90	4.0	12.6	2.4	0.0
Total 0% Greek with Blueberries, Total, Fage*	1 Serving/150g	123	0.0	82	8.3	12.3	0.0	0.0
Tropical Crunch, Healthy Balance, Fruit Corner, Muller*	1 Pot/150g	170	3.2	113	4.7	18.2	2.1	0.5
Tropical Fruit, Bio, Granola, Corner, Muller*	1 Pot/135g	161	3.2	119	5.4	18.2	2.4	0.6
Tropical Fruit, HL, Tesco*	1 Pot/125g	56	0.2	45	4.1	6.6	0.2	0.9
Vanilla & Chocolate, Muller*	1 Pot/165g	86	0.8	52	4.0	7.2	0.5	0.1
Vanilla Choco Balls, Crunch Corner, Muller*	1 Pot/135g	201	7.4	149	4.1	20.2	5.5	0.2
Vanilla Flavour, Healthy Living, Light, Tesco*	1 Pot/200g	90	0.2	45	4.1	7.0	0.1	0.0
Vanilla Flavour, Organic, Low Fat, Tesco*	1 Pot/125g	114	1.2	91	5.3	15.3	1.0	0.0
Vanilla Flavour, Weight Watchers*	1 Pot/120g	47	0.1	39	4.2	5.2	0.1	0.2
Vanilla Toffee, Low Fat, Sainsbury's*	1 Pot/125g	145	2.2	116	4.3	20.6	1.8	0.0
Vanilla with Dark Chocolate Flakes, Light, Brooklea*	1 Pot/180g	104	1.8	58	4.9	7.0	1.0	0.5
Vanilla, & Chocolate Sprinkles, Fat Free, Milbona, Lidl*	1 Pot/175g	93	0.9	53	3.9	7.6	0.5	0.1
Vanilla, Average	*1 Serving/120g*	*100*	*5.4*	*83*	*4.5*	*12.4*	*4.5*	*0.8*
Vanilla, BGTY, Sainsbury's*	1 Pot/200g	98	0.2	49	4.5	7.5	0.1	0.0
Vanilla, Bio Live, Wicked, Wholemilk, Rachel's Organic*	1 Pot/125g	125	4.4	100	5.2	12.1	3.5	0.0
Vanilla, Bio, Fat Free, Snackpot, Activia, Danone*	1 Pot/165g	87	0.2	53	5.0	8.1	0.1	0.9
Vanilla, Brooklea*	1 Pot/180g	135	0.4	75	4.8	13.4	0.2	0.0
Vanilla, Chocolate, & Black Cherry, Mullerlight, Muller*	1 Pot/175g	103	0.7	59	3.1	10.3	0.4	0.3
Vanilla, Low Fat, Probiotic, Organic, M&S*	1 Serving/100g	85	1.8	85	6.2	10.9	1.8	0.0
Vanilla, Low Fat, Tesco*	1 Pot/125g	125	2.1	100	4.9	16.3	1.7	0.0

	Measure INFO/WEIGHT	per Measure KCAL	FAT	Nutrition Values per 100g / 100ml KCAL	PROT	CARB	FAT	FIBRE
YOGHURT								
Vanilla, Madagascan, 0.06% Fat, TTD, Sainsbury's*	1 Pot/150g	210	9.0	140	3.7	17.8	6.0	0.0
Vanilla, Madagascan, Deluxe, Lidl*	1 Pot/150g	212	10.2	141	2.7	17.0	6.8	0.5
Vanilla, Madagascan, Indulgent, Dessert, Waitrose*	1 Pot/150g	240	11.4	160	3.7	19.2	7.6	0.0
Vanilla, Organic, Probiotic, Fat Free, Yeo Valley*	1 Pot/500g	400	0.5	80	5.4	14.2	0.1	0.0
Vanilla, Proviact, Milbona, Lidl*	1 Pot/150g	154	4.2	103	4.0	14.6	2.8	0.0
Vanilla, Smooth, Light, Fat Free, Muller*	1 Pot/175g	88	0.2	50	4.3	7.2	0.1	0.0
Vanilla, Thick & Creamy, Channel Island, M&S*	1 Pot/150g	188	6.6	125	4.5	17.5	4.4	1.0
Vanilla, Thick & Creamy, Probiotic, COU, M&S*	1 Pot/170g	76	0.2	45	4.2	6.9	0.1	0.6
Vanilla, Virtually Fat Free, Yeo Valley*	1 Pot/150g	122	0.2	81	5.1	15.0	0.1	0.0
Velvety Vanilla, Intensely Creamy, Activia, Danone*	1 Pot/120g	116	3.6	97	4.8	12.7	3.0	0.1
Wild Berry, Oatie Breakfast, Moma Foods*	1 Pot/235g	317	4.2	135	4.3	25.6	1.8	2.7
Wild Blueberry, Finest, Tesco*	1 Pot/150g	212	10.2	141	3.4	16.6	6.8	0.5
Wild Blueberry, Light, Fat Free, Muller*	1 Pot/175g	82	0.2	47	4.1	6.9	0.1	0.7
with Black Cherry Compote, Greek Style, M&S*	1 Pot/241g	205	3.4	85	3.4	15.0	1.4	0.5
with Golden Honey, Greek Style, Activia, Danone*	1 Pot/126g	122	3.5	97	5.0	13.0	2.8	0.1
with Reduced Sugar Rhubarb Jam, Bonne Maman*	1 Pot/125g	141	4.8	113	2.4	16.8	3.8	0.4
Yellow Fruit, Yoplait*	1 Pot/125g	139	3.6	111	3.3	18.0	2.9	0.0
Zesty Lemon, Intensely Creamy, Activia, Danone*	1 Pot/110g	110	3.3	100	4.8	13.3	3.0	0.1
YOGHURT DRINK								
Average	*1fl oz/30ml*	*19*	*0.0*	*62*	*3.1*	*13.1*	*0.0*	*0.0*
Ayran, Gazi*	1 Can/330ml	34	1.9	10	0.5	0.8	0.6	0.0
Cholesterol Lowering, Asda*	1 Bottle/100g	76	1.4	76	2.9	13.0	1.4	1.0
Fruit, Mixed, Actimel, Danone*	1 Bottle/100ml	88	1.5	88	2.7	16.0	1.5	0.0
Light, Benecol*	1 Bottle/68g	40	1.4	60	2.8	7.3	2.1	0.1
Light, Yakult*	1 Bottle/65ml	27	0.0	42	1.4	10.2	0.0	1.8
Multi Fruit, Actimel, Danone*	1 Bottle/100g	85	1.5	85	2.7	14.4	1.5	0.1
Orange, Actimel, Danone*	1 Bottle/100g	74	1.5	74	2.9	11.5	1.5	0.0
Orange, Pro Activ, Cholesterol, Flora*	1 Bottle/100g	45	1.5	45	3.2	5.6	1.5	1.1
Orange, Probiotic, Lidl*	1 Serving/125ml	105	2.0	84	2.5	14.7	1.6	0.0
Original, 0.1% Fat, Actimel, Danone*	1 Bottle/100g	28	0.1	28	2.8	3.3	0.1	1.9
Original, Actimel, Danone*	1 Bottle/100g	80	1.6	80	2.8	12.8	1.6	0.0
Original, Benecol*	1 Serving/70g	62	1.6	88	2.6	14.2	2.3	0.0
Original, Pro Activ, Cholesterol, Flora*	1 Bottle/100g	45	1.5	45	2.6	4.8	1.5	1.1
Original, Probiotic, Tesco*	1 Bottle/100g	68	1.0	68	1.7	13.1	1.0	1.4
Peach & Apricot, Benecol*	1 Bottle/68g	38	1.5	56	2.8	6.2	2.2	0.0
Peach & Mango, Actimel, Danone*	1 Bottle/100g	28	0.1	28	2.7	3.1	0.1	0.4
Pomeganate & Raspberry Pro Active, Mini Drink, Flora*	1 Serving/100g	45	1.5	45	2.6	4.7	1.5	1.1
Strawberry, Actimel, Danone*	1 Bottle/100g	74	1.5	74	2.9	11.5	1.5	0.0
Strawberry, Benecol*	1 Bottle/68g	38	1.4	56	3.2	6.2	2.0	0.0
Strawberry, Low Fat, Pre & Probiotic, Muller*	1 Pot/100g	67	1.4	67	2.5	10.7	1.4	2.4
Strawberry, Pro Activ, Cholesterol, Flora*	1 Bottle/100g	45	1.5	45	2.6	4.7	1.5	0.0
Strawberry, Yop, Yoplait*	1 Bottle/330g	261	4.3	79	2.8	14.0	1.3	0.0
Yakult*	1 Pot/65ml	43	0.1	66	1.3	14.7	0.1	0.0
YORKIE								
Original, Nestle*	1 Bar/55g	302	17.4	546	6.2	57.9	31.5	1.9
Peanut, Rowntree*	1 Bar/43g	248	16.5	576	10.8	45.4	38.3	3.1
Raisin & Biscuit, Nestle*	1 Bar/67g	338	16.9	508	5.3	61.9	25.4	1.7
YORKSHIRE PUDDING								
& Beef Dripping, M&S*	4 Puddings/100g	410	30.4	410	9.4	25.2	30.4	3.2
3", Baked, Aunt Bessie's*	1 Pudding/36g	91	2.8	252	9.0	36.4	7.9	1.7
4 Minute, Aunt Bessie's*	1 Pudding/18g	52	2.0	291	10.5	36.6	11.3	2.2
7", Baked, Aunt Bessie's*	1 Pudding/110g	290	9.9	264	8.5	37.4	9.0	2.0
Average	*1 Pudding/30g*	*62*	*3.0*	*208*	*6.6*	*24.7*	*9.9*	*0.9*

Y

INFO/WEIGHT	Measure	per Measure KCAL	FAT	Nutrition Values per 100g / 100ml KCAL	PROT	CARB	FAT	FIBRE
YORKSHIRE PUDDING								
Baked, Frozen, 4 Pack, Morrisons*	1 Pudding/34g	82	2.3	241	8.4	36.7	6.7	1.6
Batters, in Foils, Ready to Bake, Frozen, Aunt Bessie's*	1 Pudding/17g	47	1.8	276	9.1	32.6	10.8	1.4
Beef Dripping, Oven Baked, Asda*	1 Pudding/32g	87	3.4	268	9.3	33.0	10.4	2.6
Filled with Beef, Tesco*	1 Pudding/300g	408	15.6	136	6.1	16.2	5.2	1.1
Filled with Chicken & Vegetable, GFY, Asda*	1 Pack/380g	376	9.9	99	6.0	13.0	2.6	1.1
Frozen, Ovenbaked, Iceland*	1 Pudding/12g	36	1.0	290	9.7	45.1	7.9	4.1
Fully Prepared, M&S*	1 Pudding/22g	63	2.9	285	9.4	31.6	13.2	1.2
Giant VLH Kitchens	1 Serving/110g	284	9.1	259	8.5	33.6	10.0	2.3
Heat & Serve, Waitrose*	1 Pudding/30g	86	3.5	288	9.5	35.3	11.7	1.7
Home Bake, Rise in 20 Minutes, Baked, Aunt Bessie's*	1 Pudding/25g	43	1.7	174	6.0	20.0	7.0	3.1
Large, The Real Yorkshire Pudding Co*	1 Pudding/34g	103	4.1	304	11.5	37.3	12.1	2.5
Mini, Co-Op*	1 Serving/16g	50	2.0	312	6.2	43.8	12.5	2.5
Mini, Farmfoods*	1 Pudding/3g	8	0.2	281	9.6	43.2	7.7	1.9
Premium, Bisto*	1 Pudding/30g	74	3.3	248	7.3	30.3	10.9	2.1
Ready to Bake, Baked, Aunt Bessie's*	1 Pudding/17g	42	1.4	246	8.5	35.1	8.0	1.7
Ready to Bake, Sainsbury's*	1 Pudding/18g	48	1.6	263	9.9	35.9	8.9	1.3
Sage & Onion, Tesco*	1 Pudding/19g	53	2.3	280	8.0	35.0	12.0	2.6
Sainsbury's*	1 Pudding/14g	43	2.0	309	7.9	37.5	14.1	2.9
Steak & Red Wine, Filled, COU, M&S*	1 Pack/162g	211	3.6	130	12.4	15.6	2.2	1.8
The Best, Morrisons*	1 Pudding/22g	60	1.8	271	8.3	43.0	8.0	1.6
Traditional Style, Medium, Asda*	1 Pudding/36g	86	3.2	241	9.0	31.0	9.0	2.4
Traditional Style, Small, Asda*	1 Pudding/20g	52	2.0	262	8.0	35.0	10.0	2.9
Traditional, Giant, Asda*	1 Pudding/110g	310	11.0	282	10.0	38.0	10.0	2.3
Value, Tesco*	1 Pudding/16g	45	1.9	282	9.7	34.3	11.8	1.6
with Beef in Gravy, Asda*	1 Serving/290g	406	10.2	140	7.0	20.0	3.5	0.7
YULE LOG								
Chocolate, Sainsbury's*	1 Slice/35g	153	7.7	432	5.0	51.6	21.8	4.6
Christmas Range, Tesco*	1 Serving/30g	131	6.4	442	4.9	56.8	21.7	2.8
Mini, M&S*	1 Cake/36g	165	8.4	460	5.7	56.9	23.3	1.1

BURGER KING

	Measure INFO/WEIGHT	per Measure KCAL	FAT	Nutrition Values per 100g / 100ml KCAL	PROT	CARB	FAT	FIBRE
BACON								
Applewood, Burger King*	1 Serving/10g	44	3.0	442	38.0	5.0	30.0	1.0
BAGUETTE								
Chicken, BLT, Burger King*	1 Baguette/228g	578	26.0	254	10.1	27.2	11.4	1.8
Monterey Melt, Burger King*	1 Baguette/252g	687	38.0	273	13.9	19.4	15.1	1.6
BITES								
Cheese, Chilli, Burger King*	4 Bites/78g	238	13.3	305	9.0	32.2	17.0	30.7
BROWNIES								
Chocolate, Hottie, with Real Ice Cream, Burger King*	1 Serving/140g	449	36.0	321	4.5	31.9	25.7	1.1
BURGERS								
Angus, 3 Pepper, Burger King*	1 Burger/246g	684	41.0	278	15.0	17.9	16.7	1.2
Angus, Bacon, Smoked, & Cheese, Burger King*	1 Burger/281g	701	38.1	249	13.9	17.4	13.6	1.0
Angus, Bacon, Smoked, & Cheese, Double, Burger King*	1 Burger/367g	927	54.1	253	16.1	13.5	14.7	0.8
Angus, Classic, Burger King*	1 Burger/248g	579	28.8	234	12.5	19.2	11.6	1.0
Angus, Classic, Double, Burger King*	1 Burger/337g	819	45.7	243	15.4	14.4	13.6	0.8
Angus, Mini, Burger King*	1 Burger/97g	272	10.7	280	14.0	31.0	11.0	1.0
Angus, Mini, with Cheese, Burger King*	1 Burger/110g	321	15.4	292	15.0	27.0	14.0	1.0
Angus, Patty, Burger King*	1 Patty/83g	238	16.8	287	25.3	0.8	20.2	0.0
Bacon, Double Cheese, Burger King*	1 Burger/139g	376	17.9	271	15.0	24.2	12.9	1.2
Bacon, Double Cheese, XL, Burger King*	1 Burger/312g	890	52.9	285	18.3	14.5	17.0	0.8
Bean Burger, Veggie, Kids, Burger King*	1 Burger/184g	469	18.8	255	7.8	34.2	10.2	2.9
Beef, Angus, Smoky Blue, Burger King*	1 Burger/256g	650	39.0	254	13.3	16.8	15.2	0.8
Big King, Burger King*	1 Burger/232g	587	30.8	253	12.4	21.2	13.3	1.1
Big King, XL, Burger King*	1 Burger/338g	902	54.1	267	16.0	14.0	16.0	1.0
Cheeseburger, Bacon Double, Burger King*	1 Burger/138g	376	22.2	271	15.0	24.2	16.0	1.2
Cheeseburger, Bacon Double, Extra Lge, Burger King*	1 Burger/312g	890	52.9	285	18.3	14.5	17.0	0.8
Cheeseburger, Burger King*	1 Burger/119g	303	12.3	254	13.2	27.4	10.3	1.3
Cheeseburger, Double, Burger King*	1 Burger/161g	431	21.9	268	16.0	20.6	13.6	1.0
Cheeseburger, Kids, Burger King*	1 Burger/106g	301	12.2	285	14.7	30.8	11.5	1.4
Cheeseburger, Quarter Pound, Burger King*	1 Burger/242g	569	27.8	235	13.1	19.3	11.5	1.2
Cheeseburger, Supreme, Burger King*	1 Burger/147g	385	20.0	262	12.9	20.4	13.6	1.4
Chicken, Burger King*	1 Burger/131g	392	19.8	299	8.6	32.1	15.1	1.5
Chicken, Chargrilled, Mini, Burger King*	1 Burger/109g	214	3.3	196	15.0	28.0	3.0	1.0
Chicken, Kids, Burger King*	1 Burger/100g	282	10.8	282	9.4	37.0	10.8	1.8
Chicken, King, Burger King*	1 Burger/172g	465	23.7	270	10.0	26.5	13.8	1.3
Chicken, Piri Piri, Sandwich, Burger King*	1 Sandwich/196g	335	5.9	171	13.0	21.0	3.0	1.0
Chicken, Sweet Chilli, King, Burger King*	1 Burger/142g	411	19.8	289	8.0	32.9	13.9	1.5
Chicken, Tendercrisp, Burger King*	1 Burger/270g	639	31.6	237	11.3	20.7	11.7	1.3
Chicken Royale, Burger King*	1 Burger/209g	567	30.7	271	10.8	23.4	14.7	1.2
Chicken Royale, Sweet Chilli, Burger King*	1 Burger/209g	506	21.6	242	10.8	23.2	10.3	1.2
Chicken Royale, with Cheese, Burger King*	1 Burger/233g	647	37.2	278	11.6	21.4	16.0	1.1
Chicken Royale, with Cheese & Bacon, Burger King*	1 Burger/264g	759	45.9	288	13.0	19.4	17.4	1.0
Chicken Tendercrisp, with Cheese, Burger King*	1 Burger/287g	715	37.8	249	12.1	19.7	13.2	1.2
Hamburger, Burger King*	1 Burger/107g	263	9.0	245	12.6	30.1	8.4	1.5
Hamburger, Kids, Burger King*	1 Burger/94g	260	8.9	278	14.2	34.3	9.5	1.5
Hamburger, Patty, Burger King*	1 Patty/100g	289	20.7	289	25.6	0.0	20.7	0.0
King Fish, Burger King*	1 Burger/197g	502	28.0	254	8.8	22.4	14.2	1.4
Patty, Whopper, Burger King*	1 Patty/81g	229	17.1	283	23.3	0.0	21.1	0.0
Rodeo BBQ, Burger King*	1 Burger/125g	360	13.4	287	11.9	35.9	10.7	1.9
Rodeo BBQ, Double, Burger King*	1 Burger/168g	485	23.0	289	14.8	26.6	13.7	1.6
Sausage, Pork, Patty, Breakfast, Burger King*	1 Patty/48g	135	4.3	281	20.2	1.0	9.0	0.0
Steakhouse, Burger King*	1 Burger/283g	763	44.0	270	13.0	19.0	15.5	1.1
Steakhouse, Double, Burger King*	1 Burger/364g	993	61.1	273	15.3	14.8	16.8	0.9

INFO/WEIGHT	Measure	per Measure		Nutrition Values per 100g / 100ml				
		KCAL	FAT	KCAL	PROT	CARB	FAT	FIBRE

BURGER KING
BURGERS

Veggie Bean, Burger King*	1 Burger/247g	547	25.6	222	6.1	24.8	10.4	2.4
Whopper, Bacon & Cheese, Burger King*	1 Burger/318g	723	43.3	227	10.9	14.8	13.6	1.0
Whopper, Burger King*	1 Burger/280g	611	34.6	218	9.8	16.4	12.4	1.0
Whopper, Double, Burger King*	1 Burger/361g	840	51.7	233	12.8	12.7	14.3	0.8
Whopper, Junior, Burger King*	1 Burger/165g	335	16.2	203	8.4	20.4	9.8	1.2

BURGERS VEGETARIAN

Burger King*	1 Burger/222g	409	15.0	184	5.9	24.3	6.8	2.7

CHEESE

American, Slice, Lge, Burger King*	1 Slice/24g	81	6.5	336	18.8	3.8	27.1	0.4
American, Slice, Sm, Burger King*	1 Slice/12g	41	3.3	336	18.7	4.1	26.8	0.8
Bites, Chilli, Burger King*	3 Bites/60g	183	10.2	305	9.0	32.1	17.0	3.1
Edam, Slice, Burger King*	1 Slice/22g	68	5.1	311	25.9	0.0	23.2	0.0
Pepperjack, Slice, Burger King*	1 Slice/25g	84	6.9	342	19.9	2.4	28.0	0.0

CHICKEN

Bites, Burger King*	14 Bites/112g	317	15.0	283	16.1	25.0	13.4	0.9
Bites, Kids, Burger King*	1 Serving/56g	158	7.3	282	16.0	25.0	13.0	2.0
Fillet, Strips, Chargrilled, Burger King*	3 Strips/75g	95	2.2	127	25.0	0.1	3.0	0.1
Nuggets, with Dip, Burger King*	6 Nuggets/143g	331	17.5	233	12.1	18.0	12.3	0.8
Strips, Breaded, Burger King*	1 Portion/132g	342	16.0	259	21.2	18.2	12.1	0.0
Wings, Burger King*	1 Portion/85g	222	15.0	261	20.0	7.1	17.6	1.2

COFFEE

Black, Lge, Burger King*	1 Serving/284ml	6	0.0	2	0.0	0.0	0.0	0.0
Cappuccino, Lge, Burger King*	1 Serving/482ml	387	7.8	80	2.0	14.1	1.6	0.5
Cappuccino, Regular, Burger King*	1 Serving/371g	308	7.2	83	2.0	14.2	1.9	0.5
Latte, Regular, Burger King*	1 Serving/62g	82	3.1	132	10.0	15.0	5.0	0.0

COLA

Coca-Cola, Burger King*	1 Reg/400g	168	0.0	42	0.0	11.0	0.0	0.0
Coke, Diet, Burger King*	1 Reg/400g	1	0.0	0	0.0	0.0	0.0	0.0

DIP

Barbeque Sauce, Heinz, Pot, Burger King*	1 Pot/40g	48	0.0	120	0.1	28.0	0.1	0.1
Chocolate, Pot, Burger King*	1 Pot/20g	57	2.0	285	5.0	50.0	10.0	0.0
Mexican Salsa, Heinz, Pot, Burger King*	1 Pot/25g	22	0.0	88	0.1	20.0	0.1	0.1
Raspberry, Pot, Burger King*	1 Pot/20g	58	0.0	290	0.0	70.0	0.0	0.0
Sweet Chilli, Heinz, Pot, Burger King*	1 Pot/40g	96	0.0	240	0.0	60.0	0.0	0.0

DOUGHNUTS

Diddy, Burger King*	1 Serving/84g	256	8.0	305	6.0	48.8	9.5	1.2

DRESSING

Thousand Island, Burger King*	1 Sachet/40g	65	6.0	162	0.0	7.5	15.0	0.0

EGGS

Patty, Burger King*	1 Patty/100g	189	13.2	189	11.6	6.0	13.2	0.6

FANTA

Orange, Burger King*	1 Reg/400g	116	0.4	29	0.1	7.1	0.1	0.0

FLATBREAD

Lamb, Burger King*	1 Serving/330g	708	39.7	214	11.0	16.0	12.0	1.0

FRIES

Apple, Burger King*	1 Portion/60g	28	0.1	47	0.3	11.8	0.2	1.8
Lge, Burger King*	1 Serving/160g	395	17.8	247	3.2	32.5	11.1	2.3
Regular, Burger King*	1 Serving/112g	277	12.4	247	3.2	32.5	11.1	2.3
Sm, Burger King*	1 Serving/90g	222	10.0	247	3.2	32.6	11.1	2.3
Super, Burger King*	1 Serving/190g	469	21.1	247	3.2	32.5	11.1	2.3

HASH BROWNS

Regular, Burger King*	1 Regular/72g	276	19.2	383	3.3	30.7	26.7	3.3

BURGER KING

	Measure INFO/WEIGHT	per Measure KCAL	FAT	Nutrition Values per 100g / 100ml KCAL	PROT	CARB	FAT	FIBRE
HOT CHOCOLATE								
Burger King*	1 Serving/200ml	78	2.0	39	0.5	7.5	1.0	0.5
ICE CREAM								
Cone, Burger King*	1 Cone/78g	120	4.1	153	3.4	24.1	5.2	0.1
Kit Kat, Fusions, Burger King*	1 Fusion/160g	343	12.7	214	3.6	32.7	7.9	0.5
Oreo, Fusions, Burger King*	1 Serving/140g	264	10.2	188	3.4	28.1	7.3	0.5
MILK								
Semi Skimmed, Kids, Burger King*	1 Carton/258g	117	3.9	47	3.5	4.6	1.6	0.0
MILK SHAKE								
Chocolate, Lge, Burger King*	1 Serving/519g	626	12.0	121	2.8	21.9	2.3	0.2
Chocolate, Regular, Burger King*	1 Serving/401g	455	9.6	114	2.9	19.9	2.4	0.1
Strawberry, Lge, Burger King*	1 Lge/519g	583	11.5	112	2.8	20.1	2.2	0.0
Strawberry, Regular, Burger King*	1 Serving/401g	433	8.0	108	3.0	19.0	2.0	0.0
Vanilla, Lge, Burger King*	1 Shake/519g	519	3.1	100	3.1	16.0	0.6	0.0
Vanilla, Regular, Burger King*	1 Regular/371g	371	2.2	100	3.1	16.0	0.6	0.0
MUFFIN								
Blueberry Filled, Burger King*	1 Muffin/100g	430	24.0	430	5.4	48.3	24.0	0.8
Chocolate Filled, Burger King*	1 Muffin/100g	482	30.6	482	4.0	47.1	30.6	3.3
ONION RINGS								
Lge, Burger King*	1 Serving/180g	535	26.5	297	5.1	34.2	14.7	3.7
Regular, Burger King*	1 Serving/120g	356	17.6	297	5.1	34.2	14.7	3.7
Super, Burger King*	1 Serving/240g	713	35.3	297	5.1	34.2	14.7	3.7
ONIONS								
Burger King*	1 Serving/14g	5	0.0	36	1.4	7.9	0.0	1.4
Crispy, Burger King*	1 Serving/14g	81	6.2	580	5.7	40.0	44.3	4.3
PANCAKE								
& Maple Syrup, Mini, Burger King*	6 Pancakes/78g	268	10.1	346	3.7	53.0	13.1	1.3
PICKLE								
Burger King*	1 Serving/21g	0	0.0	2	0.0	0.0	0.0	0.0
PIE								
Apple, Burger King*	1 Pie/150g	330	13.5	220	2.0	33.0	9.0	1.0
Apple, Dutch, Burger King*	1 Pie/113g	339	13.9	300	1.7	46.0	12.3	0.8
POTATO WEDGES								
Burger King*	1 Portion/100g	147	3.0	147	2.0	21.0	3.0	3.0
SALAD								
Chicken, Warm & Crispy, Burger King*	1 Salad/218g	249	12.5	114	7.4	8.4	5.7	0.9
Garden, Burger King*	1 Serving/72g	14	0.4	19	0.8	3.0	0.6	1.2
SANDWICH								
Butty, Bacon, Egg & Cheese, with Ketchup, Burger King*	1 Butty/133g	333	14.0	250	11.4	27.9	10.5	1.6
Butty, Bacon, with Heinz Ketchup, Burger King*	1 Butty/76g	218	5.5	287	11.8	44.3	7.2	2.5
Butty, Bacon, with HP Sauce, Burger King*	1 Butty/77g	222	6.0	288	13.0	41.6	7.8	2.0
Butty, Big Beefy, with Heinz Ketchup, Burger King*	1 Butty/284g	677	35.9	238	13.9	16.8	12.6	1.0
Butty, Big Breakfast, Burger King*	1 Butty/301g	832	49.0	276	15.6	16.3	16.3	0.7
Butty, Breakfast in Bread, with Ketchup, Burger King*	1 Butty/184g	470	24.4	255	13.6	20.7	13.2	1.4
Butty, Egg & Cheese, with Heinz Ketchup, Burger King*	1 Butty/126g	300	11.8	238	9.9	29.0	9.4	1.7
Butty, Sausage, Egg & Cheese, Ketchup, Burger King*	1 Butty/174g	435	22.2	250	12.8	21.3	12.8	1.4
Butty, Sausage, with Heinz Ketchup, Burger King*	1 Butty/112g	300	12.3	268	12.7	30.1	11.0	1.9
Chicken, Burger King*	1 Sandwich/224g	659	39.0	294	11.2	23.6	17.4	1.3
Chicken, Flame Grilled, Burger King*	1 Sandwich/240g	284	7.0	118	9.6	13.8	2.9	0.0
Chicken, Royale, with Cheese, Burger King*	1 Sandwich/263g	660	39.0	251	11.8	17.5	14.8	1.9
SMOOTHIE								
Strawberry, Banana, Iced Fruit, Lge, Burger King*	1 Smoothie/459g	279	0.8	61	0.4	14.3	0.2	0.2
Strawberry, Banana, Iced Fruit, Regular, Burger King*	1 Smoothie/346g	208	0.6	60	0.4	14.2	0.2	0.2

	Measure INFO/WEIGHT	per Measure KCAL	FAT	Nutrition Values per 100g / 100ml KCAL	PROT	CARB	FAT	FIBRE

BURGER KING
SMOOTHIE

	Measure INFO/WEIGHT	KCAL	FAT	KCAL	PROT	CARB	FAT	FIBRE
Tropical Mango, Iced Fruit, Lge, Burger King*	1 Smoothie/459g	295	1.0	64	0.4	15.1	0.2	0.3
Tropical Mango, Iced Fruit, Regular, Burger King*	1 Smoothie/346g	221	0.7	64	0.4	15.0	0.2	0.3
SPRITE*								
Burger King*	1 Reg/400g	112	0.0	28	0.0	6.6	0.0	0.0
SUNDAE								
Caramel, Burger King*	1 Sundae/150g	252	8.5	168	2.7	27.6	5.7	0.0
Chocolate, Burger King*	1 Sundae/150g	237	6.7	158	2.8	27.7	4.5	0.3
Strawberry, Burger King*	1 Sundae/150g	223	6.5	149	7.1	25.8	4.3	0.1
TEA								
Regular, White, no Sugar, Burger King*	1 Reg/200ml	22	4.0	11	1.0	1.0	2.0	0.0
WAFFLES								
Belgian, Whipped Cream, & Choc Sauce, Burger King*	1 Serving/90g	364	19.3	405	4.3	47.7	21.4	1.7
Belgian, with Ice Cream, & Choc Sauce, Burger King*	1 Serving/135g	294	12.7	294	4.0	40.9	12.7	1.1
WRAP								
Chicken, BLT, Burger King*	1 Wrap/214g	384	17.4	179	10.5	16.2	8.1	1.0
Chicken, Sweet Chilli, Burger King*	1 Wrap/160g	298	6.9	186	14.4	22.1	4.3	1.3
Chicken, Sweet Chilli, King, Burger King*	1 Wrap/212g	356	13.8	168	8.8	18.6	6.5	1.0
Veggie, Burger King*	1 Wrap/244g	495	21.0	203	4.0	26.2	8.6	2.6

CAFFE NERO
BARS

	Measure INFO/WEIGHT	KCAL	FAT	KCAL	PROT	CARB	FAT	FIBRE
Granola, Organic, Caffe Nero*	1 Serving/64g	278	14.3	434	6.7	51.5	22.4	4.8
BISCUITS								
Amaretti, Caffe Nero*	1 Biscuit/10g	40	1.2	401	3.9	70.1	11.7	10.6
Biscotti, Almond, Organic, Caffe Nero*	1 Serving/37g	147	5.9	397	9.0	54.6	15.9	2.7
Biscotti, Chocolate, Organic, Caffe Nero*	1 Serving/37g	136	4.3	369	7.0	59.1	11.6	2.7
Double Chocolate, Caffe Nero*	1 Biscuit/25g	126	6.8	505	5.5	57.4	27.3	3.7
Rocco Reindeer, Christmas Special, Caffe Nero*	1 Biscuit/72g	338	13.8	469	5.1	68.4	19.2	1.2
Stem Ginger, Caffe Nero*	1 Pack/60g	264	8.4	438	4.9	72.3	14.0	1.6
BREAD								
Ciabatta, Roll, Caffe Nero*	1 Roll/70g	180	2.7	257	8.7	46.9	3.9	1.7
BREAKFAST CEREAL								
Porridge, Semi Skimmed, no Topping, Caffe Nero*	1 Serving/239g	234	6.7	98	4.8	13.9	2.8	1.5
Porridge, with Skimmed, no Topping, Caffe Nero*	1 Serving/239g	210	3.8	88	4.8	14.0	1.6	1.5
Porridge, with Soya, no Topping, Caffe Nero*	1 Serving/239g	232	7.7	97	4.9	12.1	3.2	2.0
BROWNIES								
Chocolate, Belgian, Caffe Nero*	1 Brownie/70g	324	20.1	463	4.6	44.8	28.7	2.5
Chocolate, Double, GF, Caffe Nero*	1 Brownie/75g	319	12.4	426	4.6	51.4	16.5	0.7
CAKE								
Bruno Bear, Milk & White Chocolate, Caffe Nero*	1 Bear/46g	250	15.8	544	7.1	53.1	34.3	1.9
Cappuccino, Caffe Nero*	1 Serving/120g	486	22.7	405	3.7	56.2	18.9	0.5
Carrot, & Raisin, Organic, Wrapped, Caffe Nero*	1 Serving/70g	290	17.5	414	4.5	43.4	25.0	3.9
Carrot, Caffe Nero*	1 Portion/103g	421	23.9	409	4.1	46.9	23.2	1.1
Carrot & Raisin, Wheat Free, Caffe Nero*	1 Portion/67g	292	17.4	436	3.7	45.9	25.9	2.8
Chocolate Crunch, Caffe Nero*	1 Serving/65g	308	16.5	473	6.2	54.3	25.3	4.2
Chocolate Fudge, Caffe Nero*	1 Serving/124g	500	25.3	403	5.8	49.1	20.4	2.9
Chocolate Fudge, Festive, Caffe Nero*	1 Portion/128g	547	27.5	427	6.0	52.4	21.5	3.3
Lemon Drizzle, Organic, Caffe Nero*	1 Serving/73g	247	9.9	338	3.3	50.5	13.6	0.5
Lemon Drizzle, Slice, Organic, Wrapped, Caffe Nero*	1 Pack/70g	248	11.1	354	4.2	48.5	15.9	0.8
Panettone, Classic, Mini, Caffe Nero*	1 Cake/100g	374	14.7	374	7.8	51.5	14.7	1.2
Panettone, Mini Chocolate, Caffe Nero*	1 Serving/100g	404	18.8	404	9.5	49.0	18.8	1.2
Raspberry & Vanilla Sponge, Caffe Nero*	1 Cake/85g	385	25.0	453	5.0	41.8	29.4	0.7
Red Velvet, Caffe Nero*	1 Slice/100g	414	19.9	414	4.2	54.7	19.9	0.9

CAFFE NERO

	Measure INFO/WEIGHT	per Measure KCAL	per Measure FAT	Nutrition Values per 100g / 100ml KCAL	PROT	CARB	FAT	FIBRE
CAKE								
Red Velvet, Caffe Nero*	1 Cake/100g	408	19.6	408	4.1	55.5	19.6	0.8
Rocky Road, Caffe Nero*	1 Portion/80g	371	18.7	464	4.5	57.8	23.4	3.5
CHEESECAKE								
Lemon, Sicilian, Caffe Nero*	1 Portion/108g	341	18.7	316	6.4	32.8	17.3	1.5
White & Dark Chocolate, Caffe Nero*	1 Portion/116g	420	23.3	362	6.1	38.1	20.1	2.0
CHOCOLATE								
Bar, Dark, 50% Cocoa, Caffe Nero*	1 Bar/40g	213	12.4	534	6.4	53.6	31.1	7.0
Bar, Milk, Caffe Nero*	1 Serving/40g	223	13.5	561	8.0	55.0	34.0	1.5
Bar, Milk, with Hazelnuts, Caffe Nero*	1 Serving/40g	229	15.2	572	8.0	49.5	38.0	1.8
Coins, Caffe Nero*	1 Portion/21g	109	5.7	517	5.6	61.6	26.8	2.5
Dark, Venezuelan Gold, Willies Cacao, Bar, Caffe Nero*	1 Portion/26g	139	9.3	535	9.0	40.8	35.6	0.0
Milk, of the Gods, Willies Cacao, Bar, Caffe Nero*	1 Portion/26g	146	9.9	560	9.0	46.0	38.0	0.1
White, El Blanco, Willies Cacao, Bar, Caffe Nero*	1 Portion/26g	159	11.9	612	8.6	41.3	45.7	0.1
COFFEE								
Cappuccino, Grande, Semi Skimmed, Caffe Nero*	1 Grande/263g	92	3.4	35	2.7	3.6	1.3	0.0
Cappuccino, Grande, Skimmed, Caffe Nero*	1 Grande/262g	68	0.5	26	2.7	3.7	0.2	0.0
Cappuccino, Grande, Soya, Caffe Nero*	1 Grande/258g	90	4.4	35	2.8	1.9	1.7	0.5
Cappuccino, Regular, Semi Skimmed, Caffe Nero*	1 Regular/142g	37	1.4	26	2.0	2.7	1.0	0.0
Cappuccino, Regular, Skimmed, Caffe Nero*	1 Regular/142g	27	0.3	19	2.0	2.7	0.2	0.0
Cappuccino, Regular, Soya, Caffe Nero*	1 Regular/138g	36	1.8	26	2.1	1.4	1.3	0.3
Caramelatte, Semi Skimmed, Caffe Nero*	1 Serving/422g	485	25.3	115	2.3	12.3	6.0	0.0
Latte, Grande, Semi Skimmed, Caffe Nero*	1 Grande/363g	138	5.1	38	2.9	3.9	1.4	0.0
Latte, Grande, Skimmed, Caffe Nero*	1 Grande/364g	102	1.1	28	2.9	4.0	0.3	0.0
Latte, Grande, Soya, Caffe Nero*	1 Grande/355g	135	6.4	38	3.1	2.1	1.8	1.8
Latte, Iced, Semi Skimmed, Caffe Nero*	1 Latte/397g	155	4.0	39	2.0	5.9	1.0	0.0
Latte, Iced, with SF Vanilla Syrup, Caffe Nero*	1 Latte/420g	84	0.8	20	1.9	3.3	0.2	0.0
Latte, Iced, with Vanilla Syrup, Caffe Nero*	1 Latte/418g	205	3.8	49	1.9	8.6	0.9	0.0
Latte, Regular, Semi Skimmed, Caffe Nero*	1 Regular/209g	69	2.5	33	2.5	3.4	1.2	0.0
Latte, Regular, Semi Skimmed, Shot of Syrup, Caffe Nero*	1 Regular/245g	191	2.4	78	2.1	15.2	1.0	0.0
Latte, Regular, Semi Skimmed, Shot SF Syrup, Caffe Nero*	1 Regular/247g	74	2.5	30	2.1	4.4	1.0	0.0
Latte, Regular, Skimmed, Caffe Nero*	1 Regular/212g	51	0.4	24	2.5	3.4	0.2	0.0
Latte, Regular, Soya, Caffe Nero*	1 Regular/212g	68	3.4	32	2.6	1.8	1.6	0.4
Latte, Spiced Orange, Grande, Caffe Nero*	1 Grande/446g	455	25.4	102	2.6	10.4	5.7	0.0
Latte, Spiced Orange, Regular, Caffe Nero*	1 Regular/297g	386	22.9	130	2.1	13.2	7.7	0.0
Latte, Winter Berry, Grande, Caffe Nero*	1 Grande/484g	557	25.2	115	2.4	14.8	5.2	0.0
Latte, Winter Berry, Regular, Caffe Nero*	1 Regular/337g	488	22.9	145	1.9	19.3	6.8	0.0
Mocha, Regular, no Cream, Semi Skim, Caffe Nero*	1 Regular/231g	150	3.2	65	2.8	10.3	1.4	0.8
Mocha, Regular, no Cream, Skimmed, Caffe Nero*	1 Serving/232g	132	1.2	57	2.8	10.3	0.5	0.8
Mocha, Regular, no Cream, Soya, Caffe Nero*	1 Regular/231g	148	3.9	64	2.9	8.8	1.7	1.1
Mocha, Regular, Whipped Cream, Semi Skim, Caffe Nero*	1 Regular/272g	302	19.3	111	2.7	9.2	7.1	0.6
Mocha, White Chocolate, Semi Skimmed, Caffe Nero*	1 Serving/402g	414	25.3	103	2.4	6.1	6.3	0.0
COFFEE BEANS								
Chocolate Coated, Caffe Nero*	1 Portion/25g	133	8.0	534	8.0	48.0	32.0	8.3
COOKIES								
Chocolate, Triple, Caffe Nero*	1 Cookie/71g	336	15.8	473	5.9	61.4	22.2	1.8
Chocolate Chip, Wrapped, Caffe Nero*	1 Cookie/60g	266	12.3	444	4.6	60.0	20.5	1.4
Chocolate Chunk, Milk, Caffe Nero*	1 Cookie/71g	344	17.3	485	5.6	59.7	24.4	2.1
Oat & Raisin, Caffe Nero*	1 Cookie/81g	332	11.4	410	4.9	64.3	14.1	3.1
Oat & Raisin, Wrapped, Caffe Nero*	1 Cookie/60g	241	10.4	401	4.8	57.0	17.3	2.8
CRISPS								
Cheddar & Spring Onion, Mature, Caffe Nero*	1 Pack/40g	202	11.4	507	6.1	54.0	28.6	4.4
Sea Salt, Caffe Nero*	1 Pack/40g	205	11.6	514	6.2	54.0	29.1	5.4

	Measure INFO/WEIGHT	per Measure KCAL	FAT	Nutrition Values per 100g / 100ml KCAL	PROT	CARB	FAT	FIBRE

CAFFE NERO

CRISPS

	Measure INFO/WEIGHT	KCAL	FAT	KCAL	PROT	CARB	FAT	FIBRE
Sea Salt & Balsamic Vinegar, Caffe Nero*	1 Pack/40g	199	11.0	496	6.3	54.0	27.5	3.8

CROISSANT

Almond, Caffe Nero*	1 Serving/83g	350	19.8	422	10.0	41.7	23.9	2.6
Apricot, Caffe Nero*	1 Serving/100g	260	11.2	258	5.6	34.0	11.1	1.6
Butter, Caffe Nero*	1 Serving/50g	204	11.6	408	8.5	40.9	23.3	1.7
Cheddar & Tomato, Caffe Nero*	1 Serving/97g	305	18.2	314	12.9	22.4	18.8	1.7
Cheese Twist, Caffe Nero*	1 Serving/76g	316	18.4	416	13.4	36.1	24.2	2.6
Chocolate Twist, Caffe Nero*	1 Serving/79g	320	15.4	405	7.7	49.7	19.5	1.6
Ham & Cheddar Cheese, Caffe Nero*	1 Croissant/112g	354	20.7	316	16.3	20.8	18.5	0.8
Pain au Chocolat, Caffe Nero*	1 Serving/65g	270	15.1	415	8.1	43.4	23.2	1.7
Pain au Raisin, Caffe Nero*	1 Serving/100g	320	13.9	320	5.7	42.5	13.9	1.8

CUPCAKES

Chocolate, Caffe Nero*	1 Serving/68g	311	19.1	457	3.1	48.7	28.1	0.5
Lemon, Caffe Nero*	1 Serving/72g	340	19.6	472	2.9	54.0	27.2	0.3
Raspberry, Caffe Nero*	1 Serving/67g	295	15.1	440	3.4	55.7	22.5	0.5

DANISH PASTRY

Maple Pecan, Caffe Nero*	1 Pastry/82g	312	25.0	381	5.2	42.3	30.5	2.1

DESSERT

Triple Chocolate Cup, Luxury, Caffe Nero*	1 Cup/105g	315	14.0	300	4.0	40.6	13.3	0.8

FLATBREAD

Mozzarella, & Chargrilled Vegetable, Caffe Nero*	1 Flatbread/134g	274	7.1	204	7.6	30.4	5.3	2.2
Mozzarella, Tomato & Pesto, Caffe Nero*	1 Flatbread/116g	306	11.8	265	9.2	33.2	10.2	1.9

FRUIT SALAD

Caffe Nero*	1 Portion/170g	78	0.2	46	0.5	9.9	0.1	1.5

GINGERBREAD

Man, Ginger Giovanni, Iced, Caffe Nero*	1 Man/27g	189	2.3	689	5.8	66.4	8.3	2.0

HOT CHOCOLATE

Luxury, no Cream, Regular, Caffe Nero*	1 Regular/269g	199	6.7	74	3.9	12.2	2.5	1.6
Luxury, with Cream, Regular, Caffe Nero*	1 Regular/309g	352	22.9	114	3.7	11.0	7.4	1.4
Milano, with Whipped Cream, Caffe Nero*	1 Serving/241g	424	22.6	176	3.5	19.3	9.4	2.0
Mint, Regular, Whipped Cream, Semi Skim, Caffe Nero*	1 Serving/250g	437	20.5	175	4.0	21.6	8.2	0.6
Regular, no Cream, Semi Skimmed, Caffe Nero*	1 Serving/235g	235	4.0	100	3.3	17.5	1.7	1.5
Regular, no Cream, Skimmed, Caffe Nero*	1 Serving/236g	217	1.9	92	3.3	17.6	0.8	1.5
Regular, no Cream, Soya, Caffe Nero*	1 Serving/234g	229	4.4	98	3.4	15.9	1.9	1.9
Regular, Whipped Cream, Semi Skimmed, Caffe Nero*	1 Serving/250g	352	18.2	141	3.1	15.3	7.3	1.3
Regular, with Whipped Cream, Caffe Nero*	1 Regular/275g	388	20.1	141	3.1	15.3	7.3	1.3

JUICE

Apple, Organic, Carton, Caffe Nero*	1 Carton/200g	94	0.0	47	0.5	11.2	0.0	0.0
Mango & Passionfruit, Booster, Caffe Nero*	1 Booster/629g	220	0.6	35	0.3	8.3	0.1	0.3
Orange, 100% Squeezed, Fresh, Caffe Nero*	1 Serving/250g	95	0.0	38	0.5	8.8	0.0	0.1
Orange, Lemon & Lime, Booster, Caffe Nero*	1 Serving/591g	207	0.6	35	0.5	7.6	0.1	0.9
Raspberry & Orange, Booster, Caffe Nero*	1 Booster/621g	236	0.6	38	0.2	9.4	0.1	0.3
Strawberry & Raspberry, Booster, Caffe Nero*	1 Serving/589g	206	1.8	35	0.4	7.5	0.3	1.6

LEMONADE

Iced, Italian, Caffe Nero*	1 Serving/619g	328	0.0	53	0.0	13.4	0.0	0.1

MARSHMALLOWS

for Hot Chocolate, Caffe Nero*	1 Portion/6g	20	0.0	340	3.0	81.4	0.2	0.5

MILK SHAKE

Frappe, Banana, Caffe Nero*	1 Frappe/420g	315	4.6	75	3.0	13.5	1.1	0.0
Frappe, Banana, Skimmed, Caffe Nero*	1 Frappe/418g	284	1.3	68	3.0	13.6	0.3	0.0
Frappe, Banana, with Cream & Sprinkles, Caffe Nero*	1 Frappe/347g	402	21.8	116	2.9	12.2	6.3	0.0
Frappe, Chocolate, Caffe Nero*	1 Frappe/345g	386	21.4	112	2.8	11.2	6.2	0.5

CAFFE NERO

	INFO/WEIGHT	KCAL	FAT	KCAL	PROT	CARB	FAT	FIBRE
MILK SHAKE								
Frappe, Coffee & Caramel, Creme, Caffe Nero*	1 Frappe/465g	367	22.3	79	1.9	6.4	4.8	0.0
Frappe, Double Chocolate, Cream, Sprinkles, Caffe Nero*	1 Frappe/345g	411	21.4	119	2.9	13.4	6.2	0.2
Frappe, Double Chocolate, Cream, Sprinkles, Caffe Nero*	1 Frappe/345g	386	21.4	112	2.8	11.2	6.2	0.5
Frappe, Double Chocolate, Skimmed, Caffe Nero*	1 Frappe/453g	290	1.4	64	2.9	12.3	0.3	0.5
Frappe, Latte, Caramel, Caffe Nero*	1 Frappe/428g	274	3.9	64	2.8	11.4	0.9	0.1
Frappe, Latte, Caramel, Cream, Sprinkles, Caffe Nero*	1 Frappe/345g	369	21.0	107	2.7	10.4	6.1	0.1
Frappe, Latte, Caramel, Semi Skimmed, Caffe Nero*	1 Frappe/428g	274	3.9	64	2.8	11.4	0.9	0.1
Frappe, Latte, Cream, & Sprinkles, Caffe Nero*	1 Frappe/344g	334	21.0	97	2.7	7.9	6.1	0.1
Frappe, Latte, Semi Skimmed, Caffe Nero*	1 Frappe/424g	225	3.8	53	2.8	8.5	0.9	0.1
Frappe, Latte, Skimmed, Caffe Nero*	1 Frappe/430g	198	0.9	46	2.8	8.6	0.2	0.1
Frappe, Latte, Soya, Caffe Nero*	1 Frappe/388g	101	5.0	26	2.2	1.5	1.3	0.4
Frappe, Mint, Caffe Nero*	1 Frappe/347g	399	21.9	115	2.9	12.0	6.3	0.0
Frappe, Mint, Semi Skimmed, Caffe Nero*	1 Frappe/419g	310	4.6	74	3.0	13.3	1.1	0.0
Frappe, Mint, Skimmed, Caffe Nero*	1 Frappe/419g	281	1.3	67	3.0	13.3	0.3	0.0
Frappe, Mocha Frappe Latte, Skimmed, Caffe Nero*	1 Frappe/453g	290	1.4	64	2.9	12.3	0.3	0.5
Frappe, Mocha Latte, Cream, & Sprinkles, Caffe Nero*	1 Frappe/345g	386	21.4	112	2.8	11.2	6.2	0.5
Frappe, Mocha Latte, Semi Skimmed, Caffe Nero*	1 Frappe/459g	317	4.5	70	2.9	12.3	1.0	0.5
Frappe, Raspberry & White Chocolate, Creme, Caffe Nero*	1 Frappe/443g	452	21.7	102	2.0	11.9	4.9	0.0
Frappe, Strawberry, Caffe Nero*	1 Frappe/416g	316	4.6	76	3.0	13.6	1.1	0.0
Frappe, Strawberry, Caffe Nero*	1 Frappe/419g	285	1.3	68	3.0	13.6	0.3	0.0
Frappe, Strawberry, Cream, & Sprinkles, Caffe Nero*	1 Frappe/347g	403	21.9	116	2.9	12.3	6.3	0.0
Frappe, Vanilla, Caffe Nero*	1 Frappe/420g	315	4.6	75	3.0	13.6	1.1	0.0
Frappe, Vanilla, Caffe Nero*	1 Frappe/416g	266	4.6	64	3.0	10.9	1.1	0.0
Frappe, Vanilla, Cream, & Sprinkles, Caffe Nero*	1 Frappe/347g	402	21.8	116	2.9	12.3	6.3	0.0
Frappe, Vanille, Skimmed, Caffe Nero*	1 Frappe/419g	285	1.3	68	3.0	13.6	0.3	0.0
Frappe Cream, Banana & Caramel, Caffe Nero*	1 Frappe/446g	460	22.3	103	2.0	11.7	5.0	0.0
Frappe Creme, Coconut & Chocolate, Caffe Nero*	1 Frappe/473g	516	25.1	109	2.2	13.2	5.3	0.4
Frappe Creme, Strawberry & Vanilla, Caffe Nero*	1 Frappe/446g	469	21.4	105	2.0	13.7	4.8	0.0
MINTS								
Peppermints, SF, Caffe Nero*	1 Serving/14g	35	0.1	249	0.6	97.0	0.8	0.0
MUFFIN								
Apple, & Pecan, Spiced, Caffe Nero*	1 Muffin/120g	522	31.1	435	5.2	44.2	25.9	1.8
Bacon, & Tomato Sauce, English, Caffe Nero*	1 Muffin/106g	277	7.5	261	13.4	34.8	7.1	2.2
Blueberry, Caffe Nero*	1 Muffin/120g	415	19.0	346	5.8	44.4	15.8	1.5
Blueberry, Reduced Fat, Caffe Nero*	1 Muffin/115g	351	11.0	305	5.6	47.3	9.6	3.3
Chocolate, Triple, Caffe Nero*	1 Muffin/120g	503	26.6	419	6.7	45.1	22.2	1.6
Cranberry & Orange, Reduced Fat, Caffe Nero*	1 Muffin/120g	322	9.8	269	4.5	44.3	8.2	3.1
Egg Mayo, with Cheese & Mustard, Caffe Nero*	1 Muffin/134g	314	12.2	234	11.3	25.9	9.1	1.7
Gingerbread Filled, Caffe Nero*	1 Muffin/120g	516	27.4	430	5.3	49.6	22.8	1.2
Ham, & Egg Mayo, with Cheese, English, Caffe Nero*	1 Muffin/134g	314	12.2	234	11.3	25.9	9.1	1.7
Lemon Poppyseed, Caffe Nero*	1 Muffin/120g	461	22.0	384	5.7	48.4	18.3	1.4
Raisin, Multiseed, Caffe Nero*	1 Muffin/120g	475	21.9	396	7.6	49.9	18.3	2.9
Raspberry & White Chocolate, Caffe Nero*	1 Muffin/120g	422	19.1	352	5.9	45.7	15.9	1.6
PANINI								
All Day Breakfast, Caffe Nero*	1 Panini/210g	480	19.8	228	10.8	24.3	9.4	1.4
Bacon, & Tomato Sauce, Breakfast, Caffe Nero*	1 Panini/105g	263	9.7	251	11.1	30.6	9.3	1.4
Brie, Bacon, & Caramelised Onion, Caffe Nero*	1 Panini/200g	624	24.2	312	12.8	37.3	12.1	1.6
Chicken, Bacon, & Arrabiata Sauce, Caffe Nero*	1 Panini/209g	422	11.1	202	13.1	24.5	5.3	2.2
Chicken, Pesto Genovese, Caffe Nero*	1 Panini/185g	424	16.9	229	14.1	22.1	9.1	1.3
Chicken Milanese, Caffe Nero*	1 Panini/249g	428	13.9	172	8.5	21.9	5.6	1.2
Chorizo, & Mozzarella, Spicy, Caffe Nero*	1 Panini/169g	461	18.1	273	12.9	30.7	10.7	1.3
Four Cheese, & Cranberry Chutney, Caffe Nero*	1 Panini/187g	544	22.6	291	11.6	33.3	12.1	1.3

	Measure INFO/WEIGHT	per Measure		Nutrition Values per 100g / 100ml				
		KCAL	FAT	KCAL	PROT	CARB	FAT	FIBRE

CAFFE NERO

PANINI

	Measure INFO/WEIGHT	KCAL	FAT	KCAL	PROT	CARB	FAT	FIBRE
Goats Cheese & Grilled Red Pepper, Caffe Nero*	1 Panini/174g	426	15.5	245	11.0	28.9	8.9	2.8
Ham, & Egg Mayo, Breakfast, Caffe Nero*	1 Panini/146g	326	16.4	223	10.8	19.9	11.2	1.2
Ham, & Mozzarella, Caffe Nero*	1 Panini/182g	447	15.9	245	14.2	27.0	8.7	1.1
Ham, Mozzarella, & Emmental, Tostati, Caffe Nero*	1 Panini/97g	225	8.1	232	13.9	24.9	8.3	1.2
Il Genovese, Caffe Nero*	1 Panini/185g	424	16.8	229	14.1	22.1	9.1	1.3
Meatball, & Mozzarella, Napoletana, Caffe Nero*	1 Panini/213g	511	23.8	240	11.7	22.6	11.2	1.2
Mozzarella, & Tomato, with Pesto, Caffe Nero*	1 Panini/191g	438	17.2	229	10.2	26.1	9.0	1.4
Mozzarella, Cheddar, & Tomato, Tostati, Caffe Nero*	1 Panini/92g	220	8.4	239	11.5	27.0	9.1	1.3
Mozzarella, Red Pepper, & Roast Tomato, Caffe Nero*	1 Panini/213g	432	19.4	203	8.5	21.0	9.1	1.5
Mushroom, Mozzarella & Cheddar, Caffe Nero*	1 Panini/195g	348	11.9	178	8.4	21.8	6.1	1.3
Mushroom, with Gorgonzola Cheese, Caffe Nero*	1 Panini/181g	377	17.4	208	7.0	23.4	9.6	1.5
Pepperoni, Mozzarella, & Tomato, Caffe Nero*	1 Panini/193g	472	23.4	244	11.1	22.1	12.1	1.1
Salami, & Grilled Peppers, Caffe Nero*	1 Panini/185g	451	23.5	244	8.3	23.2	12.7	1.6
Three Cheese, & Roasted Tomato, Tostati, Caffe Nero*	1 Panini/71g	170	8.4	240	11.8	21.5	11.8	1.1
Tuna, & Mozzarella, Melt, Caffe Nero*	1 Panini/187g	431	14.6	231	13.2	26.3	7.8	1.4
Turkey & Cranberry, Caffe Nero*	1 Panini/200g	383	6.2	192	11.7	28.7	3.1	1.2

PASTA

Bolognese, Beef, Oven Bake, Caffe Nero*	1 Portion/279g	521	25.1	187	9.9	15.8	9.0	1.8
Chicken Pesto, Oven Bake, Caffe Nero*	1 Portion/245g	524	29.6	214	9.1	16.5	12.1	1.6
Vegetable Arrabbiata, Caffe Nero*	1 Portion/319g	434	8.3	136	3.5	22.9	2.6	3.3

PIE

Lemon Meringue, Caffe Nero*	1 Serving/90g	299	12.1	332	3.8	49.1	13.4	1.3
Mince, Caffe Nero*	1 Pie/93g	361	12.2	388	3.1	63.4	13.1	2.3

POPCORN

Sea Salt, Propercorn, Caffe Nero*	1 Portion/20g	88	2.9	438	9.3	61.4	14.5	11.8
Sea Salt & Sweet Brown Sugar, Caffe Nero*	1 Portion/30g	129	4.7	431	6.5	64.4	15.8	9.9

RISOTTO

Mushroom & Spinach, Creamy, Caffe Nero*	1 Portion/342g	503	22.2	147	2.9	18.7	6.5	1.0

SALAD

Chicken with Caesar Dressing, Caffe Nero*	1 Serving/170g	156	9.8	92	6.2	3.2	5.8	0.9
Falafel & Tabbouleh, Caffe Nero*	1 Salad/269g	390	16.7	145	4.2	16.7	6.2	3.1
Mozzarella, Cherry Tom, & Red Pesto Dressing, Caffe Nero*	1 Serving/178g	276	14.1	155	5.4	14.8	7.9	1.6

SANDWICH

BLT, Caffe Nero*	1 Sandwich/179g	442	21.1	247	10.2	23.7	11.8	2.2
Cheddar, & Pickle, Malted Wheatgrain Bread, Caffe Nero*	1 Sandwich/199g	434	18.5	218	9.7	23.0	9.3	2.0
Chicken, Salad, & pesto, Roll, GF, Caffe Nero*	1 Roll/154g	359	19.4	233	10.0	18.2	12.6	3.5
Chicken, Salad, Malted Wheatgrain Bread, Caffe Nero*	1 Sandwich/199g	309	5.8	155	9.9	21.5	2.9	1.8
Chicken, with Rosemary Mayonnaise, Caffe Nero*	1 Pack/199g	309	5.8	155	9.9	21.5	2.9	1.8
Egg Mayonnaise, Free Range, Caffe Nero*	1 Serving/157g	323	13.7	205	9.4	21.2	8.7	2.5
Festive Selection, Caffe Nero*	1 Pack/164g	412	14.9	251	10.7	30.9	9.1	1.5
Ham, & Cheddar, Malted Wheatgrain Bread, Caffe Nero*	1 Sandwich/187g	454	19.2	243	14.8	22.0	10.3	1.7
Tuna Mayo, & Cucumber, Caffe Nero*	1 Sandwich/166g	258	4.7	155	10.5	21.0	2.8	2.0
Tuna Salad, Caffe Nero*	1 Serving/147g	268	5.3	182	11.7	25.8	3.6	1.8

SAUCE

Berry Compote, Topping, for Porridge, Caffe Nero*	1 Serving/40g	47	0.1	117	0.6	29.3	0.2	1.9
Maple, Topping, for Porridge, Caffe Nero*	1 Serving/40g	94	0.0	234	0.0	58.4	0.1	0.1

SCONE

Fruit, Sultana, Caffe Nero*	1 Scone/94g	287	10.1	305	6.4	46.1	10.7	1.2

SHORTBREAD

Bars, Crunchy, All Butter, Caffe Nero*	1 Bar/50g	264	14.2	526	5.4	62.3	28.2	0.6

SLICES

Caramel Shortcake, Caffe Nero*	1 Slice/65g	330	18.4	507	4.4	59.9	28.3	0.7

	Measure INFO/WEIGHT	per Measure KCAL	FAT	Nutrition Values per 100g / 100ml KCAL	PROT	CARB	FAT	FIBRE
CAFFE NERO								
SLICES								
Coconut & Raspberry, Gluten & Dairy Free, Caffe Nero*	1 Slice/63g	286	16.4	454	3.8	51.5	26.1	5.1
SOUP								
Carrot & Coriander, Caffe Nero*	1 Portion/300g	162	12.0	54	0.9	4.1	4.0	1.1
Potato & Leek, Low Fat, Caffe Nero*	1 Serving/300g	114	4.2	38	1.0	4.9	1.4	0.6
Tomato, Sundried, & Basil, Caffe Nero*	1 Portion/300g	192	12.9	64	1.4	4.8	4.3	0.5
SYRUP								
Vanilla, Caffe Nero*	1 Shot/36g	122	0.0	339	0.0	84.2	0.0	0.0
Vanilla, SF, Caffe Nero*	1 Shot/38g	5	0.0	13	0.0	10.2	0.0	0.0
TART								
Apple & Blackcurrant, Caffe Nero*	1 Serving/101g	279	12.9	276	2.9	37.4	12.8	2.2
Custard, Portuguese, Caffe Nero*	1 Serving/69g	184	6.5	266	3.9	41.5	9.4	2.4
Lemon, Caffe Nero*	1 Tart76g	331	19.3	433	3.8	47.3	25.2	0.9
TEA								
Chai Latte, Semi Skimmed, Caffe Nero*	1 Serving/401g	281	10.0	70	3.8	8.6	2.5	0.1
Chai Latte, Skimmed, Caffe Nero*	1 Serving/405g	239	5.3	59	3.8	8.4	1.3	0.0
WAFFLES								
Caramel, Caffe Nero*	1 Pack/78g	356	16.4	457	3.5	63.0	21.0	1.0
WRAP								
Chicken, Fajita, Caffe Nero*	1 Wrap/205g	418	13.9	204	10.0	24.9	6.8	1.9
Chicken Caesar, Caffe Nero*	1 Serving/165g	434	22.8	263	12.8	21.9	13.8	0.8
Houmous, & Falafel, Caffe Nero*	1 Wrap/217g	455	14.1	210	5.9	29.9	6.5	4.0
YOGHURT								
Berry & Granola, Caffe Nero*	1 Pot/160g	223	6.8	140	5.9	18.6	4.3	1.1
Blackcurrant, Greek Style, Bio, Caffe Nero*	1 Yoghurt/150g	224	12.6	149	4.8	14.2	8.4	0.2
Blueberry, Greek Style, Brunch Pot, Caffe Nero*	1 Serving/130g	198	6.1	152	6.2	20.8	4.7	1.2
Blueberry Bircher Muesli, Greek Style, Half Fat, Caffe Nero*	1 Yoghurt/180g	236	5.2	131	4.8	20.6	2.9	1.6
Honey, Greek Style, Bio, Caffe Nero*	1 Yoghurt/150g	227	12.9	151	4.9	14.2	8.6	0.1
COSTA								
BARS								
Fruit, Seed, Nut & Honey, Costa*	1 Serving/75g	317	15.2	423	7.5	52.5	20.3	0.0
Granola, Traybake, Costa*	1 Bar/75g	312	14.7	416	7.1	48.3	19.6	0.0
BISCUITS								
Biscotti, Almond, Costa*	1 Pack/17g	77	3.0	452	11.8	60.4	17.5	1.0
Bourbon, The Ultimate, Costa*	1 Biscuit/85g	427	22.8	502	6.0	57.3	26.8	3.7
Custard Cream, The Ultimate, Costa*	1 Biscuit/85g	410	18.2	482	4.4	67.2	21.4	1.4
Fruit & Oat, Costa*	1 Biscuit/30g	139	5.5	464	4.9	69.2	18.2	2.0
Gingerbread, Under the Sea, Costa*	1 Serving/61g	250	5.0	410	5.9	76.7	8.2	0.0
Gingerbread George, Costa*	1 Biscuit/55g	234	5.7	425	5.9	77.8	10.4	0.0
Jammy, The Ultimate, Costa*	1 Biscuit/65g	309	14.6	475	4.7	61.5	22.5	2.3
Linzer, Raspberry, Costa*	1 Serving/65g	308	14.8	474	4.1	63.1	22.8	0.0
Raisin, Cranberry, & Hazelnut, Costa*	1 Serving/23g	84	4.2	364	2.7	47.5	18.2	0.0
Stem Ginger, Costa*	1 Serving/30g	142	5.7	471	5.3	68.8	18.9	0.0
BREAD								
Loaf, Breakfast, Banana & Pecan, Costa*	1 Loaf/98g	394	18.8	402	5.7	50.2	19.2	0.0
Loaf, Breakfast, Costa*	1 Cake/128g	443	18.6	346	5.0	48.9	14.5	0.0
BREAKFAST								
Bacon Roll, Costa*	1 Pack/120g	377	15.6	315	17.0	33.0	13.0	1.7
Bloomer, All Day, Costa*	1 Bloomer/194g	564	22.9	291	24.1	21.3	11.8	0.0
Egg & Mushroom Roll, Costa*	1 Pack/155g	354	12.3	228	8.4	30.9	7.9	1.8
Teacake, Toasted, Costa*	1 Teacake/107g	312	5.0	292	6.1	55.0	4.7	0.0
BREAKFAST CEREAL								
Porridge, Costa*	1 Pack/80g	299	5.7	374	10.3	62.7	7.1	0.0

COSTA

	Measure INFO/WEIGHT	per Measure KCAL	FAT	Nutrition Values per 100g / 100ml KCAL	PROT	CARB	FAT	FIBRE
BROWNIES								
Belgian Chocolate, Costa*	1 Portion/85g	373	19.5	439	5.0	52.3	23.0	0.0
Bites, Costa*	1 Serving/72g	342	22.1	475	5.4	44.3	30.7	0.0
Double Chocolate, Costa*	1 Brownie/80g	372	21.0	465	5.3	51.6	26.3	0.0
GF, Costa*	1 Bar/80g	418	28.3	523	7.5	42.3	35.4	3.9
Raspberry, Mini, Bites, Costa*	1 Bite/30g	140	8.2	465	4.8	49.9	27.1	0.0
CAKE								
Belgian Chocolate, Jaffa, Costa*	1 Cake/100g	351	18.6	351	4.0	40.9	18.6	0.0
Blackcurrant & Apple, Almond, Costa*	1 Cake/30g	126	7.5	418	7.7	40.5	24.8	0.0
Caramel Crisp, Traybake, Costa*	1 Cake/75g	383	22.5	511	5.3	54.1	30.0	0.0
Carrot, Costa*	1 Slice/153g	593	26.1	388	4.6	52.8	17.1	0.0
Chocolate, Christmas, Costa*	1 Serving/162g	616	25.8	380	4.9	53.0	15.9	2.5
Chocolate, Costa*	1 Slice/150g	575	23.6	383	4.8	76.7	15.7	0.0
Chocolate, Orange, Window, Costa*	1 Cake/100g	291	10.9	291	2.8	44.6	10.9	1.7
Chocolate Mint, Fancy, Costa*	1 Cake/80g	365	20.6	456	6.1	49.8	25.7	0.0
Christmas, GF, Costa*	1 Portion/98g	403	12.0	411	3.9	70.3	12.2	1.2
Coffee & Walnut, Costa*	1 Slice/135g	637	37.7	472	4.9	50.3	27.9	0.0
Eton Mess, Very Berry, Slice, Costa*	1 Slice/70g	321	17.3	459	5.0	53.1	24.8	0.0
Fruit, GF, Costa*	1 Pack/65g	254	10.2	390	4.0	56.6	15.7	3.1
Lemon, Costa*	1 Slice/144g	576	25.4	399	3.6	56.0	17.6	0.0
Lemon & Coconut, Slice, Traybake, Costa*	1 Serving/85g	381	22.0	448	5.8	48.0	25.9	0.0
Lemon & Raspberry, Mini, Costa*	1 Cake/132g	497	19.5	377	3.2	57.1	14.8	0.0
Lemon Drizzle, Costa*	1 Serving/100g	374	20.7	374	4.9	41.4	20.7	1.2
Morello Cherry & Vanilla, Costa*	1 Cake/128g	504	22.6	394	3.5	54.8	17.7	0.0
Raspberry & Almond, Traybake, Costa*	1 Cake/95g	445	29.6	469	8.2	34.8	31.2	0.0
Raspberry & White Chocolate Chip, Fancy, Costa*	1 Cake/80g	373	20.1	466	4.8	54.8	25.1	0.0
Teacake, Belgian Chocolate, Mallow, Costa*	1 Cake/90g	399	18.6	443	5.2	58.2	20.7	1.4
Tiffin, Chocolate, Triangle, Traybake, Costa*	1 Serving/112g	460	34.5	411	4.9	51.8	30.8	0.0
Victoria Sandwich, Costa*	1 Slice/136g	546	25.6	401	3.5	54.0	18.8	0.0
Victoria Sponge, Mini, Costa*	1 Serving/100g	483	20.0	483	3.9	71.8	20.0	0.0
Viennese Finger, Mini, Costa*	1 Cake/28g	147	6.0	530	4.9	55.3	21.8	0.0
CHAI								
Powder, Costa*	1 Serving/13g	50	0.0	386	0.8	94.6	0.3	0.0
CHOCOLATE								
Belgian, Blossoms, Costa*	1 Serving/2g	10	0.6	518	5.0	51.9	30.3	0.0
Belgian, Dark, Coveture, Costa*	1 Serving/50g	279	19.7	557	6.0	39.8	39.4	0.0
Belgian, Lattice, Costa*	1 Serving/6g	32	2.0	533	5.0	50.2	32.7	0.0
Dusting, Costa*	1 Dusting/2g	8	0.1	391	5.5	74.8	5.7	0.0
Magic Dust, Powder, Costa*	1 Dusting/2g	8	0.1	385	2.9	88.3	3.0	0.0
CHOCOLATES								
Belgian, Pieces, Costa*	1 Serving/50g	278	19.5	555	6.0	39.8	38.9	0.0
Dark, Belgian, Stirrer, Costa*	1 Stirrer/10g	55	3.6	545	4.8	46.7	36.1	0.0
COFFEE								
Americano, Full Fat, Massimo, Costa*	1 Massimo/158ml	38	1.9	24	1.3	2.2	1.2	0.0
Americano, Full Fat, Medio, Costa*	1 Medio/93ml	25	1.2	27	1.5	2.5	1.3	0.0
Americano, Full Fat, Primo, Costa*	1 Primo/126mlml	24	1.1	19	1.1	1.7	0.9	0.0
Americano, Massimo, Iced, Costa*	1 Massimo/577ml	75	0.0	13	0.1	3.1	0.0	0.0
Americano, Medio, Iced, Costa*	1 Medio/475ml	57	0.0	12	0.1	2.8	0.0	0.0
Americano, no Added Milk, Massimo, Costa*	1 Massimo/120ml	12	0.1	10	0.8	1.6	0.1	0.0
Americano, no Added Milk, Medio, Costa*	1 Medio/125ml	10	0.4	8	0.5	1.1	0.3	0.0
Americano, no Added Milk, Primo, Costa*	1 Primo/166ml	10	0.3	6	0.4	0.8	0.2	0.0
Americano, Primo, Iced, Costa*	1 Primo/364ml	40	0.4	11	0.1	2.5	0.1	0.0
Americano, Skimmed, Medio, Costa*	1 Medio/94ml	17	0.3	18	1.6	2.6	0.3	0.0

COSTA
COFFEE

	INFO/WEIGHT	KCAL	FAT	KCAL	PROT	CARB	FAT	FIBRE
Americano, Skimmed, Primo, Costa*	1 Primo/123ml	16	0.4	13	1.4	2.3	0.3	0.0
Americano, Soya, Massimo, Costa*	1 Massimo/580ml	30	1.3	5	0.4	0.5	0.2	0.0
Americano, Soya, Medio, Costa*	1 Medio/373ml	21	0.9	6	0.4	0.5	0.2	0.0
Americano, Soya, Primo, Costa*	1 Primo/200ml	14	0.6	7	0.5	0.6	0.3	0.0
Babyccino, Chocolate, Full Fat, Solo, Costa*	1 Solo/65ml	85	2.4	130	3.8	20.1	3.6	0.0
Babyccino, Chocolate, Skimmed, Solo, Costa*	1 Solo/65ml	70	0.6	107	3.9	20.3	0.9	0.0
Babyccino, Chocolate, Soya, Solo, Costa*	1 Solo/66ml	75	1.5	114	3.8	18.7	2.3	0.0
Babyccino, Full Fat, Solo, Costa*	1 Solo/58ml	57	1.8	98	3.5	14.0	3.1	0.0
Babyccino, Soya, Solo, Costa*	1 Solo/59ml	47	1.0	80	3.5	12.5	1.7	0.0
Caffe Latte, Full Fat, Massimo, Costa*	1 Massimo/471ml	259	14.6	55	2.9	4.2	3.1	0.0
Caffe Latte, Full Fat, Medio, Costa*	1 Medio/365ml	201	11.3	55	2.9	4.1	3.1	0.0
Caffe Latte, Full Fat, Primo, Costa*	1 Primo/225ml	128	7.2	57	3.0	4.3	3.2	0.0
Caffe Latte, Skimmed, Massimo, Costa*	1 Massimo/470ml	141	0.5	30	3.0	4.4	0.1	0.0
Caffe Latte, Skimmed, Medio, Costa*	1 Medio/363ml	109	0.4	30	2.9	4.4	0.1	0.0
Caffe Latte, Skimmed, Primo, Costa*	1 Primo/226ml	70	0.2	31	3.0	4.5	0.1	0.0
Caffe Latte, Soya, Massimo, Costa*	1 Massimo/474ml	180	7.6	38	2.9	2.7	1.6	0.0
Caffe Latte, Soya, Medio, Costa*	1 Medio/368ml	140	5.9	38	2.9	2.7	1.6	0.0
Caffe Latte, Soya, Primo, Costa*	1 Primo/228ml	89	3.9	39	3.0	2.8	1.7	0.0
Cappuccino, Caramel, Full Fat, Massimo, Costa*	1 Massimo/474ml	308	13.7	65	3.0	7.0	2.9	0.0
Cappuccino, Caramel, Full Fat, Medio, Costa*	1 Medio/363ml	243	10.9	67	3.0	7.2	3.0	0.0
Cappuccino, Caramel, Full Fat, Primo, Costa*	1 Primo/239ml	158	6.9	66	3.0	7.3	2.9	0.0
Cappuccino, Caramel, Skimmed, Massimo, Costa*	1 Massimo/473ml	208	1.9	44	3.0	7.2	0.4	0.0
Cappuccino, Caramel, Skimmed, Medio, Costa*	1 Medio/362ml	163	1.4	45	3.1	7.4	0.4	0.0
Cappuccino, Caramel, Skimmed, Primo, Costa*	1 Primo/240ml	108	1.0	45	3.0	7.5	0.4	0.0
Cappuccino, Caramel, Soya, Massimo, Costa*	1 Massimo/473ml	241	8.0	51	3.0	5.7	1.7	0.0
Cappuccino, Caramel, Soya, Medio, Costa*	1 Medio/365ml	190	6.2	52	3.0	5.9	1.7	0.0
Cappuccino, Caramel, Soya, Primo, Costa*	1 Primo/240ml	125	4.1	52	3.0	6.1	1.7	0.0
Cappuccino, Full Fat, Massimo, Costa*	1 Massimo/408ml	204	11.0	50	2.6	4.1	2.7	0.0
Cappuccino, Full Fat, Massimo, Iced, Costa*	1 Massimo/536ml	150	4.3	28	0.8	4.4	0.8	0.0
Cappuccino, Full Fat, Medio, Costa*	1 Medio/313ml	163	8.8	52	2.6	4.3	2.8	0.0
Cappuccino, Full Fat, Medio, Iced, Costa*	1 Medio/410ml	119	3.7	29	0.9	4.4	0.9	0.0
Cappuccino, Full Fat, Primo, Costa*	1 Primo/208ml	106	5.6	51	2.6	4.4	2.7	0.0
Cappuccino, Full Fat, Primo, Iced, Costa*	1 Primo/304ml	85	2.7	28	0.9	4.2	0.9	0.0
Cappuccino, Skimmed, Massimo, Costa*	1 Massimo/407ml	118	0.8	29	2.6	4.3	0.2	0.0
Cappuccino, Skimmed, Massimo, Iced, Costa*	1 Massimo/532ml	117	0.5	22	0.9	4.5	0.1	0.0
Cappuccino, Skimmed, Medio, Costa*	1 Medio/313ml	94	0.6	30	2.7	4.5	0.2	0.0
Cappuccino, Skimmed, Medio, Iced, Costa*	1 Medio/413ml	91	0.4	22	0.9	4.4	0.1	0.0
Cappuccino, Skimmed, Primo, Costa*	1 Primo/210ml	63	0.4	30	2.6	4.6	0.2	0.0
Cappuccino, Skimmed, Primo, Iced, Costa*	1 Primo/305ml	64	0.3	21	0.9	4.2	0.1	0.0
Cappuccino, Soya, Massimo, Costa*	1 Massimo/408ml	147	6.1	36	2.5	2.9	1.5	0.0
Cappuccino, Soya, Massimo, Iced, Costa*	1 Massimo/533ml	128	2.7	24	0.8	4.1	0.5	0.0
Cappuccino, Soya, Medio, Costa*	1 Medio/307ml	117	4.6	38	2.6	3.0	1.5	0.0
Cappuccino, Soya, Medio, Iced, Costa*	1 Medio/417ml	100	2.1	24	0.9	4.0	0.5	0.0
Cappuccino, Soya, Primo, Costa*	1 Primo/280ml	77	3.1	37	2.6	3.2	1.5	0.0
Cappuccino, Soya, Primo, Iced, Costa*	1 Primo/296ml	71	1.5	24	0.9	3.8	0.5	0.0
Cooler, Full Fat, Massimo, Costa*	1 Massimo/522g	188	4.7	36	0.9	6.2	0.9	0.0
Cooler, Full Fat, Medio, Costa*	1 Medio/458ml	151	4.1	33	0.8	5.5	0.9	0.0
Cooler, Full Fat, Primo, Costa*	1 Primo/374ml	116	3.4	31	0.9	4.7	0.9	0.0
Cooler, Latte, Caramel, Full Fat, Massimo, Costa*	1 Massimo/562ml	326	5.6	58	1.2	10.9	1.0	0.0
Cooler, Latte, Caramel, Full Fat, Medio, Costa*	1 Medio/488ml	254	4.9	52	1.1	9.6	1.0	0.0
Cooler, Latte, Caramel, Full Fat, Primo, Costa*	1 Primo/400ml	184	4.0	46	1.1	8.2	1.0	0.0
Cooler, Latte, Caramel, Skimmed, Massimo, Costa*	1 Massimo/569ml	290	1.7	51	1.2	11.0	0.3	0.0

COSTA

COFFEE

	Measure INFO/WEIGHT	per Measure KCAL	FAT	Nutrition Values per 100g / 100ml KCAL	PROT	CARB	FAT	FIBRE
Cooler, Latte, Caramel, Skimmed, Medio, Costa*	1 Medio/496ml	223	1.0	45	1.2	9.7	0.2	0.0
Cooler, Latte, Caramel, Skimmed, Primo, Costa*	1 Primo/400ml	156	0.8	39	1.1	8.2	0.2	0.0
Cooler, Latte, Caramel, Soya, Massimo, Costa*	1 Massimo/570g	302	4.0	53	1.2	10.6	0.7	0.0
Cooler, Latte, Caramel, Soya, Medio, Costa*	1 Medio/485ml	233	2.9	48	1.1	9.3	0.6	0.0
Cooler, Latte, Caramel, Soya, Primo, Costa*	1 Primo/393ml	165	2.4	42	1.1	7.8	0.6	0.0
Cooler, Mocha, Full Fat, Massimo, Costa*	1 Massimo/585ml	392	7.6	67	1.0	12.5	1.3	0.0
Cooler, Mocha, Full Fat, Medio, Costa*	1 Medio/505ml	303	6.6	60	1.0	11.1	1.3	0.0
Cooler, Mocha, Full Fat, Primo, Costa*	1 Primo/409ml	217	5.3	53	1.0	9.4	1.3	0.0
Cooler, Mocha, Skimmed, Massimo, Costa*	1 Massimo/584ml	356	3.5	61	1.1	12.6	0.6	0.0
Cooler, Mocha, Skimmed, Medio, Costa*	1 Medio/504ml	272	2.5	54	1.0	11.1	0.5	0.0
Cooler, Mocha, Skimmed, Primo, Costa*	1 Primo/411ml	189	1.4	46	1.0	9.4	0.3	0.0
Cooler, Mocha, Soya, Massimo, Costa*	1 Massimo/584ml	368	5.8	63	1.0	12.2	1.0	0.0
Cooler, Mocha, Soya, Medio, Costa*	1 Medio/504ml	282	4.5	56	1.0	10.7	0.9	0.0
Cooler, Mocha, Soya, Primo, Costa*	1 Primo/404ml	198	3.6	49	1.0	9.0	0.9	0.0
Cooler, Skimmed, Medio, Costa*	1 Medio/458ml	119	0.5	26	0.9	5.5	0.1	0.0
Cooler, Skimmed, Primo, Costa*	1 Primo/378ml	87	0.4	23	0.9	4.8	0.1	0.0
Cooler, Soya, Massimo, Costa*	1 Massimo/529ml	164	2.6	31	0.9	5.8	0.5	0.0
Cooler, Soya, Medio, Costa*	1 Medio/464ml	130	2.3	28	0.8	5.1	0.5	0.0
Cooler, Soya, Primo, Costa*	1 Primo/373ml	97	1.9	26	0.9	4.3	0.5	0.0
Cooler, Toffee, Full Fat, Medio, Creamy, Costa*	1 Medio/480ml	572	21.9	119	1.4	18.1	4.6	0.0
Cooler, Toffee, Skimmed, Medio, Creamy, Costa*	1 Medio/480ml	522	16.2	109	1.4	18.2	3.4	0.0
Cooler, Toffee, Skimmed, Primo, Creamy, Costa*	1 Primo/360ml	383	12.2	106	1.5	17.5	3.4	0.0
Cooler, Toffee, Soya, Medio, Creamy, Costa*	1 Medio/480ml	529	19.0	110	1.3	17.3	4.0	0.0
Cooler, Toffee, Soya, Primo, Creamy, Costa*	1 Primo/360ml	388	14.4	108	1.3	16.6	4.0	0.0
Cooler, Vanilla, Full Fat, Medio, Creamy, Costa*	1 Medio/480ml	316	6.0	66	1.2	12.5	1.2	0.0
Cooler, Vanilla, Full Fat, Primo, Creamy, Costa*	1 Primo/360ml	220	4.5	61	1.2	11.3	1.2	0.0
Cooler, Vanilla, Skimmed, Medio, Creamy, Costa*	1 Medio/480ml	266	0.2	55	1.2	12.6	0.0	0.0
Cooler, Vanilla, Soya, Medio, Creamy, Costa*	1 Medio/480ml	256	3.0	53	1.0	10.8	0.6	0.0
Cooler, Vanilla, Soya, Primo, Creamy, Costa*	1 Primo/360ml	188	2.3	52	1.1	10.5	0.6	0.0
Cortado, Full Fat, Solo, Costa*	1 Solo/144ml	82	4.5	57	2.9	4.2	3.1	0.0
Cortado, Full Fat, Solo, Iced, Costa*	1 Solo/192ml	75	3.5	39	1.5	4.4	1.8	0.0
Cortado, Skimmed, Solo, Costa*	1 Solo/145ml	45	0.1	31	3.0	4.5	0.1	0.0
Cortado, Skimmed, Solo, Iced, Costa*	1 Solo/192ml	46	0.2	24	1.6	4.3	0.1	0.0
Cortado, Soya, Solo, Costa*	1 Solo/146ml	57	2.5	39	2.9	2.8	1.7	0.0
Cortado, Soya, Solo, Iced, Costa*	1 Solo/187ml	56	1.7	30	1.5	3.7	0.9	0.0
Espresso, Doppio, Iced, Costa*	1 Doppio/138ml	40	0.1	29	0.3	6.8	0.1	0.0
Espresso, Ristretto, Doppio, Costa*	1 Doppio/60ml	6	0.2	10	0.7	1.3	0.3	0.0
Espresso, Ristretto, Solo, Costa*	1 Solo/30ml	3	0.1	10	0.7	1.3	0.3	0.0
Espresso, Ristretto, Solo, Iced, Costa*	1 Solo/90ml	19	0.1	21	0.2	5.0	0.1	0.0
Espresso, Solo, Iced, Costa*	1 Solo/100ml	20	0.1	20	0.2	4.6	0.1	0.0
Espresso Macchiato, Full Fat, Doppio, Iced, Costa*	1 Doppio/137ml	41	0.3	30	0.3	6.8	0.2	0.0
Espresso Macchiato, Full Fat, Solo, Iced, Costa*	1 Solo/100ml	21	0.2	21	0.3	4.6	0.2	0.0
Espresso Macchiato, Skimmed, Doppio, Iced, Costa*	1 Doppio/138ml	40	0.1	29	0.3	6.8	0.1	0.0
Espresso Macchiato, Skimmed, Solo, Iced, Costa*	1 Solo/100ml	20	0.1	20	0.3	4.6	0.1	0.0
Espresso Macchiato, Soya, Doppio, Iced, Costa*	1 Doppio/137ml	41	0.3	30	0.3	6.8	0.2	0.0
Espresso Macchiato, Soya, Solo, Iced, Costa*	1 Solo/105ml	21	0.1	20	0.3	4.6	0.1	0.0
Flat White, Full Fat, Primo, Costa*	1 Primo/255ml	148	8.2	58	3.0	4.3	3.2	0.0
Flat White, Skimmed, Primo, Costa*	1 Primo/258ml	80	0.3	31	3.1	4.6	0.1	0.0
Flat White, Soya, Primo, Costa*	1 Primo/257ml	103	4.4	40	3.0	2.8	1.7	0.0
Latte, Caramel, Ful Fat, Medio, Costa*	1 Medio/480ml	251	11.2	52	2.2	5.7	2.3	0.0
Latte, Caramel, Full Fat, Massimo, Costa*	1 Massimo/477ml	310	13.8	65	2.7	7.2	2.9	0.0
Latte, Caramel, Full Fat, Massimo, Iced, Costa*	1 Massimo/630ml	252	10.7	40	1.6	4.7	1.7	0.0

COSTA
COFFEE

INFO/WEIGHT	Measure INFO/WEIGHT	per Measure KCAL	FAT	Nutrition Values per 100g / 100ml KCAL	PROT	CARB	FAT	FIBRE
Latte, Caramel, Full Fat, Medio, Costa*	1 Medio/368ml	239	10.7	65	2.7	7.1	2.9	0.0
Latte, Caramel, Full Fat, Medio, Iced, Costa*	1 Medio/503ml	196	8.0	39	1.5	4.5	1.6	0.0
Latte, Caramel, Full Fat, Primo, Costa*	1 Primo/226ml	154	6.8	68	2.8	7.4	3.0	0.0
Latte, Caramel, Full Fat, Primo, Iced, Costa*	1 Primo/406ml	146	6.5	36	1.5	4.1	1.6	0.0
Latte, Caramel, SF, Full Fat, Massimo, Costa*	1 Massimo/600ml	263	14.4	44	2.2	3.6	2.4	0.0
Latte, Caramel, SF, Full Fat, Massimo, Iced, Costa*	1 Massimo/585ml	199	11.1	34	1.7	2.8	1.9	0.0
Latte, Caramel, SF, Full Fat, Medio, Costa*	1 Serving/480ml	205	11.2	43	2.2	3.5	2.3	0.0
Latte, Caramel, SF, Full Fat, Medio, Iced, Costa*	1 Medio/476ml	157	9.0	33	1.6	2.6	1.9	0.0
Latte, Caramel, SF, Full Fat, Primo, Iced, Costa*	1 Primo/200ml	26	1.4	13	0.6	1.0	0.7	0.0
Latte, Caramel, SF, Skimmed, Massimo, Costa*	1 Massimo/600ml	153	0.7	26	2.4	4.0	0.1	0.0
Latte, Caramel, SF, Skimmed, Massimo, Iced, Costa*	1 Massimo/606ml	103	0.6	17	1.7	2.7	0.1	0.0
Latte, Caramel, SF, Skimmed, Medio, Iced, Costa*	1 Medio/476ml	81	0.5	17	1.7	2.6	0.1	0.0
Latte, Caramel, SF, Skimmed, Primo, Costa*	1 Primo/360ml	88	0.3	24	2.4	3.8	0.1	0.0
Latte, Caramel, SF, Skimmed, Primo, Iced, Costa*	1 Primo365ml	62	0.4	17	1.7	2.5	0.1	0.0
Latte, Caramel, SF, Soya, Massimo, Costa*	1 Massimo/600ml	169	7.7	28	2.2	2.1	1.3	0.0
Latte, Caramel, SF, Soya, Massimo, Iced, Costa*	1 Massimo/200ml	46	2.0	23	1.7	2.0	1.0	0.0
Latte, Caramel, SF, Soya, Massimo, Iced, Costa*	1 Massimo/200ml	46	2.0	23	1.7	2.0	1.0	0.0
Latte, Caramel, SF, Soya, Medio, Costa*	1 Medio/480ml	127	5.8	26	2.0	2.0	1.2	0.0
Latte, Caramel, SF, Soya, Medio, Iced, Costa*	1 Medio/470ml	108	4.2	23	1.6	1.9	0.9	0.0
Latte, Caramel, SF, Soya, Primo, Costa*	1 Primo/360ml	95	4.4	26	2.0	1.9	1.2	0.0
Latte, Caramel, SF, Soya, Primo, Iced, Costa*	1 Primo/361ml	83	3.2	23	1.6	1.9	0.9	0.0
Latte, Caramel, Skimmed, Massimo, Costa*	1 Massimo/471ml	198	0.5	42	2.8	7.4	0.1	0.0
Latte, Caramel, Skimmed, Massimo, Iced, Costa*	1 Massimo/638ml	166	0.6	26	1.6	4.8	0.1	0.0
Latte, Caramel, Skimmed, Medio, Costa*	1 Medio/371ml	152	0.4	41	2.8	7.3	0.1	0.0
Latte, Caramel, Skimmed, Medio, Iced, Costa*	1 Medio/516ml	129	0.5	25	1.6	4.6	0.1	0.0
Latte, Caramel, Skimmed, Primo, Costa*	1 Primo/228ml	98	0.2	43	2.9	7.7	0.1	0.0
Latte, Caramel, Skimmed, Primo, Iced, Costa*	1 Primo/413ml	95	0.4	23	1.5	4.2	0.1	0.0
Latte, Caramel, Soya, Massimo, Costa*	1 Massimo/480ml	235	7.7	49	2.7	5.8	1.6	0.0
Latte, Caramel, Soya, Massimo, Iced, Costa*	1 Massimo/629ml	195	5.7	31	1.6	3.9	0.9	0.0
Latte, Caramel, Soya, Medio, Costa*	1 Medio/369ml	181	5.9	49	2.7	5.7	1.6	0.0
Latte, Caramel, Soya, Medio, Iced, Costa*	1 Medio/503ml	151	4.5	30	1.5	3.7	0.9	0.0
Latte, Caramel, Soya, Primo, Costa*	1 Primo/229ml	117	3.7	51	2.8	6.0	1.6	0.0
Latte, Caramel, Soya, Primo, Iced, Costa*	1 Primo/200ml	56	1.6	28	1.5	3.3	0.8	0.0
Latte, Cinnamon, Full Fat, Massimo, Costa*	1 Massimo/476ml	314	13.8	66	2.7	7.3	2.9	0.0
Latte, Cinnamon, Full Fat, Medio, Costa*	1 Medio/367ml	242	10.6	66	2.7	7.2	2.9	0.0
Latte, Cinnamon, Full Fat, Primo, Costa*	1 Primo/229ml	156	6.9	68	2.8	7.6	3.0	0.0
Latte, Cinnamon, Skimmed, Medio, Costa*	1 Medio/367ml	154	0.4	42	2.8	7.5	0.1	0.0
Latte, Cinnamon, Skimmed, Primo, Costa*	1 Primo/227ml	100	0.2	44	2.9	7.8	0.1	0.0
Latte, Cinnamon, Soya, Massimo, Costa*	1 Massimo/478ml	239	7.6	50	2.7	6.0	1.6	0.0
Latte, Cinnamon, Soya, Medio, Costa*	1 Medio/368ml	184	5.9	50	2.7	5.9	1.6	0.0
Latte, Cinnamon, Soya, Primo, Costa*	1 Primo/229ml	119	3.7	52	2.8	6.2	1.6	0.0
Latte, Full Fat, Massimo, Costa*	1 Massimo/600ml	240	10.5	40	1.6	4.5	1.8	0.0
Latte, Full Fat, Massimo, Iced, Costa*	1 Massimo/627ml	257	6.3	41	1.6	4.9	1.0	0.0
Latte, Full Fat, Medio, Iced, Costa*	1 Medio/515ml	201	8.2	39	1.5	4.7	1.6	0.0
Latte, Full Fat, Primo, Iced, Costa*	1 Primo/403ml	149	6.4	37	1.5	4.2	1.6	0.0
Latte, Gingerbread, Full Fat, Massimo, Costa*	1 Massimo/473ml	116	5.0	67	2.7	7.4	2.9	0.0
Latte, Gingerbread, Full Fat, Massimo, Iced, Costa*	1 Massimo/587ml	264	11.1	45	1.7	5.2	1.9	0.0
Latte, Gingerbread, Full Fat, Medio, Costa*	1 Serving/364ml	244	10.6	67	2.7	7.4	2.9	0.0
Latte, Gingerbread, Full Fat, Medio, Iced, Costa*	1 Medio/479ml	206	9.1	43	1.6	4.9	1.9	0.0
Latte, Gingerbread, Full Fat, Primo, Costa*	1 Serving/229ml	158	6.9	69	2.8	7.7	3.0	0.0
Latte, Gingerbread, Full Fat, Primo, Iced, Costa*	1 Primo/362ml	152	6.9	42	1.6	4.6	1.9	0.0
Latte, Gingerbread, SF, Full Fat, Massimo, Iced, Costa*	1 Massimo/582ml	198	11.1	34	1.7	2.7	1.9	0.0

COSTA
COFFEE

	Measure INFO/WEIGHT	per Measure KCAL	per Measure FAT	Nutrition Values per 100g / 100ml KCAL	PROT	CARB	FAT	FIBRE
Latte, Gingerbread, SF, Full Fat, Medio, Iced, Costa*	1 Medio/473ml	156	9.0	33	1.6	2.6	1.9	0.0
Latte, Gingerbread, SF, Full Fat, Primo, Iced, Costa*	1 Primo/364ml	120	6.9	33	1.6	2.6	1.9	0.0
Latte, Gingerbread, SF, Skimmed, Massimo, Iced, Costa*	1 Massimo/600ml	102	0.6	17	1.7	2.6	0.1	0.0
Latte, Gingerbread, SF, Skimmed, Medio, Iced, Costa*	1 Medio/471ml	80	0.5	17	1.7	2.6	0.1	0.0
Latte, Gingerbread, SF, Skimmed, Primo, Iced, Costa*	1 Primo/365ml	62	0.4	17	1.7	2.5	0.1	0.0
Latte, Gingerbread, SF, Soya, Massimo, Iced, Costa*	1 Massimo/591ml	136	5.9	23	1.7	2.0	1.0	0.0
Latte, Gingerbread, SF, Soya, Medio, Iced, Costa*	1 Medio/465ml	107	4.2	23	1.6	1.9	0.9	0.0
Latte, Gingerbread, SF, Soya, Primo, Iced, Costa*	1 Primo/357ml	82	3.2	23	1.6	1.9	0.9	0.0
Latte, Gingerbread, Skimmed, Massimo, Costa*	1 Massimo/474ml	204	0.5	43	2.8	7.7	0.1	0.0
Latte, Gingerbread, Skimmed, Massimo, Iced, Costa*	1 Massimo/596ml	167	0.6	28	1.7	5.2	0.1	0.0
Latte, Gingerbread, Skimmed, Medio, Costa*	1 Medoi/365ml	157	0.4	43	2.8	7.6	0.1	0.0
Latte, Gingerbread, Skimmed, Medio, Iced, Costa*	1 Medio/478ml	129	0.5	27	1.7	4.9	0.1	0.0
Latte, Gingerbread, Skimmed, Primo, Costa*	1 Primo/230ml	101	0.2	44	2.9	8.0	0.1	0.0
Latte, Gingerbread, Skimmed, Primo, Iced, Costa*	1 Primo/365ml	95	0.4	26	1.7	4.6	0.1	0.0
Latte, Gingerbread, Soya, Massimo, Costa*	1 Massimo/475ml	242	7.6	51	2.7	6.1	1.6	0.0
Latte, Gingerbread, Soya, Massimo, Iced, Costa*	1 Massimo/591ml	201	5.9	34	1.7	4.5	1.0	0.0
Latte, Gingerbread, Soya, Medio, Costa*	1 Medio/365ml	186	5.8	51	2.7	6.0	1.6	0.0
Latte, Gingerbread, Soya, Medio, Iced, Costa*	1 Medio/473ml	156	4.3	33	1.6	4.2	0.9	0.0
Latte, Gingerbread, Soya, Primo, Costa*	1 Primo/226ml	120	3.6	53	2.8	6.3	1.6	0.0
Latte, Gingerbread, Soya, Primo, Iced, Costa*	1 Primo/359ml	115	3.2	32	1.6	3.9	0.9	0.0
Latte, Roasted Hazelnut, Full Fat, Massimo, Costa*	1 Massimo/480ml	312	13.9	65	2.7	7.2	2.9	0.0
Latte, Roasted Hazelnut, Full Fat, Massimo, Iced, Costa*	1 Massimo/589ml	259	11.2	44	1.7	5.1	1.9	0.0
Latte, Roasted Hazelnut, Full Fat, Medio, Costa*	1 Medio/369ml	240	10.7	65	2.7	7.2	2.9	0.0
Latte, Roasted Hazelnut, Full Fat, Medio, Iced, Costa*	1 Medio/470ml	202	8.9	43	1.6	4.8	1.9	0.0
Latte, Roasted Hazelnut, Full Fat, Primo, Costa*	1 Primo/228ml	155	6.8	68	2.8	7.5	3.0	0.0
Latte, Roasted Hazelnut, Full Fat, Primo, Iced, Costa*	1 Primo/366ml	150	7.0	41	1.6	4.5	1.9	0.0
Latte, Roasted Hazelnut, Skimmed, Masimo, Iced, Costa*	1 Massimo/578ml	162	0.6	28	1.7	5.0	0.1	0.0
Latte, Roasted Hazelnut, Skimmed, Massimo, Costa*	1 Massimo/474ml	199	0.5	42	2.8	7.5	0.1	0.0
Latte, Roasted Hazelnut, Skimmed, Massimo, Iced, Costa*	1 Massimo/586ml	164	0.6	28	1.7	5.0	0.1	0.0
Latte, Roasted Hazelnut, Skimmed, Medio, Costa*	1 Medio/364ml	153	0.4	42	2.8	7.4	0.1	0.0
Latte, Roasted Hazelnut, Skimmed, Medio, Iced, Costa*	1 Medio/470ml	127	0.5	27	1.7	4.8	0.1	0.0
Latte, Roasted Hazelnut, Skimmed, Medio, Iced, Costa*	1 Medio/481ml	125	0.5	26	1.7	4.7	0.1	0.0
Latte, Roasted Hazelnut, Skimmed, Primo, Costa*	1 Primo/230ml	99	0.2	43	2.9	7.7	0.1	0.0
Latte, Roasted Hazelnut, Skimmed, Primo, Iced, Costa*	1 Primo/358ml	93	0.4	26	1.7	4.5	0.1	0.0
Latte, Roasted Hazelnut, Skimmed, Primo, Iced, Costa*	1 Primo/368ml	92	0.4	25	1.7	4.4	0.1	0.0
Latte, Roasted Hazelnut, Soya, Massimo, Costa*	1 Massimo/474ml	237	7.6	50	2.7	5.9	1.6	0.0
Latte, Roasted Hazelnut, Soya, Massimo, Iced, Costa*	1 Massimo/594ml	202	5.9	34	1.7	4.4	1.0	0.0
Latte, Roasted Hazelnut, Soya, Medio, Costa*	1 Medio/364ml	182	5.8	50	2.7	5.8	1.6	0.0
Latte, Roasted Hazelnut, Soya, Medio, Iced, Costa*	1 Medio/475ml	152	4.3	32	1.6	4.1	0.9	0.0
Latte, Roasted Hazelnut, Soya, Primo, Costa*	1 Primo/229ml	117	3.7	51	2.8	6.1	1.6	0.0
Latte, Roasted Hazelnut, Soya, Primo, Iced, Costa*	1 Primo/361ml	112	3.3	31	1.6	3.8	0.9	0.0
Latte, Skimmed, Massimo, Iced, Costa*	1 Massimo/637ml	172	0.6	27	1.6	5.1	0.1	0.0
Latte, Skimmed, Medio, Iced, Costa*	1 Medio/512ml	133	0.5	26	1.6	4.8	0.1	0.0
Latte, Skimmed, Primo, Iced, Costa*	1 Primo/408ml	98	0.4	24	1.5	4.4	0.1	0.0
Latte, Soya, Massimo, Iced, Costa*	1 Massimo/625ml	200	5.6	32	1.6	4.2	0.9	0.0
Latte, Soya, Medio, Iced, Costa*	1 Medio/503ml	156	4.5	31	1.5	4.0	0.9	0.0
Latte, Soya, Primo, Iced, Costa*	1 Primo/411ml	115	3.3	28	1.5	3.5	0.8	0.0
Latte, Vanilla, Full Fat, Massimo, Iced, Costa*	1 Massimo/591ml	260	11.2	44	1.7	5.1	1.9	0.0
Latte, Vanilla, Full Fat, Medio, Costa*	1 Medio/365ml	241	10.6	66	2.7	7.2	2.9	0.0
Latte, Vanilla, Full Fat, Medio, Iced, Costa*	1 Medio/472ml	203	9.0	43	1.6	4.8	1.9	0.0
Latte, Vanilla, Full Fat, Primo, Costa*	1 Primo/229ml	156	6.9	68	2.8	7.6	3.0	0.0
Latte, Vanilla, Full Fat, Primo, Iced, Costa*	1 Primo/368ml	151	7.0	41	1.6	4.5	1.9	0.0

	Measure	per Measure		Nutrition Values per 100g / 100ml				
INFO/WEIGHT		KCAL	FAT	KCAL	PROT	CARB	FAT	FIBRE

COSTA
COFFEE

	Measure	KCAL	FAT	KCAL	PROT	CARB	FAT	FIBRE
Latte, Vanilla, Skimmed, Massimo, Costa*	1 Massimo/479ml	201	0.5	42	2.8	7.5	0.1	0.0
Latte, Vanilla, Skimmed, Massimo, Iced, Costa*	1 Massimo/586ml	164	0.6	28	1.7	5.0	0.1	0.0
Latte, Vanilla, Skimmed, Medio, Costa*	1 Medio/367ml	154	0.4	42	2.8	7.5	0.1	0.0
Latte, Vanilla, Skimmed, Medio, Iced, Costa*	1 Medio/470ml	127	0.5	27	1.7	4.8	0.1	0.0
Latte, Vanilla, Skimmed, Primo, Costa*	1 Primo/225ml	99	0.2	44	2.9	7.8	0.1	0.0
Latte, Vanilla, Skimmed, Primo, Iced, Costa*	1 Primo/372ml	93	0.4	25	1.7	4.5	0.1	0.0
Latte, Vanilla, Soya, Massimo, Costa*	1 Massimo/476ml	238	7.6	50	2.7	6.0	1.6	0.0
Latte, Vanilla, Soya, Massimo, Iced, Costa*	1 Massimo/582ml	198	5.8	34	1.7	4.4	1.0	0.0
Latte, Vanilla, Soya, Medio, Costa*	1 Medio/366ml	183	5.9	50	2.7	5.9	1.6	0.0
Latte, Vanilla, Soya, Medio, Iced, Costa*	1 Medio/481ml	154	4.3	32	1.6	4.1	0.9	0.0
Latte, Vanilla, Soya, Primo, Costa*	1 Primo/227ml	118	3.6	52	2.8	6.2	1.6	0.0
Latte, Vanilla, Soya, Primo, Iced, Costa*	1 Primo/365ml	113	3.3	31	1.6	3.8	0.9	0.0
Light, Medio, Costa*	1 Medio/480ml	88	0.4	18	1.8	2.7	0.1	0.0
Light, Primo, Costa*	1 Primo/360ml	65	0.3	18	1.8	2.7	0.1	0.0
Macchiato, Full Fat, Solo, Costa*	1 Solo/71ml	12	0.6	17	1.0	1.9	0.9	0.0
Macchiato, Skimmed, Solo, Costa*	1 Solo/69ml	9	0.2	13	1.0	1.9	0.3	0.0
Macchiato, Soya, Solo, Costa*	1 Solo/71ml	10	0.4	14	1.0	1.6	0.6	0.0
Mocha, Full Fat, Massimo, Costa*	1 Massimo/473ml	435	15.1	92	3.1	12.2	3.2	0.0
Mocha, Full Fat, Massimo, Iced, Costa*	1 Massimo/569ml	347	11.4	61	1.6	9.0	2.0	0.0
Mocha, Full Fat, Medio, Costa*	1 Medio/346ml	301	11.1	87	3.0	10.9	3.2	0.0
Mocha, Full Fat, Medio, Iced, Costa*	1 Medio/456ml	269	9.1	59	1.6	8.7	2.0	0.0
Mocha, Full Fat, Primo, Costa*	1 Primo/230ml	198	7.4	86	3.0	11.0	3.2	0.0
Mocha, Full Fat, Primo, Iced, Costa*	1 Primo/328ml	190	6.6	58	1.6	8.2	2.0	0.0
Mocha, Italia, Espresso, Doppio, Costa*	1 Doppio/60ml	60	1.8	10	0.7	1.3	0.3	0.0
Mocha, Italia, Espresso, Solo, Costa*	1 Solo/30ml	3	0.1	10	0.7	1.3	0.3	0.0
Mocha, Skimmed, Massimo, Costa*	1 Massimo/470ml	348	5.2	74	3.1	12.4	1.1	0.0
Mocha, Skimmed, Massimo, Iced, Costa*	1 Massimo/600ml	272	2.8	45	1.6	8.6	0.5	0.0
Mocha, Skimmed, Massimo, Iced, Costa*	1 Massimo/569ml	279	4.0	49	1.6	9.0	0.7	0.0
Mocha, Skimmed, Medio, Costa*	1 Medio/346ml	232	3.1	67	3.1	11.1	0.9	0.0
Mocha, Skimmed, Medio, Iced, Costa*	1 Medio/453ml	213	3.2	47	1.6	8.6	0.7	0.0
Mocha, Skimmed, Primo, Costa*	1 Primo/242ml	155	2.2	64	3.1	10.5	0.9	0.0
Mocha, Skimmed, Primo, Iced, Costa*	1 Primo/329ml	148	2.0	45	1.6	8.1	0.6	0.0
Mocha, Soya, Massimo, Costa*	1 Massimo/471ml	377	10.4	80	3.1	11.2	2.2	0.0
Mocha, Soya, Massimo, Iced, Costa*	1 Massimo/572ml	303	7.4	53	1.6	8.5	1.3	0.0
Mocha, Soya, Medio, Iced, Costa*	1 Medio/457ml	233	5.9	51	1.6	8.1	1.3	0.0
Mocha, Soya, Primo, Iced, Costa*	1 Primo/333ml	163	4.3	49	1.6	7.6	1.3	0.0
Mocha Cordato, Skimmed, Solo, Costa*	1 Solo/30ml	78	0.8	260	16.0	42.3	2.7	0.0
Mocha Cortado, Full Fat, Solo, Costa*	1 Solo/153ml	110	5.2	72	3.1	7.3	3.4	0.0
Mocha Cortado, Full Fat, Solo, Iced, Costa*	1 Solo/189ml	102	3.8	54	1.6	7.3	2.0	0.0
Mocha Cortado, Skimmed, Solo, Costa*	1 Solo/152ml	73	0.8	48	3.2	7.6	0.5	0.0
Mocha Cortado, Skimmed, Solo, Iced, Costa*	1 Solo/192ml	77	1.0	40	1.6	7.3	0.5	0.0
Mocha Cortado, Soya, Solo, Costa*	1 Solo/152g	85	3.0	56	3.1	5.9	2.0	0.0
Mocha Cortado, Soya, Solo, Iced, Costa*	1 Solo/191ml	86	2.3	45	1.6	6.7	1.2	0.0
Mocha Flake, Soya, Massimo, Costa*	1 Massimo/600ml	464	23.7	77	2.6	7.5	4.0	0.0
Mocha Flake, Soya, Primo, Costa*	1 Primo/360ml	319	17.1	89	2.6	8.4	4.8	0.0
Mocha Latte, Full Fat, Massimo, Costa*	1 Massimo/534ml	497	18.7	93	3.3	11.3	3.5	0.0
Mocha Latte, Full Fat, Medio, Costa*	1 Medio/403ml	347	14.1	86	3.2	10.2	3.5	0.0
Mocha Latte, Full Fat, Medio, Iced, Costa*	1 Medio/503ml	307	11.1	61	1.8	8.3	2.2	0.0
Mocha Latte, Full Fat, Primo, Costa*	1 Primo/250ml	228	9.0	91	3.3	10.9	3.6	0.0
Mocha Latte, Full Fat, Primo, Iced, Costa*	1 Primo/386ml	220	8.5	57	1.8	7.5	2.2	0.0
Mocha Latte, Skimmed, Massimo, Costa*	1 Massimo/535ml	380	4.8	71	3.4	11.5	0.9	0.0
Mocha Latte, Skimmed, Massimo, Iced, Costa*	1 Massimo/629ml	302	3.8	48	1.9	8.7	0.6	0.0

	Measure INFO/WEIGHT	per Measure KCAL	FAT	Nutrition Values per 100g / 100ml KCAL	PROT	CARB	FAT	FIBRE
COSTA								
COFFEE								
Mocha Latte, Skimmed, Medio, Costa*	1 Medio/398ml	255	3.2	64	3.3	10.4	0.8	0.0
Mocha Latte, Skimmed, Medio, Iced, Costa*	1 Medio/502ml	231	3.0	46	1.8	8.2	0.6	0.0
Mocha Latte, Skimmed, Primo, Costa*	1 Primo/293ml	170	2.1	58	3.2	9.4	0.7	0.0
Mocha Latte, Skimmed, Primo, Iced, Costa*	1 Primo/386ml	162	2.3	42	1.8	7.5	0.6	0.0
Mocha Latte, Soya, Massimo, Costa*	1 Massimo/537ml	419	12.4	78	3.3	10.3	2.3	0.0
Mocha Latte, Soya, Massimo, Iced, Costa*	1 Massimo/622ml	336	8.7	54	1.8	8.1	1.4	0.0
Mocha Latte, Soya, Medio, Costa*	1 Medio/403ml	286	8.9	71	3.2	8.9	2.2	0.0
Mocha Latte, Soya, Medio, Iced, Costa*	1 Medio/506ml	258	7.1	51	1.8	7.6	1.4	0.0
Mocha Latte, Soya, Primo, Iced, Costa*	1 Primo/389ml	183	5.1	47	1.8	6.9	1.3	0.0
Old Paradise Street, Espresso, Doppio, Costa*	1 Doppio60ml	6	0.2	10	0.7	1.3	0.3	0.0
Old Paradise Street, Espresso, Solo, Costa*	1 Solo/30ml	3	0.1	10	0.7	1.3	0.3	0.0
Shot, Costa*	1 Shot/40g	4	0.1	10	0.7	1.3	0.3	0.0
Strawberry, Skimmed, Primo, Costa*	1 Primo/360ml	310	7.5	86	1.3	15.6	2.1	0.0
COOKIES								
Choc Chunk, Double, Costa*	1 Pack/60g	296	15.2	493	5.2	61.1	25.3	3.7
Fruit & Oat, Costa*	1 Pack/60g	283	12.7	472	5.1	65.2	21.2	2.0
CREAM								
Whipping, Costa*	1 Serving/25g	79	8.1	314	1.7	4.2	32.4	0.0
CROISSANT								
Almond, Costa*	1 Croissant/85g	313	12.9	369	8.4	48.4	15.2	0.0
Butter, Costa*	1 Croissant/57g	248	15.4	435	8.4	38.9	27.0	0.0
Ham & Cheese, Costa*	1 Serving/105g	358	20.4	341	13.2	27.2	19.4	0.0
CUPCAKES								
Banoffee, Costa*	1 Cupcake/112g	431	17.7	385	3.7	56.7	15.8	0.0
Lemon, Costa*	1 Cupcake/97g	512	32.5	528	2.8	53.2	33.5	0.0
Rocky Road, Costa*	1 Cupcake/101g	427	17.7	421	5.1	58.9	17.5	0.0
DESSERT								
Mango Frostino, Light, Primo, Costa*	1 Primo/481ml	154	0.5	32	1.8	6.0	0.1	0.0
Strawberry Frostino, Light, Medio, Costa*	1 Medio/571ml	200	0.6	35	1.8	6.5	0.1	0.0
Strawberry Frostino, Light, Primo, Costa*	1 Primo/488ml	156	0.5	32	1.8	6.0	0.1	0.0
FLAPJACK								
Fruity, Costa*	1 Serving/90g	380	15.6	423	5.0	59.5	17.4	12.5
Nutty, Costa*	1 Serving/90g	425	23.2	472	7.7	50.0	25.8	5.0
FLATBREAD								
Cajun Chicken, Costa*	1 Pack/168g	310	5.1	184	12.7	26.6	3.0	0.0
Cheddar & Caramelised Onion Chutney, Costa*	1 Pack/118g	340	13.3	288	11.9	34.8	11.3	0.0
Chicken, Green Thai, Costa*	1 Pack/173g	325	6.4	188	12.2	26.6	3.7	0.0
Emmenthal & Mushroom, Costa*	1 Pack/158g	391	16.1	248	13.1	25.9	10.2	0.0
FRESCATO								
Coffee, Full Fat, Medio (Coffee Only), Costa*	1 Medio454ml	423	7.9	93	1.5	17.9	1.7	0.0
Coffee, Full Fat, Primo, (Coffee Only), Costa*	1 Primo/340ml	302	5.6	89	1.4	17.1	1.6	0.0
Coffee, Skimmed, Medio (Coffee Only), Costa*	1 Medio/454ml	359	0.5	79	1.6	18.0	0.1	0.0
Coffee Caramel, Full Fat, Medio, Costa*	1 Medio/454ml	488	7.9	107	1.5	21.5	1.7	0.0
Coffee Caramel, Skimmed, Medio, Costa*	1 Medio/454ml	425	0.7	94	1.6	21.6	0.2	0.0
Coffee Caramel, Skimmed, Primo, Costa*	1 Primo/340ml	289	0.5	85	1.5	19.6	0.2	0.0
Coffee Caramel, Soya, Medio, Costa*	1 Medio/454ml	441	3.9	97	1.5	20.6	0.9	0.0
Coffee Mocha, Full Fat, Medio, Costa*	1 Medio/454ml	540	8.3	119	1.6	24.0	1.8	0.0
Coffee Mocha, Full Fat, Primo, Costa*	1 Primo/340ml	380	5.9	112	1.6	22.5	1.7	0.0
Coffee Mocha, Soya, Primo, Costa*	1 Primo/340ml	346	3.1	102	1.6	21.7	0.9	0.0
Coffee Vanilla, Soya, Primo, Costa*	1 Primo/340ml	301	2.8	89	1.4	18.7	0.8	0.0
Mango & Passionfruit, Costa*	1 Medio/400ml	219	0.6	55	0.1	13.2	0.2	0.0

COSTA

FRUIT

Tropical Sticks, Costa*	1 Pack/210g	86	0.0	41	0.8	8.4	0.0	1.9

FRUIT & NUT MIX

Costa*	1 Packr/40g	205	13.6	512	15.0	34.0	34.0	0.0

FRUIT MIX

Tropical, Dried, Costa*	1 Pack/40g	135	0.7	338	3.4	72.1	1.8	0.0

FRUIT PUREE

Strawberry, Costa*	1 Serving/15g	38	0.0	256	0.5	63.1	0.1	0.0

FRUIT SALAD

Classic, Costa*	1 Serving/160g	83	0.2	52	0.6	11.2	0.1	0.0
Tropical Medley, Costa*	1 Pack/200g	84	0.4	42	0.5	8.9	0.2	2.9

HOT CHOCOLATE

Black Forest, Full Fat, Medio, Costa*	1 Medio/480ml	548	25.2	114	3.0	13.3	5.2	0.0
Black Forest, Full Fat, Primo, Costa*	1 Primo/360ml	383	17.9	106	2.8	12.4	5.0	0.0
Full Fat, Massimo, Costa*	1 Massimo/426ml	464	17.5	109	3.8	13.6	4.1	0.0
Full Fat, Medio, Costa*	1 Medio/319ml	319	12.8	100	3.7	11.9	4.0	0.0
Full Fat, Primo, Costa*	1 Primo/201ml	205	8.0	102	3.7	12.3	4.0	0.0
Skimmed, Massimo, Costa*	1 Massimo/404ml	335	4.4	83	3.9	13.9	1.1	0.0
Skimmed, Medio, Costa*	1 Medio/316ml	234	2.8	74	3.8	12.1	0.9	0.0
Skimmed, Primo, Costa*	1 Primo/200ml	152	2.0	76	3.8	12.6	1.0	0.0
Soya, Massimo, Costa*	1 Massimo/425ml	391	11.5	92	3.8	12.2	2.7	0.0
Soya, Medio, Costa*	1 Medio/320ml	262	8.0	82	3.7	10.4	2.5	0.0
Soya, Primo, Costa*	1 Primo/200ml	170	5.0	85	3.7	10.8	2.5	0.0
with Marshmallows & Cream, F/F, Massimo, Costa*	1 Massimo/450ml	639	28.4	142	3.7	17.2	6.3	0.0
with Marshmallows & Cream, F/F, Medio, Costa*	1 Medio/353ml	462	20.5	131	3.6	15.8	5.8	0.0
with Marshmallows & Cream, F/F, Primo, Costa*	1 Primo230ml	326	15.8	142	3.6	16.0	6.9	0.0
with Marshmallows & Cream, Skim, Massimo, Costa*	1 Massimo/448ml	538	16.6	120	3.8	17.4	3.7	0.0
with Marshmallows & Cream, Skim, Medio, Costa*	1 Medio/354ml	382	11.0	108	3.7	16.0	3.1	0.0
with Marshmallows & Cream, Skim, Primo, Costa*	1 Primo/230ml	276	10.1	120	3.6	16.2	4.4	0.0
with Marshmallows & Cream, Soya, Medio, Costa*	1 Medio/352ml	408	15.8	116	3.6	14.5	4.5	0.0
with Marshmallows & Cream, Soya, Primo, Costa*	1 Primo/230ml	293	13.1	127	3.6	14.7	5.7	0.0

ICE DESSERTS

Double Choc Flake, Full Fat Milk, Primo, Costa*	1 Primo/340ml	559	24.8	164	1.9	22.9	7.3	0.0
Double Choc Flake, Skimmed, Medio, Costa*	1 Medio/454ml	722	22.7	159	2.2	26.5	5.0	0.0
Double Choc Flake, Skimmed, Primo, Costa*	1 Primo/340ml	514	19.7	151	2.0	23.0	5.8	0.0
Double Choc Flake, Soya, Medio, Costa*	1 Medio/454ml	738	25.9	163	2.1	25.6	5.7	0.0
Double Choc Flake, Soya, Primo, Costa*	1 Primo/340ml	525	21.9	154	1.9	22.0	6.4	0.0
Simply Vanilla, Full Fat, Primo, Costa*	1 Primo/340ml	301	5.6	89	1.4	17.1	1.6	0.0
Simply Vanilla, Skimmed, Medio, Costa*	1 Medio/454ml	357	0.7	79	1.5	18.0	0.2	0.0
Simply Vanilla, Soya, Primo, Costa*	1 Primo/340ml	267	2.7	79	1.4	16.2	0.8	0.0
Strawberry Shortcake, Full Fat, Medio, Costa*	1 Medio/454ml	757	26.1	167	1.8	27.1	5.8	0.0
Strawberry Shortcake, Skimmed, Primo, Costa*	1 Primo/340ml	524	18.8	154	1.9	24.4	5.5	0.0
Strawberry Shortcake, Soya, Medio, Costa*	1 Medio/454ml	710	22.1	156	1.8	26.2	4.9	0.0
Strawberry Shortcake, Soya, Primo, Costa*	1 Primo/340ml	535	21.0	157	1.8	23.5	6.2	0.0

JUICE DRINK

Blackberry & Raspberry, Fruit Cooler, Massimo, Costa*	1 Massimo/588ml	312	0.0	53	0.0	12.6	0.0	0.0
Blackberry & Raspberry, Fruit Cooler, Medio, Costa*	1 Medio/496ml	248	0.0	50	0.2	11.7	0.0	0.0
Blackberry & Raspberry, Fruit Cooler, Primo, Costa*	1 Primo/406ml	187	0.0	46	0.2	10.8	0.0	0.0
Mango & Passionfruit, Fruit Cooler, Massimo, Costa*	1 Massimo584ml	321	0.6	55	0.2	13.2	0.1	0.0
Mango & Passionfruit, Fruit Cooler, Medio, Costa*	1 Medio/498ml	254	0.5	51	0.1	12.2	0.1	0.0
Mango & Passionfruit, Fruit Cooler, Primo, Costa*	1 Primo/409ml	192	0.4	47	0.1	11.3	0.1	0.0
Orange & Raspberry, Fruit Cooler, Medio, Costa*	1 Medio/480ml	320	0.2	67	0.2	15.9	0.0	0.0
Orange & Raspberry, Fruit Cooler, Primo, Costa*	1 Primo/360ml	241	0.2	67	0.2	16.1	0.1	0.0

COSTA

	Measure INFO/WEIGHT	per Measure KCAL	FAT	Nutrition Values per 100g / 100ml KCAL	PROT	CARB	FAT	FIBRE
JUICE DRINK								
Orange & Raspberry, Juice Drink, Massimo, Costa*	1 Massimo/600ml	403	0.3	67	0.2	16.1	0.0	0.0
Sicilian Lemonade, Fruit Cooler, Primo, Costa*	1 Primo/340ml	197	0.2	58	0.1	14.0	0.1	0.0
Tropical Fruit, Fruit Cooler, Medio, Costa*	1 Medio/504ml	232	2.5	46	0.2	10.4	0.5	0.0
Tropical Fruit, Fruit Cooler, Primo, Costa*	1 Primo/407ml	175	1.6	43	0.1	9.6	0.4	0.0
Watermelon & Strawberry, Fruit Cooler, Massimo, Costa*	1 Massimo/588ml	247	0.6	42	0.1	10.2	0.1	0.0
Watermelon & Strawberry, Fruit Cooler, Medio, Costa*	1 Medio/503ml	196	0.5	39	0.1	9.5	0.1	0.0
Watermelon & Strawberry, Fruit Cooler, Primo, Costa*	1 Primo/411ml	148	0.4	36	0.1	8.7	0.1	0.0
LEMONADE								
Base, Costa*	1 Serving/15g	42	0.0	283	0.0	74.3	0.0	0.0
Iced, Massimo, Costa*	1 Massimo/597ml	179	0.0	30	0.0	7.4	0.0	0.0
Iced, Medio, Costa*	1 Medio/500ml	135	0.0	27	0.0	6.8	0.0	0.0
Iced, Primo, Costa*	1 Serving/375ml	90	0.0	24	0.0	6.0	0.0	0.0
Peach, Iced, Massimo, Costa*	1 Massimo/600ml	174	0.0	29	0.0	7.1	0.0	0.0
Peach, Iced, Medio, Costa*	1 Medio/485ml	131	0.0	27	0.1	6.5	0.0	0.0
Peach, Iced, Primo, Costa*	1 Primo/366ml	88	0.0	24	0.0	5.8	0.0	0.0
Raspberry & Cranberry, Iced, Massimo, Costa*	1 Massimo/600ml	179	0.0	30	0.0	7.3	0.0	0.0
Raspberry & Cranberry, Iced, Medio, Costa*	1 Medio/480ml	134	0.0	28	0.0	6.8	0.0	0.0
Raspberry & Cranberry, Iced, Primo, Costa*	1 Primo/360ml	89	0.0	25	0.0	6.1	0.0	0.0
Strawberry, Iced, Massimo, Costa*	1 Massimo/600ml	175	0.0	29	0.0	7.1	0.0	0.0
Strawberry, Iced, Medio, Costa*	1 Medio/480ml	131	0.0	27	0.0	6.7	0.0	0.0
Strawberry, Iced, Primo, Costa*	1 Primo/360ml	87	0.0	24	0.0	5.9	0.0	0.0
Summer Punch, Medio, Costa*	1 Medio/496ml	139	0.0	28	0.0	7.0	0.0	0.0
Summer Punch, Primo, Costa*	1 Primo/368ml	92	0.0	25	0.0	6.2	0.0	0.0
MANGO								
Dried, Costa*	1 Pack/30g	94	0.3	314	1.9	69.5	0.9	0.0
MARMALADE								
Costa*	1 Portion/28g	75	0.0	268	0.0	67.0	0.0	0.0
MARMITE								
Costa*	1 Portion/8g	20	0.0	252	38.7	24.1	0.1	0.0
MARSHMALLOWS								
Crispie Bites, Costa*	1 Bite/13g	60	2.8	476	5.6	63.7	22.0	0.0
MILK								
Full Fat, Whole, Costa*	1 Sm Jug/40g	25	1.4	63	3.5	4.3	3.5	0.0
Semi Skimmed, Costa*	1 Sm Jug/40g	18	0.6	45	3.1	4.5	1.5	0.0
Skimmed, Costa*	1 Sm Jug/40g	13	0.0	33	3.4	46.0	0.1	0.0
Soya, Costa*	1 Sm Jug/40g	18	0.8	44	3.3	3.0	1.9	0.0
MILK DRINK								
Chocolate, Full Fat, Massimo, Iced, Costa*	1 Massimo/450ml	351	11.7	78	2.0	11.4	2.6	0.0
Chocolate, Full Fat, Medio, Iced, Costa*	1 Medio/357ml	271	9.3	76	2.0	10.9	2.6	0.0
Chocolate, Full Fat, Primo, Iced, Costa*	1 Primo/269ml	194	7.0	72	2.0	9.9	2.6	0.0
Chocolate, Skimmed, Massimo, Iced, Costa*	1 Massimo/451ml	275	3.6	61	2.0	11.3	0.8	0.0
Chocolate, Skimmed, Medio, Iced, Costa*	1 Medio/356ml	210	2.8	59	2.0	10.9	0.8	0.0
Chocolate, Skimmed, Primo, Iced, Costa*	1 Primo/272ml	147	1.9	54	2.0	9.9	0.7	0.0
Chocolate, Soya, Massimo, Iced, Costa*	1 Massimo/451ml	303	7.7	67	2.0	10.6	1.7	0.0
Chocolate, Soya, Medio, Iced, Costa*	1 Medio/357ml	232	5.7	65	2.0	10.2	1.6	0.0
Chocolate, Soya, Primo, Iced, Costa*	1 Primo/272ml	163	4.3	60	2.0	9.2	1.6	0.0
MILK SHAKE								
Belgian Chocolate, Cooler, Soya, Medio, Costa*	1 Medio/538ml	414	15.6	77	1.3	11.1	2.9	0.0
Belgian Chocolate, Cooler, Soya, Primo, Costa*	1 Primo/441ml	304	12.3	69	1.2	9.5	2.8	0.0
Belgian Chocolate, Full Fat, Cooler, Medio, Costa*	1 Medio/539ml	447	18.3	83	1.3	11.6	3.4	0.0
Belgian Chocolate, Full Fat, Cooler, Primo, Costa*	1 Primo/439ml	329	14.5	75	1.2	10.0	3.3	0.0
Belgian Chocolate, Skimmed, Cooler, Medio, Costa*	1 Medio/536ml	397	12.3	74	1.4	11.7	2.3	0.0

	INFO/WEIGHT	KCAL	FAT	KCAL	PROT	CARB	FAT	FIBRE
COSTA								
MILK SHAKE								
Belgian Chocolate, Skimmed, Cooler, Primo, Costa*	1 Primo/434ml	291	10.0	67	1.3	10.1	2.3	0.0
Mango, Full Fat, Cooler, Medio, Costa*	1 Medio/552ml	453	16.6	82	1.1	12.5	3.0	0.0
Mango, Full Fat, Cooler, Primo, Costa*	1 Primo/454ml	345	13.2	76	1.1	11.3	2.9	0.0
Mango, Skimmed, Cooler, Medio, Costa*	1 Medio/551ml	397	10.5	72	1.2	12.5	1.9	0.0
Mango, Skimmed, Cooler, Primo, Costa*	1 Primo/452ml	303	8.6	67	1.1	11.3	1.9	0.0
Mango, Soya, Cooler, Medio, Costa*	1 Medio/555ml	416	13.3	75	1.1	12.1	2.4	0.0
Mango, Soya, Cooler, Primo, Costa*	1 Primo/454ml	318	10.9	70	1.1	10.9	2.4	0.0
Mint Choc Chip, Full Fat, Cooler, Medio, Costa*	1 Medio/569ml	615	29.6	108	1.4	13.5	5.2	0.0
Mint Choc Chip, Full Fat, Cooler, Primo, Costa*	1 Primo/460ml	442	22.1	96	1.3	11.6	4.8	0.0
Mint Choc Chip, Skimmed, Cooler, Medio, Costa*	1 Medio/570ml	559	23.4	98	1.5	13.4	4.1	0.0
Mint Choc Chip, Skimmed, Cooler, Primo, Costa*	1 Primo/459ml	399	17.4	87	1.4	11.6	3.8	0.0
Mint Choc Chip, Soya, Cooler, Medio, Costa*	1 Medio/573ml	579	26.4	101	1.4	13.0	4.6	0.0
Mint Choc Chip, Soya, Cooler, Primo, Costa*	1 Primo/460ml	414	19.8	90	1.3	11.2	4.3	0.0
Raspberry & White Choc, Full Fat, Cooler, Medio, Costa*	1 Medio/556ml	517	18.3	93	1.3	14.7	3.3	0.0
Raspberry & White Choc, Full Fat, Cooler, Primo, Costa*	1 Primo/452ml	393	14.0	87	1.2	13.4	3.1	0.0
Raspberry & White Choc, Skimmed, Cooler, Medio, Costa*	1 Medio/557ml	468	12.3	84	1.4	14.8	2.2	0.0
Raspberry & White Choc, Skimmed, Cooler, Primo, Costa*	1 Primo/455ml	355	10.0	78	1.2	13.5	2.2	0.0
Raspberry & White Choc, Soya, Cooler, Medio, Costa*	1 Medio/556ml	484	15.6	87	1.3	14.2	2.8	0.0
Raspberry & White Choc, Soya, Cooler, Primo, Costa*	1 Primo/454ml	368	12.3	81	1.2	13.0	2.7	0.0
Strawberry, Full Fat, Cooler, Medio, Costa*	1 Medio/540ml	405	15.7	75	1.2	11.1	2.9	0.0
Strawberry, Full Fat, Cooler, Primo, Costa*	1 Primo/441ml	300	12.8	68	1.1	9.6	2.9	0.0
Strawberry, Skimmed, Cooler, Medio, Costa*	1 Medio/539ml	356	9.7	66	1.2	11.2	1.8	0.0
Strawberry, Soya, Cooler, Medio, Costa*	1 Medio/539ml	372	12.9	69	1.2	10.6	2.4	0.0
Strawberry, Soya, Cooler, Primo, Costa*	1 Primo/437ml	275	10.5	63	1.1	9.1	2.4	0.0
MUFFIN								
Banana & Nut, Costa*	1 Muffin/122g	482	27.3	395	6.3	41.8	22.4	2.8
Banana & Pecan Breakfast Loaf, Costa*	1 Muffin/113g	442	23.4	391	5.1	44.0	20.7	0.0
Banana & Toffee, Costa*	1 Muffin/117g	462	23.8	395	4.4	49.1	20.3	0.0
Blackcurrant & White Chocolate, Costa*	1 Muffin/124g	474	21.1	382	4.3	53.0	17.0	0.0
Blueberry, Costa*	1 Muffin/125g	452	22.5	362	4.5	44.4	18.0	0.0
Breakfast, Egg & Mushroom, Costa*	1 Muffin/150g	311	11.0	207	7.4	27.8	7.3	1.5
Cherry & Almond, Costa*	1 Muffin/132g	473	20.5	358	13.5	40.9	15.5	0.0
Chocolate, Mini, Costa*	1 Muffin/19g	73	3.9	383	4.3	44.5	20.5	0.0
Cookies & Cream, Costa*	1 Muffin/122g	517	26.5	424	4.1	51.8	21.7	0.0
Lemon, Costa*	1 Muffin/115g	452	21.4	393	4.6	50.6	18.6	0.0
Lemon & Orange, Low Fat, Costa*	1 Muffin/135g	319	3.1	236	4.6	49.4	2.3	1.1
Raspberry & White Chocolate, Costa*	1 Muffin/135g	511	26.0	376	4.8	46.4	19.1	0.0
Red Berry, Low Fat, Costa*	1 Muffin/124g	381	4.2	307	6.2	63.0	3.4	0.0
Salted Caramel, Costa*	1 Muffin/1123g	459	17.4	373	4.0	56.6	14.1	0.0
Triple Chocolate, Costa*	1 Muffin/122g	480	21.5	393	6.1	50.2	17.6	0.0
Very Berry, Skinny, Costa*	1 Muffin/117g	319	2.5	273	4.1	58.1	2.1	0.0
PAIN AU RAISIN								
Costa*	1 Pastry/80g	277	13.4	346	5.4	42.5	16.7	0.0
PANETTINO								
Chocolate, Costa*	1 Cake/100g	423	19.8	423	9.7	50.8	19.8	0.0
Classic, Costa*	1 Serving/100g	365	12.7	365	7.6	54.3	12.7	0.0
PANETTONE								
Classic, Costa*	1 Serving/100g	374	14.7	374	7.8	51.5	14.7	0.0
PANINI								
Brie & Bacon, Soughdough, Costa*	1 Panni/178g	503	17.8	283	1.3	33.0	10.0	0.0
Brie & Tomato Chutney, Costa*	1 Panini/177g	453	16.5	256	9.8	33.3	9.3	2.8
Chicken, Red Chilli, Costa*	1 Panini/207g	370	5.6	179	13.5	25.1	2.7	0.0

COSTA

INFO/WEIGHT	Measure	per Measure KCAL	FAT	Nutrition Values per 100g / 100ml KCAL	PROT	CARB	FAT	FIBRE
PANINI								
Chicken & Baby Spinach, Costa*	1 Panini/440g	832	11.0	189	9.8	32.5	2.5	0.0
Chicken & Chorizo, Sourdough, Costa*	1 Panini/176g	393	8.5	223	12.6	30.8	4.8	0.0
Chicken & Pesto, Costa*	1 Panini/209g	419	21.4	200	22.5	57.9	10.2	0.0
Chicken Arrabiata, Costa*	1 Panini/205g	377	5.5	184	13.7	26.1	2.7	0.0
Chicken Roasted Pepper & Rocket, Costa*	1 Panini/185g	338	7.6	183	10.4	26.0	4.1	3.2
Goats Cheese & Caramelised Onion Chutney, Costa*	1 Panini/172g	431	5.3	251	4.9	19.5	3.1	0.0
Goats Cheese & Pepper, Costa*	1 Panini/197g	424	11.0	215	9.9	30.3	5.6	0.0
Goats Cheese & Sweet Chilli Chutney, Costa*	1 Panini/173g	420	9.2	243	9.2	37.6	5.3	0.0
Ham & Cheese, Soughdough, Costa*	1 Panini/175g	434	12.8	248	15.0	29.6	7.3	0.0
Mozzarella & Tomato, Sourdough, Costa*	1 Panini/195g	489	18.1	251	11.3	29.7	9.3	0.0
Mushroom & Emmental, Costa*	1 Panini/187g	456	18.3	244	10.9	28.0	9.8	0.0
Ragu Meatball, Costa*	1 Panini/190g	477	15.8	251	11.7	31.2	8.3	0.0
Spicy Meatball, Costa*	1 Panini/177g	506	17.5	286	11.9	37.1	9.9	0.0
Steak & Cheese, Costa*	1 Panini/228g	492	16.4	216	11.3	25.7	7.2	0.0
Tuna Melt, Soughdough, Costa*	1 Panini/190g	484	17.1	255	15.0	27.6	9.0	0.0
PASTA								
Chicken, Tomato & Basil, Costa*	1 Pack/290g	513	13.0	177	8.4	25.7	4.5	2.1
PASTRY								
Cinnamon Swirl, Slices, Costa*	1 Pastry/92g	341	22.8	369	4.0	31.9	24.7	0.0
PIE								
Mince, Costa*	1 Pie/75g	362	13.3	483	4.5	74.9	17.7	3.2
POPCORN								
Sweet & Salty, Costa*	1 Serving/23g	119	6.5	517	6.1	56.4	28.4	0.0
SALAD								
Chargrilled Vegetable & Cous Cous, Costa*	1 Serving/291g	352	7.6	121	3.0	21.5	2.6	0.0
Chicken, Costa*	1 Serving/194g	297	4.1	153	12.4	21.2	2.1	0.0
Chicken & Pesto Pasta, Costa*	1 Pack/271g	420	11.4	155	7.8	21.3	4.2	1.7
Cous Cous, Moroccan Styles, Costa*	1 Pack/290g	392	7.3	135	3.6	24.6	2.5	2.2
Spiced Chicken, Grain, & Yoghurt & Mint Dressing, Costa*	1 Pack/285g	470	10.0	165	9.8	20.9	3.5	0.0
Sunblush Tomato & Feta Pasta, Costa*	1 Pack/266.66g	360	13.6	135	4.4	17.1	5.1	2.2
Tuna, Costa*	1 Pack/181g	274	4.0	151	10.3	22.6	2.2	0.0
SANDWICH								
Bacon, Lettuce & Tomato, Stack, Costa*	1 Sandwich/164g	405	15.4	247	10.5	29.0	9.4	0.0
Bacon & Tomato Sauce, Tostato, Costa*	1 Tostato/132g	316	6.6	239	8.5	40.2	5.0	0.0
BLT, Costa*	1 Pack/169g	397	15.7	235	11.0	26.8	9.3	0.0
Brie, Apple & Grape, Costa*	1 Serving/225g	536	24.5	238	8.3	28.7	10.9	0.0
Chicke, Chargrilled, Salad with Pesto, Stack, Costa*	1 Serving/188g	399	15.8	212	11.2	24.8	8.4	0.0
Chicken, & Lemon, Costa*	1 Pack/182g	433	19.3	238	10.9	25.9	10.6	0.0
Chicken, Coronation, Costa*	1 Pack/258g	600	26.1	232	12.5	23.0	10.1	2.5
Chicken, Roast, Costa*	1 Pack/177g	325	7.1	184	13.0	23.8	4.0	0.0
Chicken, Roast, with Lemon Mayonnaise, Costa*	1 Pack/176.6g	325	7.1	184	13.0	23.8	4.0	0.0
Chicken, Roast British, & Salad, Costa*	1 Pack/200g	342	6.8	171	11.9	21.5	3.4	1.0
Club, Chicken & Bacon, Costa*	1 Pack/213g	484	13.2	227	13.6	29.3	6.2	0.0
Egg, Free Range, Costa*	1 Pack/165g	342	13.5	207	10.2	21.8	8.2	0.0
Egg Mayonnaise, Costa*	1 Pack/206g	389	24.1	189	7.2	15.4	11.7	0.0
Egg Mayonnaise & Tomato, Free Range, Costa*	1 Pack/174g	389	24.1	223	8.6	18.3	13.8	0.0
Ham, Mascapone & Mushroom, Focaccia, Costa*	1 Pack/182g	427	20.1	234	11.1	21.7	11.0	0.0
Ham Hock & Mustard Pickle, Roll, Costa*	1 Pack/163g	286	5.2	176	10.6	26.1	3.2	0.0
Houmous, Costa*	1 Pack/165g	263	4.7	160	6.4	25.9	2.8	0.0
Italian Salami & Mozzarella, Toasted Focaccia, Costa*	1 Pack/157g	430	20.1	274	10.8	27.9	12.8	0.0
Ploughmans, Cheese, Roll, Costa*	1 Pack/175g	431	21.3	247	9.4	25.0	12.2	0.0
Prawn Mayonnaise, on Wholemeal, Costa*	1 Pack/163g	291	7.7	178	9.0	23.6	4.7	0.0

COSTA

	Measure INFO/WEIGHT	per Measure KCAL	FAT	Nutrition Values per 100g / 100ml KCAL	PROT	CARB	FAT	FIBRE
SANDWICH								
Salmon, & Salad, Poached, Oatmeal, Costa*	1 Pack/151g	224	4.2	148	7.7	22.9	2.8	0.0
Sausage, Chorizo, & Vine Ripened Tomato, Costa*	1 Pack/181g	315	3.8	174	15.5	26.1	2.1	0.0
Scottish Smoked Salmon & Soft Cheese, Costa*	1 Pack/175g	372	10.7	212	12.9	25.5	6.1	1.9
Smoked Ham & Free Range Egg, Stack, Costa*	1 Pack/219g	426	14.2	195	11.6	22.4	6.5	0.0
Tuna, & Salad, Costa*	1 Pack/177g	289	4.1	163	11.9	25.7	2.3	0.0
Turkey, & Pork & Apricot Stuffing, Costa*	1 Pack/201g	389	9.8	194	11.5	28.3	4.9	0.0
SAUCE								
Belgian Chocolate, Costa*	1 Serving/16g	54	0.8	339	2.6	68.4	5.3	0.0
Caramel, Costa*	1 Serving/15g	57	0.9	380	11.1	70.9	5.7	0.0
Cherry, Costa*	1 Serving/15g	40	0.0	265	0.3	66.0	0.1	0.0
Fruit Punch, Costa*	1 Serving/15g	46	0.0	308	0.2	76.2	0.1	0.0
Mango & Passion Fruit & Papaya, Costa*	1 Serving/15g	39	0.0	262	0.5	64.0	0.2	0.0
Peach Lemonade, Costa*	1 Serving/15g	43	0.0	289	0.5	71.1	0.3	0.0
Raspberry, Costa*	1 Serving/15g	51	0.0	339	0.0	84.9	0.0	0.0
White Chocolate, Costa*	1 Serving/15g	57	0.8	382	3.1	80.2	5.5	0.0
SCONE								
Fruit, Costa*	1 Serving/110g	370	11.8	336	5.6	55.1	10.7	0.0
SHORTBREAD								
Caramel, Traybake, Costa*	1 Serving/77g	404	26.3	525	4.3	49.4	34.2	0.0
Mini, Bag, Costa*	1 Serving/10g	52	2.8	525	5.5	61.4	27.8	0.0
SHORTCAKE								
Raspberry, Costa*	1 Shortcake/45g	215	10.7	477	2.4	63.5	23.7	0.0
SLICES								
Cheese, Twist, Pastry, Costa*	1 Twist/103g	346	20.4	336	11.1	29.5	19.8	0.0
Chocolate, Twist, Pastry, Costa*	1 Twist/102g	354	15.6	347	5.4	45.7	15.3	0.0
Pecan, Pastry, Costa*	1 Pastry/105g	465	29.9	443	5.6	42.1	28.5	3.0
SOUP								
Fish, Bouillabaisse, Costa*	1 Serving/400g	180	5.6	45	5.8	2.2	1.4	0.0
SUGAR								
Brown, Costa*	1 Portion/2.5g	10	0.0	398	0.0	99.5	0.0	0.0
White, Granulated, Costa*	1 Portion/2.5g	10	0.0	400	0.0	100.0	0.0	0.0
SWEETENER								
Sweet 'n' Low, Costa*	1 Portion/1g	4	0.0	370	1.0	92.0	0.0	0.0
SYRUP								
Blackberry, Costa*	1 Serving/10g	36	0.0	355	0.0	86.1	0.0	0.0
Caramel, Costa*	1 Serving/10g	31	0.0	309	0.0	76.5	0.0	0.0
Caramel, SF, Costa*	1 Serving/10g	2	0.0	19	0.0	10.2	0.0	0.0
Cinnamon, Costa*	1 Serving/10g	33	0.0	328	0.0	80.1	0.0	0.0
Curacao Orange, Costa*	1 Serving/10g	33	0.0	330	0.0	80.0	0.0	0.0
Gingerbread, Costa*	1 Serving/10g	34	0.0	342	0.0	83.5	0.0	0.0
Gingerbread, SF, Costa*	1 Serving/8g	1	0.0	13	0.0	9.6	0.0	0.0
Gomme, Costa*	1 Serving/10g	34	0.0	337	0.1	84.2	0.0	0.0
Mint Flavour, Costa*	1 Serving/17g	44	0.0	264	0.1	73.0	0.1	0.0
Praline, Costa*	1 Serving/10g	32	0.0	323	0.0	80.1	0.0	0.0
Roasted Hazelnut, Costa*	1 Serving/10g	1	0.0	10	0.0	78.4	0.0	0.0
Vanilla, Costa*	1 Serving/10g	32	0.0	324	0.0	80.2	0.0	0.0
Walnut Brownie, Costa*	1 Serving/10g	34	0.0	339	0.0	84.2	0.0	0.0
TART								
Apricot, Jam, Costa*	1 Tart/92g	356	11.0	387	3.9	65.3	12.0	0.0
Bakewell, GF, Costa*	1 Tart/30g	126	5.1	447	2.9	70.0	18.0	2.2
Chocolate & Orange, Costa*	1 Tart/78g	357	18.5	458	5.8	56.3	23.8	2.3
Chocolate Cherry, Mini, Costa*	1 Tart/33g	146	6.5	442	5.1	58.8	19.8	0.0

COSTA

	Measure INFO/WEIGHT	per Measure KCAL	FAT	Nutrition Values per 100g / 100ml KCAL	PROT	CARB	FAT	FIBRE
TART								
Lemon, Costa*	1 Tart/80g	378	20.5	473	4.9	54.8	25.7	0.0
Strawberry Jam, Costa*	1 Tart/92g	361	10.9	392	3.7	67.0	11.8	0.0
Treacle, Costa*	1 Tart/100g	307	8.8	307	3.3	52.9	8.8	1.1
TEA								
Citrus & Ginger Twist, Costa*	1 Primo/100ml	1	0.0	1	0.0	0.0	0.0	0.0
English Breakfast, Decaffeinated, Costa*	1 Primo/500ml	5	0.0	1	0.0	0.0	0.0	0.0
Green, Lime & Mint, Fruit Cooler, Massimo, Costa*	1 Massimo/585ml	269	0.0	46	0.0	11.0	0.0	0.0
Green, Lime & Mint, Fruit Cooler, Medio, Costa*	1 Medio/507ml	213	0.0	42	0.0	10.1	0.0	0.0
Green, Lime & Mint, Fruit Cooler, Primo, Costa*	1 Primo413ml	161	0.0	39	0.0	9.4	0.0	0.0
Green, Simply Sencha, Costa*	1 Primo/100ml	1	0.0	1	0.0	0.0	0.0	0.0
Iced, Lemon, Bottle, Costa*	1 Bottle/275ml	91	0.0	33	0.0	8.0	0.0	0.0
Iced, Lemon, Massimo, Costa*	1 Massimo/526ml	179	0.0	34	0.0	8.6	0.0	0.0
Iced, Lemon, Medio, Costa*	1 Medio/450ml	135	0.0	30	0.0	7.4	0.0	0.0
Iced, Lemon, Primo, Costa*	1 Primo/375ml	90	0.0	24	0.0	6.0	0.0	0.0
Iced, Original, Medio, Costa*	1 Medio/480ml	135	0.0	28	0.0	6.9	0.0	0.0
Iced, Peach, Massimo, Costa*	1 Massimo/527ml	174	0.0	33	0.0	8.2	0.0	0.0
Iced, Peach, Medio, Costa*	1 Medio/452ml	131	0.0	29	0.0	7.1	0.0	0.0
Iced, Peach, Primo, Costa*	1 Primo/367ml	88	0.0	24	0.0	5.8	0.0	0.0
Iced, Raspberry, Massimo, Costa*	1 Massimo/600ml	133	0.0	22	0.0	5.4	0.0	0.0
Iced, Summer Fruit, Massimo, Costa*	1 Massimo/517ml	186	0.0	36	0.0	8.8	0.0	0.0
Iced, Summer Fruit, Medio, Costa*	1 Medio/452ml	140	0.0	31	0.0	7.6	0.0	0.0
Iced, Summer Fruit, Primo, Costa*	1 Primo/372ml	93	0.0	25	0.0	6.2	0.0	0.0
Latte, Chai, Full Fat, Massimo, Costa*	1 Massimo/590ml	667	18.3	113	2.9	18.4	3.1	0.0
Latte, Chai, Full Fat, Massimo, Iced, Costa*	1 Massimo/463ml	426	8.8	92	1.7	17.0	1.9	0.0
Latte, Chai, Full Fat, Medio, Costa*	1 Medio/387ml	422	12.0	109	3.0	17.2	3.1	0.0
Latte, Chai, Full Fat, Medio, Iced, Costa*	1 Medio/363ml	327	7.3	90	1.8	16.3	2.0	0.0
Latte, Chai, Full Fat, Primo, Costa*	1 Primo/236ml	267	7.3	113	2.9	18.4	3.1	0.0
Latte, Chai, Full Fat, Primo, Iced, Costa*	1 Primo/275ml	231	5.5	84	1.8	14.6	2.0	0.0
Latte, Chai, Full Fat, Primo, Iced, Costa*	1 Primo/275ml	231	5.5	84	1.8	14.6	2.0	0.0
Latte, Chai, Skimmed, Massimo, Costa*	1 Massimo/587ml	517	0.6	88	3.0	18.7	0.1	0.0
Latte, Chai, Skimmed, Massimo, Iced, Costa*	1 Massimo/461ml	350	0.5	76	1.8	16.9	0.1	0.0
Latte, Chai, Skimmed, Medio, Costa*	1 Medio/388ml	322	0.4	83	3.0	17.5	0.1	0.0
Latte, Chai, Skimmed, Medio, Iced, Costa*	1 Medio/364ml	266	0.4	73	1.8	16.2	0.1	0.0
Latte, Chai, Skimmed, Primo, Costa*	1 Primo/235ml	207	0.2	88	3.0	17.5	0.1	0.0
Latte, Chai, Skimmed, Primo, Iced, Costa*	1 Primo/275ml	184	0.3	67	1.8	14.6	0.1	0.0
Latte, Chai, Soya, Massimo, Costa*	1 Massimo/591ml	567	10.0	96	2.9	17.0	1.7	0.0
Latte, Chai, Soya, Massimo, Iced, Costa*	1 Massimo/456ml	376	4.6	82	1.7	16.2	1.0	0.0
Latte, Chai, Soya, Medio, Costa*	1 Medio/385ml	355	6.6	92	3.0	15.8	1.7	0.0
Latte, Chai, Soya, Medio, Iced, Costa*	1 Medio/365ml	288	3.6	79	1.8	15.5	1.0	0.0
Latte, Chai, Soya, Primo, Costa*	1 Primo/236ml	227	4.0	96	2.9	17.0	1.7	0.0
Latte, Chai, Soya, Primo, Iced, Costa*	1 Primo/275ml	201	2.8	73	1.8	13.9	1.0	0.0
The Earl, Costa*	1 Primo/1ml	1	0.0	1	0.0	0.0	0.0	0.0
Thoroughly Minted, Costa*	1 Primo100ml	2	0.0	2	0.0	0.0	0.0	0.0
Traditional, Black, Primo, Costa*	1 Primo/500ml	5	0.0	1	0.0	0.0	0.0	0.0
TOAST								
Brown Bread, Costa*	2 Slices/64g	175	2.5	273	8.8	49.2	3.9	0.0
White Bread, Costa*	2 Slices/68g	166	1.8	245	8.5	46.0	2.6	0.0
TOASTIE								
Bacon, Costa*	1 Toastie/135g	338	9.0	250	12.9	34.4	6.7	5.3
Cheese & Tomato, Costa*	1 Toastie/177g	460	20.2	260	12.3	25.9	11.4	0.0
Chicken & Bacon, Costa*	1 Toastie/183g	483	22.1	264	13.6	24.1	12.1	0.0

	Measure INFO/WEIGHT	per Measure		Nutrition Values per 100g / 100ml				
		KCAL	FAT	KCAL	PROT	CARB	FAT	FIBRE
COSTA								
TOASTIE								
Ham & Cheese, Costa*	1 Toastie/138g	308	8.0	223	10.9	30.6	5.8	0.0
Sausage & Onion, Costa*	1 Pack/197g	512	22.3	260	12.9	25.3	11.3	0.0
Three Counties Cheese & Red Onion Jam, Costa*	1 Sandwich/185g	446	17.2	241	9.0	29.6	9.3	0.0
VANILLA								
Powder, Costa*	1 Serving/7g	26	0.0	398	0.1	99.1	0.1	0.0
WAFER								
Crema Milk, Balocco, Costa*	1 Serving/45g	239	13.5	531	7.6	57.0	30.0	0.0
WAFERS								
Crema Cacao, Balocco, Costa*	1 Portion/45g	224	11.6	503	6.9	58.0	26.0	0.0
WATER								
Cloudy Lemon, no Added Sugar, Feel Good, Costa*	1 Bottle/400ml	144	0.0	36	0.1	8.2	0.0	0.2
WRAP								
Chicken Caesar, Costa*	1 Pack/194g	420	15.6	216	11.8	24.1	8.0	1.4
Chicken Fajita, Costa*	1 Wrap/186g	428	16.3	229	11.7	24.3	8.7	0.0
Egg & Tomato, GF, Costa*	1 Wrap/204g	405	18.9	199	6.0	21.1	9.3	0.0
Moroccan Meatball, Costa*	1 Wrap/218g	525	17.2	241	9.0	32.3	7.9	0.0
Spicy Three Bean, Costa*	1 Pack/235g	456	14.3	194	7.1	27.7	6.1	0.0
Sweet Chilli Chicken, Costa*	1 Wrap/192g	365	8.3	190	10.7	27.1	4.3	0.0
YOGHURT								
Blueberry, Breakfast Pot, Costa*	1 Pot/190g	258	3.2	136	4.8	24.7	1.7	1.3
Honey & Granola, Costa*	1 Pot/190g	303	6.1	159	5.3	27.3	3.2	0.0
Strawberry & Granola, Costa*	1 Pot/190g	253	7.4	133	5.4	19.0	3.9	0.0
Vanilla with Mango & Passion Fruit Compote, Costa*	1 Pot/191g	162	4.2	85	4.3	11.8	2.2	0.0
DOMINO'S*								
BREAD								
Garlic, Pizza, Domino's*	2 Slices/101g	274	9.5	271	16.4	30.3	9.4	2.8
BROWNIES								
Chocolate, Domino's*	½ Portion/50g	248	14.2	496	7.1	54.7	28.4	3.2
CAKE								
Chocolate Melt, Domino's*	1 Portion/85g	418	31.0	489	4.7	36.8	36.3	2.1
CHICKEN								
Kickers, Domino's*	½ Portion/85g	204	9.6	239	15.3	19.1	11.3	0.9
Strippers, Domino's*	½ Portion/96g	220	9.7	230	16.1	19.0	10.1	0.6
Wings, BBQ, Spicy, Domino's*	½ Portion/111g	302	16.3	271	19.3	15.0	14.6	0.2
Wings, Domino's*	½ Portion/104g	254	15.3	244	23.0	4.9	14.7	0.0
Wings, Lightly Spiced, Domino's*	1 Wing/30g	65	4.4	218	18.9	2.4	14.5	2.2
Wings, Red Hot, Franks, Domino's*	½ Portion/111g	258	17.0	232	19.7	3.3	15.3	0.5
Wings, Tikka, Domino's*	½ Portion/111g	229	13.9	206	16.8	6.6	12.5	0.1
COLESLAW								
Tub, Domino's*	½ Portion/100g	161	13.8	161	0.8	9.2	13.8	1.5
COOKIES								
Domino's*	2 Cookies/38g	166	6.8	438	5.6	66.6	18.0	3.1
DIP								
BBQ, Domino's*	1 Pot/25g	44	0.1	178	1.3	41.9	0.4	0.8
Cayenne Pepper, Franks Red Hot, Domino's*	1 Pot/26g	18	1.0	69	4.2	4.3	3.9	2.7
Garlic & Herb, Domino's*	1 Pot/25g	174	18.9	693	1.1	1.9	75.4	0.1
Honey & Mustard, Domino's*	1 Pot/28g	128	13.0	459	1.8	7.5	46.5	0.2
Salsa, Tangy, Domino's*	1 Pot/25g	42	1.4	168	2.0	27.7	5.4	2.4
Sweet Chilli, Domino's*	1 Pot/25g	54	0.2	217	0.4	51.0	0.9	0.6
DOUGH BALLS								
Cheese & Herb, Twisted, Domino's*	½ Portion/86g	262	9.4	303	13.3	37.0	10.9	2.0
Chocolate, twisted, Domino's*	½ Portion/94g	346	14.8	368	8.5	49.5	15.7	2.8

	Measure INFO/WEIGHT	per Measure KCAL	FAT	Nutrition Values per 100g / 100ml KCAL	PROT	CARB	FAT	FIBRE
DOMINO'S*								
DOUGH BALLS								
Ham, Twisted, Domino's*	½ Portion/83g	236	5.9	286	13.9	40.4	7.2	2.0
Pepperoni, Twisted, Domino's*	½ Portion/81g	278	10.0	343	14.6	44.7	12.3	2.2
NACHOS								
no Jalapenos, Domino's*	½ Portion/75g	233	12.6	311	11.4	26.8	16.8	3.0
with Jalapenos, Domino's*	½ Portion/85g	234	12.6	276	10.2	23.8	14.8	2.7
PIZZA								
American Hot, Classic, Delight Mozz, Med, Domino's*	1 Slice/68g	175	6.5	255	15.2	26.1	9.5	2.0
American Hot, Classic, Delight Mozz, Personal, Domino's*	1 Slice/204g	520	19.2	254	11.3	30.0	9.4	2.1
American Hot, Classic, Delight Mozz, Sm, Domino's*	1 Slice/61g	157	6.3	259	11.7	28.9	10.4	1.9
American Hot, Classic, Lge, Domino's*	1 Slice/69g	179	7.8	261	11.0	28.5	11.4	1.9
American Hot, Classic, Med, Domino's*	1 Slice/69g	181	7.8	264	11.0	28.5	11.4	1.9
American Hot, Classic, Personal, Domino's*	1 Pizza/204g	535	19.8	262	11.2	31.4	9.7	2.2
American Hot, Classic, Sm, Domino's*	1 Slice/61g	160	6.8	263	12.2	27.7	11.1	1.9
American Hot, Dominator, Lge, Domino's*	1 Slice/110g	307	12.1	279	13.2	31.7	11.0	1.9
American Hot, GF, Delight Mozz, Sm, Domino's*	1 Slice/53g	138	5.8	258	12.2	26.8	10.9	2.1
American Hot, GF, Sm, Domino's*	1 Pizza/322g	804	38.9	250	8.7	25.5	12.1	2.4
American Hot, GF, Smal, Domino's*	1 Slice/53g	134	6.5	251	8.7	25.5	12.1	2.4
American Hot, Italian, Delight Mozz, Lge, Domino's*	1 Slice/66g	173	6.6	263	11.9	30.2	10.1	2.1
American Hot, Italian, Delight Mozz, Med, Domino's*	1 Slice/58g	155	6.2	266	12.0	29.7	10.6	2.1
American Hot, Italian, Delight Mozz, Sm, Domino's*	1 Slice/51g	137	5.8	269	12.1	28.9	11.3	2.0
American Hot, Italian, Lge, Domino's*	1 Slice/66g	153	6.7	233	10.6	24.1	10.2	1.8
American Hot, Italian, Med, Domino's*	1 Slice/58g	138	6.2	237	10.8	23.7	10.7	1.8
American Hot, Italian, Sm, Domino's*	1 Slice/51g	124	5.9	241	10.9	23.1	11.4	1.8
American Hot, Stuffed Crust, Delight Mozz, Lge, Domino's*	1 Slice/93g	230	9.9	247	11.6	25.3	10.6	2.1
American Hot, Stuffed Crust, Delight Mozz, Med, Domino's*	1 Slice/86g	216	9.3	250	11.8	25.3	10.8	2.1
American Hot, Stuffed Crust, Lge, Domino's*	1 Slice/932g	255	10.7	275	13.4	28.8	11.5	2.0
American Hot, Stuffed Crust, Med, Domino's*	1 Slice/86g	240	10.1	277	13.5	28.8	11.7	20.0
Americano, Classic, Delight Mozz, Lge, Domino's*	1 Slice/73g	213	6.7	290	15.1	36.0	9.1	2.1
Americano, Classic, Delight Mozz, Med, Domino's*	1 Slice/67g	197	6.3	292	15.1	35.8	9.4	2.1
Americano, Classic, Delight Mozz, Personal, Domino's*	1 Slice/203g	590	17.2	291	13.7	38.9	8.5	2.3
Americano, Classic, Delight Mozz, Sm, Domino's*	1 Slice/60g	182	5.9	303	14.9	37.8	9.8	2.5
Americano, Classic, Lge, Domino's*	1 Slice/73g	221	8.1	301	14.3	35.3	11.0	2.4
Americano, Classic, Med, Domino's*	1 Slice/68g	204	7.6	303	14.3	35.1	11.3	2.4
Americano, Classic, Personal, Domino's*	1 Pizza/203g	609	20.9	300	15.1	36.0	10.3	2.4
Americano, Classic, Sm, Domino's*	1 Slice/60g	183	7.3	305	15.5	32.4	12.1	2.5
Americano, Dominator, Lge, Domino's*	1 Slice/114g	334	11.4	293	14.1	37.0	10.0	1.8
Americano, GF, Delight Mozz, Sm, Domino's*	1 Slice/53g	159	5.9	302	13.7	35.5	11.2	2.5
Americano, GF, Sm, Domino's*	1 Pizza/317g	996	41.6	314	12.4	35.9	13.1	2.4
Americano, Italian, Delight Mozz, Lge, Domino's*	1 Slice/64g	192	6.7	299	18.4	31.8	10.4	2.8
Americano, Italian, Delight Mozz, Med, Domino's*	1 Slice/57g	172	6.2	302	18.5	31.3	10.9	2.8
Americano, Italian, Delight Mozz, Sm, Domino's*	1 Slice/50g	153	5.8	305	18.7	30.6	11.6	2.7
Americano, Italian, Lge, Domino's*	1 Slice/64g	197	7.8	307	15.5	33.0	12.1	2.4
Americano, Italian, Med, Domino's*	1 Slice/57g	176	7.2	310	15.6	32.5	12.6	2.4
Americano, Italian, Sm, Domino's*	1 Slice/50g	156	6.6	313	15.9	31.7	13.2	2.4
Americano, Stuffed Crust, BBQ, Lge, Domino's*	1 Slice/95g	269	10.5	284	13.4	31.4	11.1	2.7
Americano, Stuffed Crust, BBQ, Med, Domino's*	1 Slice/88g	253	10.0	285	13.3	31.4	11.3	2.7
Americano, Stuffed Crust, Delight Mozz, Lge, Domino's*	1 Slice/91g	256	9.7	280	15.1	30.0	10.6	1.9
Americano, Stuffed Crust, Delight Mozz, Med, Domino's*	1 Slice/85g	240	9.3	282	15.1	30.0	10.9	1.9
Americano, Stuffed Crust, Lge, Domino's*	1 Slice/91g	263	10.6	288	13.9	30.9	11.6	2.8
Americano, Stuffed Crust, Med, Domino's*	1 Slice/85g	247	10.1	290	13.9	30.8	11.8	2.8
Americao, Italian, Med, Domino's*	1 Slice/57g	177	7.2	310	15.6	32.5	12.6	2.4
Bacon Dbl Cheese, Classic, Delight Mozz, Domino's*	1 Pizza/232g	562	23.0	242	12.9	26.4	9.9	1.8

DOMINO'S*
PIZZA

INFO/WEIGHT	Measure	per Measure KCAL	FAT	Nutrition Values per 100g / 100ml KCAL	PROT	CARB	FAT	FIBRE
Bacon Dbl Cheese, Classic, Delight Mozz, Lge, Domino's*	1 Slice/85g	202	7.9	239	16.8	23.3	9.4	1.8
Bacon Dbl Cheese, Classic, Delight Mozz, Med, Domino's*	1 Slice/76g	183	7.1	240	16.8	23.3	9.3	1.8
Bacon Dbl Cheese, Classic, Delight Mozz, Sm, Domino's*	1 Slice/67g	160	6.5	239	13.4	26.0	9.7	1.7
Bacon Dbl Cheese, Italian, Delight Mozz, Lge, Domino's*	1 Slice/75g	185	7.6	247	14.2	26.4	10.2	1.8
Bacon Dbl Cheese, Italian, Delight Mozz, Med, Domino's*	1 Slice/66g	163	6.7	247	14.2	26.1	10.2	1.8
Bacon Dbl Cheese, Italian, Delight Mozz, Sm, Domino's*	1 Slice/57g	140	5.9	245	14.1	25.6	10.4	1.7
Bacon Dbl Cheese, Italian, Lge, Domino's*	1 Slice/75g	169	8.3	226	12.2	21.1	11.1	1.5
Bacon Dbl Cheese, Italian, Med, Domino's*	1 Slice/66g	149	7.4	226	12.2	20.8	11.2	1.5
Bacon Dbl Cheese, Italian, Sm, Domino's*	1 Slice/57g	128	6.5	224	12.1	20.5	11.3	1.5
Bacon Double Cheese, Classic, Lge, Domino's*	1 Slice/84g	212	10.0	251	12.2	25.5	11.8	1.6
Bacon Double Cheese, Classic, Med, Domino's*	1 Slice/76g	192	9.0	252	12.2	25.5	11.8	1.6
Bacon Double Cheese, Classic, Personal, Domino's*	1 Pizza/232g	585	25.1	252	12.1	27.6	10.8	1.9
Bacon Double Cheese, Classic, Sm, Domino's*	1 Slice/67g	163	7.3	246	13.1	25.0	11.1	1.7
Bacon Double Cheese, GF, Delight Mozz, Sm, Domino's*	1 Pizza/358g	846	36.2	236	14.1	23.8	10.1	1.9
Bacon Double Cheese, GF, Sm, Domino's*	1 Pizza/361g	840	43.3	233	10.1	22.7	12.0	2.1
Bacon Double Cheese, Stuffed Crust, Lge, Domino's*	1 Slice/102g	271	12.3	266	14.2	26.1	12.1	1.8
Bacon Double Cheese, Stuffed Crust, Med, Domino's*	1 Slice/94g	251	11.3	266	14.2	26.4	12.0	1.8
Bacon Double Cheese,Stuffed Crust, Med, Domino's*	1 Slice/94g	259	11.5	274	14.0	26.4	12.2	1.9
Carolina, Classic, Delight Mozz, Lge, Domino's*	1 Slice/79g	212	6.7	268	13.3	33.8	8.5	1.9
Carolina, Classic, Delight Mozz, Med, Domino's*	1 Slice/72g	194	6.2	269	13.4	33.7	8.6	1.9
Carolina, Classic, Delight Mozz, Personal, Domino's*	1 Slice/220g	605	19.9	274	11.9	35.5	9.0	2.0
Carolina, Classic, Delight Mozz, Sm, Domino's*	1 Slice/64g	176	5.5	277	12.9	35.7	8.7	2.3
Carolina, Classic, Lge, Domino's*	1 Slice/79g	220	8.2	278	12.6	33.0	10.3	2.1
Carolina, Classic, Med, Domino's*	1 Slice/72g	201	7.5	280	12.6	33.0	10.4	2.1
Carolina, Classic, Personal, Domino's*	1 Slice/220g	624	23.4	283	13.3	32.9	10.6	2.0
Carolina, GF, Delight Mozz, Sm, Domino's*	1 Slice/56g	153	5.6	273	11.6	33.3	10.0	2.3
Carolina, GF, Sm, Domino's*	1 Slice/56g	160	6.6	284	10.3	33.7	11.7	2.1
Carolina, Italian, Delight Mozz, Lge, Domino's*	1 Slice/69g	190	6.7	274	16.1	29.5	9.7	2.5
Carolina, Italian, Delight Mozz, Med, Domino's*	1 Slice/61g	169	6.1	275	16.2	29.2	9.9	2.5
Carolina, Italian, Delight Mozz, Sm, Domino's*	1 Slice/54g	147	5.5	274	16.1	28.6	10.2	2.4
Carolina, Italian, Sm, Domino's*	1 Slice/53g	150	6.2	281	13.5	29.6	11.7	2.1
Carolina, Stuffed Crust, Delight Mozz, Lge, Domino's*	1 Slice/97g	254	9.8	263	13.7	28.5	10.1	1.8
Carolina, Stuffed Crust, Delight Mozz, Med, Domino's*	1 Slice/90g	237	9.2	264	13.7	28.6	10.2	1.8
Carolina, Stuffed Crust, Lge, Domino's*	1 Slice/97g	262	10.6	271	12.5	29.3	11.0	2.6
Carolina, Thin & Crispy, Delight Mozz, Lge, Domino's*	1 Slice/58g	161	6.2	280	14.6	30.6	10.7	2.0
Cheese & Tomato, Classic, Delight Mozz, Domino's*	1 Personal/161g	419	10.6	260	11.8	37.1	6.6	2.4
Cheese & Tomato, Classic, Delight Mozz, Lge, Domino's*	1 Slice/58g	151	3.6	262	17.0	33.0	6.3	2.4
Cheese & Tomato, Classic, Delight Mozz, Med, Domino's*	1 Slice/53g	138	3.3	262	17.0	33.0	6.3	2.4
Cheese & Tomato, Classic, Delight Mozz, Sm, Domino's*	1 Slice/46g	120	3.1	263	12.3	37.3	6.7	2.3
Cheese & Tomato, Classic, Lge, Domino's*	1 Slice/58g	158	5.1	274	11.5	36.2	8.8	2.2
Cheese & Tomato, Classic, Med, Domino's*	1 Slice/53g	144	4.6	274	11.5	36.2	8.8	2.2
Cheese & Tomato, Classic, Med, Domino's*	1 Slice/53g	144	4.6	274	11.5	36.2	8.8	2.2
Cheese & Tomato, Classic, Personal, Domino's*	1 Slice/161g	435	11.3	270	11.6	38.9	7.0	2.5
Cheese & Tomato, Classic, Personal, Domino's*	1 Pizza/161g	435	11.3	270	11.6	38.9	7.0	2.5
Cheese & Tomato, Classic, Sm, Domino's*	1 Slice/45g	122	3.5	269	12.9	35.8	7.7	2.3
Cheese & Tomato, Classic, Sm, Domino's*	1 Slice/45g	122	3.5	269	12.9	35.8	7.7	2.3
Cheese & Tomato, Delight Mozz, Personal, Domino's*	1 Slice/50g	126	3.0	251	12.1	37.4	5.9	2.5
Cheese & Tomato, GF, Delight Mozz, Sm, Domino's*	1 Pizza/230g	606	15.7	263	13.1	36.0	6.8	2.7
Cheese & Tomato, GF, Sm, Domino's*	1 Slice/73g	185	6.2	252	8.2	34.2	8.4	3.0
Cheese & Tomato, GF, Sm, Domino's*	1 Pizza/231g	582	19.4	252	8.2	34.2	8.4	3.0
Cheese & Tomato, Italian, Delight Mozz, Lge, Domino's*	1 Slice/48g	135	3.4	279	13.0	39.7	7.0	2.6
Cheese & Tomato, Italian, Delight Mozz, Med, Domino's*	1 Slice/42g	117	2.9	279	13.0	39.7	7.0	2.6

	Measure INFO/WEIGHT	per Measure KCAL	FAT	Nutrition Values per 100g / 100ml KCAL	PROT	CARB	FAT	FIBRE

DOMINO'S*
PIZZA

	Measure INFO/WEIGHT	per Measure KCAL	FAT	KCAL	PROT	CARB	FAT	FIBRE
Cheese & Tomato, Italian, Delight Mozz, Sm, Domino's*	1 Sliceg/35g	99	2.5	279	13.0	39.7	7.0	2.6
Cheese & Tomato, Italian, Lge, Domino's*	1 Slice/48g	115	3.4	239	11.3	31.5	7.1	2.2
Cheese & Tomato, Italian, Med, Domino's*	1 Slice/42g	100	3.0	239	11.3	31.5	7.1	2.2
Cheese & Tomato, Italian, Med, Domino's*	1 Slice/42g	100	3.0	239	11.3	31.5	7.1	2.2
Cheese & Tomato, Italian, Sm, Domino's*	1 Slice/36g	85	2.5	239	11.3	31.5	7.1	2.2
Cheese & Tomato, Italian, Sm, Domino's*	1 Slice/36g	172	5.1	484	22.9	63.8	14.4	4.4
Cheese & Tomato, Italian, Sm, Domino's*	1 Slice/36g	85	2.5	239	11.3	31.5	7.1	2.2
Cheese & Tomato, Italian, Sm, Domino's*	1 Slice/36g	239	7.1	672	31.8	88.6	20.0	6.2
Cheese & Tomato, Italian, Sm, Domino's*	1 Slice/36g	85	2.5	239	11.3	31.5	7.1	2.2
Cheese & Tomato, Italian, Sm, Domino's*	1 Slice/35g	85	2.5	239	11.3	31.5	7.1	2.2
Cheese & Tomato, Personal, Domino's*	1 Slice/50g	140	3.6	278	15.1	38.3	7.2	2.4
Cheese & Tomato, Stuffed Crust, Lge, Domino's*	1 Slice/76g	218	7.4	288	14.4	34.6	9.8	2.3
Cheese & Tomato, Stuffed Crust, Med, Domino's*	1 Slice/69g	199	6.8	288	14.4	34.6	9.8	2.3
Cheese & Tomato, Stuffed Crust, Med, Domino's*	1 Slice/70g	203	6.9	288	14.4	34.6	9.8	2.3
Cheese & Tomato, Stuffed Crust, Med, Domino's*	1 Slice/70g	203	6.9	288	14.4	34.6	9.8	2.3
Chicken & Bacon, Classic, Delight Mozz, Domino's*	1 Personal/203g	508	15.6	250	13.6	30.5	7.7	2.1
Chicken & Bacon, Classic, Delight Mozz, Lge, Domino's*	1 Slice/73g	181	5.1	247	17.8	27.2	7.0	2.1
Chicken & Bacon, Classic, Delight Mozz, Med, Domino's*	1 Slice/67g	165	4.6	246	17.9	27.2	6.9	2.1
Chicken & Bacon, Classic, Delight Mozz, Sm, Domino's*	1 Slice/59g	145	4.3	246	14.1	30.3	7.3	2.1
Chicken & Bacon, Classic, Lge, Domino's*	1 Slice/73g	188	6.5	256	13.5	29.8	8.9	2.0
Chicken & Bacon, Classic, Med, Domino's*	1 Slice/67g	171	5.9	256	13.6	29.7	8.9	2.0
Chicken & Bacon, Classic, Personal, Domino's*	1 Pizza/203g	524	16.2	258	13.5	31.9	8.0	2.2
Chicken & Bacon, Classic, Sm, Domino's*	1 Slice/59g	147	4.7	251	14.7	29.1	8.1	2.1
Chicken & Bacon, GF, Delight Mozz, Sm, Domino's*	1 Pizza/310g	756	22.9	244	15.0	28.3	7.4	2.3
Chicken & Bacon, GF, Sm, Domino's*	1 Pizza/308g	726	26.5	236	11.4	27.0	8.6	2.6
Chicken & Bacon, Italian, Delight Mozz, Lge, Domino's*	1 Slice/64g	164	4.8	257	14.9	31.5	7.6	2.2
Chicken & Bacon, Italian, Delight Mozz, Med, Domino's*	1 Slice/56g	144	4.3	256	15.1	31.1	7.6	2.2
Chicken & Bacon, Italian, Delight Mozz, Sm, Domino's*	1 Slice/49g	124	3.7	254	15.1	30.6	7.6	2.2
Chicken & Bacon, Italian, Lge, Domino's*	1 Slice/64g	145	4.9	227	13.7	25.2	7.7	2.0
Chicken & Bacon, Italian, Med, Domino's*	1 Slice/57g	128	4.3	226	13.8	25.0	7.6	2.0
Chicken & Bacon, Italian, Med, Domino's*	1 Slice/49g	125	3.8	255	13.8	24.6	7.7	1.9
Chicken & Bacon, Stuffed Crust, Lge, Domino's*	1 Slice/91g	247	8.8	271	15.5	29.7	9.7	2.1
Chicken & Bacon, Stuffed Crust Med, Domino's*	1 Slice/85g	230	8.2	271	15.5	29.7	9.7	2.1
Chicken Feast, Classic, Delight Mozz, Lge, Domino's*	1 Slice/77g	177	4.0	231	18.5	26.7	5.2	2.2
Chicken Feast, Classic, Delight Mozz, Med, Domino's*	1 Slice/69g	161	3.6	232	18.7	26.6	5.2	2.2
Chicken Feast, Classic, Delight Mozz, Med, Domino's*	1 Pizza/207g	483	11.6	233	14.5	30.4	5.6	2.2
Chicken Feast, Classic, Delight Mozz, Sm, Domino's*	1 Slice/61g	141	3.3	232	15.1	29.8	5.5	2.1
Chicken Feast, Classic, Lge, Domino's*	1 Slice/77g	184	5.4	240	14.3	29.1	7.1	2.0
Chicken Feast, Classic, Med, Domino's*	1 Slice/69g	167	4.9	241	14.5	29.0	7.1	2.0
Chicken Feast, Classic, Personal, Domino's*	1 Pizza/207g	499	12.2	241	14.4	31.8	5.9	2.3
Chicken Feast, Classic, Sm, Domino's*	1 Slice/61g	143	3.8	236	15.6	28.6	6.3	2.1
Chicken Feast, Dominator, Lge, Domino's*	1 Slice/112g	289	9.2	258	13.9	32.3	8.2	2.0
Chicken Feast, GF, Delight Mozz, Sm, Domino's*	1 Pizza/322g	732	17.4	227	16.1	27.8	5.4	2.4
Chicken Feast, GF, Sm, Domino's*	1 Pizza/319g	702	21.1	220	12.6	26.5	6.6	2.6
Chicken Feast, Italian, Delight Mozz, Lge, Domino's*	1 Slice/67g	160	3.7	239	15.8	30.6	5.6	2.3
Chicken Feast, Italian, Delight Mozz, Med, Domino's*	1 Slice/59g	141	3.3	238	16.1	30.3	5.5	2.3
Chicken Feast, Italian, Delight Mozz, Sm, Domino's*	1 Slice/51g	120	2.8	237	16.2	30.0	5.5	2.3
Chicken Feast, Italian, Lge, Domino's*	1 Slice/67g	141	3.8	210	14.6	24.7	5.6	2.0
Chicken Feast, Italian, Med, Domino's*	1 Slice/59g	124	3.3	210	14.9	24.4	5.6	2.0
Chicken Feast, Italian, Sm, Domino's*	1 Slice/51g	106	2.8	209	15.0	24.2	5.6	2.0
Chicken Feast, Stuffed Crust, Lge, Domino's*	1 Slice/94g	243	7.7	258	16.1	29.1	8.2	2.1
Chicken Feast, Stuffed Crust, Med, Domino's*	1 Slice/87g	226	7.2	259	16.2	29.2	8.3	2.1

	Measure INFO/WEIGHT	per Measure		Nutrition Values per 100g / 100ml				
		KCAL	FAT	KCAL	PROT	CARB	FAT	FIBRE
PIZZA								
Deluxe, Classic, Delight Mozz, Lge, Domino's*	1 Slice/76g	188	6.6	246	15.0	26.1	8.6	2.1
Deluxe, Classic, Delight Mozz, Med, Domino's*	1 Slice/70g	174	6.2	248	15.1	25.9	8.9	2.1
Deluxe, Classic, Delight Mozz, Personal, Domino's*	1 Pizza/209g	513	17.9	246	11.3	29.8	8.6	2.1
Deluxe, Classic, Delight Mozz, Sm, Domino's*	1 Slice/62g	156	6.0	250	11.6	28.6	9.6	2.0
Deluxe, Classic, Lge, Domino's*	1 Slice/76g	195	8.0	255	10.9	28.5	10.5	1.9
Deluxe, Classic, Med, Domino's*	1 Slice/70g	180	7.6	257	11.0	28.3	10.8	1.9
Deluxe, Classic, Personal, Domino's*	1 Pizza/209g	530	18.6	253	11.1	31.2	8.9	2.2
Deluxe, Classic, Sm, Domino's*	1 Slice/62g	158	6.4	255	12.1	27.4	10.4	2.0
Deluxe, GF, Delight Mozz, Sm, Domino's*	1 Pizza/330g	822	33.3	249	12.1	26.5	10.1	2.2
Deluxe, GF, Sm, Domino's*	1 Pizza/331g	798	37.1	241	8.7	25.2	11.2	2.5
Deluxe, Italian, Delight Mozz, Lge, Domino's*	1 Slice/67g	171	6.3	256	11.9	30.0	9.4	2.2
Deluxe, Italian, Delight Mozz, Lge, Domino's*	1 Slice/67g	152	6.4	227	10.6	24.0	9.5	1.9
Deluxe, Italian, Delight Mozz, Med, Domino's*	1 Slice/60g	155	6.0	257	11.9	29.4	9.9	2.1
Deluxe, Italian, Delight Mozz, Sm, Domino's*	1 Slice/52g	135	5.4	259	12.0	28.5	10.4	2.1
Deluxe, Italian, Med, Domino's*	1 Slice/60g	137	5.9	229	10.7	23.6	9.9	1.9
Deluxe, Italian, Sm, Domino's*	1 Slice/52g	121	5.5	232	10.8	22.9	10.5	1.9
Deluxe, Stuffed Crust, Delight Mozz, Lge, Domino's*	1 Slice/94g	228	9.5	242	11.6	25.2	10.1	2.2
Deluxe, Stuffed Crust, Delight Mozz, Med, Domino's*	1 Slice/88g	215	9.1	244	11.7	25.2	10.3	2.1
Deluxe, Stuffed Crust, Lge, Domino's*	1 Slice/94g	254	10.3	270	13.3	28.7	11.0	2.1
Deluxe, Stuffed Crust, Med, Domino's*	1 Slice/88g	239	9.8	272	13.4	28.6	11.2	2.1
Extravaganza, Classic, Delight Mozz, Lge, Domino's*	1 Slice/87g	207	7.7	237	16.6	23.1	8.8	2.0
Extravaganza, Classic, Delight Mozz, Med, Domino's*	1 Slice/80g	190	7.1	238	16.6	23.0	8.9	2.0
Extravaganza, Classic, Delight Mozz, Personal, Domino's*	1 Pizza/245g	590	23.3	241	13.2	25.7	9.5	1.9
Extravaganza, Classic, Delight Mozz, Sm, Domino's*	1 Slice/71g	168	6.6	238	13.5	25.4	9.4	1.9
Extravaganza, Classic, Lge, Domino's*	1 Slice/87g	217	9.8	249	12.1	25.3	11.2	1.8
Extravaganza, Classic, Med, Domino's*	1 Slice/80g	199	9.0	249	12.2	25.1	11.3	1.8
Extravaganza, Classic, Personal, Domino's*	1 Pizza/245g	613	25.5	250	12.5	26.9	10.4	2.0
Extravaganza, Classic, Sm, Domino's*	1 Slice/71g	174	7.6	246	13.2	24.4	10.8	1.9
Extravaganza, GF, Delight Mozz, Sm, Domino's*	1 Pizza/381g	900	37.4	236	14.1	23.3	9.8	2.1
Extravaganza, GF, Sm, Domino's*	1 Pizza/381g	888	43.8	233	10.4	22.2	11.5	2.3
Extravaganza, Italian, Delight Mozz, Lge, Domino's*	1 Slice/78g	190	7.4	245	14.0	26.1	9.5	2.0
Extravaganza, Italian, Delight Mozz, Med, Domino's*	1 Slice/70g	170	6.8	244	14.1	25.5	9.7	2.0
Extravaganza, Italian, Delight Mozz, Sm, Domino's*	1 Slice/61g	148	6.1	244	14.1	24.9	10.0	2.0
Extravaganza, Italian, Lge, Domino's*	1 Slice/78g	174	8.1	224	12.1	21.0	10.4	1.8
Extravaganza, Italian, Med, Domino's*	1 Slice/70g	156	7.4	224	12.2	20.5	10.6	1.8
Extravaganza, Italian, Sm, Domino's*	1 Slice/61g	136	6.6	224	12.3	20.0	10.9	1.7
Extravaganza, Stuffed Crust, Delight Mozz, Lge, Domino's*	1 Slice/105g	247	10.6	235	13.3	22.9	10.1	2.0
Extravaganza, Stuffed Crust, Delight Mozz, Med, Domino's*	1 Slice/98g	231	10.0	236	13.3	22.9	10.2	2.0
Extravaganza, Stuffed Crust, Lge, Domino's*	1 Slice/105g	276	12.1	263	14.1	26.0	11.5	2.0
Extravaganza, Stuffed Crust, Med, Domino's*	1 Slice/98g	258	11.3	264	14.2	25.9	11.6	2.0
Extravaganzza, Lge Classic, Domino's*	1 Slice/104g	252	10.7	242	13.7	23.4	10.3	1.9
Extravaganzza, Lge Dominator, Domino's*	1 Slice/127g	337	14.1	266	13.3	28.2	11.1	1.9
Extravaganzza, Med Classic, Domino's*	1 Slice/95g	230	9.8	242	13.7	23.4	10.3	1.9
Extravaganzza, Sm Classic, Domino's*	1 Slice/86g	209	8.9	242	13.7	23.4	10.3	1.9
Farmhouse, Classic, Delight Mozz, Lge, Domino's*	1 Slice/76g	164	4.0	215	15.2	25.7	5.3	2.0
Farmhouse, Classic, Delight Mozz, Lge, Domino's*	1 Slice/70g	150	3.7	214	15.3	25.5	5.3	2.0
Farmhouse, Classic, Delight Mozz, Personal, Domino's*	1 Pizza/208g	453	11.6	218	11.4	29.4	5.6	2.0
Farmhouse, Classic, Lge, Domino's*	1 Slice/76g	171	5.5	224	11.0	28.1	7.2	1.9
Farmhouse, Classic, Med, Domino's*	1 Slice/70g	156	5.0	223	11.2	27.9	7.2	1.8
Farmhouse, Classic, Personal, Domino's*	1 Pizza/208g	469	12.3	225	11.3	30.8	5.9	2.1
Farmhouse, Classic, Sm, Domino's*	1 Slice/62g	135	3.9	217	12.3	27.0	6.3	1.9
Farmhouse, GF, Delight Mozz, Sm, Domino's*	1 Pizza/329g	678	18.1	206	12.4	26.0	5.5	2.1

	Measure INFO/WEIGHT	per Measure KCAL	FAT	Nutrition Values per 100g / 100ml KCAL	PROT	CARB	FAT	FIBRE
DOMINO'S*								
PIZZA								
Farmhouse, GF, Sm, Domino's*	1 Pizza/330g	654	21.8	198	9.0	24.8	6.6	2.3
Farmhouse, Italian, Delight Mozz, Lge, Domino's*	1 Slice/67g	148	3.8	220	12.1	29.5	5.6	2.1
Farmhouse, Italian, Delight Mozz, Med, Domino's*	1 Slice/60g	130	3.3	218	12.2	28.9	5.6	2.0
Farmhouse, Italian, Delight Mozz, Sm, Domino's*	1 Slice/52g	112	2.9	214	12.3	28.1	5.5	2.0
Farmhouse, Italian, Lge, Domino's*	1 Slice/67g	128	3.8	191	10.8	23.6	5.7	1.8
Farmhouse, Italian, Sm, Domino's*	1 Slice/52g	97	2.9	187	11.1	22.4	5.6	1.7
Farmhouse, Lge Classic, Domino's*	1 Slice/88g	195	6.0	222	13.4	26.8	6.8	2.1
Farmhouse, Lge Dominator, Domino's*	1 Slice/111g	283	9.4	255	13.0	31.7	8.5	2.0
Farmhouse, Stuffed Crust, Delight Mozz, Lge, Domino's*	1 Slice94g	205	7.0	217	11.8	24.9	7.4	2.1
Farmhouse, Stuffed Crust, Delight Mozz, Med, Domino's*	1 Slice/88g	191	6.5	217	11.9	24.8	7.4	2.1
Farmhouse, Stuffed Crust, Lge, Domino's*	1 Slice/94.g	230	7.8	244	13.4	28.3	8.3	2.0
Farmhouse, Stuffed Crust, Med, Domino's*	1 Slice/88g	215	7.3	245	13.5	28.3	8.3	2.0
Four Vegi, Classic, Delight Mozz, Lge, Domino's*	1 Slice/71g	159	3.7	225	14.4	29.1	5.3	2.5
Four Vegi, Classic, Delight Mozz, Med, Domino's*	1 Slice/64g	145	3.4	226	14.4	29.3	5.3	2.5
Four Vegi, Classic, Delight Mozz, Personal, Domino's*	1 Pizza/192g	442	10.8	230	10.4	33.3	5.6	2.6
Four Vegi, Classic, Delight Mozz, Sm, Domino's*	1 Slice/56g	126	3.1	224	10.4	32.3	5.5	2.4
Four Vegi, Classic, Lge, Domino's*	1 Slice/71g	166	5.2	235	9.9	31.7	7.3	2.3
Four Vegi, Classic, Med, Domino's*	1 Slice/64g	152	4.7	236	9.9	31.9	7.3	2.3
Four Vegi, Classic, Personal, Domino's*	1 Pizza/193g	459	11.4	238	10.3	34.8	5.9	2.7
Four Vegi, Classic, Sm, Domino's*	1 Slice/56g	129	3.5	229	11.0	31.1	6.3	2.4
Four Vegi, GF, Delight Mozz, Sm, Domino's*	1 Pizza/295g	642	15.9	218	10.8	30.6	5.4	2.7
Four Vegi, GF, Sm, Domino's*	1 Pizza/296g	618	19.8	209	7.0	29.2	6.7	3.0
Four Vegi, Italian, Delight Mozz, Lge, Domino's*	1 Slice/61g	142	3.4	233	10.9	33.8	5.6	2.6
Four Vegi, Italian, Delight Mozz, Med, Domino's*	1 Slice/54g	125	3.0	233	10.8	33.9	5.6	2.7
Four Vegi, Italian, Delight Mozz, Sm, Domino's*	1 Slice/46g	106	2.6	228	10.6	33.1	5.5	2.6
Four Vegi, Italian, Lge, Domino's*	1 Slice/61g	123	3.5	201	9.5	27.3	5.7	2.3
Four Vegi, Italian, Med, Domino's*	1 Slice/54g	108	3.1	201	9.5	27.4	5.7	2.4
Four Vegi, Italian, Sm, Domino's*	1 Slice/46g	91	2.6	197	9.3	26.8	5.6	2.3
Four Vegi, Stuffed Crust, Delight Mozz, Lge, Domino's*	1 Slice/88g	199	6.6	226	10.9	27.6	7.5	2.4
Four Vegi, Stuffed Crust, Delight Mozz, Med, Domino's*	1 Slice/82g	186	6.1	227	11.0	27.8	7.5	2.5
Four Vegi, Stuffed Crust, Lge, Domino's*	1 Slice/88g	225	7.5	255	12.7	31.2	8.5	2.4
Four Vegi, Stuffed Crust, Med, Domino's*	1 Slice/82g	210	7.0	256	12.8	31.5	8.5	2.4
Full House, Classic, Delight Mozz, Lge, Domino's*	1 Slice/84g	188	6.3	225	14.6	24.9	7.5	2.0
Full House, Classic, Delight Mozz, Med, Domino's*	1 Slice/77g	174	5.9	226	14.7	24.8	7.7	1.9
Full House, Classic, Delight Mozz, Personal, Domino's*	1 Pizza/239g	550	20.3	230	11.5	27.2	8.5	1.9
Full House, Classic, Delight Mozz, Sm, Domino's*	1 Slice/69g	155	5.6	226	11.5	27.1	8.2	1.8
Full House, Classic, Lge, Domino's*	1 Slice/84g	195	7.7	233	10.8	27.2	9.2	1.8
Full House, Classic, Med, Domino's*	1 Slice/77g	180	7.2	234	10.9	26.9	9.4	1.8
Full House, Classic, Personal, Domino's*	1 Pizza/239g	566	20.8	237	11.4	28.4	8.7	2.0
Full House, Classic, Sm, Domino's*	1 Slice/69g	158	6.1	230	12.0	26.1	8.9	1.9
Full House, GF, Delight Mozz, Sm, Domino's*	1 Pizza/368g	816	30.9	222	11.9	25.1	8.4	2.0
Full House, GF, Sm, Domino's*	1 Pizza/368g	792	34.6	215	8.9	24.0	9.4	2.3
Full House, Italian, Delight Mozz, Lge, Domino's*	1 Slice/74g	172	6.0	231	11.7	28.3	8.1	2.0
Full House, Italian, Delight Mozz, Med, Domino's*	1 Slice/66g	153	5.5	231	11.8	27.7	8.3	2.0
Full House, Italian, Delight Mozz, Sm, Domino's*	1 Slice/59g	135	5.0	230	11.8	26.9	8.6	1.9
Full House, Italian, Lge, Domino's*	1 Slice/75g	153	6.1	205	10.6	22.9	8.2	1.8
Full House, Italian, Med, Domino's*	1 Slice/66g	136	5.5	206	10.7	22.5	8.4	1.7
Full House, Italian, Sm, Domino's*	1 Slice/59g	120	5.1	205	10.8	21.9	8.7	1.7
Full House, Lge Classic, Domino's*	1 Slice/111g	268	9.9	241	13.2	27.0	8.9	2.1
Full House, Sm Classic, Domino's*	1 Slice/94g	227	8.6	242	13.5	26.3	9.2	2.1
Full House, Stuffed Crust, Delight Mozz, Lge, Domino's*	1 Slice/101g	229	9.2	226	11.5	24.3	9.1	2.0
Full House, Stuffed Crust, Delight Mozz, Med, Domino's*	1 Slice/95g	215	8.7	227	11.6	24.3	9.2	2.0

	Measure INFO/WEIGHT	per Measure KCAL	FAT	Nutrition Values per 100g / 100ml KCAL	PROT	CARB	FAT	FIBRE
DOMINO'S*								
PIZZA								
Full House, Stuffed Crust, Lge, Domino's*	1 Slice/102g	255	10.1	251	13.1	27.5	9.9	2.0
Ham & Pineapple, Classic, Delight Mozz, Lge, Domino's*	1 Slice/73g	165	4.0	227	15.7	27.6	5.5	1.9
Ham & Pineapple, Classic, Delight Mozz, Sm, Domino's*	1 Slice/60g	133	3.5	223	12.1	30.0	5.8	1.8
Ham & Pineapple, Classic, Lge, Domino's*	1 Slice/73g	172	5.5	236	11.4	30.1	7.5	1.7
Ham & Pineapple, Classic, Med, Domino's*	1 Slice/67g	157	5.0	235	11.5	29.8	7.5	1.7
Ham & Pineapple, Classic, Personal, Domino's*	1 Pizza/201g	472	12.3	235	11.5	32.5	6.1	2.0
Ham & Pineapple, Classic, Sm, Domino's*	1 Slice/60g	136	3.9	228	12.7	28.8	6.5	1.8
Ham & Pineapple, GF, Delight Mozz, Sm, Domino's*	1 Pizza/314g	684	17.9	218	12.8	28.1	5.7	2.0
Ham & Pineapple, GF, Sm, Domino's*	1 Pizza/314g	660	21.7	210	9.2	26.8	6.9	2.2
Ham & Pineapple, Italian, Delight Mozz, Lge, Domino's*	1 Slice/64g	149	3.8	234	12.5	31.9	5.9	2.0
Ham & Pineapple, Italian, Delight Mozz, Med, Domino's*	1 Slice/56g	131	3.3	232	12.6	31.2	5.9	1.9
Ham & Pineapple, Italian, Delight Mozz, Sm, Domino's*	1 Slice/50g	113	2.9	227	12.7	30.3	5.8	1.8
Ham & Pineapple, Italian, Lge, Domino's*	1 Slice/63g	129	3.8	204	11.2	25.6	6.0	1.7
Ham & Pineapple, Italian, Med, Domino's*	1 Slice/56g	114	3.3	202	11.3	25.1	5.9	1.6
Ham & Pineapple, Italian, Sm, Domino's*	1 Slice/49g	98	2.9	198	11.4	24.4	5.8	1.6
Ham & Pineapple, Stuffed Crust, Lge, Domino's*	1 Slice/91g	231	7.8	255	13.8	30.0	8.6	1.9
Ham & Pineapple, Stuffed Crust, Med, Domino's*	1 Slice/85g	216	7.3	255	13.9	29.8	8.6	1.9
Hawaiian, Classic, Delight Mozz, Lge, Domino's*	1 Slice/78g	166	4.1	212	14.8	25.7	5.2	1.9
Hawaiian, Classic, Delight Mozz, Lge, Domino's*	1 Slice/72g	152	3.7	212	14.9	25.5	5.2	1.8
Hawaiian, Classic, Delight Mozz, Personal, Domino's*	1 Pizza/214g	458	11.8	214	11.1	29.3	5.5	1.9
Hawaiian, Classic, Delight Mozz, Sm, Domino's*	1 Slice/63g	133	3.4	210	11.5	28.1	5.4	1.7
Hawaiian, Classic, Med, Domino's*	1 Slice/71g	158	5.0	221	10.9	27.9	7.0	1.7
Hawaiian, Classic, Personal, Domino's*	1 Pizza/214g	474	12.4	222	11.0	30.6	5.8	2.0
Hawaiian, Classic, Sm, Domino's*	1 Slice/64g	136	3.9	214	12.0	27.0	6.1	1.7
Hawaiian, Delight Mozz, Personal Pizza, Domino's*	1 Slice/66g	145	3.6	219	12.0	30.7	5.4	2.1
Hawaiian, Delight Mozz, Sm Classic, Domino's*	1 Slice/79g	173	4.2	220	15.2	27.7	5.4	2.2
Hawaiian, GF, Delight Mozz, Sm, Domino's*	1 Pizza/340g	690	18.0	203	12.0	26.0	5.3	1.9
Hawaiian, Italian, Delight Mozz, Lge, Domino's*	1 Slice/69g	149	3.8	217	11.7	29.5	5.5	1.9
Hawaiian, Italian, Delight Mozz, Med, Domino's*	1 Slice/61g	131	3.3	215	11.8	28.9	5.4	1.9
Hawaiian, Italian, Delight Mozz, Sm, Domino's*	1 Slice/54g	113	2.9	210	11.8	28.0	5.4	1.8
Hawaiian, Italian, Lge, Domino's*	1 Slice/69g	130	3.9	189	10.5	23.7	5.6	1.6
Hawaiian, Italian, Med, Domino's*	1 Slice/61g	115	3.4	187	10.6	23.2	5.5	1.6
Hawaiian, Lge Classic, Domino's*	1 Slice/78g	173	5.5	221	10.7	28.1	7.0	1.7
Hawaiian, Lge Dominator, Domino's*	1 Slice/113g	285	9.5	252	12.7	31.6	8.4	2.0
Hawaiian, Personal Pizza, Domino's*	1 Slice/63g	152	4.0	240	14.4	31.3	6.3	2.0
Hawaiian, Sm Classic, Domino's*	1 Slice/75g	168	5.0	224	13.7	27.2	6.7	2.1
Hawaiian, Stuffed Crust, Delight Mozz, Lge, Domino's*	1 Slice/96g	206	7.0	215	11.5	24.9	7.3	2.0
Hawaiian, Stuffed Crust, Delight Mozz, Med, Domino's*	1 Slice/90g	193	6.6	215	11.6	24.9	7.3	2.0
Hawaiian, Stuffed Crust, Lge, Domino's*	1 Slice/96g	232	7.8	242	13.2	28.3	8.1	1.9
Hawaiian, Stuffed Crust, Med, Domino's*	1 Slice/90g	217	7.3	242	13.3	28.3	8.1	1.9
Hot & Spicy, Classic, Delight Mozz, Lge, Domino's*	1 Slice/73g	161	4.5	220	14.7	27.2	6.2	2.1
Hot & Spicy, Classic, Delight Mozz, Med, Domino's*	1 Slice/66g	146	4.1	221	14.8	27.2	6.2	2.1
Hot & Spicy, Classic, Delight Mozz, Personal, Domino's*	1 Pizza/198g	443	12.9	224	10.8	31.2	6.5	2.2
Hot & Spicy, Classic, Delight Mozz, Sm, Domino's*	1 Slice/58g	128	3.8	220	11.0	30.4	6.5	2.0
Hot & Spicy, Classic, Lge, Domino's*	1 Slice/73g	168	5.9	230	10.4	29.7	8.1	2.0
Hot & Spicy, Classic, Med, Domino's*	1 Slice/66g	152	5.4	230	10.4	29.8	8.1	2.0
Hot & Spicy, Classic, Personal, Domino's*	1 Pizza/197g	459	13.4	233	10.7	32.7	6.8	2.3
Hot & Spicy, Classic, Sm, Domino's*	1 Slice/58g	130	4.2	225	11.5	29.1	7.3	2.0
Hot & Spicy, GF, Delight Mozz, Sm, Domino's*	1 Pizza/306g	654	19.9	214	11.4	28.4	6.5	2.3
Hot & Spicy, GF, Sm, Domino's*	1 Pizza/306g	630	23.9	206	7.7	27.1	7.8	2.5
Hot & Spicy, Italian, Delight Mozz, Lge, Domino's*	1 Slice/63g	144	4.3	227	11.4	31.4	6.7	2.2
Hot & Spicy, Italian, Delight Mozz, Med, Domino's*	1 Slice/56g	126	3.7	226	11.3	31.2	6.7	2.2

	Measure INFO/WEIGHT	per Measure		Nutrition Values per 100g / 100ml				
		KCAL	FAT	KCAL	PROT	CARB	FAT	FIBRE

DOMINO'S*
PIZZA

	Measure INFO/WEIGHT	KCAL	FAT	KCAL	PROT	CARB	FAT	FIBRE
Hot & Spicy, Italian, Delight Mozz, Med, Domino's*	1 Slice/48g	107	3.2	223	11.3	30.7	6.7	2.2
Hot & Spicy, Italian, Lge, Domino's*	1 Slice/63g	125	4.3	197	10.1	25.1	6.8	1.9
Hot & Spicy, Italian, Med, Domino's*	1 Slice/56g	109	3.7	196	10.0	25.0	6.7	1.9
Hot & Spicy, Lge Dominator, Domino's*	1 Slice/107g	282	9.8	264	12.2	33.0	9.2	2.2
Hot & Spicy, Stuffed Crust, Delight Mozz, Lge, Domino's*	1 Slice/91g	201	7.4	222	11.3	26.1	8.2	2.2
Hot & Spicy, Stuffed Crust, Delight Mozz, Med, Domino's*	1 Slice/84g	187	6.9	223	11.3	26.2	8.2	2.2
Hot & Spicy, Stuffed Crust, Lge, Domino's*	1 Slice/91g	227	8.3	250	13.0	29.6	9.1	2.1
Hot & Spicy, Stuffed Crust, Med, Domino's*	1 Slice/84g	211	7.6	251	13.1	29.8	9.1	2.1
House Special, Chicken, Classic, Lge, Domino's*	1 Slice/87g	231	10.4	267	14.4	24.9	12.0	1.7
House Special, Chicken, Classic, Med, Domino's*	1 Slice/79g	213	9.7	269	14.5	24.8	12.2	1.7
House Special, Chicken, Classic, Personal, Domino's*	1 Pizza/242g	662	28.8	274	14.4	26.7	11.9	1.9
House Special, Chicken, GF, Delight Mozz, Sm, Domino's*	1 Pizza/375g	972	40.5	259	16.7	22.9	10.8	1.9
House Special, Chicken, GF, Sm, Domino's*	1 Pizza/375g	960	47.2	256	12.8	21.9	12.6	2.1
House Special, Chicken, Stuffed Crust, Lge, Domino's*	1 Slice/104g	291	12.7	279	16.0	25.7	12.2	1.8
House Special, Chicken, Stuffed Crust, Med, Domino's*	1 Slice/97g	271	11.9	280	16.1	25.7	12.3	1.8
House Special, Roast Chicken, Classic, Sm, Domino's*	1 Slice/70g	186	8.2	266	15.4	24.1	11.7	1.7
House Special, Roast Chicken, Italian, Lge, Domino's*	1 Slice/77g	189	8.7	245	14.6	20.6	11.3	1.6
House Special, Tandoori, Classic, Lge, Domino's*	1 Slice/87g	233	10.4	269	14.3	25.2	12.0	1.7
House Special, Tandoori, Classic, Med, Domino's*	1 Slice/79g	214	9.7	270	14.4	25.1	12.2	1.6
House Special, Tandoori, Classic, Sm, Domino's*	1 Slice/67g	177	7.5	266	15.0	25.5	11.2	1.8
House Special, Tandoori, GF, Sm, Domino's*	1 Pizza/358g	912	43.3	255	12.2	23.3	12.1	2.2
House Special, Tandoori, Italian, Lge, Domino's*	1 Slice/77g	190	8.7	246	14.5	20.9	11.3	1.5
House Special, Tandoori, Italian, Med, Domino's*	1 Slice/69g	170	8.0	248	14.7	20.5	11.7	1.6
House Special, Tandoori, Italian, Sm, Domino's*	1 Slice/57g	140	6.5	247	14.3	21.1	11.4	1.6
House Special, Tandoori, Stuffed Crust, Lge, Domino's*	1 Slice/104g	292	12.7	280	15.9	25.9	12.2	1.8
Meat Lovers, Classic, Delight Mozz, Lge, Domino's*	1 Slice/76g	202	8.2	265	17.3	25.5	10.8	1.8
Meat Lovers, Classic, Delight Mozz, Med, Domino's*	1 Slice/70g	186	7.6	266	17.3	25.2	10.9	1.8
Meat Lovers, Classic, Delight Mozz, Personal, Domino's*	1 Pizza/206g	546	22.3	265	13.1	29.4	10.8	1.9
Meat Lovers, Classic, Delight Mozz, Sm, Domino's*	1 Slice63g	167	7.3	267	13.9	27.7	11.6	1.7
Meat Lovers, Classic, Lge, Domino's*	1 Slice/76g	209	9.6	275	13.1	27.9	12.6	1.7
Meat Lovers, Classic, Med, Domino's*	1 Slice/70g	192	8.9	275	13.2	27.6	12.8	1.7
Meat Lovers, Classic, Personal, Domino's*	1 Pizza/206g	562	22.9	273	12.9	30.8	11.1	2.0
Meat Lovers, Classic, Sm, Domino's*	1 Slice/63g	170	7.7	272	14.4	26.5	12.3	1.7
Meat Lovers, GF, Delight Mozz, Sm, Domino's*	1 Pizza/331g	888	40.8	268	14.7	25.5	12.3	1.9
Meat Lovers, GF, Sm, Domino's*	1 Pizza/332g	864	44.5	260	11.4	24.3	13.4	2.1
Meat Lovers, Italian, Delight Mozz, Lge, Domino's*	1 Slice/67g	185	7.9	278	14.4	29.3	11.9	1.9
Meat Lovers, Italian, Delight Mozz, Med, Domino's*	1 Slice/60g	166	7.3	279	14.6	28.6	12.2	1.8
Meat Lovers, Italian, Delight Mozz, Sm, Domino's*	1 Slice/53g	147	6.7	279	14.8	27.5	12.7	1.8
Meat Lovers, Italian, Lge, Domino's*	1 Slice/67g	166	8.0	249	13.2	23.3	12.0	1.6
Meat Lovers, Italian, Med, Domino's*	1 Slice/60g	149	7.3	250	13.4	22.8	12.3	1.6
Meat Lovers, Italian, Sm, Domino's*	1 Slice/52g	132	6.7	252	13.6	21.9	12.8	1.5
Meat Lovers, Stuffed Crust, Delight Mozz, Lge, Domino's*	1 Slice/94g	243	11.1	258	13.5	24.7	11.8	1.9
Meat Lovers, Stuffed Crust, Delight Mozz, Med, Domino's*	1 Slice/88g	227	10.4	259	13.5	24.6	11.9	1.9
Meat Lovers, Stuffed Crust, Lge, Domino's*	1 Slice/94g	268	11.9	286	15.2	28.2	12.7	1.9
Meat Lovers, Stuffed Crust, Med, Domino's*	1 Slice/88g	251	11.2	286	15.2	28.1	12.8	1.9
Meateor, Classic, Delight Mozz, Lge, Domino's*	1 Slice/78g	224	8.8	286	13.4	33.5	11.2	1.8
Meateor, Classic, Delight Mozz, Med, Domino's*	1 Slice/72g	207	8.2	287	13.4	33.2	11.4	1.8
Meateor, Classic, Delight Mozz, Personal, Domino's*	1 Pizza/235g	682	28.2	290	12.5	33.3	12.0	1.8
Meateor, Classic, Delight Mozz, Sm, Domino's*	1 Slice/65g	191	7.6	295	13.2	34.7	11.7	2.1
Meateor, Classic, Lge, Domino's*	1 Slice/78g	232	10.1	296	12.7	32.8	12.9	2.0
Meateor, Classic, Med, Domino's*	1 Slice/72g	214	9.4	297	12.7	32.4	13.1	2.0
Meateor, Classic, Personal, Domino's*	1 Pizza/235g	701	31.8	298	13.7	30.9	13.5	1.8

	Measure INFO/WEIGHT	per Measure KCAL	FAT	Nutrition Values per 100g / 100ml KCAL	PROT	CARB	FAT	FIBRE
DOMINO'S*								
PIZZA								
Meateor, Classic, Sm, Domino's*	1 Slice/65g	192	9.0	297	13.7	29.7	13.9	2.1
Meateor, GF, Delight Mozz, Sm, Domino's*	1 Pizza/346g	1014	46.0	293	11.9	32.1	13.3	2.0
Meateor, GF, Sm, Domino's*	1 Pizza/345g	1050	51.8	304	10.7	32.5	15.0	1.9
Meateor, Italian, Delight Mozz, Lge, Domino's*	1 Slice/69g	203	8.8	294	16.3	29.2	12.7	0.0
Meateor, Italian, Delight Mozz, Med, Domino's*	1 Slice/62g	182	8.1	295	16.3	28.6	13.1	2.3
Meateor, Italian, Delight Mozz, Sm, Domino's*	1 Slice/55g	162	7.5	296	16.3	27.5	13.7	2.2
Meateor, Italian, Lge, Domino's*	1 Slice/69g	207	9.8	301	13.5	30.4	14.3	2.0
Meateor, Italian, Med, Domino's*	1 Slice/62g	186	9.1	302	13.6	29.7	14.7	1.9
Meateor, Italian, Sm, Domino's*	1 Slice/55g	166	8.4	302	13.7	28.5	15.2	1.9
Meateor, Stuffed Crust, Delight Mozz, Lge, Domino's*	1 Slice/96g	266	11.8	277	13.8	28.3	12.3	1.6
Meateor, Stuffed Crust, Delight Mozz, Med, Domino's*	1 Slice/90g	250	11.2	278	13.8	28.2	12.4	1.6
Meateor, Stuffed Crust, Lge, Domino's*	1 Slice/96g	274	12.6	285	12.6	29.1	13.1	2.5
Meateor, Stuffed Crust, Med, Domino's*	1 Slice/90g	257	11.9	285	12.6	28.9	13.2	2.5
Meatilicious, Classic, Delight Mozz, Lge, Domino's*	1 Slice/72g	195	6.7	269	18.6	26.9	9.2	2.0
Meatilicious, Classic, Delight Mozz, Med, Domino's*	1 Slice/67g	180	6.2	269	18.6	26.7	9.3	2.0
Meatilicious, Classic, Delight Mozz, Personal, Domino's*	1 Pizza/214g	578	22.0	270	14.5	28.8	10.3	2.0
Meatilicious, Classic, Delight Mozz, Sm, Domino's*	1 Slice/60g	161	6.0	270	15.0	29.4	10.0	1.9
Meatilicious, Classic, Lge, Domino's*	1 Slice/73g	202	8.1	278	14.2	29.5	11.2	1.9
Meatilicious, Classic, Med, Domino's*	1 Slice/67g	186	7.6	278	14.2	29.2	11.3	1.9
Meatilicious, Classic, Personal, Domino's*	1 Plzza/214g	594	22.7	277	14.4	30.1	10.6	2.1
Meatilicious, Classic, Sm, Domino's*	1 Slice/60g	164	6.4	275	15.6	28.2	10.7	1.9
Meatilicious, GF, Delight Mozz, Sm, Domino's*	1 Pizza/314g	852	33.0	271	16.0	27.3	10.5	2.1
Meatilicious, GF, Sm, Domino's*	1 Pizza/315g	828	36.8	263	12.5	26.0	11.7	2.4
Meatilicious, Italian, Delight Mozz, Lge, Domino's*	1 Slice/63g	179	6.5	283	15.7	31.2	10.2	2.1
Meatilicious, Italian, Delight Mozz, Med, Domino's*	1 Slice/56g	159	5.8	283	15.9	30.5	10.4	2.1
Meatilicious, Italian, Delight Mozz, Sm, Domino's*	1 Slice/50g	141	5.4	283	16.1	29.5	10.8	2.0
Meatilicious, Italian, Lge, Domino's*	1 Slice/63g	160	6.5	252	14.5	24.9	10.2	1.8
Meatilicious, Italian, Med, Domino's*	1 Slice/57g	143	5.9	253	14.6	24.4	10.5	1.8
Meatilicious, Italian, Sm, Domino's*	1 Slice/49g	126	5.4	255	14.9	23.6	10.9	1.8
Meatilicious, Stuffed Crust, Delight Mozz, Lge, Domino's*	1 Slice/90g	236	9.6	261	14.3	25.9	10.6	2.1
Meatilicious, Stuffed Crust, Delight Mozz, Med, Domino's*	1 Slice/85g	221	9.1	261	14.3	25.8	10.7	2.1
Meatilicious, Stuffed Crust, Lge, Domino's*	1 Slice/91g	262	10.5	289	16.1	29.5	11.6	2.0
Meatilicious, Stuffed Crust, Med, Domino's*	1 Slice/85g	245	9.8	289	16.1	29.3	11.6	2.0
Meatzza, Classic, Delight Mozz, Lge, Domino's*	1 Slice/76g	198	7.6	261	17.4	25.9	10.0	1.9
Meatzza, Classic, Delight Mozz, Med, Domino's*	1 Slice/70g	184	7.2	262	17.5	25.5	10.2	1.9
Meatzza, Classic, Delight Mozz, Personal, Domino's*	1 Pizza/207g	537	20.5	259	13.2	29.8	9.9	2.0
Meatzza, Classic, Delight Mozz, Sm, Domino's*	1 Slice/63g	166	6.9	263	14.1	27.9	11.0	1.8
Meatzza, Classic, Lge, Domino's*	1 Slice/76g	205	9.0	270	13.3	28.4	11.9	1.5
Meatzza, Classic, Med, Domino's*	1 Slice/70g	190	8.5	271	13.4	27.9	12.1	1.6
Meatzza, Classic, Personal, Domino's*	1 Pizza/207g	553	21.1	267	13.1	31.2	10.2	2.1
Meatzza, Classic, Sm, Domino's*	1 Slice/63g	168	7.3	268	14.6	26.8	11.7	1.8
Meatzza, GF, Delight Mozz, Med, Domino's*	1 Pizza/335g	882	38.9	263	14.9	25.8	11.6	2.0
Meatzza, GF, Sm, Domino's*	1 Pizza/335g	858	42.6	256	11.6	24.6	12.7	2.2
Meatzza, Italian, Delight Mozz, Lge, Domino's*	1 Slice/67g	182	7.4	273	14.6	29.8	11.1	2.0
Meatzza, Italian, Delight Mozz, Med, Domino's*	1 Slice/600g	163	6.8	274	14.7	29.0	11.4	1.9
Meatzza, Italian, Delight Mozz, Med, Domino's*	1 Slice/53g	145	6.3	274	14.9	11.9	11.9	1.8
Meatzza, Italian, Lge, Domino's*	1 Slice/66g	162	7.4	244	13.4	23.8	11.1	1.6
Meatzza, Italian, Med, Domino's*	1 Slice/60g	147	6.9	246	13.5	23.2	11.5	1.7
Meatzza, Italian, Sm, Domino's*	1 Slice/53g	131	6.4	247	13.8	22.3	12.0	1.6
Meatzza, Stuffed Crust, Delight Mozz, Lge, Domino's*	1 Slice/94g	239	10.6	255	13.6	25.1	11.3	2.0
Meatzza, Stuffed Crust, Delight Mozz, Med, Domino's*	1 Slice/88g	225	10.0	256	13.6	24.9	11.4	2.0
Meatzza, Stuffed Crust, Lge, Domino's*	1 Slice/94g	265	11.4	282	15.3	26.6	12.1	1.6

	Measure INFO/WEIGHT	per Measure KCAL	FAT	Nutrition Values per 100g / 100ml KCAL	PROT	CARB	FAT	FIBRE
DOMINO'S*								
PIZZA								
Meatzza, Stuffed Crust, Med, Domino's*	1 Slice/89g	249	10.7	283	15.3	28.3	12.2	1.9
Mexican Hot, Classic, Delight Mozz, Lge, Domino's*	1 Slice/80g	196	6.9	245	16.5	24.7	8.6	1.9
Mexican Hot, Classic, Delight Mozz, Med, Domino's*	1 Slice/73g	180	6.4	247	13.6	24.6	8.8	1.9
Mexican Hot, Classic, Delight Mozz, Personal, Domino's*	1 Pizza/210g	513	17.2	244	12.5	29.2	8.2	2.0
Mexican Hot, Classic, Delight Mozz, Sm, Domino's*	1 Slice/64g	159	6.0	249	13.1	27.4	9.4	1.8
Mexican Hot, Classic, Lge, Domino's*	1 Slice/80g	206	8.9	258	11.7	27.0	11.2	1.8
Mexican Hot, Classic, Med, Domino's*	1 Slice/73g	189	8.3	260	11.8	26.9	11.4	1.8
Mexican Hot, Classic, Personal, Domino's*	1 Pizza/210g	536	19.3	255	11.7	30.5	9.2	2.1
Mexican Hot, Classic, Sm, Domino's*	1 Slice/64g	164	7.0	257	12.8	26.3	10.9	1.9
Mexican Hot, GF, Delight Mozz, Sm, Domino's*	1 Pizza/339g	840	33.2	248	13.8	25.3	9.8	2.0
Mexican Hot, GF, Sm, Domino's*	1 Pizza/339g	828	39.7	244	9.6	24.1	11.7	2.3
Mexican Hot, Italian, Delight Mozz, Lge, Domino's*	1 Slice/70g	179	6.5	255	13.7	28.2	9.3	2.0
Mexican Hot, Italian, Delight Mozz, Med, Domino's*	1 Slice/63g	160	6.1	256	13.8	27.7	9.7	2.0
Mexican Hot, Italian, Delight Mozz, Sm, Domino's*	1 Slice/54g	139	5.5	257	13.8	27.2	10.1	1.9
Mexican Hot, Italian, Lge, Domino's*	1 Slice/70g	163	7.2	232	11.6	22.5	10.3	1.7
Mexican Hot, Italian, Med, Domino's*	1 Slice/62g	146	6.7	234	11.7	22.1	10.7	1.7
Mexican Hot, Italian, Sm, Domino's*	1 Slice/54g	127	5.9	235	11.7	21.7	11.0	1.7
Mexican Hot, Stuffed Crust, Delight Mozz, Lge, Domino's*	1 Slice/98g	236	9.8	242	13.0	24.1	10.0	2.0
Mexican Hot, Stuffed Crust, Delight Mozz, Med, Domino's*	1 Slice/91g	221	9.2	244	13.0	24.1	10.2	2.0
Mexican Hot, Stuffed Crust, Lge, Domino's*	1 Slice/97g	265	11.2	272	13.9	27.4	11.5	1.9
Mexican Hot, Stuffed Crust, Med, Domino's*	1 Slice/91g	248	10.6	274	14.0	27.5	11.7	1.9
Mighty Meaty, Classic, Delight Mozz, Lge, Domino's*	1 Slice/83g	200	7.6	241	16.1	24.1	9.2	1.9
Mighty Meaty, Classic, Delight Mozz, Med, Domino's*	1 Slice/77g	186	7.2	243	16.2	23.8	9.4	1.8
Mighty Meaty, Classic, Delight Mozz, Personal, Domino's*	1 Pizza/223g	542	20.5	243	12.4	28.0	9.2	1.9
Mighty Meaty, Classic, Delight Mozz, Sm, Domino's*	1 Slice/68g	167	6.9	244	13.0	26.0	10.1	1.7
Mighty Meaty, Classic, Lge, Domino's*	1 Slice/83g	207	9.1	250	23.3	26.3	11.0	1.7
Mighty Meaty, Classic, Med, Domino's*	1 Slice/76g	192	8.6	251	12.4	26.0	11.2	1.7
Mighty Meaty, Classic, Personal, Domino's*	1 Pizza/223g	558	21.2	250	12.3	29.3	9.5	2.0
Mighty Meaty, GF, Delight Mozz, Sm, Domino's*	1 Pizza/368g	888	38.7	241	13.7	23.9	10.5	1.9
Mighty Meaty, GF, Sm, Domino's*	1 Pizza/369g	864	42.5	234	10.6	22.7	11.5	2.1
Mighty Meaty, Italian, Delight Mozz, Lge, Domino's*	1 Slice/74g	184	7.4	250	13.4	27.4	10.0	1.9
Mighty Meaty, Italian, Delight Mozz, Med, Domino's*	1 Slice/66g	165	6.9	250	13.5	26.7	10.4	1.9
Mighty Meaty, Italian, Delight Mozz, Sm, Domino's*	1 Slice/59g	147	6.4	250	13.6	25.6	10.8	1.8
Mighty Meaty, Italian, Lge, Domino's*	1 Slice/73g	164	7.4	224	12.2	22.0	10.1	1.7
Mighty Meaty, Italian, Med, Domino's*	1 Slice/66g	148	6.8	225	12.4	21.4	10.4	1.6
Mighty Meaty, Stuffed Crust, Delight Mozz, Lge, Domino's*	1 Slice/101g	241	10.6	239	12.7	23.7	10.5	2.0
Mighty Meaty, Stuffed Crust, Delight Mozz, Med, Domino's*	1 Slice/95g	227	10.0	240	12.8	23.5	10.6	1.9
Mighty Meaty, Stuffed Crust, Lge, Domino's*	1 Slice/100g	266	11.3	265	14.3	26.9	11.3	1.9
Mighty Meaty, Stuffed Crust, Med, Domino's*	1 Slice/94g	250	10.8	266	14.4	26.7	11.5	1.9
Mixed Grill, Classic, Delight Mozz, Lge, Domino's*	1 Slice/80g	197	7.2	245	15.0	25.0	9.0	2.1
Mixed Grill, Classic, Delight Mozz, Med, Domino's*	1 Slice/74g	182	6.8	246	15.1	24.9	9.2	2.0
Mixed Grill, Classic, Delight Mozz, Personal, Domino's*	1 Pizza/223g	554	21.4	248	11.4	28.1	9.6	2.0
Mixed Grill, Classic, Delight Mozz, Sm, Domino's*	1 Slice/66g	163	6.4	246	11.7	27.3	9.7	2.0
Mixed Grill, Classic, Lge, Domino's*	1 Slice/80g	204	8.7	254	11.1	27.3	10.8	1.9
Mixed Grill, Classic, Med, Domino's*	1 Slice/74g	188	8.1	254	11.1	27.1	10.9	1.9
Mixed Grill, Classic, Personal, Domino's*	1 Pizza/224g	570	22.1	255	11.3	29.4	9.9	2.1
Mixed Grill, Classic, Sm, Domino's*	1 Slice/66g	166	6.9	251	12.2	26.2	10.4	2.0
Mixed Grill, GF, Delight Mozz, Med, Domino's*	1 Pizza/354g	864	36.1	244	12.2	25.2	10.2	2.2
Mixed Grill, GF, Sm, Extravaganza, Domino's*	1 Pizza/354g	840	39.7	237	9.0	24.0	11.2	2.4
Mixed Grill, Italian, Delight Mozz, Lge, Domino's*	1 Slice/71g	181	7.0	254	12.0	28.6	9.8	2.1
Mixed Grill, Italian, Delight Mozz, Med, Domino's*	1 Slice/64g	162	6.4	255	12.1	28.0	10.1	2.1

	INFO/WEIGHT	KCAL	FAT	KCAL	PROT	CARB	FAT	FIBRE
DOMINO'S*								
PIZZA								
Mixed Grill, Italian, Delight Mozz, Med, Domino's*	1 Slice/56g	143	5.9	254	12.1	27.0	10.4	2.1
Mixed Grill, Italian, Lge, Domino's*	1 Slice/71g	161	7.0	227	10.9	23.0	9.9	1.9
Mixed Grill, Italian, Med, Domino's*	1 Slice/64g	145	6.5	228	11.0	22.5	10.2	1.9
Mixed Grill, Italian, Sm, Domino's*	1 Slice/57g	129	5.9	228	11.0	21.8	10.5	1.8
Mixed Grill, Stuffed Crust, Delight Mozz, Lge, Domino's*	1 Slice/98g	238	10.2	242	11.8	24.4	10.4	2.1
Mixed Grill, Stuffed Crust, Delight Mozz, Med, Domino's*	1 Slice/92g	223	9.5	243	11.8	24.4	10.4	2.1
Mixed Grill, Stuffed Crust, Lge, Domino's*	1 Slice/99g	264	11.0	268	13.4	27.7	11.2	2.0
Mixed Grill, Stuffed Crust, Med, Domino's*	1 Slice/92g	247	10.4	269	13.4	27.7	11.3	2.0
New Yorker, Classic, Delight Mozz, Lge, Domino's*	1 Slice/75g	196	7.4	261	16.6	25.6	9.8	1.9
New Yorker, Classic, Delight Mozz, Med, Domino's*	1 Slice/69g	180	6.9	262	16.6	25.3	10.0	1.9
New Yorker, Classic, Delight Mozz, Personal, Domino's*	1 Pizza/202g	530	20.2	262	12.3	29.7	10.0	2.0
New Yorker, Classic, Lge, Domino's*	1 Slice/75g	203	8.9	270	12.3	28.1	11.8	1.8
New Yorker, Classic, Med, Domino's*	1 Slice/69g	187	8.2	271	12.4	27.8	11.9	1.7
New Yorker, Classic, Personal, Domino's*	1 Pizza/202g	546	20.8	270	12.2	31.1	10.3	2.1
New Yorker, Classic, Sm, Domino's*	1 Slice/61g	164	7.0	268	13.6	26.7	11.4	1.8
New Yorker, GF, Delight Mozz, Sm, Domino's*	1 Pizza/326g	858	36.9	263	13.9	25.7	11.3	2.0
New Yorker, GF, Sm, Domino's*	1 Pizza/326g	834	40.4	256	10.4	24.4	12.4	2.2
New Yorker, Italian, Delight Mozz, Lge, Domino's*	1 Slice/65g	179	7.1	274	13.5	29.5	10.9	2.0
New Yorker, Italian, Delight Mozz, Med, Domino's*	1 Slice/58g	160	6.5	274	13.7	28.8	11.2	1.9
New Yorker, Italian, Delight Mozz, Sm, Domino's*	1 Slice/51g	141	6.0	274	13.8	27.7	11.6	1.9
New Yorker, Italian, Lge, Domino's*	1 Slice/66g	160	7.1	244	12.3	23.4	10.9	1.7
New Yorker, Italian, Med, Domino's*	1 Slice/58g	143	6.5	245	12.5	22.9	11.2	1.7
New Yorker, Italian, Sm, Domino's*	1 Slice/51g	127	6.0	247	12.7	22.0	11.7	1.6
New Yorker, Stuffed Crust, Delight Mozz, Lge, Domino's*	1 Slice/93g	236	10.3	255	12.8	24.8	11.1	2.0
New Yorker, Stuffed Crust, Delight Mozz, Med, Domino's*	1 Slice/89g	226	9.9	255	12.9	24.7	11.2	2.0
New Yorker, Stuffed Crust, Lge, Domino's*	1 Slice/93g	262	11.1	282	14.5	28.3	12.0	1.9
New Yorker, Stuffed Crust, Med, Domino's*	1 Slice/87g	245	10.5	283	14.6	28.2	12.1	1.9
Pepperoni Passion, Classic, Delight Mozz, Domino's*	1 Personal/203g	600	25.6	295	14.7	29.5	12.6	1.9
Pepperoni Passion, Classic, Delight Mozz, Lge, Domino's*	1 Slice/73g	216	8.9	294	19.0	26.0	12.1	1.9
Pepperoni Passion, Classic, Delight Mozz, Med, Domino's*	1 Slice/68g	201	8.6	296	19.1	25.7	12.6	1.9
Pepperoni Passion, Classic, Delight Mozz, Sm, Domino's*	1 Slice/60g	180	8.1	302	15.4	28.6	13.6	1.8
Pepperoni Passion, Classic, Lge, Domino's*	1 Slice/74g	166	11.0	226	13.8	28.5	15.0	1.7
Pepperoni Passion, Classic, Med, Domino's*	1 Slice/68g	210	10.4	310	13.9	28.2	15.4	1.7
Pepperoni Passion, Classic, Personal, Domino's*	1 Pizza/204g	623	27.9	306	13.8	31.0	13.7	2.0
Pepperoni Passion, Classic, Sm, Domino's*	1 Slice/60g	185	9.1	310	15.1	27.4	15.2	1.8
Pepperoni Passion, GF, Delight Mozz, Med, Domino's*	1 Pizza/315g	966	45.9	307	16.5	26.4	14.6	2.0
Pepperoni Passion, GF, Sm, Domino's*	1 Pizza/317g	960	52.9	303	11.9	25.2	16.7	2.2
Pepperoni Passion, Italian, Delight Mozz, Lge, Domino's*	1 Slice/64g	200	8.7	311	16.3	30.1	13.5	1.9
Pepperoni Passion, Italian, Delight Mozz, Med, Domino's*	1 Slice/57g	181	8.2	315	16.5	29.3	14.2	1.9
Pepperoni Passion, Italian, Delight Mozz, Med, Domino's*	1 Slice/50g	160	7.5	321	16.6	28.6	15.1	1.8
Pepperoni Passion, Italian, Lge, Domino's*	1 Slice/64g	184	9.4	286	14.0	23.9	14.6	1.7
Pepperoni Passion, Italian, Med, Domino's*	1 Slice/57g	167	8.8	291	14.2	23.3	15.3	1.6
Pepperoni Passion, Italian, Sm, Domino's*	1 Slice/50g	148	8.1	297	14.3	22.7	16.2	1.6
Pepperoni Passion, Stuffed Crust, Lge, Domino's*	1 Slice/92g	286	13.4	312	15.7	28.7	14.6	1.9
Pepperoni Passion, Stuffed Crust, Med, Domino's*	1 Slice/86g	269	12.7	314	15.8	28.5	14.8	1.9
Ranch BBQ, Classic, Delight Mozz, Lge, Domino's*	1 Slice/75g	217	7.7	288	15.6	34.2	10.2	1.8
Ranch BBQ, Classic, Delight Mozz, Personal, Domino's*	1 Pizza/207g	592	19.7	286	14.0	36.7	9.5	1.9
Ranch BBQ, Classic, Delight Mozz, Sm, Domino's*	1 Slice/61g	183	6.5	300	15.4	36.0	10.7	2.2
Ranch BBQ, Classic, Lge, Domino's*	1 Slice/75g	225	9.1	299	14.8	33.4	12.1	1.6
Ranch BBQ, Classic, Med, Domino's*	1 Slice/69g	207	8.5	301	14.8	33.3	12.3	2.1
Ranch BBQ, Classic, Personal, Domino's*	1 Pizza/207g	612	23.2	295	15.4	33.9	11.2	2.0
Ranch BBQ, Classic, Sm, Domino's*	1 Slice/61g	184	7.9	301	16.0	30.7	13.0	2.2

DOMINO'S*
PIZZA

	Measure INFO/WEIGHT	per Measure KCAL	FAT	Nutrition Values per 100g / 100ml KCAL	PROT	CARB	FAT	FIBRE
Ranch BBQ, ClassicCrust, Delight Mozz, Med, Domino's*	1 Slice/69g	286	10.3	290	15.6	34.1	10.4	1.8
Ranch BBQ, GF, Delight Mozz, Sm, Domino's*	1 Pizza/322g	960	39.6	298	14.3	33.4	12.3	2.1
Ranch BBQ, GF, Sm, Domino's*	1 Pizza/323g	1002	45.6	310	13.0	33.8	14.1	2.0
Ranch BBQ, Italian, Delight Mozz, Lge, Domino's*	1 Slice/66g	196	7.7	297	18.9	29.8	11.7	2.4
Ranch BBQ, Italian, Delight Mozz, Med, Domino's*	1 Slice/58g	174	7.0	299	19.0	29.4	12.1	2.4
Ranch BBQ, Italian, Delight Mozz, Sm, Domino's*	1 Slice/51g	154	6.5	301	19.2	28.5	12.7	2.3
Ranch BBQ, Italian, Lge, Domino's*	1 Slice/66g	201	8.8	305	16.0	31.0	13.4	1.7
Ranch BBQ, Italian, Med, Domino's*	1 Slice/58g	178	8.0	307	16.1	30.5	13.8	2.0
Ranch BBQ, Italian, Sm, Domino's*	1 Slice/51g	157	7.3	308	16.4	29.6	14.3	2.0
Ranch BBQ, Stuffed Crust, Delight Mozz, Lge, Domino's*	1 Slice/93g	260	10.8	279	15.5	28.6	11.6	1.7
Ranch BBQ, Stuffed Crust, Delight Mozz, Med, Domino's*	1 Slice/86g	242	10.1	280	15.5	28.7	11.7	1.7
Ranch BBQ, Stuffed Crust, Lge, Domino's*	1 Slice/93g	267	11.6	287	14.3	29.4	12.5	1.5
Ranch BBQ, Stuffed Crust, Med, Domino's*	1 Slice/86g	249	10.9	288	14.3	29.5	12.6	2.6
Rustica, Classic, Delight Mozz, Lge, Domino's*	1 Slice/73g	186	5.7	256	15.1	30.6	7.8	2.3
Rustica, Classic, Delight Mozz, Med, Domino's*	1 Slice/66g	174	5.7	265	15.3	30.5	8.7	2.3
Rustica, Classic, Delight Mozz, Personal, Domino's*	1 Pizza/201g	551	16.5	274	12.6	36.7	8.2	2.0
Rustica, Classic, Delight Mozz, Sm, Domino's*	1 Slice/58g	153	5.0	265	15.1	30.8	8.7	2.1
Rustica, Classic, Lge, Domino's*	1 Slice/72g	191	6.7	264	13.0	31.6	9.3	1.8
Rustica, Classic, Med, Domino's*	1 Slice/66g	180	6.7	273	13.2	31.4	10.2	1.8
Rustica, Classic, Sm, Domino's*	1 Slice/58g	158	6.0	273	13.3	30.9	10.4	2.1
Rustica, GF, Delight Mozz, Sm, Domino's*	1 Pizza/305g	804	29.8	264	12.7	30.6	9.8	1.9
Rustica, GF, Sm, Domino's*	1 Pizza/304g	846	35.6	278	11.3	31.2	11.7	2.3
Rustica, Italian, Delight Mozz, Lge, Domino's*	1 Slice/63g	164	5.6	261	15.7	28.7	8.9	2.4
Rustica, Italian, Delight Mozz, Med, Domino's*	1 Slice/55g	149	5.5	270	15.9	28.4	9.9	2.3
Rustica, Italian, Delight Mozz, Sm, Domino's*	1 Slice/48g	128	4.7	267	15.9	27.9	9.9	2.3
Rustica, Italian, Lge, Domino's*	1 Slice/63g	166	6.6	265	14.5	27.3	10.5	2.2
Rustica, Italian, Med, Domino's*	1 Slice/55g	151	6.4	273	14.8	27.0	11.5	2.2
Rustica, Italian, Sm, Domino's*	1 Slice/48g	130	5.5	271	14.8	26.5	11.4	2.2
Rustica, Personal, Domino's*	1 Pizza/201g	567	19.3	282	13.0	35.3	9.6	1.8
Rustica, Stuffed Crust, Delight Mozz, Lge, Domino's*	1 Slice/90g	220	7.2	244	14.6	27.6	8.0	2.1
Rustica, Stuffed Crust, Delight Mozz, Med, Domino's*	1 Slice/84g	210	7.3	251	14.7	27.6	8.7	2.0
Rustica, Stuffed Crust, Lge, Domino's*	1 Slice/90g	237	10.2	263	14.1	25.5	11.3	2.2
Rustica, Stuffed Crust, Med, Domino's*	1 Slice/84g	226	10.0	2701402.02505.0		12.0		2.2
Scrummy, Classic, Delight Mozz, Lge, Domino's*	1 Slice/81g	227	9.2	282	18.9	24.8	11.4	1.8
Scrummy, Classic, Delight Mozz, Med, Domino's*	1 Slice/74g	209	8.5	282	19.0	24.5	11.5	1.7
Scrummy, Classic, Delight Mozz, Personal, Domino's*	1 Pizza/236g	662	28.7	281	15.2	26.6	12.2	1.7
Scrummy, Classic, Delight Mozz, Sm, Domino's*	1 Slice/66g	189	8.2	284	15.7	26.8	12.3	1.6
Scrummy, GF, Delight Mozz, Sm, Domino's*	1 Pizza/355g	1020	46.2	287	16.7	24.7	13.0	1.8
Scrummy, Italian, Delight Mozz, Lge, Domino's*	1 Slice/71g	210	8.9	296	16.5	28.3	12.6	1.8
Scrummy, Italian, Delight Mozz, Med, Domino's*	1 Slice/64g	189	8.2	296	16.7	27.6	12.8	1.7
Scrummy, Italian, Delight Mozz, Sm, Domino's*	1 Slice/57g	169	7.6	298	16.8	26.5	13.4	1.7
Scrummy, Stuffed Crust, Delight Mozz, Lge, Domino's*	1 Slice/98g	267	12.1	272	15.0	24.2	12.3	1.9
Scrummy, Stuffed Crust, Delight Mozz, Med, Domino's*	1 Slice/92g	250	11.3	272	15.0	24.1	12.3	1.9
Spanish Sizzler, Classic, Delight Mozz, Lge, Domino's*	1 Slice/75g	191	5.8	255	18.2	27.1	7.8	2.1
Spanish Sizzler, Classic, Delight Mozz, Med, Domino's*	1 Slice/68g	174	5.3	255	18.3	27.1	7.8	2.1
Spanish Sizzler, Classic, Delight Mozz, Personal, Domino's*	1 Pizza/202g	518	16.2	256	14.1	30.9	8.0	2.1
Spanish Sizzler, Classic, Delight Mozz, Sm, Domino's*	1 Slice/60g	153	4.9	257	14.7	30.3	8.2	2.0
Spanish Sizzler, GF, Delight Mozz, Sm, Domino's*	1 Pizza/314g	804	26.7	256	15.7	28.3	8.5	2.3
Spanish Sizzler, Italian, Delight Mozz, Lge, Domino's*	1 Slice/66g	175	5.6	267	15.5	31.2	8.5	2.2
Spanish Sizzler, Italian, Delight Mozz, Med, Domino's*	1 Slice/57g	153	4.9	267	15.6	30.9	8.5	2.2
Spanish Sizzler, Italian, Delight Mozz, Sm, Domino's*	1 Slice/50g	133	4.3	267	15.7	30.6	8.7	2.2
Tandoori Hot, Classic, Delight Mozz, Lge, Domino's*	1 Slice/77g	168	3.9	218	18.3	26.0	5.0	2.1

DOMINO'S*

PIZZA

	Measure INFO/WEIGHT	per Measure KCAL	FAT	Nutrition Values per 100g / 100ml KCAL	PROT	CARB	FAT	FIBRE
Tandoori Hot, Classic, Delight Mozz, Med, Domino's*	1 Slice/70g	153	3.5	219	16.4	26.1	5.0	2.1
Tandoori Hot, Classic, Delight Mozz, Personal, Domino's*	1 Pizza/207g	461	11.2	223	12.5	30.1	5.4	2.1
Tandoori Hot, Classic, Delight Mozz, Sm, Domino's*	1 Slice/61g	134	3.3	218	12.8	29.1	5.3	2.0
Tandoori Hot, Classic, Lge, Domino's*	1 Slice/89g	198	5.6	223	13.4	28.1	6.3	2.2
Tandoori Hot, Classic, Med, Domino's*	1 Slice/81g	176	5.0	217	13.0	27.2	6.2	2.2
Tandoori Hot, GF, Delight Mozz, Sm, Domino's*	1 Pizza/325g	690	16.6	212	13.5	27.0	5.1	2.3
Tandoori Hot, Italian, Delight Mozz, Med, Domino's*	1 Slice/60g	133	3.1	223	13.5	29.6	5.2	2.2
Tandoori Hot, Italian, Delight Mozz, Sm, Domino's*	1 Slice/52g	114	2.7	220	13.5	29.1	5.2	2.1
Tandoori Hot, Stuffed Crust, Delight Mozz, Lge, Domino's*	1 Slice/95g	209	6.7	220	12.7	25.2	7.1	2.2
Tandoori Hot, Stuffed Crust, Delight Mozz, Med, Domino's*	1 Slice/88g	194	6.3	221	12.8	25.3	7.2	2.2
Texas BBQ, Classic, Delight Mozz, Lge, Domino's*	1 Slice/74g	191	4.8	259	14.1	35.2	6.5	2.0
Texas BBQ, Classic, Delight Mozz, Med, Domino's*	1 Slice/67g	174	4.3	259	14.2	35.2	6.4	2.0
Texas BBQ, Classic, Delight Mozz, Personal, Domino's*	1 Pizza/205g	538	13.3	263	12.7	37.4	6.5	2.1
Texas BBQ, Classic, Delight Mozz, Sm, Domino's*	1 Slice/59g	157	3.8	267	13.8	37.6	6.4	2.4
Texas BBQ, Classic, Lge, Domino's*	1 Slice/87g	240	7.0	276	14.4	36.6	8.0	1.8
Texas BBQ, Classic, Med, Domino's*	1 Slice/79g	218	6.3	276	14.4	36.6	8.0	1.8
Texas BBQ, Classic, Sm, Domino's*	1 Slice/71g	196	5.7	276	14.4	36.6	8.0	1.8
Texas BBQ, GF, Delight Mozz, Sm, Domino's*	1 Pizza/312g	810	23.1	260	12.4	35.1	7.4	2.4
Texas BBQ, Italian, Delight Mozz, Lge, Domino's*	1 Slice/65g	170	4.8	263	17.2	30.8	7.4	2.7
Texas BBQ, Italian, Delight Mozz, Med, Domino's*	1 Slice/57g	149	4.2	263	17.4	30.5	7.4	2.6
Texas BBQ, Stuffed Crust, Delight Mozz, Lge, Domino's*	1 Slice/92g	234	7.8	255	14.3	29.4	8.5	1.8
Texas BBQ, Stuffed Crust, Delight Mozz, Med, Domino's*	1 Slice/85g	217	7.2	255	14.4	29.5	8.5	1.8
Texas BBQ, Stuffed Crust, Lge, Domino's*	1 Slice/97g	252	8.8	261	15.3	28.6	9.1	2.0
Texas BBQ, Stuffed Crust, Med, Domino's*	1 Slice/90g	234	8.2	261	15.3	28.6	9.1	2.0
The Sizzler, Classic, Delight Mozz, Lge, Domino's*	1 Slice/76g	206	7.2	272	15.4	30.3	9.5	2.3
The Sizzler, Classic, Delight Mozz, Med, Domino's*	1 Slice/69g	190	6.7	274	15.6	30.1	9.7	2.3
The Sizzler, Classic, Delight Mozz, Personal, Domino's*	1 Pizza/203g	565	16.3	278	12.9	37.7	8.0	2.2
The Sizzler, Classic, Delight Mozz, Sm, Domino's*	1 Slice/61g	169	6.1	277	15.5	30.4	10.0	2.1
The Sizzler, Classic, Lge, Domino's*	1 Slice/95g	271	10.6	285	14.7	31.5	11.2	2.2
The Sizzler, Classic, Med, Domino's*	1 Slice/87g	248	9.7	285	14.7	31.5	11.2	2.2
The Sizzler, Classic, Sm, Domino's*	1 Slice/78g	222	8.7	285	14.7	31.5	11.2	2.2
The Sizzler, GF, Delight Mozz, Sm, Domino's*	1 Pizza/324g	900	36.6	278	13.3	30.1	11.3	1.9
The Sizzler, Italian, Delight Mozz, Lge, Domino's*	1 Slice/66g	184	7.1	279	16.0	28.4	10.8	2.4
The Sizzler, Italian, Delight Mozz, Med, Domino's*	1 Slice/59g	165	6.5	281	16.2	28.0	11.1	2.4
The Sizzler, Italian, Delight Mozz, Sm, Domino's*	1 Slice/51g	145	5.9	282	16.3	27.6	11.4	2.4
The Sizzler, Stuffed Crust, Delight Mozz, Lge, Domino's*	1 Slice/93g	240	8.8	257	14.9	27.4	9.4	2.1
The Sizzler, Stuffed Crust, Delight Mozz, Med, Domino's*	1 Slice/90g	231	8.3	256	14.4	28.1	9.2	2.0
The Sizzler, Stuffed Crust, Delight Mozz, Med, Domino's*	1 Slice/87g	226	8.3	259	14.9	17.4	9.5	2.1
Tuna Delight, Classic, Delight Mozz, Lge, Domino's*	1 Slice/74g	170	4.3	231	15.9	27.8	5.8	2.2
Tuna Delight, Classic, Delight Mozz, Med, Domino's*	1 Slice/67g	154	3.9	231	15.9	27.9	5.8	2.2
Tuna Delight, Classic, Delight Mozz, Personal, Domino's*	1 Pizza/199g	464	12.1	233	11.8	31.8	6.1	2.2
Tuna Delight, Classic, Delight Mozz, Sm, Domino's*	1 Slice/58g	135	3.6	232	12.1	31.2	6.2	2.1
Tuna Delight, GF, Delight Mozz, Sm, Domino's*	1 Pizza/307g	696	18.7	227	12.8	29.3	6.1	2.4
Tuna Delight, Italian, Delight Mozz, Lge, Domino's*	1 Slice/64g	154	4.1	239	12.7	32.1	6.3	2.3
Tuna Delight, Italian, Delight Mozz, Med, Domino's*	1 Slice/56g	134	3.5	238	12.7	32.0	6.3	2.3
Tuna Delight, Italian Style, Delight Mozz, Sm, Domino's*	1 Slice/48g	114	3.0	237	12.7	31.7	6.2	2.3
Tuna Delight, Stuffed Crust, Delight Mozz, Lge, Domino's*	1 Slice/92g	211	7.2	230	12.2	26.6	7.9	2.2
Tuna Delight, Stuffed Crust, Delight Mozz, Med, Domino's*	1 Slice/84g	195	6.7	231	12.2	26.7	7.9	2.2
Veg-A-Roma, Classic, Delight Mozz, Lge, Domino's*	1 Slice/74g	171	4.9	230	11.1	30.5	6.6	2.5
Veg-A-Roma, Classic, Delight Mozz, Med, Domino's*	1 Slice/68g	156	4.5	231	11.2	30.6	6.6	2.5
Veg-A-Roma, Classic, Delight Mozz, Personal, Domino's*	1 Pizza/202g	490	11.7	242	9.0	37.7	5.8	2.3
Veg-A-Roma, Delight Mozz, Sm Classic, Domino's*	1 Slice/59g	137	3.9	231	11.0	31.2	6.6	2.4

	Measure INFO/WEIGHT	per Measure KCAL	FAT	Nutrition Values per 100g / 100ml KCAL	PROT	CARB	FAT	FIBRE

DOMINO'S*
PIZZA

	Measure INFO/WEIGHT	KCAL	FAT	KCAL	PROT	CARB	FAT	FIBRE
Veg-A-Roma, GF, Delight Mozz, Sm, Domino's*	1 Pizza/311g	702	23.0	226	8.1	31.0	7.4	2.2
Veg-A-Roma, Italian, Delight Mozz, Lge, Domino's*	1 Slice/65g	150	4.9	230	11.1	28.6	7.5	2.6
Veg-A-Roma, Italian, Delight Mozz, Med, Domino's*	1 Slice/49g	112	3.6	227	11.0	28.4	7.3	2.6
Veg-A-Roma, Italian, Delight Mozz, Med, Domino's*	1 Slice/57g	131	4.2	229	11.1	28.6	7.4	2.6
Veg-A-Roma, Stuffed Crust, Delight Mozz, Lge, Domino's*	1 Slice/92g	206	6.5	223	11.4	27.5	7.0	2.2
Veg-A-Roma, Stuffed Crust, Delight Mozz, Med, Domino's*	1 Slice/85g	191	6.1	224	11.4	27.7	7.1	2.2
Vegetarian Supreme, Classic, Lge, Domino's*	1 Slice/88g	192	5.5	218	11.5	29.1	6.3	2.3
Vegetarian Supreme, Classic, Med, Domino's*	1 Slice/80g	170	4.9	213	11.0	28.3	6.1	2.3
Vegetarian Supreme, Classic, Sm, Domino's*	1 Slice/72g	156	4.5	217	11.5	28.9	6.2	2.3
Vegi Lite, Classic, Delight Mozz, Lge, Domino's*	1 Slice/72g	155	3.7	214	13.8	27.1	5.1	2.2
Vegi Lite, Classic, Delight Mozz, Med, Domino's*	1 Slice/66g	141	3.4	214	13.9	27.2	5.1	2.2
Vegi Lite, Classic, Delight Mozz, Personal, Domino's*	1 Pizza/196g	428	10.8	218	10.0	31.2	5.5	2.3
Vegi Lite, Classic, Delight Mozz, Sm, Domino's*	1 Slice/58g	123	3.1	213	10.0	30.4	5.4	2.1
Vegi Lite, GF, Delight Mozz, Sm, Domino's*	1 Pizza/303g	624	16.1	206	10.3	28.4	5.3	2.4
Vegi Lite, Italian, Delight Mozz, Lge, Domino's*	1 Slice/63g	139	3.4	219	10.3	31.4	5.4	2.3
Vegi Lite, Italian, Delight Mozz, Med, Domino's*	1 Slice/131g	286	12.1	218	10.2	31.3	9.2	2.3
Vegi Lite, Italian, Delight Mozz, Sm, Domino's*	1 Slice/48g	103	2.5	215	10.1	30.8	5.3	2.3
Vegi Lite, Stuffed Crust, Delight Mozz, Lge, Domino's*	1 Slice/90g	196	6.6	216	10.5	26.0	7.3	2.3
Vegi Lite, Stuffed Crust, Delight Mozz, Med, Domino's*	1 Slice/83g	182	6.2	218	10.6	26.2	7.4	2.3
Vegi Supreme, Classic, Delight Mozz, Lge, Domino's*	1 Slice/76g	159	3.7	208	13.3	26.6	4.9	2.2
Vegi Supreme, Classic, Delight Mozz, Med, Domino's*	1 Slice/69g	144	3.4	208	13.3	26.7	4.9	2.2
Vegi Supreme, Classic, Delight Mozz, Personal, Domino's*	1 Pizza/205g	436	10.8	213	9.6	30.6	5.3	2.2
Vegi Supreme, Classic, Delight Mozz, Sm, Domino's*	1 Slice/61g	126	3.2	207	9.6	29.7	5.2	2.1
Vegi Supreme, GF, Delight Mozz, Sm, Domino's*	1 Pizza/323g	642	16.5	199	9.9	27.7	5.1	2.4
Vegi Supreme, Italian, Delight Mozz, Lge, Domino's*	1 Slice/67g	142	3.5	212	9.9	30.6	5.2	4.7
Vegi Supreme, Italian, Delight Mozz, Med, Domino's*	1 Slice/59g	124	3.1	211	9.8	30.4	5.2	2.3
Vegi Supreme, Italian Style, Delight Mozz, Sm, Domino's*	1 Slice/51g	105	2.6	207	9.6	29.9	5.1	2.3
Vegi Supreme, Stuffed Crust, Delight Mozz, Lge, Domino's*	1 Slice/94g	199	6.7	211	10.2	25.7	7.1	2.3
Vegi Volcano, Classic, Delight Mozz, Lge, Domino's*	1 Slice/80g	173	4.7	217	15.4	24.8	5.9	2.0
Vegi Volcano, Classic, Delight Mozz, Med, Domino's*	1 Slice/72g	157	4.3	217	15.4	24.8	5.9	2.0
Vegi Volcano, Classic, Delight Mozz, Personal, Domino's*	1 Pizza/213g	468	13.0	220	11.5	28.9	6.1	2.1
Vegi Volcano, Classic, Delight Mozz, Sm, Domino's*	1 Slice/63g	136	3.8	216	11.8	27.8	6.1	1.9
Vegi Volcano, GF, Delight Mozz, Sm, Domino's*	1 Pizza/337g	708	20.6	210	12.3	25.7	6.1	2.1
Vegi Volcano, Italian, Delight Mozz, Lge, Domino's*	1 Slice/70g	157	4.5	222	12.4	28.3	6.3	2.1
Vegi Volcano, Italian, Delight Mozz, Med, Domino's*	1 Slice/62g	137	3.9	221	12.4	28.0	6.3	2.0
Vegi Volcano, Italian, Delight Mozz, Med, Domino's*	1 Slice/53g	116	3.3	218	12.2	27.6	6.2	2.0
Vegi Volcano, Stuffed Crust, Delight Mozz, Lge, Domino's*	1 Slice/98g	214	7.6	219	12.0	24.2	7.8	2.1

POTATO WEDGES

Fajita, Domino's*	½ Portion/114g	168	7.0	146	2.4	20.4	6.1	2.1
Plain, Domino's*	½ Portion/112g	168	7.0	149	2.4	20.8	6.2	2.1

WRAP

Meatball Mayhem, Wrapzz, Domino's*	1 Wrap/137g	384	17.4	280	9.6	30.7	12.7	1.8
Tandoori Hot, Wrapzz, Domino's*	1 Wrap/115g	267	9.7	232	12.5	25.7	8.4	2.1
Vegetarian Supreme, Wrapzz, Domino's*	1 Wrap/110g	234	8.0	211	8.3	27.0	7.2	2.6

EAT
BAGEL

BLT, EAT*	1 Bagel/222g	567	20.5	255	14.7	28.8	9.2	1.8
Cheese & Chilli Jam, EAT*	1 Bagel/224g	583	21.1	260	11.1	33.5	9.4	1.8
Egg, Free Range & Chorizo, EAT*	1 Bagel/240g	561	24.0	234	10.7	25.9	10.0	1.6
Pastrami, New York, EAT*	1 Bagel/217g	468	11.7	216	13.6	29.1	5.4	1.5
Smoked Salmon & Cream Cheese, EAT*	1 Bagel/199g	444	10.8	223	13.0	31.2	5.4	1.7

EAT

	Measure INFO/WEIGHT	per Measure KCAL	FAT	Nutrition Values per 100g / 100ml KCAL	PROT	CARB	FAT	FIBRE
BAGUETTE								
Beef, & Tomato, Rustic, EAT*	1 Baguette/114g	247	8.3	217	11.3	25.5	7.3	2.8
Beef & Rocket, EAT*	1 Baguette/228g	556	18.2	244	13.2	29.2	8.0	1.8
Brie, Tomato & Basil, EAT*	1 Baguette/191g	455	17.2	238	9.2	29.1	9.0	1.9
Chicken, & Herb Salad, Roast, Rustic, EAT*	1 Baguette/253g	622	27.3	246	11.9	24.1	10.8	2.7
Chicken, Bacon & Avocado, EAT*	1 Baguette/252g	552	19.9	219	13.2	23.8	7.9	1.9
Chicken, Thai, EAT*	1 Baguette/201g	432	12.3	215	11.9	28.4	6.1	1.8
Chicken Banh Mi, EAT*	1 Pack/282g	454	8.2	161	9.0	24.0	2.9	1.6
Eat Club, EAT*	1 Baguette/270g	550	22.8	203	11.0	21.0	8.4	1.4
Egg & Bacon, Half, EAT*	1 Serving/112g	311	12.2	278	13.5	30.5	10.9	1.8
Egg & Tomato, EAT*	1 Serving/140g	304	12.2	217	9.0	24.8	8.7	1.7
Full Works, Festive, EAT*	1 Baguette/267g	536	13.6	201	12.4	26.0	5.1	1.4
Ham, & Jarlsberg, Smoked, Rustic, EAT*	1 Baguette/243g	622	26.2	256	14.8	23.0	10.8	2.4
Ham & Jarlsberg, EAT*	1 Baguette/218g	566	23.3	260	15.4	24.9	10.7	1.4
Ham & Tomato, EAT*	1 Baguette/245g	422	10.3	172	9.6	23.2	4.2	1.6
Ham Brie & Cranberry, EAT*	1 Baguette/245g	583	25.1	239	11.0	25.8	10.3	1.4
Houmous, & Avocado, EAT*	1 Baguette/262g	584	23.8	223	6.6	27.8	9.1	3.7
Mature Cheddar, & Sweet Chilli Jam, EAT*	1 Baguette/201g	577	25.1	287	10.4	33.1	12.5	1.7
Red Pepper Tapenade, Avocado, & Feta, Rustic, EAT*	1 Baguette/220g	526	22.5	239	7.2	28.9	10.2	4.4
Smoked Salmon & Soft Cheese, Half, EAT*	1 Pack/93g	218	6.7	235	11.0	30.2	7.2	1.7
Sticky BBQ Banh Mi, EAT*	1 Roll/269g	473	2.4	176	7.9	33.1	0.9	1.8
The Big Salami, EAT*	1 Baguette/254g	569	26.9	224	9.2	22.5	10.6	1.5
Tuna, & Cucumber, EAT*	1 Baguette/235g	583	27.0	248	11.1	24.0	11.5	1.5
BARS								
Cereal, Fruity Granola, EAT*	1 Bar/67g	282	14.7	421	5.5	51.7	22.0	4.8
BREAD								
Brioche, Fruited without Butter, Toasted, EAT*	1 Serving/120g	414	13.4	345	7.3	50.2	11.2	2.2
Brown Roll, for Soup, EAT*	1 Roll/69g	187	3.5	271	8.5	47.4	5.1	2.0
Chunk of Freshly Baked Brown Bread, EAT*	1 Serving/67g	141	1.3	211	7.4	44.0	1.9	2.7
Chunk of Freshly Baked White Bread, EAT*	1 Serving/67g	162	2.9	242	7.3	46.4	4.3	1.9
Rolls, Crusty, EAT*	1 Roll/80g	198	1.0	247	8.3	48.3	1.3	2.6
Rolls, White, for Soup, EAT*	1 Roll/100g	244	0.9	244	7.2	50.1	0.9	3.4
Wheat Free Seeded Rye Bread, EAT*	1 Serving/144g	331	6.0	230	6.7	48.0	4.2	6.7
BREAKFAST								
Poached Egg, Beans & Ham, Hot Pot, EAT*	1 Big/269g	420	10.8	156	8.0	12.3	4.0	2.6
Poached Egg, Our Beans, & Mushrooms, Pot, EAT*	1 Sm/168g	215	6.3	144	6.3	11.8	4.2	2.5
Poached Egg, Our Beans, Ham Hock, & Mushroom, EAT*	1 Big/389g	572	14.0	147	6.9	12.5	3.6	2.7
Toast, Cheese & Marmite, Sourdough, EAT*	1 Serving/150g	458	21.2	305	13.9	29.7	14.1	2.7
BREAKFAST CEREAL								
Bircher, Mango & Passionfruit, EAT*	1 Serving/225g	336	9.2	149	3.1	25.2	4.1	2.2
Granola & Full Fat, EAT*	1 Serving/230g	476	17.7	207	5.7	29.9	7.7	4.1
Granola & Full Fat, with Chocolate Syrup, EAT*	1 Serving/239g	509	18.4	213	5.7	31.2	7.7	4.4
Granola & Skimmed, EAT*	1 Serving/230g	435	13.3	189	5.7	30.0	5.8	4.1
Granola & Soya, EAT*	1 Serving/230g	435	15.9	189	5.8	27.3	6.9	4.5
Granola & Soya, with Chocolate Syrup, EAT*	1 Serving/239g	468	16.7	196	5.9	28.7	7.0	4.7
Grapenuts, Banana & Honey, EAT*	1 Serving/228g	349	6.4	153	6.3	25.4	2.8	1.5
Muesli, Apple, Almond & Cinnamon, Bircher, EAT*	1 Serving/210g	361	12.2	172	6.1	23.3	5.8	2.3
Muesli, Apple & Cinnamon, Super Bircher, EAT*	1 Serving/205g	232	5.1	113	4.3	17.6	2.5	2.2
Muesli, Swiss, Bircher, EAT*	1 Serving/205g	246	3.1	120	4.7	21.7	1.5	2.0
Porridge, Plain, Big, EAT*	1 Serving/280g	213	3.1	76	4.4	11.9	1.1	1.1
Porridge, Plain, Sm, EAT*	1 Serving/180g	137	2.0	76	4.4	11.9	1.1	1.2
Porridge, Plain, Super, Big, EAT*	1 Serving/342g	205	5.5	60	2.4	9.0	1.6	1.8
Porridge, with Apple & Blackberry, Compote, Big, EAT*	1 Serving/331g	291	3.6	88	3.9	16.0	1.1	1.5

	Measure INFO/WEIGHT	per Measure KCAL	FAT	Nutrition Values per 100g / 100ml KCAL	PROT	CARB	FAT	FIBRE

EAT
BREAKFAST CEREAL

	Measure INFO/WEIGHT	KCAL	FAT	KCAL	PROT	CARB	FAT	FIBRE
Porridge, with Apple & Blackberry, Compote, Sm, EAT*	1 Serving/231g	210	2.3	91	3.6	17.2	1.0	1.7
Porridge, with Banana, & Maple Syrup, Big, EAT*	1 Serving/315g	308	6.9	98	4.0	15.1	2.2	1.2
Porridge, with Banana, & Maple Syrup, Sm, EAT*	1 Serving194g	177	1.9	91	4.1	16.0	1.0	1.0
Porridge, with Banana, & Maple Syrup, Super, EAT*	1 Serving/364g	266	5.5	73	2.2	12.0	1.5	1.8
Porridge, with Banana, Big, EAT*	1 Serving/300g	234	0.9	78	4.1	12.8	0.3	1.2
Porridge, with Banana, Sm, EAT*	1 Serving/200g	162	2.2	81	4.0	13.5	1.1	1.3
Porridge, with Banana, Super, Big, EAT*	1 Serving/350g	224	5.2	64	2.3	9.8	1.5	1.8
Porridge, with Banana, Super, Sm, EAT*	1 Serving/240g	156	3.6	65	2.3	10.1	1.5	1.9
Porridge, with Berry Compote, Big, EAT*	1 Serving/330g	271	3.0	82	3.8	14.3	0.9	1.1
Porridge, with Berry Compote, Sm, EAT*	1 Serving/230g	196	2.1	85	3.6	15.3	0.9	1.1
Porridge, with Berry Compote, Super, Big, EAT*	1 Serving/330g	284	3.3	86	3.8	15.5	1.0	1.2
Porridge, with Berry Compote, Super, Sm, EAT*	1 Serving/30g	205	2.3	89	3.6	16.4	1.0	1.2
Porridge, with Maple Syrup, Big, EAT*	1 Serving/294g	253	3.2	86	4.2	14.6	1.1	1.0
Porridge, with Maple Syrup, Sm, EAT*	1 Serving/195g	185	2.1	95	4.1	17.3	1.1	1.1

BROWNIES

Belgian Chocolate, Bites, Mini, EAT*	1 Pack/18g	84	5.0	464	4.8	47.3	27.7	4.5
Belgian Chocolate, EAT*	1 Brownie/73g	339	20.2	464	4.8	47.3	27.7	4.5

BUNS

Chelsea, EAT*	1 Bun/100g	350	9.7	350	5.8	60.3	9.7	2.1

CAKE

Carrot, Bar, EAT*	1 Bar/100g	319	20.0	319	2.8	33.1	20.0	1.6
Chocolate Caramel Crispie, Slice, EAT*	1 Slice/61g	279	17.4	458	3.9	53.6	28.5	0.9
Lamington, EAT*	1 Cake/90g	324	15.8	360	4.0	47.7	17.5	2.1
Lemon Curd, Slice, EAT*	1 Slice/75g	300	12.9	400	3.2	59.0	17.2	1.6

CHEESECAKE

Lemon, Sicilian, EAT*	1 Portion/80g	308	24.1	385	4.6	23.7	30.1	0.4

CHILLI

Texan, with Rice, Pot, EAT*	1 Sm/382g	386	9.9	101	5.8	13.3	2.6	1.8

COFFEE

Cappuccino, Skimmed, EAT*	1 Tall/12oz	118	4.0	33	2.4	3.4	1.1	0.0
Cappuccino, Soya, EAT*	1 Tall/12oz	131	4.9	37	3.2	3.5	1.4	0.9
Cappuccino, Whole, Big, EAT*	1 Big/474ml	159	8.4	34	2.3	2.3	1.8	0.0
Cappuccino, Whole, Sm, EAT*	1 Tall/12oz	130	6.5	37	2.6	2.4	1.8	0.0
Espresso, Macchiato, Skimmed, EAT*	1 Espresso/4oz	8	0.3	7	0.5	0.6	0.3	0.0
Espresso, Macchiato, Whole, Double, EAT*	1 Double/8oz	20	0.4	8	1.4	0.4	0.2	0.0
Espresso, Macchiato, Whole, Single, EAT*	1 Single/4oz	13	0.3	11	1.5	0.6	0.2	0.0
Latte, Chai, Skimmed, EAT*	1 Tall/12oz	305	1.0	86	3.2	17.7	0.3	0.0
Latte, Chai, Whole, Big, EAT*	1 Big/16oz	332	12.8	70	2.7	9.0	2.7	0.0
Latte, Iced, Skimmed, EAT*	1 Tall/12oz	95	3.2	27	1.9	2.7	0.9	0.0
Latte, Iced, Whole, EAT*	1 Latte (12oz)	135	7.3	38	1.9	2.7	2.0	0.0
Latte, Matcha, Soya, EAT*	1 Tall/12oz	201	5.8	57	3.0	7.4	1.6	0.3
Latte, Skimmed, EAT*	1 Sm/12oz	99	3.4	42	3.0	4.2	1.4	0.0
Latte, Soya, EAT*	1 Tall/12oz	157	5.9	46	4.0	4.3	1.7	1.1
Latte, Whole, Sm, EAT*	1 Sm/12oz	173	9.0	49	3.3	3.2	2.5	0.0
Mocha, Soya, EAT*	1 Tall/12oz	173	6.1	49	4.0	5.0	1.7	1.2
Mocha, Whole, EAT*	1 Tall/12oz	219	11.4	62	3.0	4.8	3.2	0.0
White, Flat, Skimmed, EAT*	1 Tall/341ml	87	0.3	26	2.6	3.7	0.1	0.0
White, Flat, Soya, EAT*	1 Tall/341ml	147	4.8	43	5.1	2.3	1.4	0.4
White, Flat, Whole, EAT*	1 Sm 8oz/227ml	122	6.2	52	3.8	3.5	2.6	0.0

COOKIES

Chocolate, Triple, EAT*	1 Cookie/90g	394	15.3	438	5.6	64.7	17.0	1.8
Oat & Fruit, EAT*	1 Pack/84g	329	12.0	392	5.6	59.6	14.3	4.1

EAT

INFO/WEIGHT	Measure	per Measure		Nutrition Values per 100g / 100ml				
		KCAL	FAT	KCAL	PROT	CARB	FAT	FIBRE
CROISSANT								
Almond, EAT*	1 Serving/83g	350	19.8	422	10.0	41.7	23.9	2.9
Chocolate, EAT*	1 Serving/81g	361	21.3	445	6.9	45.4	26.2	3.0
EAT*	1 Serving/71g	305	17.1	427	9.4	43.4	23.9	2.7
Egg, Cheese & Tomato, EAT*	1 Pack/149g	434	25.1	291	9.0	20.8	16.8	1.6
Ham, & Cheese, EAT*	1 Croissant/126g	339	21.2	269	15.2	22.1	16.8	0.0
Ham & Jarlsberg Croissant, EAT*	1 Serving/128g	339	21.1	265	15.6	20.8	16.5	0.0
CURRY								
Chicken, Green Thai, with Rice, Pot, EAT*	1 Sm/416g	491	19.1	118	4.0	13.2	4.6	1.1
Chicken, Vietnamese, EAT*	1 Sm/390g	402	12.1	103	4.9	12.6	3.1	1.0
Chicken, with Rice, Burmese, Hot Pot, EAT*	1 Sm/398g	462	19.1	116	5.3	12.3	4.8	1.2
DANISH PASTRY								
Maple Pecan, Plait, EAT*	1 Serving/83g	377	26.0	454	4.7	38.4	31.3	5.2
DESSERT								
Bag of Cherries, EAT*	1 Serving/125g	55	0.1	44	0.8	9.0	0.1	1.8
Banana Toffee & Pecan Cake, EAT*	1 Serving/79g	247	10.8	313	3.3	45.1	13.7	0.9
Belgian Chocolate Brownie, EAT*	1 Serving/73g	330	20.0	452	5.1	46.2	27.4	1.0
Big Fruit Salad, EAT*	1 Serving/279g	120	0.3	43	0.6	10.9	0.1	1.8
Caramel Tiffin, EAT*	1 Serving/73g	351	18.9	481	3.6	60.0	25.9	0.7
Chilli & Herb Olives, EAT*	1 Serving/75g	99	10.1	132	0.8	1.8	13.5	3.5
Chocolate Cookie, EAT*	1 Serving/90g	401	16.8	446	6.6	61.4	18.7	2.7
Coconut & Raspberry, Slice, EAT*	1 Slice/75g	306	17.6	408	5.9	44.1	23.4	4.5
Coconut & Raspberry Slice, EAT*	1 Serving/75g	306	17.6	408	5.9	44.1	23.4	4.5
Fresh Fruit Salad, EAT*	1 Serving/160g	77	0.2	48	0.6	11.3	0.1	0.5
Grape Bag, EAT*	1 Serving/133g	80	0.1	60	0.4	15.4	0.1	1.0
Haagen Das Belgian Chocolate, EAT*	1 Serving/100g	227	18.4	227	3.9	23.8	18.4	1.7
Haagen Das Cookies & Cream, EAT*	1 Serving/100g	225	14.4	225	3.7	20.0	14.4	0.7
Haagen Das Strawberries & Cream, EAT*	1 Serving/100g	221	14.1	221	3.5	20.0	14.1	0.3
Haagen Das Vanilla, EAT*	1 Serving/100g	225	15.2	225	3.8	18.1	15.2	0.0
Honey & Chilli Nuts, EAT*	1 Serving/100g	496	31.7	496	15.9	44.4	31.7	5.6
Jelly, Elderflower & Berry, EAT*	1 Pack/150g	110	0.2	73	1.1	16.3	0.1	0.9
Jelly, Plum & Apple Jelly, EAT*	1 Pot/130g	143	0.1	110	1.8	25.7	0.1	0.5
Lemon Drizzle Cake, EAT*	1 Serving/70g	232	10.8	332	3.5	44.8	15.5	0.8
Millionares Shortcake, EAT*	1 Cake/85g	396	21.2	466	3.5	57.6	25.0	0.8
Muesli Cookie, EAT*	1 Serving/90g	376	13.4	418	5.7	63.5	14.9	3.6
Oat & Fruit Slice, EAT*	1 Serving/73g	292	11.7	400	4.1	61.2	16.0	3.3
Pineapple & Lime, EAT*	1 Serving/181g	76	0.4	42	0.4	9.2	0.2	1.1
Rainbow Fruit Salad, EAT*	1 Serving/141g	86	0.6	61	0.8	12.5	0.4	2.6
Red Velvet Cake, EAT*	1 Pack/128g	500	24.3	391	4.7	50.0	19.0	0.9
Summer Berries, EAT*	1 Serving/130g	48	0.3	37	0.8	6.8	0.2	3.1
Tiffin, Milk Chocolate & Brazil Nut, EAT*	1 Tiffin/80g	374	19.2	468	4.6	58.6	24.0	1.8
Toffee Waffles, EAT*	1 Serving/65g	301	11.7	463	3.5	71.7	18.0	2.2
Victoria Sponge Cake, EAT*	1 Serving/72g	166	7.9	230	2.5	30.5	10.9	0.6
Wasabi Peas, EAT*	1 Serving/38g	158	4.6	416	20.0	57.0	12.0	7.0
FROZEN YOGHURT								
Plain, EAT*	1 Serving/140g	169	0.3	121	3.5	29.0	0.2	2.0
with Blueberry & Pomegranate Compote, EAT*	1 Serving/180g	232	0.4	129	3.0	30.9	0.2	2.2
with Fresh Berries, EAT*	1 Serving/200g	190	0.4	95	2.7	22.0	0.2	2.5
FRUIT & NUT MIX								
& Seeds, Snack, EAT*	1 Pack/40g	186	14.9	465	18.2	11.5	37.2	5.2
FRUIT SALAD								
Mango & Lime, EAT*	1 Pot/125g	76	0.3	60	0.7	12.9	0.2	1.7

	Measure INFO/WEIGHT	per Measure KCAL	FAT	Nutrition Values per 100g / 100ml KCAL	PROT	CARB	FAT	FIBRE
EAT								
FUDGE								
Scottish, Handmade, EAT*	1 Pack/45g	194	4.1	431	1.5	85.8	9.0	0.6
GOULASH								
Sweet Potato & Bell Pepper, EAT*	1 Sm/383g	322	6.5	84	2.3	14.6	1.7	1.4
HOT CHOCOLATE								
Whole, Sm, EAT*	1 Sm/12oz	298	12.5	84	3.3	9.9	3.5	1.2
HOT POT								
BBQ Pulled Pork, EAT*	1 Pack/340g	510	15.0	150	9.7	17.3	4.4	0.8
Cumberland Sausage, Mash & Onion Gravy, EAT*	1 Pack/470g	658	40.4	140	4.8	10.1	8.6	1.2
Full Works, Chestnut, Festive, EAT*	1 Sm/439g	386	13.6	88	1.6	12.9	3.1	2.0
Moroccan Vegetable, Slow Cooked, EAT*	1 Sm/394g	335	4.7	85	2.2	14.6	1.2	1.8
Pork, BBQ, Pulled, with Cold Slaw, & Rice, EAT*	1 Sm/360g	486	20.9	135	6.1	13.5	5.8	0.9
Slow Cooked Beef & Moroccan Vegetable, EAT*	1 Big/680g	646	12.9	95	4.8	12.7	1.9	1.5
Texan Chilli, EAT*	1 Pack/378g	386	9.5	102	5.8	13.6	2.5	1.9
Thai Green Chicken Curry, EAT*	1 Pack/386g	491	22.0	127	5.9	11.3	5.7	0.9
Turkey, festive Full Works, EAT*	1 Sm/475g	413	18.5	87	3.6	8.6	3.9	1.5
JUICE								
Apple, EAT*	1 Bottle/250ml	128	0.2	51	0.1	11.8	0.1	0.1
JUICE DRINK								
Mango & Lime, Blast, EAT*	1 Tall/12oz	253	0.3	71	0.3	17.7	0.1	0.1
Peach & Mint, Blast, EAT*	1 Tall/12oz	216	0.2	61	0.2	15.1	0.1	0.0
MACARONI CHEESE								
Hot Pot, EAT*	1 Sm/394g	544	28.0	138	5.0	13.9	7.1	0.7
MASH & GRAVY								
EAT*	1 Serving/220g	178	6.6	81	1.5	10.9	3.0	1.8
MUFFIN								
Bacon Butty, Hot Toasted, EAT*	1 Serving/90g	291	10.9	324	17.1	36.1	12.1	0.8
Bacon Butty, Toasted, Hot, Lge, EAT*	1 Serving/190g	589	18.4	310	15.4	39.7	9.7	0.9
Blueberry, Low Fat, EAT*	1 Muffin/119g	383	13.4	322	5.8	47.9	11.3	2.5
Chocolate, Belgian, EAT*	1 Serving/124g	511	26.4	412	5.0	48.9	21.3	2.1
Chocolate, Double, EAT*	1 Muffin/118g	472	23.7	400	5.1	48.9	20.1	1.5
Egg, Mushroom & Cheddar, Hot Toasted, EAT*	1 Serving/125g	240	6.9	192	9.1	26.2	5.5	1.0
Eggs Benedict, Hot Toasted, EAT*	1 Serving/120g	265	8.9	220	10.2	27.6	7.4	0.8
Fruit & Bran, EAT*	1 Muffin/124g	498	25.1	402	5.7	47.2	20.3	3.8
Full English Breakfast, EAT*	1 Serving/295g	687	24.5	233	10.7	28.4	8.3	0.7
Smoked Salmon & Egg, Hot Toasted, EAT*	1 Serving/126g	325	10.0	258	11.8	37.1	7.9	1.5
PAIN AU CHOCOLAT								
EAT*	1 Serving/78g	329	18.4	422	9.8	42.6	23.6	3.6
PANCAKE								
American Buttermilk, with Maple, EAT*	1 Serving/100g	239	2.2	238	3.6	55.5	2.2	1.0
American Buttermilk, with Maple & Bacon, EAT*	1 Serving/106g	292	4.9	275	8.5	50.0	4.6	0.8
American Buttermilk, with Maple & Banana, EAT*	1 Serving/113g	260	2.1	231	3.2	50.0	1.9	1.2
American Buttermilk, with Maple & Berry Compote, EAT*	1 Serving/171g	328	3.2	192	3.4	40.0	1.9	0.9
PASTRY								
Cinnamon Swirl, Slices, EAT*	1 Serving/77g	360	24.5	470	5.1	40.4	32.0	4.4
PIE								
Banoffee, EAT*	1 Serving/112g	395	24.1	353	3.7	36.0	21.5	1.4
Beef, & Ale, EAT*	1 Pie/250g	553	27.5	221	8.7	23.5	11.0	1.5
Beef, & Ale, with Mash, & Gravy, EAT*	1 Portion/548g	800	36.7	146	4.8	16.7	6.7	1.7
Beef & Stilton, Pie Only, EAT*	1 Pie/270g	629	31.6	233	10.2	21.1	11.7	1.6
Butternut Squash, & Feta, EAT*	1 Pie/250g	630	43.8	252	7.3	16.3	17.5	1.7
Butternut Squash, & Feta, with Mash, & Gravy, EAT*	1 Portion/548g	877	53.2	160	4.2	13.5	9.7	1.8
Cheese & Onion, EAT*	1 Pie/270g	856	58.9	317	8.5	21.5	21.8	1.8

	INFO/WEIGHT	per Measure KCAL	per Measure FAT	KCAL	PROT	CARB	FAT	FIBRE
EAT								
PIE								
Cheese & Onion, Pie Only, EAT*	1 Pie/270g	856	58.9	317	8.5	21.5	21.8	1.8
Cheese & Onion, with Mash, & Gravy, EAT*	1 Portion/560g	1086	67.2	194	4.9	16.0	12.0	1.8
Cheese & Onion with Mash & Gravy, EAT*	1 Pie/560g	1098	67.8	196	4.9	16.2	12.1	1.9
Chicken, & Mushroom, EAT*	1 Pie/250g	685	37.8	274	11.3	22.6	15.1	1.4
Chicken, & Mushroom, with Mash, & Gravy, EAT*	1 Portion/548g	932	47.1	170	6.0	16.3	8.6	1.7
Chicken, Bacon, & Stuffing, EAT*	1 Pie/250g	705	41.5	282	10.8	22.0	16.6	1.4
Chicken, Bacon, & Stuffing, with Mash, & Gravy, EAT*	1 Portion/548g	954	51.0	174	5.8	16.1	9.3	1.7
Chicken & Mushroom with Mash & Gravy, EAT*	1 Pie/540g	929	47.0	172	6.1	16.5	8.7	1.7
Goats Cheese & Sweet Potato, Pie Only, EAT*	1 Pie/270g	694	36.7	257	6.6	26.2	13.6	1.9
Goats Cheese & Sweet Potato with Mash & Gravy, EAT*	1 Pie/560g	946	45.9	169	4.1	18.4	8.2	2.0
Mince, EAT*	1 Pie/101g	376	38.0	372	15.1	58.2	37.6	2.3
Steak, & Red Wine, EAT*	1 Pie/250g	635	35.2	254	10.7	20.4	14.1	1.2
Steak, & Red Wine, with Mash, & Gravy, EAT*	1 Portion/548g	882	44.9	161	5.7	15.3	8.2	1.6
Steak & Ale, Pie Only, EAT*	1 Pie/250g	670	37.8	268	10.4	22.1	15.1	1.5
Steak & Ale with Mash & Gravy, EAT*	1 Pie/540g	913	47.0	169	5.7	16.3	8.7	1.7
POPCORN								
& Almonds, Smokey, EAT*	1 Pack/30g	141	5.9	470	13.0	55.7	19.7	0.0
Cheese & Jalapeno, EAT*	1 Pack/25g	137	9.0	549	6.0	46.1	35.9	8.9
Salt & Vinegar, EAT*	1 Pack/25g	111	4.3	445	10.4	57.6	17.3	8.2
Salted, Rock Salt, EAT*	1 Bag/23g	122	7.2	532	9.4	50.4	31.1	6.4
QUICHE								
Cheddar & Bacon, with Coleslaw, EAT*	1 Pack/235g	529	37.9	225	7.1	13.5	16.1	1.0
Mature Cheddar & Bacon, EAT*	1 Quiche/160g	426	28.2	266	9.9	18.1	17.6	0.6
Smoked Bacon & Cheddar, EAT*	1 Quiche/155g	468	33.8	302	11.1	15.3	21.8	1.0
Smoked Bacon & Cheddar, with Coleslaw, EAT*	1 Pack/230g	573	43.5	249	7.9	11.5	18.9	1.3
Spinach, Feta & Tomato, EAT*	1 Pack/155g	398	27.4	257	9.3	15.2	17.7	1.1
Spinach, Feta & Tomato, with Coleslaw, EAT*	1 Pack/230g	504	37.1	219	6.7	11.5	16.1	1.4
RICE CAKES								
Berry Yoghurt, EAT*	1 Pack/33g	170	8.3	508	6.4	62.9	24.9	1.5
Dark Chocolate, EAT*	1 Pack/33g	163	7.7	488	6.3	61.0	23.1	5.1
ROLL								
Bacon, & Poached Egg, Back, British, EAT*	1 Roll/160g	336	8.8	210	14.7	24.9	5.5	0.0
Bacon, Back, British, EAT*	1 Roll/140g	321	6.6	229	17.6	28.2	4.7	0.0
Beef, & Horseradish, Slow Cooked, EAT*	1 Roll/213g	413	13.4	194	13.7	19.5	6.3	0.2
Poached Egg, Mushroom, & Cheese, EAT*	1 Roll/173g	337	11.2	195	10.3	23.6	6.5	0.2
Sausage, Pigs in Blankets, Crusty, EAT*	1 Roll/1710g	425	20.1	250	11.5	23.7	11.8	0.0
Turkey, Festive Full Works, EAT*	1 Roll/213g	379	10.0	178	10.0	23.5	4.7	0.3
SALAD								
Beef, Teriyaki, Pot, no Dressing, EAT*	1 Salad/122g	111	3.3	91	6.9	14.4	2.7	2.4
Beef, Thai, Noodle, Rare, no Dressing, EAT*	1 Salad/260g	169	4.4	65	4.8	18.7	1.7	1.8
Beef, Thai, Noodle, Rare, with Dressing, EAT*	1 Salad/311g	261	7.5	84	4.5	20.6	2.4	1.6
Bold Chipotle, Chicken Tortilla,without Dressing, EAT*	1 Pack/345g	515	19.4	149	9.0	16.2	5.6	2.7
Bold Mediterranean Serrano Ham, no Dressing, EAT*	1 Pack/304g	368	14.9	121	9.3	9.1	4.9	2.1
Bold Mediterranean Serrano Ham, with Dressing, EAT*	1 Pack/331g	501	28.2	151	8.6	9.1	8.5	2.0
Bold Salmon Sushi, with Dressing, EAT*	1 Pack/340g	493	11.9	145	5.5	24.1	3.5	1.0
Bold Salmon Sushi, without Dressing, EAT*	1 Pack/308g	434	9.8	141	6.0	23.2	3.2	1.1
Chicken, & Riced Cauliflower, Harissa, EAT*	1 Pack/378g	287	14.0	76	6.2	4.7	3.7	1.4
Chicken, Simple, no Dressing, EAT*	1 Salad/338g	362	18.9	107	6.3	7.5	5.6	1.2
Chicken, Simple, with Dressing, EAT*	1 Salad/366g	494	32.2	135	5.9	7.6	8.8	1.1
Greek, Pot, EAT*	1 Pot/156g	131	6.1	84	3.5	8.0	3.9	2.1
Greens, & Feta, Super, Side, no Dressing, EAT*	1 Salad/162g	172	6.0	106	8.3	3.7	3.7	3.0
Greens, & Feta, Super, Side, with Dressing, EAT*	1 Salad/180g	243	12.1	135	7.5	7.8	6.7	2.7

EAT
SALAD

	Measure INFO/WEIGHT	per Measure KCAL	per Measure FAT	Nutrition Values per 100g / 100ml KCAL	PROT	CARB	FAT	FIBRE
Ham Hock & Egg, with Dressing, Side, EAT*	1 Serving/166g	227	15.6	137	9.7	2.7	9.4	1.0
Ham Hock & Egg, without Dressing, Side, EAT*	1 Serving/148g	142	7.1	96	10.7	1.9	4.8	1.1
Houmous, Detox Box, with Dressing, EAT*	1 Pack/254g	478	40.9	188	3.1	7.4	16.1	3.3
Houmous, Detox Box, without Dressing, EAT*	1 Pack/262g	414	33.3	158	3.3	7.5	12.7	3.6
Houmous & Falafel Mezze with Dressing, Bold, EAT*	1 Box/378g	491	24.5	130	3.0	13.7	6.5	4.3
Houmous & Falafel Mezze without Dressing, EAT*	1 Box/353g	395	16.9	112	3.2	12.8	4.8	4.6
Mexican Bean, Less Than 5% Fat, Pot, Vegetarian, EAT*	1 Salad/172g	192	4.0	111	5.2	17.1	2.3	4.1
Mezze, with Dressing, EAT*	1 Serving/306g	425	26.6	139	3.6	12.0	8.7	2.7
Mezze, without Dressing, EAT*	1 Serving/286g	349	20.3	122	3.8	11.0	7.1	2.9
Pea & Mint Pot, no Dressing, EAT*	1 Salad/106g	98	2.6	92	6.8	7.4	2.4	3.0
Pea & Mint Pot with Dressing, EAT*	1 Salad/125g	171	9.8	136	5.9	7.5	7.8	2.7
Prawn Cocktail, Side, EAT*	1 Serving/166g	345	29.4	208	9.4	2.4	17.7	0.7
Prawn Cocktail Pot, EAT*	1 Salad/129g	218	17.2	169	9.9	2.1	13.3	0.6
Quinoa, & Vegetable, Rainbow, no Dressing, EAT*	1 Salad/315g	416	19.9	132	6.2	12.3	6.3	2.7
Quinoa, & Vegetable, Rainbow, with Dressing, EAT*	1 Salad/355g	575	33.0	162	5.6	13.8	9.3	2.5
Rainbow, Side, with Dressing, EAT*	1 Salad/188g	320	12.4	170	7.5	18.3	6.6	3.0
Rainbow Side,without Dressing, EAT*	1 Pack/170g	247	6.5	145	8.2	17.6	3.8	3.2
Rainbow Superfood, with Dressing, EAT*	1 Serving/340g	520	24.8	153	5.4	15.2	7.3	2.6
Salmon, & Potato, Hot Smoked, no Dressing, EAT*	1 Salad/183g	249	13.5	136	7.8	7.9	7.4	1.6
Salmon, & Potato, Hot Smoked, with Dressing, EAT*	1 Salad/201g	334	22.1	166	7.2	8.0	11.0	1.5
Salmon, Omega Booster, no Dressing, Box, EAT*	1 Pack/173g	281	23.6	162	7.4	1.3	13.6	2.1
Salmon, Omega Booster, with Dressing, Box, EAT*	1 Pack/194g	392	34.9	202	6.6	2.3	18.0	1.9
Salmon, Poached, & Potato Salad, no Dressing, EAT*	1 Serving/231g	254	15.7	110	6.7	5.3	6.8	1.0
Salmon, Poached, & Potato Salad, with Dressing, EAT*	1 Serving/251g	354	26.4	141	6.2	5.2	10.5	0.9
Smoked Chicken, Potato & Watercress, no Dressing, EAT*	1 Salad/316g	395	25.6	125	6.5	6.0	8.1	1.2
Smoked Chicken, Potato & Watercress, with Dressing, EAT*	1 Salad/346g	516	37.7	149	6.0	6.2	10.9	1.1
Spicy Chicken Noodles Less Than 5% fat, EAT*	1 Serving/325g	419	9.1	129	8.9	16.8	2.8	1.6
Spicy Crayfish Noodles, Less Than 5% Fat, EAT*	1 Serving/285g	348	8.0	122	6.6	18.2	2.8	1.6
Summer Ham & Potato, with Dressing, EAT*	1 Serving/331g	480	36.7	145	6.0	4.9	11.1	0.8
Tandoori Chicken, Mango & Rice, with Dressing, EAT*	1 Serving/206g	251	5.6	122	8.3	15.6	2.7	1.6
Tuna, Simple, no Dressing, EAT*	1 Salad/292g	193	5.8	66	7.4	4.3	2.0	0.9
Tuna, Simple, with Dressing, EAT*	1 Salad/322g	316	17.7	98	6.9	4.6	5.5	0.8
Vietnamese Slaw, Side, with Dressing, EAT*	1 Pack/156g	150	9.1	96	3.0	7.2	5.8	2.2
Vietnamese Slaw, Side, without Dressing, EAT*	1 Pack/137g	81	2.9	59	2.4	7.4	2.1	2.3

SANDWICH

	Measure INFO/WEIGHT	per Measure KCAL	per Measure FAT	Nutrition Values per 100g / 100ml KCAL	PROT	CARB	FAT	FIBRE
Bacon, Lettuce & Tomato, EAT*	1 Pack/204g	479	25.1	235	11.1	19.9	12.3	1.7
Bacon Butty, EAT*	1 Butty/170g	600	15.5	353	17.8	53.3	9.1	2.2
Beef, & Pink Onion Chutney, White Bloomer, EAT*	1 Sandwich/222g	462	10.4	208	11.2	30.0	4.7	1.6
Cheese, Two, & Chive Slaw, Malted Bread, Simple, EAT*	1 Sandwich/201g	519	30.6	258	10.1	20.4	15.2	1.8
Chicken, & Bacon, Caesar, White Bloomer, EAT*	1 Sandwich/261g	543	24.8	208	11.2	19.9	9.5	1.5
Chicken, Pork, Sage & Onion, White Bloomer, EAT*	1 Sandwich/238g	569	25.9	239	11.8	24.7	10.9	1.8
Chicken & Bacon, EAT*	1 Pack/229g	472	21.5	206	12.3	18.0	9.4	1.6
Chicken & Chorizo, EAT*	1 Sandwich/209g	416	17.4	199	12.3	19.7	8.3	1.7
Club, EAT*	1 Pack/296g	624	28.7	211	12.9	17.7	9.7	1.3
Crayfish, Lemon & Rocket, EAT*	1 Pack/188g	333	13.9	177	9.5	20.9	7.4	1.6
Egg, Free Range & Roast Tomato, Bloomer, EAT*	1 Pack/215g	525	25.6	244	11.1	23.4	11.9	2.8
Egg Mayonnaise, & Watercress, Chunky, EAT*	1 Sandwich/204g	462	25.2	227	8.8	20.0	12.4	1.7
Full Works, Festive, White Bloomer, EAT*	1 Sandwich/292g	599	19.9	205	12.2	23.7	6.8	2.2
Full Works, White Bloomer, EAT*	1 Sandwich/322g	541	27.0	168	11.5	15.8	8.4	1.2
Ham, & Egg, Free Range, EAT*	1 Pack/250g	580	29.0	232	13.2	19.2	11.6	2.0
Ham, Tomato & Mustard, EAT*	1 Pack/203g	394	17.5	194	9.8	19.3	8.6	1.6
Ham & Cheese, Simply, Toastie, EAT*	1 Serving/240g	588	31.2	245	11.8	21.4	13.0	1.0

EAT

SANDWICH

	INFO/WEIGHT	KCAL	FAT	KCAL	PROT	CARB	FAT	FIBRE
Ham & Free Range Egg, White Bloomer, EAT*	1 Sandwich/246g	573	28.5	233	13.0	19.4	11.6	2.0
Ham & Pickle, Malted Bread, Simple, EAT*	1 Sandwich/233g	354	11.6	152	7.3	20.5	5.0	1.6
Mature Cheddar Salad, Simple, EAT*	1 Pack/188g	405	18.8	215	9.4	21.7	10.0	1.8
Pastrami, New York, EAT*	1 Pack/224g	358	11.4	160	9.9	18.6	5.1	1.3
Pastrami, New York, White Bloomer, EAT*	1 Sandwich/240g	513	20.7	213	11.3	22.3	8.6	0.3
Pork & Apple Sauce, Hot Roll, EAT*	1 Roll/230g	467	19.1	203	7.3	25.2	8.3	0.6
Pulled Pork, Brioche Bun, EAT*	1 Pack/235g	456	12.5	194	12.7	24.6	5.3	0.8
Simple Chicken Salad less than 5% fat, EAT*	1 Pack/203g	327	9.7	161	10.1	19.3	4.8	1.9
Skipjack Tuna & Cucumber less than 5% fat, EAT*	1 Pack/187g	305	7.1	163	10.8	21.3	3.8	1.7
Smoked Chicken, Tomato & Pesto Bloomer, EAT*	1 Pack/244g	454	15.4	186	12.4	20.4	6.3	2.2
Smoked Salmon, Egg & Watercress, EAT*	1 Pack/211g	477	25.3	226	10.8	18.7	12.0	1.6
Smoked Scottish Salmon & Soft Cheese, EAT*	1 Pack/165g	380	16.5	230	12.1	22.9	10.0	1.6
Steak & Cheese Melt, Toastie, EAT*	1 Pack/265g	552	24.9	208	10.8	21.2	9.4	1.3
The Hot Cubano, Toastie, EAT*	1 Pack/270g	521	22.4	193	10.8	20.0	8.3	0.9
Tuna & Cheddar Melt, Toastie, EAT*	1 Pack/255g	594	28.6	233	13.9	20.7	11.2	1.0
Tuna & Mayo, Simple, Kids, EAT*	1 Sandwich/138g	371	17.0	269	12.4	27.4	12.3	1.9
Tuna & Rocket, EAT*	1 Pack/250g	577	29.9	230	11.1	19.8	11.9	2.3
Tuna Mayonnaise, & Cucumber, Malted Bread, EAT*	1 Sandwich/199g	334	10.7	168	9.5	20.3	5.4	1.6
Turkey & Cranberry, less than 5% Fat, EAT*	1 Pack/223g	381	10.0	171	11.8	22.2	4.5	1.5
Very Sm Chicken & Bacon, EAT*	1 Pack/114g	241	11.5	211	12.2	17.7	10.1	1.6
Very Sm Crayfish, Lemon & Rocket, EAT*	1 Pack/99g	174	6.8	176	9.4	19.9	6.9	1.4

SAUSAGE

	INFO/WEIGHT	KCAL	FAT	KCAL	PROT	CARB	FAT	FIBRE
Pigs in Blankets, Pot, EAT*	1 Serving/114g	290	21.6	255	12.9	8.4	19.0	0.3

SAUSAGE ROLL

	INFO/WEIGHT	KCAL	FAT	KCAL	PROT	CARB	FAT	FIBRE
Great British, EAT*	1 Pack/130g	442	28.2	340	12.1	25.0	21.7	1.9

SHORTBREAD

	INFO/WEIGHT	KCAL	FAT	KCAL	PROT	CARB	FAT	FIBRE
Millionaires, EAT*	1 Slice/97g	441	25.2	455	3.5	52.4	26.0	1.0
Millionaires, Peanut Butter, EAT*	1 Slice/75g	284	14.8	378	11.4	36.6	19.7	1.9

SLICES

	INFO/WEIGHT	KCAL	FAT	KCAL	PROT	CARB	FAT	FIBRE
Bakewell, EAT*	1 Slice/88g	359	19.8	408	4.8	47.1	22.5	1.5

SMOOTHIE

	INFO/WEIGHT	KCAL	FAT	KCAL	PROT	CARB	FAT	FIBRE
Almond, Four Berries, EAT*	1 Bottle/250g	232	14.0	93	1.9	8.8	5.6	0.5

SOUP

	INFO/WEIGHT	KCAL	FAT	KCAL	PROT	CARB	FAT	FIBRE
Bacon, & Potato, Fully Loaded, EAT*	1 Sm/315g	258	12.6	82	4.3	7.7	4.0	0.5
Beef, Chilli, Salsa, with Garnish, EAT*	1 Sm/349g	244	6.6	70	4.7	6.6	1.9	0.6
Beef, Rendang, Malaysian, no Garnish, EAT*	1 Sm/300g	261	12.6	87	4.2	7.5	4.2	1.1
Beef, Rendang, Malaysian, with Garnish, EAT*	1 Sm/302g	263	12.7	87	4.2	7.5	4.2	1.1
Beef Ragu, EAT*	1 Sm/310g	217	8.4	70	5.2	5.9	2.7	1.0
Butternut Squash, Thai, EAT*	1 Sm/300g	168	6.6	56	1.0	6.9	2.2	1.5
Cauliflower Cheese, EAT*	1 Sm/300	219	13.5	73	3.0	4.7	4.5	1.1
Chicken, & Barley, Hearty, EAT*	1 Sm/317g	187	2.9	59	4.4	7.4	0.9	1.5
Chicken, & Egg, Noodle, Old Fashioned, EAT*	1 Sm/303g	109	1.5	36	4.2	3.5	0.5	0.5
Chicken, & Vegetable, Garden, no Granish, EAT*	1 Sm/300g	123	1.5	41	4.5	4.5	0.5	0.7
Chicken, & Vegetable, Garden, with Garnish, EAT*	1 Sm/320g	131	1.6	41	4.5	4.5	0.5	0.7
Chicken, Gyoza, Miso, Pot, EAT*	1 Pot/657g	322	3.3	49	2.5	8.8	0.5	0.7
Chicken, Hot & Sour, with Garnish, EAT*	1 Sm/300g	102	1.5	34	3.7	3.6	0.5	0.4
Chicken, Jerk, no Garnish, EAT*	1 Sm/300g	282	12.9	94	5.1	9.2	4.3	1.1
Chicken, Jerk, with Garnish, EAT*	1 Sm/340g	340	13.9	100	4.8	11.6	4.1	1.1
Chicken, Laksa, no Garnish, EAT*	1 Sm/300g	273	15.0	91	5.0	5.1	5.0	0.1
Chicken, Laksa, with Garnish, EAT*	1 Sm/307g	276	15.0	90	4.9	5.0	4.9	0.2
Chicken, Pot Pie, no Garnish, EAT*	1 Sm/300g	216	9.0	72	4.6	6.8	3.0	1.0
Chicken, Pot Pie, with Garnish, EAT*	1 Sm/390g	343	16.4	88	4.7	7.9	4.2	1.0

EAT

	Measure INFO/WEIGHT	per Measure KCAL	FAT	Nutrition Values per 100g / 100ml KCAL	PROT	CARB	FAT	FIBRE
SOUP								
Chicken, Thai Green Curry, no Garnish, EAT*	1 Sm/300g	252	13.2	84	4.6	5.2	4.4	0.5
Chicken, Thai Green Curry, with Garnish, EAT*	1 Sm/355g	309	14.9	87	4.3	7.9	4.2	0.6
Chicken, Tortilla, no Garnish, EAT*	1 Sm/300g	120	0.9	40	4.6	4.4	0.3	1.0
Chicken, Tortilla, with Garnish, EAT*	1 Sm/378g	189	3.8	50	4.8	5.0	1.0	1.0
Chicken & Rice Noodles, Pho, Pot, EAT*	1 Pot/875g	315	1.8	36	3.0	5.2	0.2	0.4
Chicken Noodle, Coconut, EAT*	1 Sm/340g	313	17.0	92	4.2	6.5	5.0	0.5
Chicken Pho, EAT*	1 Serving/786ml	291	4.7	37	3.7	3.6	0.6	0.3
Chilli, non Carne, EAT*	1 Sm/300g	156	2.4	52	2.1	8.0	0.8	2.0
Chorizo & Chickpea, EAT*	1 Serving/402ml	358	16.5	89	5.0	8.1	4.1	1.6
Creamy Sweetcorn, Simple, EAT*	1 Sm/300g	315	15.3	105	2.5	12.1	5.1	1.3
Duck, Gyoza, & Egg Noodle, Pot, EAT*	1 Pot/900g	387	3.6	43	2.3	7.5	0.4	0.6
Duck Gyoza Dumpling & Egg Noodles Pho, Pot, EAT*	1 Pot/849g	382	5.1	45	2.1	7.8	0.6	0.6
French Onion, with Garnish, EAT*	1 Serving/316ml	136	3.8	43	1.6	6.2	1.2	0.5
French Onion, without Garnish, EAT*	1 Serving/400ml	112	1.2	28	0.7	5.4	0.3	0.5
Goulash, Hungarian, no Garnish, EAT*	1 Sm/300g	234	6.3	78	7.7	7.2	2.1	0.8
Goulash, Hungarian, with Garnish, EAT*	1 Sm/303g	236	6.4	78	7.7	7.2	2.1	0.8
Ham, Pea & Mint, with garnish, EAT*	1 Serving/321ml	202	4.5	63	4.8	7.5	1.4	1.1
Ham, Pea & Mint, without garnish, EAT*	1 Serving/626ml	388	8.8	62	4.7	7.4	1.4	0.6
Ham Hock, Pea, & Barley, no Granish, EAT*	1 Sm/300g	129	3.6	43	3.4	4.1	1.2	3.4
Ham Hock, Pea, & Barley, with Garnish, EAT*	1 Sm/320g	144	3.8	45	3.5	4.4	1.2	1.2
Hoisin Duck Gyoza Dumpling, EAT*	1 Serving/847ml	432	7.6	51	2.3	8.4	0.9	0.5
Leek & Potato, EAT*	1 Sm/300g	210	11.7	70	1.8	6.4	3.9	1.1
Lobster Bisque, Simple, EAT*	1 Sm/300g	267	21.6	89	1.5	4.1	7.2	1.1
Meatball, Italian, no Garnish, EAT*	1 Sm/300g	225	6.0	75	4.1	9.5	2.0	2.2
Meatball, Italian, with Garnish, EAT*	1 Sm/322g	254	7.4	79	4.4	9.4	2.3	2.2
Mexican Chicken Chilli with garnish, EAT*	1 Serving/300ml	264	7.5	88	6.1	10.2	2.5	1.4
Mexican Chicken Chilli without garnish, EAT*	1 Serving/300ml	282	8.1	94	6.5	10.8	2.7	1.4
Minestrone, Vegetable, Chunky, EAT*	1 Sm/300g	126	3.6	42	1.7	6.0	1.2	1.4
Prawn Tom Yum, EAT*	1 Serving/814ml	285	9.0	35	1.8	4.1	1.1	0.5
Prawn Tom Yum Pho, Pot, EAT*	1 Pack/839g	369	10.1	44	3.0	5.3	1.2	0.7
Ramen, Shitake, Miso & Udon Noodles, EAT*	1 Pot/625g	250	4.4	40	2.3	5.4	0.7	0.8
Red Pepper, & Goats Cheese, Fire Roasted, EAT*	1 Sm/300g	141	6.9	47	1.9	4.6	2.3	0.9
Spicy Rare Beef, Noodle Pot, EAT*	1 Pack/645g	316	7.7	49	3.4	6.1	1.2	0.6
Steak & Ale Pot Pie with Garnish, EAT*	1 Serving/415ml	415	13.3	100	8.3	9.2	3.2	1.2
Steak & Ale Pot Pie without Garnish, EAT*	1 Serving/625ml	550	13.8	88	8.4	8.3	2.2	1.2
Super Chana Dal, Sm, EAT*	1 Sm/300g	198	3.6	66	3.9	10.0	1.2	3.0
Sweet Potato, & Chilli, EAT*	1 Sm/300g	261	13.2	87	1.3	9.6	4.4	1.7
Tomato, & Basil, Spicy, EAT*	1 Sm/300g	78	0.9	26	0.9	4.6	0.3	0.9
Tomato, Slow Roasted, Creamy, EAT*	1 Sm/300g	240	18.3	80	1.2	4.7	6.1	1.1
Vegetable, Moroccan, Spicy, EAT*	1 Sm/300g	138	2.1	46	1.7	7.8	0.7	1.9
Vegetable Gyoza Dumpling & Egg Noodles Pho, Pot, EAT*	1 Pot/855g	402	9.4	47	2.1	6.9	1.1	0.6
Vegetarian Gyoza Dumpling, EAT*	1 Serving/798ml	431	11.2	54	2.3	7.6	1.4	0.6
Wild Forest Mushroom, EAT*	1 Serving/300ml	150	8.7	50	2.0	3.7	2.9	0.8
Wild Mushroom & Chestnut, Simple, EAT*	1 Sm/300g	240	14.1	80	1.4	8.1	4.7	1.1
TEA								
Chai Latte, Soya, EAT*	1 Cup/355ml	208	6.4	59	4.2	7.1	1.8	0.0
TOAST								
Cheese & Tomato, EAT*	1 Toast/148g	305	10.4	206	10.0	25.6	7.0	2.1
Nutella & Banana, EAT*	1 Serving/153g	393	10.9	257	6.0	41.8	7.1	2.4
TOASTIE								
Chicken, Firecracker, EAT*	1 Toastie/252g	433	10.8	172	11.2	21.0	4.3	1.7
Chicken, Smoked, & Basil, EAT*	1 Toastie/215g	490	18.3	228	13.1	22.8	8.5	1.2

	Measure INFO/WEIGHT	per Measure KCAL	per Measure FAT	Nutrition Values per 100g / 100ml KCAL	PROT	CARB	FAT	FIBRE
EAT								
TOASTIE								
Four Cheese, Ultimate, Sourdough, EAT*	1 Toastie/168g	480	24.3	286	10.9	26.8	14.5	2.4
Ham, & Mature Cheddar, Hot Smoked, EAT*	1 Toastie/151g	553	20.2	367	12.7	21.0	13.4	1.0
Mozzarella, Tomato, & Pesto, EAT*	1 Toastie/224g	508	23.9	227	10.2	20.0	10.7	1.2
Reuben, Sourdough, EAT*	1 Toastie/261g	493	19.8	189	10.5	18.0	7.6	1.5
WRAP								
Chicken, & Roast Pepper, Smoked, Hot, EAT*	1 Wrap/241g	427	30.9	177	12.8	25.1	12.8	1.1
Chicken, Roast, Simple, EAT*	1 Wrap/185g	409	20.5	221	10.0	19.9	11.1	1.2
Chicken, Satay, EAT*	1 Wrap/205g	408	14.1	199	11.2	18.6	6.9	1.4
Halloumi, & Red Pepper Tapenade, Hot, EAT*	1 Wrap/197g	550	23.8	279	12.6	30.6	12.1	1.0
Ham Hock & Cheddar Salad, EAT*	1 Pack/221g	455	22.7	206	12.7	17.2	10.3	0.8
Houmous & Falafel, EAT*	1 Wrap/244g	471	21.2	193	5.9	22.9	8.7	3.7
Houmous & Falafel, Half, EAT*	1 Pack/122g	235	10.6	193	5.9	22.9	8.7	3.7
Mexican Chicken, EAT*	1 Pack/215g	396	13.6	184	9.9	22.1	6.3	2.0
Mexican Chicken, Half, EAT*	1 Pack/108g	198	6.8	184	9.9	22.1	6.3	2.0
Peking Duck, EAT*	1 Wrap/208g	433	16.2	208	11.3	22.9	7.8	1.3
Prawn, King, Thai, EAT*	1 Wrap/220g	361	13.9	164	6.7	19.9	6.3	4.4
Simple Houmous & Salad, EAT*	1 Wrap/202g	362	17.0	179	4.9	21.1	8.4	2.6
Tuna Nicoise, Naked, EAT*	1 Wrap/238g	457	19.0	192	10.6	19.2	8.0	1.8
YOGHURT								
& Granola, EAT*	1 Bowl/197g	313	11.4	159	7.7	19.6	5.8	1.9
Granola & Mixed Red Berries, EAT*	1 Serving/180g	306	8.8	170	5.8	26.1	4.9	2.4
Honey, Grapenuts, & Banana, EAT*	1 Pot/300g	378	6.0	126	4.0	23.3	2.0	1.0
Mango & Passionfruit, EAT*	1 Serving/124g	145	3.6	117	5.6	17.1	2.9	0.2
Mixed Red Berries, EAT*	1 Serving/124g	131	3.6	106	5.6	14.1	2.9	0.3
FIVE GUYS								
BURGERS								
Bacon, Bunless, Five Guys*	1 Burger/238g	628	54.0	264	16.8	0.0	22.7	0.0
Bacon, Five Guys*	1 Burger/315g	888	63.0	282	14.9	12.4	20.0	0.6
Bacon, Little, Bunless, Five Guys*	1 Burger/144g	383	33.0	266	16.7	0.0	22.9	0.0
Bacon, Little, Five Guys*	1 Burger/221g	643	42.0	291	14.0	17.6	19.0	0.9
Cheeseburger, Bacon, Bunless, Five Guys*	1 Burger/262g	708	60.0	270	17.2	0.4	22.9	0.0
Cheeseburger, Bacon, Five Guys*	1 Burger/339g	968	69.0	286	15.3	11.8	20.4	0.6
Cheeseburger, Bacon, Little, Bunless, Five Guys*	1 Burger/156g	423	36.0	271	17.0	0.3	23.1	0.0
Cheeseburger, Bacon, Little, Five Guys*	1 Burger/233g	683	45.0	293	14.4	17.0	19.3	0.9
Cheeseburger, Bunless, Five Guys*	1 Burger/212g	570	48.0	269	17.4	0.5	22.6	0.0
Cheeseburger, Five Guys*	1 Burger/289g	830	57.0	287	15.2	13.8	19.7	0.7
Cheeseburger, Little, Bunless, Five Guys*	1 Burger/106g	285	24.0	269	17.4	0.5	22.6	0.0
Cheeseburger, Little, Five Guys*	1 Burger/183g	545	33.0	298	13.9	21.6	18.0	1.1
Hamburger, Bunless, Five Guys*	1 Burger/188g	490	42.0	261	17.0	0.0	22.3	0.0
Hamburger, Bunless, Little, Five Guys*	1 Burger/94g	245	21.0	261	17.0	0.0	22.3	0.0
Hamburger, Five Guys*	1 Burger/265g	750	51.0	283	14.7	14.7	19.2	0.8
Hamburger, Little, Five Guys*	1 Burger/171g	505	30.0	295	13.4	22.8	17.5	1.2
FRIES								
Lge, Five Guys*	1 Portion/567g	1314	57.0	232	3.5	31.9	10.0	3.7
Little, Five Guys*	1 Portion/227g	526	23.0	232	3.5	31.7	10.1	3.5
Regular, Five Guys*	1 Portion/411g	953	41.0	232	3.6	31.9	10.0	3.6
HOT DOG								
Bacon, & Cheese, Bunless, Five Guys*	1 Hot Dog/152g	388	33.0	255	14.8	1.3	21.7	0.0
Bacon, & Cheese, Five Guys*	1 Hot Dog/229g	648	42.0	283	12.9	17.9	18.3	0.9
Bacon, Bunless, Five Guys*	1 Hot Dog/140g	348	30.0	249	14.3	1.1	21.4	0.0
Bacon, Five Guys*	1 Hot Dog/217g	608	39.0	280	12.4	18.7	18.0	0.9
Cheese, Bunless, Five Guys*	1 Hot Dog/102g	250	21.0	245	14.2	2.0	20.6	0.0

	Measure INFO/WEIGHT	per Measure KCAL	FAT	Nutrition Values per 100g / 100ml KCAL	PROT	CARB	FAT	FIBRE
FIVE GUYS								
HOT DOG								
Cheese, Five Guys*	1 Hot Dog/179g	510	30.0	285	12.0	22.9	16.8	1.1
Original, Bunless, Five Guys*	1 Hot Dog/90g	210	18.0	233	13.3	1.7	20.0	0.0
Original, Five Guys*	1 Hot Dog/167g	470	27.0	281	11.4	24.2	16.2	1.2
SANDWICH								
BLT, Five Guys*	1 Sandwich/273g	642	43.0	235	8.6	15.4	15.8	1.0
Cheese, Grilled, Five Guys*	1 Sandwich/115g	470	22.0	409	8.3	35.6	19.1	2.2
Veggie, Cheese, Five Guys*	1 Sandwich/255g	372	15.0	146	5.1	18.0	5.9	1.4
Veggie, Five Guys*	1 Sandwich/231g	292	9.0	126	3.5	19.9	3.9	1.5
GREGGS								
BAGUETTE								
Bacon, Breakfast, Greggs*	1 Baguette/188g	540	17.7	287	16.0	38.0	9.4	0.0
Bacon & Sausage, Greggs*	1 Baguette/225g	617	22.5	274	15.0	33.0	10.0	0.0
Chicken, & Sweetcorn, Greggs*	1 Baguette/235g	480	11.0	204	10.2	29.8	4.7	0.0
Chicken, BBQ, Greggs*	1 Pack/247g	460	2.9	186	10.1	36.0	1.2	0.0
Chicken, Club, Chargrilled, Hot, Greggs*	1 Roll/167g	510	23.5	305	15.9	27.0	14.1	0.0
Chicken, Club, Greggs*	1 Baguette/265g	600	18.5	226	10.6	29.1	7.0	0.0
Chicken, Fajita, Hot, Greggs*	1 Roll/165g	410	11.0	248	12.7	33.3	6.7	0.0
Chicken, Pesto, Greggs*	1 Baguette/214g	520	16.0	243	11.7	32.5	7.5	0.0
Chicken, Sweet Chilli, Greggs*	1 Baguette/237g	520	3.0	219	10.3	39.7	1.3	0.0
Chicken, Tandoori, Greggs*	1 Baguette/200g	490	16.0	245	10.5	36.0	8.0	0.0
Chicken, Tikka, Greggs*	1 Baguette/250g	490	10.5	196	10.2	29.0	4.2	0.0
Chicken Mayonnaise, Greggs*	1 Baguette/200g	510	16.0	255	10.5	33.8	8.0	0.0
Egg Mayonnaise, & Tomato, Free Range, Greggs*	1 Baguette/237g	480	13.0	203	8.2	29.3	5.5	0.0
Ham, & Cheese, Greggs*	1 Baguette/216g	580	19.0	269	14.4	32.2	8.8	0.0
Ham, & Cheese, Hot, Greggs*	1 Roll/156g	430	17.5	276	16.4	26.9	11.2	0.0
Ham, & Coleslaw, Greggs*	1 Baguette/193g	450	10.5	233	9.3	35.8	5.4	0.0
Meatball Melt, Hot, Greggs*	1 Roll/175g	390	12.5	223	9.4	29.1	7.1	0.0
Mozzarella, & Tomato, Hot, Greggs*	1 Roll/149g	460	20.5	309	12.8	31.2	13.8	0.0
Omelette, Breakfast, Greggs*	1 Baguette/210g	454	12.2	216	9.2	35.0	5.8	0.0
Prawn Mayonnaise, Greggs*	1 Baguette/235g	500	15.0	213	8.7	4.5	6.4	0.0
Sausage, Breakfast, Greggs*	1 Baguette/234g	604	22.7	258	12.0	34.0	9.7	0.0
Tuna Crunch, Greggs*	1 Baguette/235g	530	12.5	226	10.6	32.6	5.3	0.0
Tuna Crunch Melt, Hot, Greggs*	1 Roll/187g	440	13.0	235	13.4	30.0	7.0	0.0
BAKE								
BBQ Pulled Pork, Lattice, Greggs*	1 Lattice/150g	429	26.0	286	5.4	27.3	17.3	0.0
Chicken, Greggs*	1 Bake/150g	426	27.0	284	8.9	20.0	18.0	0.0
Chicken Curry, Greggs*	1 Bake/131g	400	25.5	305	7.6	21.4	19.5	0.0
Festive, Greggs*	1 Slice/141g	480	32.0	340	8.2	24.5	22.7	0.0
Sausage, Bean & Cheese, Melt, Greggs*	1 Bake/140g	430	27.5	307	7.1	25.4	19.6	0.0
Steak, Greggs*	1 Bake/136g	404	25.8	297	10.0	21.0	19.0	0.0
The Spicy One, Fajita Flavour Chicken, Greggs*	1 Bake/143g	430	27.1	301	7.3	24.0	19.0	0.0
BISCUITS								
Bunny, Greggs*	1 Biscuit/52g	269	12.1	513	5.5	72.0	23.0	0.0
Caramel & Pecan Momento, Greggs*	1 Serving/62g	308	17.0	497	5.0	58.1	27.4	0.0
Caramel Heart, Greggs*	1 Biscuit/63g	307	15.7	488	5.7	61.0	25.0	0.0
Jammy Heart, Greggs*	1 Serving/60g	305	16.0	508	5.2	61.7	26.7	0.0
Spikey Mikey, Greggs*	1 Biscuit/38g	204	10.3	536	5.3	70.0	27.0	0.0
Toffee Crunch, Greggs*	1 Biscuit/75g	375	21.0	500	5.0	56.0	28.0	0.0
BREAD								
Brown, Bloomer, Greggs*	1 Serving/36g	98	1.3	272	9.6	50.6	3.5	0.0
Oatmeal, Loaf, Greggs*	1 Serving/80g	190	2.0	238	10.0	38.8	2.5	0.0
Rolls, Corn Topped, Greggs*	1 Roll/76g	190	2.5	250	9.9	44.7	3.3	0.0

GREGGS

INFO/WEIGHT	Measure	per Measure		Nutrition Values per 100g / 100ml				
		KCAL	FAT	KCAL	PROT	CARB	FAT	FIBRE
BREAD								
Rolls, Oval Bite, Greggs*	1 Roll/79g	230	5.0	291	10.1	45.6	6.3	0.0
Rolls, Sub, Seeded, Greggs*	1 Roll/97g	270	4.0	278	11.3	46.9	4.1	0.0
Rolls, Sub, White, Greggs*	1 Roll/89g	230	2.5	258	10.7	46.6	2.8	0.0
Stottie, Greggs*	1 Serving/156g	347	2.2	222	8.6	4.2	1.4	0.0
White, Bloomer, Loaf, Greggs*	1 Serving/56g	138	1.0	247	10.2	46.2	1.7	3.0
BREAKFAST CEREAL								
Porridge, Golden Syrup, Greggs*	1 Pot/234g	252	3.0	108	3.5	20.0	1.3	0.0
Porridge, Red Berry, Greggs*	1 Pot/234g	250	3.3	107	3.8	20.8	1.4	0.0
BROWNIES								
Chocolate, Mini, Greggs*	1 Brownie/18g	90	5.0	500	8.3	58.3	27.8	0.0
BUNS								
Belgian, Greggs*	1 Bun/130g	406	4.7	312	4.5	65.0	3.6	0.0
Easter Ring, Greggs*	1 Bun/61g	246	11.0	404	3.4	57.0	18.0	0.0
Hot Cross, Greggs*	1 Bun/66g	176	1.5	265	7.1	54.1	2.3	0.0
Iced, Christmas Ring, Greggs*	1 Bun/60g	210	5.0	350	4.2	62.5	8.3	0.0
Iced, Finger, Greggs*	1 Bun/35g	111	3.0	316	7.0	52.4	8.7	1.6
CAKE								
Christmas Slice, Greggs*	1 Slice/86g	360	11.5	419	5.8	67.4	13.4	0.0
Crispy Cornfake, Greggs*	1 Cake/100g	280	11.7	280	3.0	38.0	11.7	0.0
Easter, Crispy nest, Greggs*	1 Cake/70g	326	13.3	466	3.9	71.0	19.0	0.0
Vanilla Slice, Greggs*	1 Slice/138g	359	17.0	260	3.6	34.8	12.3	0.7
Victoria Sponge, Mini, Greggs*	1 Sponge/129g	497	31.0	385	3.6	37.0	24.0	0.0
COFFEE								
Black, Regular, Greggs*	1 Cup/455ml	20	0.6	4	0.3	0.3	0.1	0.0
Cappuccino, no Chocolate Topping, Regular, Greggs*	1 Regular/455ml	110	4.0	24	1.8	2.5	0.9	0.0
Cappuccino, no Chocolate Topping, Sm, Greggs*	1 Sm/340ml	90	3.0	26	1.8	2.5	0.9	0.0
White, Regular, Greggs*	1 Regular/455ml	40	1.5	9	0.7	0.8	0.3	0.0
White, Sm, Greggs*	1 Sm/340ml	30	0.9	9	0.6	0.7	0.3	0.0
COLA								
Coca-Cola, Greggs*	1 Serving/330ml	139	0.0	42	0.0	10.6	0.0	0.0
Coke Zero, Coca-Cola, Greggs*	1 Serving/500ml	3	0.0	1	0.0	0.0	0.0	0.0
Diet, Coca-Cola, Greggs*	1 Serving/500ml	3	0.0	1	0.0	0.0	0.0	0.0
COOKIES								
Fruit & Oat, Greggs*	1 Cookie/77g	341	15.4	444	5.8	60.0	20.0	0.0
Fruit & Oatie, Greggs*	1 Cookie/76g	338	15.2	445	5.8	60.0	20.0	0.0
Milk Chocolate Chunk, Greggs*	1 Cookie/75g	380	20.3	506	7.0	58.5	27.0	2.8
Triple Chocolate Chunk, Greggs*	1 Cookie/75g	374	20.3	498	6.5	56.0	27.0	4.2
White Chocolate Chunk, Greggs*	1 Cookie/75g	383	20.3	510	6.8	59.0	27.0	0.0
CROISSANT								
All Butter, Greggs*	1 Croissant/55g	288	16.5	524	10.0	53.0	30.0	0.0
CUPCAKES								
Chocolate, Greggs*	1 Cupcake/74g	280	10.0	378	4.0	59.5	13.5	0.0
Easter, Greggs*	1 Cake/87g	393	22.6	452	3.7	52.0	26.0	0.0
Foundation, Greggs*	1 Cupcake/79g	320	13.0	405	3.2	60.1	16.5	0.0
Ice Cream, Greggs*	1 Cupcake/73g	270	11.0	370	4.1	51.4	15.1	0.0
Sweet Lemon, Greggs*	1 Cake/81g	380	16.0	469	0.0	71.6	19.8	0.0
DOUGHNUTS								
Blueberry Burst, Greggs*	1 Doughnut/95.7g	340	10.5	355	6.3	57.0	11.0	0.0
Caramel Custard, Greggs*	1 Doughnut/102g	306	11.2	301	4.8	45.0	11.0	0.0
Cinnamon, Greggs*	1 Doughnut/96g	380	16.5	396	6.2	54.7	17.2	0.0
Cream Finger, Greggs*	1 Finger/101g	325	19.2	322	5.6	30.0	19.0	0.0
Easter, Greggs*	1 Doughnut/78g	305	14.0	391	5.9	50.0	18.0	0.0

	Measure INFO/WEIGHT	per Measure KCAL	FAT	Nutrition Values per 100g / 100ml KCAL	PROT	CARB	FAT	FIBRE
GREGGS								
DOUGHNUTS								
Finger, Creamed Filled, Topped with Jam, Greggs*	1 Finger/109g	390	26.5	358	5.5	27.5	24.3	0.0
Jaffa Cake, Greggs*	1 Doughnut/95g	320	8.5	337	5.3	58.4	9.0	0.0
Jam Filled, Greggs*	1 Doughnut/74g	242	8.1	329	6.6	51.0	11.0	0.0
Lemon Drizzle, Greggs*	1 Doughnut/105g	360	11.5	343	5.2	55.7	11.0	0.0
Strawberry Milkshake Filled, Greggs*	1 Doughnut/91g	360	15.0	396	6.3	53.8	16.5	0.0
Sugar, Mini, Greggs*	1 Doughnut/17g	64	3.0	363	5.9	47.1	17.0	0.0
Sugar Strand, Greggs*	1 Doughnut/79g	276	7.3	347	5.9	60.0	9.2	0.0
Triple Chocolate, Vanilla Filled, Greggs*	1 Doughnut/91g	341	14.5	376	5.4	52.0	16.0	0.0
Yum Yum, Greggs*	1 Yum Yum/73g	294	16.8	403	5.2	43.0	23.0	0.0
Yum Yum, Toffee Topping, Greggs*	1 Yum Yum/73g	290	16.5	397	5.5	43.2	22.6	0.0
Yum Yums, Mini, Greggs*	1 Portion/30g	121	6.9	404	5.2	43.0	23.0	0.0
DR PEPPER*								
Greggs*	1 Serving/500ml	210	0.0	42	0.0	2.1	0.0	0.0
ECLAIR								
Chocolate, with Cream, Greggs*	1 Eclair/86g	325	19.8	378	4.7	35.0	23.0	0.0
FANTA								
Fanta, Greggs*	1 Serving/500ml	150	0.0	30	0.0	7.1	0.0	0.0
FLAPJACK								
Fruity, Mini, Greggs*	1 Flapjack/22g	110	5.0	500	6.8	59.1	22.7	0.0
FLATBREAD								
Cajun Chicken, Balanced Choice, Greggs*	1 Wrap/180g	326	6.0	181	10.0	27.8	3.3	0.0
Chilli Chicken, Soy, Greggs*	1 Portion/165g	285	1.5	173	20.0	47.0	0.9	0.0
Mexican Five Bean, Greggs*	1 Flatbread/186g	327	7.1	176	5.0	29.0	3.8	0.0
FRUIT								
Tropical, Greggs*	1 Serving/150g	80	0.0	53	0.7	11.3	0.0	0.0
GINGERBREAD								
Man, with Chocolate Beans, Greggs*	1 Biscuit/42g	180	4.6	428	7.1	76.0	11.0	0.0
IRN BRU								
Diet, Greggs*	1 Serving/330ml	2	0.0	1	0.0	0.0	0.0	0.0
Greggs*	1 Serving/500ml	215	0.0	43	0.0	10.5	0.0	0.0
JUICE								
Apple, Fairtrade, Greggs*	1 Serving/500ml	220	0.0	44	0.0	11.0	0.0	0.0
Orange, Fairtrade, Greggs*	1 Serving/500ml	220	0.0	44	0.1	10.2	0.0	0.0
JUICE DRINK								
Citrus Punch, Oasis, Greggs*	1 Serving/500ml	90	0.0	18	0.0	4.1	0.0	0.0
Summer Fruits, Oasis, Greggs*	1 Serving/500ml	90	0.0	18	0.0	4.2	0.0	0.0
LUCOZADE								
Energy Orange, Greggs*	1 Serving/500ml	350	0.0	70	0.0	17.2	0.0	0.0
Sport, Greggs*	1 Serving/500ml	140	0.0	28	0.0	6.4	0.0	0.0
MUFFIN								
Chocolate, Triple, Greggs*	1 Muffin/129g	511	28.4	396	4.2	45.0	22.0	0.0
Jam & Toast, Breakfast, Greggs*	1 Muffin/110g	381	13.2	346	5.7	54.0	12.0	0.0
Lemon, Sicilian, Greggs*	1 Muffin/126g	500	24.5	397	5.2	48.8	19.4	0.0
Sticky Toffee, Greggs*	1 Muffin/128g	530	27.0	414	5.1	49.2	21.1	0.0
PAIN AU CHOCOLAT								
with Belgian Chocolate, Greggs*	1 Pain/82g	393	21.3	479	9.6	51.0	26.0	0.0
PASTA								
Cheese & Tomato, with Mixed Herbs, Pot, Greggs*	1 Pack/300g	381	10.2	127	5.0	19.0	3.4	0.0
Fajita Chicken, in Tomato Sauce, Spicy, Pot, Greggs*	1 Pack/300g	345	7.2	115	5.2	18.0	2.4	0.0
PASTY								
Cheese & Onion, Freshly Baked, Greggs*	1 Pasty/126g	390	26.0	310	6.0	23.4	20.6	0.0
Cheese & Onion, Roll, Greggs*	1 Roll/105g	317	21.0	302	6.2	22.0	20.0	0.0

GREGGS

	INFO/WEIGHT	KCAL	FAT	KCAL	PROT	CARB	FAT	FIBRE
PASTY								
Cornish, Greggs*	1 Pasty/190g	560	32.0	295	7.4	21.0	16.8	0.0
Ham & Cheese Past, Greggs*	1 Pasty/140g	420	28.0	300	7.0	22.0	20.0	0.0
Steak & Cheese, Roll, Greggs*	1 Roll/108g	340	22.7	315	12.0	20.0	21.0	0.0
PIE								
Mince, Sweet, Greggs*	1 Pie/70g	290	11.0	414	4.3	61.4	15.7	0.0
Mince, Sweet, Iced, Greggs*	1 Pie/63g	230	6.5	365	2.4	62.7	10.3	0.0
PIZZA								
Cheese & Tomato, Greggs*	1 Serving/111g	290	10.5	261	9.5	32.0	9.5	0.0
Chicken, Chargrilled, Greggs*	1 Serving/111g	340	11.5	306	14.9	36.5	10.4	0.0
Chicken, Spicy, Greggs*	1 Serving/183g	450	11.5	246	12.3	36.9	6.3	0.0
Pepperoni, Greggs*	1 Serving/121g	350	14.0	289	11.6	33.1	11.6	0.0
PUDDING								
Bread, Greggs*	1 Portion/50g	118	3.9	236	4.6	38.0	7.8	0.0
RIBENA*								
Greggs*	1 Serving/500ml	215	0.0	43	0.0	10.5	0.0	0.0
ROLL								
Bacon, & Sausage, Corn Topped, Breakfast, Greggs*	1 Roll/162g	439	21.1	271	15.0	23.0	13.0	0.0
Bacon, Corn Topped Roll, Breakfast, Greggs*	1 Roll/124g	360	14.9	289	17.0	27.0	12.0	0.0
Omelette, Breakfast, Greggs*	1 Roll/161g	322	13.0	200	9.5	22.0	8.1	0.0
Sausage, Corn Topped Roll, Breakfast, Greggs*	1 Roll/159g	410	19.1	258	12.0	25.0	12.0	0.0
SALAD								
Chicken & Bacon, Layered, Greggs*	1 Pack/211g	262	11.0	124	6.8	13.0	5.2	0.0
Chicken & Bacon, Pasta, Greggs*	1 Portion/235g	327	14.1	139	7.0	13.0	6.0	0.0
Tuna, Layered, Greggs*	1 Box/211g	230	8.2	109	5.5	14.0	3.9	0.0
Tuna Crunch, Pasta, Greggs*	1 Serving/250g	282	8.0	113	6.0	14.0	3.2	0.0
SANDWICH								
Beef, & Dijon Mustard, Rye Oval Bite, Greggs*	1 Pack166g	340	7.0	205	13.0	28.0	4.2	3.2
BLT, Sweetcure Bacon, Malted Brown, Classic, Greggs*	1 Serving/100g	258	13.2	258	8.9	24.2	13.2	0.0
Cheese, & Tomato, Mature Cheddar, Oatmeal, Greggs*	1 Sandwich/187g	490	23.0	262	9.9	26.7	12.3	0.0
Cheese, Savoury, on Seeded White, Greggs*	1 Pack/166g	480	22.0	289	10.8	31.0	13.2	0.0
Cheese Ploughman's, Oval Bite, Greggs*	1 Pack/201g	420	20.0	209	8.7	20.9	10.0	0.0
Chicken, & Mango, on Malted Brown, Bloomer, Greggs*	1 Bloomer/217g	510	18.5	235	11.3	28.3	8.5	0.0
Chicken, & Mango, on White, Bloomer, Greggs*	1 Bloomer/217g	510	19.5	235	11.3	26.7	9.0	0.0
Chicken, & Salsa, Chargrilled, on Oatmeal, Greggs*	1 Sandwich/216g	340	3.5	157	12.0	22.2	1.6	0.0
Chicken, & Sweetcorn, Red Fat Mayo, Oatmeal, Greggs*	1 Sandwich/166g	310	5.5	187	11.4	25.9	3.3	0.0
Chicken, Bacon, & Sweetcorn, Brown Bloomer, Greggs*	1 Bloomer/235g	520	18.0	221	11.3	26.8	7.7	0.0
Chicken, Bacon, & Sweetcorn, White, Bloomer, Greggs*	1 Bloomer/235g	520	18.5	221	11.1	27.0	7.9	0.0
Chicken, BBQ, Oval Bite, Greggs*	1 Roll/204g	340	6.0	167	10.8	23.0	2.9	0.0
Chicken, Brie & Bacon Rustic, Greggs*	1 Pack/211g	549	22.0	260	15.2	24.6	10.4	0.0
Chicken, Chargrilled, Oval Bite, Greggs*	1 Roll/211g	440	19.0	209	11.6	19.2	9.0	0.0
Chicken, Chilli, Double, Oval Bite, Greggs*	1 Roll/219g	390	9.5	178	11.0	22.4	4.3	0.0
Chicken, Mexican, Oval Bite, Greggs*	1 Roll/179g	420	15.0	235	14.2	24.0	8.4	0.0
Chicken, Sweet Chilli, on White, Bloomer, Greggs*	1 Sandwich/255g	460	3.0	180	10.8	31.0	1.2	0.0
Chicken, Sweet Chilli, White, no Mayo, Bloomer, Greggs*	1 Bloomer/242g	430	3.5	178	11.0	29.8	1.4	0.0
Chicken & Chorizo Rustic, Greggs*	1 Pack/226g	566	24.0	250	15.0	23.4	10.6	0.0
Chicken Salad, Classic, on Malted Brown, Greggs*	1 Sandwich/248g	520	23.0	210	9.9	20.6	9.3	0.0
Chicken Salad, Low Fat Mayo, Malted Brown, Greggs*	1 Pack/218g	380	7.0	174	10.8	25.2	3.2	0.0
Christmas Dinner, Greggs*	1 Pack/205g	570	18.5	278	12.2	35.4	9.0	0.0
Egg Mayonnaise, on Seeded White, Greggs*	1 Pack/174g	420	17.5	241	11.2	26.7	10.1	0.0
Egg Mayonnaise, with Cracked Black Pepper, Greggs*	1 Sandwich/166g	420	12.0	253	9.9	35.5	7.2	0.0
Ham, & Egg, Honey Roast, Salad, on Oatmeal, Greggs*	1 Sandwich/243g	450	15.5	185	9.9	21.0	6.4	0.0
Ham, Cheese, & Pickle, Malted Brown, Bloomer, Greggs*	1 Bloomer/228g	540	19.0	237	11.2	29.0	8.3	0.0

GREGGS

	INFO/WEIGHT	KCAL	FAT	KCAL	PROT	CARB	FAT	FIBRE
SANDWICH								
Ham, Cheese, & Pickle, on White, Bloomer, Greggs*	1 Bloomer/228g	510	18.0	224	11.2	27.4	7.9	0.0
Ham Salad, Honey Roast, no Mayo, Greggs*	1 Pack/212g	400	13.0	189	9.0	23.8	6.1	0.0
Ham Salad, Oval Bite, Greggs*	1 Sandwich/175g	320	10.5	183	9.1	21.7	6.0	0.0
Prawn Mayonnaise, Reduced Fat, on Oatmeal, Greggs*	1 Sandwich/166g	300	7.5	181	10.2	23.8	4.5	0.0
Southern Fried Chicken Rustic, Greggs*	1 Pack/268g	563	16.0	210	11.2	27.2	6.0	0.0
Steak & Cheese Rustic, Greggs*	1 Pack/237g	512	16.0	216	13.5	24.9	6.8	0.0
Sub, Chicken, & Mayonnaise, on White, Greggs*	1 Sub/186g	400	15.0	215	11.6	22.3	8.1	0.0
Sub, Egg Mayonnaise, & Bacon, on Plain White, Greggs*	1 Roll/181g	430	16.5	238	12.2	26.2	9.1	0.0
Sub, Ham, & Egg, with Salad, on White, Greggs*	1 Sub/220g	390	14.5	177	9.8	19.1	6.6	0.0
Sub, Tuna Mayonnaise, on Seeded White, Greggs*	1 Sub/222g	410	12.0	185	11.7	21.0	5.4	0.0
Sub, Tuna Mayonnaise, on White, Greggs*	1 Roll/202g	350	10.0	173	11.6	19.6	5.0	0.0
Tuna, Sweet Chilli, & Red Pepper, on Oatmeal, Greggs*	1 Sandwich/206g	370	4.5	180	11.2	27.2	2.2	0.0
Tuna Crunch, on Brown, Bloomer, Greggs*	1 Sandwich/235g	520	15.0	221	11.1	28.9	6.4	0.0
Tuna Crunch, on White, Bloomer, Greggs*	1 Bloomer/217g	430	13.5	198	10.8	24.6	6.2	0.0
Tuna Mayo, & Cucumber, Malted Brown, Low Fat, Greggs*	1 Sandwich/201g	360	5.0	179	10.7	27.6	2.5	0.0
Tuna Mayo, & Sweetcorn, Low Fat, on Oatmeal, Greggs*	1 Sandwich/166g	310	5.5	187	13.0	24.7	3.3	0.0
Tuna Mayonnaise, & Cucumber, on Oatmeal, Greggs*	1 Sandwich/194g	400	11.0	206	12.1	25.5	5.7	0.0
Tuna Mayonnaise, on Malted Brown, Greggs*	1 Sandwich/203g	440	13.5	217	12.3	26.6	6.6	0.0
SAUSAGE ROLL								
Freshly Baked, Greggs*	1 Serving/103g	360	25.5	350	8.2	22.8	24.8	0.0
Mini, Greggs*	1 Roll/26g	81	6.5	310	8.5	21.5	25.0	0.0
SCONE								
Derby, Greggs*	1 Scone/60g	268	13.1	447	5.3	58.0	21.8	0.0
SLICES								
Toffee Apple, Lattice, Greggs*	1 Slice/77g	277	15.0	360	4.0	41.0	19.5	0.0
SMOOTHIE								
Mango & Orange, Greggs*	1 Serving/250ml	145	0.0	58	0.6	13.2	0.0	0.0
Raspberry & Banana, Greggs*	1 Serving/250ml	135	0.0	54	0.6	12.2	0.0	0.0
SOUP								
Cajun Chicken, Greggs*	1 Serving/300g	159	3.0	53	3.1	7.4	1.0	0.0
Lentil & Bacon, Greggs*	1 Serving/300g	177	4.2	59	3.4	7.9	1.4	0.0
Tomato, Heinz, Greggs*	1 Pot/300g`	240	9.9	80	1.0	11.0	3.3	0.0
SPRITE*								
Greggs*	1 Serving/500ml	220	0.0	44	0.0	10.6	0.0	0.0
TART								
Egg Custard, Greggs*	1 Tart/90g	257	13.0	286	5.5	33.2	14.5	0.0
Strawberry, Greggs*	1 Tart/65g	180	7.5	277	2.3	41.5	11.5	0.0
Strawberry, with Fresh Cream, Greggs*	1 Tart/94g	300	16.5	319	3.2	35.1	17.6	0.0
TEACAKES								
Bakery, Greggs*	1 Teacake/74g	206	3.4	278	7.4	52.0	4.6	0.0
TURNOVER								
Apple, Fresh Cream, Greggs*	1 Turnover/176g	540	32.5	307	2.8	34.1	18.5	0.0
WATER								
Cranberry or Raspberry, Greggs*	1 Serving/500ml	5	0.0	1	0.0	0.0	0.0	0.0
WRAP								
Bacon & Cheese, Greggs*	1 Wrap/91g	382	28.2	420	14.0	21.0	31.0	0.0
Chicken, & Bacon, Caesar, Greggs*	1 Wrap/189g	450	23.5	238	10.8	20.4	12.4	0.0
Chicken, Chargrilled, Greggs*	1 Wrap/192g	410	18.5	214	10.2	20.8	9.6	0.0
Moroccan Tagine Chicken, Greggs*	1 Wrap/175g	354	10.2	202	5.6	31.4	5.8	2.3
YOGHURT								
Greek Style, Greggs*	1 Pot/190g	230	7.0	121	5.5	16.0	3.7	0.0
Raspberry, & Granola, Natural, Greggs*	1 Pot/190g	228	4.8	120	5.0	18.5	2.5	0.0

	INFO/WEIGHT	KCAL	FAT	KCAL	PROT	CARB	FAT	FIBRE
ITSU								
BEANS								
Edamame, Itsu*	1 Pack/100g	124	3.8	124	9.9	11.5	3.8	0.0
Edamame, Yoghurt Coated, Itsu*	½ Pack/35g	110	6.9	314	6.3	43.4	19.7	2.6
CHICKEN &								
Coconut, Noodle Pot, Itsu*	1 Pot/500g	299	12.6	60	4.1	5.9	2.5	0.3
CHICKEN TERIYAKI								
On a Bed, Low Carb, Itsu*	1 Pack/150g	423	10.6	282	16.1	37.3	7.1	2.6
Potsu, Hot, Itsu*	1 Serving/334g	446	7.3	134	11.8	16.1	2.2	0.9
DRESSING								
for Salad Boxes, Itsu*	Sm Pot/10g	41	4.0	410	5.0	30.0	40.0	0.0
DRIED FRUIT & NUTS								
Superseeds, Frogo, Itsu*	1 Portion/100g	359	12.7	359	10.9	53.3	12.7	7.7
DUMPLINGS								
Vegetable, with Rice, Itsu*	1 Serving/100g	382	6.2	382	9.4	69.1	6.2	5.2
FRUIT								
Fresh, Pot, Itsu*	1 Pot/150g	102	0.4	68	0.9	14.7	0.3	0.0
FRUIT COCKTAIL								
Melon, Pineapple, Mango, Apple & Red Grapes, Itsu*	1 Pot/166g	80	0.2	48	0.5	10.4	0.1	0.0
FRUIT SALAD								
Hawaii 5 0, Itsu*	1 Pot/100g	113	0.5	113	1.5	24.3	0.5	2.8
MIXED FRUIT								
Yoghurt Fruit & Goji Berries, Itsu*	1 Pack/70g	211	12.6	302	2.0	66.0	18.0	0.0
NOODLES								
Pot, Chicken, Itsu*	1 Pot/744g	409	3.7	55	2.0	9.9	0.5	1.2
Vegetable Festival, Crystal Noodle Cup, Itsu*	1 Cup/364g	160	2.9	44	1.2	7.9	0.8	0.5
POPCORN								
Sea Salt Flavour, Itsu*	1 Bag/23g	115	6.5	501	8.2	53.6	28.2	10.9
Wasabi, Itsu*	1 Pack/25g	121	6.6	484	8.4	54.1	26.2	9.7
POTSU								
Ricebowl, Superbowl, Lge, Itsu*	1 Lge Potsu/470g	525	17.8	112	1.8	6.4	3.8	1.0
Superbowl, 7 Vegetables with Rice, Itsu*	1 Potsu/380g	525	17.8	138	2.3	8.0	4.7	1.2
PUDDING								
Lemon Zinger, Itsu*	1 Pudding/70g	234	16.3	334	1.3	29.8	23.3	0.3
White Chocolate Dream, Pot, Itsu*	1 Pot/100g	293	22.7	293	1.7	20.2	22.7	0.0
RICE CAKES								
Chocolate, Dark, Itsu*	1 Slice/17g	85	4.1	500	6.1	63.4	24.0	2.8
Chocolate, Milk, Itsu*	1 Pack/50g	249	11.4	498	6.0	65.4	22.8	3.0
Yoghurt, Itsu*	1 Pack/50g	240	9.6	480	9.0	66.0	19.2	3.0
RICE CRACKERS								
Peanut, Snack, Itsu*	1 Pack/70g	239	16.1	342	17.0	55.0	23.0	0.0
SALAD								
Box, Smoked Chicken, Itsu*	1 Box/250g	425	6.5	170	16.1	19.8	2.6	2.2
Chicken, Smoked, Low Carb, Box, Itsu*	1 Box/250g	269	9.3	108	15.4	2.9	3.7	0.0
Chicken & Avocado, Itsu*	1 Serving/250g	340	19.8	136	11.8	3.9	7.9	2.1
Duck Hoisin & Quinoa, Itsu*	1 Pack/200g	488	12.2	244	12.3	34.2	6.1	8.7
Egg, Avo & Quinoa, with Spicy Sauce, Go Go Pot, Itsu*	1 Serving/100g	192	11.8	192	8.1	14.0	11.8	2.3
Ham Hock, Itsu*	1 Pack/200g	404	15.0	202	11.0	22.2	7.5	1.2
Hip & Healthy, Box, Itsu*	1 Pack/371g	230	9.4	62	1.7	8.6	2.5	0.9
Low Carb Salmon & Tuna Tartar, Box, Itsu*	1 Box/137g	173	5.3	126	8.2	3.6	3.9	0.8
Salmon & Tuna Tartare on a Bed, Itsu*	1 Pack/100g	347	10.2	347	20.3	41.9	10.2	2.0
Salmon Supreme, Omega 3, Itsu*	1 Pack/400g	367	15.5	92	5.3	9.2	3.9	0.0
Side, Itsu*	1 Serving/100g	21	0.2	21	1.1	2.8	0.2	1.4
Special Salmon, Itsu*	1 Meal/200g	402	13.4	201	12.2	22.2	6.7	2.3

ITSU

INFO/WEIGHT	Measure	per Measure KCAL	FAT	Nutrition Values per 100g / 100ml KCAL	PROT	CARB	FAT	FIBRE
SALAD								
Tuna, Low Carb, Itsu*	1 Serving/100g	169	8.1	169	20.9	9.1	8.1	0.0
Tuna, no Lettuce, Itsu*	1 Serving/250g	169	8.1	68	8.4	3.6	3.2	0.0
Tuna Rice Oise, Itsu*	1 Pack/300g	268	5.3	89	11.8	33.0	1.8	3.3
SALMON								
& Avocado, Spicy, Maki Box, Itsu*	1 Box/172g	458	19.9	266	5.5	6.2	11.6	1.2
& Egg, Special, Go Go Pot, Itsu*	1 Pot/140g	219	12.6	156	14.0	4.6	9.0	2.0
Poached, Cooked Rare, Itsu*	1 Pack/100g	370	23.5	370	32.6	5.9	23.5	2.4
Sashimi, Muki Beans, Wakame & Wasabi, Itsu*	1 Pack/127g	198	8.0	156	13.1	12.5	6.3	3.3
SANDWICH								
Chicken & Avocado Salad with Bread, Itsu*	1 Pack/250g	441	12.1	176	10.2	18.4	4.8	3.1
Crab, California, Maki Boxes & Sushi Sandwiches, Itsu*	1 Pack/138g	327	14.6	237	6.1	6.0	10.6	1.0
Salmon Supreme, Sushi, Itsu*	1 Pack/114g	202	13.3	177	6.6	6.2	11.7	1.2
Tangy Tuna, Salad, no Mayo, Itsu*	1 Pack/150g	256	9.8	171	16.3	11.5	6.5	2.1
Tuna Sushi, Sushi, Itsu*	1 Pack/116g	179	7.9	154	6.3	7.2	6.8	1.0
Veggie Club, Sushi, Itsu*	1 Pack/161g	175	5.1	109	3.6	16.0	3.2	2.2
SAUCE								
Hot Su Potsu, Itsu*	1 Serving/7g	6	0.0	86	0.1	20.0	0.1	0.1
SEAWEED								
Crispy Thins, Snack, Itsu*	1 Pack/5g	24	1.6	470	27.0	7.7	32.8	18.1
Crispy Thins, Wasabi Flavour, Itsu*	1 Pack/5g	22	1.4	433	29.8	7.0	27.3	20.2
SMOOTHIE								
Raw Veg Cleanse, Itsu*	1 Glass/400ml	162	5.5	40	0.8	6.7	1.4	1.1
SOUP								
Chicken Jaipur, Itsu*	1 Pot/386g	299	8.4	77	6.2	8.4	2.2	0.4
Chicken Noodle, Classic, Itsu*	1 Pot/386g	219	6.8	57	4.2	6.1	1.8	0.3
Miso, Itsu*	1 Pot/309ml	96	8.0	31	5.9	12.2	2.6	3.1
Miso, Noodle, Detox, Itsu*	1 Pot/100g	183	3.1	183	5.3	32.2	3.1	2.7
Miso, Original, from Supermarket, Itsu*	1 Serving/25g	44	1.2	175	10.2	20.5	4.9	3.8
Teriyaki Chicken with Rice, Potsu, Itsu*	1 Serving/450g	627	20.0	139	6.6	7.3	4.4	1.0
Thai Duck Hot, Potsu, Itsu*	1 Serving/200g	397	16.9	198	8.1	22.0	8.4	1.6
SUSHI								
Best of Its, Itsu*	1 Pack/250g	413	12.2	165	10.6	21.1	4.9	2.6
Crab, California Rolls, Itsu*	1 Pack/200g	194	5.2	97	3.6	12.4	2.6	2.8
Health & Happiness, Box, Itsu*	1 Serving/100g	447	17.2	447	28.7	46.1	17.2	4.5
It Box, Itsu*	1 Box/100g	284	9.6	284	15.8	36.2	9.6	5.6
Maki, Spicy Tuna, Itsu*	1 Pack/162g	151	1.3	93	7.4	12.8	0.8	0.9
Maki Roll, Duck Hoisin, Itsu*	1 Box/162g	197	2.1	122	6.4	20.5	1.3	1.4
Omega 3 Salmon Supreme, Itsu*	1 Pack/100g	459	25.7	459	25.5	32.3	25.7	2.9
Salmon & Avo, Maki Rolls, Itsu*	1 Pack/171g	242	10.8	142	6.9	13.9	6.3	1.8
Salmon & Salmon, Itsu*	1 Serving/200g	518	13.4	259	7.0	6.6	6.7	0.7
Salmon & Tuna, Junior Pack, Itsu*	1 Pack/170g	165	4.1	97	8.0	11.9	2.4	0.6
Salmon Sushi, Itsu*	1 Serving/100g	203	8.4	203	14.2	17.8	8.4	0.4
Slim Salmon, Itsu*	1 Serving/150g	288	11.2	192	10.9	20.5	7.5	0.0
Super Salmon 3 Ways, Itsu*	1 Serving/100g	474	21.0	474	29.1	44.3	21.0	4.2
Tuna, Lots of Ginger, Itsu*	1 Pack/185g	141	0.8	76	7.8	11.0	0.4	0.6
Tuna & Salmon, Sashimi Box, Itsu*	1 Box/250g	240	5.5	96	7.7	12.2	2.2	0.8
Tuna & Salmon Junior, Itsu*	1 Serving/100g	174	4.7	174	15.3	18.0	4.7	0.4
Tuna & Salmon Sushi, Itsu*	1 Serving/100g	245	6.4	245	12.6	14.9	6.4	1.3
WATER								
Vitsu Water, Lemon Ninja, Itsu*	1 Bottle/500ml	60	0.5	12	0.1	2.7	0.1	0.1

JD WETHERSPOON

	INFO/WEIGHT	KCAL	FAT	KCAL	PROT	CARB	FAT	FIBRE
BAGUETTE								
BLT, Malted Grain, Wetherspoons*	1 Baguette/399g	823	45.5	206	8.3	17.8	11.4	1.3
Cheddar Cheese & Pickle, Malted Grain, Wetherspoons*	1 Baguette/361g	696	29.9	193	7.9	21.9	8.3	1.6
Chicken, BBQ & Bacon, Melt, Malted Grain, Wetherspoons*	1 Baguette/342g	1271	49.3	371	20.6	37.4	14.4	2.9
Chicken, Southern Fried, Creole Mayo, Wetherspoons*	1 Meal/250g	817	35.7	327	12.6	37.7	14.3	2.0
Crayfish, Malted Grain, Wetherspoons*	1 Baguette/314g	594	25.5	189	6.1	23.2	8.1	1.7
Hot Sausage & Tomato Chutney, Wetherspoons*	1 Meal/250g	839	33.4	336	14.1	40.7	13.4	3.8
Ploughmans, Lloyds, Wetherspoons*	1 Baguette/346g	778	34.3	225	8.6	25.5	9.9	2.2
Tuna Mayonnaise, Malted Grain, Wetherspoons*	1 Baguette/401g	710	31.3	177	8.9	18.1	7.8	1.3
Wiltshire Ham, Wetherspoons*	1 Baguette/346g	536	13.1	155	9.9	20.4	3.8	1.5
BALTI								
Chicken, Rice, Naan, Chutney, Poppadoms, Wetherspoons*	1 Meal/650g	927	27.1	143	6.0	21.0	4.2	1.3
BEEF DINNER								
Roast, Roast Potatoes, Yorkshire Pud & Veg, Wetherspoons*	1 Meal/837g	1305	62.7	156	6.1	17.7	7.5	2.3
BEEF WITH								
Chips, Ribeye, & Side Salad, Wetherspoons*	1 Meal/562g	1006	71.9	179	8.0	8.9	12.8	0.3
Chips, Ribeye, Peas, Tomato & Mushroom, Wetherspoons*	1 Meal/531g	945	63.7	178	9.3	9.3	12.0	0.3
Chips, Ribeye, Prawn Skewer, & Salad, Wetherspoons*	1 Meal/714g	1093	56.4	153	11.0	7.7	7.9	0.3
Chips, T-Bone, & Salad, Wetherspoons*	1 Meal/673g	1313	97.6	195	9.4	7.4	14.5	0.2
Jacket Potato, Ribeye, 8oz, & Salad, Wetherspoons*	1 Meal/620g	850	43.4	137	8.2	10.1	7.0	1.1
Jacket Potato, T-Bone, 12oz, & Salad, Wetherspoons*	1 Meal/756g	1496	96.7	198	9.1	12.3	12.8	1.2
Salad, Rump Steak, Skinny, Wetherspoons*	1 Serving/200g	461	41.3	230	22.2	2.4	20.6	0.8
BHAJI								
Onion, Wetherspoons*	1 Bhaji/30g	43	2.2	143	5.3	18.7	7.3	5.7
BIRYANI								
Chicken, with Naan Bread, Curry Club, Wetherspoons*	1 Meal/706g	897	26.8	127	5.1	18.1	3.8	1.3
Chicken, without Naan, Wetherspoons*	1 Meal/614g	700	24.6	114	4.7	14.8	4.0	1.3
BREAD								
Garlic, Ciabatta, Wetherspoons*	1 Serving/142g	406	17.9	286	8.0	1.0	12.6	1.5
Naan, Wetherspoons*	1 Naan/90g	197	2.5	219	7.6	41.0	2.8	1.4
BREAKFAST								
Baguette, Quorn Sausage, Wetherspoons*	1 Baguette/285g	622	18.3	218	10.5	29.4	6.4	3.4
Blueberry Muffin, Wetherspoons*	1 Muffin/124g	467	25.8	374	4.7	43.2	20.7	0.4
Bran, Fruit & Nut Muffin, Wetherspoons*	1 Serving/145g	571	31.7	394	7.2	43.0	21.9	1.1
Children's, Wetherspoons*	1 Serving/341g	613	37.1	180	10.4	10.8	10.9	2.3
Eggs Benedict, Wetherspoons*	1 Serving/100g	573	30.9	573	38.7	33.6	30.9	2.4
Farmhouse, with Toast, Wetherspoons*	1 Serving/796g	1647	101.8	207	9.4	14.0	12.8	1.9
Morning Roll, with Bacon, Wetherspoons*	1 Roll/183g	546	34.6	298	11.1	21.7	18.9	1.1
Morning Roll, with Fried Egg, Wetherspoons*	1 Roll/143g	400	21.3	280	9.7	27.8	14.9	1.4
Morning Roll, with Quorn Sausage, Wetherspoons*	1 Roll/143g	367	16.1	257	10.1	29.5	11.3	2.6
Morning Roll, with Sausage, Wetherspoons*	1 Roll/158g	517	28.0	327	13.8	30.1	17.7	2.3
Sausage, Bacon & Egg Bloomer, Wetherspoons*	1 Serving/100g	653	34.9	653	35.6	46.9	34.9	3.6
Sausage, Bacon & Egg Sandwich, Wetherspoons*	1 Sandwich/357g	840	55.8	235	12.6	11.3	15.6	1.5
Scrambled Egg, on Toast, Wetherspoons*	1 Serving/265g	503	24.9	190	8.4	17.4	9.4	1.1
Toast & Preserves, Wetherspoons*	1 Serving/148g	420	15.2	284	5.7	41.8	10.3	3.2
Traditional, Wetherspoons*	1 Breakfast/523g	904	60.1	173	8.4	9.4	11.5	1.8
Vegetarian, Wetherspoons*	1 Breakfast/562g	984	57.1	175	6.7	14.3	10.2	2.1
BREAKFAST CEREAL								
Porridge, Strawberry & Blueberry Compote, Wetherspoons*	1 Portion/100g	311	4.9	311	12.3	51.9	4.9	6.4
BROWNIES								
Chocolate, Fudge, & Vanilla Ice Cream, Wetherspoons*	1 Portion/108.1g	334	17.5	309	4.5	35.6	16.2	1.5
BURGERS								
Beef, Double, & Chips, Wetherspoons*	1 Serving/598g	1382	81.6	231	16.8	11.4	13.6	0.5

JD WETHERSPOON

	Measure INFO/WEIGHT	per Measure KCAL	FAT	Nutrition Values per 100g / 100ml KCAL	PROT	CARB	FAT	FIBRE
BURGERS								
Beef, Double, Bacon, Cheese, & Chips, Wetherspoons*	1 Serving/729g	1891	119.3	259	18.1	9.4	16.4	0.4
Beef, Double, Cheese, & Chips, Wetherspoons*	1 Serving/654g	1565	91.4	239	17.2	10.7	14.0	0.5
Beef, with Bacon, Cheese & Chips, Wetherspoons*	1 Serving/531g	1295	78.9	244	15.2	12.6	14.8	0.5
Beef, with Cheese, & Chips, Wetherspoons*	1 Serving/456g	966	53.8	212	13.7	13.8	11.8	0.5
Beef, with Chips, Wetherspoons*	1 Serving/428g	881	46.4	206	12.8	15.7	10.8	0.6
Chicken, Butterfly Breast with Chips, Wetherspoons*	1 Portion/440g	893	23.4	203	11.0	23.3	5.3	1.5
Chicken, Fillet, with Chips, Wetherspoons*	1 Serving/465g	727	17.1	156	10.9	16.7	3.7	0.8
Lamb, Minted, with Chips, Wetherspoons*	1 Serving/428g	712	27.8	166	11.3	17.2	6.5	0.9
Skinny Chicken, Wetherspoons*	1 Serving/320g	613	17.3	192	14.0	14.0	5.4	1.5
Vegetable, with Chips, Wetherspoons*	1 Meal/488g	839	25.9	172	4.7	27.2	5.3	2.0
BUTTY								
Bacon, Brown Bloomer, Wetherspoons*	1 Serving/309g	869	39.6	281	23.3	18.3	12.8	1.2
Bacon, White Poppy Seed, Wetherspoons*	1 Serving/309g	856	41.1	277	21.9	18.2	13.3	1.0
Bacon & Egg, Brown Bloomer, Wetherspoons*	1 Serving/269g	702	31.1	261	18.2	21.0	11.6	1.4
Bacon & Egg, White Bloomer, Wetherspoons*	1 Serving/269g	689	32.7	256	16.7	20.9	12.2	1.2
Chip, Brown Bloomer, Wetherspoons*	1 Serving/204g	478	14.7	234	7.6	35.7	7.2	1.9
Chip, White Bloomer, Wetherspoons*	1 Serving/204g	465	16.3	228	5.6	35.6	8.0	1.6
Chip & Cheese, Brown Bloomer, Wetherspoons*	1 Serving/232g	593	24.4	256	9.7	31.4	10.5	1.6
Chip & Cheese, White Bloomer, Wetherspoons*	1 Serving/232g	580	26.0	250	7.9	31.3	11.2	1.4
CAKE								
Chocolate Fudge, & Ice Cream, Wetherspoons*	1 Serving/239g	822	47.3	344	4.0	37.6	19.8	0.4
CARBONARA								
Bacon, Wetherspoons*	1 Portion/100g	1096	56.1	1096	32.5	91.2	56.1	5.5
CHEESECAKE								
Chocolate Chip, Wetherspoons*	1 Serving/100g	270	11.5	270	4.9	36.8	11.5	0.5
Salted Caramel, Eli's, Wetherspoons*	1 Serving/110g	315	20.6	315	4.3	28.9	20.6	0.6
Vanilla with Compote, Baked, Eli's, Wetherspoons*	1 Portion/189g	454	27.9	240	3.3	24.0	14.8	0.6
White Chocolate & Raspberry, Wetherspoons*	1 Serving/175g	656	36.9	375	5.6	40.8	21.1	0.9
CHICKEN								
Peri-Peri, Salad, Dressing & Coleslaw, Wetherspoons*	1 Serving/100g	447	43.6	447	39.0	16.6	43.6	3.6
Skewers, Piri Piri, with Peppers, & Salad, Wetherspoons*	1 Serving/210g	449	8.3	214	10.5	4.9	4.0	2.3
Strips, Southern Fried, Wetherspoons*	1 Meal/100g	1065	49.5	1065	43.4	108.8	49.5	7.6
Wings, Buffalo, Wetherspoons*	1 Portion/328g	636	42.9	194	15.2	4.0	13.1	0.5
CHICKEN ALFREDO								
Pasta, with Dressed Side Salad, Wetherspoons*	1 Meal/576g	950	52.4	165	8.7	12.0	9.1	0.3
Pasta, with Garlic Bread, Wetherspoons*	1 Meal/501g	1007	47.6	201	10.8	13.0	9.5	0.3
Pasta, without Garlic Bread, Wetherspoons*	1 Meal/430g	804	38.7	187	11.3	15.0	9.0	0.1
CHICKEN PIRI PIRI								
& Wedges, Wetherspoons*	1 Serving/100g	574	22.5	574	26.2	72.6	22.5	5.1
Roast, Wetherspoons*	1 Serving/994g	994	47.1	100	8.4	5.8	4.7	0.8
CHICKEN VINDALOO								
Wetherspoons*	1 Meal/500g	704	19.0	141	6.4	21.0	3.8	1.3
CHICKEN WITH								
BBQ Sauce, & Salad, Roast, Wetherspoons*	1 Meal/666g	913	46.0	137	12.2	6.0	6.9	0.9
Chips & BBQ Sauce, Roast, Wetherspoons*	1 Meal/768g	1183	53.0	154	11.5	12.2	6.9	0.9
Chips & Salad, Roast, Wetherspoons*	1 Meal/695g	983	52.1	141	13.1	5.9	7.5	0.6
Jacket Potato, Salad, & Salsa, Roast, Wetherspoons*	1 Meal/785g	1193	57.3	152	12.2	10.2	7.3	1.3
CHILLI								
Con Carne, Wetherspoons*	1 Meal/500g	744	20.0	149	7.5	20.8	4.0	1.5
Con Carne, with Chips, Wetherspoons*	1 Serving/465g	500	14.9	108	4.8	16.7	3.2	0.7
Con Carne, with Rice, & Tortilla Chips, Wetherspoons*	1 Serving/585g	744	20.0	127	6.5	17.8	3.4	1.6
Five Bean, with Rice & Tortilla Chips, Wetherspoons*	1 Portion/390g	568	10.5	146	4.1	25.4	2.7	2.4

JD WETHERSPOON

	Measure INFO/WEIGHT	per Measure KCAL	FAT	Nutrition Values per 100g / 100ml KCAL	PROT	CARB	FAT	FIBRE
CHIPS								
Bowl, Wetherspoons*	1 Serving/300g	750	30.4	250	3.5	36.5	10.1	2.9
with Cheese, Wetherspoons*	1 Serving/501g	1002	51.6	200	5.2	21.9	10.3	1.8
with Roast Gravy, Wetherspoons*	1 Serving/400g	392	12.4	98	2.5	17.6	3.1	0.0
CHUTNEY								
Mango, Wetherspoons*	1 Serving/25g	47	0.2	188	0.4	44.8	0.8	0.4
CRUMBLE								
Apple, Pear, & Raspberry, with Custard, Wetherspoons*	1 Serving/372g	648	23.8	174	2.5	26.3	6.4	0.0
Apple, Pear, & Raspberry, with Ice Cream, Wetherspoons*	1 Serving/300g	579	24.3	193	2.6	27.0	8.1	2.1
CURRY								
Beef, Malaysian, Rendang, no Naan, Wetherspoons*	1 Meal/615g	947	38.1	154	6.7	17.0	6.2	1.0
Chicken, The Flaming Dragon, Wetherspoons*	1 Serving/640g	1041	24.7	163	9.0	22.6	3.9	2.2
Chicken Phaal, Meal, Wetherspoons*	1 Serving/720g	1234	46.1	171	7.5	21.0	6.4	1.6
Daal Masala Meal, no Naan, Curry Club, Wetherspoons*	1 Meal/640g	627	16.6	98	2.8	16.1	2.6	1.1
Kashmiri, Lamb, with Naan, Wetherspoons*	1 Meal/704g	1021	33.1	145	7.2	19.5	4.7	1.2
Kashmiri, Lamb, without Naan, Wetherspoons*	1 Meal/615g	824	30.7	134	7.1	16.3	5.0	1.1
Kerala, Fish, with Naan, Wetherspoons*	1 Meal/706g	1066	36.0	151	7.0	20.0	5.1	1.0
Kerala, Fish, without Naan, Wetherspoons*	1 Meal/616g	869	33.3	141	6.9	16.9	5.4	0.9
Mushroom Dopiaza, no Naan Bread, Wetherspoons*	1 Meal/617g	580	14.2	94	2.6	16.7	2.3	1.4
Mushroom Dopiaza, with Naan Bread, Wetherspoons*	1 Serving/719g	899	24.5	125	3.5	21.5	3.4	1.5
Royal Thali, with Naan, Wetherspoons*	1 Meal/948g	1336	48.3	141	7.1	16.8	5.1	1.3
Thai, Green, Chicken, with Naan, Wetherspoons*	1 Portion/705g	1234	49.4	175	7.5	20.6	7.0	0.6
Thai, Green Chicken, no Naan, Wetherspoons*	1 Meal/617g	1037	46.9	168	7.5	17.6	7.6	0.5
Vegetable, Goan, with Naan Bread, Wetherspoons*	1 Meal/707g	1032	36.8	146	3.6	21.2	5.2	1.3
Vegetarian, Thali, with Naan, Wetherspoons*	1 Meal/950g	1320	42.7	139	5.3	20.3	4.5	2.4
DHANSAK								
Lamb, Meal, Wetherspoons*	1 Serving/720g	983	26.1	137	7.2	19.6	3.6	0.8
FISH & CHIPS								
Haddock, Wetherspoons*	1 Meal/496g	806	40.7	162	7.2	14.4	8.2	2.4
Plaice, Breaded, & Peas, Wetherspoons*	1 Serving/460g	550	15.6	120	6.8	15.0	3.4	1.7
Traditional, Wetherspoons*	1 Serving/495g	804	40.6	162	7.2	14.4	8.2	2.4
GAMMON &								
Chips, Peas, Tomato, & Egg, Wetherspoons*	1 Meal/564g	844	41.2	150	15.0	6.7	7.3	1.3
Chips, Peas, Tomato, & Pineapple, Wetherspoons*	1 Meal/575g	799	36.2	139	13.6	7.8	6.3	1.4
Jacket Potato, Peas, Tomato, & Pineapple, Wetherspoons*	1 Serving/665g	1009	38.6	152	12.3	12.4	5.8	1.9
HAGGIS								
with Neeps & Tatties, Wetherspoons*	1 Meal/682g	982	52.5	144	4.6	15.0	7.7	1.9
HAM								
& Eggs, Wetherspoons*	1 Serving/396g	253	12.7	64	4.9	3.5	3.2	0.0
& Eggs, with Chips, Wetherspoons*	1 Serving/100g	683	33.4	683	40.2	55.2	33.4	4.4
ICE CREAM								
Bombe, Mint Chocolate, Wetherspoons*	1 Portion/135g	300	13.4	222	2.6	30.6	9.9	0.8
Chocolate, Bomb, Wetherspoons*	1 Portion/100g	259	13.4	259	5.9	34.3	13.4	5.4
Neopolitan, Movenpick, Wetherspoons*	1 Bowl/100g	181	9.6	181	3.0	20.0	9.6	0.0
Wetherspoons*	1 Serving/100ml	146	7.2	146	3.0	15.6	7.2	0.0
JALFREZI								
Chicken, Meal, with Naan Bread, Wetherspoons*	1 Meal/705g	916	19.7	130	6.8	19.9	2.8	1.3
Chicken, without Naan Bread, Wetherspoons*	1 Meal/614.5g	719	17.2	117	6.7	16.9	2.8	1.3
KORMA								
Chicken, Meal, without Naan, Wetherspoons*	1 Meal/617g	944	38.2	153	6.4	17.0	6.2	0.8
Chicken, with Naan, Wetherspoons*	1 Meal/704g	1141	40.8	162	6.6	20.1	5.8	0.9
LAMB								
Braised, Mashed Potato & Vegetables, Wetherspoons*	1 Meal/843.9g	1114	66.7	132	8.9	6.8	7.9	1.0

	Measure INFO/WEIGHT	per Measure		Nutrition Values per 100g / 100ml				
		KCAL	FAT	KCAL	PROT	CARB	FAT	FIBRE
JD WETHERSPOON								
LAMB								
Shank, with Rosemary Sauce, Wetherspoons*	1 Portion/949g	1166	66.3	123	9.7	6.8	7.0	0.6
LASAGNE								
Al Forno with Dressed Side Salad, Wetherspoons*	1 Meal/658g	823	40.8	125	5.5	11.4	6.2	0.8
MASALA								
Prawn, Sri Lankan, with Naan, Wetherspoons*	1 Meal/708g	1027	36.1	145	5.7	19.7	5.1	0.8
Prawn, Sri Lankan, without Naan, Wetherspoons*	1 Meal/617g	827	33.3	134	5.4	16.6	5.4	1.0
Vegetable, Tandoori, Meal, Wetherspoons*	1 Serving/720g	1020	36.0	142	3.4	20.7	5.0	2.3
MEATBALLS								
with Linguine Pasta, Wetherspoons*	1 Serving/512g	614	24.0	120	6.3	13.1	4.7	1.9
MIXED GRILL								
Chips, & Salad, Wetherspoons*	1 Serving/784g	1324	87.0	169	12.0	5.6	11.1	0.3
Chips, Peas, Tomato, & Mushrooms, Wetherspoons*	1 Serving/777g	1250	81.0	161	11.0	4.7	10.4	0.8
Jacket Potato, & Salad, Wetherspoons*	1 Serving/874g	1534	91.8	176	11.4	9.5	10.5	0.9
Tikka, Starter, Wetherspoons*	1 Portion/374g	460	23.9	123	13.4	3.2	6.4	0.9
NACHOS								
Wetherspoons*	1 Serving/366g	1139	67.3	311	7.0	29.2	18.4	3.2
with Chilli Con Carne, Wetherspoons*	1 Meal/570g	1505	88.9	264	8.6	22.2	15.6	1.8
with Fajita Chicken, Wetherspoons*	1 Serving/486g	1225	70.5	252	5.7	24.7	14.5	2.9
with Five Bean Chilli, Wetherspoons*	1 Serving/571g	1399	81.1	245	7.3	21.8	14.2	2.7
NOODLES								
Sweet Chilli, Wetherspoons*	1 Serving/360g	356	11.4	99	1.9	15.8	3.2	1.2
Sweet Chilli, with Chicken, Wetherspoons*	1 Portion/400g	486	13.5	122	10.4	12.4	3.4	0.9
Thai, with Chicken, Wetherspoons*	1 Serving/100g	516	20.8	516	20.8	39.0	20.8	4.4
NUT ROAST								
Roast Potatoes, Yorkshire Pud & Veg, Wetherspoons*	1 Serving/746g	1045	61.2	140	5.2	13.7	8.2	2.5
ONION RINGS								
Beer Battered, Portion of 12, Wetherspoons*	1 Portion/144g	571	28.3	397	5.3	49.6	19.6	2.8
PANINI								
BBQ Chicken & Bacon, Melt, Wetherspoons*	1 Panini/337g	650	27.6	193	9.9	19.9	8.2	1.7
Cheese, Tomato, & Bacon, Wetherspoons*	1 Panini/261g	630	29.0	241	14.3	21.6	11.1	0.8
Cheese & Tuna, Wetherspoons*	1 Panini/221g	551	22.3	249	15.5	24.9	10.1	0.7
Club, Wetherspoons*	1 Panini/378g	734	38.6	194	9.7	16.1	10.2	1.6
Fajita Chicken, Wetherspoons*	1 Panini/235g	359	6.1	153	4.4	28.8	2.6	1.7
Gouda & Ham, Wetherspoons*	1 Panini/215g	581	23.1	270	13.2	24.3	10.8	1.3
Ham & Cheddar Cheese, Wetherspoons*	1 Panini/354g	868	49.9	245	12.7	16.7	14.1	1.5
Mature, Cheddar Cheese & Tomato, Wetherspoons*	1 Panini/330g	750	27.1	227	10.4	18.0	8.2	1.7
Pepperoni & Mozzarella, Wetherspoons*	1 Panini/205g	617	33.4	301	11.6	27.5	16.3	1.0
Tomato, Mozzarella & Green Pesto, Wetherspoons*	1 Panini/245g	502	22.9	205	7.3	23.0	9.4	1.4
PASTA								
5 Cheese & Bacon, with Salad, Wetherspoons*	1 Meal/544g	506	28.8	93	2.3	9.1	5.3	1.3
Alfredo, Wetherspoons*	1 Serving/500g	830	52.6	166	4.1	13.2	10.5	0.7
Pesto, Chargrilled Chicken, Wholewheat, Wetherspoons*	1 Serving/350g	770	36.2	220	15.2	14.7	10.3	4.2
Spiral, Chargrilled Veg & Sundried Tomato, Wetherspoons*	1 Meal/500g	600	2.5	120	3.6	15.2	0.5	0.7
PASTA BAKE								
Mediterranean, Wetherspoons*	1 Serving/450g	577	22.1	128	4.3	16.4	4.9	0.9
PASTA SALAD								
Superfood, Wetherspoons*	1 Serving/300g	471	18.2	157	5.0	19.6	6.1	2.1
PIE								
Aberdeen Angus, Chips, & Vegetables, Wetherspoons*	1 Serving/780g	1356	86.6	174	5.5	15.7	11.1	0.9
Beef & Abbot Ale, Chips, Veg & Gravy, Wetherspoons*	1 Meal/850g	1258	68.0	148	4.0	14.9	8.0	1.0
Cottage, with Chips & Peas, Wetherspoons*	1 Meal/682g	846	33.4	124	3.7	15.6	4.9	1.9
Fish, Carrot & Broccoli, in Herb Butter, Wetherspoons*	1 Serving/550g	612	38.0	111	4.6	9.7	6.9	2.4

JD WETHERSPOON

	INFO/WEIGHT	KCAL	FAT	KCAL	PROT	CARB	FAT	FIBRE
PIE								
Ice Cream, Toffee & Chocolate, Wetherspoons*	1 Serving/140g	542	29.5	387	5.2	51.2	21.1	2.3
Scotch, Wetherspoons*	1 Serving/145g	302	15.4	208	13.1	7.8	10.6	0.9
Scotch, with Chips & Beans, Wetherspoons*	1 Serving/435g	603	22.2	139	6.8	14.9	5.1	1.5
PLATTER								
Italian Style, Wetherspoons*	1 Platter/1020g	1985	75.5	195	10.4	22.9	7.4	0.6
Mexican, Chilli, Sour Cream, Wetherspoons*	1 Platter/1062g	2560	141.2	241	7.5	22.6	13.3	2.8
Western, Wetherspoons*	1 Platter/1454g	2973	168.7	204	16.9	9.1	11.6	0.4
POPPADOMS								
& Dips, Wetherspoons*	1 Serving/134g	425	10.9	317	4.6	28.4	8.1	2.5
Wetherspoons*	1 Poppadom/12g	35	0.2	281	6.7	45.0	1.9	10.0
PORK DINNER								
Roast Potatoes, Yorkshire Pud & Veg, Wetherspoons*	1 Meal/659g	995	40.9	151	10.4	14.6	6.2	2.1
POTATO BOMBAY								
Wetherspoons*	1 Serving/300g	285	14.7	95	1.8	10.8	4.9	2.5
POTATO SKINS								
Cheese & Bacon, Loaded, Wetherspoons*	1 Serving/439g	949	58.4	216	8.9	15.2	13.3	1.5
Cheese & Red Onion, Loaded, Wetherspoons*	1 Serving/414g	835	51.3	202	6.0	16.5	12.4	1.6
Chilli Con Carne, Loaded, Wetherspoons*	1 Serving/503g	735	35.7	146	5.0	15.7	7.1	1.9
POTATO WEDGES								
Spicy, Wetherspoons*	1 Serving/270g	434	15.7	161	2.2	27.7	5.8	1.8
Spicy, with Sour Cream, Wetherspoons*	1 Serving/330g	558	27.4	169	2.3	23.4	8.3	1.5
POTATOES								
Diced, Garlic & Herb, with Dip, Wetherspoons*	1 Serving/320g	586	33.9	183	2.0	19.9	10.6	2.9
Jacket, Baked Beans, & Salad, Wetherspoons*	1 Meal/575g	725	24.7	126	3.3	19.6	4.3	2.4
Jacket, BBQ Pulled Pork, Wetherspoons*	1 Serving/420g	482	7.1	115	1.7	13.1	1.7	2.3
Jacket, Cheese, & Salad, Wetherspoons*	1 Serving/486g	761	41.8	157	5.0	15.8	8.6	1.6
Jacket, Chilli Con Carne, Sour Cream, Wetherspoons*	1 Meal/615g	775	30.1	126	4.4	17.0	4.9	1.9
Jacket, Coleslaw, Wetherspoons*	1 Meal/596g	918	48.9	154	2.3	17.1	8.2	1.8
Jacket, Fajita Chicken, & Salad, Wetherspoons*	1 Serving/550g	617	25.8	112	2.3	16.3	4.7	1.8
Jacket, Five Bean Chilli, & Salad, Wetherspoons*	1 Meal/597g	705	25.7	118	3.0	17.9	4.3	2.4
Jacket, Mature, Cheddar Cheese, Wetherspoons*	1 Meal/496g	858	44.6	173	5.6	18.7	9.0	1.8
Jacket, Poached Salmon, Mayo, & Salad, Wetherspoons*	1 Serving/471g	800	47.1	170	4.8	16.2	10.0	1.5
Jacket, Prawn Mayonnaise & Salad, Wetherspoons*	1 Serving/486g	682	39.4	140	2.2	15.7	8.1	1.5
Jacket, Tuna Mayonnaise, & Salad, Wetherspoons*	1 Meal/645g	845	39.6	131	5.4	14.6	6.1	1.4
Mashed, Creamy, Wetherspoons*	1 Portion/279g	349	21.2	125	1.5	15.0	7.6	1.1
Roast, Wetherspoons*	1 Portion/200g	290	9.4	145	2.5	23.0	4.7	2.3
RIBS								
Double, Wetherspoons*	1 Serving/350g	767	41.0	219	16.7	11.9	11.7	0.4
Double, with Chips, Wetherspoons*	1 Serving/500g	949	46.5	190	12.5	14.9	9.3	0.3
RICE								
Basmati, Yellow, Wetherspoons*	1 Portion/200g	286	1.2	143	3.4	31.1	0.6	0.2
Wetherspoons*	1 Serving/200g	274	0.4	137	2.9	30.9	0.2	0.2
ROGAN JOSH								
Lamb, Meal, without Naan, Wetherspoons*	1 Meal/617g	820	27.7	133	7.1	17.0	4.5	1.0
Lamb, with Naan, Wetherspoons*	1 Meal/706g	1017	30.4	144	7.2	20.1	4.3	1.1
SALAD								
Caesar, Chicken, Wetherspoons*	1 Meal/230g	384	13.9	167	18.5	6.4	6.0	0.9
Caesar, Wetherspoons*	1 Meal/211g	448	38.0	212	6.8	5.8	18.0	1.1
Chicken, & Balsamic Vinaigrette, Wetherspoons*	1 Serving/100g	468	26.6	468	42.3	13.5	26.6	5.1
Chicken, BBQ, Croutons & Dressing, Wetherspoons*	1 Portion/350g	315	8.4	90	9.4	7.5	2.4	0.8
Chicken & Bacon, Warm, Wetherspoons*	1 Meal/426g	600	41.3	141	9.8	3.8	9.7	0.6
Chicken & Bacon, Warm, Wetherspoons*	1 Serving/150g	688	33.4	459	46.1	18.3	22.3	1.5

JD WETHERSPOON

	Measure INFO/WEIGHT	per Measure KCAL	FAT	Nutrition Values per 100g / 100ml KCAL	PROT	CARB	FAT	FIBRE
SALAD								
Crayfish, Wetherspoons*	1 Meal/317g	247	18.0	78	4.4	2.7	5.7	0.6
Salmon, & Balsamic Vinaigrette, Wetherspoons*	1 Serving/350g	470	30.2	134	10.8	2.8	8.6	1.5
Salmon & Prawn, no Croutons, Wetherspoons*	1 Serving/150g	404	30.2	269	19.5	2.7	20.1	1.2
Salmon & Prawn, with Croutons, Wetherspoons*	1 Serving/150g	481	34.5	321	20.6	7.9	23.0	1.3
Side, no Dressing, Wetherspoons*	1 Salad/195g	125	4.5	64	2.0	8.9	2.3	1.1
Side, with Dressing, Wetherspoons*	1 Salad/215g	263	19.6	122	2.2	8.1	9.1	1.0
Side, with Dressing & Croutons, Wetherspoons*	1 Portion/140g	221	18.3	158	2.1	8.6	13.1	1.1
Side, with Dressing & no Croutons, Wetherspoons*	1 Portion/129g	145	14.0	112	1.0	3.2	10.8	0.9
Superfood, & Balsamic Vinaigrette, Wetherspoons*	1 Serving/100g	279	22.6	279	6.3	11.2	22.6	5.1
Thai Noodle, Wetherspoons*	1 Portion/394g	433	21.3	110	2.7	12.7	5.4	1.4
Thai Noodle, with Chicken, Wetherspoons*	1 Meal/554g	637	27.7	115	9.2	9.6	5.0	1.4
Tiger Prawn, Dressing, & Chilli Jam, Wetherspoons*	1 Portion/340g	500	33.0	147	4.7	10.1	9.7	0.9
Tuna, with Eggs, Olives, & Croutons, Wetherspoons*	1 Portion/395g	679	51.7	172	10.3	3.2	13.1	0.7
SAMOSAS								
Lamb, Wetherspoons*	1 Samosa/90g	160	3.8	178	7.9	29.9	4.2	3.9
Vegetable, Wetherspoons*	1 Samosa/50g	92	3.1	184	5.4	28.4	6.2	2.2
SANDWICH								
BBQ Chicken & Bacon Melt, Ciabatta, Wetherspoons*	1 Ciabatta/333g	716	33.6	215	11.3	20.4	10.1	1.8
Beef, Hot, Brown Bloomer, Wetherspoons*	1 Sandwich/299g	618	27.2	207	11.4	19.9	9.1	1.3
Beef, Hot, White Poppy Seed Bloomer, Wetherspoons*	1 Sandwich/299g	605	28.7	202	10.0	19.8	9.6	1.1
BLT, Brown Bloomer, Wetherspoons*	1 Sandwich/404g	885	39.6	219	18.0	14.6	9.8	1.2
BLT, Ciabatta, Wetherspoons*	1 Ciabatta/390g	789	47.3	202	8.2	15.4	12.1	1.5
BLT, White Bloomer, Wetherspoons*	1 Sandwich/404g	872	32.7	216	17.0	14.6	8.1	1.0
Cheddar, & Pickle, Brown Bloomer, Wetherspoons*	1 Sandwich/260g	665	31.9	256	11.0	25.4	12.3	1.9
Cheese & Pickle, Ciabatta, Wetherspoons*	1 Ciabatta/350g	662	31.5	189	7.8	19.4	9.0	1.7
Chicken, Cheese, Bacon, Mayo, Brown, Wetherspoons*	1 Sandwich/312g	763	38.1	245	14.8	18.9	12.2	1.4
Chicken, Cheese, Bacon, Mayo, White, Wetherspoons*	1 Sandwich/312g	710	39.6	228	13.5	18.8	12.7	1.2
Chicken, Half Fat Mayo, Brown, Hot, Wetherspoons*	1 Sandwich/289g	628	28.3	217	11.8	20.7	9.8	1.7
Club, Ciabatta, Wetherspoons*	1 Ciabatta/378g	734	38.6	194	9.7	16.1	10.2	1.6
Crayfish, Ciabatta, Wetherspoons*	1 Ciabatta/305g	561	27.4	184	5.8	20.3	9.0	1.9
Egg Mayonnaise, Brown Bloomer, Wetherspoons*	1 Sandwich/295g	704	39.5	239	10.1	19.7	13.4	1.3
Egg Mayonnaise, White Bloomer, Wetherspoons*	1 Sandwich/295g	692	41.0	235	8.7	19.6	13.9	1.1
Ham, & Tomato, Brown Bloomer, Wetherspoons*	1 Sandwich/239g	514	17.2	215	11.4	24.4	7.2	1.8
Ham, & Tomato, White Bloomer, Wetherspoons*	1 Sandwich/239g	501	18.6	210	9.7	24.4	7.8	1.5
Prawn Mayonnaise, Brown Bloomer, Wetherspoons*	1 Sandwich/244g	579	26.6	237	11.0	23.8	10.9	1.6
Salmon, Lemon Mayo, Brown Bloomer, Wetherspoons*	1 Sandwich/229g	637	33.7	278	11.4	25.4	14.7	1.7
Tuna Mayonnaise, Ciabatta, Wetherspoons*	1 Ciabatta/391g	676	32.8	173	8.8	15.8	8.4	1.5
Tuna Mayonnaise, Half Fat Mayo, Brown, Wetherspoons*	1 Sandwich/389g	841	45.5	216	12.3	15.7	11.7	1.1
Tuna Mayonnaise, Half Fat Mayo, White, Wetherspoons*	1 Sandwich/389g	828	47.1	213	11.2	15.6	12.1	1.0
Wiltshire Ham, Ciabatta, Wetherspoons*	1 Ciabatta/335g	503	14.8	150	9.8	17.7	4.4	1.7
SAUSAGE								
with Bacon & Egg, Wetherspoons*	1 Serving/582g	1040	57.6	179	11.7	11.3	9.9	1.0
with Chips, & Beans, Wetherspoons*	1 Meal/554g	897	42.6	162	7.3	16.4	7.7	2.3
SAUSAGE & MASH								
with Red Wine Gravy, Wetherspoons*	1 Portion/677g	887	50.8	131	6.0	10.2	7.5	1.8
SCAMPI								
Breaded, Chips, Peas, Tartare Sauce, Wetherspoons*	1 Serving/561g	987	43.7	176	5.2	19.9	7.8	2.3
SORBET								
Mango & Passionfruit, Wetherspoons*	1 Serving/135g	115	0.1	85	0.2	20.0	0.1	0.2
SOUP								
Leek & Potato, without Bread & Butter, Wetherspoons*	1 Bowl/420	105	0.8	25	0.9	5.1	0.2	1.0
Mushroom, with Brown Bloomer, Wetherspoons*	1 Serving/429g	561	23.7	131	3.4	16.0	5.5	1.2

	Measure INFO/WEIGHT	per Measure KCAL	FAT	Nutrition Values per 100g / 100ml KCAL	PROT	CARB	FAT	FIBRE
JD WETHERSPOON								
SOUP								
Tomato, no Bread, Wetherspoons*	1 Serving/305g	198	14.0	65	0.9	3.9	4.6	0.6
Tomato, with Brown Bloomer, Wetherspoons*	1 Serving/429g	576	25.8	134	3.7	15.7	6.0	1.3
Tomato, with White Bloomer, Wetherspoons*	1 Serving/429g	563	27.3	131	2.8	15.6	6.4	1.2
Tomato & Basil, Organic, no Bread, Wetherspoons*	1 Bowl/350g	200	15.0	57	0.7	3.0	4.3	0.6
Tomato & Basil, Organic, with Bread, Wetherspoons*	1 Bowl/450g	396	8.6	88	1.0	6.0	1.9	1.1
SPONGE PUDDING								
Treacle, with Hot Custard, Wetherspoons*	1 Serving/515g	1267	71.1	246	2.3	41.8	13.8	0.2
SQUASH								
Butternut, Roast Dinner, Wetherspoons*	1 Meal/847g	1211	55.9	143	4.9	17.5	6.6	2.9
STEW								
Irish, Wetherspoons*	1 Serving/600g	516	23.4	86	7.3	5.6	3.9	0.9
STUFFING BALLS								
Sage & Onion, Wetherspoons*	1 Portion/70g	137	1.1	196	6.6	32.3	1.6	3.6
TAGLIATELLE								
Ham & Mushroom, Wetherspoons*	1 Serving/400g	392	12.0	98	5.6	12.1	3.0	0.7
TART								
Apple, with Ice Cream, Wetherspoons*	1 Serving/235g	464	20.0	197	1.6	29.8	8.5	0.4
TIKKA MASALA								
Chicken, with Rice & Naan Bread, Wetherspoons*	1 Serving/708g	1069	36.1	151	7.0	19.9	5.1	1.2
Chicken, with Rice & no Naan Bread, Wetherspoons*	1 Meal/614g	872	33.2	142	6.9	16.9	5.4	1.2
VEGETABLES								
Side Serving, Wetherspoons*	1 Serving/160g	54	0.8	34	0.8	5.2	0.5	2.4
WAFFLES								
Belgian, Ice Cream & Maple Syrup, Wetherspoons*	1 Serving/395g	934	33.6	236	13.8	28.4	8.5	0.8
WRAP								
Breakfast, Wetherspoons*	1 Wrap/100g	681	38.8	681	32.8	51.2	38.8	4.0
Chicken, Cheese, Tortilla Chips, Salsa, Wetherspoons*	1 Serving/356g	699	32.4	196	8.8	20.6	9.1	1.5
Chicken, Guacamole, Tortillas, Salsa, Wetherspoons*	1 Serving/273g	474	16.9	174	8.2	21.9	6.2	2.0
Chicken, Reggae Reggae, Wetherspoons*	1 Meal/100g	364	9.6	364	24.4	42.0	9.6	2.7
Chicken, Southern Fried, & Creole Mayo, Wetherspoons*	1 Wrap/320g	553	30.0	173	7.1	16.3	9.4	1.4
Chicken, with Chicken Breast, Wetherspoons*	1 Wrap/292g	450	21.6	154	9.4	14.5	7.4	1.5
Chicken, with Potato Wedges, Wetherspoons*	1 Serving/373g	647	24.2	174	6.7	23.9	6.5	1.7
Chicken, with Sweet Chilli Sauce, Wetherspoons*	1 Portion/100g	339	7.0	339	23.9	47.1	7.0	2.4
Chicken, with Tortilla Chips & Salsa, Wetherspoons*	1 Serving/328g	584	23.0	178	7.5	22.3	7.0	1.6
Chicken & Cheese, Wetherspoons*	1 Wrap/271g	553	26.3	204	10.7	19.6	9.7	1.4
Club Wetherwrap, & Potato Wedges, Wetherspoons*	1 Serving/381g	822	43.1	216	10.9	19.2	11.3	1.2
Fajita Chicken, Tortilla Chips, Salsa, Wetherspoons*	1 Serving/313g	491	20.3	157	3.5	21.9	6.5	1.9
Fajita Chicken, Wetherspoons*	1 Wrap/228g	345	14.1	151	3.8	21.2	6.2	1.9
Fajita Chicken, with Potato Wedges, Wetherspoons*	1 Serving/358g	554	21.8	155	3.2	23.5	6.1	1.9
YORKSHIRE PUDDING								
Wetherspoons*	2 Puddings/56g	132	4.6	236	8.2	32.9	8.2	1.1
KFC								
BEANS								
Baked, BBQ, Lge, KFC*	1 Portion/292g	245	1.7	84	4.1	18.0	0.6	0.0
Baked, BBQ, Regular, KFC*	1 Portion/126g	105	0.7	83	4.1	17.8	0.6	0.0
BURGERS								
Chicken, Big Daddy, KFC*	1 Burger/250g	655	29.0	262	13.6	26.0	11.6	0.0
Chicken, Fillet, KFC*	1 Burger/245g	440	15.0	180	11.8	19.4	6.1	0.0
Chicken, Fillet, Mini, KFC*	1 Burger/114g	280	9.9	246	15.2	26.3	8.7	0.0
Chicken, Fillet, Tower, KFC*	1 Burger/263g	384	16.2	236	12.2	24.7	10.0	0.0
Chicken, Kids, KFC*	1 Burger/114g	260	7.0	228	15.2	27.5	6.1	0.0
Chicken, Zinger, Tower, KFC*	1 Burger/264g	620	28.7	235	11.0	24.0	10.9	0.0

	Measure INFO/WEIGHT	per Measure KCAL	FAT	Nutrition Values per 100g / 100ml KCAL	PROT	CARB	FAT	FIBRE
KFC								
BURGERS								
Zinger, KFC*	1 Burger/219g	450	17.5	205	11.7	21.7	8.0	0.0
CHICKEN								
Breast, Original Recipe, KFC*	1 Piece/137g	260	11.7	190	24.0	4.2	8.5	0.0
Drumstick, Original Recipe, KFC*	1 Piece/95g	170	9.7	179	14.4	7.7	10.2	0.0
Popcorn, Lge, KFC*	1 Portion/170g	465	25.9	274	20.2	14.6	15.2	0.0
Popcorn, Regular, KFC*	1 Portion/105g	285	16.0	271	20.2	14.7	15.2	0.0
Popcorn, Sm, KFC*	1 Portion/50g	135	7.6	270	20.2	14.6	15.2	0.0
Rib, Original Recipe, KFC*	1 Piece/126g	340	19.3	270	26.1	6.7	15.3	0.0
Thigh, Original Recipe, KFC*	1 Piece/134g	285	20.6	213	16.3	4.9	15.4	0.0
Wing, Original Recipe, KFC*	1 Piece/48g`	185	10.5	385	35.0	11.2	21.9	0.0
Wings, Hot, KFC*	1 Portion/58g	85	5.6	147	7.8	6.6	9.7	0.0
COLESLAW								
Lge, KFC*	1 Portion/200g	290	24.6	145	0.8	7.7	12.3	0.0
Regular, KFC*	1 Portion/100g	145	12.3	145	0.8	7.7	12.3	0.0
CORN								
Cobette, KFC*	1 Portion/141g	85	1.4	60	2.0	11.2	1.0	0.0
FRIES								
Lge, KFC*	1 Portion/193g	450	21.3	233	3.2	31.5	11.0	0.0
Regular, KFC*	1 Portion/133g	310	14.6	233	3.2	31.4	11.0	0.0
GRAVY								
Lge, KFC*	1 Portion/204g	275	14.6	135	4.3	13.3	7.2	0.0
Regular, KFC*	1 Portion/102g	120	6.5	118	3.8	11.8	6.4	0.0
MILK SHAKE								
Maltesers, Krushems, KFC*	1 Portion/380g	315	9.3	83	1.9	12.8	2.4	0.0
Milky Bar, Krushems, KFC*	1 Portion/380g	435	17.1	114	2.3	15.8	4.5	0.0
Oreo, Krushems, KFC*	1 Portion/380g	380	13.5	100	1.7	14.8	3.6	0.0
SALAD								
Chicken, Original Recipe, no Dressing, KFC*	1 Portion/292g	265	9.6	91	8.2	6.9	3.3	0.0
Chicken, Zinger, no dressing, KFC*	1 Portion/285g	275	12.1	96	7.4	7.1	4.2	0.0
WRAP								
Chicken, Original Recipe, Toasted, Twister, KFC*	1 Wrap/217g	480	20.0	221	12.9	21.4	9.2	0.0
KRISPY KREME								
DOUGHNUTS								
Apple Pie, Krispy Kreme*	1 Doughnut/80g	311	17.6	389	6.0	41.0	22.0	1.9
Blueberry, Powdered, Filled, Krispy Kreme*	1 Doughnut/86g	307	17.2	357	7.0	36.0	20.0	5.0
Butterscotch Fudge, Krispy Kreme*	1 Doughnut/93g	372	16.7	400	6.0	53.0	18.0	0.0
Chocolate, Glazed, Krispy Kreme*	1 Doughnut/80g	309	13.6	387	4.0	55.0	17.0	3.0
Chocolate, Krispy Kreme*	1 Doughnut/80g	340	18.0	425	3.8	52.5	22.5	1.2
Chocolate Dreamcake, Krispy Kreme*	1 Doughnut/95g	390	19.0	411	6.0	51.0	20.0	2.0
Chocolate Iced, Creme Filled, Krispy Kreme*	1 Doughnut/87g	372	20.0	428	6.0	46.0	23.0	2.0
Chocolate Iced, Custard Filled, Krispy Kreme*	1 Doughnut/87g	318	16.5	366	5.0	41.0	19.0	1.8
Chocolate Iced, Ring, Glazed, Krispy Kreme*	1 Doughnut/66g	278	13.2	422	5.0	54.0	20.0	1.5
Chocolate Iced, with Creme Filling, Krispy Kreme*	1 Doughnut/87g	350	20.9	402	3.0	42.0	24.0	1.0
Chocolate Iced, with Sprinkles, Krispy Kreme*	1 Doughnut/71g	298	12.7	421	6.0	55.0	18.0	1.6
Chocolate Praline Fudge Cake, Krispy Kreme*	1 Doughnut/73g	346	21.2	474	6.0	43.0	29.0	5.6
Cinnamon Apple, Filled, Krispy Kreme*	1 Doughnut/81g	269	14.6	332	7.0	37.0	18.0	5.0
Cookie Crunch, Krispy Kreme*	1 Doughnut/73g	316	14.6	433	4.0	56.0	20.0	5.0
Cookies & Kreme, Krispy Kreme*	1 Doughnut/93g	379	16.7	408	4.0	57.0	18.0	0.0
Cruller, Glazed, Krispy Kreme*	1 Doughnut/54g	254	15.6	471	4.0	49.0	29.0	3.0
Glazed, with a Creme Filling, Krispy Kreme*	1 Doughnut/86g	309	15.5	359	5.0	44.0	18.0	4.0
Lemon Filled, Glazed, Krispy Kreme*	1 Doughnut/66g	218	10.5	331	5.0	41.0	16.0	4.0
Maple Iced, Krispy Kreme*	1 Doughnut/66g	279	15.2	422	5.0	49.0	23.0	3.0

KRISPY KREME

DOUGHNUTS

	INFO/WEIGHT	KCAL	FAT	KCAL	PROT	CARB	FAT	FIBRE
Millionaires Shortbread, Krispy Kreme*	1 Doughnut/90g	349	16.2	388	6.0	47.0	18.0	2.1
Orange Sundae Gloss, Krispy Kreme*	1 Doughnut/81g	338	17.0	418	5.0	50.0	21.0	3.0
Original, Glazed, Krispy Kreme*	1 Doughnut/52g	222	11.9	428	6.0	48.0	23.0	1.1
Raspberry, Glazed, Krispy Kreme*	1 Doughnut/86g	350	17.2	407	6.0	48.0	20.0	1.8
Salted Caramel, Cheesecake, Krispy Kreme*	1 Doughnut/91g	380	18.6	418	5.5	52.0	20.4	2.0
Strawberries & Kreme, Krispy Kreme*	1 Doughnut/91g	381	20.9	419	5.0	47.0	23.0	1.8
Strawberry Filled, Powdered, Krispy Kreme*	1 Doughnut/74g	248	13.3	335	7.0	36.0	18.0	5.0
Strawberry Gloss, Krispy Kreme*	1 Doughnut/62g	253	12.4	409	5.0	50.0	20.0	1.6
Vanilla, Krispy Kreme*	1 Doughnut/80g	315	13.7	391	4.0	57.0	17.0	2.0
White Chocolate & Almond, Krispy Kreme*	1 Doughnut/93g	421	24.2	453	8.0	45.0	26.0	1.9

LEON RESTAURANTS

AUBERGINE

	INFO/WEIGHT	KCAL	FAT	KCAL	PROT	CARB	FAT	FIBRE
Chilled Roasted, Leon*	1 Portion/125g	138	13.0	110	1.6	3.2	10.4	0.0

BISCUITS

Lemon & Ginger, Crunch, Leon*	1 Serving/160g	562	39.8	351	5.4	28.1	24.9	0.0

BREAKFAST

Full English, Pot, Leon*	1 Portion/228g	416	30.3	182	11.4	3.9	13.3	0.0
New York Breakfasts, Classic, Leon*	1 Serving/130g	229	8.7	176	8.5	22.2	6.7	0.0
Poached Egg & Truffle Gruyere, Leon*	1 Portion/76g	139	11.7	183	10.7	0.5	15.3	0.0
Poached Egg with Chorizo & Saucy Beans, Leon*	1 Portion/131g	168	10.0	128	9.4	4.7	7.7	0.0
Poached Egg with Chorizo & Truffle Gruere, Leon*	1 Portion/96g	177	13.5	184	13.7	0.8	14.0	0.0
Poached Egg with Ham & Saucy Beans, Leon*	1 Portion/136g	164	9.5	121	9.4	4.4	7.0	0.0
Poached Egg with Ham & Truffle Gruyere, Leon*	1 Portion/96g	164	12.5	171	12.9	0.5	13.1	0.0
Pot, Full English, Leon*	1 Pot/228g	416	30.3	182	11.4	3.9	13.3	0.0
Toast, Wholemeal, Hot, Buttered, Leon*	1 Serving/92g	355	12.2	386	9.9	48.1	13.2	0.0
Toast, Wholemeal & Marmalade, Leon*	1 Portion/116g	418	14.1	360	7.9	51.8	12.1	0.0
Toast, Wholemeal with Blossom Honey, Leon*	1 Portion/106g	396	14.1	374	8.6	51.3	13.3	0.0

BREAKFAST CEREAL

Compote Only, Leon*	1 Serving/40g	42	0.0	105	0.8	27.2	0.0	0.0
Porridge, Blueberry, & Toasted Seeds, Organic, Leon*	1 Serving/320g	401	14.4	125	4.0	16.4	4.5	0.0
Porridge, of the Gods, Sm, Leon*	1 Serving/290g	374	8.4	129	3.4	21.0	2.9	0.0
Porridge, Plain, Organic, Leon*	1 Serving/270g	273	9.2	101	3.7	13.2	3.4	0.0
Porridge, Plain, Organic, Sm, Leon*	1 Serving/235g	329	13.1	140	3.9	17.5	5.6	0.0
Porridge, with Compote & Granola, Leon*	1 Serving/335g	430	16.5	128	3.8	16.2	4.9	0.0
Porridge, with Compote & Granola, Sm, Leon*	1 Serving/235g	329	13.1	140	3.9	17.5	5.6	0.0
Seeds Only, Leon*	1 Serving/20g	112	9.6	560	20.0	11.5	48.0	0.0

BROCCOLI

Garlic & Chilli, Grazing Dishes, Leon*	1 Serving/130g	113	9.0	87	4.1	2.1	6.9	0.0

BROWNIES

Better, Bits in Between, Leon*	1 Serving/85g	403	26.0	474	7.0	41.2	30.6	2.4

BURGERS

Chorizo, Leon*	1 Serving/247g	548	16.5	222	16.7	22.0	6.7	0.0
Halloumi, Leon*	1 Serving/206g	423	19.7	205	9.0	19.3	9.6	0.0
Meatball, Leon*	1 Serving/245g	518	18.6	212	9.6	24.6	7.6	0.0

CAKE

Carrot, Bits in Between, Leon*	1 Portion/114g	458	29.1	402	3.7	37.9	25.5	0.0
Orange & Walnut, Bits in Between, Leon*	1 Portion/100g	360	21.0	360	10.4	30.6	21.0	0.0

CHEESE

Halloumi, Grilled, Grazing Dishes, Leon*	1 Serving/140g	538	45.1	384	22.9	0.6	32.2	0.0

CHICKEN

Chargrilled, Chilli, Hot Boxes, Leon*	1 Serving/437g	655	29.0	150	8.5	13.5	6.6	1.1
Garlic, Rice Box, Leon*	1 Serving/422g	172	8.0	172	9.1	15.0	8.0	0.0

LEON RESTAURANTS

	Measure INFO/WEIGHT	per Measure KCAL	FAT	Nutrition Values per 100g / 100ml KCAL	PROT	CARB	FAT	FIBRE
CHICKEN								
Kids Menu, Leon*	1 Serving/240g	351	6.9	146	13.6	15.8	2.9	0.0
Nuggets, Grilled, Sides, Leon*	1 Serving/100g	247	13.7	247	29.0	2.0	13.7	0.0
CHICKEN CHILLI								
Rice Box, Leon*	1 Serving/442g	723	33.1	164	8.7	14.7	7.5	0.0
CHICKEN WITH								
Aioli, Chargrilled, Hot Boxes, Leon*	1 Serving/417g	648	29.0	155	8.9	13.7	7.0	1.2
Aoili, Chargrilled, Hot Box, Leon*	1 Serving/165g	276	12.6	167	21.5	2.8	7.6	0.0
CHILLI								
Con Carne, Black Bean, Leon*	1 Serving/518g	731	30.9	141	5.5	15.6	6.0	0.0
CHOCOLATE								
Dark, & Raspberry, Bits in Between, Leon*	1 Serving/25g	135	9.3	540	6.0	40.4	37.2	8.0
Dark, Bits in Between, Leon*	1 Serving/25g	136	9.9	544	8.4	32.4	39.6	12.4
Dark, Orange & Almond, Bits in Between, Leon*	1 Serving/25g	142	10.3	568	8.0	36.4	41.2	8.4
COFFEE								
Americano, Leon*	1 Serving/320ml	1	0.0	0	0.0	0.0	0.0	0.0
Cappucino, with Full Fat, Leon*	1 Serving/200ml	122	7.2	61	3.1	4.3	3.6	0.0
Filter, Leon*	1 Serving/324ml	6	0.0	2	0.2	0.3	0.0	0.0
Latte, Full Fat, Leon*	1 Serving/340ml	185	10.9	54	2.7	3.6	3.2	0.0
Macchiato, with Full Fat, Leon*	1 Serving/70ml	8	0.4	11	0.6	0.8	0.5	0.0
COLESLAW								
Fresh, Grazing Dishes, Leon*	1 Serving/115g	156	13.0	136	3.0	5.6	11.3	0.0
Slaw, Fresh, Sides, Leon*	1 Serving/110g	158	13.6	143	2.3	4.3	12.4	0.0
COOKIES								
Almond & Orange, Bits in Between, Leon*	1 Cookie/74g	400	25.0	541	14.9	41.9	33.8	5.4
Triple Chocolate, Bits in Between, Leon*	1 Cookie/50g	250	16.0	500	14.0	38.0	32.0	8.0
CROISSANT								
Pain au Chocolat, Leon*	1 Serving/75g	321	21.0	428	5.3	38.7	28.0	0.0
Pain Aux Raisins, Leon*	1 Serving/110g	483	22.8	439	4.6	40.4	20.7	0.0
Plain, Leon*	1 Serving/75g	287	20.0	383	5.3	30.7	26.7	0.0
CURRY								
Chicken, Hot Boxes, Leon*	1 Serving/505g	799	42.0	158	7.6	14.5	8.3	0.0
Leon Gobi, Hot Boxes, Leon*	1 Serving/524g	709	37.6	135	2.9	14.8	7.2	0.0
Mamta's Pea & Squash, Leon*	1 Serving/437g	517	19.2	118	2.8	18.5	4.4	1.9
Thai Green, Pot, Leon*	1 Pot/200g	143	5.0	72	8.0	4.0	2.5	0.5
DRESSING								
Chimmichuri, Leon*	1 Pot/25g	76	8.0	304	0.0	4.0	32.0	0.0
EGGS								
Poached, & Saucy Beans, Leon*	1 Portion/116g	137	8.5	118	7.3	5.1	7.3	0.0
FALAFEL								
Sweet Potato, Grazing Dishes, Leon*	1 Serving/146g	261	10.0	179	5.4	26.6	6.8	0.0
Sweet Potato, Hot Boxes, Leon*	1 Pack/423g	671	33.0	159	3.1	17.7	7.8	2.1
FLAPJACK								
Cranberry & Pecan, Bits in Between, Leon*	1 Serving/83g	385	22.7	464	4.6	48.4	27.4	0.0
FLATBREAD								
Sides, Leon*	1 Portion/80g	205	0.8	256	9.6	50.5	1.0	0.0
FRIES								
Baked, Sides, Leon*	1 Portion/100g	303	14.7	303	4.1	36.8	14.7	0.0
HOT CHOCOLATE								
with Full Fat, Leon*	1 Serving/165ml	313	17.3	190	3.7	19.6	10.5	0.0
HOUMOUS								
& Flatbread, Sides, Leon*	1 Serving/215g	713	39.5	331	8.8	30.8	18.4	0.0
Hummus, without Flatbread, Sides, Leon*	1 Serving/130g	283	20.4	218	6.6	12.5	15.7	0.0

LEON RESTAURANTS

	Measure INFO/WEIGHT	per Measure KCAL	FAT	Nutrition Values per 100g / 100ml KCAL	PROT	CARB	FAT	FIBRE
JUICE								
Blackcurrant, Quencher, Leon Kids Menu, Sm, Leon*	1 Serving/250ml	100	0.0	40	0.1	10.1	0.0	0.0
Blackcurrant, Quencher, Leon*	1 Serving/315ml	114	0.0	36	0.1	8.6	0.0	0.0
Lemon, Ginger & Mint, Quencher, Leon*	1 Serving/300ml	54	0.0	18	0.1	4.1	0.0	0.0
Lemon, Lime & Ginger, Quencher, Leon*	1 Serving/315ml	123	0.0	39	0.1	9.7	0.0	0.0
Orange, Freshly Squeezed, Leon*	1 Serving/315ml	106	0.0	34	0.6	7.7	0.0	0.0
LAMB								
Rhubarb Koresh, Hot Boxes, Leon*	1 Portion/498g	644	27.0	129	5.4	13.6	5.4	1.5
LEMONADE								
Fresh, Leon*	1 Serving/307ml	105	0.0	34	0.1	8.4	0.0	0.0
Raspberry, Leon*	1 Serving/315ml	110	0.2	35	0.2	7.8	0.0	0.0
MEATBALLS								
Grilled, Rice Box, Leon*	1 Box/505g	880	49.0	174	6.0	15.0	9.7	0.0
Hot Boxes, Lunchbox, Leon*	1 Serving/308g	462	15.4	150	5.5	19.2	5.0	1.0
Moroccan, Grazing Dishes, Leon*	1 Serving/165g	243	15.4	147	11.8	4.6	9.3	0.0
Moroccan, Hot Boxes, Leon*	1 Serving/480g	767	42.0	160	5.4	14.0	8.8	1.2
Moroccan, Sides, Leon*	1 Serving/140g	198	11.5	141	12.4	5.0	8.2	0.0
MILK SHAKE								
Banana & Cinnamon, Milk Free, Leon*	1 Portion/250g	98	2.0	39	0.8	6.8	0.8	0.0
MUFFIN								
Bacon, Breakfast, Leon*	1 Serving/214g	566	25.8	264	12.0	25.2	12.1	0.0
Mushroom & Egg, Breakfast, Leon*	1 Muffin/200g	366	18.0	183	7.5	17.5	9.0	0.5
NUTS								
Chilli Roasted, Bar Snacks, Leon*	1 Serving/80g	489	49.7	611	19.0	6.4	62.1	0.0
PIE								
Banoffi, Grab & Go, Bits in Between, Leon*	1 Serving/70g	278	12.4	397	6.6	54.3	17.7	0.0
Pecan, Leon*	1 Serving/153g	572	37.0	374	5.9	31.4	24.2	2.0
POPCORN								
Sea Salt, Propercorn, Bits in Between, Leon*	1 Portion/20g	87	3.1	435	8.0	59.5	15.5	0.0
Sweet Salty, Propercorn, Bits in Between, Leon*	1 Portion/30g	128	4.1	427	5.7	63.3	13.7	0.0
POTATOES								
Mashed, Grazing Dishes, Leon*	1 Serving/215g	384	14.6	179	5.4	25.8	6.8	0.0
PUDDING								
Banana Split, Puds, Leon*	1 Serving/525g	1196	84.8	228	2.8	18.8	16.2	0.0
Chocolate Tart, Dark, Puds, Leon*	1 Serving/226g	823	46.9	364	5.0	40.6	20.8	0.0
RICE								
with Sweet Potato & Falafel, Rice Box, Leon*	1 Box/423g	718	35.7	170	3.2	19.2	8.4	0.0
SALAD								
Chicken, & Chorizo, Club, Leon*	1 Salad/317g	463	23.8	146	12.4	6.5	7.5	0.0
Chicken, Garlic, Leon*	1 Salad/292g	460	25.1	158	12.8	6.4	8.6	0.0
Chicken, Grilled, Leon*	1 Serving/400g	619	34.3	155	13.5	6.2	8.6	0.0
Chicken, Grilled, Superfood, Leon*	1 Pack/287g	435	23.1	152	12.7	6.4	8.0	0.0
Chicken, Persian, & Avocado, Leon*	1 Salad/323g	486	33.1	150	8.8	4.8	10.3	0.0
Green, Sunshine, Sides, Leon*	1 Serving/147g	294	24.9	200	6.3	5.6	16.9	0.0
Green Sunshine, without Vinaigrette, Leon*	1 Serving/117g	85	3.0	73	6.7	5.2	2.6	0.0
Lamb Kofte, with Houmous, Leon*	1 Serving/412g	579	37.0	141	6.3	7.3	9.0	1.9
Mackerel, Smoked, & Beetroot, Magic, Leon*	1 Serving/395g	601	31.8	152	7.6	11.1	8.1	0.0
Pea, Crushed, Sides, Leon*	1 Serving/127g	171	10.9	134	5.1	7.2	8.6	0.0
Quinoa & Chicken, Superclean, Leon*	1 Serving/263g	344	15.0	131	8.8	11.0	5.7	0.8
Roasted Cauliflower Salad, Leon*	1 Portion/279g	286	21.0	102	2.9	7.5	7.5	2.2
Salmon, Superfood, Leon*	1 Salad/315g	486	37.5	154	7.9	2.6	11.9	0.0
Sunshine, Grazing Dishes, Leon*	1 Serving/127g	145	9.6	114	6.2	6.5	7.6	0.0
Superclean Quinoa Pot, Leon*	1 Pot/110g	141	7.0	128	4.6	13.6	6.4	0.9

LEON RESTAURANTS

	Measure INFO/WEIGHT	per Measure KCAL	FAT	Nutrition Values per 100g / 100ml KCAL	PROT	CARB	FAT	FIBRE
SALAD								
Superfood, Original, Leon*	1 Serving/346g	526	36.9	152	5.6	7.2	10.7	0.0
Wrap, Persian Chicken, Leon*	1 Serving/235g	517	15.9	220	14.6	24.3	6.8	0.0
SANDWICH								
Bacon, Egg & Mushroom, Breakfast, Leon*	1 Serving/215g	452	23.5	210	11.3	17.6	10.9	0.0
Bacon & Cheese, Breakfast, Leon*	1 Serving/132g	377	18.2	286	15.9	26.0	13.8	0.0
Egg & Mushroom, Breakfast, Leon*	1 Serving/191g	370	19.1	194	9.0	18.1	10.0	0.0
SAUCE								
Aioli, Leon*	1 Serving/30g	126	12.5	420	4.0	1.3	41.7	0.0
Chilli, Hot, Leon*	1 Serving/30g	14	0.5	47	1.3	7.7	1.7	0.0
SAUSAGE								
Chorizo, Hot, Grilled, Grazing Dishes, Leon*	1 Serving/189g	227	10.6	120	15.8	1.6	5.6	0.0
SHORTBREAD								
Billionaire's, Bits in Between, Leon*	1 Serving/43g	228	15.0	530	7.0	51.2	34.9	0.0
SMOOTHIE								
Banana, Power, Leon*	1 Serving/325ml	398	16.7	122	4.4	14.1	5.1	0.0
Power, Seasonal, Leon*	1 Serving/325ml	398	16.7	122	4.4	14.1	5.1	0.0
Strawberry, Power, Leon*	1 Serving/300ml	348	14.4	116	4.1	14.1	4.8	0.0
SOUP								
Chicken, Roast, & Sweetcorn, Meaty, Leon*	1 Serving/360ml	288	11.9	80	4.2	8.8	3.3	0.0
Chicken Noodle, Leon*	1 Portion/295g	99	2.0	34	3.4	2.7	0.7	0.0
Harira, Moroccan, Harira, Veggie, Leon*	1 Serving/375ml	211	5.1	56	3.1	8.2	1.4	0.0
Lentil & Bacon, Leon*	1 Serving/312g	211	13.7	68	2.7	3.7	4.4	0.0
Pea, Bacon & Basil, Meaty, Leon*	1 Serving/370ml	199	7.0	54	4.0	5.5	1.9	0.0
Pea, French, & Mint, Veggie, Leon*	1 Serving/370ml	249	14.2	67	2.5	6.0	3.8	0.0
Potato, Shallot & Thyme, Leon*	1 Serving/312g	178	8.4	57	1.1	6.5	2.7	0.0
Tomato, Roy's, Veggie, Leon*	1 Serving/360ml	108	3.6	30	1.1	4.3	1.0	0.0
TART								
Cranberry Bakewell, Bits in Between, Leon*	1 Serving/84g	362	26.0	431	7.1	29.8	31.0	3.6
Lemon Ginger Crunch, Bits in Between, Leon*	1 Serving/83g	425	31.5	512	8.2	33.0	38.0	0.0
TEA								
Cammomile, Leon*	1 Serving/324ml	0	0.0	0	0.0	0.0	0.0	0.0
Earl Grey, no Milk, Leon*	1 Serving/324ml	0	0.0	0	0.0	0.0	0.0	0.0
English Breakfast, no Milk, Leon*	1 Serving/324ml	0	0.0	0	0.0	0.0	0.0	0.0
Ginger, Steeper, Leon*	1 Serving/324ml	4	0.1	1	0.0	0.2	0.0	0.0
Mint, Steeper, Leon*	1 Serving/324ml	4	0.1	1	0.1	0.2	0.0	0.0
Rooibus, Leon*	1 Serving/324ml	0	0.0	0	0.0	0.0	0.0	0.0
VINAIGRETTE								
Leon Restaurants*	1 Serving/30g	183	20.1	610	0.7	0.3	67.0	0.0
WRAP								
Chicken, & Chorizo, Club, Hot, Leon*	1 Serving/261g	563	20.9	216	16.0	19.2	8.0	0.0
Chicken, Garlic, Leon*	1 Serving/224g	461	12.0	206	16.8	21.8	5.4	0.0
Chicken, Grilled, Hot, Leon*	1 Serving/280g	429	11.1	153	12.9	17.5	4.0	0.0
Chicken Chilli, Hot, Leon*	1 Serving/256g	473	7.0	185	14.8	16.0	2.7	0.0
Falafel, Sweet Potato, Hot, Leon*	1 Serving/226g	489	16.3	217	6.1	30.3	7.2	0.0
Fish Finger, Hot, Leon*	1 Serving/274g	619	23.9	226	8.9	27.0	8.7	0.0
Halloumi, Grilled, Leon*	1 Wrap/220g	531	25.0	241	10.4	26.4	11.4	1.8
YOGHURT								
Greek, of the Gods, Leon*	1 Serving/255g	382	14.9	150	4.8	18.4	5.8	0.0
Greek, Simple, Leon*	1 Serving/135g	179	12.3	133	6.3	6.4	9.1	0.0
Greek, with Blueberries & Seeds, Leon*	1 Serving/185g	307	17.5	166	6.0	13.8	9.4	0.0
Greek, with Compote & Granola, Leon*	1 Serving/200g	336	19.7	168	5.7	13.7	9.8	0.0
Yoghurt & Fruit, Blueberry Boost, Leon*	1 Serving/230g	328	18.8	143	5.6	11.6	8.2	0.0

MCDONALD'S

	Measure INFO/WEIGHT	per Measure KCAL	FAT	Nutrition Values per 100g / 100ml KCAL	PROT	CARB	FAT	FIBRE
APPLES								
McDonald's*	1 Apple/140g	59	0.0	42	0.3	10.0	0.0	2.2
BAGEL								
Toasted, with Strawberry Jam, McDonald's*	1 Bagel/105g	260	1.0	248	8.0	52.0	1.0	3.0
with Bacon, Egg & Cheese, McDonald's*	1 Bagel/182g	480	23.7	263	13.0	26.0	13.0	2.0
with Butter & Jam, McDonald's*	1 Bagel/122g	399	10.2	326	5.9	58.8	8.3	2.2
with Flora & Jam, McDonald's*	1 Bagel/120g	369	6.9	305	6.0	59.4	5.7	2.2
with Philadelphia, McDonald's*	1 Bagel/125g	318	5.9	254	7.7	47.5	4.7	2.1
with Sausage, Egg & Cheese, McDonald's*	1 Bagel/211g	562	29.6	266	14.0	22.0	14.0	2.0
with Sausage & Egg, McDonald's*	1 Bagel/207g	551	26.5	266	13.3	23.3	12.8	1.6
BREAD								
Bagel, Plain, Toasted, McDonald's*	1 Bagel/87g	216	0.9	248	9.0	50.0	1.0	3.0
BREAKFAST								
Big Breakfast, McDonald's*	1 Breakfast/272g	611	38.0	225	11.0	15.0	14.0	1.0
Big Breakfast, with Bun, McDonald's*	1 Bun/242g	571	32.2	236	13.0	15.1	13.3	0.9
BREAKFAST CEREAL								
Porridge, Oat So Simple, & Jam, McDonald's*	1 Serving/232g	246	5.3	106	4.0	17.0	2.3	0.9
Porridge, Oat So Simple, & Sugar, McDonald's*	1 Serving/215g	205	5.4	95	4.3	13.7	2.5	0.9
Porridge, Oat So Simple, Plain, McDonald's*	1 Serving/211g	194	4.2	92	5.0	13.0	2.0	1.0
BROWNIES								
Belgian Bliss, McDonald's*	1 Serving/85g	390	22.1	459	6.0	51.0	26.0	2.0
BURGERS								
1955 Burger, McDonald's*	1 Burger/281g	655	33.7	233	14.0	18.0	12.0	2.0
Arizona, Grande, McDonald's*	1 Burger/251g	655	40.2	261	16.0	15.0	16.0	2.0
Bacon, Chicken & Onion, McDonald's*	1 Burger/255g	660	33.1	259	14.0	22.0	13.0	2.0
Bacon Cheeseburger, McDonald's*	1 Burger/136g	368	16.6	270	16.0	23.6	12.2	2.3
Bacon McDouble, with Cheese, McDonald's*	1 Burger/141g	372	19.0	264	16.1	19.6	13.5	2.2
Beef, Deluxe, McDonald's*	1 Burger/265g	650	34.5	245	14.0	18.0	13.0	2.0
Beef, Deluxe, with Bacon, McDonald's*	1 Burger/274g	689	38.4	252	15.0	18.0	14.0	2.0
Big Mac, Bigger, McDonald's*	1 Burger/324g	714	34.0	220	12.9	18.5	10.5	1.6
Big Mac, McDonald's*	1 Burger/220g	508	26.6	229	13.0	19.0	12.0	2.0
Big Mac, no Sauce, no Cheese, McDonald's*	1 Burger/181g	400	16.0	221	12.2	23.8	8.8	1.1
Big Tasty, McDonald's*	1 Burger/346g	835	52.0	241	13.0	14.0	15.0	1.0
Big Tasty, with Bacon, McDonald's*	1 Burger/359g	890	57.4	248	14.0	14.0	16.0	1.0
Cheeseburger, Bacon, McDonald's*	1 Burger/127g	336	15.3	264	16.0	24.0	12.0	2.0
Cheeseburger, Double, McDonald's*	1 Burger/170g	445	24.0	260	17.0	19.0	14.0	1.0
Cheeseburger, McDonald's*	1 Burger/119g	301	12.0	253	14.4	26.2	10.1	2.5
Chicago Works, McDonald's*	1 Burger/261g	680	39.2	260	15.0	16.0	15.0	1.0
Chicken, BLC, McDonald's*	1 Burger/250g	394	18.0	158	6.8	15.6	7.2	1.1
Chicken & Cheddar Classic, McDonald's*	1 Burger/500g	640	32.0	128	7.0	10.6	6.4	0.5
Chicken Fiesta, McDonald's*	1 Burger/240g	610	26.4	254	14.0	24.0	11.0	2.0
Chicken Legend, Bacon, Spicy Tomato Salsa, McDonald's*	1 Serving/233g	555	16.3	238	15.0	29.0	7.0	2.0
Chicken Legend, Spicy Tomato Salsa, McDonald's*	1 Burger/218g	501	13.1	230	13.0	30.0	6.0	2.0
Chicken Legend, with Bacon, Cool Mayo, McDonald's*	1 Burger/227g	590	22.7	260	15.0	27.0	10.0	2.0
Chicken Legend, with Cool Mayo, McDonald's*	1 Burger/215g	541	21.5	252	14.0	28.0	10.0	2.0
Filet-O-Fish, McDonald's*	1 Burger/150g	350	18.1	232	10.0	24.0	12.0	1.0
Filet-O-Fish, no Tartar Sauce, McDonald's*	1 Burger/124g	290	9.0	234	12.1	30.6	7.3	0.8
Grilled Chicken Caprese, McDonald's*	1 Burger/275g	470	21.2	171	12.5	15.0	7.7	2.1
Hamburger, McDonald's*	1 Burger/104g	250	8.3	240	13.0	29.0	8.0	2.0
Mayo Chicken, McDonald's*	1 Burger/126g	319	13.8	254	10.0	30.0	11.0	2.0
McChicken Grill with BBQ Sauce, McDonald's*	1 Sandwich/215g	309	5.5	144	12.1	18.1	2.6	2.2
McChicken Premiere, McDonald's*	1 Burger/221g	464	17.0	210	10.4	24.4	7.7	1.4
McChicken Sandwich, McDonald's*	1 Sandwich/173g	388	17.3	224	9.0	26.0	10.0	2.0

MCDONALD'S

	Measure INFO/WEIGHT	per Measure KCAL	FAT	Nutrition Values per 100g / 100ml KCAL	PROT	CARB	FAT	FIBRE
BURGERS								
New York Special, McDonald's*	1 Burger/255g	680	43.3	267	16.0	14.0	17.0	2.0
Quarter Pounder, Bacon with Cheese, McDonald's*	1 Burger/230g	592	33.2	259	16.5	15.4	14.5	1.3
Quarter Pounder, Deluxe, Bacon & Cheese, McDonald's*	1 Burger/229g	592	33.2	259	16.5	15.4	14.5	1.3
Quarter Pounder, Deluxe, McDonald's*	1 Burger/253g	521	26.8	206	11.4	16.1	10.6	1.7
Quarter Pounder, Double, with Cheese, McDonald's*	1 Burger/275g	710	40.3	259	19.5	12.2	14.7	1.1
Quarter Pounder, McDonald's*	1 Burger/178g	424	19.0	238	14.5	20.9	10.7	2.1
Quarter Pounder, with Cheese, McDonald's*	1 Burger/205g	518	26.7	252	16.0	19.0	13.0	2.0
Smokehouse, McDonald's*	1 Burger/300g	638	29.0	213	13.0	18.0	9.7	1.2
Summer Chorizo, McDonald's*	1 Burger/238g	650	35.7	273	17.0	17.0	15.0	1.0
The M with Bacon, McDonald's*	1 Serving/249g	620	32.4	249	17.0	18.0	13.0	1.0
The Texas Grande, McDonald's*	1 Burger/242g	585	31.4	242	15.0	16.0	13.0	2.0
BURGERS VEGETARIAN								
Vegetable, Deluxe, McDonald's*	1 Burger/181g	411	16.3	227	6.0	30.0	9.0	6.0
CARROTS								
Sticks, McDonald's*	1 Bag/89g	34	0.0	38	0.0	8.0	0.0	2.0
CHEESE								
Melt, Dippers, McDonald's*	1 Serving/72g	265	18.7	368	12.0	21.0	26.0	1.0
Mozzarella, Dippers, McDonald's*	3 Dippers/85g	271	13.6	319	13.0	27.0	16.0	1.0
Soft, Philadelphia, Light, McDonald's*	1 Serving/33g	50	3.5	157	9.0	3.0	11.0	0.0
CHICKEN								
McBites, McDonald's*	1 Portion/85g	180	8.0	212	17.6	11.8	9.4	1.2
McNuggets, 4 Pieces, McDonald's*	4 Pieces/70g	170	9.1	243	13.0	19.0	13.0	1.0
McNuggets, 6 Pieces, McDonald's*	6 Pieces/109g	259	14.1	238	13.0	19.0	13.0	1.0
McNuggets, 9 Pieces, McDonald's*	9 Pieces/163g	388	21.2	238	13.0	19.0	13.0	1.0
Selects, 3 Pieces, McDonald's*	3 Pieces/128g	359	19.2	280	16.0	20.0	15.0	1.0
Selects, 5 Pieces, McDonald's*	5 Pieces/214g	599	32.1	280	16.0	20.0	15.0	1.0
COFFEE								
Black, Lge, McDonald's*	1 Lge/417ml	8	0.0	2	0.0	0.0	0.0	0.0
Black, Med, McDonald's*	1 Med/312ml	6	0.0	2	0.0	0.0	0.0	0.0
Cappuccino, Lge, McDonald's*	1 Serving/317ml	124	3.2	39	3.0	4.0	1.0	0.0
Cappuccino, Med, McDonald's*	1 Med241ml	94	2.4	39	3.0	4.0	1.0	0.0
Caramel Frappe, Iced, McDonald's*	1 Med/268ml	387	16.3	144	2.2	20.5	6.1	0.0
Espresso, Double Shot, McDonald's*	1 Double/60ml	1	0.0	2	0.0	0.0	0.0	0.0
Espresso, Single Shot, McDonald's*	1 Serving/30ml	1	0.0	3	0.0	0.0	0.0	0.0
Latte, Lge, McDonald's*	1 Lge/468ml	192	4.7	41	3.0	4.0	1.0	0.0
Latte, Med, McDonald's*	1 Med/355ml	142	3.6	40	3.0	4.0	1.0	0.0
Mocha, Frappe, Iced, McDonald's*	1 Med/268ml	396	20.0	148	2.1	17.5	7.5	0.9
Mocha, Freshly Ground, Lge, McDonald's*	1 Lge/450ml	368	13.0	82	3.6	10.2	2.9	0.4
Mocha, Freshly Ground, Med, McDonald's*	1 Serving/335ml	318	11.0	95	3.6	12.2	3.3	0.6
White, Lge, McDonald's*	1 Lge/500ml	40	0.0	8	0.0	1.0	0.0	0.0
White, Med, McDonald's*	1 Med/375ml	30	0.0	8	1.0	1.0	0.0	0.0
COLA								
Coca-Cola, Diet, McDonald's*	1 Med/405ml	2	0.0	0	0.0	0.0	0.0	0.0
Coca-Cola, McDonald's*	1 Med/405ml	170	0.0	42	0.0	10.0	0.0	0.0
COOKIES								
Triple Chocolate, McDonald's*	1 Pack/60g	368	19.0	613	7.0	73.3	31.7	3.2
CREAMER								
Uht, McDonald's*	1 Cup/14ml	17	1.4	123	4.2	4.2	10.0	0.0
DIP								
Barbeque, Smokey, McDonald's*	1 Portion/50g	84	1.0	170	0.0	38.0	2.0	0.0
BBQ, McDonald's*	1 Pot/30g	49	0.2	168	0.9	39.0	0.8	0.0
Curry, Sweet, McDonald's*	1 Portion/30g	50	0.9	171	0.0	38.0	3.0	3.0

MCDONALD'S

	Measure INFO/WEIGHT	per Measure KCAL	FAT	Nutrition Values per 100g / 100ml KCAL	PROT	CARB	FAT	FIBRE
DIP								
Salsa, McDonald's*	1oz/28g	38	0.0	135	3.4	30.4	0.0	3.4
Sour Cream & Chive, McDonald's*	1 Pot/50g	158	16.9	300	2.0	2.0	32.0	4.0
Sweet & Sour, McDonald's*	1 Portion/30g	44	0.0	172	0.0	38.0	0.0	0.0
Sweet Chilli, McDonald's*	1 Pot/50g	115	1.3	256	0.0	58.0	3.0	0.0
DOUGHNUTS								
Chocolate Donut, McDonald's*	1 Donut/79g	345	16.2	437	5.7	43.8	20.5	1.0
Chocolate Donut, McMini, McDonald's*	1 Donut/17g	64	3.0	375	6.8	46.9	17.8	1.6
Cinnamon Donut, McDonald's*	1 Donut/72g	302	18.1	419	5.1	43.1	25.1	3.8
Sugared Donut, McDonald's*	1 Donut/49g	189	10.0	386	6.9	40.8	20.4	2.6
DRESSING								
Balsamic, Low Fat, McDonald's*	1 Sachet/30g	26	0.8	87	0.3	14.7	2.7	0.0
Caesar, Low Fat, McDonald's*	1 Sachet/80g	55	1.6	68	2.0	10.0	2.0	0.0
Fajita Style, McDonald's*	1 Portion/30g	21	0.8	70	1.0	10.0	2.7	1.3
Ranch, Salad, McDonald's*	1 Sachet/79ml	107	6.5	136	3.1	12.3	8.3	0.8
FANTA								
Orange, McDonald's*	1 Sm/250ml	105	0.0	42	0.0	10.0	0.0	0.0
FISH FINGERS								
McDonald's*	3 Fingers/84g	195	9.2	232	15.0	19.0	11.0	1.0
FLATBREAD								
Chicken Salsa, McDonald's*	1 Serving/100g	480	15.5	480	27.3	57.6	15.5	0.0
FRIES								
Chunky, McDonald's*	1oz/28g	47	1.7	169	3.0	25.5	6.0	2.5
French, Lge, McDonald's*	1 Serving/160g	444	22.4	278	3.0	38.0	14.0	4.0
French, Med, McDonald's*	1 Serving/114g	337	16.0	296	3.0	37.0	14.0	4.0
French, Sm, McDonald's*	1 Serving/80g	237	11.2	296	2.0	38.0	14.0	4.0
FRUIT								
Bag, Apple & Grape, McDonald's*	1 Bag/85g	46	0.1	54	0.3	13.0	0.1	2.3
Bag, Happy Meal, McDonald's*	1 Bag/80g	43	0.1	54	0.3	13.0	0.1	2.3
Bag, McDonald's*	1 Pack/80g	40	0.8	50	0.0	12.0	1.0	2.0
Bag, Pineapple & Grape, McDonald's*	1 Pack/80g	38	0.2	47	0.4	11.1	0.2	1.2
FRUIT DRINK								
Fruitizz, Sparkling, McDonald's*	1 Drink/250ml	160	0.0	64	0.4	15.6	0.0	0.0
FRUIT SHOOT								
Robinsons, McDonald's*	1 Bottle/200ml	10	0.0	5	0.1	0.8	0.0	0.0
HAPPY MEAL								
Cheeseburger with Carrot Sticks, McDonald's*	1 Meal/190g	335	12.2	176	8.7	19.6	6.4	2.5
Cheeseburger with Fruit Bag, McDonald's*	1 Meal/100g	347	12.1	347	16.3	41.0	12.1	4.2
Cheeseburger with Sm Fries, McDonald's*	1 Meal/199g	538	24.0	270	9.2	30.2	12.1	2.5
Chicken McNuggets with Carrot Sticks, McDonald's*	1 Meal/150g	207	9.1	138	7.7	12.1	6.1	1.9
Chicken McNuggets with Fruit Bag, McDonald's*	1 Meal/150g	219	9.0	146	7.5	14.7	6.0	1.5
Chicken McNuggets with Sm Fries, McDonald's*	1 Meal/150g	410	20.9	273	8.9	27.3	13.9	2.0
Fish Fingers with Carrot Sticks, McDonald's*	1 Meal/184g	228	8.7	124	7.3	12.1	4.7	1.7
Fish Fingers with Fruit Bag, McDonald's*	1 Meal/184g	240	8.6	130	7.2	14.1	4.7	1.4
Fish Fingers with Sm Fries, McDonald's*	1 Meal/184g	234	11.1	234	8.3	24.5	11.1	1.8
Hamburger with Carrot Sticks, McDonald's*	1 Meal/180g	284	8.5	158	7.5	20.1	4.7	2.7
Hamburger with Fruit bag, McDonald's*	1 Meal/190g	296	8.4	156	7.0	21.0	4.4	2.2
Hamburger with Sm Fries, McDonald's*	1 Meal/184g	487	20.3	265	8.3	32.1	11.0	2.7
HASH BROWNS								
McDonald's*	1 Hash Brown/52g	136	8.8	264	2.0	26.0	17.0	2.0
HOT CHOCOLATE								
McDonald's*	1 Med/349ml	173	3.8	50	0.7	8.8	1.1	0.0

	Measure	per Measure		Nutrition Values per 100g / 100ml				
	INFO/WEIGHT	KCAL	FAT	KCAL	PROT	CARB	FAT	FIBRE

MCDONALD'S
ICE CREAM CONE
McDonald's*	1 Cone/93g	145	4.7	156	4.5	24.4	5.0	0.0
with Flake, McDonald's*	1 Cone/99g	190	7.2	191	4.8	27.0	7.2	0.6

JAM
Strawberry, McDonald's*	1 Pack/15g	39	0.0	250	0.0	60.0	0.0	0.0

JUICE
Orange, Pure, McDonald's*	1 Regular/200ml	86	2.0	43	1.0	9.0	1.0	0.1
Tropicana, McDonald's*	1 Bottle/250ml	120	0.0	48	1.6	10.0	0.0	0.4

KETCHUP
Tomato, McDonald's*	1 Portion/17ml	21	0.0	109	0.0	26.0	0.0	0.0

LEMONADE
Sprite, McDonald's*	1 Regular/251ml	108	0.0	43	0.0	10.5	0.0	0.0
Sprite, Zero, McDonald's*	1 Lge/500ml	5	0.0	1	0.0	0.0	0.0	0.0

MCFLURRY
After Eight, McDonald's*	1 McFlurry/206g	400	16.5	194	3.0	27.0	8.0	1.0
Cadbury, Shortcake, Limited Edition, McDonald's*	1 McFlurry/206g	385	14.4	187	3.0	28.0	7.0	1.0
Chocolate, Cornetto, McDonald's*	1 Serving/207g	400	16.6	193	3.0	29.0	8.0	1.0
Cornetto, Mint Choc, McDonald's*	1 Serving/207g	400	16.6	193	3.0	29.0	8.0	1.0
Creme Egg, Cadbury's, McDonald's*	1 McFlurry/203g	381	12.9	188	2.9	29.8	6.3	0.5
Crunchie, McDonald's*	1 McFlurry/181g	323	10.9	178	3.0	28.0	6.0	1.0
Dairy Milk, Deluxe, McDonald's*	1 McFlurry/205g	392	14.4	191	3.2	28.6	7.0	0.1
Dairy Milk, McDonald's*	1 McFlurry/180g	332	12.6	184	3.0	28.0	7.0	1.0
Dairy Milk, with Caramel, McDonald's*	1 McFlurry/206g	385	13.0	187	2.9	29.1	6.3	0.0
Flake, Chocolate, McDonald's*	1 McFlurry/206ml	400	14.4	194	3.0	29.0	7.0	0.0
Flake, Raspberry, McDonald's*	1 McFlurry/205ml	370	12.3	180	3.0	27.0	6.0	0.0
Galaxy Ripple, McDonald's*	1 Serving/206g	408	16.0	198	3.2	28.2	7.8	0.6
Raspberry, McDonald's*	1 McFlurry/206ml	370	12.3	180	3.0	27.0	6.0	0.0
Rolo, McDonald's*	1 McFlurry/205g	390	13.3	190	4.0	29.2	6.5	0.1
Smarties, McDonald's*	1 McFlurry/181g	322	10.9	178	3.0	28.0	6.0	1.0
Toffee Swirl, Oreo Cookie, McDonald's*	1 McFlurry/206ml	400	12.4	194	3.0	31.0	6.0	1.0
Triple Caramel, McDonald's*	1 McFlurry/237g	398	14.0	168	2.4	26.2	5.9	0.4
Wispa Gold, McDonald's*	1 McFlurry/206g	395	14.0	192	2.9	29.1	6.8	0.5
Yorkie, McDonald's*	1 McFlurry/204g	379	14.9	186	3.4	27.0	7.3	0.8

MCMUFFIN
Bacon & Egg, Double, McDonald's*	1 McMuffin/161g	401	20.9	249	15.0	16.0	13.0	1.0
Bacon & Egg, McDonald's*	1 McMuffin/146g	348	17.5	238	14.0	18.0	12.0	1.0
Egg, McDonald's*	1 McMuffin/127g	281	12.8	221	12.2	20.4	10.1	3.2
Sausage, no Egg, no Cheese, McDonald's*	1 Sandwich/96g	310	18.0	323	12.5	29.2	18.8	4.2
Sausage & Egg, Double, McDonald's*	1 McMuffin/222g	565	35.5	254	16.0	12.0	16.0	1.0
Sausage & Egg, Double, no Muffin, McDonald's*	1 Serving/100g	416	33.5	416	27.6	0.2	33.5	0.0
Sausage & Egg, McDonald's*	1 McMuffin/174g	430	24.4	247	14.0	16.0	14.0	1.0

MCRIB
McDonald's*	1 Sandwich/100g	428	15.0	428	26.0	46.0	15.0	2.7

MILK
Fresh, Portion, McDonald's*	1 Portion/14ml	10	0.0	69	0.0	7.0	0.0	0.0
Organic, McDonald's*	1 Bottle/250ml	125	4.5	50	3.6	4.8	1.8	0.0

MILK SHAKE
Banana, Lge, McDonald's*	1 Lge/393ml	495	11.8	126	3.0	21.0	3.0	0.0
Banana, Med, McDonald's*	1 Med/306ml	386	9.2	126	3.0	21.0	3.0	0.0
Banana, Sm, McDonald's*	1 Sm/160ml	203	4.8	127	3.0	21.0	3.0	0.0
Cadbury Dairy Milk, Caramel Flavour, Sm, McDonald's*	1 Med/177ml	220	5.3	124	3.0	20.0	3.0	1.0
Cadburys Dairy Milk, Caramel, Lge, McDonald's*	1 Lge/417ml	505	16.7	121	3.0	19.0	4.0	1.0
Chocolate, Lge, McDonald's*	1 Lge/397ml	488	11.9	123	3.0	20.0	3.0	0.0

MCDONALD'S

	Measure INFO/WEIGHT	per Measure KCAL	FAT	Nutrition Values per 100g / 100ml KCAL	PROT	CARB	FAT	FIBRE
MILK SHAKE								
Chocolate, Med, McDonald's*	1 Med/301ml	380	9.0	126	3.0	21.0	3.0	0.0
Chocolate, Sm, McDonald's*	1 Sm/157ml	200	4.7	127	3.0	21.0	3.0	0.0
Strawberry, Lge, McDonald's*	1 Lge/390ml	488	11.7	125	3.0	21.0	3.0	0.0
Strawberry, Med, McDonald's*	1 Med/303ml	379	9.1	125	3.0	21.0	3.0	0.0
Strawberry, Sm, McDonald's*	1 Sm/161ml	200	4.8	124	3.0	21.0	3.0	0.0
Vanilla, Lge, McDonald's*	1 Lge/390ml	483	11.7	124	3.0	21.0	3.0	0.0
Vanilla, Med, McDonald's*	1 Med/302ml	377	9.0	125	3.0	21.0	3.0	0.0
Vanilla, Sm, McDonald's*	1 Sm/160ml	198	4.8	124	3.0	21.0	3.0	0.0
MUFFIN								
Blueberry, Low Fat, McDonald's*	1 Muffin/126g	300	3.8	238	5.0	50.0	3.0	2.0
Blueberry, McDonald's*	1 Muffin/125g	401	14.0	321	5.1	49.6	11.2	1.3
Buttered, McDonald's*	1 Muffin/63g	158	3.7	250	8.6	40.7	5.9	2.9
Buttered, with Preserve, McDonald's*	1 Muffin/93g	234	3.7	252	5.9	48.1	4.0	2.0
Carrot, McDonald's*	1 Muffin/135g	360	3.9	267	4.8	55.4	2.9	1.6
Chocolate, McDonald's*	1 Muffin/125g	515	29.0	412	5.8	45.6	23.2	1.4
Double Chocolate, McDonald's*	1 Muffin/123g	515	28.3	419	6.0	46.0	23.0	2.0
Triple Chocolate, McDonald's*	1 Muffin/138g	581	33.6	420	4.7	45.7	24.3	0.9
OASIS								
McDonald's*	1 Sm/250ml	42	0.0	17	0.0	4.0	0.0	0.0
ONION RINGS								
McDonald's*	1 Serving/99g	245	11.9	247	4.0	31.0	12.0	3.0
PANCAKE								
& Sausage, with Syrup, McDonald's*	1 Portion/241g	664	21.7	275	8.0	42.0	9.0	2.0
& Syrup, McDonald's*	1 Pack/180g	529	14.4	294	4.0	52.0	8.0	2.0
PIE								
Apple, Hot, McDonald's*	1 Pie/86g	250	13.8	289	2.0	35.0	16.0	0.0
Festive, McDonald's*	1 Pie/84g	310	17.6	369	4.0	42.0	21.0	1.0
POTATO WEDGES								
McDonald's*	1 Portion/177g	349	17.7	197	3.3	23.3	10.0	2.8
ROLL								
Bacon, McBacon, McDonald's*	1 Roll/122g	349	14.0	286	13.5	30.5	11.5	1.7
Bacon, with Brown Sauce, McDonald's*	1 Roll/116g	323	8.1	278	15.0	37.0	7.0	2.0
Bacon, with Tomato Ketchup, McDonald's*	1 Roll/116g	319	8.2	273	15.0	36.0	7.0	2.0
SALAD								
Caesar, Crispy Chicken, Croutons, McDonald's*	1 Salad/295g	385	18.2	131	9.4	8.8	6.2	1.3
Caesar, Crispy Chicken, Dressing, Croutons, McDonald's*	1 Salad/371g	530	30.0	143	8.0	9.1	8.1	1.2
Caesar, Crispy Chicken, Dressing, McDonald's*	1 Salad/316g	472	28.9	149	8.8	7.5	9.2	1.2
Caesar, Grilled Chicken, Croutons, McDonald's*	1 Salad/294g	280	9.6	95	11.5	4.2	3.3	1.3
Caesar, Grilled Chicken, Dressing, McDonald's*	1 Salad/305g	367	20.3	120	11.0	3.3	6.7	1.2
Caesar, Grilled Chicken, Dressing & Croutons, McDonald's*	1 Salad/370g	425	21.4	115	9.6	5.4	5.8	1.1
Caesar, Grilled Chicken, Plain, McDonald's*	1 Salad/298g	304	14.3	102	8.4	6.4	4.8	1.4
Chicken, no Bacon, Grilled, McDonald's*	1 Salad/274g	123	2.7	45	7.0	2.0	1.0	1.0
Chicken, with Bacon, Grilled, McDonald's*	1 Salad/260g	160	5.2	62	9.0	2.0	2.0	1.0
Crispy Chicken, no Bacon, McDonald's*	1 Salad/281g	265	13.0	94	7.5	5.7	4.6	0.6
Crispy Chicken, with Bacon, McDonald's*	1 Serving/271g	302	13.6	111	10.0	7.0	5.0	1.0
Garden, Side, Balsamic Dressing, McDonald's*	1 Salad/128g	91	3.8	71	1.0	11.0	3.0	1.0
Garden, Side, Low Fat Caesar Dressing, McDonald's*	1 Salad/63g	40	1.3	63	2.0	8.0	2.0	2.0
Garden, Side, no Dressing, McDonald's*	1 Salad/164g	18	0.0	11	1.0	2.0	0.0	1.0
Grilled Chicken, Newmans Own Balsamic, McDonald's*	1 Salad/320g	227	8.6	71	8.9	2.8	2.7	1.2
Ranch, Grilled Chicken, Dressing, McDonald's*	1 Salad/400g	396	20.0	99	9.8	3.1	5.0	1.1
Ranch, Grilled Chicken, no Dressing, McDonald's*	1 Salad/298g	268	12.5	90	11.4	1.4	4.2	1.0

MCDONALD'S

	Measure INFO/WEIGHT	per Measure KCAL	FAT	Nutrition Values per 100g / 100ml KCAL	PROT	CARB	FAT	FIBRE
SANDWICH								
Cheese, Ham & Pepperoni, Brown Roll, McDonald's*	1 Sandwich/300g	616	32.0	208	10.4	18.5	10.8	1.6
Chicken, Grilled, McDonald's*	1 Serving/211g	367	14.0	174	11.9	16.9	6.6	0.0
Chicken, Salad, McDonald's*	1 Sandwich/216g	350	8.6	162	7.0	24.0	4.0	2.0
Chicken, Sweet Chilli, McDonald's*	1 Sandwich/150g	342	13.5	228	12.0	28.0	9.0	2.0
Chicken & Bacon, Cheese, no Salad, White, McDonald's*	1 Sandwich/194g	547	23.4	281	14.0	30.0	12.0	2.0
Chicken & Bacon, Cheese & Salad, Brown, McDonald's*	1 Sandwich/228g	556	22.8	243	11.0	26.0	10.0	1.0
Chicken & Bacon, Cheese & Salad, White, McDonald's*	1 Sandwich/228g	551	22.8	241	12.0	25.0	10.0	1.0
Chicken & Bacon, McDonald's*	1 Sandwich/192g	405	13.4	211	10.0	27.0	7.0	2.0
Chicken & Bacon, Salad, no Cheese, White, McDonald's*	1 Sandwich/207g	486	18.7	234	11.0	28.0	9.0	1.0
Chicken Salad, no Cheese, Toasted, Brown, McDonald's*	1 Sandwich/222g	366	6.7	164	9.0	26.0	3.0	2.0
Chicken Salad, no Cheese, Toasted, White, McDonald's*	1 Sandwich/222g	360	4.4	162	10.0	25.0	2.0	1.0
Chicken Salad & Mayo, Brown, McDonald's*	1 Sandwich/292g	391	7.9	134	8.6	20.3	2.7	1.7
Chicken Salad & Mayo, White, McDonald's*	1 Sandwich/293g	375	6.7	128	8.5	19.5	2.3	1.5
Chicken Snack Wrap, Honey Mustard, McDonald's*	1 Wrap/111g	320	15.5	289	10.0	29.0	14.0	2.0
Chicken Tikka, White Roll, McDonald's*	1 Sandwich/266g	341	4.8	128	9.6	20.3	1.8	1.5
Crispy Chicken & Bacon, Deli Choices, McDonald's*	1 Sandwich/130g	591	28.0	455	23.1	55.4	21.5	2.5
Grilled Chicken Salad, McDonald's*	1 Sandwich/120g	406	8.1	338	22.5	45.8	6.8	22.5
Ham Salad, Toasted, Brown Roll, McDonald's*	1 Sandwich/209g	346	8.0	166	9.1	25.0	3.8	1.4
Ham Salad, Toasted, White Roll, McDonald's*	1 Sandwich/207g	344	5.0	166	9.2	27.5	2.4	1.9
Meatball Melt, Cheese, White Roll, McDonald's*	1 Sandwich/216g	455	14.0	211	11.1	27.8	6.5	2.3
Roast Beef & Cheddar, White Roll, McDonald's*	1 Sandwich/280g	464	16.5	166	9.8	19.5	5.9	1.3
Sausage & Bacon, McDonald's*	1 Sandwich/200g	458	20.0	229	11.5	22.5	10.0	1.6
Spicy Veggie, Cheese, Toasted, Brown, McDonald's*	1 Sandwich/248g	606	17.4	243	8.0	37.0	7.0	4.0
Spicy Veggie, Cheese, Toasted, White, McDonald's*	1 Serving/248g	606	17.4	243	8.0	37.0	7.0	4.0
Spicy Veggie, McDonald's*	1 Sandwich/216g	555	21.6	257	6.0	36.0	10.0	4.0
Spicy Veggie, McDonald's*	1 Sandwich/195g	511	15.0	262	6.7	39.5	7.7	3.5
Sweet Chilli, Crispy, Chicken, Delli, McDonald's*	1 Sandwich/130g	555	18.0	427	21.5	53.1	13.8	2.5
Sweet Chilli Chicken, Cheese, Toasted, Brown, McDonald's	1 Sandwich/292g	678	20.7	229	12.0	29.0	7.0	2.0
Veggie Melt, Grilled, Brown Roll, McDonald's*	1 Sandwich/249g	458	17.2	184	8.4	23.6	6.9	2.1
Veggie Melt, Grilled, White Roll, McDonald's*	1 Sandwich/250g	445	16.0	178	8.4	22.8	6.4	1.7
SMOOTHIE								
Mango & Pineapple, Iced, McDonald's*	1 Med/170ml	187	0.8	110	1.5	24.5	0.5	1.0
Mango & Strawberry, Iced, McDonald's*	1 Serving/200ml	190	1.0	95	1.0	20.5	0.5	1.5
Peach & Passion Fruit, Iced Fruit, McDonald's*	1 Med/245ml	195	1.0	80	1.2	16.7	0.4	1.4
Strawberry & Banana, Iced, McDonald's*	1 Med/170g	180	0.7	106	1.3	23.5	0.4	1.3
SUNDAE								
Hot Caramel, McDonald's*	1 Sundae/189g	357	8.3	189	3.8	33.9	4.4	0.0
Hot Fudge, McDonald's*	1 Sundae/187g	352	10.7	188	4.5	30.0	5.7	0.0
Strawberry, McDonald's*	1 Sundae/174g	292	7.0	168	2.0	33.0	4.0	0.0
Toffee, McDonald's*	1 Sundae/179g	344	9.0	192	3.0	34.0	5.0	1.0
SYRUP								
Pancake, McDonald's*	1 Pot/55g	183	0.0	345	0.0	84.0	0.0	0.0
TEA								
with Milk, McDonald's*	1 Serving/400ml	12	4.0	3	0.0	1.0	1.0	0.0
WRAP								
Bacon & Egg, Ketchup or Brown Sauce, McDonald's*	1 Wrap/205g	293	13.0	143	7.8	13.7	6.3	1.0
Breakfast, with Brown Sauce, McDonald's*	1 Wrap/229g	609	30.0	266	10.9	23.6	13.1	1.7
Breakfast, with Tomato Ketchup, McDonald's*	1 Wrap/229g	605	30.0	264	10.9	23.6	13.1	1.7
Chicken, BBQ, Snack, McDonald's*	1 Wrap/115g	300	12.0	261	10.4	30.4	10.4	1.7
Chicken, Cajun, McDonald's*	1 Wrap/222g	585	33.4	263	9.0	22.0	15.0	2.0
Chicken, Cheese & Bacon Snack, McDonald's*	1 Wrap/100g	360	18.0	360	14.0	33.0	18.0	2.0
Chicken, Fajita, McDonald's*	1 Wrap/259g	647	31.1	250	8.9	26.7	12.0	1.2

	Measure INFO/WEIGHT	per Measure KCAL	per Measure FAT	Nutrition Values per 100g / 100ml KCAL	PROT	CARB	FAT	FIBRE

MCDONALD'S
WRAP
	Measure INFO/WEIGHT	KCAL	FAT	KCAL	PROT	CARB	FAT	FIBRE
Chicken, Grilled, Salad, McDonald's*	1 Wrap/212g	322	10.6	152	7.2	19.9	5.0	1.8
Chicken, Snack, McDonald's*	1 Wrap/112g	266	11.2	237	10.0	29.0	10.0	2.0
Chicken & Bacon, McDonald's*	1 Wrap/100g	495	20.0	495	23.0	55.0	20.0	2.0
Chicken Poivre, France, McDonald's*	1 Wrap/280g	610	27.4	218	9.8	22.0	9.8	1.1
Crispy Chicken & Bacon, Deli Choices, McDonald's*	1 Wrap/240g	510	21.0	212	10.4	22.9	8.8	1.4
Egg & Cheese, Ketchup or Brown Sauce, McDonald's*	1 Serving/100g	253	10.0	253	12.0	28.0	10.0	2.0
Garlic & Herb, Snack, McDonald's*	1 Serving/121g	335	18.2	276	12.0	25.0	15.0	2.0
Oriental, Snack, McDonald's*	1 Wrap/127g	265	10.1	209	10.0	25.0	8.0	2.0
Paneer Salsa, McDonald's*	1 Wrap/178g	439	24.2	247	7.1	24.1	13.6	0.0
Sausage & Egg, Ketchup or Brown Sauce, McDonald's*	1 Wrap/212g	323	14.8	152	7.5	14.0	7.0	1.0
Sweet Chilli Crispy Chicken, McDonald's*	1 Wrap/213g	474	19.1	223	10.0	26.0	9.0	1.0
Vegetable, Spicy, McDonald's*	1 Wrap/195g	428	15.6	219	5.0	29.0	8.0	5.0

NANDO'S
BEANS
	Measure INFO/WEIGHT	KCAL	FAT	KCAL	PROT	CARB	FAT	FIBRE
Luso, Nando's*	1 Serving/200g	242	4.0	121	3.7	14.6	2.0	2.8

BREAD
Garlic, Nando's*	1 Regular/100g	336	16.4	336	6.7	39.0	16.4	2.7

BURGERS
Chicken Breast Fillet, Nando's*	1 Burger/232g	367	6.3	158	15.1	17.9	2.7	1.3
Double Chicken Breast, Nando's*	1 Burger/308g	494	8.1	160	20.4	13.3	2.6	1.0
Portobello Mushroom & Halloumi Cheese, Nando's*	1 Burger/308g	649	39.1	210	6.1	17.4	12.7	1.2
Veggie, Nando's*	1 Burger/265g	442	11.7	167	6.7	24.3	4.4	2.0

BURGERS VEGETARIAN
Bean, Nando's*	1 Burger/265g	533	19.6	201	7.9	24.5	7.4	2.3

CHEESE
Cheddar, Nando's*	1 Portion/20g	78	6.4	390	26.0	0.0	32.0	0.0
Halloumi, Grilled, Nando's*	1 Portion/54g	177	13.8	328	22.0	2.4	25.6	0.0

CHICKEN
¼ Breast, Peri Peri, Nando's*	¼ Breast/193g	309	7.2	160	29.9	1.8	3.7	0.0
¼ Leg, Peri Peri, Nando's*	1 Portion/125g	314	19.6	251	27.1	0.3	15.7	0.0
½ Peri Peri, Nando's*	½ Chicken/318g	623	26.9	196	28.8	1.2	8.4	0.0
Breast, Fillet Strips, Nandinos, Nando's*	1 Serving/92g	130	1.8	141	30.6	0.2	2.0	0.0
Butterfly, Peri Peri, Flame Grilled, Nando's*	1 Portion/190g	310	8.9	163	30.1	0.1	4.7	0.5
Butterfly, Peri Peri, Nando's*	1 Serving/190g	310	8.9	163	30.1	0.1	4.7	0.5
Thigh, Peri-Peri, Nando's*	4 Thighs/232g	561	30.6	242	30.5	0.4	13.2	0.5
Whole, Nando's*	1 Chicken/636g	1245	53.7	196	28.8	1.2	8.4	0.0
Wings, 10, Nando's*	10 Wings/236g	630	37.6	267	30.8	0.1	15.9	0.5
Wings, 3, Nando's*	3 Wings/71g	190	11.3	268	30.8	0.1	15.9	0.6
Wings, 5, Nando's*	5 Wings/118g	315	18.8	267	30.8	0.1	15.9	0.5

CHIPS
Lge, Nando's*	1 Serving/551g	1424	57.0	259	2.8	36.8	10.4	3.8
Per Peri, Regular, Nando's*	1 Portion/246g	548	22.3	223	2.9	33.5	9.1	2.6
Regular, Nando's*	1 Serving/211g	546	21.8	258	2.8	36.8	10.3	3.8

COLESLAW
Fino, Nando's*	1 Serving/150g	75	4.5	50	1.1	3.0	3.0	1.1
Lge, Nando's*	1 Serving/300g	528	48.0	176	0.8	8.0	16.0	1.7
Regular, Nando's*	1 Serving/150g	264	24.0	176	0.8	8.0	16.0	1.7

CORN
Cobs, Lge, Nando's*	1 Lge Cob/138g	190	5.1	138	7.9	30.4	3.7	6.3
Cobs Regular, Nando's*	1 Reg Cob/70g	144	2.7	206	8.1	31.4	3.8	6.6

CRISPS
Hot Peri Peri, Nando's*	1 Bag/40g	206	10.8	514	5.1	57.4	27.0	3.4

NANDO'S

	Measure INFO/WEIGHT	per Measure KCAL	FAT	Nutrition Values per 100g / 100ml KCAL	PROT	CARB	FAT	FIBRE
CRISPS								
Peri Peri Chicken, Nando's*	½ Bag/75g	410	20.2	547	5.1	57.4	27.0	3.4
Smoky Barbeque Peri Peri, Nando's*	½ Pack/75g	375	20.2	500	5.1	57.4	27.0	3.4
Spicy Chicken, Peri Peri Grooves, Nando's*	1 Serving/25g	130	7.2	521	5.1	58.6	28.8	3.4
DESSERT								
Caramel Cheesecake, with Double Cream, Nando's*	1 Serving/158g	564	42.1	357	5.1	27.0	26.6	0.8
Carrot Cake, Nando's*	1 Serving/215g	839	62.0	390	3.7	26.7	28.8	0.9
Cheesecake, White Choc Raspberry Swirl, Nando's*	1 Serving/162g	623	48.2	385	4.5	23.1	29.8	0.8
Choc-a-Lot Cake, Nando's*	1 Serving/182g	650	44.0	357	4.5	33.0	24.2	1.7
Chocolate Cheesecake, with Double Cream, Nando's*	1 Serving/153g	612	48.8	400	5.5	24.8	31.9	0.8
Mango & Passion Fruit Cheesecake, Nando's*	1 Serving/131g	419	26.2	320	50.4	29.0	20.0	0.0
Naughty Natas, Custard Tart, Nando's*	1 Serving/62g	174	6.7	280	5.5	40.3	10.8	2.0
DIP								
Red Pepper, Nando's*	1 Serving/260g	490	7.2	188	5.2	35.2	2.8	1.6
FROZEN YOGHURT								
Banana, Nando's*	1 Serving/100g	87	0.1	87	3.3	18.2	0.1	0.1
Chocolate, Nando's*	1 Serving/100g	88	0.3	88	3.1	18.4	0.3	0.6
Strawberry, Nando's*	1 Serving/100g	71	0.2	71	2.5	15.2	0.2	0.1
Vanilla, Nando's*	1 Serving/100ml	70	0.1	70	2.5	15.0	0.1	0.1
Very Berry, Nando's*	1 Serving/100g	72	0.2	72	2.5	15.2	0.2	0.1
HOUMOUS								
with Peri Peri Drizzle & Pitta, Nando's*	1 Serving/305g	791	34.7	259	7.2	30.8	11.4	2.6
ICE CREAM								
Chocolate, Nando's*	1 Serving/90g	191	10.0	212	2.2	24.0	11.1	1.0
Passion Fruit, Nando's*	1 Serving/90g	122	0.0	136	0.3	32.9	0.0	2.5
Strawberries & Cream, Nando's*	1 Serving/90g	164	6.3	182	2.4	24.8	7.0	0.5
Toffee, Nando's*	1 Serving/90g	178	7.3	198	3.9	20.8	8.1	1.0
Vanilla, Nando's*	1 Serving/90g	191	10.4	212	3.8	20.7	11.6	0.0
ICE LOLLY								
Chilly Billy, Nando's*	1 Lolly/70g	30	0.1	43	0.1	10.1	0.1	0.0
MARINADE								
Lemon & Rosemary, Nando's*	1fl oz/30ml	44	3.9	147	1.0	11.8	13.0	0.2
Lime & Coriander with Peri Peri, Nando's*	1 Tsp/5g	9	0.8	182	0.0	13.1	16.6	0.2
Peri Peri, Hot, Nando's*	1 Serving/40g	46	2.2	115	1.4	15.2	5.4	0.9
Peri Peri, Portuguese BBQ, Nando's*	1 Serving/40g	36	0.6	90	1.1	17.7	1.6	1.0
Sun Dried Tomato & Basil with Peri-Peri, Nando's*	1 Bottle/270g	319	25.6	118	0.1	15.3	9.5	0.8
MASH								
Creamy, Nando's*	1 Regular/200g	270	15.8	135	1.7	13.0	7.9	2.5
Sweet Potato, Fino Side, Nando's*	1 Serving/100g	126	2.1	126	2.2	23.2	2.1	2.8
MAYONNAISE								
Perinaise, Nando's*	1 Serving/50g	159	14.3	316	0.6	13.8	28.4	0.2
NUTS								
Peri-Peri, Nando's*	1 Serving/100g	784	66.0	784	26.3	17.1	66.0	8.3
OLIVES								
Spicy, Mixed, Nando's*	1 Bowl/125g	138	13.5	110	1.0	0.6	10.8	3.0
PEAS								
Macho, Lge, Nando's*	1 Serving/280g	336	20.7	120	4.7	7.0	7.4	4.2
Macho, Regular, Nando's*	1 Serving/140g	168	10.4	120	4.7	7.0	7.4	4.2
PITTA								
Bean, Nando's*	1 Pitta/240g	516	17.9	215	8.6	27.0	7.4	2.3
Chicken Breast, Nando's*	1 Pitta/200g	351	4.6	176	16.7	22.0	2.3	1.0
Double Chicken, Nando's*	1 Serving/275g	460	6.1	167	20.0	16.6	2.2	0.7
Mushroom & Halloumi Cheese, Nando's*	1 Serving/305g	614	29.1	201	5.9	18.2	9.6	1.0

	Measure INFO/WEIGHT	per Measure KCAL	FAT	Nutrition Values per 100g / 100ml KCAL	PROT	CARB	FAT	FIBRE
NANDO'S								
PITTA								
Veggie, Nando's*	1 Pitta/233g	426	9.9	183	7.1	28.5	4.2	1.8
POTATO WEDGES								
Sweet, Roasted, Nando's*	1 Serving/100g	357	13.9	357	8.8	54.5	13.9	10.9
RATATOUILLE								
Fino Side, Nando's*	1 Serving/180g	108	6.5	60	1.3	3.8	3.6	3.4
RICE								
Spicy, Lge, Nando's*	1 Serving/250g	453	9.0	182	3.0	32.8	3.6	3.4
Spicy, Regular, Nando's*	1 Serving/150g	275	5.4	182	3.0	32.8	3.6	3.4
ROLL								
Portuguese with Chicken Livers, Nando's*	1 Serving/213g	469	14.4	220	17.5	23.2	6.8	2.0
Prego Steak, Nando's*	1 Roll/150g	391	16.4	260	19.4	22.2	11.0	2.6
SALAD								
Avocado & Green Bean, Nando's*	1 Serving/245g	305	25.8	124	2.4	3.4	10.5	3.3
Caesar, no Chicken, Nando's*	1 Salad/226g	285	22.0	126	3.4	6.5	9.8	1.1
Caesar, with Chicken, Nando's*	1 Serving/326g	415	23.3	127	11.1	4.4	7.2	1.0
Chicken, Grilled, Nando's*	1 Serving/363g	219	5.5	60	9.1	2.6	1.5	0.0
Chicken, with Quinoa, Nando's*	1 Serving182g	382	14.6	210	17.5	15.5	8.0	4.6
Mediterranean, without Chicken, Nando's*	1 Salad/180g	266	21.8	148	5.1	4.5	12.1	2.4
Mediterranean with Chicken, Nando's*	1 Portion/250g	395	23.6	158	15.0	3.3	9.4	1.8
Mixed Leaf, Nando's*	1 Regular/100g	13	0.2	13	0.9	1.6	0.2	1.0
SAUCE								
Coconut, Lime & Coriander, Cooking, Nando's*	1 Serving/65g	88	6.5	135	1.5	12.2	10.0	1.2
Peri Peri, Marinade, Med, Nando's*	1 Serving/24g	15	2.4	61	0.3	2.1	10.1	0.2
Peri Peri, Med, Nando's*	1 Serving/50g	34	1.8	69	0.5	8.4	3.7	0.8
Peri-Peri, Extra, Extra Hot, Nando's*	1 Serving/5g	2	0.1	50	0.6	8.2	1.6	1.2
Peri-Peri, Extra Hot, Nando's*	1 Serving/5g	4	0.2	71	0.7	8.8	3.7	1.4
Peri-Peri, Hot, Nando's*	1 Serving/5g	4	0.2	75	0.6	9.6	3.8	1.3
Peri-Peri, Sweet, Nando's*	1 Tbsp/25g	36	0.5	142	0.5	30.7	2.1	0.0
VINAIGRETTE								
Portuguese, Nando's*	1 Tbsp/15g	61	6.6	409	1.0	2.0	44.0	0.3
WRAP								
Beanie, Nando's*	1 Wrap/339g	759	31.9	224	7.2	26.2	9.4	2.1
Chicken, Breast, Fillet, Double, Nando's*	1 Wrap/389g	724	24.9	186	16.2	16.8	6.4	1.0
Chicken, Breast, Fillet, Nando's*	1 Wrap/288g	594	22.1	206	12.1	21.5	7.7	1.2
Portabello Mushroom & Halloumi Cheese, Nando's*	1 Wrap/322g	792	52.0	246	6.5	18.0	16.2	1.2
Veggie, Nando's*	1 Wrap/316g	669	25.8	212	7.0	26.9	8.2	2.5
PAPA JOHNS								
BREAD								
Bacon & Cheese, Sticks, Sides, Papa Johns*	1 Serving/35g	118	5.8	335	12.4	33.3	16.5	1.9
Garlic & Cheese, Sticks, Sides, Papa Johns*	1 Serving/69g	229	11.2	333	11.2	34.3	16.3	2.0
Garlic Pizza, Sticks, Sides, Papa Johns*	1 Serving/54g	181	7.6	336	8.4	42.5	14.1	2.5
CHICKEN								
Poppers, Sides, Papa Johns*	1.Serving/198g	436	18.8	220	17.0	16.6	9.5	0.5
Wings, BBQ, Sides, Papa Johns*	1 Serving/300g	712	38.8	237	20.4	9.2	12.9	0.5
Wings, Buffalo, Sides, Papa Johns*	1 Serving/300g	635	40.1	212	20.5	1.7	13.4	0.5
Wings, Plain, Sides, Papa Johns*	1 Serving/240g	600	38.6	250	25.4	0.1	16.1	0.5
DESSERT								
Chocolate Cookie, Papa Johns*	1 Serving/41g	160	6.9	394	3.6	57.1	16.9	0.0
Chocolate Lava Cake, Papa Johns*	1 Serving/90g	337	20.4	374	4.9	37.7	22.6	1.6
Cinna Pie, Papa Johns*	1 Portion/46g	176	7.9	379	6.1	49.4	17.0	0.9
PEPPERS								
Jalapeno, Breaded, Bites, Sides, Papa Johns*	1 Serving/167	516	35.2	309	5.0	25.5	21.1	1.3

PAPA JOHNS

PIZZA

	Measure	per Measure KCAL	per Measure FAT	KCAL	PROT	CARB	FAT	FIBRE
All The Meats, Original Base, Lge, Papa Johns*	1 Slice/101g	272	11.0	270	12.8	29.2	10.9	1.7
All the Meats, Original Base, Med, Papa Johns*	1 Slice/90g	243	9.7	271	12.7	29.7	10.8	1.7
All The Meats, Original Base, Sm, Papa Johns*	1 Slice/82g	220	8.5	268	12.3	30.3	10.4	1.8
All the Meats, Original Base, XXL, Papa Johns*	1 Slice/115g	312	12.2	271	12.7	30.5	10.6	1.8
All the Meats, Stuffed Crust, Lge, Papa Johns*	1 Slice/115g	320	14.6	279	13.8	26.4	12.7	1.5
All the Meats, Stuffed Crust, Med, Papa Johns*	1 Slice/105g	295	13.6	281	14.0	26.2	13.0	1.5
All the Meats, Stuffed Crust, XXL, Papa Johns*	1 Slice/128g	356	15.6	279	13.5	27.9	12.2	1.6
All the Meats, Thin, Lge, Papa Johns*	1 Slice/85g	237	10.6	279	13.8	27.8	12.5	1.6
All the Meats, Thin, Med, Papa Johns*	1 Slice/72g	202	8.8	279	13.6	27.8	12.2	1.6
All the Meats, Thin, XXL, Papa Johns*	1 Slice/94g	266	11.7	282	13.8	27.9	12.4	1.6
American Hot, Original Base, Lge, Papa Johns*	1 Slice/93g	216	7.9	232	9.5	28.6	8.5	1.7
American Hot, Original Base, Med, Papa Johns*	1 Slice/83g	195	7.2	235	9.6	28.7	8.7	1.7
American Hot, Original Base, Sm, Papa Johns*	1 Slice/84g	194	7.1	231	9.4	28.7	8.4	1.7
American Hot, Original Base, XXL, Papa Johns*	1 Slice/104g	243	8.4	233	9.4	29.9	8.1	1.8
American Hot, Stuffed Crust, Lge, Papa Johns*	1 Slice/106g	257	11.0	242	10.8	25.5	10.4	1.5
American Hot, Stuffed Crust, Med, Papa Johns*	1 Slice/98g	242	10.7	246	11.2	25.0	10.9	1.5
American Hot, Stuffed Crust, XXL, Papa Johns*	1 Slice/117g	284	11.5	242	10.5	27.1	9.8	1.6
American Hot, Thin, Lge, Papa Johns*	1 Slice/68g	152	5.9	223	9.1	26.4	8.7	1.7
American Hot, Thin, Med, Papa Johns*	1 Slice/68g	153	5.9	224	9.0	26.7	8.7	1.7
American Hot, Thin, XXL, Papa Johns*	1 Slice/82g	184	7.0	225	9.1	27.2	8.5	1.7
Cheese & Tomato, Original Base, Lge, Papa Johns*	1 Slice/86g	226	7.5	262	11.0	33.9	8.7	2.0
Cheese & Tomato, Original Base, Med, Papa Johns*	1 Slice/79g	210	7.6	267	11.7	32.4	9.7	1.9
Cheese & Tomato, Original Base, XXL, Papa Johns*	1 Slice/101g	268	8.8	266	11.2	34.6	8.7	2.0
Cheese & Tomato, Stuffed Crust, Lge, Papa Johns*	1 Slice/101g	268	8.8	266	11.2	34.6	8.7	2.0
Cheese & Tomato, Stuffed Crust, Med, Papa Johns*	1 Slice/95g	262	11.2	277	13.0	28.9	11.8	1.6
Cheese & Tomato, Stuffed Crust, XXL, Papa Johns*	1 Slice/111g	302	11.4	273	12.1	32.0	10.3	1.8
Cheese & Tomato, Thin, Lge, Papa Johns*	1 Slice/68g	172	5.9	253	10.7	31.9	8.7	1.9
Cheese & Tomato, Thin, Med, Papa Johns*	1 Slice/60g	160	5.7	266	11.4	33.0	9.4	2.0
Cheese & Tomato, Thin, XXL, Papa Johns*	1 Slice/75g	200	6.7	267	11.1	34.5	8.9	2.1
Chicken BBQ, Original Base, Lge, Papa Johns*	1 Slice/102g	253	8.1	249	11.7	31.4	8.0	1.8
Chicken BBQ, Original Base, Med, Papa Johns*	1 Slice/92g	230	7.5	250	11.9	31.2	8.2	1.8
Chicken BBQ, Original Base, Sm, Papa Johns*	1 Slice/95g	213	6.8	224	10.5	28.4	7.2	1.6
Chicken BBQ, Original Base, XXL, Papa Johns*	1 Slice/115g	288	8.9	251	11.6	32.8	7.8	1.9
Chicken BBQ, Stuffed Crust, Lge, Papa Johns*	1 Slice/116g	267	10.1	231	11.7	25.8	8.7	1.5
Chicken BBQ, Stuffed Crust, Med, Papa Johns*	1 Slice/105g	275	10.9	262	13.2	28.0	10.4	1.6
Chicken BBQ, Stuffed Crust, XXL, Papa Johns*	1 Slice/125g	324	11.6	259	12.4	30.6	9.3	1.7
Chicken BBQ, Thin, Lge, Papa Johns*	1 Slice/83g	205	6.7	248	12.0	30.8	8.1	1.8
Chicken BBQ, Thin, Med, Papa Johns*	1 Slice/75g	178	5.8	236	11.6	29.3	7.7	1.7
Chicken BBQ, Thin, XXL, Papa Johns*	1 Slice/91g	230	7.4	252	12.0	31.6	8.1	1.8
Chicken Club, Original Base, Lge, Papa Johns*	1 Slice/100g	236	7.5	235	11.3	29.5	7.5	1.9
Chicken Club, Original Base, Med, Papa Johns*	1 Slice/92g	216	7.0	236	11.5	29.4	7.6	1.9
Chicken Club, Original Base, Sm, Papa Johns*	1 Slice/85g	199	6.4	235	11.3	29.7	7.5	1.9
Chicken Club, Original Base, XXL, Papa Johns*	1 Slice/113g	271	8.3	239	11.2	31.1	7.3	2.0
Chicken Club, Stuffed Crust, Lge, Papa Johns*	1 Slice/115g	284	11.2	248	12.6	26.6	9.8	1.7
Chicken Club, Stuffed Crust, Med, Papa Johns*	1 Slice/107g	268	10.9	251	13.0	25.9	10.2	1.6
Chicken Club, Stuffed Crust, XXL, Papa Johns*	1 Slice/126g	315	11.6	250	12.3	28.4	9.2	1.8
Chicken Club, Thin, Lge, Papa Johns*	1 Slice/84g	188	6.4	223	11.3	26.4	7.6	1.8
Chicken Club, Thin, Med, Papa Johns*	1 Slice/74g	164	5.5	222	11.4	26.2	7.5	1.8
Chicken Club, Thin, XXL, Papa Johns*	1 Slice/93g	211	7.2	227	11.4	27.3	7.7	1.8
Double Pepperoni, Original Base, Lge, Papa Johns*	1 Slice/97g	279	12.3	289	12.1	30.5	12.7	1.8
Double Pepperoni, Original Base, Med, Papa Johns*	1 Slice/89g	261	11.8	293	12.4	29.9	13.3	1.7
Double Pepperoni, Original Base, XXL, Papa Johns*	1 Slice/108g	311	13.0	288	11.8	32.3	12.0	1.9

PAPA JOHNS

PIZZA

	Measure INFO/WEIGHT	per Measure KCAL	per Measure FAT	Nutrition Values per 100g / 100ml KCAL	PROT	CARB	FAT	FIBRE
Double Pepperoni, Stuffed Crust, Lge, Papa Johns*	1 Slice/110g	340	16.6	309	13.9	28.7	15.1	1.6
Double Pepperoni, Stuffed Crust, Med, Papa Johns*	1 Slice/104g	313	15.8	300	13.8	26.4	15.1	1.5
Double Pepperoni, Stuffed Crust, XXL, Papa Johns*	1 Slice/121g	355	16.3	294	12.9	29.4	13.5	1.7
Double Pepperoni, Thin, Lge, Papa Johns*	1 Slice/78g	234	11.2	300	12.6	29.3	14.3	1.8
Double Pepperoni, Thin, Med, Papa Johns*	1 Slice/70g	213	10.5	305	12.9	28.6	15.0	1.7
Double Pepperoni, Thin, XXL, Papa Johns*	1 Slice/85g	256	11.8	300	12.5	30.5	13.8	1.8
Garden Party, Original Base, Lge, Papa Johns*	1 Slice/101g	223	6.7	220	9.0	30.1	6.6	2.0
Garden Party, Original Base, Med, Papa Johns*	1 Slice/90g	202	6.1	224	9.2	30.5	6.8	2.0
Garden Party, Original Base, Sm, Papa Johns*	1 Slice/79g	193	5.8	243	9.9	33.3	7.3	2.1
Garden Party, Original Base, XXL, Papa Johns*	1 Slice/115g	257	7.4	223	8.9	31.3	6.4	2.0
Garden Party, Stuffed Crust, Lge, Papa Johns*	1 Slice/115g	270	10.3	234	10.5	27.2	8.9	1.8
Garden Party, Stuffed Crust, Med, Papa Johns*	1 Slice/105g	254	10.0	241	11.0	26.8	9.5	1.7
Garden Party, Stuffed Crust, XXL, Papa Johns*	1 Slice/128g	301	10.8	235	10.2	28.7	8.4	1.8
Garden Party, Thin, Lge, Papa Johns*	1 Slice/83g	177	5.3	212	8.6	28.9	6.4	2.0
Garden Party, Thin, Med, Papa Johns*	1 Slice/71g	145	4.4	203	8.2	28.0	6.1	1.9
Garden Special, Papa Johns*	1 Slice/155g	286	9.0	185	7.7	25.8	5.8	1.9
Hawaiian Chicken BBQ, Original Base, Lge, Papa Johns*	1 Slice/100g	231	7.0	232	10.6	30.9	7.0	1.5
Hawaiian Chicken BBQ, Original Base, Med, Papa Johns*	1 Slice/89g	205	6.0	230	10.5	31.3	6.7	1.6
Hawaiian Chicken BBQ, Original Base, Sm, Papa Johns*	1 Slice/81g	187	5.3	231	10.4	31.7	6.6	1.6
Hawaiian Chicken BBQ, Original Base, XXL, Papa Johns*	1 Slice/113g	265	7.6	234	10.4	32.2	6.7	1.6
Hawaiian Chicken BBQ, Stuffed Crust, Lge, Papa Johns*	1 Slice/110g	266	9.9	242	11.7	27.7	9.0	1.4
Hawaiian Chicken BBQ, Stuffed Crust, Med, Papa Johns*	1 Slice/104g	251	9.4	242	11.8	27.4	9.1	1.3
Hawaiian Chicken BBQ, Stuffed Crust, XXL, Papa Johns*	1 Slice/124g	297	10.0	240	11.1	29.9	8.1	1.5
Hawaiian Chicken BBQ, Thin, Lge, Papa Johns*	1 Slice/80g	180	5.4	224	10.5	29.7	6.7	1.4
Hawaiian Chicken BBQ, Thin, Med, Papa Johns*	1 Slice/71g	158	4.6	222	10.4	29.6	6.5	1.4
Hawaiian Chicken BBQ, Thin, XXL, Papa Johns*	1 Slice/90g	204	6.0	226	10.3	30.5	6.6	1.4
Hawaiian Special, Original Base, Lge, Papa Johns*	1 Slice/92g	211	6.8	229	10.2	29.6	7.4	1.8
Hawaiian Special, Original Base, Med,, Papa Johns*	1 Slice/90g	205	6.3	228	10.0	30.3	7.0	1.9
Hawaiian Special, Original Base, Sm, Papa Johns*	1 Slice/84g	199	6.0	237	10.4	31.6	7.2	1.9
Hawaiian Special, Original Base, XXL, Papa Johns*	1 Slice/113g	260	7.7	231	10.0	31.7	6.8	1.9
Hawaiian Special, Stuffed Crust, Lge, Papa Johns*	1 Slice/114g	274	9.9	241	11.6	28.3	8.7	1.4
Hawaiian Special, Stuffed Crust, Med, Papa Johns*	1 Slice/106g	257	9.7	242	11.8	27.4	9.1	1.3
Hawaiian Special, Stuffed Crust, XXL, Papa Johns*	1 Slice/125g	304	11.0	243	11.2	29.0	8.8	1.7
Hawaiian Special, Thin, Lge, Papa Johns*	1 Slice/81g	180	5.5	221	9.9	29.0	6.8	1.8
Hawaiian Special, Thin, Med, Papa Johns*	1 Slice/71g	148	4.5	209	9.2	27.9	6.4	1.8
Hawaiian Special, Thin, XXL, Papa Johns*	1 Slice/89g	201	6.1	226	10.0	29.9	6.9	1.9
Hot Pepper Passion, Original Base, Lge, Papa Johns*	1 Slice/95g	218	6.6	230	9.3	31.3	7.0	2.0
Hot Pepper Passion, Original Base, Med, Papa Johns*	1 Slice/85g	198	6.1	233	9.5	31.5	7.2	2.0
Hot Pepper Passion, Original Base, Sm, Papa Johns*	1 Slice/76g	191	5.8	250	10.1	34.1	7.6	2.2
Hot Pepper Passion, Original Base, XXL, Papa Johns*	1 Slice/110g	257	7.9	234	9.6	31.8	7.2	2.0
Hot Pepper Passion, Stuffed Crust, Lge, Papa Johns*	1 Slice/107g	258	9.4	241	10.9	28.4	8.8	1.8
Hot Pepper Passion, Stuffed Crust, Med, Papa Johns*	1 Slice/100g	250	10.0	249	11.4	27.5	10.0	1.7
Hot Pepper Passion, Thin, Lge, Papa Johns*	1 Slice/77g	171	5.3	223	9.0	30.2	6.9	2.1
Hot Pepper Passion, Thin, Med, Papa Johns*	1 Slice/66g	141	4.3	214	8.6	29.2	6.5	2.0
Hot Pepper Passion, Thin, XXL, Papa Johns*	1 Slice/85g	192	5.9	226	9.1	30.8	6.9	2.1
Meatball Pepperoni, Authentic Crust, Lge, Papa Johns*	1 Slice/86g	218	10.4	253	11.9	23.4	12.1	1.4
Meatball Pepperoni, Authentic Crust, Med, Papa Johns*	1 Slice/77g	196	9.5	255	12.1	23.0	12.4	1.4
Meatball Pepperoni, Authentic Crust, XXL, Papa Johns*	1 Slice/93g	236	10.9	254	11.8	24.5	11.7	1.4
Meatball Pepperoni, Original Base, Lge, Papa Johns*	1 Slice/102g	262	11.5	256	11.6	26.3	11.2	1.5
Meatball Pepperoni, Original Base, Med, Papa Johns*	1 Slice/94g	241	10.7	257	11.8	26.0	11.4	1.5
Meatball Pepperoni, Original Base, Sm, Papa Johns*	1 Slice/88g	224	9.9	254	11.7	26.0	11.2	1.5
Meatball Pepperoni, Original Base, XXL, Papa Johns*	1 Slice/114g	291	12.1	255	11.4	27.7	10.6	1.6

PAPA JOHNS

PIZZA

	Measure INFO/WEIGHT	per Measure KCAL	FAT	Nutrition Values per 100g / 100ml KCAL	PROT	CARB	FAT	FIBRE
Meatball Pepperoni, Stuffed Crust, Lge, Papa Johns*	1 Slice/116g	304	14.6	262	12.6	23.7	12.6	1.4
Meatball Pepperoni, Stuffed Crust, Med, Papa Johns*	1 Slice/109g	288	14.2	264	12.9	23.0	13.0	1.3
Meatball Pepperoni, Stuffed Crust, XXL, Papa Johns*	1 Slice/127g	331	15.1	261	12.2	25.4	11.9	1.5
Mexican, Original Base, Lge, Papa Johns*	1 Slice/100g	237	8.0	237	10.0	30.2	8.0	2.0
Mexican, Original Base, Med, Papa Johns*	1 Slice/90g	214	7.3	238	10.2	30.1	8.1	2.0
Mexican, Original Base, Sm, Papa Johns*	1 Slice/74g	157	5.2	213	9.0	27.3	7.1	1.8
Mexican, Original Base, XXL, Papa Johns*	1 Slice/114g	278	9.3	243	10.3	31.1	8.1	2.0
Mexican, Stuffed Crust, Lge, Papa Johns*	1 Slice/113g	282	11.5	250	11.5	27.2	10.2	1.8
Mexican, Stuffed Crust, Med, Papa Johns*	1 Slice/91g	220	7.9	242	10.1	29.8	8.7	2.0
Mexican, Stuffed Crust, XXL, Papa Johns*	1 Slice/124g	312	11.9	252	11.2	29.0	9.6	1.9
Mexican, Thin, Lge, Papa Johns*	1 Slice/73g	173	6.3	236	10.3	28.5	8.6	2.0
Mexican, Thin, Med, Papa Johns*	1 Slice/72g	159	5.5	222	9.5	27.6	7.7	2.0
Mexican, Thin, XXL, Papa Johns*	1 Slice/83g	200	7.2	240	10.4	29.4	8.6	2.1
Piri Piri Chicken, Original Base, Lge, Papa Johns*	1 Slice/102g	234	6.9	229	10.8	30.2	6.8	2.0
Piri Piri Chicken, Original Base, Med, Papa Johns*	1 Slice/92g	213	6.4	231	10.7	30.3	6.9	2.0
Piri Piri Chicken, Original Base, Sm, Papa Johns*	1 Slice/81g	192	5.8	237	10.6	31.8	7.1	2.0
Piri Piri Chicken, Original Base, XXL, Papa Johns*	1 Slice/117g	270	7.7	231	10.6	31.2	6.6	2.1
Piri Piri Chicken, Stuffed Crust, Lge, Papa Johns*	1 Slice/116g	295	11.0	254	12.6	28.5	9.5	1.9
Piri Piri Chicken, Stuffed Crust, Med, Papa Johns*	1 Slice/108g	265	10.3	246	12.3	26.8	9.6	1.7
Piri Piri Chicken, Stuffed Crust, XXL, Papa Johns*	1 Slice/130g	315	11.1	242	11.7	28.6	8.5	1.9
Piri Piri Chicken, Thin, Lge, Papa Johns*	1 Slice/84g	188	5.6	224	10.9	29.0	6.7	2.1
Piri Piri Chicken, Thin, Med, Papa Johns*	1 Slice/73g	163	4.8	223	10.7	29.2	6.6	2.1
Piri Piri Chicken, Thin, XXL, Papa Johns*	1 Slice/94g	213	6.3	226	10.9	29.4	6.7	2.1
Sausage & Pepperoni, Original Base, Lge, Papa Johns*	1 Slice/100g	295	14.3	294	14.4	26.5	14.3	1.5
Sausage & Pepperoni, Original Base, Med, Papa Johns*	1 Slice/93g	275	13.1	296	14.3	27.0	14.1	1.6
Sausage & Pepperoni, Original Base, Sm, Papa Johns*	1 Slice/87g	264	11.8	302	14.0	30.1	13.5	1.8
Sausage & Pepperoni, Original Base, XXL, Papa Johns*	1 Slice/122g	355	15.8	292	13.9	29.1	13.0	1.7
Sausage & Pepperoni, Stuffed Crust, Lge, Papa Johns*	1 Slice/124g	368	18.8	297	14.9	24.5	15.2	1.4
Sausage & Pepperoni, Stuffed Crust, Med, Papa Johns*	1 Slice/114g	340	17.5	299	15.1	24.4	15.4	1.4
Sausage & Pepperoni, Stuffed Crust, XXL, Papa Johns*	1 Slice/134g	399	19.2	297	14.6	26.8	14.3	1.5
Sausage & Pepperoni, Thin, Lge, Papa Johns*	1 Slice/100g	305	16.0	305	15.4	23.0	16.0	1.4
Sausage & Pepperoni, Thin, Med, Papa Johns*	1 Slice/83g	245	13.1	296	15.0	23.0	15.8	1.4
Sausage & Pepperoni, Thin, XXL, Papa Johns*	1 Slice/99g	303	14.9	306	15.1	26.9	15.0	1.6
Spicy Italian, Original Base, Lge, Papa Johns*	1 Slice/97g	273	11.5	280	12.1	30.5	11.8	1.8
Spicy Italian, Original Base, Med, Papa Johns*	1 Slice/87g	245	10.3	281	12.1	30.6	11.8	1.8
Spicy Italian, Original Base, Sm, Papa Johns*	1 Slice/82g	229	9.7	280	12.0	30.7	11.8	1.8
Spicy Italian, Original Base, XXL, Papa Johns*	1 Slice/110g	309	12.4	281	11.9	32.0	11.3	1.9
Spicy Italian, Papa Johns*	1 Slice/103g	260	8.0	252	10.7	26.2	7.8	1.9
Spicy Italian, Stuffed Crust, Lge, Papa Johns*	1 Slice/111g	321	15.2	288	13.2	27.4	13.6	1.6
Spicy Italian, Stuffed Crust, Med, Papa Johns*	1 Slice/103g	298	14.2	290	13.6	26.9	13.8	1.5
Spicy Italian, Stuffed Crust, XXL, Papa Johns*	1 Slice/122g	350	15.6	288	12.9	29.2	12.8	1.7
Spicy Italian, Thin, Lge, Papa Johns*	1 Slice/80g	219	9.9	276	12.0	28.0	12.5	1.7
Spicy Italian, Thin, Med, Papa Johns*	1 Slice/69g	189	8.5	275	12.0	28.1	12.4	1.7
Spicy Italian, Thin, XXL, Papa Johns*	1 Slice/87g	242	10.7	278	12.0	28.9	12.3	1.7
Spicy Pulled Pork, Original Base, Lge, Papa Johns*	1 Slice/94g	245	9.1	261	11.1	31.6	9.7	1.5
Spicy Pulled Pork, Original Base, Med, Papa Johns*	1 Slice/86g	224	8.4	261	11.2	31.4	9.8	1.5
Spicy Pulled Pork, Original Base, Sm, Papa Johns*	1 Slice/76g	200	7.3	262	11.2	31.9	9.6	1.5
Spicy Pulled Pork, Original Base, XXL, Papa Johns*	1 Slice/108g	281	9.8	260	10.8	32.9	9.1	1.6
Spicy Pulled Pork, Stuffed Crust, Lge, Papa Johns*	1 Slice/107g	286	12.3	268	12.2	28.2	11.5	1.3
Spicy Pulled Pork, Stuffed Crust, Med, Papa Johns*	1 Slice/101g	271	11.9	268	12.5	27.4	11.8	1.3
Spicy Pulled Pork, Stuffed Crust, Med, Papa Johns*	1 Slice/101g	271	11.9	268	12.5	27.4	11.8	1.3
Spicy Pulled Pork, Stuffed Crust, XXL, Papa Johns*	1 Slice/121g	321	13.0	265	11.7	29.9	10.7	1.4

	Measure INFO/WEIGHT	per Measure KCAL	FAT	Nutrition Values per 100g / 100ml KCAL	PROT	CARB	FAT	FIBRE

PAPA JOHNS

PIZZA

	Measure INFO/WEIGHT	per Measure KCAL	FAT	KCAL	PROT	CARB	FAT	FIBRE
Spicy Pulled Pork, Thin, Lge, Papa Johns*	1 Slice/75g	196	7.6	260	11.2	30.3	10.1	1.4
Spicy Pulled Pork, Thin, Med, Papa Johns*	1 Slice/66g	172	6.7	259	11.1	30.2	10.1	1.3
Spicy Pulled Pork, Thin, XXL, Papa Johns*	1 Slice/85g	221	8.4	259	11.0	31.0	9.8	1.4
Tandoori Spice, Original Base, Lge, Papa Johns*	1 Slice/104g	248	8.8	238	10.6	28.7	8.4	1.7
Tandoori Spice, Original Base, Med, Papa Johns*	1 Slice/93g	225	8.1	242	10.7	29.0	8.7	1.7
Tandoori Spice, Original Base, Sm, Papa Johns*	1 Slice/82g	205	7.4	249	10.5	30.2	9.0	1.7
Tandoori Spice, Original Base, XXL, Papa Johns*	1 Slice/118g	283	9.6	239	10.6	29.9	8.1	1.8
Tandoori Spice, Stuffed Crust, Lge, Papa Johns*	1 Slice/118g	295	12.4	250	11.9	25.9	10.5	1.5
Tandoori Spice, Stuffed Crust, Med, Papa Johns*	1 Slice/108g	277	12.0	256	12.2	25.7	11.1	1.5
Tandoori Spice, Stuffed Crust, XXL, Papa Johns*	1 Slice/131g	327	12.8	250	11.6	27.5	9.8	1.6
Tandoori Spice, Thin, Lge, Papa Johns*	1 Slice/86g	193	7.2	225	10.2	25.9	8.4	1.6
Tandoori Spice, Thin, Med, Papa Johns*	1 Slice/74g	168	6.3	227	10.1	26.3	8.5	1.6
Tandoori Spice, Thin, XXL, Papa Johns*	1 Slice/96g	216	7.8	226	10.3	26.6	8.2	1.6
The Greek, Original Base, Lge, Papa Johns*	1 Slice/103g	233	7.8	227	9.3	29.4	7.6	2.0
The Greek, Original Base, Med, Papa Johns*	1 Slice/93g	212	7.1	227	9.3	29.3	7.6	2.0
The Greek, Original Base, Sm, Papa Johns*	1 Slice/85g	193	6.5	228	9.5	29.2	7.7	2.0
The Greek, Original Base, XXL, Papa Johns*	1 Slice/116g	268	8.6	231	9.3	30.8	7.4	2.0
The Greek, Stuffed Crust, Lge, Papa Johns*	1 Slice/117g	281	11.3	241	10.7	26.5	9.7	1.7
The Greek, Stuffed Crust, Med, Papa Johns*	1 Slice/109g	264	11.0	243	11.1	25.9	10.1	1.7
The Greek, Stuffed Crust, XXL, Papa Johns*	1 Slice/128g	312	11.9	243	10.5	28.3	9.3	1.8
The Greek, Thin, Lge, Papa Johns*	1 Slice/85g	179	6.2	211	8.6	26.8	7.3	1.9
The Greek, Thin, Med, Papa Johns*	1 Slice/74g	154	5.3	208	8.4	26.7	7.1	1.9
The Greek, Thin, XXL, Papa Johns*	1 Slice/94g	202	6.9	216	8.8	27.6	7.4	1.9
The Works, Original Base, Lge, Papa Johns*	1 Slice/107g	260	10.2	243	10.7	27.9	9.5	1.8
The Works, Original Base, Med, Papa Johns*	1 Slice/95g	232	8.9	245	10.8	28.4	9.4	1.8
The Works, Original Base, Sm, Papa Johns*	1 Slice/85g	212	8.0	250	10.9	29.4	9.4	1.9
The Works, Original Base, XXL, Papa Johns*	1 Slice/122g	298	11.2	245	10.6	29.1	9.2	1.9
The Works, Stuffed Crust, Lge, Papa Johns*	1 Slice/120g	322	14.4	267	12.5	26.5	11.9	1.7
The Works, Stuffed Crust, Med, Papa Johns*	1 Slice/110g	284	12.8	259	12.3	25.2	11.7	1.6
The Works, Stuffed Crust, XXL, Papa Johns*	1 Slice/134g	342	14.5	255	11.7	26.8	10.8	1.7
The Works, Thin, Med, Papa Johns*	1 Slice/77g	190	8.0	247	11.0	26.4	10.4	1.8
The Works, Thin, XXL, Papa Johns*	1 Slice/101g	251	10.6	249	11.2	26.4	10.5	1.8
Thin Crust, Cheese, Papa Johns*	1 Slice/96g	240	3.5	250	0.0	22.9	3.6	0.0

POTATO WEDGES

Sides, Papa Johns*	1 Serving/266g	420	12.2	158	2.5	27.8	4.6	2.5

RIBS

Memphis BBQ, Papa Johns*	1 Serving/240g	658	49.7	274	17.8	3.9	20.7	0.1

PIZZA EXPRESS

ANTIPASTO

Italian, Classic, Sharing Starter, Pizza Express*	½ Serving/278g	656	42.2	236	10.8	19.0	15.2	2.3

ARRABIATA

Pollo, Pizza Express*	100g	98	1.7	98	6.2	14.5	1.7	1.2

AUBERGINE

Parmigiana, Melanzane, Main, Pizza Express*	1 Serving/434g	607	45.1	140	5.1	6.1	10.4	1.7

BREAD

Garlic, Starter, Pizza Express*	1 Serving/105g	239	4.9	228	7.8	39.8	4.7	2.5
Garlic, with Mozzarella, Starter, Pizza Express*	1 Serving/131g	304	9.3	232	11.2	32.1	7.1	2.0

BROCCOLINI

Side, Pizza Express*	1 Serving/120g	167	14.9	139	4.7	2.4	12.4	2.9

BROWNIES

Chocolate Dessert, Pizza Express*	1 Serving/173g	552	28.4	319	4.5	37.9	16.4	0.2
GF, Dolcetti, Pizza Express*	1 Serving/55g	215	11.8	392	4.6	43.6	21.6	0.1

	Measure INFO/WEIGHT	per Measure KCAL	FAT	Nutrition Values per 100g / 100ml KCAL	PROT	CARB	FAT	FIBRE
PIZZA EXPRESS								
BROWNIES								
Piccolo, Pizza Express*	1 Serving/55g	215	11.8	392	4.6	43.6	21.6	0.1
BRUSCHETTA								
Con Funghi, Starter, Pizza Express*	1 Serving/272g	367	13.3	135	4.0	19.2	4.9	1.3
Originale, Starter, Pizza Express*	1 Serving/218g	393	19.6	180	4.5	21.2	9.0	1.6
CAKE								
Chocolate, Fresh Strawberry, Mini, Piccolo, Pizza Express*	1 Serving/85g	251	11.2	295	4.5	39.1	13.2	1.6
Chocolate Fudge, & Ice Cream, Pizza Express*	1 Serving/161g	424	18.5	263	4.7	34.9	11.5	1.2
Chocolate Fudge, Mini, Dolcetti, Pizza Express*	1 Serving/85g	251	11.2	295	4.5	39.1	13.2	1.6
Chocolate Fudge, Pizza Express*	1 Serving/101g	311	14.0	308	4.9	40.4	13.9	1.6
CALZONE								
Calabrese, Main, Pizza Express*	1 Calzone/574g	1165	58.5	203	10.7	17.8	10.2	1.3
Classico, Pizza Express*	1 Calzone/532g	953	43.1	179	8.8	18.8	8.1	1.5
Salami E Salsiccia, Main, Pizza Express*	1 Calzone/518g	984	50.8	190	8.7	17.5	9.8	1.4
Verdure, Main, Pizza Express*	1 Calzone/564g	1280	80.7	227	6.4	19.0	14.3	1.4
CAVATAPPI								
Formaggi, Main, Pizza Express*	1 Serving/544g	1093	56.0	201	9.0	17.9	10.3	0.9
CHEESECAKE								
Strawberry & Mint Fool, Pizza Express*	1 Serving/34g	133	9.9	392	3.3	29.5	29.2	0.9
Vanilla & Ice Cream, Pizza Express*	1 Serving/201g	549	31.8	273	4.4	28.9	15.8	1.4
CHIPS								
Polenta, Side, Pizza Express*	1 Serving/120g	328	20.3	273	4.5	24.9	16.9	1.7
COLESLAW								
Side, Pizza Express*	1 Serving/125g	213	19.9	170	1.2	6.3	15.9	0.0
CRUMBLE								
Fruit, Winter, Mulled, Pizza Express*	1 Serving/160g	333	10.2	208	3.3	34.0	6.4	0.0
DESSERT								
Caffe Reale, Dolcetti, Pizza Express*	1 Serving/65g	191	11.7	293	3.1	29.9	18.0	1.9
Chocolate Glory, Pizza Express*	1 Serving/309g	687	23.5	222	4.2	34.1	7.6	1.1
Dough balls with Nutella, Pizza Express*	1 Serving/100g	480	0.0	480	0.0	0.0	0.0	0.0
Dough Balls with Nutella Docetti, Pizza Express*	1 Serving/100g	241	0.0	241	0.0	0.0	0.0	0.0
Posset, Lemon Crunch, Dolcetti, Pizza Express*	1 Serving/33g	146	11.8	442	0.0	30.0	35.6	0.5
Semi Freddo Reale, Dolcetti, Pizza Express*	1 Serving/40g	134	8.8	336	2.6	29.0	22.1	0.3
Summer Pudding, Pizza Express*	1 Serving/140g	255	37.6	182	3.2	26.1	26.9	1.6
Toffee Fudge Glory, Pizza Express*	1 Serving/295g	631	20.1	214	3.7	34.6	6.8	0.4
DIP								
Garlic Butter, Pizza Express*	¼ Pot/9g	67	7.3	741	0.9	1.4	81.3	0.3
DOUGH BALLS								
Doppio, Sharing Starter, Pizza Express*	½ Serving/129g	321	17.4	249	6.9	33.8	13.5	2.3
Formaggi, Starter, Pizza Express*	1 Serving/140g	419	21.4	299	11.0	30.4	15.3	1.9
Garlic Butter, Side Salad, Piccolo, Pizza Express*	1 Serving/158g	187	8.2	118	3.1	15.1	5.2	1.4
Mini, Side, Pizza Express*	1 Serving/60g	125	1.1	209	8.1	41.4	1.8	2.6
Side Salad, Olive Oil & Balsamic, Piccolo, Pizza Express*	1 Serving/158g	177	7.0	112	3.5	15.0	4.4	1.4
Starter, Pizza Express*	1 Serving/120g	347	16.8	289	7.0	35.0	14.0	2.2
DRESSING								
House, Pizza Express*	1 Tbsp/10ml	44	4.7	442	1.3	4.1	47.0	0.2
Light, Pizza Express*	1 fl oz/30ml	89	9.2	297	1.3	4.2	30.5	0.3
FRESELLA								
Starter, Pizza Express*	1 Serving/370g	630	41.5	170	6.3	11.5	11.2	1.0
ICE CREAM								
Chocolate, Gelato, Coppa, Pizza Express*	1 Serving/125g	253	10.5	202	4.5	27.6	8.4	1.8
Strawberry, Gelato, Coppa, Pizza Express*	1 Serving/125g	215	3.4	172	0.7	35.8	2.7	0.3
Vanilla, Chocolate Sauce, Piccolo, Pizza Express*	1 Serving/70g	146	4.6	209	4.1	33.3	6.6	0.9

PIZZA EXPRESS

	Measure INFO/WEIGHT	per Measure KCAL	FAT	Nutrition Values per 100g / 100ml KCAL	PROT	CARB	FAT	FIBRE
ICE CREAM								
Vanilla, Chocolate Sauce & Cone, Piccolo, Pizza Express*	1 Serving/72g	154	4.8	213	4.2	34.3	6.6	0.9
Vanilla, Cone, Piccolo, Pizza Express*	1 Serving/62g	120	4.6	194	4.6	27.0	7.5	0.6
Vanilla, Fresh Strawberry, Piccolo, Pizza Express*	1 Serving/62g	120	4.6	194	4.6	27.0	7.5	0.6
Vanilla, Fruit Coulis, & Cone, Piccolo, Pizza Express*	1 Serving/72g	132	4.7	183	4.0	27.4	6.5	0.7
Vanilla, Fruit Coulis, Piccolo, Pizza Express*	1 Serving/70g	125	4.6	178	3.9	26.3	6.5	0.7
Vanilla, Fruit Coulis, Strawberry, Piccolo, Pizza Express*	1 Serving/82g	134	4.7	164	3.6	24.8	5.7	0.8
Vanilla, Fudge Cubes, Piccolo, Pizza Express*	1 Serving/70g	153	5.8	219	4.1	32.0	8.3	0.4
Vanilla, Gelato, Coppa, Pizza Express*	1 Serving/125g	245	9.1	196	4.7	28.1	7.3	0.5
Vanilla, Gelato, Piccolo, Pizza Express*	1 Serving/60g	113	4.5	188	4.5	25.7	7.5	0.5
Vanilla, Toffee Sauce, Piccolo, Pizza Express*	1 Serving/70g	143	4.5	204	3.9	32.7	6.4	0.4
Vanilla, Toffee Sauce & Cone, Piccolo, Pizza Express*	1 Serving/72g	150	4.6	208	3.9	35.7	6.4	0.5
ICE LOLLY								
Ice Pop, Pizza Express*	1 Serving/35g	22	0.0	63	0.2	14.5	0.1	0.1
LASAGNE								
Classica, Main, Pizza Express*	1 Serving/427g	623	32.9	146	9.0	10.4	7.7	0.1
Verde, Main, Pizza Express*	1 Serving/468g	744	52.4	159	4.4	9.7	11.2	0.2
Verdi, Pizza Express*	1 Serving/468g	744	52.4	159	4.4	9.7	11.2	0.2
MELANZANINE								
Starter, Pizza Express*	1 Serving/154g	223	16.6	145	5.9	5.8	10.8	1.5
NOCI								
Harissa Mix, Pizza Express*	1 Serving/60g	319	18.9	531	18.5	48.6	31.5	10.2
OLIVES								
Marinate, Pizza Express*	1 Serving/80g	122	10.7	153	1.4	8.3	13.4	3.6
PASTA								
Bianca, Piccolo, Main, Pizza Express*	1 Serving/220g	389	15.6	177	4.6	23.3	7.1	0.8
Bolognese, Piccolo, Main, Pizza Express*	1 Serving/260g	387	11.7	149	7.6	19.1	4.5	1.0
Burro, Piccolo, Main, Pizza Express*	1 Serving/115g	311	12.1	270	6.3	37.7	10.5	2.2
Napoletana, Piccolo, Main, Pizza Express*	1 Serving/218g	309	7.2	142	4.1	24.5	3.3	1.1
Pollo, Main, Pizza Express*	1 Serving/573g	923	47.0	161	7.9	14.0	8.2	0.8
Pollo Pesto, Pizza Express*	1 Serving/586g	1136	68.5	194	7.4	14.7	11.7	0.6
PIADINA								
Bread, Pizza Express*	1 Serving/106g	232	3.5	219	9.2	39.4	3.3	2.5
Caesar, Pizza Express*	1 Serving/201g	426	18.1	212	12.7	20.5	9.0	1.6
Capresse, Pizza Express*	1 Serving/220g	460	23.1	209	9.3	20.5	10.5	1.5
Chicken & Avocado, Pizza Express*	1 Serving/275g	493	26.2	179	7.0	17.0	9.5	2.1
Italian Meat, Pizza Express*	1 Serving/219g	532	30.2	243	11.9	19.0	13.8	1.2
PLT, Pizza Express*	1 Serving/211g	432	21.6	216	8.9	21.3	10.8	1.6
PIE								
Banoffee, & Ice Cream, Pizza Express*	1 Serving/142g	524	38.9	369	2.1	28.4	27.4	2.6
PIZZA								
American, Classic, GF, Pizza Express*	1 Pizza/381g	1020	45.5	268	6.6	33.4	12.0	0.8
American, Classic, Main, Pizza Express*	1 Pizza/376g	804	33.4	214	10.3	24.2	8.9	1.6
American, Hot, HGP, Romanita, Lunch, Pizza Express*	1 Pizza/255g	493	22.7	193	10.3	18.9	8.9	1.3
American, Hot, Leggera, Main, Pizza Express*	1 Pizza/269g	396	15.6	147	8.1	16.5	5.8	1.3
American, Light Mozz, Piccolo, GF, Pizza Express*	1 Pizza/180g	408	14.8	227	7.0	31.2	8.2	0.8
American, Light Mozz, Piccolo, Pizza Express*	1 Pizza/190g	338	9.7	178	10.4	24.0	5.1	1.6
American, Piccolo, Pizza Express*	1 Pizza/181g	354	11.9	196	9.9	25.3	6.6	1.7
American, Romanita, Lunch, Pizza Express*	1 Pizza/234g	490	22.5	209	11.1	20.3	9.6	1.4
American, Simple, Pepperoni, Pizza Express*	½ Pizza/255g	551	18.9	216	9.1	28.1	7.4	2.0
American Hot, Classic, Main, Pizza Express*	1 Pizza/396g	807	33.2	204	9.8	23.2	8.4	1.6
American Hot, Romana, Main, Pizza Express*	1 Pizza/417g	863	37.5	207	10.4	22.1	9.0	1.5
American Hot, Supermarket, 8 inch, Pizza Express*	1 Half/145g	293	10.0	202	8.7	26.2	6.9	2.0

PIZZA EXPRESS

PIZZA

	Measure INFO/WEIGHT	per Measure KCAL	FAT	Nutrition Values per 100g / 100ml KCAL	PROT	CARB	FAT	FIBRE
American Hottest, Romana 65, Pizza Express*	1 Pizza/536g	1222	74.0	228	8.0	18.4	13.8	1.3
Caprina Rossa, Romana, Main, Pizza Express*	1 Pizza/524g	901	39.3	172	7.7	19.4	7.5	1.5
Caronara, Romana, Main, Pizza Express*	1 Pizza/478g	1057	55.5	221	11.3	18.8	11.6	1.1
Da Morire, Romana, Main, Pizza Express*	1 Pizza/537g	940	44.0	175	7.7	17.9	8.2	2.1
Diavolo, Romana, Main, Pizza Express*	1 Pizza/477g	978	42.9	205	11.0	20.2	9.0	1.6
Etna, Romana, Main, Pizza Express*	1 Pizza/502g	1039	46.7	207	11.3	20.1	9.3	1.4
Fiorentina, Classic, GF, Pizza Express*	1 Pizza/493g	1045	45.1	212	6.2	26.2	9.1	0.7
Fiorentina, Classic, Main, Pizza Express*	1 Pizza/488g	830	32.7	170	9.0	19.1	6.7	1.4
Four Seasons, Classic, GF, Pizza Express*	1 Pizza/380g	894	35.0	235	4.3	33.4	9.2	1.0
Four Seasons, Classic, Main, Pizza Express*	1 Pizza/375g	679	22.9	181	8.0	24.4	6.1	1.9
Giardiniera, Classic, GF, Pizza Express*	1 Pizza/525g	1115	55.8	212	4.1	25.0	10.6	1.3
Giardiniera, Classic, Main, Pizza Express*	1 Pizza/520g	900	43.7	173	6.7	18.4	8.4	1.9
Il Padrino, Romana, Main, Pizza Express*	1 Pizza/513g	1032	49.8	201	10.0	19.1	9.7	1.5
La Regina, Romana 65, Pizza Express*	1 Pizza/464g	993	52.4	214	9.4	19.3	11.3	1.5
La Reine, Classic, Main, Pizza Express*	1 Pizza/413g	740	26.0	179	9.4	22.1	6.3	1.7
La Reine, Light Mozz, Piccolo, GF, Pizza Express*	1 Pizza/203g	396	12.9	195	6.7	27.8	6.4	0.8
La Reine, Light Mozz, Piccolo, Pizza Express*	1 Pizza/213g	326	7.7	153	9.7	21.6	3.6	1.6
La Reine, Piccolo, GF, Pizza Express*	1 Pizza/193g	411	15.2	213	6.1	29.2	7.9	0.9
La Reine, Piccolo, Pizza Express*	1 Pizza/203g	341	9.9	168	9.3	22.6	4.9	1.7
La Reine, Romanita, Lunch, Pizza Express*	1 Pizza/250g	405	14.2	162	9.2	19.4	5.7	1.5
Leggera Gustova (Approximate), Pizza Express*	1 Pizza/500g	550	0.0	110	0.0	0.0	0.0	0.0
Margherita, Classic, GF, Pizza Express*	1 Pizza/359g	899	45.5	250	5.5	35.1	12.7	0.8
Margherita, Classic, Main, Pizza Express*	1 Pizza/354g	683	22.6	193	9.4	25.7	6.4	1.7
Margherita, Light Mozz, Piccolo, GF, Pizza Express*	1 Pizza/170g	359	10.6	211	6.1	32.9	6.2	0.8
Margherita, Light Mozz, Piccolo, Pizza Express*	1 Pizza/180g	290	5.4	161	9.6	25.3	3.0	1.6
Margherita, Piccolo, GF, Pizza Express*	1 Pizza/165g	388	14.0	235	5.9	33.8	8.5	0.8
Margherita, Piccolo, Pizza Express*	1 Pizza/175g	319	8.8	182	9.5	25.9	5.0	1.7
Margherita, Romana, Light Mozz, Piccolo, Pizza Express	1 Pizza/240g	367	9.6	153	11.0	19.8	4.0	1.3
Margherita, Romana, Piccolo, GF, Pizza Express*	1 Pizza/220g	495	21.4	225	8.2	26.3	9.7	0.6
Margherita, Romana, Piccolo, Pizza Express*	1 Pizza/230g	426	16.1	185	10.9	20.6	7.0	1.4
Margherita, Romano, Light Mozz, Piccolo, Pizza Express*	1 Pizza/240g	367	9.6	153	11.0	19.8	4.0	1.3
Margherita Bufala, Romana 65, Pizza Express*	1 Pizza/415g	814	36.1	196	7.8	22.2	8.7	1.5
Melsnzane, Romana, Main, Pizza Express*	1 Pizza/464g	840	36.2	181	11.1	20.7	7.8	2.1
Mushroom, Light Mozz, Piccolo, GF, Pizza Express*	1 Pizza/191g	363	10.7	190	5.6	29.4	5.6	0.8
Mushroom, Light Mozz, Piccolo, Pizza Express*	1 Pizza/201g	293	5.6	146	8.9	22.8	2.8	1.6
Mushroom, Piccolo, GF, Pizza Express*	1 Pizza/180g	377	13.0	210	4.9	31.0	7.2	0.8
Mushroom, Piccolo, Pizza Express*	1 Pizza/190g	308	7.8	162	8.4	23.2	4.1	1.7
Nicoise Romana, Main, Pizza Express*	1 Pizza/601g	1135	54.6	189	11.8	15.6	9.1	1.3
Padana, Leggera, Main, Pizza Express*	1 Pizza/349g	450	10.8	129	4.1	21.6	3.1	1.4
Padana, Romanita, Lunch, Pizza Express*	1 Pizza/327g	546	18.6	167	7.2	22.6	5.7	1.3
Padana Romana, Main, Pizza Express*	1 Pizza/459g	830	27.1	181	7.4	25.4	5.9	1.5
Pianta, Classic, Pizza Express*	1 Pizza/528g	824	38.0	156	4.3	18.8	7.2	2.1
Pianta Romana, Main, Pizza Express*	1 Pizza/528g	824	38.0	156	4.3	18.8	7.2	2.1
Pollo, Light Mozz, Piccolo, GF, Pizza Express*	1 Pizza/190g	382	10.8	201	8.1	29.4	5.7	0.7
Pollo, Light Mozz, Piccolo, Pizza Express*	1 Pizza/200g	312	5.6	156	11.2	22.8	2.8	1.5
Pollo, Piccolo, GF, Pizza Express*	1 Pizza/180g	396	13.1	220	7.5	31.0	7.3	0.7
Pollo, Piccolo, Pizza Express*	1 Pizza/190g	327	7.8	172	10.8	23.9	4.1	1.6
Pollo Ad Astra, Leggera, Main, Pizza Express*	1 Pizza/367g	418	8.8	114	9.6	14.1	2.4	1.1
Pollo Ad Astra, Romana, Main, Pizza Express*	1 Pizza/491g	800	22.1	163	11.2	20.1	4.5	1.4
Pollo Ad Astra, Romanita, Lunch, Pizza Express*	1 Pizza/337g	479	12.8	142	11.3	16.3	3.8	1.2
Pollo Forza, Pizza Express*	1 Pizza/487g	877	31.2	180	11.1	20.1	6.4	1.6
Pollo Forza, Romana, Pizza Express*	1 Pizza/547g	984	36.6	180	12.1	18.3	6.7	1.5

PIZZA EXPRESS

INFO/WEIGHT	per Measure KCAL	per Measure FAT	Nutrition Values per 100g / 100ml KCAL	PROT	CARB	FAT	FIBRE

PIZZA

	Measure INFO/WEIGHT	per Measure KCAL	per Measure FAT	KCAL	PROT	CARB	FAT	FIBRE
Polpette Bolognese, Romana, Main, Pizza Express*	1 Pizza/580g	1160	58.6	200	10.1	17.6	10.1	1.0
Pomodoro, Pesto, Leggera, Main, Pizza Express*	1 Pizza/316g	401	17.4	127	5.7	14.7	5.5	1.3
Pomodoro, Pesto, Romana, Main, Pizza Express*	1 Pizza/543g	1151	60.3	212	11.5	17.1	11.1	1.1
Porchetta, Pizza Express*	1 Serving/524g	1207	54.6	230	13.8	21.0	10.4	1.0
Prosciutto Fichi, Pizza Express*	1 Pizza/476g	1014	44.3	213	10.7	22.3	9.3	1.2
Quattro Formaggi, Romana, Main, Pizza Express*	1 Pizza/424g	886	39.0	209	10.9	21.6	9.2	1.4
Romana, Melanzane, Pizza Express*	¼ Pizza/116g	222	10.4	191	7.2	20.7	9.0	2.1
Rustichella, Romana, Main, Pizza Express*	1 Pizza/511g	1022	46.5	200	9.8	20.5	9.1	1.8
Sloppy Giuseppe, Classic, Main, Pizza Express*	1 Pizza/469g	952	39.4	203	11.3	20.9	8.4	1.7
Sloppy Giuseppe, Leggera, Pizza Express*	1 Pizza/319g	450	16.9	141	9.0	15.0	5.3	1.1
Sloppy Guiseppe, Classic, GF, Pizza Express*	1 Pizza/474g	1167	51.3	246	8.3	28.1	10.8	1.1
Spinach & Mascarpone, Sienese, Pizza Express*	½ Pizza/333g	703	24.0	211	7.8	28.8	7.2	2.2
Toscana Romana, Main, Pizza Express*	1 Pizza/524g	1169	62.4	223	11.9	17.8	11.9	1.2
Trifolata, Mushroom, Pizza Express*	1 Serving/495g	914	43.0	185	8.8	18.1	8.7	1.3
Veneziana, Romana, Main, Pizza Express*	1 Pizza/423g	796	30.1	188	9.1	23.0	7.1	1.7
Veneziana, Romanita, Lunch, Pizza Express*	1 Pizza/265g	440	54.1	166	8.3	6.1	20.4	1.7

PIZZA BASE

	Measure INFO/WEIGHT	per Measure KCAL	per Measure FAT	KCAL	PROT	CARB	FAT	FIBRE
Main Base, GF, Pizza Express*	1 Base/195g	444	2.3	228	2.6	52.5	1.2	1.3
Main Base, Pizza Express*	1 Base/200g	410	2.4	205	8.2	41.7	1.2	2.6
Piccolo, GF, Pizza Express*	1 Base/90g	206	1.1	228	2.6	52.5	1.2	1.3
Piccolo, Pizza Express*	1 Base/100g	205	1.2	205	8.2	41.7	1.2	2.6

RISOTTO

	Measure INFO/WEIGHT	per Measure KCAL	per Measure FAT	KCAL	PROT	CARB	FAT	FIBRE
Arancini, Ragu, Rice, Pizza Express*	1 Serving/165g	371	12.9	225	7.5	30.3	7.8	1.9
Fresco, Main, Pizza Express*	1 Serving/431g	659	36.6	153	7.0	11.7	8.5	0.2
Fresco, Pizza Express*	1 Serving/182g	324	20.4	178	7.5	11.7	11.2	0.2
Pollo Funghi, Starter, Pizza Express*	1 Serving/237g	367	21.8	155	6.4	11.3	9.2	0.4
Prosciutto Piselli, Main, Pizza Express*	1 Serving/465g	767	45.1	165	6.6	12.8	9.7	1.0
Prosciutto Piselli, Pizza Express*	1 Serving/232g	383	22.5	165	6.6	12.8	9.7	1.0

RUCOLA

	Measure INFO/WEIGHT	per Measure KCAL	per Measure FAT	KCAL	PROT	CARB	FAT	FIBRE
Pizza Express*	1 Serving/50g	140	13.2	281	9.7	1.0	26.5	0.7

SALAD

	Measure INFO/WEIGHT	per Measure KCAL	per Measure FAT	KCAL	PROT	CARB	FAT	FIBRE
Bosco, Main, Pizza Express*	1 Serving/361g	603	32.9	167	7.2	14.7	9.1	2.1
Bosco, Mini, Lunch, Pizza Express*	1 Serving/264g	444	33.3	168	5.3	8.5	12.6	2.3
Bosco, with Chicken, Pizza Express*	1 Serving/432g	687	34.6	159	10.0	12.4	8.0	1.8
Caesar, Side, Pizza Express*	1 Serving/129g	313	25.4	243	8.1	8.1	19.7	0.9
Chicken Caesar, Grande, Main, Pizza Express*	1 Serving/350g	630	25.9	180	12.1	16.5	7.4	1.4
Fichi Fresca, Pizza Express*	1 Serving/406g	788	47.9	194	7.6	15.1	11.8	1.5
Leggera, with Chicken, Superfood, Main, Pizza Express*	1 Serving/443g	385	25.2	87	6.0	3.5	5.7	1.4
Leggera Superfood, Main, Pizza Express*	1 Serving/401g	337	24.5	84	4.1	3.8	6.1	1.5
Mixed Leaf, Side, Pizza Express*	1 Serving/411g	185	14.4	45	0.8	2.9	3.5	0.8
Mozzarella & Tomato, Starter, Pizza Express*	1 Serving/190g	311	28.4	164	4.7	2.6	15.0	0.5
Nicoise, Mini, Lunch, Pizza Express*	1 Serving/290g	340	17.4	117	7.4	8.6	6.0	0.9
Nicoise, Pizza Express*	1 Serving/419g	532	23.0	127	9.1	10.7	5.5	1.0
Pollo, Main, Pizza Express*	1 Serving/393g	644	29.8	164	8.7	15.4	7.6	1.3
Pollo, Mini, Lunch, Pizza Express*	1 Serving/247g	363	17.5	147	8.1	13.0	7.1	1.2
Pollo, Verdure, Pizza Express*	1 Serving/388g	862	55.5	222	7.5	16.2	14.3	1.4
Pollo Pancetta, Main, Pizza Express*	1 Serving/445g	784	42.3	176	9.4	13.7	9.5	1.2
Primavera, Pizza Express*	1 Serving/467g	934	63.0	200	8.5	11.5	13.5	1.5
Salmon, Leggera, Pizza Express*	1 Serving/409g	413	27.0	101	6.7	4.3	6.6	1.2
Superfood, Mini, Lunch, Pizza Express*	1 Serving/316g	272	19.9	86	4.4	3.2	6.3	1.4
Vegetable, & Goats Cheese, Warm, Main, Pizza Express*	1 Serving/406g	690	43.4	170	4.3	14.1	10.7	1.8

	Measure INFO/WEIGHT	per Measure KCAL	FAT	Nutrition Values per 100g / 100ml KCAL	PROT	CARB	FAT	FIBRE
PIZZA EXPRESS								
SORBET								
Lemon Curd, Dolcetti, Pizza Express*	1 Serving/65g	84	1.9	129	0.5	24.9	2.9	0.0
Lemon Curd, Main, Pizza Express*	1 Serving/129g	167	3.8	129	0.5	24.9	2.9	0.0
Raspberry, Dolcetti, Pizza Express*	1 Serving/65g	86	1.9	132	1.0	25.4	2.9	1.6
Raspberry, Piccolo, Pizza Express*	1 Serving/60g	61	0.2	101	0.6	23.7	0.4	1.1
Raspberry, Pizza Express*	1 Serving/127g	147	2.2	116	0.9	24.3	1.7	1.4
SOUP								
Butternut, Pizza Express*	1 Serving/427g	529	27.7	124	2.6	13.9	6.5	1.4
Tomato, Pizza Express*	1 Serving/425g	514	28.5	121	2.4	12.9	6.7	1.3
STEW								
Contadino, Sausage & Lentil, Pizza Express*	1 Serving/352g	483	18.7	137	6.0	16.7	5.3	1.2
TALEGGIO								
Oven Baked, Sharing Starter, Pizza Express*	½ Serving/164g	377	16.6	230	11.3	24.0	10.1	1.6
TIRAMISU								
Pizza Express*	1 Serving/100g	242	8.6	242	3.0	37.2	8.6	1.7
TORTA								
Double Chocolate Espresso, Dolcetti, Pizza Express*	1 Serving/81g	374	28.2	461	3.8	33.1	34.8	3.1
Lemon, & Mascarpone, Pizza Express*	1 Serving/167g	529	32.7	317	5.1	32.1	19.6	0.3
Lemon Meringue, Dolcetti, Pizza Express*	1 Serving/51g	185	10.0	362	5.9	40.6	19.6	0.9
PIZZA HUT								
BREAD								
Garlic, Fingers, Pizza Hut*	1 Portion/136g	511	30.7	376	6.4	36.7	22.6	0.0
Garlic, Pizza Hut*	1 Portion/136g	511	30.7	376	6.4	36.7	22.6	0.0
Garlic, with Cheese, & Bacon, Pizza Hut*	1 Portion/217g	754	47.4	347	12.3	24.2	21.8	0.0
Garlic, with Cheese, Pizza Hut*	1 Portion/197g	689	43.4	350	10.0	26.6	22.0	0.0
CHEESE								
Triangles, Fried, Pizza Hut*	1 Portion/151g	535	35.0	354	15.1	22.1	23.2	0.0
Triangles, Oven Baked, Pizza Hut*	1 Portion/153g	21	13.0	14	20.4	1.1	8.5	0.0
CHICKEN								
Bites, BBQ, Pizza Hut*	1 Portion/241g	459	17.3	190	10.0	21.2	7.2	0.0
Bites, Plain, Pizza Hut*	1 Portion/191g	397	17.2	208	12.3	19.4	9.0	0.0
Bites, Sweet Chilli, Pizza Hut*	1 Portion/241g	500	17.2	207	9.8	26.0	7.1	0.0
Wings, BBQ, Texan Style, Pizza Hut*	1 Portion/215g	409	23.2	190	17.0	5.7	10.8	0.0
DIP								
BBQ, Texan, Pizza Hut*	1 Serving/50g	62	1.0	124	2.0	28.4	2.0	0.0
Ketchup, Tomato, Pizza Hut*	1 Serving/50g	45	0.2	90	2.0	22.2	0.4	0.0
Mayonnaise, Garlic, Pizza Hut*	1 Serving/50g	243	25.9	486	1.2	3.6	51.8	0.0
Mayonnaise, Light, Pizza Hut*	1 Serving/50g	186	17.9	372	0.8	11.8	35.8	0.0
Sour Cream, & Chive, Dressing, Pizza Hut*	1 Serving/50g	148	15.6	296	0.8	3.6	31.2	0.0
Sweet Chilli, Pizza Hut*	1 Serving/50g	103	0.0	206	0.4	51.4	0.0	0.0
FRIES								
Fried, Bucket, Pizza Hut*	1 Portion/330g	888	39.9	269	3.3	38.3	12.1	0.0
Oven Baked, Bucket, Pizza Hut*	1 Portion/330g	498	19.1	151	2.4	22.9	5.8	0.0
LASAGNE								
Main, Pizza Hut*	1 Portion/490g	801	43.0	163	8.4	12.4	8.8	0.0
ONION RINGS								
Crispy, Fried, Pizza Hut*	1 Portion/180g	520	28.4	289	4.4	33.9	15.8	0.0
Crispy, Oven Baked, Pizza Hut*	1 Portion/180g	338	14.8	188	2.9	32.9	8.2	0.0
PASTA								
Bolognese, Happy Hour, Pizza Hut*	1 Portion/225g	248	6.3	110	4.6	16.3	2.8	0.0
Four Cheese, & Spinach, Happy Hour, Pizza Hut*	1 Portion/225g	286	10.0	112	4.3	14.4	3.9	0.0
Vegetable, Roasted, Pizza Hut*	1 Portion/460g	607	26.3	132	5.0	14.4	5.7	0.0

PIZZA HUT

	Measure INFO/WEIGHT	per Measure KCAL	FAT	Nutrition Values per 100g / 100ml KCAL	PROT	CARB	FAT	FIBRE

PASTA BAKE

	Measure INFO/WEIGHT	per Measure KCAL	FAT	KCAL	PROT	CARB	FAT	FIBRE
Chicken, Herby, Pizza Hut*	1 Portion/472g	735	31.0	156	8.7	14.7	6.6	0.0
Salmon, Pizza Hut*	1 Portion/400g	664	37.1	166	6.7	13.9	9.3	0.0

PIZZA

	Measure INFO/WEIGHT	per Measure KCAL	FAT	KCAL	PROT	CARB	FAT	FIBRE
BBQ Deluxe, Cheesy Bites, Pizza Hut*	1 Slice/143g	358	11.6	251	11.7	34.4	8.1	0.0
BBQ Deluxe, Italian, Individual, Pizza Hut*	1 Slice/78g	185	6.1	238	10.9	34.3	7.9	0.0
BBQ Deluxe, Italian, Lge, Pizza Hut*	1 Slice/95g	239	8.0	252	14.3	29.7	8.4	0.0
BBQ Deluxe, Italian, Med, Pizza Hut*	1 Slice/105g	253	8.0	241	12.0	31.1	7.6	0.0
BBQ Deluxe, Pan, Individual, Pizza Hut*	1 Slice/79g	200	7.9	253	12.7	28.0	10.0	0.0
BBQ Deluxe, Pan, Lge, Pizza Hut*	1 Slice/122g	306	12.1	251	11.8	28.6	9.9	0.0
BBQ Deluxe, Pan, Med, Pizza Hut*	1 Slice/107g	276	11.3	257	11.7	28.8	10.5	0.0
BBQ Deluxe, Stuffed Crust, Pizza Hut*	1 Slice/155g	337	10.4	217	11.6	31.9	6.7	0.0
Cajun Chicken, Hot One, Italian, Med, Pizza Hut*	1 Slice/100g	250	9.3	250	12.5	29.1	9.3	0.0
Cajun Chicken, Hot One, Pan, Lge, Pizza Hut*	1 Slice/125g	321	14.7	257	12.9	24.7	11.8	0.0
Cajun Chicken, Hot One, Pan, Med, Pizza Hut*	1 Slice/105g	273	12.3	259	12.7	25.6	11.7	0.0
Cheese Feast, Italian, Med, Pizza Hut*	1 Slice/96g	260	11.3	272	12.3	29.1	11.8	0.0
Cheese Feast, Pan, Med, Pizza Hut*	1 Slice/106g	299	15.0	283	14.6	24.2	14.2	0.0
Cheese Feast, Stuffed Crust, Pizza Hut*	1 Slice/132g	361	13.8	273	14.3	30.5	10.4	0.0
Chicken, Hi Light, Med, Pizza Hut*	1 Slice/83g	189	5.5	230	13.2	29.2	6.7	0.0
Chicken Feast, Italian, Med, Pizza Hut*	1 Slice/100g	249	8.6	248	14.1	28.6	8.6	0.0
Chicken Feast, Pan, Med, Pizza Hut*	1 Slice/109g	283	12.0	259	15.5	24.6	11.0	0.0
Chicken Feast, Stuffed Crust, Pizza Hut*	1 Slice/133g	337	12.6	254	14.8	27.3	9.5	0.0
Chicken Supreme, Express, Pizza Hut*	1 Slice/65g	143	5.8	221	10.1	28.1	9.0	0.0
Chicken Supreme, Italian, Individual, Pizza Hut*	1 Slice/74g	169	4.4	229	10.7	35.4	5.9	0.0
Chicken Supreme, Italian, Lge, Pizza Hut*	1 Slice/111g	217	6.4	196	9.8	29.3	5.8	0.0
Chicken Supreme, Italian, Med, Pizza Hut*	1 Slice/102g	220	6.3	215	10.3	31.9	6.2	0.0
Chicken Supreme, Pan, Individual, Pizza Hut*	1 Slice/81g	186	8.0	231	11.6	26.9	9.9	0.0
Chicken Supreme, Pan, Lge, Pizza Hut*	1 Slice/124g	271	11.6	219	10.9	26.1	9.4	0.0
Chicken Supreme, Pan, Med, Pizza Hut*	1 Slice/115g	251	9.9	219	11.2	26.6	8.6	0.0
Chicken Supreme, Stuffed Crust, Pizza Hut*	1 Slice/153g	367	11.0	240	11.6	34.8	7.2	0.0
Express, Supreme, Pizza Hut*	1 Slice/68g	165	7.6	242	10.7	27.8	11.2	0.0
Farmhouse, Italian, Lge, Pizza Hut*	1 Slice/92g	206	6.7	224	10.2	34.0	7.3	0.0
Farmhouse, Italian, Med, Pizza Hut*	1 Slice/59g	113	3.4	190	11.0	23.1	5.7	1.8
Farmhouse, Pan, Individual, Pizza Hut*	1 Slice/70g	179	7.4	256	11.3	31.6	10.6	0.0
Farmhouse, Pan, Lge, Pizza Hut*	1 Slice/106g	257	11.0	242	11.4	29.7	10.4	0.0
Farmhouse, Pan, Med, Pizza Hut*	1 Slice/100g	242	10.4	242	11.3	28.6	10.4	0.0
Happy Hour, Chicken & Mushroom, Pizza Hut*	1 Slice/80g	165	5.4	207	9.6	27.6	6.8	0.0
Happy Hour, Pepperoni & Onion, Pizza Hut*	1 Slice/80g	179	6.9	224	9.4	28.2	8.6	0.0
Hawaiian, Express, Pizza Hut*	1 Slice/60g	147	6.4	245	10.5	29.9	10.6	0.0
Hawaiian, Italian, Individual, Pizza Hut*	1 Slice/71g	164	4.2	229	9.8	37.9	5.8	0.0
Hawaiian, Italian, Lge, Pizza Hut*	1 Slice/99g	221	7.0	223	10.0	33.2	7.1	0.0
Hawaiian, Italian, Med, Pizza Hut*	1 Slice/92g	201	5.6	219	9.8	33.3	6.1	0.0
Hawaiian, Pan, Individual, Pizza Hut*	1 Slice/73g	175	6.5	240	10.9	32.2	8.9	0.0
Hawaiian, Pan, Lge, Delivery, Pizza Hut*	1 Slice/89g	234	10.2	262	10.6	32.6	11.4	0.0
Hawaiian, Pan, Lge, Pizza Hut*	1 Slice/112g	293	12.7	262	10.6	32.6	11.4	0.0
Hawaiian, Pan, Med, Pizza Hut*	1 Slice/109g	245	9.7	224	10.1	28.5	8.9	0.0
Hawaiian, Stuffed Crust, Pizza Hut*	1 Slice/141g	306	10.3	217	11.0	30.7	7.3	0.0
Hot 'n' Spicy, Italian, Individual, Pizza Hut*	1 Slice/66g	180	6.9	272	11.0	36.5	10.4	0.0
Hot 'n' Spicy, Italian, Lge, Pizza Hut*	1 Slice/93g	236	9.4	254	11.2	32.7	10.1	0.0
Hot 'n' Spicy, Italian, Med, Pizza Hut*	1 Slice/86g	222	8.4	259	11.0	34.5	9.8	0.0
Hot 'n' Spicy, Pan, Individual, Pizza Hut*	1 Slice/71g	183	7.9	259	10.9	30.4	11.2	0.0
Hot 'n' Spicy, Pan, Lge, Pizza Hut*	1 Slice/105g	266	11.4	254	12.0	30.2	10.9	0.0
Hot 'n' Spicy, Pan, Med, Pizza Hut*	1 Slice/93g	237	10.6	254	11.5	29.2	11.4	0.0

PIZZA HUT
PIZZA

	Measure INFO/WEIGHT	per Measure KCAL	FAT	Nutrition Values per 100g / 100ml KCAL	PROT	CARB	FAT	FIBRE
Margherita, Cheesy Bites, Pizza Hut*	1 Slice/128g	337	12.9	263	12.8	33.1	10.1	0.0
Margherita, Italian, Individual, Pizza Hut*	1 Slice/67g	177	5.4	264	11.9	39.2	8.0	0.0
Margherita, Italian, Lge, Pizza Hut*	1 Slice/91g	229	8.6	252	10.4	34.2	9.5	0.0
Margherita, Italian, Med, Pizza Hut*	1 Slice/80g	205	7.0	256	11.0	35.7	8.8	0.0
Margherita, Pan, Individual, Pizza Hut*	1 Slice/71g	189	8.1	268	11.6	32.4	11.5	0.0
Margherita, Pan, Lge, Pizza Hut*	1 Slice/105g	273	12.4	261	11.6	29.8	11.9	0.0
Margherita, Pan, Med, Pizza Hut*	1 Slice/97g	256	11.4	265	11.6	30.6	11.8	0.0
Margherita, Stuffed Crust, Pizza Hut*	1 Slice/140g	349	12.4	248	14.0	31.6	8.8	0.0
Margherita, Thick, Kids, Pizza Hut*	1 Slice/202g	506	17.9	251	9.0	33.0	8.9	0.0
Meat Feast, Italian, Individual, Pizza Hut*	1 Slice/81g	220	8.8	270	13.9	32.3	10.8	0.0
Meat Feast, Italian, Lge, Pizza Hut*	1 Slice/111g	279	12.7	251	12.9	27.3	11.4	0.0
Meat Feast, Italian, Med, Pizza Hut*	1 Slice/100g	257	11.0	258	13.0	30.0	11.0	0.0
Meat Feast, Pan, Individual, Pizza Hut*	1 Slice/84g	220	9.9	262	13.3	27.6	11.8	0.0
Meat Feast, Pan, Lge, Pizza Hut*	1 Slice/124g	344	16.4	277	12.6	29.1	13.2	0.0
Meat Feast, Pan, Med, Pizza Hut*	1 Slice/112g	294	13.9	262	12.2	28.0	12.4	0.0
Meat Feast, Stuffed Crust, Pizza Hut*	1 Slice/152g	376	15.8	247	13.5	28.0	10.4	0.0
Meaty, The Edge, Med, Pizza Hut*	1 Slice/36g	110	5.7	308	17.0	20.4	16.1	0.0
Meaty BBQ, Cheesy Bites, Delivery, Pizza Hut*	1 Slice/115g	282	10.8	245	11.3	31.1	9.4	0.0
Meaty BBQ, Italian, Med, Delivery, Pizza Hut*	1 Slice/70g	154	5.0	220	10.9	30.0	7.2	0.0
Mediterranean Meat Deluxe, Italian, Individual, Pizza Hut*	1 Slice/72g	206	8.8	288	12.6	34.7	12.3	0.0
Pepperoni Feast, Cheesy Bites, Pizza Hut*	1 Slice/135g	382	16.7	284	15.8	29.6	12.4	0.0
Pepperoni Feast, Italian, Individual, Pizza Hut*	1 Slice/72.7g	205	8.4	282	11.4	36.3	11.6	0.0
Pepperoni Feast, Italian, Lge, Delivery, Pizza Hut*	1 Slice/68g	195	9.5	286	12.0	30.8	14.0	0.0
Pepperoni Feast, Italian, Lge, Pizza Hut*	1 Slice/103g	286	13.3	278	12.2	30.9	12.9	0.0
Pepperoni Feast, Italian, Med, Pizza Hut*	1 Slice/93g	254	9.8	273	12.3	35.0	10.5	0.0
Pepperoni Feast, Pan, Individual, Pizza Hut*	1 Slice/79g	227	10.8	286	12.3	30.3	13.6	0.0
Pepperoni Feast, Pan, Lge, Pizza Hut*	1 Slice/115g	347	20.2	302	12.0	26.4	17.6	0.0
Pepperoni Feast, Pan, Med, Pizza Hut*	1 Slice/106g	297	15.9	279	12.6	26.2	14.9	0.0
Pepperoni Feast, Stuffed Crust, Pizza Hut*	1 Slice/143g	375	16.2	261	13.1	30.4	11.3	0.0
Seafood Fantastico, Italian, Individual, Pizza Hut*	1 Slice/81g	173	4.6	213	15.3	25.1	5.7	0.0
Seafood Fantastico, Italian, Lge, Pizza Hut*	1 Slice/106g	228	6.6	215	15.1	24.6	6.2	0.0
Seafood Lovers, Italian, Individual, Pizza Hut*	1 Slice/66g	170	5.4	258	9.8	38.4	8.2	0.0
Seafood Lovers, Italian, Med, Pizza Hut*	1 Slice/82g	202	6.6	245	10.1	35.3	8.0	0.0
Seafood Lovers, Pan, Med, Pizza Hut*	1 Slice/98g	233	10.4	237	9.7	28.3	10.6	0.0
Spicy, Hot One, Pan, Med, Pizza Hut*	1 Slice/115g	274	13.0	239	11.2	23.1	11.3	0.0
Super Supreme, Italian, Lge, Pizza Hut*	1 Slice/128g	281	13.2	219	10.6	24.4	10.3	0.0
Super Supreme, Italian, Med, Pizza Hut*	1 Slice/119g	267	11.5	225	11.1	26.3	9.7	0.0
Super Supreme, Pan, Lge, Pizza Hut*	1 Slice/148g	346	17.7	234	11.4	22.5	12.0	0.0
Super Supreme, Pan, Med, Pizza Hut*	1 Slice/127g	323	18.5	255	11.4	22.8	14.6	0.0
Super Supreme, Stuffed Crust, Pizza Hut*	1 Slice/165g	397	14.3	241	11.7	29.0	8.7	0.0
Supreme, Italian, Individual, Pizza Hut*	1 Slice/81g	204	7.5	251	10.9	33.5	9.2	0.0
Supreme, Italian, Lge, Pizza Hut*	1 Slice/113g	264	11.0	233	9.7	29.6	9.7	0.0
Supreme, Pan, Individual, Pizza Hut*	1 Slice/84g	209	9.6	248	11.0	28.0	11.4	0.0
Supreme, Stuffed Crust, Pizza Hut*	1 Slice/160g	371	13.8	232	11.9	29.7	8.6	0.0
The Sizzler, Cajun Chicken, Italian, Med, Pizza Hut*	1 Slice/67g	147	4.8	220	11.8	30.2	7.2	0.0
The Sizzler, Cajun Chicken, Pan, Lge, Pizza Hut*	1 Slice/90g	215	7.9	238	10.8	27.2	8.8	0.0
The Sizzler, Cajun Chicken, Pan, Med, Pizza Hut*	1 Slice/75g	166	7.0	221	10.3	27.3	9.3	0.0
The Sizzler, Spicy Beef, Italian, Med, Pizza Hut*	1 Serving/68g	163	6.1	240	10.9	31.6	9.0	0.0
The Works, The Edge, Med, Pizza Hut*	1 Slice/64g	150	6.7	235	12.7	19.5	10.4	0.0
Tortilla, Thin, Kids, Pizza Hut*	1 Slice/108g	264	14.4	245	9.1	20.9	13.4	0.0
Tuscani, Chicken & Mushroom, Pizza Hut*	1 Slice/491g	1032	55.0	210	10.5	16.9	11.2	0.0
Tuscani, Verde, Pizza Hut*	1 Slice/460g	878	42.3	191	8.0	18.6	9.2	0.0

	Measure INFO/WEIGHT	per Measure KCAL	per Measure FAT	Nutrition Values per 100g / 100ml KCAL	PROT	CARB	FAT	FIBRE
PIZZA HUT								
PIZZA								
Tuscani Caprina, Pizza Hut*	1 Pizza/474g	990	45.5	209	9.0	20.6	9.6	0.0
Vegetable Supreme, Cheesy Bites, Pizza Hut*	1 Slice/145g	312	10.0	215	10.0	30.7	6.9	0.0
Vegetable Supreme, Italian, Individual, Pizza Hut*	1 Slice/77g	160	4.7	207	8.7	32.4	6.1	0.0
Vegetable Supreme, Italian, Lge, Pizza Hut*	1 Slice/111g	222	6.3	200	7.4	32.5	5.7	0.0
Vegetable Supreme, Italian, Med, Pizza Hut*	1 Slice/99g	196	6.0	198	8.3	30.7	6.1	0.0
Vegetable Supreme, Pan, Individual, Pizza Hut*	1 Slice/84g	180	7.6	214	8.6	27.7	9.0	0.0
Vegetable Supreme, Pan, Lge, Pizza Hut*	1 Slice/126g	258	11.6	204	8.1	25.7	9.2	0.0
Vegetable Supreme, Pan, Med, Pizza Hut*	1 Slice/109g	263	11.2	241	9.9	30.0	10.3	0.0
Vegetable Supreme, Stuffed Crust, Pizza Hut*	1 Slice/156g	307	10.8	197	9.3	27.8	6.9	0.0
Vegetarian, Hi Light, Med, Pizza Hut*	1 Slice/77g	170	5.1	221	10.3	30.0	6.6	0.0
Vegetarian Hot One, Cheesy Bites, Pizza Hut*	1 Slice/142g	302	10.1	212	9.8	30.3	7.1	0.0
Vegetarian Hot One, Italian, Individual, Pizza Hut*	1 Slice/78g	164	4.5	211	8.1	34.6	5.8	0.0
Vegetarian Hot One, Italian, Lge, Pizza Hut*	1 Slice/114g	165	6.7	145	7.5	19.1	5.9	0.0
Vegetarian Hot One, Italian, Med, Pizza Hut*	1 Slice/98g	188	5.4	192	9.3	29.5	5.5	0.0
Vegetarian Hot One, Pan, Individual, Pizza Hut*	1 Slice/82g	174	6.0	211	8.8	29.6	7.3	0.0
Vegetarian Hot One, Pan, Lge, Pizza Hut*	1 Slice/126g	290	12.1	231	9.4	29.7	9.6	0.0
Vegetarian Hot One, Pan, Med, Pizza Hut*	1 Slice/115g	234	9.9	204	8.4	26.6	8.6	0.0
Vegetarian Hot One, Stuffed Crust, Pizza Hut*	1 Slice/161g	334	11.1	208	10.1	30.2	6.9	0.0
Veggie, The Edge, Med, Pizza Hut*	1 Slice/60g	136	5.4	227	11.2	22.2	9.0	0.0
PLATTER								
Favourites, Perfect for Sharing, Pizza Hut*	1 Portion/641g	1468	77.7	229	7.7	21.9	12.1	0.0
Nachos, Perfect for Sharing, Pizza Hut*	1 Portion/380g	1139	63.7	300	7.0	27.7	16.8	0.0
Vegetarian, Fried, Perfect for Sharing, Pizza Hut*	1 Portion/601g	1606	95.5	267	8.1	22.7	15.9	0.0
Vegetarian, Oven Baked, Perfect for Sharing, Pizza Hut*	1 Portion/603g	1587	94.7	263	7.7	22.3	15.7	0.0
POTATO WEDGES								
Starter, Pizza Hut*	1 Portion/253g	382	17.1	151	2.5	20.1	6.8	0.0
PRET A MANGER								
BAGUETTE								
Asparagus, & Roasted Peppers, Artisan, Pret*	1 Pack/222g	403	12.4	182	7.0	25.7	5.6	2.6
Avocado & Basil, Pret*	1 Pack/254g	163	7.2	163	4.6	19.8	7.2	2.8
Beef, Rare, & Horseradish, Artisan, Pret*	1 Pack/233g	508	15.4	218	14.9	24.6	6.6	2.1
Brie, Tomato & Basil, Pret*	1 Pack/209g	418	17.3	200	8.2	23.2	8.3	1.6
Cheddar, & Pickle, Posh, Artisan, Pret*	1 Pack/235g	660	26.8	281	10.0	32.8	11.4	2.6
Cheddar, Mature, & Roasted Tomatoes, Artisan, Pret*	1 Pack/249g	614	29.0	247	8.4	26.8	11.6	1.8
Chicken, Bang Bang, Pret*	1 Pack/229g	451	14.8	197	11.0	23.4	6.5	1.8
Chicken, Sweet Chilli, & Coriander, Pret*	1 Pack/210g	390	11.4	186	10.2	23.8	5.4	1.5
Chicken Caesar & Bacon on Artisan, Pret*	1 Pack/230g	584	25.8	254	13.5	24.3	11.2	1.8
Egg, & Roasted Tomatoes, Pret*	1 Pack/227g	514	25.8	226	9.4	51.6	11.4	1.2
Egg, Mayo, & Bacon Breakfast, Pret*	1 Pack/147g	307	9.3	209	8.8	28.3	6.3	1.2
Egg Mayo, & Roasted Tomatoes, Breakfast, Pret*	1 Pack/147g	318	14.5	216	8.4	22.4	9.9	2.0
Ham, & Chutney, Festive, Artisan, Pret*	1 Pack/227g	491	16.8	216	10.9	26.7	7.4	2.0
Ham, & Greve Cheese, Pret*	1 Pack/225g	535	24.0	238	13.9	21.4	10.7	1.5
Prosciutto, Italian, Artisan, Pret*	1 Pack/246g	545	24.7	222	9.8	25.8	10.0	2.0
Salmon, Poached, & Watercress, on Artisan, Pret*	1 Pack/234g	472	12.9	202	12.1	27.4	5.5	2.3
Salmon, Smoked, & Free Range Egg, Breakfast, Pret*	1 Pack/153g	350	17.8	229	10.6	20.5	11.6	1.2
Salmon, Smoked, & Prawn, on Artisan, Pret*	1 Pack/246g	449	12.4	183	12.0	22.2	5.0	1.8
Tuna Mayo, & Cucumber Baguette, Pret*	1 Pack/228g	500	22.6	219	11.0	22.0	9.9	1.3
BARS								
Chocolate Brownie, Pret*	1 Bar/60g	320	19.1	500	6.2	49.3	29.8	4.7
Love Bar, Pret*	1 Bar/70g	324	18.3	463	6.1	50.6	26.1	3.6
Pret Bar, Pret*	1 Bar/65g	279	12.5	429	6.2	55.4	19.2	4.5

	Measure INFO/WEIGHT	per Measure KCAL	per Measure FAT	Nutrition Values per 100g / 100ml KCAL	PROT	CARB	FAT	FIBRE
PRET A MANGER								
BISCUITS								
Fruit & Oat, Pret*	1 Pack/40g	187	9.8	468	8.2	50.0	24.5	6.2
BITES								
Mini Florentine, Pret*	1 Pack/108g	545	28.4	505	9.9	54.4	26.3	4.7
BREAD								
Artisan Soup, Pret*	1 Serving/80g	168	0.6	210	7.0	43.8	0.8	2.0
Baguette, White, for Soup, Pret*	1 Baguette/64g	177	1.6	277	8.4	53.1	2.5	2.5
BREAKFAST CEREAL								
Bircher Muesli Bowl, Pret*	1 Bowl/206g	304	9.7	148	6.3	20.2	4.7	1.4
Honey & Granola Pret Pot, Pret*	1 Pot/133g	263	7.8	198	7.3	28.8	5.9	1.3
Porridge, 5 Grain, Pret*	1 Pot/300g	204	4.2	68	2.0	11.4	1.4	1.3
Porridge, no Topping, Pret*	1 Serving/300g	243	8.4	81	3.0	9.6	2.8	1.7
Porridge, with Compote, Pret*	1 Serving/332g	276	8.4	83	2.8	11.1	2.5	1.6
Porridge, with Honey, Pret*	1 Serving/335g	350	8.4	104	2.7	16.6	2.5	1.5
CAKE								
Apple, Slice, Pret*	1 Slice/100g	303	14.7	303	3.8	38.8	14.7	1.9
Banana, Slice, Pret*	1 Slice/82g	275	11.9	335	3.5	47.3	14.5	1.5
Carrot, Slice, Pret*	1 Slice/112g	400	22.2	357	3.9	40.6	19.8	2.4
Choc Bar, Pret*	1 Slice/70g	380	21.7	543	5.1	59.0	31.0	3.8
Chocolate, Slice, Pret*	1 Slice/88g	354	20.9	402	5.3	41.7	23.8	1.4
Lemon Cake Slice, Pret*	1 Slice/70g	257	10.6	367	4.1	52.4	15.1	2.1
Mince Pie, Pret*	1 Pack/60g	241	11.6	402	3.5	55.0	19.3	2.3
CHEESECAKE								
Lemon, Pot, Pret*	1 Pot/120g	390	25.9	325	2.7	29.3	21.6	1.4
CHICKEN &								
Humous, Protein Pot, Pret*	1 Pack/217g	370	15.0	171	10.7	16.5	6.9	5.5
CHOCOLATE								
Dark with Sea Salt, Pret*	1 Bar/25g	136	9.0	544	4.0	44.0	36.0	8.0
COFFEE								
Americano, Pret*	1 Serving/360ml	35	1.3	10	0.7	0.9	0.4	0.0
Americano White, Semi Skimmed, Pret*	1 Cup/350g	14	0.5	4	0.3	0.4	0.1	0.0
Cappuccino, Pret*	1 Serving/231ml	88	3.1	38	2.7	3.8	1.3	0.0
Espresso, Pret*	1 Serving/137ml	0	0.0	0	0.0	0.0	0.0	0.0
Filter Coffee, Semi Skimmed, Pret*	1 Serving/350ml	14	0.5	4	0.3	0.4	0.1	0.0
Flat White, Pret*	1 Serving/210ml	75	2.7	36	2.6	3.4	1.3	0.0
Latte, Merry, Very Berry, Pret*	1 Regular/295g	145	0.6	49	2.4	9.1	0.2	0.0
Latte, Skimmed, Pret*	1 Serving/285ml	110	4.0	39	2.8	3.7	1.4	0.0
Macchiato, Pret*	1 Serving/60ml	5	0.2	8	0.5	0.8	0.3	0.0
Mocha, Semi Skimmed, Pret*	1 Serving/293ml	175	5.0	60	3.0	8.0	1.7	0.0
Mocha, Skimmed, Pret*	1 Regular/293ml	145	1.4	49	2.9	8.4	0.5	0.0
COOKIES								
Chocolate Chunk, Pret*	1 Cookie/90g	381	13.9	423	5.3	64.6	15.4	2.6
Oat, Apple & Raisin, Pret*	1 Cookie/90g	353	10.3	392	6.3	62.2	11.4	3.1
White Chocolate & Orange, Pret*	1 Cookie/90g	365	11.6	406	5.4	65.7	12.9	2.4
CRISPS								
Croxton Manor Cheese & Red Onion, Pret*	1 Pack/40g	210	12.8	525	6.2	49.8	32.0	5.2
Double Cheddar & Onion Topcorn, Pret*	1 Pack/25g	123	6.5	492	8.0	55.6	26.0	9.6
Kale, Pret*	1 Pack/25g	105	6.6	420	14.4	30.8	26.4	17.2
Maldon Sea Salt Crisps, Pret*	1 Pack/40g	218	14.3	545	5.2	48.0	35.8	5.5
Parsnip, Beetroot & Carrot Crisps, Pret*	1 Pack/25g	120	8.6	480	4.4	38.4	34.4	15.2
Sea Salt & Organic Cider Vinegar Crisps, Pret*	1 Pack/40g	204	12.2	510	5.2	51.8	30.5	5.5
Sweet Potato & Chipotle Chilli Crisps, Pret*	1 Pack/25g	123	8.2	492	5.2	44.8	32.8	9.6

PRET A MANGER

	Measure INFO/WEIGHT	per Measure KCAL	FAT	Nutrition Values per 100g / 100ml KCAL	PROT	CARB	FAT	FIBRE
CROISSANT								
Almond, Pret*	1 Croissant/95g	387	20.1	407	8.7	47.0	21.2	3.5
Chocolate, Pret*	1 Croissant/95g	420	23.2	442	7.7	46.5	24.4	2.9
Egg & Bacon, Pret*	1 Croissant/167g	483	20.1	289	11.3	20.6	12.0	1.8
French, Butter, Pret*	1 Croissant/80g	324	18.9	405	8.2	39.5	23.6	2.4
Ham, Bacon & Cheese, Pret*	1 Croissant/110g	351	22.7	319	12.2	19.8	20.6	1.2
Mozzarella & Tomato, Pret*	1 Croissant/110g	373	24.6	339	13.4	20.2	22.4	1.3
Pain au Raisin, Pret*	1 Croissant/110g	311	13.5	283	5.1	37.4	12.3	1.6
CURRY								
Sweet Potato & Cauli, Quinoa, Rice Pot, Pret*	1 Pot/320g	432	16.2	135	3.3	19.0	5.1	0.5
DRESSING								
for Chef's Italian Chicken Salad, Pret*	1 Pot/45g	231	23.8	513	0.7	8.0	52.9	0.0
for Crayfish & Avocado, Pret*	1 Serving/28g	144	14.8	514	0.7	8.2	52.9	0.0
for Greens & Grains, no Bread, Pret*	1 Pot/45g	41	3.0	91	4.0	3.8	6.7	0.2
for Pole & Line Caught Tuna Nicoise, Pret*	1 Pot/45g	231	23.8	513	0.7	8.0	52.9	0.0
for Roasted Vegetable & Feta, Pret*	1 Pot/45g	231	23.8	513	0.7	8.0	52.9	0.0
for Sesame Chicken & Noodle Salad, Pret*	1 Pot/45g	140	9.8	311	12.0	16.0	21.8	0.0
for Superfood Salad, Pret*	1 Pot/45g	231	23.8	513	0.7	8.0	52.9	0.0
for Teriyaki Salmon Salad, Pret*	1 Pack/28g	46	0.0	164	3.9	36.4	0.1	0.0
FLAT BREAD								
Chipotle Chicken with Avocado, Pret*	1 Pack/326g	567	18.3	174	9.0	20.2	5.6	2.2
Mediterranean Tuna, Pret*	1 Pack/312g	418	4.1	134	11.5	18.9	1.3	1.7
Mexican Avocado, Pret*	1 Pack/325g	487	20.8	150	3.8	17.3	6.4	2.6
Mezze, Pret*	1 Pack/242g	554	27.6	229	7.9	22.8	11.4	4.0
FRUIT								
British Berries, Pret*	1 Pot/130g	34	0.1	26	0.9	5.4	0.1	1.6
Five Berry Bowl, Pret*	1 Bowl/220g	379	12.4	172	6.7	23.3	5.6	1.7
Five Berry Pot, Pret*	1 Pot/148g	152	4.7	103	6.0	12.6	3.2	0.3
Fruit Salad, Pret's, Pret*	1 Serving/180g	106	0.5	59	0.9	12.2	0.3	2.2
Kid's Fruit Pot, Pret*	1 Pot/140g	43	0.1	31	0.5	7.4	0.1	1.0
Mango & Lime, Pret*	1 Serving/150g	91	0.3	61	0.7	13.0	0.2	1.9
Nectarine & Raspberries, Pret*	1 Serving/56g	24	0.1	43	1.4	7.8	0.2	2.7
Pomegranate & Orange, Pret*	1 Serving/116g	54	0.0	47	1.2	10.0	0.0	0.0
Seedless Grapes, Pret*	1 Serving/165g	109	0.0	66	0.4	15.4	0.0	1.0
Strawberries, Coconut & Chocolate, Pret*	1 Serving/125g	194	15.8	155	2.0	8.2	12.6	4.6
Superfruit Bowl, Pret*	1 Serving/155g	71	0.2	46	0.8	11.0	0.1	2.0
Tropical Fruit Sticks, Pret*	1 Serving/200g	78	0.4	39	0.6	8.9	0.2	1.4
FRUIT & NUTS								
Pret a Manger*	1 Bag/40g	175	9.2	438	8.5	46.5	23.0	6.2
GINGER BEER								
Pure Pret, Pret*	1 Serving/330ml	152	0.0	46	0.0	11.4	0.0	0.0
GINGERBREAD								
Godfrey, Pret's Gingerbread Man, Pret*	1 Biscuit/54g	195	7.3	361	4.6	55.4	13.5	1.7
Hansel the Snowman, Pret*	1 Biscuit/48g	206	7.6	429	7.3	64.6	15.8	2.3
HOT CHOCOLATE								
Pret a Manger*	1 Serving/285ml	237	5.9	83	3.4	12.7	2.1	0.0
JUICE								
Apple, Pret*	1 Bottle/250g	120	0.3	48	0.1	11.8	0.1	0.0
Carrot, Pret*	1 Serving/250ml	60	0.3	24	0.5	5.7	0.1	0.0
Green Goodness, Pret*	1 Bottle/400ml	176	0.0	44	0.4	10.7	0.0	0.0
Orange, Freshly Squeezed, Natural, Super, Pret*	1 Bottle/250ml	123	0.3	49	0.6	10.2	0.1	0.1
Orange, Lge, Pret*	1 Serving/500ml	229	0.6	46	0.6	10.2	0.1	0.1
Orange, Pret*	1 Serving/260ml	114	0.0	44	0.6	11.0	0.0	0.1

PRET A MANGER

	Measure INFO/WEIGHT	per Measure KCAL	FAT	Nutrition Values per 100g / 100ml KCAL	PROT	CARB	FAT	FIBRE
JUICE DRINK								
Berry Shot, Pomegranate & Blueberry, Pret*	1 Shot/110ml	55	0.2	50	0.9	10.5	0.2	1.5
Ginseng & Echinacea, Sparking, Yoga Bunny Detox, Pret*	1 Can/330g	132	0.0	40	0.0	9.7	0.0	0.0
Grape & Elderflower, Sparkling, Pure Pret, Pret*	1 Serving/330ml	146	0.0	44	0.0	10.6	0.0	0.0
Mandarin & Lychee, Pure, Still, Pret*	1 Serving/500g	103	0.0	21	0.1	4.9	0.0	0.0
Mango & Passion Fruit, Still, Pret*	1 Bottle/500ml	106	0.0	21	0.0	5.2	0.0	0.0
Orange, Pure Pret, Pret*	1 Serving/330ml	200	0.0	61	0.1	3.1	0.0	0.0
Pomegranate, Still, Pret Pure, Pret*	1 Bottle/500ml	105	0.0	21	0.0	5.1	0.0	0.0
Pure Pret Apple, Pret*	1 Serving/330ml	159	0.0	48	0.1	11.6	0.0	0.0
LEMONADE								
Pink, Pret*	1 Serving/250ml	75	0.0	30	0.1	7.1	0.0	0.0
Still, Pure Pret, Pret*	1 Bottle/500ml	171	0.0	34	0.0	8.3	0.0	0.0
MACARONI CHEESE								
Kale & Cauli, Pret*	1 Portion/360g	451	25.7	125	6.4	8.8	7.1	0.9
Prosciutto, Pret*	1 Pack/360g	488	27.8	136	7.5	8.9	7.7	0.9
MACAROONS								
Coconut in Milk Chocolate, Pret*	1 Pack/108g	523	34.0	484	6.9	40.7	31.5	4.1
MILK SHAKE								
Banana & Cashew, Almond, Dairy Free, Pret*	1 Pack/264g	232	13.4	88	2.6	8.4	5.1	0.0
Cacao & Date, Almond, Dairy Free, Pret*	1 Pack/264g	192	8.7	73	2.6	9.1	3.3	0.0
MOUSSE								
Chocolate, Pret*	1 Pack/306g	1170	117.4	382	3.8	22.2	38.4	1.6
Chocolate Mousse, Pret*	1 Serving/100g	375	29.2	375	3.4	24.6	29.2	1.2
MUFFIN								
Double Berry, Pret*	1 Muffin/145g	498	23.8	343	5.2	44.5	16.4	2.3
High Fibre Muffin, Pret*	1 Muffin/130g	442	24.4	340	8.0	28.6	18.8	9.0
NUTS								
Naked, Pret*	1 Pack/40g	262	23.4	655	17.8	11.2	58.5	6.0
POPCORN								
Bar, Pret*	1 Bar/34g	173	8.9	508	5.8	61.6	26.2	0.0
Chocolate Crackle Topcorn, Pret*	1 Serving/55g	220	8.4	400	5.1	59.6	15.3	7.1
Double Cheese & Onion, Skinny, Topcorn, Pret*	1 Pack/23g	98	3.3	424	10.5	63.2	14.4	12.2
Rock Salt, Light, Pret*	1 Pack/29g	138	7.1	476	6.6	63.8	24.5	15.2
Savoury, Skinny, Topcorn, Pret*	1 Pack/23g	96	3.0	417	9.6	65.3	12.9	12.0
Sweet & Salt, Light, Pret*	1 Pack/30g	138	5.8	460	7.1	64.3	19.3	6.7
Wasabi, Pret*	1 Pack/29g	137	6.4	472	7.2	55.2	22.1	10.7
PRETZELS								
Pret a Manger*	1 Serving/105g	333	7.6	317	8.7	52.8	7.2	3.0
RICE								
Korean BBQ Pulled Pork, Quinoa, Rice Pot, Pret*	1 Pot/320g	468	9.4	146	8.8	21.0	2.9	0.5
RICE CAKES								
Dark Chocolate Coated, Pret*	1 Pack/50g	250	12.0	500	6.0	63.4	24.0	2.8
ROLL								
Focaccia, Ham & Egg, Breakfast, Pret*	1 Muffin/157g	389	18.4	248	14.0	21.7	11.7	1.0
Focaccia, with Bacon, Breakfast, Pret*	1 Muffin/120g	381	21.2	318	15.0	24.9	17.7	1.3
SALAD								
Asian Beef & Noodle, no Dressing, Pret*	1 Pack/266g	309	6.3	116	7.3	16.4	2.4	1.4
Asian Beef & Noodle, with Dressing, Pret*	1 Serving/311g	449	16.1	144	8.0	16.4	5.2	1.2
Beets, Squash & Feta, Superbowl, Pret*	1 Bowl/279g	330	10.3	118	6.1	13.3	3.7	3.4
Chefs Chipotle Chicken, no Dressing, Pret*	1 Pack/308g	301	17.7	98	8.8	2.5	5.7	1.6
Chefs Chipotle Chicken, with Dressing, Pret*	1 Pack/329g	436	32.5	132	8.3	3.0	9.9	1.5
Chicken, Bacon & Avocado with Dressing, Pret*	1 Serving/272g	212	11.3	78	7.6	2.4	4.2	1.8

PRET A MANGER

	Measure INFO/WEIGHT	per Measure KCAL	FAT	Nutrition Values per 100g / 100ml KCAL	PROT	CARB	FAT	FIBRE
SALAD								
Chicken & Broccoli, Super Noodle, Pret*	1 Pack/273g	385	17.5	141	7.6	12.5	6.4	2.1
Chicken & Pasta Salad, Pret*	1 Serving/267g	507	21.9	190	7.4	21.0	8.2	1.3
Chicken Ceasar, Pret*	1 Pack/252g	370	16.0	147	11.9	9.1	6.4	0.8
Chipotle Chicken & Avocado, Superbowl, Pret*	1 Bowl/383g	502	23.4	131	7.1	9.9	6.1	3.6
Crayfish, Mango & Cashew, Superbowl, Pret*	1 Bowl/310g	468	9.0	151	5.8	24.9	2.9	0.5
Crayfish & Avocado, no Bread, Pret*	1 Pack/205g	203	15.0	99	7.1	1.2	7.3	2.1
Crayfish & Quinoa, Protein Pot, Pret*	1 Pack/168g	210	7.4	125	9.4	12.0	4.4	2.0
Crayfish & Thai Noodle Salad, Pret*	1 Serving/239g	174	5.2	73	4.7	8.4	2.2	1.6
Edamame, Bowl, Pret*	1 Pot/125g	94	4.2	75	6.3	4.9	3.4	0.0
Edamame Bowl, Pret*	1 Serving/125g	94	4.2	76	6.3	4.9	3.4	0.0
Greens & Grains, no Bread, no Dressing, Pret*	1 Serving/253g	293	18.5	116	3.6	9.0	7.3	3.0
Hoisin Duck, no Bread, Pret*	1 Pack/202g	138	10.6	68	7.5	7.5	5.2	1.7
Italian Proscuitto & Puy Lentil, no Bread, Pret*	1 Pack/250g	554	18.4	222	14.2	18.2	7.4	3.8
Korean Chicken & Kimchi, Superbowl, Pret*	1 Pack/292g	482	11.4	165	8.9	22.9	3.9	0.8
No Bread, Moroccan Chickpea, Pret*	1 Serving/322g	610	28.0	189	9.1	18.8	8.7	7.5
Pasta & Roasted Nut Pesto, with Dressing, Pret*	1 Pack/223g	622	41.0	279	7.5	20.2	18.4	2.4
Pole & Line Caught Tuna Nicoise, no Dressing, Pret*	1 Serving/275g	168	5.8	61	9.2	1.4	2.1	0.9
Prosciutto, Asparagus & Egg, with Dressing, Pret*	1 Pack/338g	520	36.9	154	6.0	8.0	10.9	1.6
Prosciutto, Egg & Asparagus, no Dressing, Pret*	1 Pack/293g	289	13.1	99	6.8	8.0	4.5	1.8
Roasted Vegetable & Feta, no Dressing, Pret*	1 Pack/285g	187	7.6	66	3.1	6.7	2.7	1.3
Salmon & Baby Kale, Superbowl, no Dressing, Pret*	1 Serving/304g	462	16.1	152	12.4	11.3	5.3	3.7
Sesame Chicken & Noodle, no Dressing, Pret*	1 Pack/293g	323	5.2	110	8.7	14.8	1.8	1.3
Sesame Chicken Sushi, without Dressing, Pret*	1 Pack/238g	273	5.0	115	8.0	15.8	2.1	0.4
Smoke Roast Salmon Salad, Pret*	1 Serving/323g	455	30.5	141	5.8	8.4	9.4	1.6
Smoked Salmon & King Prawn with Potato Salad, Pret*	1 Pack/273g	272	38.0	100	13.0	15.0	13.9	3.6
Superfood, no Dressing, Pret*	1 Serving/337g	375	17.8	111	4.3	11.9	5.3	4.2
Teriyaki Salmon, no Dressing, Pret*	1 Pack/239g	294	7.9	123	9.5	13.6	3.3	0.5
Vietnamese Pulled Pork, Pret*	1 Pack296g	334	14.4	113	5.8	11.3	4.9	1.3
Wiltshire Cured Ham & Potato Salad, Pret*	1 Serving/294g	272	14.2	93	6.4	6.0	4.8	1.1
SANDWICH								
Beech Smoked BLT, Pret*	1 Pack/232g	444	20.0	191	8.4	20.0	8.6	1.9
Bloomer, Naked Avocado, Pret*	1 Pack/225g	460	21.5	204	7.2	21.7	9.6	5.0
Brie, & Cranberry, on Granary Bread, Christmas, Pret*	1 Pack/205g	567	33.3	277	10.2	22.5	16.2	2.5
Chicken, Coronation, & Fruit Chutney, Pret*	1 Pack/290g	529	27.3	182	7.9	16.5	9.4	1.7
Chicken, Ham & Swiss Cheese Club, Pret*	1 Pack/318g	492	20.0	155	11.5	12.9	6.3	1.3
Chicken & Pesto Bloomer, Pret*	1 Pack/273g	477	17.1	175	10.2	18.0	6.3	1.9
Chicken Avocado, Pret*	1 Pack/246g	469	23.4	191	9.7	16.1	9.5	2.7
Chicken Caesar, Slim, Pret*	1 Pack/214g	350	16.7	164	8.5	0.0	7.8	0.0
Christmas Lunch, Pret*	1 Pack/247g	542	23.2	220	11.2	22.9	9.4	2.1
Christmas Lunch, Veggie, Pret*	1 Pack/231g	525	23.1	227	5.9	28.1	10.0	2.8
Classic Ham & Eggs Bloomer, Pret*	1 Pack/225g	547	25.2	243	14.7	20.9	11.2	1.9
Classic Super Club, Pret*	1 Pack/255g	505	24.8	198	11.1	15.7	9.7	1.5
Corned Beef, Bloomer, Pret*	1 Pack/289g	536	21.4	185	10.7	18.5	7.4	1.5
Coronation Turkey, Pret*	1 Pack/290g	477	20.7	164	8.3	16.9	7.1	1.8
Cracking Egg Salad, Pret*	1 Pack/241g	430	23.1	178	7.0	16.2	9.6	1.5
Edam Salad, Pret*	1 Pack/212g	473	26.6	223	8.8	18.7	12.6	1.8
Egg & Tomato, Roasted, Roll, Pret*	1 Roll/163g	346	15.9	212	9.2	21.8	9.8	1.1
Egg Mayo, & Roasted Tomato, Breakfast Roll, Pret*	1 Roll/147g	318	14.5	216	8.4	22.4	9.9	2.0
Eggs Florentine, Bloomer, Pret*	1 Pack/254g	545	26.8	215	9.8	19.4	10.6	2.1
Emmental Cheese Salad, Pret*	1 Pack/239g	494	28.2	207	8.3	16.9	11.8	1.8
Falafel & Humous, Moroccan, Pret*	1 Pack/285g	525	17.6	184	5.8	23.0	6.2	3.3
Free-Range Egg Mayo, Pret*	1 Pack/189g	426	23.5	225	8.9	19.6	12.4	1.6

PRET A MANGER

	Measure INFO/WEIGHT	per Measure KCAL	per Measure FAT	Nutrition Values per 100g / 100ml KCAL	PROT	CARB	FAT	FIBRE
SANDWICH								
Ham, & Pickle, Wiltshire Cured, on Granary, Pret*	1 Pack/240g	367	12.2	153	7.4	18.8	5.1	1.7
Jalapeno, Tomato & Soft Cheese, Bloomer, Pret*	1 Pack/243g	371	9.8	153	6.8	21.9	4.0	2.5
Jambon Beurre,, Pret*	1 Pack/144g	359	13.1	249	11.3	29.6	9.1	1.9
Kid's Cheese Sandwich, Pret*	1 Pack/127g	399	20.2	314	13.9	28.9	15.9	2.2
Kid's Ham Sandwich, Pret*	1 Pack/127g	289	8.2	228	13.4	28.9	6.5	2.2
Kid's Tuna Mayo, Pret*	1 Pack/150g	372	17.3	248	10.9	24.9	11.5	1.9
King Prawn Cocktail, Pret*	1 Pack/199g	362	14.4	182	9.0	19.4	7.2	1.8
Mature Cheddar & Pret Pickle, Pret*	1 Pack/246g	479	24.3	195	7.6	18.4	9.9	1.7
Moroccan Falafel Salad, Pret*	1 Pack/278g	417	8.8	150	5.5	21.2	3.2	1.4
New York on Rye, Pret*	1 Pack/214g	444	20.4	207	11.8	19.9	9.5	2.0
Pole & Line Caught Tuna & Cucumber, Baguette, Pret*	1 Pack/228g	483	20.8	212	10.2	22.0	9.1	1.3
Pole & Line Caught Tuna & Rocket Bloomer, Pret*	1 Pack/233g	552	26.3	237	12.9	21.4	11.3	2.0
Pole & Line Caught Tuna Nicoise on Granary, Pret*	1 Pack/305g	481	24.5	158	7.9	13.4	8.0	1.9
Pret's All Day Breakfast, Pret*	1 Pack/329g	654	37.7	199	9.9	14.1	11.5	1.4
Scottish Smoked Salmon, Pret*	1 Pack/156g	366	14.2	235	14.5	23.6	9.1	1.8
Scottish Smoked Salmon & Soft Cheese Baguette, Pret*	1 Pack/150g	300	7.8	200	12.5	25.1	5.2	1.5
Spring Houmus & Feta, Granary, Pret*	1 Pack/216g	404	17.4	187	7.4	21.5	8.1	3.2
Super Greens, Pret*	1 Pack/239g	389	19.5	163	5.0	17.1	8.2	3.6
The New York Bloomer, Pret*	1 Pack/227g	507	22.0	223	13.0	22.0	9.7	2.2
Wensleydale Cheese & Chutney Bloomer, Pret*	1 Pack/276g	564	26.1	204	9.0	20.9	9.5	2.2
Wild Crayfish & Rocket, Pret*	1 Pack/194g	374	15.0	193	10.6	19.4	7.7	1.5
SMOOTHIE								
Berry Blast, Pret*	1 Pack/362g	186	2.4	51	0.6	10.9	0.7	1.7
Coconut Crush, Pret*	1 Pack/218g	102	2.3	47	0.5	8.6	1.1	1.6
Mango Smoothie, Pret*	1 Serving/250ml	143	0.5	57	0.6	13.7	0.2	3.0
Passion Pop, Pret*	1 Pack/390g	169	0.3	43	0.4	10.1	0.1	0.6
Strawberry Smoothie, Pret*	1 Serving/250ml	128	0.8	51	0.9	11.2	0.3	0.0
Vitamin Volcano Smoothie, Pret*	1 Serving/250ml	138	0.8	55	0.6	12.4	0.3	1.3
SOUP								
Asian Pepper, Pret*	1 Serving/370g	178	9.3	48	0.7	5.3	2.5	0.0
Beef, Ale & Barley, Pret*	1 Serving/370g	230	6.7	62	3.3	6.3	1.8	1.4
Beetroot & Horseradish Soup, Pret*	1 Serving/370g	122	1.9	33	1.2	6.2	0.5	0.0
Broccoli & Italian Cheese, Pret*	1 Pack/370g	226	14.1	61	2.2	3.8	3.8	1.3
Butternut Squash, Spiced, Pret*	1 Serving/380g	171	6.1	45	1.4	6.2	1.6	0.2
Butternut Squash & Sage, Pret*	1 Pot/370g	104	3.0	28	0.9	3.9	0.8	0.0
Butternut Squash & Spinach, Pret*	1 Serving/370g	156	8.9	42	0.8	4.3	2.4	0.9
Carrot, Butternut & Spice, Pret*	1 Pot/370g	199	8.9	54	1.3	6.1	2.4	0.0
Carrot & Coriander Soup, Pret*	1 Serving/370g	181	10.7	49	0.9	4.5	2.9	0.7
Cauliflower Cheese, Pret*	1 Serving/370g	293	13.5	79	3.3	5.2	3.6	1.0
Celeriac & Smoked Pancetta, Pret*	1 Pot/370g	215	15.6	58	2.5	2.1	4.2	0.9
Chicken, Asian, Aromatic, Pret*	1 Pack/370g	199	7.0	54	2.4	6.4	1.9	0.0
Chicken, Broccoli, & Brown Rice, Pret*	1 Serving/370g	134	2.2	36	2.7	4.6	0.6	0.0
Chicken, Cream of, Pret*	1 Carton/370g	292	19.6	79	2.5	5.4	5.3	0.5
Chicken, Edamame Bean & Ginger, Pret*	1 Pack/370g	137	1.9	37	2.4	5.4	0.5	0.0
Chicken & Mushroom Soup, Pret*	1 Serving/370g	269	14.4	73	6.6	2.7	3.9	0.5
Chicken & Roasted Corn, Chowder, Pret*	1 Soup/370g	259	8.9	70	3.5	7.6	2.4	1.0
Garden Pea & Mint, Pret*	1 Pack320g	253	17.6	79	2.4	4.0	5.5	0.0
Gazpacho, Pret*	1 Pack/320g	131	7.5	41	1.2	3.7	2.3	1.1
Ham Hock, Pret*	1 Serving/370g	410	18.9	111	6.0	8.9	5.1	2.6
Italian Meatball Soup, Pret*	1 Serving/370g	263	15.5	71	2.4	5.8	4.2	1.0
Kale & Garden Vegetable, Pret*	1 Pack/370g	229	14.8	62	1.9	3.9	4.0	1.0
Leek & Potato Soup, Pret*	1 Serving/370g	189	9.3	51	1.2	5.5	2.5	0.9

PRET A MANGER

	INFO/WEIGHT	KCAL	FAT	KCAL	PROT	CARB	FAT	FIBRE
SOUP								
Lentil & Coconut Curry, Pret*	1 Pack/370g	403	15.9	109	5.4	11.5	4.3	1.5
Lentil & Quinoa, Pret*	1 Pot/370g	199	6.3	54	1.7	7.0	1.7	0.0
Lentil & Smoked Bacon Soup, Pret*	1 Serving/370g	274	11.5	74	5.9	6.3	3.1	1.2
Malaysian Chicken Curry Soup, Pret*	1 Serving/370g	270	14.8	73	2.7	5.5	4.0	2.0
Mexican Chilli with a Hint of Chocolate, Pret*	1 Pack/370g	344	8.9	93	3.8	12.4	2.4	3.2
Miso Soup, Pret*	1 Serving/20g	32	1.0	160	10.0	0.0	5.0	0.0
Moroccan Chicken Soup, Pret*	1 Serving/370g	304	9.9	82	4.5	8.8	2.7	2.4
Mushroom, Cream of, Pret*	1 Pack/370g	159	8.9	43	1.3	3.2	2.4	0.6
Mushroom Risotto Soup, Pret*	1 Serving/370g	259	13.7	70	2.4	6.4	3.7	0.0
Pea & ham, Pret*	1 Pack/370g	233	10.7	63	4.5	3.8	2.9	2.0
Pork, BBQ, Pulled & Bean, Pret*	1 Pack/370g	341	7.4	92	6.4	10.8	2.0	2.4
Pret's Classic Tomato Soup, Pret*	1 Serving/370g	218	10.7	59	1.8	6.0	2.9	0.8
Red Pepper & Creme Fraiche, Pret*	1 Pack/370g	215	15.2	58	1.1	3.7	4.1	0.9
Sag Aloo, Pret*	1 Serving/375g	245	11.5	65	1.6	7.9	3.1	0.2
Sausage Hot Pot, Pret*	1 Serving/370g	230	13.0	62	4.0	2.6	3.5	2.0
Smoky Root Veg & Bean, Pret*	1 Serving/370g	192	3.0	52	2.3	7.4	0.8	3.2
Spanish Chorizo & Butter Bean Soup, Pret*	1 Serving/370g	233	8.9	63	3.8	6.1	2.4	1.1
Spicy Chicken & Bean, Pret*	1 Pot/370g	281	5.9	76	5.2	8.3	1.6	3.8
Sweet Tomato & Saffron, Pret*	1 Pack/370g	255	14.8	69	1.7	5.9	4.0	0.7
Thai Chicken Curry, Pret*	1 Pack/370g	259	16.7	70	2.7	4.2	4.5	1.1
Thai Corn, Pret*	1 Pack/370ml	213	9.3	58	1.5	7.6	2.5	1.0
Tomato, South Indian, & Spice, Pret*	1 Pack/370g	181	3.3	49	2.6	7.1	0.9	0.0
Tuscan Minestrone, Pret*	1 Pot/370g	203	6.7	55	2.5	7.1	1.8	0.0
SUSHI								
California Rolls, Pret*	1 Pack/206g	354	9.3	172	5.1	27.5	4.5	1.4
Deluxe, Pret*	1 Pack/232g	382	9.3	165	6.2	25.8	4.0	1.3
Deluxe Bento Box, Pret*	1 Serving/256g	353	10.0	138	6.4	19.5	3.9	1.7
Maki & Nigiri, Pret*	1 Serving/200g	314	8.4	157	5.4	23.4	4.2	1.0
Salmon, Prawn & Crab, Pret*	1 Box/230g	359	8.3	156	6.2	23.7	3.6	0.0
Salmon & Prawn Sushi, Pret*	1 Serving/232g	382	9.3	165	6.2	25.8	4.0	1.3
Veggie, Pret*	1 Pack/226g	333	5.8	147	3.6	27.7	2.6	2.0
Veggie, Protein Pot, Pret*	1 Pot/149g	149	6.6	100	5.4	8.2	4.4	2.6
TART								
Pret's Bakewell Tart, Pret*	1 Serving/68g	318	18.1	468	7.6	49.7	26.6	2.5
TEA								
Ceylon, Breakfast, Pret*	1 Serving/360ml	14	0.5	4	0.3	0.4	0.1	0.0
Earl Grey, Black, Pret*	1 Serving/360ml	14	0.5	4	0.3	0.4	0.1	0.0
Pure Pret Still - Peach Iced Tea, Pret*	1 Serving/500ml	78	0.0	16	0.0	3.8	0.0	0.0
Red Berries Tea, Pret*	1 Serving/60ml	0	0.0	0	0.0	0.0	0.0	0.0
Tropical Green Tea, Pret*	1 Serving/60ml	0	0.0	0	0.0	0.0	0.0	0.0
Vanilla Chai, Pret*	1 Cup/360g	14	0.5	4	0.3	0.4	0.1	0.0
TOASTIE								
Brie, Tomato & Basil, Pret*	1 Toastie/209g	451	18.0	216	10.0	23.1	8.6	2.7
Chicken & Bacon, Pret*	1 Pack/254g	533	21.2	210	14.2	19.1	8.4	2.0
Halloumi & Red Pepper, Pret*	1 Pack/233g	543	25.5	233	11.7	21.6	10.9	2.9
Ham, Cheese & Mustard Toastie, Pret*	1 Serving/215g	588	27.6	273	17.8	21.8	12.8	2.0
Italian Mozzarella & Pesto Toastie, Pret*	1 Serving/234g	511	24.3	218	10.3	20.8	10.4	2.2
New York Deli Toastie, Pret*	1 Serving/233g	586	28.0	252	15.2	21.3	12.0	2.4
Tuna Melt Toastie, Pret*	1 Serving/219g	555	24.0	253	16.8	21.5	11.0	2.4
WRAP								
Avocado, Pine Nut, Tomato, Spinach, Basil & Mayo, Pret*	1 Wrap/212.13g	341	2.8	161	3.2	14.5	1.3	3.7
Avocado & Herb Salad, Pret*	1 Wrap/246g	460	30.5	187	4.8	13.6	12.4	2.6

	Measure INFO/WEIGHT	per Measure KCAL	FAT	Nutrition Values per 100g / 100ml KCAL	PROT	CARB	FAT	FIBRE

PRET A MANGER
WRAP

	Measure INFO/WEIGHT	KCAL	FAT	KCAL	PROT	CARB	FAT	FIBRE
Beef Samosa, Hot, Pret*	1 Wrap/235g	531	29.1	226	8.3	20.2	12.4	2.3
Chicken, Harissa, Pret*	1 Pack/214g	427	19.3	200	9.6	18.4	9.0	3.4
Chicken, Jalapeno, Hot, Pret*	1 Wrap/262g	430	14.5	164	12.7	15.1	5.5	1.9
Chicken, Raita, with Salad, Pret*	1 Wrap/233g	314	7.1	135	9.7	16.3	3.0	2.2
Chickpea Salad, Indian Spiced, Pret*	1 Wrap/243g	361	7.5	149	4.9	22.5	3.1	3.7
Coronation Cauliflower, Pret*	1 Wrap/220g	394	20.0	179	4.1	19.6	9.1	3.2
Crayfish, Sweet Chilli, & Salad, Pret*	1 Wrap/223g	282	10.1	126	5.9	15.5	4.5	1.4
Crayfish & Chipotle, Salad, Pret*	1 Wrap/239g	416	18.6	174	5.5	17.7	7.8	3.4
Duck, Hoisin, Pret*	1 Wrap/212g	341	19.5	161	8.4	19.8	9.2	1.5
Falafel & Halloumi, Hot, Pret*	1 Wrap/244g	578	22.8	237	7.4	24.8	9.3	1.7
Guacamole, Mexican, GF, Pret*	1 Pack/234g	389	20.1	166	2.9	17.4	8.6	4.3
Houmous, Chunky, & Salad, Pret*	1 Pack/209g	446	20.9	213	7.2	24.0	10.0	5.8
Houmous, Chunky, & Salad, Pret*	1 Wrap/210g	449	21.0	214	7.2	24.0	10.0	5.8
Meatball, Swedish, Hot, Pret*	1 Wrap/233g	674	41.3	289	14.1	17.9	17.7	1.8
Nori, Super Veg, Pret*	1 Pack/187g	347	13.5	186	5.6	23.5	7.2	0.0
Prawn, Sweet Chilli, & Salad, Pret*	1 Wrap/219g	298	10.3	136	7.7	15.5	4.7	1.5
Salmon, & Salad, O'mega, Pret*	1 Pack/200g	319	13.2	160	9.2	15.8	6.6	1.6

YOGHURT

	Measure INFO/WEIGHT	KCAL	FAT	KCAL	PROT	CARB	FAT	FIBRE
Coconut, Dairy Free, Pot, Pret*	1 Pot/109g	269	27.2	247	3.4	4.1	25.0	0.0
Fruit & Nuts, Greek Style, Yoga Bunny Bowl, Pret*	1 Bowl/238g	265	5.0	111	5.4	18.2	2.1	1.2
Honey & Granola, Greek Style, Pot, Pret*	1 Serving/130g	265	7.8	204	7.2	30.5	6.0	1.4

YOGHURT DRINK

	Measure INFO/WEIGHT	KCAL	FAT	KCAL	PROT	CARB	FAT	FIBRE
Blueberry, Probiotic, Pret*	1 Serving/250ml	185	4.3	74	2.3	12.4	1.7	0.0
Vanilla, Probiotic, Pret*	1 Serving/250ml	203	6.3	81	2.9	9.7	2.5	0.0

STARBUCKS
BAGEL

	Measure INFO/WEIGHT	KCAL	FAT	KCAL	PROT	CARB	FAT	FIBRE
Smoked Salmon with Cream Cheese, Starbucks*	1 Bagel/155g	358	10.7	231	12.4	28.9	6.9	1.6

BARS

	Measure INFO/WEIGHT	KCAL	FAT	KCAL	PROT	CARB	FAT	FIBRE
Chocolate, Dark, Fairtrade, Starbucks*	1 Bar/40g	238	18.5	594	6.7	32.2	46.3	10.7
Chocolate, Milk, Fairtrade, Starbucks*	1 Bar/30g	170	10.9	567	6.2	52.7	36.5	1.9
Cranberry, Pumpkin Seed & Blueberry, Starbucks*	1 Bar/50g	235	12.4	470	12.3	49.5	24.8	1.0
Granola, Starbucks*	1 Bar/80g	350	16.1	435	6.6	56.4	20.0	4.7
Millionaire Shortbread, Starbucks*	1 Bar/80g	399	22.3	499	5.5	57.5	27.9	0.0
Peanut & Cashew, Starbucks*	1 Bar/45g	209	12.4	466	15.7	36.1	27.6	8.2
Raw Raspberry & Nut, Starbucks*	1 Bar/55g	185	4.1	337	6.0	59.6	7.4	6.0
Rocky Road, Starbucks*	1 Bar/75g	401	24.8	535	5.6	56.1	33.1	4.2

BISCUITS

	Measure INFO/WEIGHT	KCAL	FAT	KCAL	PROT	CARB	FAT	FIBRE
Almond Biscotto, Starbucks*	1 Pack/38g	169	6.7	446	10.4	61.6	17.6	11.4
Biscotti, Almond, Starbucks*	1 Biscuit/45g	201	7.9	447	10.3	61.9	17.5	4.5
Dolcetto al Cacao, Starbucks*	1 Pack/28g	148	8.8	530	6.7	54.8	31.6	1.4
Ginger Snaps, Starbucks*	1 Biscuit/25g	115	4.3	459	4.8	70.0	17.3	1.8

BREAD

	Measure INFO/WEIGHT	KCAL	FAT	KCAL	PROT	CARB	FAT	FIBRE
Fruit, Toasted, Luxury, Starbucks*	1 Portion/145g	481	11.6	332	7.5	55.7	8.0	3.4
Pumpkin, Starbucks*	1 Portion/100g	322	11.6	322	5.0	50.4	11.6	1.6

BREAKFAST CEREAL

	Measure INFO/WEIGHT	KCAL	FAT	KCAL	PROT	CARB	FAT	FIBRE
Berry Good Bircher, Starbucks*	1 Pot/190g	251	3.6	132	5.9	21.7	1.9	2.6
Bircher Muesli, Pod Good Food, Starbucks*	1 Pot/220g	249	4.8	113	3.9	19.3	2.2	11.9
Maple & Honey Granola, Topping, Starbucks*	1 Serving/25g	112	4.0	448	9.0	64.5	15.9	5.6
Porridge, Dairy, Starbucks*	1 Serving/230g	244	6.2	106	4.1	17.4	2.7	1.8
Porridge, Soy, Starbucks*	1 Serving/230g	205	4.8	89	4.6	13.9	2.1	2.2
Very Berry Compote, Topping, Starbucks*	1 Serving/50g	59	0.1	119	0.6	29.7	0.2	2.1

	Measure INFO/WEIGHT	per Measure KCAL	FAT	Nutrition Values per 100g / 100ml KCAL	PROT	CARB	FAT	FIBRE
STARBUCKS								
BROWNIES								
Belgian Chocolate, GF, Fairtrade, Starbucks*	1 Cake/71g	300	20.0	425	4.9	37.2	28.3	2.7
Caramel, Pecan, Starbucks*	1 Serving/80g	368	21.0	460	5.6	51.6	26.3	0.0
CAKE								
Carrot, Starbucks*	1 Slice/150g	580	34.5	387	4.7	40.2	23.0	1.0
Chocolate, Layered Fudge & Vanilla Icing, Starbucks*	1 Slice/146g	624	32.1	428	5.9	52.0	22.0	2.9
Chocolate Chilli, Petite, Starbucks*	1 Piece/38g	170	8.7	448	5.3	57.6	22.8	4.4
Chocolate Swirl, Starbucks*	1 Swirl/133g	427	13.6	321	7.2	47.4	10.2	2.6
Cinnamon Swirl, Starbucks*	1 Swirl/146g	472	14.9	323	7.4	49.1	10.2	2.6
Loaf, Banana Nut, Starbucks*	1 Cake/103g	431	25.8	418	6.5	40.5	25.0	2.8
Loaf, Lemon, Starbucks*	1 Cake/86g	365	20.2	424	5.0	47.3	23.5	1.6
Loaf, Raspberry & Coconut, Starbucks*	1 Cake/89g	402	22.8	452	4.5	49.9	25.6	2.1
Loaf Cake Chocolate Hazelnut, Starbucks*	1 Cake/85g	331	20.8	389	4.0	38.4	24.5	3.2
Marshmallow Twizzle, Chocolate, Starbucks*	1 Cake/40g	193	8.6	483	4.4	66.9	21.6	1.8
Marshmallow Twizzle, Red White & Blue, Starbucks*	1 Cake/35g	147	4.9	421	4.4	68.8	13.9	1.6
Pumpkin, Loaf, Starbucks*	1 Slice/102g	381	19.0	374	4.8	42.0	18.7	0.5
Rocky Road, Starbucks*	1 Cake/78g	423	27.1	542	4.3	51.5	34.8	2.7
Strawberry Shortcake, Petites, Starbucks*	1 Cake/41g	207	11.3	501	4.7	60.2	27.4	2.5
COFFEE								
Americano, Grande, Starbucks*	1 Grande/454ml	17	0.0	4	0.2	0.7	0.0	0.0
Americano, Short, Starbucks*	1 Short/227ml	6	0.0	3	0.2	0.4	0.0	0.0
Americano, Tall, Starbucks*	1 Tall/340ml	11	0.0	3	0.2	0.6	0.0	0.0
Americano, Venti, Starbucks*	1 Venti/568ml	23	0.0	4	0.2	0.7	0.0	0.0
Cappuccino, Grande, Semi Skimmed, Starbucks*	1 Grande/454ml	115	4.1	25	1.7	2.6	0.9	0.0
Cappuccino, Grande, Skimmed, Starbucks*	1 Grande/454ml	82	0.2	18	1.7	2.7	0.0	0.0
Cappuccino, Grande, Soy, Starbucks*	1 Grande/454ml	92	3.2	20	1.4	1.9	0.7	0.2
Cappuccino, Grande, Whole, Starbucks*	1 Grande/454ml	136	6.8	30	1.6	2.5	1.5	0.0
Cappuccino, Short, Semi Skimmed, Starbucks*	1 Short/227ml	78	2.8	34	2.2	3.4	1.2	0.0
Cappuccino, Short, Skimmed, Starbucks*	1 Short/227ml	55	0.1	24	2.3	3.6	0.0	0.0
Cappuccino, Short, Soy, Starbucks*	1 Short/227ml	62	2.2	27	1.9	2.4	1.0	0.3
Cappuccino, Short, Whole, Starbucks*	1 Short/227ml	92	4.7	41	2.2	3.3	2.1	0.0
Cappuccino, Tall, Semi Skimmed, Starbucks*	1 Tall/340ml	97	3.4	29	1.9	3.0	1.0	0.0
Cappuccino, Tall, Skimmed, Starbucks*	1 Tall/340ml	70	0.1	21	1.9	3.1	0.0	0.0
Cappuccino, Tall, Soy, Starbucks*	1 Tall/340ml	727	24.7	22	1.5	2.1	0.7	0.2
Cappuccino, Tall, Whole, Starbucks*	1 Tall/340ml	116	5.6	34	1.8	3.0	1.6	0.0
Cappuccino, Venti, Semi Skimmed, Starbucks*	1 Venti/568ml	161	5.7	28	1.9	3.0	1.0	0.0
Cappuccino, Venti, Skimmed, Starbucks*	1 Venti/568ml	115	0.2	20	1.9	3.0	0.0	0.0
Cappuccino, Venti, Soy, Starbucks*	1 Venti/568ml	123	4.2	22	1.5	2.0	0.7	0.2
Cappuccino, Venti, Whole, Starbucks*	1 Venti/568ml	192	9.3	34	1.8	3.0	1.6	0.0
Caramel Macchiato, Short, Soy, Starbucks*	1 Short/227ml	104	3.0	46	2.0	6.1	1.3	0.3
Caramel Macchiato, Short, Whole, Starbucks*	1 Short/227g	137	5.7	60	2.3	7.1	2.5	0.0
Chocolate Mocha Flavour, Discoveries, Starbucks*	1 Cup/220ml	139	3.5	63	2.9	9.4	1.6	0.0
Espresso, Con Panna, Doppio, Starbucks*	1 Doppio/60ml	36	0.9	60	4.2	4.5	1.5	0.0
Espresso, Con Panna, Solo, Starbucks*	1 Solo/30g	30	0.5	103	8.3	5.7	1.7	0.0
Espresso, Doppio, Starbucks*	1 Doppio/60ml	11	0.7	18	0.0	3.3	1.2	0.0
Espresso, Solo, Starbucks*	1 Solo/30ml	6	0.0	20	0.0	0.0	0.0	0.0
Espresso Macchiato, Doppio, Soy, Starbucks*	1 Doppio/60ml	14	0.1	22	1.5	3.3	0.2	0.0
Espresso Macchiato, Doppio, Whole, Starbucks*	1 Doppio/60ml	15	0.2	24	1.5	3.8	0.3	0.0
Espresso Macchiato, Doppio, Semi Skim, Starbucks*	1 Doppio/60ml	14	0.1	23	1.5	3.8	0.2	0.0
Espresso Macchiato, Doppio, Skimmed, Starbucks*	1 Doppio/60ml	13	0.0	22	1.7	4.0	0.0	0.0
Espresso Macchiato, Doppio, Soy, Starbucks*	1 Doppio/60g	13	0.9	22	0.0	3.3	1.5	0.0
Espresso Macchiato, Doppio, Whole, Starbucks*	1 Doppio/60g	15	0.9	25	0.3	3.8	1.5	0.0
Espresso Macchiato, Solo, Semi Skim, Starbucks*	1 Solo/30ml	8	0.1	27	1.7	4.0	0.3	0.0

STARBUCKS
COFFEE

INFO/WEIGHT	Measure	per Measure KCAL	FAT	KCAL	PROT	CARB	FAT	FIBRE
Espresso Macchiato, Solo, Skimmed, Starbucks*	1 Solo/30ml	7	0.0	23	1.7	4.0	0.0	0.0
Espresso Macchiato, Solo, Soy, Starbucks*	1 Solo/30g	7	0.5	23	0.3	3.7	1.7	0.0
Espresso Macchiato, Solo, Whole, Starbucks*	1 Solo/30ml	8	0.2	27	1.7	4.0	0.7	0.0
Filter, Grande, Starbucks*	1 Grande/454ml	5	0.1	1	0.0	0.0	0.0	0.0
Filter, Short, Starbucks*	1 Short/227ml	3	0.3	1	0.0	0.0	0.1	0.0
Filter, Tall, Starbucks*	1 Tall/340ml	4	0.1	1	0.0	0.0	0.0	0.0
Filter, Venti, Starbucks*	1 Venti/568ml	6	0.1	1	0.0	0.0	0.0	0.0
Flat White, Short, as Standard, Whole, Starbucks*	1 Short/227ml	119	5.8	52	2.9	4.4	2.6	0.0
Green, Very Berry Hibiscus, Cool, Grande, Starbucks*	1 Grande/454ml	70	0.0	15	0.0	3.7	0.0	0.2
Green, Very Berry Hibiscus, Cool, Tall, Starbucks*	1 Tall/340ml	60	0.0	18	0.0	4.1	0.0	0.3
Green, Very Berry Hibiscus, Cool, Trenta, Starbucks*	1 Trenta/880ml	120	0.0	14	0.0	3.3	0.0	0.1
Iced, Caffe Americano, Grande, Starbucks*	1 Grande/454ml	17	0.0	4	0.2	0.7	0.0	0.0
Iced, Caffe Americano, Tall, Starbucks*	1 Tall/340ml	11	0.0	3	0.2	0.6	0.0	0.0
Iced, Caffe Americano, Venti, Starbucks*	1 Venti/568ml	23	0.0	4	0.2	0.7	0.0	0.0
Iced, Caffe Mocha, & Whip, Grande, Semi Skim, Starbucks*	1 Grande/454ml	316	16.8	70	2.1	8.5	3.7	0.4
Iced, Caffe Mocha, & Whip, Grande, Skim, Starbucks*	1 Grande/454ml	289	13.6	64	2.1	8.6	3.0	0.4
Iced, Caffe Mocha, & Whip, Grande, Soy, Starbucks*	1 Grande/454ml	300	16.1	66	1.9	8.0	3.6	0.6
Iced, Caffe Mocha, & Whip, Grande, Whole, Starbucks*	1 Grande/454ml	333	18.9	73	2.0	8.4	4.2	0.4
Iced, Caffe Mocha, & Whip, Tall, Semi Skim, Starbucks*	1 Tall/335ml	225	11.8	67	1.9	8.4	3.5	0.4
Iced, Caffe Mocha, & Whip, Tall, Skim, Starbucks*	1 Tall/335ml	208	9.8	62	2.0	8.5	2.9	0.4
Iced, Caffe Mocha, & Whip, Tall, Whole, Starbucks*	1 Tall/335ml	236	13.1	71	1.9	8.4	3.9	0.4
Iced, Caffe Mocha, & Whip, Venti, Semi Skim, Starbucks*	1 Venti/568ml	340	17.0	60	1.7	7.9	3.0	0.4
Iced, Caffe Mocha, & Whip, Venti, Skimmed, Starbucks*	1 Venti/568ml	315	14.1	55	1.8	8.0	2.5	0.4
Iced, Caffe Mocha, & Whip, Venti, Soy, Starbucks*	1 Venti/568ml	325	16.4	57	1.6	7.5	2.9	0.5
Iced, Caffe Mocha, & Whip, Venti, Whole, Starbucks*	1 Venti/568ml	357	19.0	63	1.7	7.9	3.4	0.4
Iced, Caramel Macchiato, Grande, Semi Skim, Starbucks*	1 Grande/454ml	231	6.3	51	2.1	7.4	1.4	0.0
Iced, Caramel Macchiato, Grande, Skimmed, Starbucks*	1 Grande/454ml	188	1.3	41	2.2	7.5	0.3	0.0
Iced, Caramel Macchiato, Grande, Soy, Starbucks*	1 Grande/454ml	206	5.3	45	1.9	6.5	1.2	0.2
Iced, Caramel Macchiato, Grande, Whole, Starbucks*	1 Grande/454ml	257	9.8	57	2.1	7.3	2.2	0.0
Iced, Caramel Macchiato, Tall, Semi Skim, Starbucks*	1 Tall/340ml	146	3.7	43	1.6	6.7	1.1	0.0
Iced, Caramel Macchiato, Tall, Skimmed, Starbucks*	1 Tall/340ml	124	1.1	36	1.6	6.7	0.3	0.0
Iced, Caramel Macchiato, Tall, Soy, Starbucks*	1 Tall/340ml	134	3.3	39	1.4	6.1	1.0	0.2
Iced, Caramel Macchiato, Tall, Whole, Starbucks*	1 Tall/340ml	161	5.5	47	1.5	6.7	1.6	0.0
Iced, Caramel Macchiato, Venti, Semi Skim, Starbucks*	1 Venti/568ml	221	5.0	39	1.4	6.4	0.9	0.0
Iced, Caramel Macchiato, Venti, Skimmed, Starbucks*	1 Venti/568ml	189	1.2	33	1.4	6.4	0.2	0.0
Iced, Caramel Macchiato, Venti, Soy, Starbucks*	1 Venti/568ml	201	4.2	35	1.2	5.8	0.7	0.1
Iced, Caramel Macchiato, Venti, Whole, Starbucks*	1 Venti/568ml	243	7.5	43	1.3	6.4	1.3	0.0
Iced, Grande, Starbucks*	1 Grande/454ml	4	0.1	1	0.1	0.0	0.0	0.0
Iced, Tall, Starbucks*	1 Tall/340ml	3	0.1	1	0.1	0.0	0.0	0.0
Iced, Venti, Starbucks*	1 Venti/591ml	5	0.1	1	0.1	0.0	0.0	0.0
Iced, Venti, Starbucks*	1 Venti/568ml	5	0.1	1	0.1	0.0	0.0	0.0
Iced Caffe Latte, Grande, Semi Skimmed, Starbucks*	1 Grande/454ml	126	4.5	28	1.8	2.8	1.0	0.0
Iced Caffe Latte, Grande, Skimmed, Starbucks*	1 Grande/454ml	90	0.2	20	1.9	3.0	0.0	0.0
Iced Caffe Latte, Grande, Soy, Starbucks*	1 Grande/454ml	104	3.6	23	1.6	2.1	0.8	0.2
Iced Caffe Latte, Grande, Whole, Starbucks*	1 Grande/454ml	149	7.5	33	1.8	2.7	1.6	0.0
Iced Caffe Latte, Tall, Semi Skimmed, Starbucks*	1 Tall/340ml	87	3.0	26	1.7	2.7	0.9	0.0
Iced Caffe Latte, Tall, Skimmed, Starbucks*	1 Tall/340ml	63	0.1	19	1.7	2.8	0.0	0.0
Iced Caffe Latte, Tall, Soy, Starbucks*	1 Tall/340ml	71	2.4	21	1.4	2.0	0.7	0.2
Iced Caffe Latte, Tall, Whole, Starbucks*	1 Tall/334ml	104	4.9	31	1.6	2.7	1.4	0.0
Iced Caffe Latte, Venti, Semi Skimmed, Starbucks*	1 Venti/568ml	132	4.6	23	1.5	2.5	0.8	0.0
Iced Caffe Latte, Venti, Skimmed, Starbucks*	1 Venti/568ml	95	0.2	17	1.6	2.5	0.0	0.0
Iced Caffe Latte, Venti, Soy, Starbucks*	1 Venti/568ml	109	3.7	19	1.3	1.8	0.6	0.2

STARBUCKS
COFFEE

INFO/WEIGHT	Measure	per Measure		Nutrition Values per 100g / 100ml				
		KCAL	FAT	KCAL	PROT	CARB	FAT	FIBRE
Iced Caffe Latte, Venti, Whole, Starbucks*	1 Venti/568ml	158	7.5	28	1.5	2.5	1.3	0.0
Iced Cappuccino, Grande, Semi Skimmed, Starbucks*	1 Grande/454ml	130	4.7	29	1.9	2.9	1.0	0.0
Iced Cappuccino, Grande, Skimmed, Starbucks*	1 Grande/454ml	92	0.2	20	1.9	3.0	0.0	0.0
Iced Cappuccino, Grande, Soy, Starbucks*	1 Grande/454ml	111	4.0	24	1.7	2.2	0.9	0.2
Iced Cappuccino, Grande, Whole, Starbucks*	1 Grande/4543ml	156	7.8	34	1.8	2.9	1.7	0.0
Iced Cappuccino, Tall, Semi Skimmed, Starbucks*	1 Tall/340ml	94	3.3	28	1.8	2.9	1.0	0.0
Iced Cappuccino, Tall, Skimmed, Starbucks*	1 Tall/340ml	68	0.1	20	1.8	3.0	0.0	0.0
Iced Cappuccino, Tall, Whole, Starbucks*	1 Tall/340ml	113	5.4	33	1.8	2.9	1.6	0.0
Iced Cappuccino, Venti, Semi Skimmed, Starbucks*	1 Venti/568ml	141	4.9	25	1.6	2.6	0.9	0.0
Iced Cappuccino, Venti, Skimmed, Starbucks*	1 Venti/568ml	101	0.2	18	1.6	2.7	0.0	0.0
Iced Cappuccino, Venti, Soy, Starbucks*	1 Venti/568ml	116	3.9	20	1.4	1.9	0.7	0.2
Iced Cappuccino, Venti, Whole, Starbucks*	1 Venti/568ml	168	8.1	30	1.6	2.6	1.4	0.0
Latte, Coconut Milk, Tall, Starbucks*	1 Tall/340g	121	8.0	36	0.0	3.4	2.4	0.3
Latte, Eggnog, Starbucks*	1 Tall/340ml	182	7.2	54	0.7	6.7	2.1	0.0
Latte, Grande, Coconut Milk, Starbucks*	1 Grande/454g	163	10.2	36	0.0	3.4	2.2	0.3
Latte, Grande, Semi Skimmed, Starbucks*	1 Grande/454ml	188	7.0	41	2.7	4.1	1.5	0.0
Latte, Grande, Skimmed, Starbucks*	1 Grande/454ml	131	0.3	29	2.8	4.3	0.1	0.0
Latte, Grande, Soy, Starbucks*	1 Grande/454ml	148	5.3	33	2.3	2.8	1.2	0.3
Latte, Grande, Whole, Starbucks*	1 Grande/454ml	223	11.5	49	2.7	3.9	2.5	0.0
Latte, Pumpkin Spice, Whipped Cream, Short, Starbucks*	1 Short/227ml	172	8.2	76	2.9	7.4	3.6	0.0
Latte, Pumpkin Spice, Whipped Cream, Starbucks*	1 Grande/454ml	311	13.3	68	2.8	7.2	2.9	0.0
Latte, Pumpkin Spice, Whipped Cream, Tall, Starbucks*	1 Tall/340ml	249	11.1	73	3.1	7.4	3.3	0.0
Latte, Pumpkin Spice, Whipped Cream, Venti, Starbucks*	1 Venti/568ml	380	15.3	67	3.0	7.3	2.7	0.0
Latte, Short, Coconut Milk, Starbucks*	1 Short/227g	81	5.5	36	0.0	3.4	2.4	0.3
Latte, Short, Semi Skimmed, Starbucks*	1 Short/227ml	95	3.5	42	2.8	4.1	1.5	0.0
Latte, Short, Skimmed, Starbucks*	1 Short/227ml	67	0.1	30	2.8	4.4	0.0	0.0
Latte, Short, Soy, Starbucks*	1 Short/227ml	75	2.7	33	2.3	2.9	1.2	0.3
Latte, Short, Whole, Starbucks*	1 Short/227ml	113	5.6	50	2.7	4.0	2.5	0.0
Latte, Skimmed, Tall, Starbucks*	1 Tall/340ml	102	0.2	30	2.9	4.4	0.1	0.0
Latte, Skinny, Iced, Discoveries, Starbucks*	1 Pot/220g	101	2.0	46	2.8	5.3	0.9	0.0
Latte, Soy, Tall, Starbucks*	1 Tall/340ml	110	4.0	32	2.3	2.9	1.2	0.3
Latte, Tall, Semi Skimmed, Starbucks*	1 Tall/340ml	143	5.1	42	2.8	4.4	1.5	0.0
Latte, Tall, Whole, Starbucks*	1 Tall/340ml	172	8.4	51	2.7	4.4	2.5	0.0
Latte, Venti, Coconut, Starbucks*	1 Venti/568g	204	14.6	36	2.4	3.4	2.6	0.3
Latte, Venti, Semi Skimmed, Starbucks*	1 Venti/568ml	248	9.2	44	2.9	4.4	1.6	0.0
Latte, Venti, Skimmed, Starbucks*	1 Venti/568ml	174	0.4	31	2.9	4.4	0.1	0.0
Latte, Venti, Soy, Starbucks*	1 Venti/568ml	185	6.7	33	2.2	2.9	1.2	0.3
Latte, Venti, Whole, Starbucks*	1 Venti/568ml	299	15.0	53	2.8	4.4	2.6	0.0
Macchiato, Caramel, Grande, Semi Skim, Starbucks*	1 Grande/454ml	240	6.7	53	2.3	7.5	1.5	0.0
Macchiato, Caramel, Grande, Skimmed, Starbucks*	1 Grande/454ml	191	1.1	42	2.4	7.7	0.2	0.0
Macchiato, Caramel, Grande, Whole, Starbucks*	1 Grande/454ml	269	10.5	59	2.3	7.4	2.3	0.0
Macchiato, Caramel, Short, Semi Skimmed, Starbucks*	1 Short/227ml	122	3.8	54	2.4	7.2	1.7	0.0
Macchiato, Caramel, Short, Skimmed, Starbucks*	1 Short/227ml	97	0.9	43	2.5	7.4	0.4	0.0
Macchiato, Caramel, Tall, Semi Skimmed, Starbucks*	1 Tall/340ml	209	6.3	61	2.9	8.3	1.8	0.0
Macchiato, Caramel, Tall, Skimmed, Starbucks*	1 Tall/340ml	165	1.0	49	3.0	8.4	0.3	0.0
Macchiato, Caramel, Tall, Soy, Starbucks*	1 Tall/340ml	167	4.6	49	2.2	6.8	1.4	0.3
Macchiato, Caramel, Tall, Whole, Starbucks*	1 Tall/340ml	240	9.8	71	2.8	8.3	2.9	0.0
Macchiato, Caramel, Venti, Semi Skimmed, Starbucks*	1 Venti/568ml	329	9.3	58	2.7	8.2	1.6	0.0
Macchiato, Caramel, Venti, Skimmed, Starbucks*	1 Venti/568ml	261	1.2	46	2.7	8.3	0.2	0.0
Macchiato, Caramel, Venti, Soy, Starbucks*	1 Venti/568ml	280	7.4	49	2.2	6.9	1.3	0.3
Macchiato, Caramel, Venti, Whole, Starbucks*	1 Venti/568ml	376	14.6	66	2.6	8.2	2.6	0.0
Misto, Grande, Semi Skimmed, Starbucks*	1 Grande/454ml	106	4.1	23	1.6	2.1	0.9	0.0

STARBUCKS

COFFEE

	Measure INFO/WEIGHT	per Measure KCAL	FAT	Nutrition Values per 100g / 100ml KCAL	PROT	CARB	FAT	FIBRE
Misto, Grande, Skimmed, Starbucks*	1 Grande/454ml	73	0.2	16	1.6	2.3	0.0	0.0
Misto, Grande, Soy, Starbucks*	1 Grande/454g	82	3.2	18	1.3	1.4	0.7	0.2
Misto, Grande, Whole, Starbucks*	1 Grande/454ml	126	6.8	28	1.5	2.1	1.5	0.0
Misto, Short, Semi Skimmed, Starbucks*	1 Short/227ml	54	2.1	24	1.6	2.2	0.9	0.0
Misto, Short, Skimmed, Starbucks*	1 Short/227g	37	0.1	16	1.6	2.3	0.0	0.0
Misto, Short, Soy, Starbucks*	1 Short/227g	42	1.6	18	1.3	1.4	0.7	0.2
Misto, Short, Whole, Starbucks*	1 Short/227ml	65	3.5	29	1.6	2.1	1.5	0.0
Misto, Tall, Semi Skimmed, Starbucks*	1 Tall/340ml	81	3.2	24	1.6	2.2	0.9	0.0
Misto, Tall, Skimmed, Starbucks*	1 Tall/340g	56	0.2	16	1.6	2.3	0.1	0.0
Misto, Tall, Soy, Starbucks*	1 Tall/340g	63	2.4	19	1.4	1.3	0.7	0.2
Misto, Tall, Whole, Starbucks*	1 Tall/340g	97	5.2	29	1.6	2.1	1.5	0.0
Misto, Venti, Semi Skimmed, Starbucks*	1 Venti/5568ml	134	5.2	24	1.6	2.2	0.9	0.0
Misto, Venti, Skimmed, Starbucks*	1 Venti/568ml	92	0.3	16	1.6	2.3	0.0	0.0
Misto, Venti, Soy, Starbucks*	1 Venti/568ml	104	4.0	18	1.3	1.4	0.7	0.2
Misto, Venti, Whole, Starbucks*	1 Venti/568g	160	8.6	28	1.6	2.1	1.5	0.0
Mocha, & Whip Cream, Grande, Semi Skim, Starbucks*	1 Grande/454ml	335	15.0	74	2.9	9.4	3.3	0.4
Mocha, & Whip Cream, Grande, Skimmed, Starbucks*	1 Grande/454ml	288	9.5	63	3.0	9.6	2.1	0.4
Mocha, & Whip Cream, Grande, Soy, Starbucks*	1 Grande/454ml	302	13.7	67	2.6	8.5	3.0	0.7
Mocha, & Whip Cream, Grande, Whole, Starbucks*	1 Grande/454ml	364	18.7	80	2.9	9.4	4.1	0.4
Mocha, & Whip Cream, Short, Semi Skim, Starbucks*	1 Short/227ml	184	9.1	81	3.0	9.7	4.0	0.4
Mocha, & Whip Cream, Short, Skim, Starbucks*	1 Short/227ml	160	6.4	70	3.0	9.9	2.8	0.4
Mocha, & Whip Cream, Short, Soy, Starbucks*	1 Short/227ml	167	8.5	74	2.6	8.7	3.7	0.7
Mocha, & Whip Cream, Short, Whole, Starbucks*	1 Short/227ml	198	11.0	87	2.9	9.6	4.8	0.4
Mocha, & Whip Cream, Tall, Semi Skim, Starbucks*	1 Tall/340ml	225	11.8	66	1.9	8.3	3.5	0.4
Mocha, & Whip Cream, Tall, Skim, Starbucks*	1 Tall/340ml	208	9.8	61	2.1	8.5	2.9	0.4
Mocha, & Whip Cream, Tall, Soy, Starbucks*	1 Tall/340ml	214	11.3	63	1.8	7.8	3.3	0.5
Mocha, & Whip Cream, Tall, Whole, Starbucks*	1 Tall/340ml	236	13.1	69	1.8	8.3	3.8	0.4
Mocha, & Whip Cream, Venti, Semi Skim, Starbucks*	1 Venti/568ml	417	17.7	73	2.8	9.6	3.1	0.4
Mocha, & Whip Cream, Venti, Skimmed, Starbucks*	1 Venti/568ml	359	10.9	63	2.9	9.7	1.9	0.4
Mocha, & Whip Cream, Venti, Soy, Starbucks*	1 Venti/568ml	373	15.8	66	2.6	8.7	2.8	0.7
Mocha, & Whip Cream, Venti, Whole, Starbucks*	1 Venti/568ml	456	22.3	80	2.8	9.6	3.9	0.4
Mocha, no Cream, Non Fat Milk, Venti, Skinny, Starbucks*	1 Venti/591ml	280	3.0	47	2.9	9.1	0.5	0.0
Mocha, White Choc, Whipped Cream, Skim, Starbucks*	1 Tall/340ml	327	10.4	96	3.4	14.2	3.1	0.0
Mocha, White Choc, Whipped Cream, Skim, Starbucks*	1 Venti/568ml	515	14.3	91	3.3	14.0	2.5	0.0
Mocha, White Choc, Whipped Cream, Soy, Starbucks*	1 Grande/454ml	439	17.0	97	2.9	12.8	3.7	0.2
Mocha, White Choc, Whipped Cream, Soy, Starbucks*	1 Short/227ml	236	10.1	104	3.0	13.0	4.4	0.3
Mocha, White Choc, Whipped Cream, Soy, Starbucks*	1 Tall/340ml	465	20.4	137	4.9	15.9	6.0	0.2
Mocha, White Choc, Whipped Cream, Soy, Starbucks*	1 Venti/568ml	531	19.5	93	2.9	12.8	3.4	0.2
Mocha, White Choc, Whipped Cream, Whole, Starbucks*	1 Grande/454ml	500	22.1	110	3.2	13.7	4.9	0.0
Mocha, White Choc, Whipped Cream, Whole, Starbucks*	1 Short/227ml	267	12.7	118	3.3	13.9	5.6	0.0
Mocha, White Choc, Whipped Cream, Whole, Starbucks*	1 Tall/340ml	385	17.1	113	3.2	14.0	5.0	0.0
Mocha, White Choc, Whipped Cream, Whole, Starbucks*	1 Venti/568ml	613	25.8	108	3.2	13.9	4.5	0.0
Mocha Chocolate Frappuccino, Bottle, Starbucks*	1 Bottle/250ml	160	3.0	64	2.9	10.0	1.2	0.0
Refresha, Cool Lime, Grande, Starbucks*	1 Grande/454ml	71	0.0	16	0.0	3.9	0.0	0.0
Refresha, Cool Lime, Tall, Starbucks*	1 Tall/340ml	53	0.0	16	0.0	4.0	0.0	0.0
Refresha, Cool Lime, Trenta, Starbucks*	1 Trenta/918ml	100	0.0	11	0.0	2.7	0.0	0.0
Refresha, Cool Lime, Venti, Starbucks*	1 Venti/568ml	89	0.0	16	0.0	3.9	0.0	0.0
Refresha, Valencia Orange, Grande, Starbucks*	1 Grande/473ml	71	0.0	15	0.0	3.8	0.0	0.0
Refresha, Valencia Orange, Short, Starbucks*	1 Short/236ml	63	0.0	27	0.0	5.9	0.0	0.0
Refresha, Valencia Orange, Tall, Starbucks*	1 Tall/254ml	93	0.0	37	0.0	7.9	0.0	0.0
Refresha, Valencia Orange, Venti, Starbucks*	1 Venti/200ml	51	0.0	26	0.0	5.6	0.0	0.0
Seattle Latte, Iced, Short, Discoveries, Starbucks*	1 Latte/220ml	154	5.7	70	2.8	9.1	2.6	0.0

STARBUCKS

	INFO/WEIGHT	KCAL	FAT	KCAL	PROT	CARB	FAT	FIBRE
COOKIES								
Chocolate, Milk, Chunk, Starbucks*	1 Cookie/79g	372	18.1	471	6.4	58.3	22.9	2.8
Chocolate Sandwich, Starbucks*	1 Cookie/72g	351	18.1	487	4.5	59.1	25.1	3.5
Fruit & Oat, Starbucks*	1 Cookie/50g	216	8.8	433	4.4	64.3	17.6	3.1
Nutella & Oat, Starbucks*	1 Cookie/82g	383	18.2	467	6.3	58.7	22.2	3.5
Salted Caramel, Starbucks*	1 Cookie/79g	346	13.3	438	5.4	64.9	16.9	2.4
CRISPS								
Sea Salt & Cider Vinegar, Potato Chips, Starbucks*	1 Pack/50g	248	14.2	496	6.2	54.2	28.3	4.3
CROISSANT								
Almond, Starbucks*	1 Croissant/127g	525	26.2	413	6.3	49.7	20.6	2.0
Butter Croissant, Starbucks*	1 Croissant/70g	272	16.5	389	5.9	37.1	23.6	1.1
Cheese & Mushroom, Starbucks*	1 Croissant/166g	519	35.2	313	7.9	21.9	21.2	1.9
Ham & Cheese, Starbucks*	1 Croissant/161g	493	25.0	306	13.9	27.1	15.5	1.5
DOUGHNUTS								
Apple Fritter, Starbucks*	1 Doughnut/115g	473	24.3	411	6.0	47.5	21.1	3.1
FLATBREAD								
Chicken, Chorizo & Egg, Starbucks*	1 Flatbread/197g	447	16.3	227	6.7	26.8	8.3	3.3
Lamb Kofte, Starbucks*	1 Flatbread/234g	531	14.3	227	8.1	34.1	6.1	1.9
Mumbai Spiced, Starbucks*	1 Flatbread/218g	510	17.4	234	5.6	33.9	8.0	2.1
FRAPPUCCINO								
Caramel, no Whip, Grande, Skimmed, Starbucks*	1 Grande/454ml	232	1.9	51	0.8	11.0	0.4	0.0
Caramel, no Whip, Light, Grande, Skimmed, Starbucks*	1 Grande/454ml	134	0.1	30	0.7	6.6	0.0	0.0
Caramel, no Whip, Light, Venti, Skimmed, Starbucks*	1 Venti/568ml	166	0.1	29	0.7	6.4	0.0	0.0
Caramel, no Whip, Tall, Skimmed, Starbucks*	1 Tall/340ml	96	0.1	28	0.7	6.2	0.0	0.1
Caramel Cream, with Whip, Grande, Semi Skim, Starbucks*	1 Grande/454ml	338	14.4	74	1.1	10.5	3.2	0.0
Caramel Cream, with Whip, Grande, Skim, Starbucks*	1 Grande/4540ml	317	11.9	70	1.1	10.6	2.6	0.0
Caramel Cream, with Whip, Grande, Soy, Starbucks*	1 Grande/454ml	325	13.9	72	1.0	10.1	3.1	0.1
Caramel Cream, with Whip, Grande, Whole, Starbucks*	1 Grande/454ml	351	16.0	77	10.8	10.5	3.5	0.0
Caramel Cream, with Whip, Tall, Semi Skim, Starbucks*	1 Tall/340ml	255	10.7	75	1.2	10.6	3.2	0.0
Caramel Cream, with Whip, Tall, Skimmed, Starbucks*	1 Tall/340ml	238	8.7	70	1.2	10.7	2.6	0.0
Caramel Cream, with Whip, Tall, Skimmed, Starbucks*	1 Tall/340ml	226	8.7	66	1.4	10.3	2.6	0.2
Caramel Cream, with Whip, Tall, Soy, Starbucks*	1 Tall/340ml	243	10.3	71	1.0	10.1	3.0	0.2
Caramel Cream, with Whip, Tall, Whole, Starbucks*	1 Tall/340ml	265	12.1	78	1.2	10.5	3.6	0.0
Caramel Cream, with Whip, Venti, Semi Skim, Starbucks*	1 Venti/568ml	393	14.0	69	1.0	10.8	2.5	0.0
Caramel Cream, with Whip, Venti, Skimmed, Starbucks*	1 Venti/568ml	368	11.0	65	1.1	10.9	1.9	0.0
Caramel Cream, with Whip, Venti, Soy, Starbucks*	1 Venti/568ml	377	13.4	66	0.9	10.4	2.4	0.1
Caramel Cream, with Whip, Venti, Whole, Starbucks*	1 Venti/568ml	409	16.0	72	1.0	10.8	2.8	0.0
Caramel with Whip, Grande, Semi Skim, Starbucks*	1 Grande/454ml	390	13.7	86	0.9	13.9	3.0	0.0
Caramel with Whip, Grande, Skimmed, Starbucks*	1 Grande/454ml	375	11.9	83	0.9	13.9	2.6	0.0
Caramel with Whip, Grande, Soy, Starbucks*	1 Grande/454ml	380	13.4	84	0.8	13.6	3.0	0.1
Caramel with Whip, Grande, Whole, Starbucks*	1 Grande/454ml	400	15.0	88	0.9	13.8	3.3	0.0
Caramel with Whip, Tall, Semi Skimmed, Starbucks*	1 Tall/340ml	286	10.2	84	1.0	13.4	3.0	0.0
Caramel with Whip, Tall, Skimmed, Starbucks*	1 Tall/340ml	273	8.7	80	1.0	13.5	2.6	0.0
Caramel with Whip, Tall, Soy, Starbucks*	1 Tall/340ml	278	9.9	82	0.8	13.1	2.9	0.1
Caramel with Whip, Tall, Whole, Starbucks*	1 Tall/340ml	294	11.2	86	0.9	13.4	3.3	0.0
Caramel with Whip, Venti, Semi Skimmed, Starbucks*	1 Venti/568ml	444	13.0	78	0.8	13.7	2.3	0.0
Caramel with Whip, Venti, Skimmed, Starbucks*	1 Venti/568ml	427	10.9	75	0.8	13.8	1.9	0.0
Caramel with Whip, Venti, Soy, Starbucks*	1 Venti/568ml	433	12.6	76	0.7	13.4	2.2	0.1
Caramel with Whip, Venti, Whole, Starbucks*	1 Venti/568ml	455	14.3	80	0.8	13.7	2.5	0.0
Chocolate Cream, & Whip, Grande, Skim, Starbucks*	1 Grande/473ml	314	12.2	66	1.3	10.3	2.6	0.2
Chocolate Cream, & Whip, Grande, Soy, Starbucks*	1 Grande/473ml	322	14.2	68	1.1	9.8	3.0	0.3
Chocolate Cream, & Whip, Grande, Whole, Starbucks*	1 Grande/473ml	349	16.3	74	1.2	10.2	3.4	0.2
Chocolate Cream, & Whip, Tall, Semi Skim, Starbucks*	1 Tall/335ml	243	10.7	72	1.3	10.3	3.2	0.2

STARBUCKS

FRAPPUCCINO

	INFO/WEIGHT	KCAL	FAT	KCAL	PROT	CARB	FAT	FIBRE
Chocolate Cream, & Whip, Tall, Skimmed, Starbucks*	1 Tall/335ml	226	8.7	67	1.4	10.4	2.6	0.2
Chocolate Cream, & Whip, Tall, Soy, Starbucks*	1 Tall/335ml	232	10.3	69	1.2	9.9	3.1	0.3
Chocolate Cream, & Whip, Tall, Whole, Starbucks*	1 Tall/335ml	253	12.0	75	1.3	10.3	3.6	0.2
Chocolate Cream, & Whip, Venti, Skim, Starbucks*	1 Venti/591ml	361	11.5	61	1.2	10.4	2.0	0.2
Chocolate Cream, & Whip, Venti, Soy, Starbucks*	1 Venti/591ml	370	13.8	63	1.0	9.9	2.3	0.3
Chocolate Cream, with Whip, Semi Skim, Starbucks*	1 Grande/454ml	335	14.7	74	1.3	10.6	3.2	0.2
Chocolate Cream, with Whip, Semi Skim, Starbucks*	1 Tall/340ml	243	10.7	71	1.3	10.2	3.2	0.2
Chocolate Cream, with Whip, Semi Skim, Starbucks*	1 Venti/568ml	386	14.4	68	1.2	10.7	2.5	0.2
Chocolate Cream, with Whip, Skim, Starbucks*	1 Grande/454ml	314	12.2	69	1.3	10.7	2.7	0.2
Chocolate Cream, with Whip, Skimmed, Starbucks*	1 Tall/340ml	226	8.7	66	1.4	10.3	2.6	0.2
Chocolate Cream, with Whip, Skimmed, Starbucks*	1 Venti/568ml	360	11.5	63	1.2	10.8	2.0	0.2
Chocolate Cream, with Whip, Soy, Starbucks*	1 Grande/340ml	322	14.2	71	1.2	10.2	3.1	0.3
Chocolate Cream, with Whip, Soy, Starbucks*	1 Tall/340ml	232	10.3	68	1.2	9.7	3.0	0.3
Chocolate Cream, with Whip, Soy, Starbucks*	1 Venti/568ml	370	13.8	65	1.1	10.3	2.4	0.3
Chocolate Cream, with Whip, Whole, Starbucks*	1 Grande/454ml	349	16.3	77	1.3	10.6	3.6	0.2
Chocolate Cream, with Whip, Whole, Starbucks*	1 Tall/340ml	253	12.0	74	1.3	10.1	3.5	0.2
Chocolate Cream, with Whip, Whole, Starbucks*	1 Venti/568ml	401	16.4	71	1.2	10.7	2.9	0.2
Coffee, Mocha, Jarva Chip, with Whip, Iced, Starbucks*	1 Grande/454ml	500	21.1	110	1.0	16.0	4.6	0.3
Coffee, Mocha, Jarva Chip, with Whip, Iced, Starbucks*	1 Tall/340ml	349	15.1	103	1.0	14.5	4.4	0.2
Coffee, Mocha, Jarva Chip, with Whip, Iced, Starbucks*	1 Venti/568ml	600	22.3	106	0.9	16.6	3.9	0.3
Coffee, no Whip, Grande, Semi Skimmed, Starbucks*	1 Grande/473ml	232	1.9	49	0.7	10.6	0.4	0.0
Coffee, no Whip, Grande, Skimmed, Starbucks*	1 Grande/454ml	118	0.1	26	0.8	5.6	0.0	0.1
Coffee, no Whip, Grande, Soy, Starbucks*	1 Grande/454ml	222	1.6	49	0.7	10.7	0.4	0.1
Coffee, no Whip, Grande, Whole, Starbucks*	1 Grande/454ml	242	3.2	53	0.8	11.0	0.7	0.0
Coffee, no Whip, Tall, Semi Skimmed, Starbucks*	1 Tall/340ml	170	1.6	50	0.8	10.6	0.5	0.0
Coffee, no Whip, Tall, Skimmed, Starbucks*	1 Tall/340ml	83	0.1	24	0.8	5.2	0.0	0.1
Coffee, no Whip, Tall, Soy, Starbucks*	1 Tall/340ml	161	1.3	47	0.7	10.2	0.4	0.1
Coffee, no Whip, Tall, Whole, Starbucks*	1 Tall/340ml	177	2.6	52	0.8	10.5	0.8	0.0
Coffee, no Whip, Venti, Semi Skimmed, Starbucks*	1 Venti/568ml	286	2.1	50	0.7	11.0	0.4	0.0
Coffee, no Whip, Venti, Skimmed, Starbucks*	1 Venti/568ml	269	11.4	47	0.7	11.1	2.0	0.0
Coffee, no Whip, Venti, Soy, Starbucks*	1 Venti/568ml	275	1.7	48	0.6	10.8	0.3	0.1
Coffee, no Whip, Venti, Whole, Starbucks*	1 Venti/568ml	296	3.5	52	0.6	11.0	0.6	0.0
Espresso, no Whip, Grande, Semi Skim, Starbucks*	1 Grande/454ml	210	1.3	46	0.6	10.3	0.3	0.0
Espresso, no Whip, Grande, Skimmed, Starbucks*	1 Grande/454ml	200	0.1	44	0.6	10.4	0.0	0.0
Espresso, no Whip, Grande, Soy, Starbucks*	1 Grande/454ml	204	1.1	45	0.5	10.1	0.2	0.1
Espresso, no Whip, Grande, Whole, Starbucks*	1 Grande/454ml	217	2.1	48	0.6	10.3	0.5	0.0
Espresso, no Whip, Tall, Semi Skimmed, Starbucks*	1 Tall/340ml	143	0.9	42	0.6	9.3	0.3	0.0
Espresso, no Whip, Tall, Skimmed, Starbucks*	1 Tall/340ml	136	0.0	40	0.6	9.4	0.0	0.0
Espresso, no Whip, Tall, Soy, Starbucks*	1 Tall/340ml	139	0.7	41	0.5	9.1	0.2	0.1
Espresso, no Whip, Tall, Whole, Starbucks*	1 Tall/340ml	148	1.5	44	0.6	9.3	0.4	0.0
Espresso, no Whip, Venti, Semi Skimmed, Starbucks*	1 Venti/568ml	262	1.5	46	0.6	10.4	0.3	FIBRE
Espresso, no Whip, Venti, Skimmed, Starbucks*	1 Venti/568ml	250	0.1	44	0.6	10.4	0.0	0.0
Espresso, no Whip, Venti, Soy, Starbucks*	1 Venti/568ml	254	1.2	45	0.5	10.2	0.2	0.1
Espresso, no Whip, Venti, Whole, Starbucks*	1 Venti/568ml	270	2.5	48	0.5	10.3	0.4	0.0
Light, no Whip, Grande, Skimmed, Starbucks*	1 Grande/473ml	118	0.1	25	0.7	5.4	0.0	0.1
Light, no Whip, Tall, Skimmed, Starbucks*	1 Tall/335ml	83	0.1	25	0.8	5.3	0.0	0.1
Mango Passion, Tea, Grande, Starbucks*	1 Grande/454ml	191	0.3	42	0.2	10.2	0.1	0.3
Mango Passion, Tea, Tall, Starbucks*	1 Tall/340ml	157	0.2	46	0.2	11.2	0.1	0.3
Mango Passion, Tea, Venti, Starbucks*	1 Venti/568ml	228	0.3	40	0.2	9.8	0.0	0.3
Mocha, no Whip, Grande, Skimmed, Starbucks*	1 Grande/454ml	143	0.8	32	0.9	7.0	0.2	0.2
Mocha, no Whip, Tall, Skimmed, Starbucks*	1 Tall/340ml	96	0.5	28	0.8	6.2	0.2	0.2
Mocha, no Whip, Venti, Skimmed, Starbucks*	1 Venti/568ml	179	0.9	32	0.9	7.0	0.2	0.2

STARBUCKS

FRAPPUCCINO

	Measure INFO/WEIGHT	per Measure KCAL	FAT	Nutrition Values per 100g / 100ml KCAL	PROT	CARB	FAT	FIBRE
Mocha with Whip, Grande, Semi Skimmed, Starbucks*	1 Grande/454ml	361	13.7	80	1.0	12.7	3.0	0.2
Mocha with Whip, Grande, Skimmed, Starbucks*	1 Grande/454ml	346	12.0	76	1.0	12.7	2.6	0.2
Mocha with Whip, Grande, Soy, Starbucks*	1 Grande/454ml	352	13.3	78	0.9	12.4	2.9	0.2
Mocha with Whip, Grande, Whole, Starbucks*	1 Grande/454ml	370	14.8	82	1.0	12.6	3.3	0.2
Mocha with Whip, Tall, Semi Skimmed, Starbucks*	1 Tall/340ml	266	10.0	78	1.1	12.4	2.9	0.2
Mocha with Whip, Tall, Skimmed, Starbucks*	1 Tall/340ml	254	8.6	75	1.1	12.5	2.5	0.2
Mocha with Whip, Tall, Soy, Starbucks*	1 Tall/340ml	258	9.7	76	1.0	12.1	2.8	0.2
Mocha with Whip, Tall, Whole, Starbucks*	1 Tall/340ml	274	11.0	81	1.1	12.4	3.2	0.2
Mocha with Whip, Venti, Semi Skimmed, Starbucks*	1 Venti/568ml	427	13.2	75	1.0	13.2	2.3	0.2
Mocha with Whip, Venti, Skimmed, Starbucks*	1 Venti/568ml	410	11.3	72	1.0	13.3	2.0	0.2
Mocha with Whip, Venti, Soy, Starbucks*	1 Venti/568ml	416	12.8	73	0.8	12.9	2.2	0.2
Mocha with Whip, Venti, Whole, Starbucks*	1 Venti/568ml	437	14.6	77	0.9	13.2	2.6	0.2
Raspberry, Blackcurrant, Zen Tea, Grande, Starbucks*	1 Grande/454ml	192	0.1	42	0.1	10.4	0.0	0.2
Raspberry, Blackcurrant, Zen Tea, Tall, Starbucks*	1 Tall/340ml	158	0.1	46	0.1	11.4	0.0	0.2
Raspberry, Blackcurrant, Zen Tea, Venti, Starbucks*	1 Venti/568ml	229	0.1	40	0.1	9.9	0.0	0.1
Raspberry, Tea, Grande, Starbucks*	1 Grande/473ml	192	0.1	41	0.1	10.0	0.0	0.2
Raspberry, Tea, Venti, Starbucks*	1 Venti/591ml	229	0.1	39	0.1	9.5	0.0	0.1
Raspberry, Tea, Tall, Starbucks*	1 Tall/335ml	158	0.1	47	0.1	11.6	0.0	0.2
Strawberries & Cream, & Whip, Semi Skim, Starbucks*	1 Grande/454ml	403	13.6	89	1.1	14.7	3.0	0.1
Strawberries & Cream, & Whip, Semi Skim, Starbucks*	1 Tall/340ml	316	9.9	93	1.2	15.8	2.9	0.1
Strawberries & Cream, & Whip, Semi Skim, Starbucks*	1 Venti/568ml	445	13.0	78	1.0	13.6	2.3	0.1
Strawberries & Cream, & Whip, Skim, Starbucks*	1 Grande/454ml	384	11.3	85	1.1	14.8	2.5	0.1
Strawberries & Cream, & Whip, Skim, Starbucks*	1 Tall/340ml	300	8.1	88	1.2	15.8	2.4	0.1
Strawberries & Cream, & Whip, Skim, Starbucks*	1 Venti/568ml	422	10.3	74	1.0	13.7	1.8	0.1
Strawberries & Cream, & Whip, Skim, Starbucks*	1 Grande/473ml	384	11.3	81	1.0	14.2	2.4	0.1
Strawberries & Cream, & Whip, Soy, Starbucks*	1 Grande/454ml	391	13.1	86	0.9	14.3	2.9	0.2
Strawberries & Cream, & Whip, Soy, Starbucks*	1 Tall/340ml	306	9.6	90	1.0	15.4	2.8	0.2
Strawberries & Cream, & Whip, Soy, Starbucks*	1 Venti/568ml	431	12.5	76	0.8	13.3	2.2	0.2
Strawberries & Cream, & Whip, Whole, Starbucks*	1 Grande/454ml	415	15.1	91	1.0	14.6	3.3	0.1
Strawberries & Cream, & Whip, Whole, Starbucks*	1 Tall/340ml	326	11.2	96	1.1	15.7	3.3	0.1
Strawberries & Cream, & Whip, Whole, Starbucks*	1 Venti/568ml	459	14.9	81	1.0	13.6	2.6	0.1
Vanilla Cream, with Whip, Semi Skimmed, Starbucks*	1 Grande/454ml	327	13.9	72	1.1	10.1	3.1	0.0
Vanilla Cream, with Whip, Skimmed, Starbucks*	1 Grande/454ml	305	11.3	67	1.2	10.2	2.5	1.5
Vanilla Cream, with Whip, Soy, Starbucks*	1 Grandeg/454ml	313	13.4	69	1.0	9.7	3.0	0.1
Vanilla Cream, with Whip, Tall, Semi Skim, Starbucks*	1 Tall/340ml	233	10.0	69	1.2	9.4	2.9	0.0
Vanilla Cream, with Whip, Tall, Skimmed, Starbucks*	1 Tall/340ml	216	8.1	64	1.2	9.5	2.4	0.0
Vanilla Cream, with Whip, Tall, Soy, Starbucks*	1 Tall/340ml	222	9.7	65	1.0	9.0	2.8	0.2
Vanilla Cream, with Whip, Tall, Whole, Starbucks*	1 Tall340ml	243	11.4	71	1.1	9.4	3.4	0.0
Vanilla Cream, with Whip, Venti, Semi Skimmed, Starbucks*	1 Venti/568ml	372	13.4	65	1.0	10.1	2.4	0.0
Vanilla Cream, with Whip, Venti, Skimmed, Starbucks*	1 Venti/568ml	347	10.4	61	1.0	10.2	1.8	0.0
Vanilla Cream, with Whip, Venti, Soy, Starbucks*	1 Venti/568ml	346	12.4	61	0.8	9.6	2.2	0.1
Vanilla Cream, with Whip, Venti, Whole, Starbucks*	1 Venti/568ml	388	15.4	68	1.0	10.1	2.7	0.0
Vanilla Cream, with Whip, Whole, Starbucks*	1 Grande/454ml	341	15.6	75	1.1	10.1	3.4	0.0
Vanilla with Whip, Grande, Skimmed, Starbucks*	1 Grande/473ml	305	11.3	65	1.1	9.8	2.4	0.0
Vanilla with Whip, Tall, Semi Skimmed, Starbucks*	1 Tall/335ml	233	10.0	69	1.2	9.6	3.0	0.0
Vanilla with Whip, Tall, Skimmed, Starbucks*	1 Tall/335ml	216	8.1	64	1.2	9.6	2.4	0.0
Vanilla with Whip, Tall, Soy, Starbucks*	1 Tall/335ml	222	9.7	66	1.0	9.1	2.9	0.1
Vanilla with Whip, Venti, Skimmed, Starbucks*	1 Venti/591ml	347	10.4	59	1.0	9.8	1.8	0.0
Vanilla with Whip, Venti, Soy, Starbucks*	1 Venti/591ml	346	12.4	59	0.7	9.2	2.1	0.1
Vanilla with Whip, Venti, Whole, Starbucks*	1 Venti/591ml	388	15.4	66	1.0	9.7	2.6	0.0

HOT CHOCOLATE

	Measure INFO/WEIGHT	per Measure KCAL	FAT	Nutrition Values per 100g / 100ml KCAL	PROT	CARB	FAT	FIBRE
Classic with Whip, Grande, Semi Skimmed, Starbucks*	1 Grande/454ml	323	15.0	71	2.8	9.0	3.3	0.4

STARBUCKS

	Measure INFO/WEIGHT	KCAL	FAT	KCAL	PROT	CARB	FAT	FIBRE
HOT CHOCOLATE								
Classic with Whip, Grande, Skimmed, Starbucks*	1 Grande/454ml	277	9.5	61	2.8	9.2	2.1	0.4
Classic with Whip, Grande, Soy, Starbucks*	1 Grande/474ml	291	13.7	64	2.4	8.0	3.0	0.7
Classic with Whip, Grande, Whole, Starbucks*	1 Grande/454ml	352	18.7	78	2.7	8.9	4.1	0.4
Classic with Whip, Short, Semi Skimmed, Starbucks*	1 Short/227ml	178	9.1	78	2.8	9.2	4.0	0.4
Classic with Whip, Short, Skimmed, Starbucks*	1 Short/227ml	155	6.4	68	2.9	9.4	2.8	0.4
Classic with Whip, Short, Soy, Starbucks*	1 Serving/227ml	162	8.5	71	2.4	8.2	3.7	0.7
Classic with Whip, Short, Whole, Starbucks*	1 Short/227ml	193	11.0	85	2.7	9.1	4.8	0.4
Classic with Whip, Tall, Semi Skimmed, Starbucks*	1 Tall/340ml	261	12.5	77	3.0	9.4	3.7	0.4
Classic with Whip, Tall, Skimmed, Starbucks*	1 Tall/340ml	222	8.0	65	3.0	9.6	2.4	0.4
Classic with Whip, Tall, Soy, Starbucks*	1 Tall/340ml	234	11.4	69	2.6	8.3	3.4	0.7
Classic with Whip, Tall, Whole, Starbucks*	1 Tall/340ml	284	15.5	84	2.9	9.3	4.6	0.4
Classic with Whip, Venti, Semi Skimmed, Starbucks*	1 Venti/68ml	398	17.5	70	2.9	9.1	3.1	0.4
Classic with Whip, Venti, Skimmed, Starbucks*	1 Venti/568ml	336	10.2	59	2.9	9.3	1.8	0.4
Classic with Whip, Venti, Soy, Starbucks*	1 Venti/568ml	355	15.7	62	2.5	8.0	2.8	0.7
Classic with Whip, Venti, Whole, Starbucks*	1 Venti/568ml	437	22.5	77	2.8	9.0	4.0	0.4
Signature with Whip, Grande, Semi Skimmed, Starbucks*	1 Grande/454ml	537	30.7	118	3.4	13.0	6.8	1.5
Signature with Whip, Grande, Skimmed, Starbucks*	1 Brande/454ml	505	27.0	111	3.4	13.1	6.0	1.5
Signature with Whip, Grande, Soy, Starbucks*	1 Grande/473ml	537	31.0	113	3.1	12.3	6.6	1.6
Signature with Whip, Grande, Whole, Starbucks*	1 Grande/454ml	556	33.5	122	3.3	13.0	7.4	1.5
Signature with Whip, Short, Semi Skimmed, Starbucks*	1 Short/227ml	283	16.9	125	3.4	13.1	7.4	1.4
Signature with Whip, Short, Skimmed, Starbucks*	1 Short/227ml	267	15.0	118	3.4	13.2	6.6	1.4
Signature with Whip, Short, Soy, Starbucks*	1 Short/227ml	272	16.4	120	3.2	12.4	7.2	1.6
Signature with Whip, Short, Whole, Starbucks*	1 Short/227ml	293	18.1	129	3.4	13.0	8.0	1.4
Signature with Whip, Tall, Semi Skimmed, Starbucks*	1 Tall/335ml	412	23.9	123	3.5	13.3	7.1	1.5
Signature with Whip, Tall, Skimmed, Starbucks*	1 Tall/340ml	393	21.3	116	3.5	13.4	6.3	1.5
Signature with Whip, Tall, Soy, Starbucks*	1 Tall/340ml	401	23.5	118	3.2	12.6	6.9	1.7
Signature with Whip, Tall, Whole, Starbucks*	1 Tall/340ml	433	26.1	127	3.4	13.2	7.7	1.5
Signature with Whip, Venti, Semi Skimmed, Starbucks*	1 Venti/568ml	665	37.2	117	3.4	13.2	6.6	1.5
Signature with Whip, Venti, Skimmed, Starbucks*	1 Venti/568ml	624	32.4	110	3.4	13.2	5.7	1.5
Signature with Whip, Venti, Soy, Starbucks*	1 Venti/568ml	637	36.0	112	3.2	12.5	6.3	1.7
Signature with Whip, Venti, Whole, Starbucks*	1 Venti/568ml	690	40.4	121	3.4	13.0	7.1	1.5
MILK								
Steamed, Grande, Semi Skimmed, Starbucks*	1 Grande/454ml	203	8.0	45	3.0	4.2	1.8	0.0
Steamed, Grande, Skimmed, Starbucks*	1 Grande/454ml	138	0.3	30	3.0	4.4	0.1	0.0
Steamed, Grande, Soy, Starbucks*	1 Grande/454ml	157	6.1	35	2.4	2.8	1.3	0.3
Steamed, Grande, Whole, Starbucks*	1 Grande/454ml	244	13.2	54	2.9	4.0	2.9	0.0
Steamed, Short, Semi Skimmed, Starbucks*	1 Short/227ml	103	4.0	45	3.0	4.2	1.8	0.0
Steamed, Short, Skimmed, Starbucks*	1 Short/227ml	70	0.2	31	3.0	4.5	0.1	0.0
Steamed, Short, Soy, Starbucks*	1 Short/227ml	80	3.1	35	2.5	2.8	1.4	0.4
Steamed, Short, Whole, Starbucks*	1 Short/227ml	123	6.7	54	2.9	4.1	3.0	0.0
Steamed, Tall, Semi Skimmed, Starbucks*	1 Tall/340ml	156	6.1	46	3.0	4.3	1.8	0.0
Steamed, Tall, Skimmed, Starbucks*	1 Tall/340ml	106	0.3	31	3.1	4.5	0.1	0.0
Steamed, Tall, Soy, Starbucks*	1 Tall/340ml	120	4.7	35	2.5	2.8	1.4	0.4
Steamed, Tall, Whole, Starbucks*	1 Tall/340ml	187	10.1	55	2.9	4.2	3.0	0.0
Steamed, Venti, Semi Skimmed, Starbucks*	1 Venti/568ml	258	10.2	45	3.0	4.2	1.8	0.0
Steamed, Venti, Skimmed, Starbucks*	1 Venti/568ml	175	0.4	31	3.1	4.5	0.1	0.0
Steamed, Venti, Soy, Starbucks*	1 Venti/568ml	199	7.8	35	2.5	2.8	1.4	0.3
Steamed, Venti, Whole, Starbucks*	1 Venti/568ml	309	16.7	54	2.9	4.1	2.9	0.0
MINTS								
After Coffee, Starbucks*	1 Mint/2g	5	0.0	250	0.0	100.0	0.0	0.0
Peppermints, SF, Starbucks*	1 Mint/2g	4	0.0	242	0.0	99.0	0.6	0.0

STARBUCKS

INFO/WEIGHT	Measure		per Measure		Nutrition Values per 100g / 100ml				
			KCAL	FAT	KCAL	PROT	CARB	FAT	FIBRE
MUFFIN									
Apple, Cinnamon & Walnut, Starbucks*	1 Muffin/126g		476	25.6	378	5.2	45.4	20.3	1.6
Banana & Nut, Starbucks*	1 Muffin/122g		481	25.7	394	5.9	46.3	21.1	1.5
Chocolate & Belgian Choc Sauce, Starbucks*	1 Muffin/119g		430	17.8	361	6.6	48.7	15.0	2.6
Classic Blueberry, Starbucks*	1 Muffin/122g		472	23.7	387	5.4	47.1	19.4	5.4
Lemon, Poppyseed, Starbucks*	1 Muffin/131g		470	17.9	359	4.7	53.4	13.7	1.8
Lemon & Poppy Seed, Skinny, Starbucks*	1 Muffin/122g		338	2.3	277	5.4	58.5	1.9	2.2
Rise & Shine, Starbucks*	1 Muffin/124g		448	18.8	361	7.1	47.8	15.2	2.3
Skinny Blueberry Muffin, Starbucks*	1 Muffin/120g		312	2.9	260	3.9	55.0	2.4	1.2
Skinny Peach & Raspberry, Starbucks*	1 Muffin/136g		369	3.9	271	6.2	53.9	2.9	2.3
Spelt & Fruit, Starbucks*	1 Muffin/114g		402	18.7	353	5.8	44.1	16.4	3.1
NUTS									
Mixed, Starbucks*	1 Pack/75g		401	25.2	535	17.7	41.1	33.6	6.7
Roasted Almonds, Starbucks*	1 Pack/440g		425	36.8	567	20.3	11.1	49.0	10.8
OMELETTE									
Feta, Spinach & Egg White, Crepe, Starbucks*	1 Crepe/119g		132	8.2	111	10.0	2.2	6.9	0.4
Kale & Smoked Cheese, Crepe, Starbucks*	1 Serving/144g		300	23.3	209	11.6	3.8	16.2	0.6
Sausage & Egg White, Crepe, Starbucks*	1 Crepe/117g		153	8.1	131	10.4	6.4	6.9	0.8
PAIN AU CHOCOLAT									
Starbucks*	1 Pastry/65g		272	16.5	418	6.2	39.9	25.4	2.7
PAIN AU RAISIN									
Starbucks*	1 Pastry/110g		370	19.5	336	4.5	39.8	17.7	1.4
PANCAKE									
Buttermilk, Starbucks*	1 Pack/90g		227	2.4	252	4.6	51.9	2.7	1.2
PANINI									
Beef & Blue Cheese, Limited Edition, Starbucks*	1 Panini/180g		436	17.8	242	13.5	24.2	9.9	1.0
Bella Mozzarella, Starbucks*	1 Panini/183g		510	28.0	279	11.4	23.3	15.3	2.4
Cheese & Marmite, Starbucks*	1 Panini/130g		378	17.8	291	14.3	27.1	13.7	1.1
Chicken, Lemon, Mediterranean, Starbucks*	1 Panini/190g		466	21.7	245	12.8	22.4	11.4	1.0
Chicken Jambalya, Starbucks*	1 Panini/211g		388	8.9	184	10.0	25.6	4.2	2.1
Chicken Jambalya, Starbucks*	1 Panini/211g		388	8.9	184	10.0	25.6	4.2	2.1
Croque Monsieur, Starbucks*	1 Panini/195g		463	21.2	238	13.1	21.4	10.9	0.8
Italian Mozzarella & Slow Roast Tomato, Starbucks*	1 Panini/178g		470	20.5	264	11.2	28.0	11.5	1.5
Meatball Melt, Starbucks*	1 Panini/215g		559	28.8	260	10.1	24.0	13.4	1.6
Pulled Pork & Bean, Starbucks*	1 Panini/210g		480	17.2	229	10.4	27.6	8.2	1.6
Roast Chicken & Tomato, Starbucks*	1 Panini/223g		375	8.0	168	10.2	23.1	3.6	1.4
Roasted Pepper & Goat's Cheese, Starbucks*	1 Panini/180g		389	16.3	215	7.2	25.3	9.0	2.0
Smokehouse Chicken & Bacon, Starbucks*	1 Panini/188g		483	21.4	257	14.1	24.0	11.4	1.1
Steak, Cheese & Caramelised Onion, Starbucks*	1 Panini/210g		525	20.4	250	14.9	25.3	9.7	1.0
Tuna Melt & Mature Cheddar, Starbucks*	1 Panini/200g		492	21.0	246	13.3	24.2	10.5	0.9
Tuna or Later, Starbucks*	1 Panini/185g		482	23.8	261	13.3	22.3	12.9	0.8
SALAD									
Chicken & Red Pesto, Bistro Box, Starbucks*	1 Salad/296g		275	13.9	93	5.1	7.1	4.7	1.1
Chicken Mango, Starbucks*	1 Serving/230g		179	4.8	78	6.4	7.2	2.1	2.4
Cured Ham Hock, Bistro Box, Starbucks*	1 Salad/302g		387	20.5	128	7.9	8.2	6.8	1.3
Falafel Mezze, Bistro Box, Starbucks*	1 Salad/329g		494	14.5	150	5.0	20.9	4.4	3.6
Feta Compli, Starbucks*	1 Serving/271g		379	34.4	140	1.4	5.6	12.7	1.7
Hail Caesar, Starbucks*	1 Pack/200g		376	26.9	189	11.9	4.8	13.5	0.6
Holy Guacamole, Starbucks*	1 Pack/290g		374	11.3	129	7.3	15.0	3.9	2.6
Meze, Moreish, Starbucks*	1 Box/325g		465	20.5	143	4.1	15.7	6.3	3.9
Tuna, Potato & Pea, Bistro Box, Starbucks*	1 Salad/286g		320	14.6	112	6.3	9.5	5.1	1.7
SANDWICH									
Egg Mayonnaise, & Cress, Starbucks*	1 Sandwich/193g		460	26.1	238	10.3	17.2	13.5	3.3

	Measure	per Measure		Nutrition Values per 100g / 100ml				
	INFO/WEIGHT	KCAL	FAT	KCAL	PROT	CARB	FAT	FIBRE

STARBUCKS
SANDWICH

All Day Breakfast, Butty, Starbucks*	1 Butty/162g	429	18.6	265	13.3	26.8	11.5	1.0
Bacon Butty, Starbucks*	1 Butty/125g	451	21.0	361	20.3	31.5	16.8	1.3
Cheese & Pickle, GF, Starbucks*	1 Sandwich/197g	552	32.5	280	7.5	23.9	16.5	2.9
Chicken, Sunshine Salad, Starbucks*	1 Pack/241g	433	18.5	180	9.3	17.6	7.7	1.7
Roasted Chicken with Herb Mayonnaise, Starbucks*	1 Sandwich/201g	314	7.2	156	10.6	19.2	3.6	2.1
Salt Beef, New York Deli, Starbucks*	1 Pack/146g	270	9.3	185	1.6	14.4	6.4	1.7
Sausage, Sarnie, Starbucks*	1 Sarnie/170g	442	18.7	260	11.7	28.0	11.0	1.5

SHORTBREAD

Chocolate Caramel, Starbucks*	1 Serving/66g	357	20.7	541	4.2	59.9	31.4	0.8
Chocolate Chunk, Fairtrade, Starbucks*	1 Shortbread/96g	497	29.0	518	6.2	53.5	30.2	3.1
Starbucks*	1 Pack/13g	68	4.0	538	5.4	57.1	31.6	1.6

SWEETS

Starbucks*	1 Sweet/6g	20	0.0	333	0.1	82.0	0.2	1.5

SYRUP

1 Pump - 1/4 fl oz 10g, Starbucks*	1 Pump/10g	20	0.0	200	0.0	50.0	0.0	0.0
2 Pumps - 1/2 fl oz - 20 g, Starbucks*	2 Pumps/20g	40	0.0	200	0.0	50.5	0.0	0.0
3 Pumps - 3/4 fl oz - 30 g, Starbucks*	3 Pumps/30g	60	0.0	200	0.0	50.3	0.0	0.0
4 Pumps - 1 fl oz - 40 g, Starbucks*	4 Pumps/40g	81	0.0	202	0.0	50.2	0.0	0.0
Bar Mocha, 1 Pump - ½ fl oz - 17 g, Starbucks*	1 Pump/17g	26	0.6	153	3.5	37.6	3.5	5.9
Bar Mocha, 2 Pumps - 1 fl oz - 34 g, Starbucks*	2 Pumps/34g	53	1.1	156	3.8	37.6	3.2	5.9
Bar Mocha, 3 Pumps - 1½ fl oz - 51 g, Starbucks*	3 Pumps/51g	79	1.7	155	3.7	37.4	3.3	5.9
Bar Mocha, 4 Pumps - 2 fl oz - 68 g, Starbucks*	4 Pumps/68g	106	2.3	156	3.7	37.5	3.4	5.7
Bar Mocha, 5 Pumps - 2 1/2 fl oz - 85 g, Starbucks*	5 Pumps/85g	132	2.8	155	3.6	37.5	3.3	5.8
SF, Starbucks*	1 Pump/10g	0	0.0	0	0.0	0.0	0.0	0.0

TEA

Brewed, Grande, Starbucks*	1 Grande/473ml	0	0.0	0	0.0	0.0	0.0	0.0
Brewed, Short, Starbucks*	1 Short/227ml	0	0.0	0	0.0	0.0	0.0	0.0
Brewed, Tall, Starbucks*	1 Tall/335ml	0	0.0	0	0.0	0.0	0.0	0.0
Brewed, Venti, Starbucks*	1 Venti/591ml	0	0.0	0	0.0	0.0	0.0	0.0
Chai, Hot Mulled Fruit, Apple, Grande, Starbucks*	1 Grande/454ml	229	0.0	50	0.1	15.2	0.0	0.1
Chai, Hot Mulled Fruit, Apple, Tall, Starbucks*	1 Tall/340ml	148	0.0	44	0.1	13.8	0.0	0.1
Chai, Hot Mulled Fruit, Apple, Venti, Starbucks*	1 Venti/568ml	310	0.0	55	0.1	15.5	0.0	0.1
Chai, Hot Mulled Fruit, Grape, Grande, Starbucks*	1 Grande454ml	257	0.0	57	0.1	16.7	0.0	0.0
Chai, Hot Mulled Fruit, Grape, Tall, Starbucks*	1 Tall/340ml	167	0.0	49	0.1	15.3	0.0	0.0
Chai, Hot Mulled Fruit, Grape, Venti, Starbucks*	1 Venti/568ml	348	0.0	61	0.1	17.4	0.0	0.0
Chai, Latte, Grande, Semi Skimmed, Starbucks*	1 Grande/454ml	236	4.0	52	1.6	9.6	0.9	0.0
Chai, Latte, Grande, Skimmed, Starbucks*	1 Grande/454ml	204	0.2	45	1.6	9.8	0.0	0.0
Chai, Latte, Grande, Soy, Starbucks*	1 Grande/454ml	213	3.2	47	1.4	8.9	0.7	0.2
Chai, Latte, Grande, Whole, Starbucks*	1 Grande/454ml	255	6.5	56	1.6	9.6	1.4	0.0
Chai, Latte, Short, Semi Skimmed, Starbucks*	1 Short/227ml	119	2.0	52	1.7	9.7	0.9	0.0
Chai, Latte, Short, Skimmed, Starbucks*	1 Short/227ml	103	0.1	45	1.7	9.8	0.0	0.00
Chai, Latte, Short, Soy, Starbucks*	1 Short/227ml	108	1.6	48	1.4	9.0	0.7	0.2
Chai, Latte, Short, Whole, Starbucks*	1 Short/227ml	129	3.3	57	1.6	9.6	1.4	0.0
Chai, Latte, Tall, Semi Skimmed, Starbucks*	1 Tall/340ml	179	3.0	53	1.7	9.7	0.9	0.3
Chai, Latte, Tall, Skimmed, Starbucks*	1 Tall/340ml	154	0.2	45	1.7	9.8	0.1	0.0
Chai, Latte, Tall, Soy, Starbucks*	1 Tall/335ml	162	2.4	48	1.4	9.1	0.7	0.2
Chai, Latte, Tall, Whole, Starbucks*	1 Tall/340ml	194	5.0	57	1.6	9.6	1.5	0.0
Chai, Latte, Venti, Semi Skimmed, Starbucks*	1 Venti/568ml	297	5.0	52	1.6	9.7	0.9	0.0
Chai, Latte, Venti, Skimmed, Starbucks*	1 Venti/568ml	256	0.3	45	1.7	9.8	0.0	0.0
Chai, Latte, Venti, Soy, Starbucks*	1 Venti/568ml	268	4.0	47	1.4	8.9	0.7	0.2
Chai, Latte, Venti, Whole, Starbucks*	1 Venti/568ml	322	8.3	57	1.6	9.6	1.5	0.0
Iced, Chai, Latte, Grande, Semi Skimmed, Starbucks*	1 Grande/454ml	238	4.2	52	1.6	9.7	0.9	0.0

STARBUCKS

	Measure INFO/WEIGHT	per Measure KCAL	FAT	Nutrition Values per 100g / 100ml KCAL	PROT	CARB	FAT	FIBRE
TEA								
Iced, Chai, Latte, Grande, Skimmed, Starbucks*	1 Grande/454ml	205	0.2	45	1.7	9.8	0.0	0.0
Iced, Chai, Latte, Grande, Soy, Starbucks*	1 Grande/454	219	3.4	48	1.4	9.0	0.8	0.2
Iced, Chai, Latte, Grande, Whole, Starbucks*	1 Grande/454ml	259	6.9	57	1.6	9.6	1.5	0.0
Iced, Chai, Latte, Tall, Semi Skimmed, Starbucks*	1 Tall/340ml	176	3.0	52	1.6	9.6	0.9	0.0
Iced, Chai, Latte, Tall, Skimmed, Starbucks*	1 Tall/340ml	152	0.2	45	1.6	9.7	0.1	0.0
Iced, Chai, Latte, Tall, Soy, Starbucks*	1 Tall/340ml	162	2.4	48	1.4	9.0	0.7	0.2
Iced, Chai, Latte, Tall, Whole, Starbucks*	1 Tall/340ml	191	5.0	56	1.6	9.5	1.5	0.0
Iced, Chai, Latte, Venti, Semi Skimmed, Starbucks*	1 Venti/568ml	277	4.4	49	1.4	9.3	0.8	0.0
Iced, Chai, Latte, Venti, Skimmed, Starbucks*	1 Venti/568ml	242	0.3	43	1.4	9.3	0.0	0.0
Iced, Chai, Latte, Venti, Soy, Starbucks*	1 Venti/568ml	256	3.5	45	1.2	8.8	0.6	0.2
Iced, Chai, Latte, Venti, Whole, Starbucks*	1 Venti/568ml	299	7.2	53	1.4	9.3	1.3	0.0
TOASTIE								
Ham & Cheese, Starbucks*	1 Toastie/151g	367	17.4	243	12.9	21.6	11.5	1.1
Triple Cheese, Starbucks*	1 Toastie/131g	404	22.2	309	13.6	24.8	17.0	1.2
TOPPING								
Whipped Cream, Cold, Grande, Starbucks*	1 Grande/35g	114	11.2	326	1.7	8.6	32.0	0.0
Whipped Cream, Cold, Venti, Starbucks*	1 Venti/32g	104	10.2	325	1.9	9.4	31.9	0.0
Caramel - 4 g, Starbucks*	1 Serving/4g	15	0.6	375	0.0	62.5	15.0	0.0
Chocolate - 4 g, Starbucks*	1 Serving/4g	6	0.1	150	2.5	37.5	2.5	2.5
Sprinkles - 1 g, Starbucks*	1 Serving/1g	4	0.0	400	0.0	100.0	0.0	0.0
Whipped Cream, Cold, Tall, Starbucks*	1 Tall/25g	81	8.0	324	1.6	8.0	32.0	0.0
Whipped Cream, Hot, Grande/Venti, Starbucks*	1 Serving/22g	72	7.0	327	1.8	9.1	31.8	0.0
Whipped Cream, Hot, Short, Beverage, Starbucks*	1 Short/16g	52	5.1	325	1.9	6.2	31.9	0.0
Whipped Cream, Hot, Tall, Beverage, Starbucks*	1 Tall/19	62	6.1	326	1.6	10.5	32.1	0.0
WAFFLES								
Caramel, Lge, Starbucks*	1 Waffle/78g	356	16.4	457	3.5	63.0	21.0	1.0
WRAP								
Chicken Caesar, Starbucks*	1 Wrap/166g	515	28.6	310	14.3	23.5	17.2	2.1
Chicken Jalapeno, Starbucks*	1 Wrap/234g	448	15.4	192	10.1	22.2	6.6	1.7
Falafel, GF, Starbucks*	1 Wrap/211g	403	13.3	191	4.7	26.9	6.3	4.3
Roast Chicken Salsa, Starbucks*	1 Wrap/195g	387	10.6	198	10.1	25.9	5.4	2.4
Veggie Good Falafel, GF, Starbucks*	1 Wrap/211g	403	13.3	191	4.7	26.9	6.3	4.3
Veggie Good Houmous, Starbucks*	1 Wrap/192g	351	10.4	183	4.3	27.1	5.4	4.3
YOGHURT								
Apple, Oats & Berries, Breakfast Pot, Starbucks*	1 Pot/180g	319	11.9	177	4.1	24.3	6.6	2.1
Greek, Raspberry & Lemon Parfait, Starbucks*	1 Pot/172g	310	7.0	180	7.6	28.5	4.1	1.7
Natural, Creamy, Starbucks*	1 Serving/140g	132	6.4	94	5.5	7.5	4.6	0.0

SUBWAY

	Measure INFO/WEIGHT	per Measure KCAL	FAT	Nutrition Values per 100g / 100ml KCAL	PROT	CARB	FAT	FIBRE
BACON								
2 Strips, Subway*	2 Strips/9g	40	2.9	444	33.3	0.0	32.2	0.0
BREAD								
Flatbread, Subway*	1 Flatbread/85g	203	2.5	239	9.4	42.4	2.9	3.1
Rolls, Sub, Honey Oat, 9 Grain, 6 Inch, Subway*	1 Sub/78g	198	1.5	254	11.5	44.9	1.9	6.7
Rolls, Sub, Italian, Hearty, 6 Inch, Subway*	1 Sub/75g	201	1.5	268	10.7	50.7	2.0	2.8
Rolls, Sub, Italian, Herbs & Cheese, 6 Inch, Subway*	1 Sub/82g	234	4.3	285	12.2	46.3	5.2	2.3
Rolls, Sub, Wheat, 9 Grain, 6 Inch, Subway*	1 Sub/78g	198	1.5	254	11.5	44.9	1.9	6.7
Rolls, Sub, White, Italian, 6 Inch, Subway*	1 Sub/71g	190	1.3	268	9.9	50.7	1.8	2.2
CHEESE								
American, Subway*	1 Serving/11g	40	3.4	364	18.2	9.1	30.9	0.0
Cheddar, Monterey, Subway*	1 Serving/14g	57	4.4	407	25.0	0.0	31.4	0.0
Peppered, Subway*	1 Serving/11g	39	3.1	355	18.2	0.0	28.2	0.0

	Measure INFO/WEIGHT	per Measure KCAL	FAT	Nutrition Values per 100g / 100ml KCAL	PROT	CARB	FAT	FIBRE
SUBWAY								
COOKIES								
Chocolate Chip, Subway*	1 Cookie/45g	218	10.3	484	4.4	64.4	22.9	2.4
Chocolate Chunk, Subway*	1 Cookie/45g	214	10.2	476	4.4	66.7	22.7	2.0
Double Choc Chip, Subway*	1 Cookie/45g	221	11.7	491	4.4	60.0	26.0	2.7
Oatmeal Raisin, Subway*	1 Cookie/45g	196	8.1	436	6.7	66.7	18.0	1.1
Rainbow, Subway*	1 Cookie/45g	211	9.7	469	4.4	66.7	21.6	2.0
White Chip Macadamia Nut, Subway*	1 Cookie/45g	218	11.0	484	4.4	62.2	24.4	1.1
DOUGHNUTS								
Chocolate, Subway*	1 Doughnut/55g	243	15.5	442	7.3	38.2	28.2	2.2
Sugared, Subway*	1 Doughnut/49g	207	11.6	422	6.1	42.9	23.7	1.0
FLATBREAD								
Bacon, Breakfast, Subway*	1 Flatbread/113g	281	7.3	249	13.9	32.4	6.5	2.4
Bacon, Egg, & Cheese, Breakfast, Subway*	1 Flatbread/145g	340	12.5	234	11.8	26.3	8.6	2.0
Beef, Low Fat, Subway*	1 Flatbread/226g	292	4.1	129	10.0	17.5	1.8	1.7
Beef, Melt, Big, Subway*	1 Flatbread/247g	418	17.9	169	8.5	16.4	7.2	2.0
Chicken, & Bacon, Ranch Melt, Subway*	1 Flatbread/299g	513	20.3	172	12.5	14.0	6.8	1.3
Chicken, Breast, Low Fat, Subway*	1 Flatbread/240g	314	4.1	131	11.1	16.9	1.7	1.6
Chicken, Tandoori, Low Fat, Subway*	1 Flatbread/261g	320	4.7	123	10.3	14.9	1.8	1.4
Chicken, Temptation, Subway*	1 Flatbread/269g	416	9.8	155	9.9	20.0	3.6	1.4
Chicken, Teriyaki, Low Fat, Subway*	1 Flatbread/261g	330	4.2	126	10.4	16.9	1.6	1.6
Chicken, Tikka, Low Fat, Subway*	1 Flatbread/240g	312	4.1	130	11.1	16.6	1.7	1.6
Club, Low Fat, Subway*	1 Flatbread/259g	320	4.5	124	11.0	15.4	1.7	1.5
Egg, & Cheese, Breakfast, Subway*	1 Flatbread/131g	304	10.1	232	10.2	29.1	7.7	2.2
Ham, & Turkey Breast, Low Fat, Subway*	1 Flatbread/235g	288	4.0	123	9.4	17.0	1.7	1.6
Ham, Low Fat, Subway*	1 Flatbread/226g	279	4.6	123	8.4	17.8	2.0	1.7
Italian, Spicy, Subway*	1 Flatbread/229g	482	26.4	210	9.0	17.3	11.5	1.8
Italian BMT, Subway*	1 Flatbread/233g	406	17.8	174	9.0	17.2	7.6	1.6
Meatball Marinara, Subway*	1 Flatbread/307g	445	16.6	145	7.6	16.6	5.4	2.2
Mega Melt, Breakfast, Subway*	1 Flatbread/221g	517	23.6	234	13.0	20.7	10.7	1.7
Melt, Includes Cheese, Subway*	1 Flatbread/256g	369	10.3	144	10.7	15.9	4.0	1.5
Pulled Pork, no BBQ, Subway*	1 Flatbread/194g	347	9.0	179	13.2	20.2	4.6	1.6
Pulled Pork, with BBQ, Subway*	1 Flatbread/215g	180	4.2	180	12.0	22.5	4.2	1.6
Sausage, Breakfast, Subway*	1 Flatbread/161g	385	13.6	239	12.3	27.4	8.4	2.2
Sausage, Egg, & Cheese, Breakfast, Subway*	1 Flatbread/207g	480	21.2	232	12.1	22.1	10.2	1.8
Steak, & Cheese, Subway*	1 Flatbread/256g	369	10.3	144	10.7	15.9	4.0	1.5
Tuna, Subway*	1 Flatbread/240g	365	12.9	152	8.4	16.8	5.4	1.6
Turkey, Breast, Low Fat, Subway*	1 Flatbread/226g	279	3.3	123	9.3	17.4	1.5	1.7
Veggie Delite, Low Fat, Subway*	1 Flatbread/169g	223	2.7	132	5.3	23.0	1.6	2.2
Veggie Patty, Subway*	1 Flatbread/254g	390	9.8	154	8.4	18.9	3.9	1.5
MAYONNAISE								
Light, Subway*	1 Serving/15g	56	6.0	373	0.0	6.7	40.0	0.0
MEATBALLS								
Bowl, Subway*	1 Bowl/206g	317	19.1	154	9.2	9.2	9.3	2.0
MUFFIN								
Blueberry, Subway*	1 Muffin/111g	352	20.6	317	4.5	36.0	18.6	2.7
Chocolate Chunk, Subway*	1 Muffin/111g	394	22.9	355	5.4	39.6	20.6	2.6
Double Chocolate Chunk, Subway*	1 Muffin/111g	389	22.0	350	5.4	40.5	19.8	2.8
NACHOS								
Cheese, Melted, Subway*	1 Serving/126g	415	24.3	329	8.7	28.6	19.3	2.1
SALAD								
Beef, Subway*	1 Salad/328g	118	2.4	36	4.9	1.8	0.7	1.1
Chicken, Breast, Subway*	1 Salad/342g	139	2.4	41	5.8	2.0	0.7	1.0
Chicken, Teriyaki, Subway*	1 Salad/364g	155	2.5	43	5.8	3.0	0.7	1.1

SUBWAY

	Measure INFO/WEIGHT	per Measure KCAL	per Measure FAT	Nutrition Values per 100g / 100ml KCAL	PROT	CARB	FAT	FIBRE
SALAD								
Chicken, Tikka, Subway*	1 Salad/342g	137	2.4	40	5.8	1.8	0.7	1.0
Club, Subway*	1 Salad/361g	145	2.8	40	6.1	1.9	0.8	1.0
Garden, Side, Subway*	1 Salad/135g	21	0.2	16	0.7	2.2	0.2	1.3
Ham, & Turkey Breast, Subway*	1 Salad/338g	113	2.3	33	4.7	1.8	0.7	1.1
Ham, Subway*	1 Salad/328g	104	2.9	32	3.7	2.1	0.9	1.1
Turkey, Breast, Subway*	1 Salad/328g	104	1.6	32	4.6	1.8	0.5	1.1
Veggie Delite, Subway*	1 Salad/271g	49	1.0	18	1.1	1.8	0.4	1.3
SAUCE								
BBQ, Low Fat, Subway*	1 Serving/21g	37	0.1	176	0.0	42.9	0.5	1.0
Chipotle Southwest, Subway*	1 Serving/21g	90	9.2	429	0.0	9.5	43.8	0.5
Honey Mustard,Low Fat, Subway*	1 Serving/21g	32	0.2	152	0.0	33.3	1.0	0.5
Sweet Onion, Low Fat, Subway*	1 Serving/21g	34	0.1	162	0.0	38.1	0.5	0.5
SOUP								
Beef Goulash, Subway*	1 Serving/250g	199	11.8	80	3.3	6.0	4.7	0.9
Carrot & Coriander, Subway*	1 Serving/250g	80	1.8	32	1.0	5.6	0.7	1.1
Chicken, & Vegetable, Country, Subway*	1 Serving/250g	168	11.0	67	2.7	4.2	4.4	0.2
Chicken, Cream of, Subway*	1 Serving/250g	160	11.3	64	2.7	3.1	4.5	0.0
Leek & Potato, Subway*	1 Serving/250g	124	3.0	50	1.7	8.0	1.2	1.1
Lentil, & Bacon, Subway*	1 Serving/250g	182	5.0	73	4.4	9.3	2.0	1.1
Lentil, & Potato, Subway*	1 Serving/250g	182	5.0	73	4.4	9.3	2.0	1.1
Minestrone, Subway*	1 Serving/250g	125	3.0	50	1.7	7.8	1.2	1.7
Mushroom, Cream of, Subway*	1 Serving/250g	150	10.8	60	1.0	4.4	4.3	0.3
Mushroom, Wild, Subway*	1 Serving/250g	101	5.5	40	1.0	4.1	2.2	0.3
Red Pepper, & Tomato, Subway*	1 Serving/250g	100	4.0	40	1.4	6.0	1.6	0.9
Tomato, Subway*	1 Serving/250g	103	3.8	41	0.8	6.0	1.5	0.3
Vegetable, Highland, Subway*	1 Serving/250g	73	0.3	29	1.5	5.5	0.1	0.9
Vegetable, Thai Style, Subway*	1 Serving/250g	87	1.0	35	1.1	6.7	0.4	0.8
SUBS								
Bacon, 9 Grain Wheat, Breakfast, Subway*	1 Sub/106g	271	6.3	256	15.1	33.0	5.9	4.9
Bacon, Egg, & Cheese, 9 Grain Wheat, Breakfast, Subway*	1 Sub/138g	330	11.4	239	13.0	26.1	8.3	3.9
Bacon, Egg, & Cheese, Hearty Italian, Breakfast, Subway*	1 Sub/135g	333	11.4	247	12.6	28.9	8.4	1.7
Bacon, Egg, & Cheese, Honey Oat, Breakfast, Subway*	1 Sub/138g	330	11.4	239	13.0	26.1	8.3	3.9
Bacon, Egg, & Cheese, Italian Herbs & Cheese, Subway*	1 Sub/142g	366	14.2	258	13.4	27.5	10.0	1.5
Bacon, Egg, & Cheese, Italian White, Breakfast, Subway*	1 Sub/207g	498	22.4	241	13.5	21.8	10.8	1.3
Bacon, Hearty Italian, Breakfast, Subway*	1 Sub/103g	274	6.3	266	14.6	36.9	6.1	2.0
Bacon, Honey Oat, Breakfast, Subway*	1 Sub/106g	271	6.3	256	15.1	33.0	5.9	4.9
Bacon, Italian Herbs & Cheese, Breakfast, Subway*	1 Sub/110g	307	9.1	279	15.4	34.6	8.3	1.7
Bacon, Italian White, Breakfast, Subway*	1 Sub/99g	263	6.1	266	15.0	36.5	6.2	1.6
Beef, 9 Grain Wheat, Kids Pak, Subway*	1 Sub/156g	210	2.2	135	10.3	18.6	1.4	3.1
Beef, 9 Grain Wheat, Low Fat, Subway*	1 Sub/219g	282	3.0	129	10.5	17.4	1.4	2.9
Beef, Big Melt, Hearty Italian, Subway*	1 Sub/230g	402	16.7	175	8.3	18.7	7.3	0.4
Beef, Big Melt, Honey Oat, Subway*	1 Sub/233g	399	16.7	171	8.6	17.2	7.2	1.8
Beef, Big Melt, Italian Herbs & Cheese, Subway*	1 Sub/237g	435	19.5	184	8.9	18.1	8.2	0.3
Beef, Hearty Italian, Low Fat, Subway*	1 Sub/216g	285	3.0	132	10.2	19.0	1.4	1.5
Beef, Honey Oat, Low Fat, Subway*	1 Sub/219g	282	3.0	129	10.5	17.4	1.4	2.9
Beef, Honey Oat, Low Fat, Subway*	1 Sub/219g	282	3.0	129	10.5	17.4	1.4	2.9
Beef, Italian Herbs & Cheese, Low Fat, Subway*	1 Sub/223g	318	5.8	143	10.8	18.4	2.6	1.4
Beef, Italian White, Kids Pak, Subway*	1 Sub/151g	184	2.0	122	9.7	17.5	1.3	1.2
Beef, Italian White, Low Fat, Subway*	1 Sub/212g	274	2.9	129	10.3	18.4	1.4	1.3
Beef, Melt, Big, 9 Grain Wheat, Subway*	1 Sub/233g	399	16.7	171	8.6	17.2	7.2	1.8
Beef, Melt, Big, Italian White, Subway*	1 Sub/233g	399	16.7	171	8.8	17.4	7.2	1.8
Chicken, & Bacon, Ranch Melt, 9 Grain Wheat, Subway*	1 Sub/292g	503	19.2	172	13.0	13.7	6.6	2.2

SUBWAY
SUBS

	Measure INFO/WEIGHT	per Measure KCAL	FAT	Nutrition Values per 100g / 100ml KCAL	PROT	CARB	FAT	FIBRE
Chicken, & Bacon, Ranch Melt, Hearty Italian, Subway*	1 Sub/289g	506	19.2	175	12.8	14.9	6.6	1.1
Chicken, & Bacon, Ranch Melt, Honey Oat, Subway*	1 Sub/292g	503	19.2	172	13.0	13.7	6.6	2.2
Chicken, & Bacon, Ranch Melt, Italian White, Subway*	1 Sub/285g	494	19.1	173	12.8	14.6	6.7	1.0
Chicken, & Chorizo, 9 Grain Wheat, Subway*	1 Sub/248g	356	7.4	144	12.4	15.8	3.0	2.5
Chicken, & Chorizo, Hearty Italian, Subway*	1 Sub/245g	359	7.4	147	12.1	17.2	3.0	1.3
Chicken, & Chorizo, Honey Oat, Subway*	1 Sub/248g	356	7.4	144	12.4	15.8	3.0	2.5
Chicken, & Chorizo, Italian Herbs & Cheese, Subway*	1 Sub/252g	392	10.2	156	12.6	16.7	4.0	1.2
Chicken, & Chorizo, Italian White, Subway*	1 Sub/241g	348	7.2	144	12.2	16.8	3.0	1.1
Chicken, & Jalapeño, Melt, Subway*	1 Sub/249g	345	6.4	139	11.7	15.7	2.6	2.6
Chicken, Breast, 9 Grain Wheat, Low Fat, Subway*	1 Sub/233g	304	3.0	130	11.6	16.7	1.3	2.7
Chicken, Breast, Hearty Italian, Low Fat, Subway*	1 Sub/230g	307	3.0	133	11.3	18.3	1.3	1.4
Chicken, Breast, Honey Oat, Low Fat, Subway*	1 Sub/233g	304	3.0	130	11.6	16.7	1.3	2.7
Chicken, Breast, Italian Herbs & Cheese, Low Fat, Subway*	1 Sub/237g	340	5.8	143	11.8	17.7	2.4	1.3
Chicken, Breast, Italian White, Low Fat, Subway*	1 Sub/226g	295	2.9	131	11.5	17.7	1.3	1.2
Chicken, Tandoori, 9 Grain Wheat, Low Fat, Subway*	1 Sub/254g	315	3.7	124	11.0	15.0	1.5	2.5
Chicken, Tandoori, Hearty Italian, Low Fat, Subway*	1 Sub/251g	318	3.7	127	10.8	16.4	1.5	1.3
Chicken, Tandoori, Honey Oat, Low Fat, Subway*	1 Sub/254g	315	3.7	124	11.0	15.0	1.5	2.5
Chicken, Tandoori, Italian Herb Cheese, Low Fat, Subway*	1 Sub/258g	351	6.5	136	11.2	15.9	2.5	1.2
Chicken, Temptation, 9 Grain Wheat, Subway*	1 Sub/262g	406	8.7	155	10.3	19.8	3.3	2.4
Chicken, Temptation, Hearty Italian, Subway*	1 Sub/259g	409	8.7	158	10.0	21.2	3.4	1.2
Chicken, Temptation, Honey Oat, Subway*	1 Sub/262g	406	8.7	155	10.3	19.8	3.3	2.4
Chicken, Temptation, Italian Herbs & Cheese, Subway*	1 Sub/266g	442	11.5	166	10.5	20.7	4.3	1.1
Chicken, Temptation, Italian White, Subway*	1 Sub/255g	398	8.6	156	10.2	20.9	3.4	1.1
Chicken, Teriyaki, 9 Grain Wheat, Low Fat, Subway*	1 Sub/254g	320	3.2	126	11.0	16.5	1.3	2.6
Chicken, Teriyaki, Hearty Italian, Low Fat, Subway*	1 Sub/251g	323	3.2	129	10.8	17.9	1.3	1.4
Chicken, Teriyaki, Honey Oat, Low Fat, Subway*	1 Sub/254g	320	3.2	126	11.0	16.5	1.3	2.6
Chicken, Teriyaki, Italian Herb Cheese, Low Fat, Subway*	1 Sub/258g	356	6.0	138	11.2	17.4	2.3	1.3
Chicken, Teriyaki, Italian White, Low Fat, Subway*	1 Sub/247g	311	3.0	126	10.7	17.6	1.2	1.2
Chicken, Teriyaki, Sweet Onion, Low Fat, Subway*	1 Sub/276g	354	3.3	128	10.1	18.1	1.2	2.4
Chicken, Tikka, 9 Grain Wheat, Low Fat, Subway*	1 Sub/233g	302	3.0	130	11.6	16.3	1.3	2.7
Chicken, Tikka, Hearty Italian, Low Fat, Subway*	1 Sub/230g	305	3.0	133	11.3	17.8	1.3	1.4
Chicken, Tikka, Honey Oat, Low Fat, Subway*	1 Sub/233g	302	3.0	130	11.6	16.3	1.3	2.7
Chicken, Tikka, Italian Herbs & Cheese, Low Fat, Subway*	1 Sub/237g	338	5.8	143	11.8	17.3	2.4	1.3
Chicken, Tikka, Italian White, Low Fat, Subway*	1 Sub/226g	293	2.9	130	11.5	17.4	1.3	1.2
Club, 9 Grain Wheat, Low Fat, Subway*	1 Sub/252g	310	3.4	123	11.5	15.1	1.4	2.5
Club, Hearty Italian, Low Fat, Subway*	1 Sub/249g	313	3.4	126	11.2	16.5	1.4	1.3
Club, Honey Oat, Low Fat, Subway*	1 Sub/252g	310	3.4	123	11.5	15.1	1.4	2.5
Club, Honey Oat, Low Fat, Subway*	1 Sub/162g	213	1.6	131	5.6	22.8	1.0	3.9
Club, Italian Herbs & Cheese, Low Fat, Subway*	1 Sub/256g	346	6.2	135	11.7	16.0	2.4	1.2
Club, Italian White, Low Fat, Subway*	1 Sub/245g	302	3.3	123	11.4	16.1	1.4	1.1
Club, with Cheese & Salad, Subway*	1 Sub/160g	311	3.7	194	18.1	23.8	2.3	3.9
Egg, & Cheese, 9 Grain Wheat, Breakfast, Subway*	1 Sub/124g	294	9.0	237	11.3	29.0	7.3	4.4
Egg, & Cheese, Hearty Italian, Breakfast, Subway*	1 Sub/121g	297	9.0	245	10.7	32.2	7.4	1.9
Egg, & Cheese, Honey Oat, Breakfast, Subway*	1 Sub/124g	294	9.0	237	11.3	29.0	7.3	4.4
Egg, & Cheese, Italian Herbs & Cheese, Subway*	1 Sub/128g	330	11.8	258	11.7	30.5	9.2	1.6
Eggs, & Cheese, Italian White, Breakfast, Subway*	1 Sub/131g	304	10.1	232	9.6	29.1	7.7	1.4
Ham, & Turkey Breast, Hearty Italian, Low Fat, Subway*	1 Sub/225g	281	3.0	125	9.3	18.2	1.3	1.4
Ham, & Turkey Breast, Honey Oat, Low Fat, Subway*	1 Sub/228g	278	3.0	122	9.6	16.7	1.3	2.8
Ham, & Turkey Breast, Italian White, Low Fat, Subway*	1 Sub/221g	269	2.8	122	9.6	17.8	1.3	1.2
Ham, 9 Grain Wheat, Kids Pak, Subway*	1 Sub/147g	192	2.2	131	8.2	19.7	1.5	3.3
Ham, 9 Grain Wheat, Low Fat, Subway*	1 Sub/219g	269	3.5	123	8.7	17.4	1.6	2.9
Ham, Hearty Italian, Low Fat, Subway*	1 Sub/216g	272	3.5	126	8.3	19.0	1.6	1.5

SUBWAY

SUBS

	Measure INFO/WEIGHT	per Measure KCAL	FAT	Nutrition Values per 100g / 100ml KCAL	PROT	CARB	FAT	FIBRE
Ham, Honey Oat, Low Fat, Subway*	1 Sub/219g	269	3.5	123	8.7	17.4	1.6	2.9
Ham, Italian Herbs & Cheese, Low Fat, Subway*	1 Sub/223g	305	6.3	137	94.2	18.4	2.8	1.4
Ham, Italian White, Kids Pak, Subway*	1 Sub/141g	166	2.0	118	7.4	18.9	1.4	1.3
Ham, Italian White, Low Fat, Subway*	1 Sub/212g	260	3.4	123	8.5	18.8	1.6	1.3
Italian BMT, 9 Grain Wheat, Subway*	1 Sub/226g	396	16.8	175	9.3	16.8	7.4	2.8
Italian BMT, Hearty Italian, Subway*	1 Sub/223g	399	16.8	179	9.0	18.4	7.5	1.4
Italian BMT, Honey Oat, Subway*	1 Sub/226g	396	16.8	175	9.3	16.8	7.4	2.8
Italian BMT, Italian Herbs & Cheese, Subway*	1 Sub/230g	432	19.6	188	9.6	17.8	8.5	1.3
Italian BMT, Italian White, Subway*	1 Sub/219g	387	16.6	177	9.2	18.0	7.6	1.2
Meatball Marinara, 9 Grain Wheat, Subway*	1 Sub/300g	435	15.5	145	8.0	16.3	5.2	3.1
Meatball Marinara, Hearty Italian, Subway*	1 Sub/297g	438	15.5	147	7.7	17.5	5.2	2.1
Meatball Marinara, Honey Oat, Subway*	1 Sub/300g	435	15.5	145	8.0	16.3	5.2	3.1
Meatball Marinara, Italian Herbs & Cheese, Subway*	1 Sub/304g	471	18.3	155	8.2	17.1	6.0	2.0
Meatball Marinara, Italian White, Subway*	1 Sub/293g	426	15.4	145	7.7	17.2	5.3	2.0
Mega Melt, 9 Grain Wheat, Breakfast, Subway*	1 Sub/214g	507	22.5	237	13.6	20.6	10.5	2.9
Mega Melt, Hearty Italian, Subway*	1 Sub/211g	510	22.5	242	13.3	22.3	10.7	1.5
Mega Melt, Honey Oat, Breakfast, Subway*	1 Sub/214g	507	22.5	237	13.6	20.6	10.5	2.9
Mega Melt, Italian herbs & Cheese, Breakfast, Subway*	1 Sub/218g	543	25.3	249	13.8	21.6	11.6	1.3
Mega Melt, Italian White, Breakfast, Subway*	1 Sub/147g	366	12.4	249	12.9	29.7	8.4	1.7
Melt, Hearty Italian, Subway*	1 Sub/246g	362	9.3	147	11.0	17.1	3.8	1.3
Melt, Honey Oat, Subway*	1 Sub/249g	359	9.3	144	11.2	15.7	3.7	2.5
Melt, Includes Cheese, Italian White, Subway*	1 Sub/242g	350	9.1	145	11.0	16.6	3.8	1.1
Melt, Italian Herbs & Cheese, Subway*	1 Sub/253g	395	12.1	156	11.5	16.6	4.8	1.2
Pulled Pork, Barbeque, Subway*	1 Sub/201g	367	7.8	183	12.5	23.8	3.9	1.1
Sausage, 9 Grain Wheat, Breakfast, Subway*	1 Sub/154g	374	12.6	243	13.0	27.3	8.2	4.0
Sausage, Egg, & Cheese, 9 Grain Wheat, Subway*	1 Sub/200g	470	20.1	235	12.5	22.0	10.0	3.1
Sausage, Egg, & Cheese, Hearty Italian, Subway*	1 Sub/197g	473	20.1	240	12.2	23.9	10.2	1.6
Sausage, Egg, & Cheese, Honey Oat, Subway*	1 Sub/200g	470	20.1	235	12.5	22.0	10.0	3.1
Sausage, Egg, & Cheese, Italian Herbs & Cheese, Subway*	1 Sub/204g	506	22.9	248	12.8	23.0	11.2	1.4
Sausage, Egg, & Cheese, Italian White, Subway*	1 Sub/193g	461	20.0	239	12.5	23.4	10.4	1.4
Sausage, Hearty Italian, Breakfast, Subway*	1 Sub/151g	377	12.6	250	12.6	29.8	8.3	2.0
Sausage, Honey Oat, Breakfast, Subway*	1 Sub/154g	374	12.6	243	13.0	27.3	8.2	4.0
Sausage, Italian Herbs & Cheese, Breakfast, Subway*	1 Sub/158g	410	15.4	259	13.3	28.5	9.8	1.8
Sausage, Italian White, Breakfast, Subway*	1 Sub/131g	322	11.3	246	12.5	28.7	8.6	1.4
Spicy Italian, 9 Grain Wheat, Subway*	1 Sub/222g	471	25.3	212	9.5	17.1	11.4	2.8
Spicy Italian, Hearty Italian, Subway*	1 Sub/219g	474	25.3	216	9.1	18.7	11.6	1.5
Spicy Italian, Honey Oat, Subway*	1 Sub/222g	471	25.3	212	9.5	17.1	11.4	2.8
Spicy Italian, Italian Herbs & Cheese, Subway*	1 Sub/226g	507	28.1	224	9.7	18.1	12.4	1.3
Spicy Italian, Italian White, Subway*	1 Sub/215g	463	25.2	215	9.2	18.2	11.7	1.3
Steak, & Cheese, Hearty Italian, Subway*	1 Sub/242g	346	8.5	143	10.3	17.8	3.5	1.5
Steak, & Cheese, Honey Oat, Subway*	1 Sub/245g	343	8.5	140	10.6	16.3	3.5	2.7
Steak, & Cheese, Italian Herbs & Cheese, Subway*	1 Sub/249g	379	11.3	152	10.8	17.3	4.5	1.4
Steak, & Cheese, Italian White, Subway*	1 Sub/238g	335	8.4	141	10.2	17.4	3.5	1.3
Steak, & Chorizo, Melt, 9 Grain Wheat, Subway*	1 Sub/252g	387	12.7	154	11.0	16.6	5.0	1.2
Steak, & Chorizo, Melt, Italian White, Subway*	1 Sub/259g	395	12.9	153	11.2	15.6	5.0	1.0
Steak, & Chorizo Melt, Hearty Italian, Subway*	1 Sub/249g	390	12.7	157	10.8	18.0	5.1	0.0
Steak, & Chorizo Melt, Honey Oat, Subway*	1 Sub/252g	387	12.7	154	11.0	16.6	5.0	1.2
Steak, & Chorizo Melt, Italian Herbs & Cheese, Subway*	1 Sub/256g	423	15.5	165	11.2	17.5	6.0	0.7
Steak & Cheese, 9 Grain Wheat, Subway*	1 Sub/245g	343	8.5	140	10.6	16.3	3.5	2.7
Tuna, 9 Grain Wheat, Subway*	1 Sub/233g	355	11.8	152	9.0	16.3	5.1	2.7
Tuna, Hearty Italian, Subway*	1 Sub/230g	358	11.8	156	8.7	17.8	5.1	1.4
Tuna, Honey Oat, Subway*	1 Sub/233g	355	11.8	152	9.0	16.3	5.1	2.7

	Measure INFO/WEIGHT	per Measure KCAL	FAT	Nutrition Values per 100g / 100ml KCAL	PROT	CARB	FAT	FIBRE

SUBWAY
SUBS

	Measure/INFO/WEIGHT	KCAL	FAT	KCAL	PROT	CARB	FAT	FIBRE
Tuna, Italian Herbs & Cheese, Subway*	1 Sub/237g	391	14.6	165	9.3	17.3	6.2	1.3
Tuna, Italian White, Subway*	1 Sub/226g	347	11.7	154	8.6	17.6	5.2	1.2
Turkey, & Ham, 9 Grain Wheat, Low Fat, Subway*	1 Sub/228g	278	3.0	122	9.6	16.7	1.3	2.8
Turkey, Breast, 9 Grain Wheat, Kids Pak, Subway*	1 Sub/156g	201	1.6	129	9.6	18.6	1.0	3.1
Turkey, Breast, 9 Grain Wheat, Low Fat, Subway*	1 Sub/219g	269	2.2	123	10.0	17.4	1.0	2.9
Turkey, Breast, Hearty Italian, Low Fat, Subway*	1 Sub/216g	272	2.2	126	9.7	19.0	1.0	1.5
Turkey, Breast, Honey Oat, Low Fat, Subway*	1 Sub/219g	269	2.2	123	10.0	17.4	1.0	2.9
Turkey, Breast, Italian Herbs & Cheese, Low Fat, Subway*	1 Sub/223g	305	5.0	137	10.3	18.4	2.2	1.4
Turkey, Breast, Italian White, Kids Pak, Subway*	1 Sub/151g	175	1.4	116	9.0	17.4	0.9	1.2
Turkey, Breast, Italian White, Low Fat, Subway*	1 Sub/212g	260	2.1	123	9.5	18.4	1.0	1.3
Veggie Delight, 9 Grain Wheat, Kids Pak, Subway*	1 Sub/118g	164	1.2	139	5.9	24.6	1.0	4.1
Veggie Delite, 9 Grain Wheat, Low Fat, Subway*	1 Sub/162g	213	1.6	131	5.6	22.8	1.0	3.9
Veggie Delite, Hearty Italian, Low Fat, Subway*	1 Sub/159g	216	1.6	136	5.0	25.2	1.0	2.0
Veggie Delite, Italian Herbs & Cheese, Low Fat, Subway*	1 Sub/166g	249	4.4	150	6.0	24.1	2.6	1.8
Veggie Delite, Italian White, Low Fat, Subway*	1 Sub/162g	213	1.6	131	5.9	22.8	1.0	3.9
Veggie Patty, 9 Grain Wheat, Subway*	1 Sub/247g	380	8.7	154	8.9	18.6	3.5	2.6
Veggie Patty, Hearty Italian, Subway*	1 Sub/244g	383	8.7	157	8.6	20.1	3.6	1.3
Veggie Patty, Honey Oat, Subway*	1 Sub/247g	380	8.7	154	8.9	18.6	3.5	2.6
Veggie Patty, Italian Herbs & Cheese, Subway*	1 Sub/251g	416	11.5	166	9.2	19.5	4.6	1.2
Veggie Patty, Italian White, Subway*	1 Sub/240g	364	10.0	152	8.4	18.9	4.2	2.9

TOASTIE

Cheese, Subway*	1 Toastie/64g	210	9.5	328	17.2	29.7	14.8	1.2
Pepperoni Pizza, Subway*	1 Toastie/93g	248	12.5	267	11.8	23.7	13.4	1.4

WRAP

Beef, Subway*	1 Wrap/242g	412	8.1	170	9.1	25.6	3.4	1.3
Chicken & Bacon Ranch Melt, Subway*	1 Wrap/315g	633	24.3	201	11.8	20.6	7.7	1.0
Chicken Breast, Subway*	1 Wrap/256g	434	8.1	170	10.2	24.6	3.2	1.2
Chicken Tikka, Subway*	1 Wrap/256g	432	8.1	169	10.2	24.6	3.2	1.2
Ham, Subway*	1 Wrap/242g	399	8.6	165	7.8	26.0	3.6	1.3
Meatball Marinara, Subway*	1 Wrap/323g	561	20.2	174	7.1	22.9	6.2	1.9
Spicy Italian, Subway*	1 Wrap/245g	602	30.4	246	8.2	25.3	12.4	1.3
Steak & Cheese, with Peppers & Onions, Subway*	1 Wrap/268g	473	13.6	176	9.3	24.2	5.1	1.3
Subway Melt with Cheese, Subway*	1 Wrap/272g	489	14.3	180	9.9	23.2	5.3	1.1
Sweet Onion Chicken Teriyaki, Subway*	1 Wrap/299g	484	8.3	162	9.0	25.1	2.8	1.2
Tuna, Subway*	1 Wrap/256g	489	17.7	191	7.8	25.0	6.9	1.2
Turkey Breast, Subway*	1 Wrap/242g	399	7.3	165	8.7	25.6	3.0	1.3
Turkey Breast & Ham, Subway*	1 Wrap/251g	408	8.1	163	8.8	25.1	3.2	1.2
Veggie Delite, Subway*	1 Wrap/185g	343	6.7	185	4.9	33.5	3.6	1.7

THE REAL GREEK FOOD COMPANY LTD
ASPARAGUS

Grilled, Hot Meze, Real Greek Food Co*	1 Serving/110g	140	9.8	127	3.3	9.3	8.9	2.4

CHEESE

Halloumi, Grilled, Hot Meze, Real Greek Food Co*	1 Portion/86g	151	11.8	175	10.3	74.5	13.7	0.9
Halloumi, Skewers, Hot Meze, Real Greek Food Co*	1 Serving/128g	118	8.5	92	6.8	49.7	6.6	0.5
Halloumi, Skewers, Kids Menu, Real Greek Food Co*	1 Skewer/128g	118	8.5	92	6.8	50.0	6.6	0.5

CHICK PEAS

Revithia, Cold Meze, Real Greek Food Co*	1 Serving/160g	286	20.1	179	4.8	11.9	12.6	4.0

CHICKEN

Skewers, Hot Meze, Real Greek Food Co*	1 Serving/144g	177	7.6	123	3.1	1.3	5.3	0.7
Skewers, Kids Menu, Real Greek Food Co*	1 Serving/72g	88	3.8	123	3.2	1.4	5.3	0.7

CHIPS

The Real Greek Food Company Ltd*	1 Serving/372g	528	19.6	142	2.7	22.3	5.3	0.0

THE REAL GREEK FOOD COMPANY LTD

	Measure INFO/WEIGHT	per Measure KCAL	per Measure FAT	Nutrition Values per 100g / 100ml KCAL	PROT	CARB	FAT	FIBRE
COD								
Salt, Hot Meze, Real Greek Food Co*	1 Serving/152g	346	1.5	227	21.1	34.2	1.0	0.6
CRUDITES								
Cold Meze, Real Greek Food Co*	1 Serving/231g	37	0.4	16	0.6	3.1	0.2	1.6
DESSERT								
Watermelon, Sweet & Salty, Real Greek Food Co*	1 Serving/365g	124	2.2	34	0.6	7.0	0.6	0.2
Yoghurt, Greek with Raspberries, Real Greek Food Co*	1 Serving/201g	223	13.1	111	3.7	10.4	6.5	0.6
DIP								
Aioli, Parsley, Real Greek Food Co*	1 Serving/35g	176	18.8	504	2.3	2.3	53.8	0.6
Dip, Selection, Real Greek Food Co*	1 Serving/140g	589	56.5	421	1.8	9.9	40.4	0.8
Mayonnaise, Lemon, Preserved, Real Greek Food Co*	1 Serving/35g	279	30.3	797	2.0	1.1	86.6	0.0
Melitzanasalata, Cold Meze, Real Greek Food Co*	1 Serving/140g	236	21.8	168	1.2	7.1	15.5	3.2
Relish, Chilli, Smoked, Real Greek Food Co*	1 Serving/35g	42	0.1	119	1.1	30.0	0.3	0.6
Relish, Sundried Tomato Red Pepper, Real Greek Food Co*	1 Serving/35g	92	7.3	263	2.0	6.0	20.9	2.0
DOLMADES								
Cold Meze, Real Greek Food Co*	1 Serving/130g	254	15.7	194	2.9	18.8	12.0	0.8
FLATBREAD								
Greek, Cold Meze, Real Greek Food Co*	1 Serving/200g	615	15.7	307	6.6	52.6	7.8	7.4
Greek, with Olive & Dukkah, Nibbles, Real Greek Food Co*	1 Serving/129g	538	32.4	417	6.4	41.3	25.1	6.4
HOUMOUS								
Cold Meze, Real Greek Food Co*	1 Serving/140g	298	19.1	213	7.6	15.6	13.6	5.2
LAMB								
Cutlets, Hot Meze, Real Greek Food Co*	1 Serving/260g	881	79.1	339	16.4	0.0	30.4	0.0
Kefte, Hot Meze, Real Greek Food Co*	1 Serving/216g	344	24.8	159	12.0	2.2	11.5	0.3
Skewers, Hot Meze, Real Greek Food Co*	1 Serving/166g	255	18.8	154	11.8	1.2	11.4	0.6
NUTS								
Mixed, Athenian, Nibbles, Real Greek Food Co*	1 Serving/75g	479	45.4	638	17.7	6.1	60.5	9.2
OCTOPUS								
Grilled, Hot Meze, Real Greek Food Co*	1 Serving/128g	447	25.4	349	39.4	3.2	19.8	0.3
OLIVES								
Nibbles, Real Greek Food Co*	1 Serving/110g	317	33.2	288	1.7	2.4	30.2	4.3
PARCELS								
Tiropitakia, Filo Pastry, Hot Meze, Real Greek Food Co*	1 Serving/120g	416	21.2	344	10.0	37.3	17.5	1.3
PORK								
Skewers, Hot Meze, Real Greek Food Co*	1 Serving/165g	281	21.7	170	11.8	1.2	13.1	0.6
POTATOES								
New, Olive Oil & Lemon Juice, Real Greek Food Co*	1 Serving/386g	293	5.2	76	1.7	15.2	1.4	1.4
RICE								
Saffron, Hot Meze, Real Greek Food Co*	1 Serving/258g	406	2.8	157	3.2	32.2	1.1	0.3
SALAD								
Cos, Real Greek Food Co*	1 Serving/117g	42	3.0	36	1.2	1.4	2.6	1.5
Tabouleh, Cold Meze, Real Greek Food Co*	1 Serving/165g	117	8.2	71	1.3	6.3	5.0	1.9
Watermelon, Mint & Feta, Real Greek Food Co*	1 Serving/192g	102	7.7	53	1.9	2.6	4.0	0.2
SARDINES								
Grilled, Hot Meze, Real Greek Food Co*	1 Serving/360g	619	32.8	172	22.2	0.3	9.1	0.1
SOUVLAKI								
Lamb, Kefte, Real Greek Food Co*	1 Serving/322g	730	39.0	227	10.7	19.0	12.1	2.7
Lamb, Real Greek Food Co*	1 Serving/270g	607	29.4	225	10.3	21.6	10.9	3.3
Pork, Real Greek Food Co*	1 Serving/271g	633	32.2	234	10.3	21.5	11.9	3.3
Souvlaki, Halloumi & Vegetable, Real Greek Food Co*	1 Serving/234g	451	18.9	193	5.6	39.1	8.1	3.6
SQUID								
Kalamari, Grilled, Hot Meze, Real Greek Food Co*	1 Serving/140g	286	135.4	203	12.4	1.6	96.1	0.2

	Measure INFO/WEIGHT	per Measure KCAL	FAT	Nutrition Values per 100g / 100ml KCAL	PROT	CARB	FAT	FIBRE

THE REAL GREEK FOOD COMPANY LTD

TARAMASALATA

	Measure INFO/WEIGHT	KCAL	FAT	KCAL	PROT	CARB	FAT	FIBRE
Cold Meze, Real Greek Food Co*	1 Serving/140g	913	99.0	652	2.5	2.1	70.7	0.0
TZATZIKI								
Cold Meze, Real Greek Food Co*	1 Serving/141g	163	14.1	116	3.5	3.1	10.0	0.4
TOBY CARVERY								
BACON								
Back, Breakfast, Toby Carvery*	1 Rasher/29g	38	2.0	132	16.9	0.0	7.1	0.0
BEANS								
Baked, Breakfast, Toby Carvery*	1 Portion/100g	91	1.4	91	4.5	12.8	1.4	0.0
Green, Toby Carvery*	1 Portion/40g	17	0.5	42	1.8	7.2	1.3	0.0
Romano, Toby Carvery*	1 Portion/40g	17	0.5	42	1.8	7.2	1.3	0.0
BEEF								
Roast, Kids, Toby Carvery*	1 Portion/80g	229	13.7	286	32.0	1.0	17.1	0.0
Roast, Tewkesbury Mustard Glazed, Toby Carvery*	1 Portion/160g	458	27.2	286	32.0	1.0	17.0	0.0
BREAD								
Garlic, Baguette, Cheesy, Toby Carvery*	1 Portion/189g	625	31.3	331	12.0	32.8	16.6	0.0
Garlic, Baguette, Quarters, Toby Carvery*	1 Portion/146g	451	16.7	310	8.2	42.6	11.5	0.0
BROCCOLI								
Toby Carvery*	1 Portion/40g	20	0.9	49	4.3	1.8	2.1	0.0
BRUSSELS SPROUTS								
Toby Carvery*	1 Portion/40g	26	1.1	64	3.4	4.0	2.6	0.0
BUTTER								
Portion, Breakfast, Toby Carvery*	1 Portion/7g	52	5.7	738	0.6	1.0	81.0	0.0
CABBAGE								
Red, with Cranberry & Orange, Toby Carvery*	1 Portion/40g	12	0.3	29	1.4	4.3	0.7	0.0
with Onions, Toby Carvery*	1 Portion/40g	8	0.2	21	1.0	2.1	0.4	0.0
CARROTS								
Toby Carvery*	1 Portion/40g	24	0.4	61	0.6	12.2	1.0	0.0
CAULIFLOWER CHEESE								
Toby Carvery*	1 Portion/40g	17	0.5	43	2.3	5.5	1.3	0.0
CHICKEN								
& Yorkshire Pudding, Breast, Roast, Kids, Toby Carvery*	1 Portion/163g	296	7.8	182	0.9	7.2	4.8	0.0
CRUMBLE								
Butternut Squash & Kale, Brown Rice, Toby Carvery*	1 Portion/371g	442	17.5	119	2.5	15.8	4.7	0.0
EGGS								
Fried, Free Range, Breakfast, Toby Carvery*	1 Egg/65g	117	9.0	180	13.6	0.0	13.9	0.0
Scrambled, Free Range, Breakfast, Toby Carvery*	1 Portion/100g	119	8.5	119	8.7	2.0	8.5	0.0
GAMMON								
Roast, Honey & Mustard Glazed, Toby Carvery*	1 Portion/160g	317	13.3	198	30.8	1.0	8.3	0.0
Roast, Klids, Toby Carvery*	1 Portion/80g	158	6.6	198	30.8	0.0	8.3	0.0
GRAVY								
Beef, & Onion, Toby Carvery*	1 Serving/100g	21	0.2	21	0.5	4.3	0.2	0.0
Breakfast, Toby Carvery*	1 Serving/100g	23	0.2	23	1.0	4.9	0.2	0.0
Onion, Vegetarian, Toby Carvery*	1 Serving/100g	23	0.0	23	0.2	5.1	0.0	0.0
Poultry, Toby Carvery*	1 Serving/100g	21	0.0	21	0.4	4.5	0.0	0.0
HASH								
Potato, Bacon, Cheese, & Onion, Breakfast, Toby Carvery*	1 Portion/100g	113	4.3	113	3.1	14.8	4.3	0.0
JAM								
Apricot, Hartleys, Portion, Breakfast, Toby Carvery*	1 Portion/6g	14	0.0	238	0.3	59.0	0.1	0.0
Blackcurrant, Hartleys, Portion, Breakfast, Toby Carvery*	1 Portion/6g	14	0.0	241	0.3	58.0	0.6	0.0
Raspberry, Hartleys, Portion, Breakfast, Toby Carvery*	1 Portion/6g	14	0.0	237	0.5	58.0	0.1	0.0
Strawberry, Hartleys, Portion, Breakfast, Toby Carvery*	1 Portion/6g	14	0.0	238	0.3	59.0	0.1	0.0

TOBY CARVERY

	Measure INFO/WEIGHT	per Measure KCAL	per Measure FAT	Nutrition Values per 100g / 100ml KCAL	PROT	CARB	FAT	FIBRE
LEEKS								
Toby Carvery*	1 Portion/40g	8	0.2	19	1.1	2.2	0.5	0.0
MUSHROOMS								
Button, Roasted, Breakfast, Toby Carvery*	1 Portion/100g	93	9.3	93	1.6	0.4	9.3	0.0
Garlic, with Warmed Bread, Toby Carvery*	1 Portion/377g	614	47.8	163	2.9	8.9	12.7	0.0
MUSTARD								
Toby Carvery*	1 Serving/15g	29	1.3	194	8.0	21.0	9.0	0.0
Wholegrain, Toby Carvery*	1 Serving/15g	32	2.1	214	9.6	10.9	14.0	0.0
ONIONS								
in Gravy, Toby Carvery*	1 Portion/40g	30	0.4	75	1.4	15.1	1.0	0.0
PARCELS								
Broccoli & Brie, Puff Pastry, Toby Carvery*	1 Portion/278g	763	51.9	275	6.3	20.0	18.7	0.0
PARSNIP								
Toby Carvery*	1 Portion/40g	134	8.8	334	2.3	31.3	22.0	0.0
PASTA								
Tomato, Garlic Bread & Veggie Sticks, Kids, Toby Carvery*	1 Portion/404g	380	14.6	94	2.3	12.5	3.6	0.0
PATE								
Chicken Liver, & Baguette, Chutney, & Salad, Toby Carvery*	1 Portion/283g	492	26.6	174	5.5	16.3	9.4	0.0
PEAS								
Toby Carvery*	1 Portion/40g	46	0.6	114	5.8	19.2	1.5	0.0
PIE								
Cottage, Lentil, Parsnip Mash, Toby Carvery*	1 Portion/353g	409	17.3	116	4.0	12.7	4.9	0.0
Shepherds, Kids, Toby Carvery*	1 Portion/251g	228	12.5	91	4.0	7.0	5.0	0.0
PORK								
Crackling, Homemade, Toby Carvery*	1 Portion/100g	670	71.4	670	6.8	0.0	71.4	0.0
Roast, Glazed Apple & Sage, no Crackling, Toby Carvery*	1 Portion/160g	424	19.2	265	38.9	1.0	12.0	0.0
Roast, Kids, Toby Carvery*	1 Portion/80g	212	9.8	265	38.9	0.0	12.2	0.0
POTATOES								
Mashed, Toby Carvery*	1 Portion/40g	46	2.2	115	1.2	15.5	5.4	0.0
Roast, Toby Carvery*	3 Potatoes/150g	258	4.4	172	3.8	32.7	2.9	0.0
PRAWN COCKTAIL								
King, Classic, & Brown Bread, Toby Carvery*	1 Portion/278g	447	27.5	161	6.9	10.3	9.9	0.0
King, Mini, with Wholemeal Bread, Kids, Toby Carvery*	1 Portion/171g	255	11.0	149	7.7	14.0	6.4	0.0
PUDDING								
After Eight Munchies Sundae, Toby Carvery*	1 Portion/248g	549	18.6	221	3.4	34.6	7.5	0.0
Apple & Cinnamon Crumble, with Custard, Toby Carvery*	1 Portion/343g	498	16.8	145	1.4	23.3	4.9	0.0
Banoffee Sundae, Toby Carvery*	1 Portion/329g	565	16.8	172	2.8	28.3	5.1	0.0
Blackcurrant Eton Mess, Toby Carvery*	1 Portion/287g	915	77.7	319	1.9	16.6	27.1	0.0
Chocolate Brownie Ice Cream Sensation, Toby Carvery*	1 Portion/306g	1296	60.0	214	4.1	26.5	9.9	0.0
Honeycomb Dream Sundae, Toby Carvery*	1 Portion/234g	489	14.3	209	3.3	35.1	6.1	0.0
Lemon Frost Sundae, Toby Carvery*	1 Portion/253g	511	10.1	202	3.2	38.3	4.0	0.0
Lemon Shortbread Cheesecake, Toby Carvery*	1 Portion/205g	714	52.9	348	2.4	26.4	25.8	0.0
Mini Rolo Sundae, Toby Carvery*	1 Portion/243g	534	18.4	220	3.7	34.0	7.6	0.0
Profiteroles with Belgian Chocolate Sauce, Toby Carvery*	1 Portion/200g	645	47.7	322	2.4	24.6	23.8	0.0
SALAD								
House, & Reduced Calorie French Dressing, Toby Carvery*	1 Portion/393g	177	7.5	45	1.2	4.9	1.9	0.0
House, with Baked Salmon Fillet, Toby Carvery*	1 Portion/586g	580	33.4	99	8.1	3.4	5.7	0.0
House, with Beef, Toby Carvery*	1 Portion/557g	635	35.1	114	10.1	3.8	6.3	0.0
House, with Gammon, Toby Carvery*	1 Portion/555g	494	21.1	89	9.7	3.8	3.8	0.0
House, with Pork, Toby Carvery*	1 Portion/566g	668	34.0	118	12.0	3.7	6.0	0.0
House, with Roast Chicken Breast, Toby Carvery*	1 Portion/540	475	22.1	88	8.8	3.7	4.1	0.0
House, with Turkey, Toby Carvery*	1 Portion/558g	430	12.8	77	10.1	3.8	2.3	0.0

TOBY CARVERY

	Measure INFO/WEIGHT	per Measure KCAL	FAT	Nutrition Values per 100g / 100ml KCAL	PROT	CARB	FAT	FIBRE
SALMON								
Fillet, Baked, Coriander & Lime Butter, Toby Carvery*	1 Portion/220g	489	34.8	222	19.4	0.2	15.8	0.0
SANDWICH								
Baguette, Beef, & Horseradish, Roast, Toby Carvery*	1 Portion/420g	1038	38.2	247	11.3	29.8	9.1	0.0
Baguette, Cheddar, with Fruity Chutney, Toby Carvery*	1 Portion/394g	1016	40.2	258	9.0	32.2	10.2	0.0
Baguette, Gammon, Roast, Toby Carvery*	1 Portion/530g	981	30.8	185	8.9	23.7	5.8	0.0
Baguette, King Prawns, in Seafood Sauce, Toby Carvery*	1 Portion/331g	1015	44.3	307	9.7	36.5	13.4	0.0
Baguette, Pork, Stuffing, & Apple Sauce, Toby Carvery*	1 Portion/490g	1063	31.8	217	10.7	28.4	6.5	0.0
Baguette, Turkey, Stuffing, Cranberry Sauce, Toby Carvery*	1 Portion/668g	948	24.7	142	7.0	19.9	3.7	0.0
Bap, Beef, & Horseradish, Roast, Toby Carvery*	1 Portion/379g	989	42.1	261	11.2	28.9	11.1	0.0
Bap, Cheddar, with Fruity Chutney, Toby Carvery*	1 Portion/354g	967	43.9	273	8.7	31.5	12.4	0.0
Bap, Gammon, Roast, Toby Carvery*	1 Portion/491g	932	28.9	190	7.1	18.6	5.9	0.0
Bap, King Prawns, in Seafood Sauce, Toby Carvery*	1 Portion/331g	966	48.3	292	8.2	31.9	14.6	0.0
Bap, Pork, Stuffing, & Apple Sauce, Toby Carvery*	1 Portion/344g	1014	35.7	295	13.9	35.9	10.4	0.0
Bap, Turkey, Stuffing, & Cranberry Sauce, Toby Carvery*	1 Portion/629g	899	28.3	143	6.7	18.8	4.5	0.0
SAUCE								
Apple, Toby Carvery*	1 Serving/30g	20	0.0	65	0.2	19.0	0.0	0.0
Bread, Toby Carvery*	1 Serving/100g	36	1.8	36	0.6	4.4	1.8	0.0
Cranberry, Toby Carvery*	1 Serving/30g	34	0.0	112	0.2	27.9	0.0	0.0
Horseradish, Toby Carvery*	1 Serving/15g	26	1.4	175	1.3	21.8	9.3	0.0
Mint, Toby Carvery*	1 Serving/30g	21	0.0	70	0.7	15.2	0.0	0.0
SAUSAGE								
King Size, Toby Carvery*	1 Portion/45g	174	14.2	389	13.2	12.4	31.8	0.0
Pork, British, Breakfast, Toby Carvery*	1 Sausage/63g	214	16.2	339	14.1	13.3	25.6	0.0
Quorn, Breakfast, Toby Carvery*	1 Sausage/75g	133	5.9	177	10.2	13.4	7.8	0.0
SAUSAGES								
Chipolata, Honey & Mustard, & Red Onion, Toby Carvery*	1 Portion/176g	603	43.4	343	10.7	19.4	24.7	0.0
SOUP								
Tomato, with Wholemeal Bread, Kids, Toby Carvery*	1 Portion/247g	232	7.2	94	2.7	13.4	2.9	0.0
SPREAD								
Sunflower, Portion, Breakfast, Toby Carvery*	1 Portion/8g	49	5.6	613	0.0	0.0	70.0	0.0
STUFFING								
Sage & Onion, Toby Carvery*	1 Portion/20g	73	0.7	359	9.8	72.5	3.3	0.0
SWEDE								
Toby Carvery*	1 Portion/40g	20	0.3	50	0.6	10.2	0.8	0.0
SWEETCORN								
Toby Carvery*	1 Portion/40g	61	1.6	152	5.2	25.3	4.0	0.0
TART								
Pear & Blue Cheese, Salad, & Dresisng, Toby Carvery*	1 Tart/232g	432	23.2	186	3.8	18.9	10.0	0.0
TOAST								
Brown, Breakfast, Toby Carvery*	1 Portion/128g	315	3.8	246	10.5	42.0	3.0	0.0
White, Breakfast, Toby Carvery*	1 Portion/128g	348	2.6	272	8.8	52.0	2.0	0.0
TOMATOES								
Plum, Breakfast, Toby Carvery*	1 Portion/100g	18	0.1	18	1.0	3.0	0.1	0.0
TURKEY								
Roast, Kids, Toby Carvery*	1 Portion/80g	126	2.6	158	32.1	0.0	3.3	0.0
Roast, Succulent, British, Toby Carvery*	1 Portion/160g	253	5.3	158	32.1	1.0	3.3	0.0
VEGETABLES								
Sticks, & Cheesy BBQ Dip, Kids, Toby Carvery*	1 Portion/168g	106	1.9	63	1.2	11.5	1.1	0.0
WELLINGTON								
Carrot & Chick Pea, Wholegrain, Toby Carvery*	1 Portion/282g	749	40.6	266	7.2	25.3	14.4	0.0
YORKSHIRE PUDDING								
Roasted Onion & Bacon Bits, Breakfast, Toby Carvery*	1 Portion/46g	187	13.7	407	7.4	27.1	29.8	0.0

	Measure INFO/WEIGHT	per Measure KCAL	per Measure FAT	Nutrition Values per 100g / 100ml KCAL	PROT	CARB	FAT	FIBRE
TOBY CARVERY								
YORKSHIRE PUDDING								
Toby Carvery*	1 Yorkshire/23g	89	3.4	387	12.3	50.7	15.0	0.0
WAGAMAMA								
BEANS								
Edamame with Salt, Wagamama*	1 Serving/202g	179	6.3	89	6.6	3.7	3.1	9.9
BROCCOLI								
& Bok Choy, in Garlic & Soy, Wok Fried, Wagamama*	1 Portion/165g	182	15.6	110	1.9	3.7	9.4	1.4
BUNS								
Beef, & Red Onion, Korean BBQ, Hirat, Wagamama*	1 Portion/111g	285	12.2	257	12.0	26.0	11.0	1.0
Mushrooms, & Auberine, Hirat, Wagamama*	1 Portion/150g	340	19.6	226	5.0	22.0	13.0	1.0
Pork Belly & Apple, Steamed, Hirata, Wagamama*	1 Portion/101g	301	17.1	298	7.5	28.0	16.9	2.1
CHICKEN								
with Sesame Soy Sauce, Tori Kara Age, Wagamama*	1 Portion/171g	494	30.4	289	25.9	6.3	17.8	0.1
CURRY								
Beef, Massaman, Wagamama*	1 Portion/742g	1338	52.7	180	7.6	21.1	7.1	0.9
Chicken, Firecracker, Wagamama*	1 Portion/718g	1149	28.7	160	7.0	25.0	4.0	1.0
Chicken, Katsu, Wagamama*	1 Portion/620g	1147	49.6	185	7.6	20.3	8.0	0.8
Chicken, Raisukaree, Wagamama*	1 Portion/774g	1253	55.7	162	5.1	18.9	7.2	0.8
Chicken, Surendras, Wagamama*	1 Portion/683g	1345	61.4	197	6.5	22.0	9.0	1.2
Prawn, Firecracker, Wagamama*	1 Portion/659g	1002	19.8	152	4.0	27.0	3.0	1.0
Prawn, Raisukaree, Wagamama*	1 Portion/753g	1129	52.7	150	2.9	18.5	7.0	0.8
Tilapia, Surendras, Wagamama*	1 Portion/693g	1352	61.0	195	5.7	22.7	8.8	1.1
Vegetable, Surendras, Yasai, Wagamama*	1 Portion/724g	1339	62.2	185	2.5	23.8	8.6	1.4
Vegetable, Yasai Katsu, Wagamama*	1 Portion/626g	1176	55.0	188	2.9	23.5	8.8	1.2
DESSERT								
Banana Katsu, Wagamama*	1 Portion/136g	298	12.4	219	2.9	30.8	9.1	0.9
Black Rice, Wagamama*	1 Portion/40g	68	3.0	169	1.7	23.9	7.4	0.1
Cake, Chocolate Fudge, Wagamama*	1 Portion/203g	664	37.0	327	3.9	36.8	18.2	0.6
Cheesecake, Passionfruit, Wagamama*	1 Portion/149g	474	28.6	318	5.1	30.7	19.2	0.9
Cheesecake, White Chocolate & Ginger, Wagamama*	1 Portion/142g	455	22.3	320	5.2	39.2	15.7	0.4
Coconut Reika, Wagamama*	1 Portion/195g	410	21.5	210	3.3	24.0	11.0	1.0
Mini Cakes, Wagamama*	1 Portion/144g	419	17.5	290	4.9	40.1	12.1	0.5
Sweet Onigiri, Wagamama*	1 Portion/114g	379	19.9	333	2.7	40.2	17.5	2.0
DONBURI								
Beef, Teriyaki, Wagamama*	1 Portion/594g	1010	23.2	170	8.9	24.4	3.9	0.8
Chicken, & Prawn, Cha Han, Wagamama*	1 Portion/778g	970	24.9	125	4.8	18.6	3.2	0.8
Chicken, Teriyaki, Wagamama*	1 Portion/580g	910	16.8	157	8.1	24.1	2.9	0.8
Tofu, & vegetable, Yasai Cha Han, Wagamama*	1 Portion/770g	1005	30.8	131	4.2	19.1	4.0	0.8
DUCK								
Cucumber, Mint, & Coriander, Yakitori, Wagamama*	1 Portion/453g	1194	71.6	264	8.9	21.3	15.8	0.3
DUMPLINGS								
Chicken, Gyoza, Steamed, Wagamama*	1 Portion/128g	245	9.0	191	8.0	23.0	7.0	1.0
Duck, Gyoza, Fried, Wagamama*	1 Portion/434g	820	45.1	189	12.5	11.0	10.4	1.1
Pork, Pulled, Gyoza, Steamed, Wagamama*	1 Portion/100g	206	4.0	206	11.0	31.0	4.0	2.0
Prawn, Gyoza, Fried, Wagamama*	1 Portion/112g	220	8.7	197	8.3	21.6	7.8	3.1
Yasai, Gyoza, Steamed, Wagamama*	1 Portion/129g	233	6.5	180	4.0	27.0	5.0	2.0
ICE CREAM								
Coconut Mochi, Wagamama*	1 Portion/92g	231	9.5	251	2.8	36.1	10.3	2.2
Mix It Up Mochi, Wagamama*	1 Portion/92g	232	8.1	252	4.1	38.2	8.8	1.6
Raspberry Mochi, Wagamama*	1 Portion/92g	193	3.8	210	2.4	40.6	4.1	0.6
Toasted Sesame Mochi, Wagamama*	1 Portion/92g	265	11.0	288	7.1	36.8	12.0	1.8
JUICE								
Blueberry Spice, Wagamama*	1 Serving/262g	139	2.6	53	0.5	9.4	1.0	2.2

	Measure INFO/WEIGHT	per Measure KCAL	FAT	Nutrition Values per 100g / 100ml KCAL	PROT	CARB	FAT	FIBRE
WAGAMAMA								
JUICE								
Carrot, Wagamama*	1 Serving/313g	72	0.3	23	0.2	5.0	0.1	1.1
Clean Green, Wagamama*	1 Serving/259g	150	3.1	58	0.6	10.1	1.2	1.9
Fruit, Wagamama*	1 Serving/312g	128	0.2	41	0.4	10.4	0.1	0.3
Orange, Wagamama*	1 Serving/275g	110	0.1	40	0.7	9.1	0.0	0.7
Raw, Wagamama*	1 Serving/268g	83	0.1	31	0.4	7.3	0.0	0.1
Super Green, Wagamama*	1 Serving/273g	153	0.2	56	0.2	13.8	0.1	0.3
Tropical, Wagamama*	1 Serving/208g	100	0.2	48	0.4	10.5	0.1	1.6
LAMB TERIYAKI								
Mushrooms, Asparagus, Kale & Mangetout, Wagamama*	1 Portion/434g	820	45.1	189	12.5	11.0	10.4	1.1
NOODLES								
Beef, Steak, Teriyaki Soba, Teppanyaki, Wagamama*	1 Portion/654g	818	28.1	125	10.4	10.8	4.3	1.1
Beef Rib, Short, Ramen, Wagamama*	1 Portion/1039g	1097	58.2	106	6.1	7.5	5.6	0.3
Chicken, & Prawn, Tamarind Sauce, Pad Thai, Wagamama*	1 Portion/632g	828	36.7	131	4.4	14.6	5.8	1.4
Chicken, & Prawn, Tamarind Sauce, Pad Thai, Wagamama*	1 Portion/650g	799	31.2	123	5.2	14.1	4.8	1.4
Chicken, & Prawn, Udon, Teppamyaki, Wagamama*	1 Portion/620g	701	26.1	113	5.4	12.7	4.2	1.6
Chicken, Chilli, Ramen, Wagamama*	1 Portion/952g	590	10.5	62	4.6	8.1	1.1	0.6
Chicken, Ginger, Udon, Teppamyaki, Wagamama*	1 Portion/606g	751	28.5	124	6.5	13.1	4.7	1.7
Chicken, Itame, Wagamama*	1 Portion/829g	820	48.9	99	3.9	7.0	5.9	1.3
Chicken, Kare Lomen, Ramen, Wagamama*	1 Portion/851g	860	37.5	101	6.9	8.0	4.4	1.0
Chicken, Pork, Prawns & Mussels, Ramen, Wagamama*	1 Portion/905g	706	21.9	78	5.7	8.4	2.4	1.2
Chicken, Prawn, Egg, Yaki Soba, Teppanyaki, Wagamama*	1 Portion/454g	586	28.3	129	6.4	11.3	6.2	1.1
Chicken, Ramen, Wagamama*	1 Portion/810g	510	10.5	63	5.0	7.5	1.3	0.4
Duck, Ramen, Wagamama*	1 Portion/884g	990	60.1	112	5.3	7.2	6.8	0.3
Mushroom, & Vegetables, Yasai Yaki Soba, Wagamama*	1 Portion/563g	664	27.6	118	4.7	13.2	4.9	1.3
Pork, Ramen, Wagamama*	1 Portion/874g	699	25.3	80	3.9	8.6	2.9	0.4
Prawn, Itame, Wagamama*	1 Portion/798g	718	45.5	90	1.8	7.3	5.7	1.3
Prawn, Kare Lomen, Ramen, Wagamama*	1 Portion/768g	707	33.8	92	3.3	9.3	4.4	1.0
Salmon, Teriyaki Soba, Teppanyaki, Wagamama*	1 Portion/598g	807	38.3	135	7.6	11.3	6.4	1.0
Seafood, Ramen, Wagamama*	1 Portion/966g	821	28.0	85	7.0	7.4	2.9	0.5
Steak, Chilli, Ramen, Wagamama*	1 Portion/1039g	665	7.3	64	6.6	7.6	0.7	0.7
Tofu, & Vegetable, Tamarind, Yasai Pad Thai, Wagamama*	1 Portion/632g	828	36.7	131	4.4	14.6	5.8	1.4
Tofu, Itame, Wagamama*	1 Portion/896g	917	61.0	102	2.1	7.4	6.8	1.3
Tofu, Omelette, & Mushroom, Yasi, Ramen, Wagamama*	1 Portion/689g	551	27.6	80	3.2	7.5	4.0	0.9
PRAWNS								
Chilli & Garlic Sauce, Ebi Katsu, Wagamama*	1 Portion/129g	291	16.8	225	9.0	17.0	13.0	1.0
Skewers, Kushiyaki, Lollipop, Grilled, Wagamama*	1 Portion/105g	170	6.5	162	12.1	14.2	6.2	0.4
RIBS								
Pork, Korean BBQ Sauce, & Sesame Seeds, Wagamama*	1 Portion/252g	702	42.8	279	15.5	15.6	17.0	0.4
RICE								
Balls, Mushroom, Onigiri, Wagamama*	1 Portion/120g	256	11.6	214	3.9	26.6	9.7	2.0
SALAD								
Beef, & Shitake, Wagamama*	1 Portion/323g	381	14.9	118	16.4	2.3	4.6	0.9
Chicken, Chilli, Warm, Wagamama*	1 Portion/322g	499	32.8	155	8.9	6.4	10.2	1.2
Raw, with Fried Shallots, Wagamama*	1 Portion/143g	219	20.2	153	1.2	3.5	14.1	0.1
Tofu, Chilli, Warm, Wagamama*	1 Portion/338g	503	36.1	149	4.1	8.4	10.7	1.4
SQUID								
Chilli, Crispy, with Shichimi, Wagamama*	1 Portion/208g	493	33.3	237	8.7	19.4	16.0	0.4
TOFU								
In Dashi Stock, Crispy, Aga Dashi, Wagamama*	1 Portion/187g	153	3.7	82	3.0	12.0	2.0	1.0
TUNA								
Quinoa, Kale, Peppers, Onions & Edamame, Wagamama*	1 Portion/477g	626	27.7	131	9.5	9.7	5.8	1.3

WIMPY

	Measure INFO/WEIGHT	per Measure KCAL	FAT	Nutrition Values per 100g / 100ml KCAL	PROT	CARB	FAT	FIBRE
BACON								
Extras, Wimpy*	1 Serving/91g	267	22.0	294	24.2	0.0	24.2	0.0
BEANS								
Baked, Heinz, Wimpy*	1 Portion/110g	85	0.2	77	4.4	12.6	0.2	3.6
BREAKFAST								
Bacon & Egg Breakfast Roll, Wimpy*	1 Roll/194g	368	12.1	190	13.4	18.3	6.2	0.0
Bacon Breakfast Roll, Wimpy*	1 Roll/144g	278	5.1	193	13.3	24.7	3.5	0.0
Hashbrown, Wimpy*	1 Serving/424g	545	41.1	129	4.1	8.7	9.7	1.9
Sausage & Egg Breakfast Roll, Wimpy*	1 Roll/211g	527	28.4	250	11.8	20.3	13.5	0.0
Sausage Breakfast Roll, Wimpy*	1 Roll/161g	437	21.5	271	11.3	26.6	13.4	0.0
The Country Breakfast, Wimpy*	1 Serving/271g	392	23.1	145	9.4	6.9	8.5	1.7
Wimpy Breakfast, Wimpy*	1 Serving/307g	503	31.2	164	11.4	6.1	10.2	1.5
BURGERS								
BBQ Burger, Wimpy*	1 Burger/236g	644	30.5	273	14.2	24.6	12.9	1.6
Bender, with Cheese, in a Bun, Wimpy*	1 Burger/170g	424	23.4	249	10.2	20.8	13.8	1.2
Chicken & Bacon Melt, Wimpy*	1 Burger/172g	443	20.2	258	12.6	25.4	11.7	0.0
Chicken Fillet, in a Bun, Savoury, Wimpy*	1 Burger/218g	356	13.8	163	10.4	16.1	6.3	1.1
Chicken Fillet, Wimpy*	1 Burger/327g	380	16.8	116	6.7	11.1	5.1	0.0
Chicken Fillet in a Bun, Hot & Spicy, Wimpy*	1 Burger/193g	398	18.5	206	10.6	19.1	9.6	1.8
Chicken in a Bun, Wimpy*	1 Burger/191g	449	21.4	235	10.4	22.7	11.2	1.3
Classic, Wimpy*	1 Burger/159g	337	15.1	212	12.4	19.9	9.5	0.0
Classic Bacon Cheeseburger, Wimpy*	1 Burger/192g	405	19.0	211	13.6	16.8	9.9	0.0
Classic with Cheese, Wimpy*	1 Burger/175g	379	18.5	217	12.7	17.3	10.6	1.1
Halfpounder with Bacon & Cheese, Wimpy*	1 Burger/312g	892	50.5	286	19.2	15.5	16.2	0.8
Quarterpounder, Wimpy*	1 Burger/200g	538	31.3	269	15.0	18.0	15.6	0.0
Quarterpounder with Bacon & Cheese, Wimpy*	1 Burger/237g	658	33.4	278	16.8	20.5	14.1	1.1
Quarterpounder with Cheese, Wimpy*	1 Burger/213g	578	34.6	271	15.1	17.2	16.2	0.0
Spicy Bean, Wimpy*	1 Burger/233g	611	29.4	262	5.9	30.5	12.6	2.7
CHEESE								
Mozzarella, Meltz 6, Extras, Wimpy*	6 Meltz/157g	506	30.8	322	15.6	25.9	19.6	2.5
CHEESEBURGER								
with Chips, Junior, Kids Meal, Wimpy*	1 Serving/191g	497	23.5	260	10.0	27.8	12.3	2.1
CHEESEBURGER								
with Salad, Junior, Kids Meal, Wimpy*	1 Serving/206g	322	14.1	156	8.5	14.8	6.8	1.1
CHICKEN								
Chunks, with Chips, Kids, Wimpy*	1 Serving/172g	440	26.1	256	8.4	22.2	15.2	1.8
Chunks, with Salad, Kids Meal, Wimpy*	1 Serving/187g	265	16.8	142	6.8	8.4	9.0	0.8
CHIPS								
Lge Portion, Extras, Wimpy*	1 Portion/143g	333	17.1	233	3.0	30.4	12.0	3.0
Standard Portion, Extras, Wimpy*	1 Portion/114g	267	13.7	234	3.0	30.5	12.0	3.0
CHOCOLATE								
Crushed Flake (for desserts), Wimpy*	1 Serving/20g	104	6.1	520	7.5	57.0	30.5	1.0
COLESLAW								
Extras, Wimpy*	1 Serving/50g	49	3.8	98	1.4	6.2	7.6	0.8
DESSERT								
Brown Derby with Dairy Ice Cream, Wimpy*	1 Serving/180g	431	20.6	239	4.5	31.3	11.4	1.4
Brownie Sundae, Wimpy*	1 Sundae/252g	574	21.8	228	3.8	34.7	8.6	0.6
Chocolate Waffle with Dairy Ice Cream, Wimpy*	1 Serving/178g	691	37.0	388	5.1	45.3	20.8	0.0
Chocolate Waffle with Squirty Cream, Wimpy*	1 Serving/158g	667	36.9	422	5.1	47.7	23.4	0.0
Dairy Ice Cream with Chocolate Sauce, Wimpy*	1 Serving/88g	200	8.1	227	3.4	32.5	9.2	0.0
Dairy Ice Cream with Strawberry Sauce, Wimpy*	1 Serving/88g	199	7.9	226	3.0	34.3	9.0	0.0
Deep Filled Apple Tart, Wimpy*	1 Serving/164g	339	10.2	207	1.7	36.2	6.2	0.0
Half Chocolate Waffle with Dairy Ice Cream, Wimpy*	1 Serving/116g	395	18.8	341	4.0	44.7	16.2	0.0

WIMPY

	Measure INFO/WEIGHT	per Measure KCAL	FAT	Nutrition Values per 100g / 100ml KCAL	PROT	CARB	FAT	FIBRE
DESSERT								
Ice Cream Sundae, Plain, Wimpy*	1 Sundae/170g	190	8.8	112	3.1	15.0	5.2	0.0
Mini Knickerbocker Glory with Dairy Ice Cream, Wimpy*	1 Serving/194g	190	8.5	98	1.6	13.2	4.4	0.0
FISH								
Bites, with Chips, Kids Meal, Wimpy*	1 Serving/160g	380	20.9	238	6.7	24.7	13.1	2.1
Bites, with Salad, Kids Meal, Wimpy*	1 Serving/175g	205	11.6	117	5.2	9.8	6.6	0.9
Haddock, Peas & Chips, Wimpy*	1 Serving/314g	674	37.9	215	6.6	21.2	12.1	2.4
Scampi & Chips with Peas, Wimpy*	1 Serving/303g	577	29.8	190	5.2	22.7	9.8	2.3
GRILL								
All-Day Breakfast, Wimpy*	1 Serving/410g	731	39.7	178	8.3	14.5	9.7	0.0
Burger, Pork Bender, Fried Egg, Chips & Tomato, Wimpy*	1 Serving/350g	766	55.8	219	9.7	10.7	15.9	1.1
Gourmet Chicken Platter, Wimpy*	1 Serving/392g	525	21.4	134	11.4	10.0	5.5	1.4
Sausage, with Egg & Chips, Grill, Wimpy*	1 Serving/244g	597	38.8	245	9.0	17.4	15.9	1.7
HASH BROWNS								
Extras, Wimpy*	1 Serving/55g	93	7.8	169	2.2	19.6	14.2	1.8
ICE CREAM								
Banana Longboat with Soft Ice Cream, Wimpy*	1 Serving/209g	260	6.0	124	2.3	23.9	2.9	0.0
Choc Nut Sundae, Wimpy*	1 Serving/83g	196	6.2	236	4.6	38.4	7.5	0.0
Knickerbockerglory with Soft Ice Cream, Wimpy*	1 Serving/138g	196	6.0	142	2.7	24.7	4.4	0.0
Triple Strawberry Sundae with Soft Ice Cream, Wimpy*	1 Serving/170g	123	3.3	72	1.4	13.1	1.9	0.0
MUFFIN								
Giant Blueberry, Wimpy*	1 Muffin/108g	470	25.6	435	5.9	48.9	23.7	0.0
Giant Choc Chunk, Wimpy*	1 Muffin/108g	473	26.6	438	5.5	49.7	24.6	0.0
NUTS								
Nibbed (for desserts), Wimpy*	1 Serving/5g	32	2.8	640	26.0	6.0	56.0	12.0
ONION RINGS								
Lge (12), Extras, Wimpy*	1 Portion/180g	401	23.2	223	3.2	23.6	12.9	0.0
Standard (6), Extras, Wimpy*	1 Portion/90g	201	11.6	223	3.2	23.6	12.9	3.0
PANINI								
Cheese & Tomato, Wimpy*	1 Panini/225g	694	25.1	309	14.6	37.4	11.1	2.2
Cheese with Red Onion, Wimpy*	1 Panini/205g	673	22.8	329	14.6	42.7	11.1	1.9
Ham, Tomato & Cheese, Wimpy*	1 Panini/275g	1145	39.0	417	33.0	38.4	14.2	2.2
Ham & Cheese, Wimpy*	1 Panini/235g	944	33.3	402	32.0	35.7	14.2	1.4
PEAS								
Extras, Wimpy*	1 Portion/50g	35	0.5	70	6.0	9.8	1.0	5.2
POTATOES								
Baked, Jacket, Plain, with Butter, Wimpy*	1 Serving/327g	453	7.6	139	3.5	27.7	2.3	2.4
Baked, Jacket, with Baked Beans, Wimpy*	1 Serving/452g	549	7.9	121	3.4	23.5	1.8	2.7
Baked, Jacket, with Beans & Cheese, Wimpy*	1 Serving/577g	1069	51.5	185	8.4	18.4	8.9	2.1
Baked, Jacket, with Coleslaw, Wimpy*	1 Serving/452g	576	17.1	127	2.9	21.7	3.8	2.0
Baked, Jacket, with Grated Cheese, Wimpy*	1 Serving/452g	973	51.2	215	9.6	20.0	11.3	1.8
Baked, Jacket, with Tuna Mayo, Wimpy*	1 Serving/452g	764	34.2	169	5.9	20.6	7.6	1.8
RIBS								
BBQ, Rack Platter, Grill, Wimpy*	1 Serving/439g	713	35.2	162	5.6	17.5	8.0	1.4
ROLL								
Bacon & Egg, in a Bun, Wimpy*	1 Roll/155g	702	41.7	453	29.6	22.6	26.9	1.4
Bacon in a Bun, Wimpy*	1 Roll/125g	341	16.1	273	16.0	22.6	12.9	1.4
WimpyClub, Wimpy*	1 Roll/310g	639	26.2	206	13.5	19.4	8.5	0.0
SALAD								
Fish, Wimpy*	1 Serving/356g	389	21.3	109	4.6	9.9	6.0	0.0
Gourmet Chicken, Wimpy*	1 Serving/358g	251	4.3	70	11.9	2.7	1.2	0.4
Hot & Spicy Chicken, Wimpy*	1 Serving/290g	283	15.2	98	6.1	6.7	5.2	0.9
Scampi, Wimpy*	1 Serving/356g	376	19.1	106	4.2	10.7	5.4	0.0

	Measure INFO/WEIGHT	per Measure KCAL	FAT	Nutrition Values per 100g / 100ml KCAL	PROT	CARB	FAT	FIBRE
WIMPY								
SALAD								
Side, Extras, Wimpy*	1 Portion/145g	44	0.3	30	1.4	6.1	0.2	0.8
Spicy Beanburger, Wimpy*	1 Serving/334g	406	23.0	122	1.5	13.6	6.9	0.0
Steak, Wimpy*	1 Serving/355g	329	16.9	93	10.0	2.7	4.8	0.4
SAUCE								
Chocolate (for sundae), Wimpy*	1 Serving/28g	80	0.4	286	1.4	66.1	1.4	1.1
SAUSAGE								
with Chips, Kids Meal, Wimpy*	1 Serving/160g	428	27.7	268	8.9	19.9	17.3	1.9
with Salad, Kids Meal, Wimpy*	1 Serving/175g	253	18.4	145	7.1	5.5	10.5	0.7
SWEETS								
Mini Marshmallows (for desserts), Wimpy*	1 Serving/10g	33	0.0	330	4.0	83.0	0.0	0.0
TEACAKES								
Toasted, with Butter, Wimpy*	1 Teacake/66g	227	2.3	344	1.7	10.4	3.4	0.4
TOAST								
with Jam, Extras, Wimpy*	1 Serving/89g	276	8.3	310	7.3	52.6	9.3	1.7
TOASTIE								
Cheese, with Salad, Kids, Wimpy*	1 Serving/250g	367	8.8	147	5.9	24.2	3.5	1.2
VEGETARIAN								
Spicy Beanburger, Wimpy*	1 Serving/233g	593	29.2	255	5.4	30.8	12.5	0.0

Useful Resources

Weight Loss
Weight Loss Resources is home to the UK's largest calorie and nutrition database along with diaries, tools and expert advice for weight loss and health.
Tel: 01733 345592   Email: helpteam@weightlossresources.co.uk
Website: www.weightlossresources.co.uk

Exercise Equipment for Home
Diet and Fitness Resources has a range of equipment for exercise at home, from pedometers to treadmills and fitballs to weights. As well as diet tools such as food diaries, a weight loss kit and diet plates.
Tel: 01733 345592   Email: helpteam@dietandfitnessresources.co.uk
Website: www.dietandfitnessresources.co.uk

Dietary Advice
The British Dietetic Association has helpful food fact leaflets and information on how to contact a registered dietitian.
Tel: 0121 200 8080 Email: info@bda.uk.com
Website: www.bda.uk.com

Healthy Eating
The British Nutrition Foundation has lots of in depth scientifically based nutritional information, knowledge and advice on healthy eating for all ages.
Tel: 0207 7557 7930 Email: postbox@nutrition.org.uk
Website: www.nutrition.org.uk

Healthy Heart
The British Heart Foundation provides advice and information for all on all heart aspects from being healthy, to living with heart conditions, research and fundraising.
Tel: 0207 554 000 Email: via their website
Website: www.bhf.org.uk

Cancer Research
Cancer Research UK is the leading UK charity dedicated to research, education and fundraising for all forms of cancer.
Tel: 0300 123 1022 Email: via their website
Website: www.cancerresearchuk.org

Diabetes Advice
Diabetes UK is the leading charity working for people with diabetes. Their mission is to improve the lives of people with diabetes and to work towards a future without diabetes
Tel : 0345 123 2399 Email: info@diabetes.org.uk
Website: www.diabetes.org.uk

Beating Bowel Cancer
Beating Bowel Cancer is a leading UK charity for bowel cancer patients, working to raise awareness of symptoms, promote early diagnosis and encourage open access to treatment choice for those affected by bowel cancer.Tel: 08450 719301   Email: nurse@beatingbowelcancer.org
Website: www.beatingbowelcancer.org

Safety and Standards
The Food Standards Agency is an independent watchdog, set up to protect the public's health and consumer interests in relation to food.
Tel: 0207 276 8829 Email: helpline@foodstandards.gsi.gov.uk
Website: www.food.gov.uk

Feedback

If you have any comments or suggestions about The Calorie, Carb & Fat Bible, or would like further information on Weight Loss Resources, please call, email, or write to us:

Tel:	01733 345592
Email:	helpteam@weightlossresources.co.uk
Address:	Rebecca Walton,
	Weight Loss Resources Ltd,
	2C Flag Business Exchange,
	Vicarage Farm Road,
	Peterborough,
	PE1 5TX.

Reviews for The Calorie Carb & Fat Bible

'What a brilliant book. I know I'll be sinking my teeth into it.'
GMTV Nutritionist Amanda Ursell, BSc RD

'To help you make low-cal choices everyday, invest in a copy.'
ZEST magazine

'There is no doubt that the food listings are extremely helpful
for anyone wishing to control their calorie intake in order to lose
pounds or maintain a healthy weight.'
Women's Fitness magazine

'Useful if you don't want to exclude any overall food groups.'
Easy Living magazine

'Quite simply an astonishing achievement by the authors.'
Evening Post, Nottingham

'The book gives you all the basic information so you can work out
your daily calorie needs.'
Woman magazine

'This is a welcome resource in view of the 'national epidemic of obesity.'

Bryony Philip, Bowel Cancer UK

'The authors seem to understand the problems of slimming.'

Dr John Campion

'Jam-packed with info on dieting, and full to bursting point with the calorie, carbohydrate and fat values of thousands of different foods, it's the perfect weight loss tool.'

Evening Express, Aberdeen

'Excellent resource tool - used by myself in my role as a Practice Nurse.'

Pam Boal, Sunderland

'I recently bought your book called the Calorie, Carb & Fat Bible and would love to tell you what a brilliant book it is. I have recently started a weight management programme and I honestly don't know where I'd be without your book. It has helped me a lot and given me some really good advice.'

Rachel Mitchell

About Weight Loss Resources

weightlossresources.co.uk

"What this does is put you in control with no guilt, no awful groups and no negativity! Fill in your food diary, get support on the boards and watch it fall off!"

LINDAB, Weight Loss Resources Member

How Does It Work?

Weight Loss Resources is home to the UK's biggest online calorie and nutrition database. You simply tap in your height, weight, age and basic activity level - set a weight loss goal, and the programme does all the necessary calculations.

What Does It Do?

The site enables you to keep a food diary which keeps running totals of calories, fat, fibre, carbs, proteins and portions of fruit and veg. You can also keep an exercise diary which adds the calories you use during exercise. At the end of a week, you update your weight and get reports and graphs on your progress.

How Will It Help?

You'll learn a great deal about how your eating and drinking habits affect your weight and how healthy they are. Using the diaries and other tools you'll be able to make changes that suit your tastes and your lifestyle. The result is weight loss totally tailored to your needs and preferences. A method you can stick with that will help you learn how to eat well for life!

Try It Free!

Go to **www.weightlossresources.co.uk** and take a completely free, no obligation, 24 hour trial. If you like what you see you can sign up for membership from £6.95 per month.